Every Decker book is accompanied by a CD-ROM.

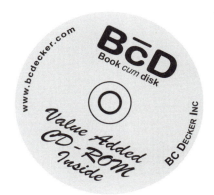

The disk appears in the front of each copy, in its own sealed jacket. Affixed to the front of the book will be a distinctive BcD sticker **"Book *cum* disk."**

The disk contains the complete text and illustrations of the book, in fully searchable PDF files. The book and disk are sold *only* as a package; neither is available independently, and no prices are available for the items individually.

BC Decker Inc is committed to providing high-quality electronic publications that complement traditional information and learning methods.

/CD package

comments

)ecker

Publisher

Holland · Frei

Oncologic Emergencies

Sai-Ching Jim Yeung, MD, PhD

Carmen P. Escalante, MD

University of Texas M.D. Anderson Cancer Center

Houston, Texas

2002

BC Decker Inc

Hamilton • London

BC Decker Inc
P.O. Box 620, L.C.D. 1
Hamilton, Ontario L8N 3K7
Tel: 800-568-7281
Fax: 888-311-4987
E-mail: info@bcdecker.com
www.bcdecker.com

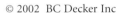

02 03 04 05 / FP / 9 8 7 6 5 4 3 2 1

ISBN 1–55009–171–9
Printed in Canada

Sales and Distribution

United States
BC Decker Inc
P.O. Box 785
Lewiston, NY 14092-0785
Tel: 905-522-7017; 800-568-7281
Fax: 905-522-7839
E-mail: info@bcdecker.com
Web site: www.bcdecker.com

Canada
BC Decker Inc
20 Hughson Street South
P.O. Box 620, LCD 1
Hamilton, Ontario L8N 3K7
Tel: 905-522-7017; 800-568-7281
Fax: 905-522-7839
E-mail: info@bcdecker.com
Web site: www.bcdecker.com

Foreign Rights
John Scott & Company
International Publishers' Agency
P.O. Box 878
Kimberton, PA 19442
Tel: 610-827-1640
Fax: 610-827-1671
E-mail: jsco@voicenet.com

Japan
Igaku-Shoin Ltd.
Foreign Publications Department
3-24-17 Hongo
Bunkyo-ku, Tokyo, Japan 113-8719
Tel: 3 3817 5680
Fax: 3 3815 6776
E-mail: fd@igaku-shoin.co.jp

U.K., Europe, Scandinavia, Middle East
Elsevier Science
Customer Service Department
Foots Cray High Street
Sidcup, Kent
DA14 5HP, UK
Tel: 44 (0) 208 308 5760
Fax: 44 (0) 181 308 5702
E-mail: cservice@harcourt.com

Singapore, Malaysia, Thailand, Philippines, Indonesia, Vietnam, Pacific Rim, Korea
Elsevier Science Asia
583 Orchard Road
#09/01, Forum
Singapore 238884
Tel: 65-737-3593
Fax: 65-753-2145

Australia, New Zealand
Elsevier Science Australia
Customer Service Department
STM Division
Locked Bag 16
St. Peters, New South Wales, 2044
Australia
Tel: 61 02 9517-8999
Fax: 61 02 9517-2249
E-mail: stmp@harcourt.com.au
Web site: www.harcourt.com.au

Mexico and Central America
Rafael Sainz
ETM SA de CV
Calle de Tula 59
Colonia Condesa
06140 Mexico DF, Mexico
Tel: 52-5-5553-6657
Fax: 52-5-5211-8468
E-mail:
editoresdetextosmex@prodigy.net.mx

CONTRIBUTORS

M. Amir Ahmadi, MD
Department of Plastic Surgery
University of Texas M.D. Anderson
    Cancer Center
Houston, Texas

Narin Apisarnthanarax, MD
Department of Dermatology
University of Texas M.D. Anderson
    Cancer Center
Houston, Texas

Noemi Badrina, MSN, RN
Department of General Internal
    Medicine, Ambulatory Treatment
    and Emergency Care
University of Texas M.D. Anderson
    Cancer Center
Houston, Texas

Lodovico Balducci, MD
Department of Interdisciplinary Oncology
University of South Florida College
    of Medicine
Tampa, Florida

Diane C. Bodurke, MD
Department of Gynecologic Oncology
University of Texas M.D. Anderson
    Cancer Center
Houston, Texas

Thomas W. Burke, MD
Department of Gynecologic Oncology
University of Texas M.D. Anderson
    Cancer Center
Houston, Texas

Gary E. Deng, MD, PhD
Department of General Internal
    Medicine, Ambulatory Treatment,
    and Emergency Care
University of Texas M.D. Anderson
    Cancer Center
Houston, Texas

Jean Bernard Durand, MD
Department of Cardiology
University of Texas M.D. Anderson
    Cancer Center
Houston, Texas

Madeleine Duvic, MD
Department of Dermatology
University of Texas M.D. Anderson
    Cancer Center
Houston, Texas

Carmen P. Escalante, MD
Department of General Internal
    Medicine, Ambulatory Treatment,
    and Emergency Care
University of Texas M.D. Anderson
    Cancer Center
Houston, Texas

Bita Esmaeli, MD
Department of Plastic Surgery
University of Texas M.D. Anderson
    Cancer Center
Houston, Texas

Michael S. Ewer, MD, MPH, JD
Department of Cardiology and
    Medical Affairs
University of Texas M.D. Anderson
    Cancer Center
Houston, Texas

Anne L. Flamm, JD
Department of Ethics
University of Texas M.D. Anderson
    Cancer Center
Houston, Texas

Arthur D. Forman, MD
Department of Neuro-Oncology
University of Texas M.D. Anderson
    Cancer Center
Houston, Texas

Robert F. Gagel, MD
Department of Endocrine Neoplasia
    and Hormonal Disorders
University of Texas M.D. Anderson
    Cancer Center
Houston, Texas

Harish K. Gagneja, MD
Department of Gastrointestinal
    Medicine and Nutrition
University of Texas M.D. Anderson
    Cancer Center
Houston, Texas

Shuwei Gao, MD
Department of General Internal
    Medicine, Ambulatory Treatment,
    and Emergency Care
University of Texas M.D. Anderson
    Cancer Center
Houston, Texas

Venera Grasso, MD
Department of Medicine
Joan and Sanford I. Weill Medical
    College of Cornell University
New York, New York

Tejpal S. Grover, MD, MBA
Department of General Internal
    Medicine, Ambulatory Treatment
    and Emergency Care
University of Texas M.D. Anderson
    Cancer Center
Houston, Texas

Richard J. Hatchett, MD
Department of Medicine
Memorial Sloan-Kettering Cancer Center
New York, New York

Tuong-Vi Ho, MSN, RN, CS
Department of General Internal
    Medicine, Ambulatory Treatment
    and Emergency Care
University of Texas M.D. Anderson
    Cancer Center
Houston, Texas

Rola Husni, MD
Department of Internal Medicine
University of Texas M.D. Anderson
    Cancer Center
Houston, Texas

Jessica P. Hwang, MD, MPH
Department of General Internal
    Medicine, Ambulatory Treatment
    and Emergency Care
University of Texas M.D. Anderson
    Cancer Center
Houston, Texas

Erik K. Johnson, MD
Department of Medicine
Joan and Sanford I. Weill Medical
    College of Cornell University
New York, New York

Adam D. Klotz, MD
Department of Medicine
Joan and Sanford I. Weill Medical
    College of Cornell University
New York, New York

Christopher J. Kripas, MD
Department of Medicine
Memorial Sloan-Kettering Cancer Center
New York, New York

Guillermo Lazo-Diaz, MD
Department of Medical Oncology
University of Texas M.D. Anderson
    Cancer Center
Houston, Texas

Eva Lu Lee, MSN, RN, CS, ANP
Department of General Internal
    Medicine, Ambulatory Treatment
    and Emergency Care
University of Texas M.D. Anderson
    Cancer Center
Houston, Texas

MARTIN LEVETT, MD
Department of General Internal
    Medicine, Ambulatory Treatment,
    and Emergency Care
University of Texas M.D. Anderson
    Cancer Center
Houston, Texas

WENLI LIU, MD
Department of General Internal
    Medicine, Ambulatory Treatment
    and Emergency Care
University of Texas M.D. Anderson
    Cancer Center
Houston, Texas

ELLEN F. MANZULLO, MD
Department of General Internal
    Medicine, Ambulatory Treatment,
    and Emergency Care
University of Texas M.D. Anderson
    Cancer Center
Houston, Texas

BRIAN A. MELTZER, MD, MBA
Urgent Care Center
Memorial Sloan-Kettering Cancer Center
New York, New York

PAUL A. MEYERS, MD
Department of Pediatrics
Joan and Sanford I. Weill Medical College
    of Cornell University
New York, New York

AIDA B. NARVIOS, MD
Department of Laboratory
    Medicine-Patient Care Services
University of Texas M.D. Anderson
    Cancer Center
Houston, Texas

AMELIA NG, BS, MD
Department of Pulmonary and
    Critical Care Medicine
University of Texas Health Science
    Center at Houston Medical School
Houston, Texas

SUSAN O'BRIEN, MD
Department of Leukemia
University of Texas M.D. Anderson
    Cancer Center
Houston, Texas

KENAN ONEL, MD, PhD
Department of Pediatrics
Joan and Sanford I. Weill Medical
    College of Cornell University
New York, New York

REBECCA D. PENTZ, PhD
Winship Cancer Institute
Emory Univeristy
Atlanta, Georgia

ISSAM I. RAAD, MD
Department of Infectious Diseases,
    Infection Control, and Employee
    Health
University of Texas M.D. Anderson
    Cancer Center
Houston, Texas

ARUN RAJAGOPAL, MD
Section of Cancer Pain Management
University of Texas M.D. Anderson
    Cancer Center
Houston, Texas

LAURENCE D. RHINES, MD
Department of Neurosurgery
University of Texas M.D. Anderson
    Cancer Center
Houston, Texas

MARGARET ROW, MD
Department of General Internal
    Medicine, Ambulatory Treatment,
    and Emergency Care
University of Texas M.D. Anderson
    Cancer Center
Houston, Texas

SINA SAFAR, BS
Department of Plastic Surgery
University of Texas M.D. Anderson
    Cancer Center
Houston, Texas

TERESITA SANJURJO-HARTMAN, MD
Department of Mental Health and
    Behavioral Science
James A. Haley Veterans Hospital
Tampa, Florida

VICKIE R. SHANNON, MD
Department of Pulmonary Medicine
University of Texas M.D. Anderson
    Cancer Center
Houston, Texas

FRANK A. SINICROPE, MD, FACP
Department of Gastrointestinal
    Medicine and Nutrition
University of Texas M.D. Anderson
    Cancer Center
Houston, Texas

JENNIFER STRICKLAND, PharmD, BCPS
Department of Interdisciplinary Oncology
University of South Florida College
    of Pharmacy
Tampa, Florida

JOSEPH SWAFFORD, MD
Department of Cardiology
University of Texas M.D. Anderson
    Cancer Center
Houston, Texas

NICOLE D. SWITZER, MD
Department of General Internal Medicine,
    Ambulatory Treatment
    and Emergency Care
University of Texas M.D. Anderson
    Cancer Center
Houston, Texas

GIAMPAOLO TALAMO, MD
Department of Emergency Medicine
Aosta General Hospital
Aosta, Italy

ROSALIE VALDRES, MSN, RN, CS
Department of General Internal
    Medicine, Ambulatory Treatment
    and Emergency Care
University of Texas M.D. Anderson
    Cancer Center
Houston, Texas

ANJALI A. VAZE, MD
Department of Medicine
Joan and Sanford I. Weill Medical College
    of Cornell University
New York, New York

MARY ANN WEISER, MD, PhD
Department of General Internal
    Medicine, Ambulatory Treatment
    and Emergency Care
University of Texas M.D. Anderson
    Cancer Center
Houston, Texas

MICHAEL A. WEITZNER, MD
Department of Interdisciplinary Oncology
University of South Florida College
    of Medicine
Tampa, Florida

JULIE BETH YELIN, MD
Department of Plastic Surgery
University of Texas M.D. Anderson
    Cancer Center
Houston, Texas

SAI-CHING JIM YEUNG, MD, PhD
Department of General Internal
    Medicine, Ambulatory Treatment,
    and Emergency Care
University of Texas M.D. Anderson
    Cancer Center
Houston, Texas

SYED WAMIQUE YUSUF, MD, MRCP
Department of Cardiology
University of Texas M.D. Anderson
    Cancer Center
Houston, Texas

Contents

PREFACE

Cancer care has become very specialized. Many centers dedicated to the treatment of cancer are located in major cities worldwide. The emergency departments of these cancer centers provide specialized care for cancer-related emergencies and acute conditions. This type of supportive care for oncology patients is evolving into a new discipline—a hybrid of oncology and emergency medicine. However, most cancer patients are not treated for their emergencies at specialized centers; rather, they go to acute care facilities or emergency rooms in general hospitals, where the treating physician needs to be aware of the cancer-related conditions and provide appropriate care.

Our purpose in preparing this text is to provide an additional resource for primary care providers (internists, family practitioners, advanced clinical practitioners), emergency physicians, oncologists, and other healthcare providers who may not see oncology patients on a regular basis. When a cancer patient requires acute symptom management, an easily accessible review for these individuals is often helpful. Our text will provide additional avenues in the approach to acute care in oncology patients, and may improve emergent and urgent care of cancer patients.

One objective is to provide a comprehensive text written by acute care oncology experts on oncologic emergencies and urgencies. The authors of this book have great expertise in the acute management of cancer patients with a majority having daily encounters with the medical problems in their respective chapters. We hope our text is informative as well as authoritative and an effective resource relating to oncologic emergencies and urgencies.

The first section includes chapters discussing triage, life and death situations, major presenting symptoms, and pathophysiology of emergency illness. The second section features 14 chapters on the organ systems (including pain emergencies and psychiatric emergencies). An additional chapter is devoted to miscellaneous emergencies and includes important aspects of acute care such as systemic side effects of cytokines and chemotherapeutic drug extravasation. There are chapters devoted to pediatric cancer patients and to geriatric cancer patients. The organ system chapters follow a general organizational structure we believe will aid the reader in quickly accessing necessary information. This structure includes an introduction, clinical manifestations, pathophysiology, etiology, diagnosis, treatment, summary, and references. The text is extensively indexed for easy access and retrieval of information. Algorithms are used throughout this book, especially for diagnostic approaches or therapeutic management.

We hope that this text provides a compact, concise and yet comprehensive guide to the management of acute and emergency situations relating to cancer.

Sai-Ching Jim Yeung
Carmen P. Escalante
Houston, Texas
April 2002

We dedicate this book to our
families for their support and faith in our abilities.

Acknowledgments

We thank Dr. Robert Bast for his encouragement and support during the planning and writing of this text.

We acknowledge our wonderful support staff in the Department of General Internal Medicine, Ambulatory Treatment, and Emergency Care for their superb clerical assistance and careful attention to detail.

We would also like to acknowledge the expert editorial staff at BC Decker for their efficiency and professionalism.

CHAPTER 1

EMERGENCY CARE AT COMPREHENSIVE CANCER CENTERS

CARMEN P. ESCALANTE, MD
BRIAN A. MELTZER, MD, MBA

During the course of their disease, many patients with cancer require emergent or urgent care for conditions related to their cancer or cancer treatment. Most such patients are evaluated in local community-based emergency centers that evaluate all patients requiring emergent and urgent care. Some patients requiring urgent care for cancer-related conditions are initially evaluated in their oncologist's office and are then either referred to the local emergency center or directly admitted to their community hospital. For example, patients with neutropenic fever may undergo initial assessment with blood culture and begin a course of antibiotics at their oncologist's office, and patients with uncontrolled pain may be given an injection of narcotics in their oncologist's office to ease their discomfort before being admitted, if necessary, to the hospital. Potential care patterns for patients who require treatment of cancer-related emergencies and acute conditions are shown in Figure 1–1.

Patients with cancer have a third option, in addition to oncologists' offices and general emergency rooms, for the treatment of cancer-related emergencies: the cancer center emergency room. Cancer care has become exceptionally specialized over the past decade, and there are now many centers throughout the world that are dedicated solely to the diagnosis and treatment of cancer. Some of these centers have emergency departments or urgent care centers that specialize in the management of cancer-related emergencies and acute medical conditions of cancer patients. This design promotes a type of supportive care for cancer patients that is a hybrid of oncology and emergency medicine.

This chapter briefly reviews the definition of an oncologic emergency, then describes the history and operations of two cancer centers' emergency rooms.

WHAT IS AN ONCOLOGIC EMERGENCY?

An oncologic emergency is often defined as a life-threatening event precipitated by malignancy or treatment of malignancy. In addition, some events that are not life threatening but that are urgent (such as superior vena cava syndrome) have traditionally been defined as oncologic emergencies. This book uses the term "oncologic emergency" to refer both to true oncologic emergencies and to events or conditions that require immediate assessment but that are not necessarily life threatening (eg, acute pain). Oncologic emergencies in patients with cancer can be divided into three basic types: (1) events due to the neoplasm itself, (2) events due to treatment of the neoplasm, and (3) events due to comorbid conditions (Figure 1–2). Any oncologic emergency may necessitate reassessment and modification of the cancer treatment plan.

OVERVIEW OF EMERGENCY DEPARTMENTS AT TWO COMPREHENSIVE CANCER CENTERS

This section describes the structure and function of the emergency departments at two comprehensive cancer centers: The University of Texas M. D. Anderson Cancer Center and Memorial Sloan-Kettering Cancer Center.

The University of Texas M. D. Anderson Cancer Center

The Emergency Center at M. D. Anderson Cancer Center is dedicated to the care of the institution's cancer patients and is the institution's urgent/emergency care center. More than 90% of the patients seen in the Emergency Center have medical problems; fewer than 10% have sur-

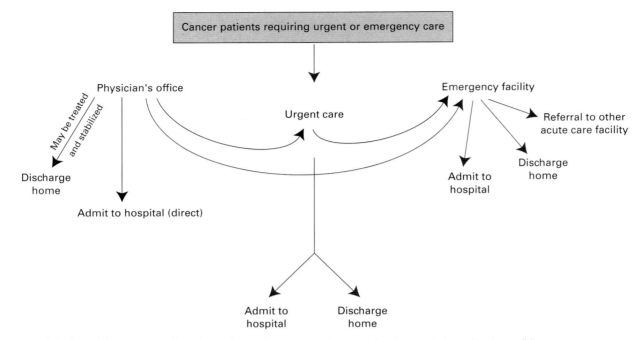

Figure 1–1. Potential care patterns for patients who require treatment of cancer-related emergencies and acute conditions.

gical issues. The center has no trauma rooms. The Emergency Center, which always has a physician on site and which provides access to consultation services, is designated a level III emergency center by the Joint Commission on Accreditation of Healthcare Organizations and by the Centrs for Medicare and Medicaid Services. Visitors and employees who require urgent care are treated in the Emergency Center and are then transferred to other medical facilities once they are medically stable.

Development of the Emergency Center. Until 1986, the emergency center was an open ward referred to as "Station 19." No faculty were assigned to the area. When a patient who required emergency or urgent care arrived, the patient's physician was notified and sent to the ward to evaluate the patient. This situation was not optimal for acutely ill patients or for patients scheduled in the clinic, and the lack of individual patient rooms made it difficult to maintain patients' privacy and confidentiality.

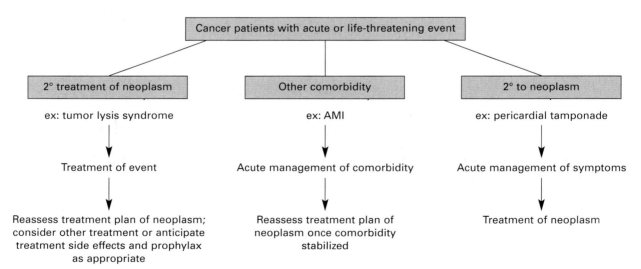

Figure 1–2. Cancer patients presenting with an acute or life-threatening events may be classified as to whether the event is directly related to treatment of the neoplasm, another comorbidity, or the neoplasm itself. Primary treatment of the neoplasm will be dependent upon the etiology of the acute event. AMI = acute myocardial infarction.

Over the past 16 years, many changes have addressed these deficiencies, including the implementation of full-time faculty staffing the area and the creation of individual patient treatment rooms. The number of patients treated and the complexity and severity of their conditions have also increased significantly over the years. These changes may be attributable partly to the trend toward treating patients on an outpatient basis even when their treatment regimens are highly complex. This trend has been driven partly by technologic advances (eg, infusion pumps and indwelling catheters) and by improvements in pharmaceutical agents for symptom control (especially antiemetics). Patients formerly treated as inpatients now are treated on an outpatient basis and often require greater outpatient support (sometimes including more frequent urgent care visits) to complete these regimens. Another trend that may help explain the increase in patient volume is the aging of the US population. Many cancers now are diagnosed in patients older than 65 years of age, many of whom have comorbid conditions (hypertension, coronary artery disease, diabetes mellitus, etc). The management and stabilization of these diseases are important to the successful initiation and completion of cancer treatment.

The Emergency Center Today. Today, the Emergency Center at M. D. Anderson has 24 rooms and 27 beds (there are three rooms with double occupancy) and is open 24 hours per day, 7 days per week. The Emergency Center is staffed around the clock by internists in the Department of General Internal Medicine, all of whom are board certified or board eligible in internal medicine and have Advanced Cardiopulmonary Life Support certification. Advanced clinical practitioners (physician assistants and advanced nurse practitioners) are also on duty in the center.

The Emergency Center registered approximately 14,000 patient visits in the year 2000, an 8% increase over the number of visits in 1999. Of the patients evaluated in 2000, 91% were from medical services; of these, approximately 65% had solid tumors, and approximately 35% had hematologic malignancies. Breast cancer and gastrointestinal cancer were the most frequent diagnoses among patients with solid tumors, reflecting the high frequency of these diagnoses in the cancer patient population. In the hematologic group, patients with leukemia and patients undergoing bone marrow transplantation had the most Emergency Center visits. Although patients with solid tumors had more Emergency Center visits, more resources were expended in caring for the patients with hematologic malignancies since they were often more acutely ill at presentation.

Of the patients who presented to the Emergency Center in 2000, approximately 4% had true emergencies (eg, code in progress, hypertensive crisis), 61% had con-

ditions requiring urgent care (eg, neutropenic fever, vomiting with hypotension), and 35% had nonurgent conditions (eg, constipation, rash). The rate of admission to the hospital from the Emergency Center was approximately 40%, much higher than the rate for a typical emergency department. Of patients admitted, approximately 94% were admitted to a floor bed, and approximately 6% were admitted to the intensive care unit. Most Emergency Center visits (65%) occurred between noon and midnight. The majority of patients required laboratory or diagnostic imaging services or both. The chief complaints of patients at triage are shown in Figure 1–3.

Urgent Care Center at Memorial Sloan-Kettering Cancer Center

The Urgent Care Center at Memorial Sloan-Kettering Cancer Center has a history very similar to that of the Emergency Center at M. D. Anderson. What began as a nurse-managed "bedholding" unit in the early 1970s has become a full-service emergency room specializing in the management of acute symptoms in cancer patients.

In the early 1970s, the unit functioned as a way station between the clinics and the inpatient unit. The staff consisted of advanced-practice registered nurses. Medical treatment was provided, but only by direct order of the patient's attending physician—a catch-as-catch-can proposition at best. Space was cramped. There were 12 stretchers separated by curtains, and there were cardiac

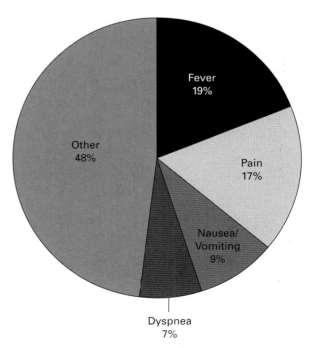

Figure 1–3. Chief complaints at triage of patients seen in the M.D. Anderson Cancer Center Emergency Center.

monitors next to some of the stretchers. There was no waiting room; patients were consigned to waiting in chairs in a long hallway.

The transition to a center staffed by physicians occurred slowly between 1990 and 1995. During these years, the patient's own attending physician would care for the patient during the day, and moonlighting residents and fellows would cover the unit at night. In 1994, full-time physicians were hired to staff the unit. However, coverage was not complete, and moonlighting physicians continued to fill in the scheduling gaps.

In 1995, the Urgent Care Center was created, and construction began on a 12-bed, 4,200-square-foot unit complete with two negative-pressure isolation rooms. A full-time medical director was appointed and given the task of creating an emergency program for Memorial Sloan-Kettering patients to function 24 hours per day, 7 days per week. Since then, the physical space has remained the same, but patient volumes have dictated that the full-time attending staff grow to seven physicians who are board certified in internal medicine and whose sole responsibility is the management of cancer-related emergencies.

As the care of cancer patients requiring complex treatment has shifted from the inpatient to the outpatient setting, the Urgent Care Center has experienced a significant growth in the volume of patients. In 1997, 8,452 patients were encountered; in 2000, more than 14,800 patients were encountered. Because of limitations in physical space, the bed turnover rate for the Urgent Care Center has increased from 1.75 times per day to 3.5 times per day. To handle this increase, the workflow process was altered to emulate a true emergency room.

Approximately half of the patients seen in the Urgent Care Center are admitted to the hospital; this proportion is much higher than is typical for a general emergency department and reflects the severity of the conditions treated in the center. Because of the increasing volume of patients and the physical-space limitations of the Urgent Care Center, a dedicated triage nurse position was created to ensure optimal management of patients. The triage nurse prioritizes the order in which physicians see patients, plans the use of resources for patients who are expected to arrive in the unit, and maintains a physical presence in the waiting area to respond to emergencies.

Upon arrival at the Urgent Care Center, patients are classified according to an adapted triage classification system (Table 1–1). The triage nurse has the authority to activate a standard intake order set consisting of a complete blood count with differential and a basic metabolic panel (Na, K, Cl, CO_2, glucose, Ca, and Mg). Other diagnostic tests (eg, venous duplex sonography, chest radiography) are ordered as needed after discussion with the attending physician.

TABLE 1–1. Triage Classification System for Memorial Sloan-Kettering Cancer Center Urgent Care Center

Emergent: A condition that requires immediate attention. The condition is life threatening, and delay in treatment would be harmful to the patient. Examples are as follows:
- Cardiac arrest
- Airway and breathing difficulties
- Chest pain
- Acute allergic reaction
- Seizure
- Shock (hypovolemic, septic, or anaphylactic)
- Uncontrolled or suspected severe bleeding
- Unresponsiveness or acute change in mental status
- Hypertension or hypotension

Urgent: A condition that requires medical attention. Failure to provide proper care could endanger the patient. Examples are as follows:
- Abdominal pain
- Abnormal results on laboratory examinations in an asymptomatic patient
- Bladder spasms or distention
- Confusion
- Signs or symptoms of epidural spinal cord compression
- Diverticulitis
- Nonspecific chest pain
- Persistent nausea, vomiting, or diarrhea with orthostatic changes
- Recent seizure activity
- Neutropenic fever
- Fracture
- Headache
- Hematemesis without orthostatic changes
- Hemoptysis
- Positive blood culture report
- Change in mental status
- Pain
- Pneumonia
- Syncope
- Thrombocytopenia or anemia
- Complications related to vascular access device

Nonurgent: A condition that is not acute and that does not threaten life or function. Examples are as follows:
- Ascites
- Cellulitis
- Constipation
- Dehydration (asymptomatic)
- Diarrhea
- Dysphagia/mucositis
- Dysuria
- Employee incident
- "Failure to thrive"
- Fatigue
- Cough
- Jaundice without fever or abdominal pain
- Needle stick
- Rash or suspected varicella-zoster virus infection (isolation of patient)
- Routine blood draw
- Flushing of vascular access device
- Scheduled blood product transfusion

The triage standards for the Urgent Care Center emphasize rapid identification of the likely diagnosis and accelerated treatment plans when appropriate. For example, the standards require that empiric treatment for neutropenic fever be started within 1 hour of confirmed neutropenia. In patients with suspected epidural spinal cord compression, the triage nurse and attending physician discuss the pretest probability of the diagnosis and administer high-dose steroids if compression is considered likely. Patients with suspected varicella-zoster infection are isolated immediately upon arrival in the unit. Patients with other diagnoses are prioritized for evaluation, according to the time of their arrival and the severity of their condition.

CANCER CENTER EMERGENCY ROOM AS A "VALUE ADDED" SERVICE

Cancer care is not truly comprehensive until the cancer center is prepared to help patients during times of great stress and need. The availability of around-the-clock emergency services provides patients and their families with the peace of mind needed during crises and provides the cancer center with a tremendous competitive advantage in the "cancer marketplace" through improved patient satisfaction and an improved revenue stream.

SUMMARY

Various approaches are available for treating emergency and acute conditions in cancer patients. Some patients will require emergency care facilities to evaluate and manage their acute events. Other patients may be appropriately stabilized in a physician's office or in an urgent care facility, thus bypassing an emergency facility completely. Some physician offices are appropriately equipped and staffed to handle various acute emergencies. Regardless of where acutely ill cancer patients are evaluated, they will require a similar approach to stabilize the acute symptom. It is expected that as life expectancy continues to increase, the number of people diagnosed with cancer will also continue to increase. A majority of those patients will require emergency or urgent care related to their cancer at some time.

CHAPTER 2

TRIAGE

WENLI LIU, MD
TUONG-VI HO, MSN, RN, CS
EVA LU LEE, MSN, RN, CS, ANP
ROSALIE VALDRES, MSN, RN, CS
NOEMI BADRINA, MSN, RN

Each visit to an emergency room requires multiple forms of assessment, beginning with triage. The word "triage" describes a priority decision-making process that is used during the care of emergency patients. The term is derived from the French word "trier," meaning "to sort"[1] and was adopted into the English language after the Napoleonic Wars. In its original use on the battlefield, triage was a process by which priority of care was assigned to soldiers with treatable wounds. These soldiers could rapidly be returned to the front whereas those with mortal wounds were set aside to die. This form of triage was guided by military needs.

The concept of wartime triage became useful in modern hospital emergency centers when the demand for emergency services outpaced available emergency resources. Specifically, Purnell suggested that triage was first used in the emergency centers of US hospitals in the 1960s.[2] Having been distanced from its historical military intent, triage is now used in emergency centers to organize available medical care and to prioritize resources according to the acuteness of the patient's condition.

PRINCIPLES OF TRIAGE

Prompt assessment of the patient and the reduction of possibly harmful delays in the waiting room are the most obvious goals of triage. Additionally, patient priority, the regulation of the flow of patients through the emergency center, and the initiation of diagnostic and treatment measures serve beneficial purposes in triage.[3]

Because emergency centers are facing increased patient volume, acuity and enormous pressure to control costs and legal risks, the determination of a triage method or system that accurately meets these needs is very important. A rich literature demonstrating a wide range of opinions on various aspects of the role of triage has evolved. It is difficult to envision a nationally or internationally accepted triage model. However, the diverse views appear to reflect local needs and the views of individuals.[3]

In the literature, the most frequently discussed and reported (although not fully validated) issue is that of triage systems, such as those from Australia,[4] Canada,[5] and England.[6] Other issues that have been covered include those of (1) who performs triage, (2) education or orientation programs, and (3) the assessment of triage system efficiency.[3]

Currently, most of emergency centers in the United States use some type of triage system despite the absence of good evidence supporting a particular triage system or protocol.[7] Whichever triage system is used must enable triage nurses to assess patients accurately, consistently, and efficiently.[8] Professional standards should be followed when creating triage systems or protocols. Additionally, the length and the level of complexity of these protocols should be realistic, accounting for the ability of the nursing staff, the type and volume of emergency center patients, the time taken to perform the assessment, and available resources. Triage nurses should use these protocols as tools and not be restricted by them. Also, triage decision making should be based on the patient's history and physical examination, with top priority placed on the patient's welfare. Finally, triage protocols should be approved and supervised by an emergency physician, who must assume the ultimate responsibility for the protocol.[9]

Triage involves the use of high-level assessment skills. Consequently, there is divided opinion as to who should perform triage.[3] The decision concerning who performs triage and the amount of training needed to do so should take into account the types and number of patients who visit the emergency center, the availability of qualified personnel, the triage provider's experience and ability, and the financial resources available for providing triage. Because of tradition and necessity, triage is frequently performed by nurses because of their training, experience, and availability.[9] Typically, during triage, a registered nurse takes an inventory of the patient's medical problems and assigns an appropriate acuteness rating to the patient's medical history. The nurse then ensures that the relevant medical intervention is initiated.

The position of a triage person is a challenging one that requires special qualifications, education, and skills. Qualifications for the triage role vary at different hospitals. Some hospitals require the completion of specific educational programs, such as advanced cardiac life support or certified emergency nursing (CEN) certification.[8] The need for triage training has been widely discussed and supported. In the literature, however, opinions on approaches to triage training are diverse. Specifically, a number of authors have recommended nonspecific training courses whereas others have suggested a nationally recognized training course.[3] Gilboy also suggested that a training course for triage nurses be accepted and mandated as the standard at all hospitals in the United States.[8] Regarding such a program, we believe that the educational content should incorporate theoretic, scientific, and empiric knowledge, with an emphasis on different patient populations. Competence should be assessed by written and/or oral examinations in conjunction with chart reviews.

Without an effective universally accepted triage system, each emergency center should oversee the practice of its individual triage system carefully and closely. Data should be collected to assess the efficiency of the system (ie, user-friendliness for triage nurses, patient waiting time, patient satisfaction, appropriateness of the patient flow through the emergency center, and cost-effectiveness).

Triage is routinely practiced in the emergency rooms of oncologic institutions as well as in general hospitals. There are few emergency centers at comprehensive cancer hospitals and centers in the United States, and little information on the triage of oncologic emergencies exists. Wherever triage is practiced, the goals and fundamental principles of triage should be followed. Triage personnel should be properly trained, especially with regard to the oncologic patient population.

Oncologic emergencies include neutropenic fever, superior vena cava syndrome, acute tumor lysis syndrome, hyperviscosity syndrome, hyperuricemia, hypercalcemia, neoplastic cardiac tamponade, spinal-cord compression, increased intracranial pressure, and reactions to chemotherapy. Each of these crises produces characteristic symptoms, physical findings, and laboratory abnormalities that the triage nurses should be properly trained to recognize.

TRIAGE PROCEDURES IN ONCOLOGY

The triage process begins when an oncology patient with a symptom or complaint presents to an emergency cen-

ter. Such a patient seeks emergency medical attention for a multitude of reasons that may be influenced by personal, cultural, financial, and social factors.[10] The process involves the collection of information pertinent to the visit and includes the gathering of demographic data, the triage interview, the classification of the patient by acuteness of condition, and the patient's transition from triage to the treatment area.

Initial Encounter

Most emergency centers have only one triage station and one triage nurse. The triage person is the first emergency center staff member the patient sees and is responsible for evaluating and prioritizing the urgency of patient care. In addition, some hospitals have a receptionist who attends the front desk. The receptionist is responsible for gathering patient information by using an individualized information sheet that is filled out by the patient and given to the triage nurse. This system provides and protects the patient's privacy and confidentiality. Also, the nurse or the receptionist informs the patient and family members about what they can expect while they are in the emergency center. A brochure containing emergency center information available at the reception area may be helpful.

When the reception area is at full capacity, the patient advocate should assist in providing basic comfort needs as well as in alleviating the anxiety of patients and their family members. Patients usually judge the service provided by the emergency center staff on the the basis of the knowledge and kindness exhibited by the staff, starting with the receptionist.[11]

The Interview

The triage interview provides substantial information about which actions and interventions should be taken. The triage nurse performs the interview by obtaining objective and subjective data. First, the triage nurse must introduce him- or herself to the patient. Next, an initial assessment of the patient's airway, breathing, and circulation should be done.[12] A brief physical assessment is performed, using the five senses.[13] Questions should be brief and easy to comprehend, and the patient's age, competency, cultural beliefs, and language should be taken into consideration when choosing the most appropriate interview technique.

The interview process is very important as a means of establishing a rapport with and alleviating the anxiety of patients and their family members. A patient advocate aids in this process by assisting new oncology patients who come to the emergency center seeking medical attention. Also, language barriers should be overcome with the help of interpreters.

Decision-Making Process. Triage nurses are expected to make a clinical judgment based on the triage interview. The same general concept in triage decision making is applied, in addition to assessment, specifically to oncologic emergencies. Therefore, a triage person must have an in-depth knowledge of oncologic emergencies and other disease processes.

Patients who become acutely ill while awaiting triage require a concise and accurate assessment. Those who arrive by ambulance and are determined to be emergency cases are taken directly to the treatment area for quick triage and immediate treatment. Most emergency centers have the triage or charge nurse coordinate room assignments for patients who need emergency care or who are critically ill.[14] The triage or charge nurse following hospital protocols, policies, and procedures can initiate diagnostic tests.

An estimated 40 to 55% of all patients who visit emergency centers represent nonurgent cases.[15] In some hospital emergency centers, nurse practitioners manage nonurgent patients. Additionally, a study of waiting time in a general hospital in Everett, Washington, revealed a reduction in waiting time from triage to discharge after a fast-track unit was opened for patients with noncritical problems.[16] Finally, both urgent and nonurgent patients who are taken to the waiting area need periodic reassessment by the triage person.

Documentation. The triage interview is not complete until all the information obtained is documented in the emergency center record. The oncology emergency center record should contain the following triage information:

- Date
- Time
- Mode of transportation
- Accompanying person
- Acuity classification
- Primary physician
- Chief complaint and history of present illness
- Vital signs (orthostatic if indicated)
- Allergies
- Past medical history
- Current cancer treatment
- Medications being taken

Revision

The triage process requires periodic review and revision for improvement. Benchmarking is one of the ways of reviewing a current triage process to determine the best practice. A continuous quality improvement of the triage process can be accomplished through satisfaction surveys, waiting-time analysis, patient volume and acuity measurement, nurse-to-patient ratio analysis, and reviews of logistics, physical layout, new-employee orientation, and Joint Commission on Accreditation of Healthcare Organization (JCAHO) recommendations. An annual review of the process should be done by a focus group, comparing the current practice with what is considered the best practice.

Compliance with Antidumping Laws

Under the 1986 patient antidumping laws, also known as the Emergency Medical Treatment and Active Labor Act (EMTALA)[17]/Consolidated Omnibus Budget Reconciliation Act (COBRA)[17] of 1985, all Medicare participant hospitals with emergency rooms must provide appropriate medical screening to all patients requesting emergency care, to determine whether the patient has a condition that requires immediate medical attention. If so, the hospital must, within its capabilities, provide stabilizing care. The transfer of an unstable patient to another facility is allowed only when an informed patient requests the transfer or a physician certifies that the medical benefits of this action outweigh the risks. Violators of the antidumping law face significant penalties. Doctors and large hospitals that violate any requirement of the law are subject to a civil penalty of up to $50,000 per offense. Hospitals that violate this law can also face termination from the Medicare program, and physicians who are found to be responsible for repeated or flagrant violations can be excluded from participation in all federal health care programs.[17]

Under the EMTALA/COBRA statute, hospitals are required to maintain a list of on-call physicians.[17] After performing an initial examination, the emergency center physician may determine that a patient requires the service of a listed on-call physician and may notify that physician. If the on-call physician fails or refuses to appear within a reasonable period and the emergency center physician determines that the benefits of transferring the patient to another facility outweigh the risks, the emergency center physician may authorize the transfer and shall not be subject to penalty.[17] However, the statute does not exempt from liability either the hospital or the on-call physician who fails or refuses to appear.

Patient Departure before Treatment

Patients who present with non-life-threatening problems in the emergency center often have to wait for several hours and sometimes get tired of waiting and leave. If such a patient became seriously ill because he or she did not receive medical attention, the nurse could be held accountable if the delay in treatment was unwarranted or if the patient was not informed of the risk incurred by leaving. Patients in the emergency center must be re-evaluated at reasonable intervals, and their status must be documented each time. This documentation shows that the nurse monitored the patient throughout his or her stay. If the patient wants to leave before being treated, the nurse should inform the patient of the risks and procure documentation that the patient has been so informed. If the patient still wants to leave, he or she should be asked to sign an Against Medical Advice Form, which should be filed in the patient's chart. If the patient refuses to sign, refusal should be documented in the chart.

Maintaining medical records and a medical records library is mandated by the federal government, non-governmental agencies such as JCAHO, and state and local rules. The American Legal System suggests that to chart entries correctly, medical personnel should (1) make an entry for every observation; (2) always make an entry, even if it is late; (3) make an entry after and not before each event; (4) use clear and objective language; (5) make entries that are realistic and factual; (6) chart a patient's refusal of care, including refusal of patient education; (7) never alter a record at someone else's request; (8) provide a signature after each entry; and (9) leave no room for liability.[18]

Telephone Triage

Since its invention in 1876, the telephone has been linked to medicine. Alexander Graham Bell made the first telephone call to his assistant for medical assistance when he spilled sulfuric acid on himself. By 1887, a telephone consultation had been described in the medical literature (after listening to a child cough over the telephone, a physician reassured the mother that her child did not have croup).[19] Since then, telephone triage has become an integral part of health care in the United States and around the world. Emergency and urgent care centers and physician's offices receive such telephone inquiries from a wide range of patients.

Telephone triage is the process in which a health care provider communicates with the patient via telephone and thereby assesses the presenting concerns, develops a working diagnosis, and determines a suitable plan of management.[20] In emergency centers, telephone triage is a way to give patients information on demand, assess and prioritize the need for treatment, and direct the patient to the most appropriate service available.

The purpose of telephone triage is similar to that of face-to-face triage: to determine the level of care required and to assign an acuity level.[21] Telephone triage provides patients with advice when the office or clinic is closed, enables physicians to practice demand management, and decreases the costs for insurance companies.[22]

The telephone system is critical to the success of cancer patient care. The system must be accessible, capable of handling an adequate volume of calls, and user-friendly. Also, the telephone triage staff members must understand the difference between routine calls and emergency calls. The role of the triage nurse is to make decisions about the acuity of each case. The four main telephone triage outcomes are *emergency*, which should

be handled by interrupting the physician or by calling 911; *urgent*, which should be responded to within 1 to 2 hours with a decision for care; *same day*, which should be responded to with an appointment or a later call back; and *routine*, which can be dealt with when convenient.

Systematic patient assessment is critical in providing safe and effective patient care by telephone. Nurses and other health care professionals who care for patients by telephone know that the essence of telephone triage lies in the ability to make accurate decisions based on verbal communication only. Therefore, communication skills are of paramount importance.

The following processes must be carried out for effective telephone triage:

1. *Definition of the scope of the problem.* Whether the institution in question is a cancer center or a general medical center, identification of the scope of the problem being reported will help prioritize the most common complaints received via telephone.

2. *Development of clinical protocols.* Protocols designed to address the most frequently reported problems can be developed after a prospective study identifies the types of calls received. Telephone protocols are organized guidelines used to evaluate, classify, advise, educate, and intervene. Two major content areas must be addressed in the protocol: assessment, which includes evaluation and classification; and disposition, which consists of information related to advice, education, self-care, and treatment.[23]

3. *Documentation.* Documenting each call is vital because it provides a written record, thereby minimizing the legal risk involved with giving advice over the telephone. In addition, written documentation will assist other professionals involved in telephone triage when people call back with further questions. The documentation should be clear, concise, detailed, and measurable. It should include the patient's own words as well as the following information:

   - Name of the caller/patient
   - Date and time of the call
   - Demographic information about the caller/patient
   - Brief statement about the illness
   - History, signs, and symptoms
   - Brief statement about the advice given
   - Protocol followed and any warnings given to the caller/patient

   Also, the patient's disposition, assessment, clinic appointment, compliance, warnings, consultation with the physician, and signature must be documented.[22]

4. *Quality assurance.* A written or computer-based documentation log provides a means of tracking call trends and critiquing the quality of information recorded by the nurse. Also, frequent audits by the

TABLE 2–1. Triage Urgency Classification of Presenting Problems

Emergent
    Cardiac arrest
    Respiratory distress or dyspnea
    Chest pain
    Drug overdose
    Anaphylaxis
    Symptomatic arrhythmia
    Severe abdominal pain
    Fever with known/suspected neutropenia or unstable vital signs
    Major bleeding (hematemesis, hemoptysis, epistaxis, vaginal bleeding, hematochezia, or melena)
    Unresponsiveness, obtundation
    Suspected spinal-cord compression
    Active or recent seizures
    Severe cancer-related pain (8 to 10 on 0–10 pain scale)
    Intractable nausea, vomiting, and/or diarrhea with severe dehydration
    Acute leukemia with high white blood cell counts
    Syncope with orthostatic change or other symptoms such as dyspnea or palpitations
Urgent
    Palpitations without symptoms
    Mental status changes
    Nausea, vomiting, and/or diarrhea without orthostatic change
    Mild to moderate cancer pain
    Fever in a patient known not to be neutropenic
    Headache without nausea/vomiting or neurologic changes
    Dysuria or hematuria
    Minor bleeding (hematemesis, hemoptysis, epistaxis, vaginal bleeding, hematochezia, or melena)
    Stomatitis/mucositis
    Fatigue or weakness without orthostatic change
    Abnormal but not critical laboratory values
Nonurgent
    Failure to thrive
    Lower back pain
    Sore throat, cough
    Constipation
    Rash
    Anxiety with no associated symptoms
    Scheduled procedures: analysis of blood products, electrolyte replacement
    Ascites

quality assurance committee, using an audit checklist, can help maintain consistent standards. Suggestions for protocols or for changes in protocols should be submitted to this committee and reviewed.

Although the best legal recommendation is to avoid giving advice over the telephone, patients will still call emergency centers and request information. In today's cancer care environment, many people have very limited financial resources, which prevents them from seeking medical care in an emergency center. Therefore, their only link to health care professionals may be through the telephone. Telephone triage can provide the cancer care community easy access to information for the management of specific problems.

Management of telephone triage (or advice calls) is controversial. Although formal policies and procedures on handling these calls are scarce, the pertinent literature usually directs that advice should not be given and that the decision to visit the emergency center should be left to the caller. Giving generic advice such as "call 911" or "come to the emergency center" may be medically correct but inadequate. Establishing formal policies and procedures with protocols for specific situations may be a proactive method of handling this difficult situation. Policies and procedures set standards, which can be used to implement protocols to guide interviewers.[24] If telephone advice is given, calls should be logged with the caller's name, location, and callback number; a description of the medical concern; and a description of the advice given. It is important to realize that callers may be noncompliant with any advice given via telephone. Documentation is very important in protecting the health care provider and institution from liability.

FAST-TRACK PROGRAMS IN ONCOLOGY EMERGENCY CENTERS

Data from the 1995 US Department of Health and Human Services Emergency Department Survey indicate that approximately 96.5 million emergency department visits were made in 1995.[25] The number of visits by patients to emergency centers (ECs) across the country has been increasing in recent years, owing to the use of ECs for primary care after regular office hours, to shorter hospitalization stays and earlier discharges, to increased acuity, and to the use of the EC as the "front door" of the hospital. In the early 1980s, numerous urgent care clinics were established in communities to provide care for patients with nonurgent minor injuries and illnesses. Compared with traditional ECs, urgent care clinics can treat patients more quickly and economically. Traditional ECs are often criticized for incurring high cost, subjecting patients to long waiting times, and focusing mainly on patients who are critically ill or in need of urgent care.[26] Traditionally, the sickest and most unstable patients are examined first whereas patients who do not require urgent care usually have to wait for hours before they are examined. This prioritizing resulted in poor satisfaction among patients who did not require urgent care.[27]

The problems with general ECs, as described above, also apply to oncology ECs although the patient populations of oncology ECs are more limited. The chief complaints of patients who visit oncology ECs are mostly cancer-related problems (such as neutropenic fever, nausea and vomiting, dehydration, pneumonia, and constipation) and rarely involve trauma. Throughout the United States, many alternative programs have been developed to solve these problems as well as to compete with ECs for patients. One solution is the fast-track (FT) program, whereby a nonurgent care facility is housed adjacently to the EC.

Various health care providers who schedule time to meet the nonurgent care needs of a particular EC often create the FT program informally and by necessity via innovative methods. These efforts are made to respond to the increasing demand for ECs by quickly assigning patients to their level of care, thus reducing waiting times and ultimately saving some unnecessary expenses.

Facility Staffing

In most ECs, the use of midlevel providers such as nurse practitioners (NPs) or physician assistants (PAs) has become a cost- and time-efficient measure[27,28] and is becoming more popular. A written protocol would serve as a guide to assist these personnel in their practice. This approach would allow physicians more time to devote to patients with more emergent problems. Overall, the use of NPs in the FT facilities of ECs has proved beneficial, providing a high quality of patient care.[21,29]

Since most FT facilities are located near an EC, supervision by or consultation with a physician is readily available. In some FT facilities, the use of physicians may be more cost- and time-efficient than would be the use of midlevel providers,[27] owing to reimbursement issues as well as to physician supervision.

Triage Process and Criteria

All patients presenting at an EC should undergo triage as described above. Patients that meet certain criteria (Table 2–2) can be transferred from EC triage to the FT area. Patients whose condition becomes unstable can be moved back to the main EC at any time.

The criteria for FT assignment emphasizes the complaint and the patient's conditions in the context of the cancer. For instance, sore throat and fever in a neutropenic oncology patient may be more serious and may necessitate more laboratory testing and medication intervention than in a patient without cancer. Another example is that nausea and vomiting in an oncology patient raise the possibility of bowel obstruction and may thus require radiologic study and laboratory testing. Furthermore, most oncology patients also have chronic diseases, such as heart disease, diabetes mellitus, chronic obstructive pulmonary disease, or hypertension. These conditions make the overall assessment of these patients more time-consuming and complex. Because of this complexity, an FT system in an oncology EC may differ from an FT system in a general EC.

TABLE 2–2. Presenting Criteria for Fast-Track Triage

Presenting Symptom	Criteria*
Allergic reaction	• No respiratory distress, no chest pains
Conjunctivitis	• No eye pain; no visual changes; no fever
Constipation	• No abdominal pain, nausea, or vomiting
Cough	• T < 38.5°C; new onset (5 days); O$_2$ saturation > 92%
Employee/visitor illness or injury	• No chest pain
	• On-the-job injury
	• Needle stick (if not treated already by employee health care)
	• High blood pressure without chest pain or syncope
	• Fall without fracture or deep laceration
	• Superficial abrasion or laceration
	• Acute minor strain or sprain
	• Superficial cut without tendon involvement
	• First- or second-degree or superficial burn from chemical, heat, or ice
Fever	• No septic symptoms: SBP > 100 mm Hg; DBP > 50 mm Hg; P < 120 bpm; R < 24/min; T < 39.5°C; no bleeding
Foley catheter problems	• Catheter does not drain or contains hematuria/sediments
	• No mental status change, no edema, no elevation of blood pressure
Hypertension	• SBP < 210 mm Hg; DPB < 110 mm Hg; no chest pain; no shortness of breath
Mucositis/cold sore	• Grade 1 or 2; T < 38.3°C; no bleeding
Nasal congestion	• T < 38.3°C; no facial swelling
Otitis media	• Ear pain; no mental status change; T < 38.3°C
Rash/dermatitis	• No shortness of breath; no chest pain
Upper respiratory infection/sore throat	• No stridor; no shortness of breath
Urinary tract infection	• No hematuria
Reflux	• No acute nausea/vomiting
Cellulitis	• No fever, no signs of sepsis
Foreign body	• No perforation of tympanic membrane

DBP = diastolic blood pressure; P = pulse; R = respiration; SBP = systolic blood pressure; T = temperature.
*Table 2–1 shows conditions that could be considered fast-track criteria in oncology emergency centers.

Conclusion

The success of the FT program also depends on other supportive factors, such as radiology and laboratory turnaround time, transportation, and nursing and medical staffs. Once an FT program has been implemented, it can be redesigned later to correct problem areas in radiology departments[30] or in laboratories, for example.

The FT programs in oncology ECs may improve patient satisfaction and decrease waiting time. A pilot study using midlevel providers to examine and treat patients in the EC of M. D. Anderson Cancer Center (unpublished data) indicated that the average waiting time of patients treated in the FT program was 49 minutes less than that of patients treated in the general EC.

However, FT programs may not solve other problems such as space constraints and long waiting times for ancillary services such as laboratory testing and radiology.

REFERENCES

1. Webster's Encyclopedic Unabridged Dictionary. New York: Gramercy Books; 1996.
2. Purnell LD. A survey of emergency department triage in 185 hospitals: physical facilities, fast-track systems, patient-classification systems, waiting times, and qualification, training, and skills of triage personnel, J Emerg Nurs 1991;17:402–7.
3. McDonald L, Butterworth T, Yates DW. Triage: a literature review 1985–1993. Accid Emerg Nurs 1995;3:201–7.
4. Policy document—triage. Australasian College for Emergency Medicine; 1993. http://www.acem.org.au/open/documents/triage.htm.
5. Beveridge R. Implementation guidelines for the Canadian Emergency Department Triage and Acuity Scale. Canadian Association of Emergency Physicians; 1998. http://www.caep.ca/caep/plsql/get?page=index3.html.
6. The Manchester Triage Group. Emergency triage. Mackway-Jones K. editor. London: BMJ Publishing Group; 1997.
7. Femandes CM, Wuerz R, Clark S, Djurdjev O. How reliable is emergency department triage? Am Emerg Med 1999;34:141–147.
8. Gilboy N, Travers D, Wuerz R. Re-evaluating triage in the new millennium: a comprehensive look at the need for standardization and quality. J Emerg Nurs 1999;25:468–73.
9. Rice MM. Legal issues in emergency medicine. In: Rosen P, editor. Emergency medicine. 4th ed. Vol. 1. St. Louis: Mosby; 1998. p. 233–44.
10. Williams RM. Triage and emergency department services. Ann Emerg Med 1996;27:506–8.
11. Baker S. Managing patient expectations: the art of finding and keeping loyal patients. San Francisco: Jossey-Bass Publishers; 1998.
12. Handysides G. Triage: critical skills, complexities and challenges. In: Handysides G, editor. Triage in emergency practice. St. Louis: Mosby Publishing; 1996. p. 1–27.
13. Rice M, Abel C. Triage. In: Sheeby SB, editor. Emergency nursing principles and practice. 3rd ed. Philadelphia: Mosby Year Book; 1992. p. 23–31.
14. Mayer TA. Triage: history and horizons. Top Emerg Med 1997;19:1–11.
15. Kellermann AL. Nonurgent emergency department visits: meeting an unmet need. JAMA 1994;271:1953–4.
16. Romanelli N. We put ED patients on the fast track. RN 1992;55:17–20.
17. Policy Document: COBRA statute 42 USC 1395 dd (1985). http://medlaw.com/statute.htm.
18. Guido GW. Documentation and confidentiality. Legal and ethical issues in nursing. 3rd ed. Upper Saddle River (NJ): Prentice Hall; 2001. p. 169–99.
19. Elnicki DM, Ogden P, Flannery M, et al. Telephone medicine for internists. J Gen Intern Med 2000;15:337–43.
20. DeVore NE. Telephone triage. A challenge for practicing midwives. J Nurse Midwifery 1999;44:471–9.
21. Grossman VGA. Triage process. Quick reference to triage. 1st ed. Philadelphia: Lippincott; 1999.
22. Princiotta CM. Telephone triage: good business. Adv Nurse Pract 1999;7:21.
23. Robinson DL, Anderson MM, Acheson PM. Telephone advice: lessons learned and considerations for starting programs. J Emerg Nurs 1996;22:409–15.
24. Trandel-Korenchuk DM, Trandel-Korenchuk KM. Nursing and the law. 5th ed. Gaitherburg (MD): Aspen Publications; 1997. p. 179–180.
25. Blunt E. Role and productivity of nurse practitioners in one urban emergency department. J Emerg Nurs 1998;24:234–9.
26. Meislin HW, Coates SA, Cyr J, Valenzuela T. Fast track: urgent care within a teaching hospital emergency department: can it work? Ann Emerg Med 1988;17:453–6.
27. Docimo AB, Pronovost PJ, Davis RO, et al. Using the online and offline change model to improve efficiency for fast-track patients in an emergency department. Jt Comm J Qual Improv 2000;26:503–14.
28. Counselman FL, Schafermeyer RW, Perina DG. Academic departments of emergency medicine: the effects of managed care. Acad Emerg Med 1998;5:1095–100.
29. Wright SW, Erwin TL, Blanton DM, Covington CM. Fast track in the emergency department: a one-year experience with nurse practitioners. J Emerg Med 1992;10:367–73.
30. Espinosa JA, Treiber PM, Kosnik LA. Reengineering success story: process improvement in emergency department x-ray cycle time, leading to breakthrough performance in the ED ambulatory care (fast track) process. Ambul Outreach 1997;19:24–7.

CHAPTER 3

ETHICAL EMERGENCY CARE

REBECCA D. PENTZ, PhD
ANNE L. FLAMM, JD
ELLEN F. MANZULLO, MD

ALGORITHM FOR ETHICAL MEDICAL EMERGENCY CARE

The ethical principles of emergency medicine are the same as those of medicine in general: beneficence, nonmaleficence, justice, and respect for personal autonomy, with the correlative requirement of truth telling.[1,2] (This list of ethical principles is intended not to be exhaustive but rather to include the principles that are most relevant to the ethical exigencies of emergency medicine.) However, the exigencies of the emergency environment, the frequent absence of a developed physician-patient relationship, patients' need for immediate treatment, and the high quotient of unknown factors require the nuanced application of each principle in the emergency setting. The algorithm outlined in Figure 3–1 and summarized in Table 3–1 provides a general ethical framework for medical emergency care, with special attention to cancer patients. In the following description, each step of the algorithm is accompanied by a discussion of the relevant ethical principles and considerations.

Step I: Determine whether an Emergent Medical Condition Exists

The open access of emergency centers and the specialized training of their staffs enable professionals in these centers to attend to patients whose immediate condition, if not remedied, threatens death or serious impairment. While these characteristics reflect the premium societal value placed on preserving human life, they also contribute to the high costs of maintaining emergency centers. Health professionals, as well as the patients who depend on emergency centers for care, have an ethical obligation to act as stewards of health care resources and to reserve emergency resources for the patients for whom they are designed and staffed. Thus, the emergency center staff's first obligation is to determine whether a patient requires immediate medical care.

If an Emergency Condition Exists. Most of this chapter concerns ethical issues that may arise once physicians assume care of a patient who presents to the emergency center. However, an ethical dilemma may arise the moment a patient who cannot pay for treatment walks through the doors. Although physicians have a duty to treat the patient, providing "free" care threatens the viability of institutions, in turn threatening the well-being of citizens whose community hospitals may be forced to shut down their emergency centers. This conundrum illustrates the convergence of and conflict between physicians' and hospitals' obligations of beneficence toward patients who present to the emergency center and the broader principle of justice, which requires health care resources to be distributed fairly and evenly to a community's residents.

In 1986, Congress enacted the Emergency Medical Treatment and Active Labor Act (EMTALA)[3] to prevent the arbitrary refusal of treatment to uninsured people presenting to emergency departments (referred to as "patient dumping"). This act mandates that any person who presents at a qualifying hospital (ie, any hospital with a Medicare contract) is entitled to appropriate medical screening to determine whether he or she has an emergency medical condition. Thus, if the physician's examination indicates that such a condition exists, an emergency center must, using the staff and facilities available, provide the examination and treatment necessary to stabilize the person's emergency medical condition. "Stabilization" includes ensuring that no material deterioration of the patient's condition is likely to occur (within reasonable medical probability) as a result of the transfer of the patient from a facility. Once stabilized, the patient may be safely discharged home or transferred to another medical facility, as appropriate. The act ensures compliance by hospitals and physicians through various enforcement mechanisms, including civil causes of action, monetary penalties, and exclusion from Medicare. Because it obligates hospitals to

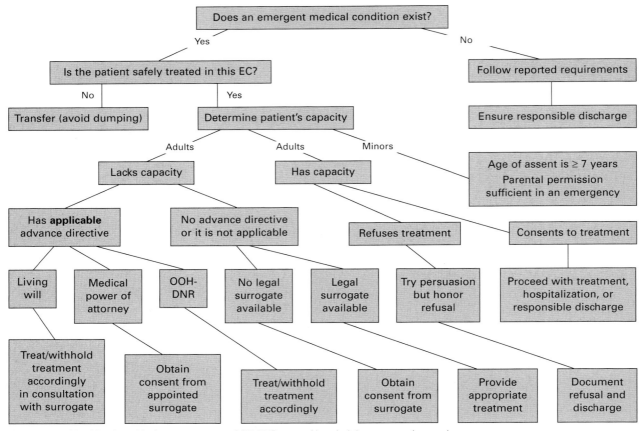

Figure 3–1. Algorithm for ethical emergency care. OOH-DNR = out of hospital do-not-resuscitate order.

screen and treat patients without providing a mechanism by which to pay for the emergency care, EMTALA has been criticized for leaving hospitals at the mercy of "free-riding"[4] managed-care companies and patients. The dilemma created by requiring hospitals to provide emergency care to nonpaying patients remains unresolved.

If the benefits of treating the patient at another facility that is better prepared to treat the patient's condition outweigh the risks of transfer, the beneficent physician will recommend transfer. Recognizing that this situation does not constitute dumping, EMTALA specifies a procedure for certifying an unstable patient's transfer based on a physician's assessment that the benefits of transfer outweigh the risks. An unstable patient may also request to be transferred if he or she has the capacity to decide and voluntarily chooses transfer. If the unstable patient chooses transfer even after the physician has informed the patient of the hospital's obligation to treat and the risks of transfer, EMTALA will not impose liability for dumping.

In any transfer, the patient's health and well-being are the overriding concerns. The transferring physician should obtain the agreement of the receiving institution, communicating all relevant clinical information and sending pertinent records along with the patient. As with

any discharge from an emergency center, staff members are responsible for the patient's safety during transport.

Although reportable conditions are not typically coincident with cancer, emergency personnel must be familiar with local reporting requirements that often apply in cases of communicable diseases (such as tuberculosis) and the abuse of children or elderly persons. In addition, state law may require health professionals to report to the state cancer registry those patients who present to the emergency center and who are diagnosed with a new malignancy.[5]

If No Emergency Condition Exists. The duty of beneficence imposes obligations on physicians in the discharge of patients from the emergency center, whether or not the physicians have provided emergency care. If there is no emergent condition, then the physician should follow the procedure for responsible release outlined in step III, below.

Step II: Determine the Patient's Capacity, and Proceed with Treatment

An adult is judged to have the capacity to make medical decisions if the physician determines that the patient can (1) understand the treatment options, (2) grasp the consequences of choosing one option or another, (3) relate the options to her or his own values and life priorities, and (4) communicate these choices.

> Case 1: Frank Slade comes to the emergency room short of breath. The medical record shows that a year ago, he was treated for squamous cell carcinoma of the lung with radiation and chemotherapy, that he recently relapsed, and that he was again receiving standard chemotherapy. In spite of his hypoxic condition, Mr. Slade is oriented to time and place and knows why he is in the emergency center, namely, to be relieved of shortness of breath.

The bioethical underpinning of the requirement to determine a patient's capacity is respect for personal autonomy—specifically, the right to control over one's body. In the United States, US Supreme Court Justice Benjamin Cardozo first explicitly articulated the principle of patients' autonomy in health care in 1914, writing, "Every human being of adult years and sound mind has a right to determine what shall be done with his own body."[6] Gaining prominence following the Civil Rights movement of the 1960s,[7,8] the principle supported the development of a shared decision-making model in which the physician recommends the treatment that promises the most benefit to the patient yet expects the patient to make the ultimate choice. This practice, which incorporates the physician's duty of beneficence and respect for the patient's autonomy, has become the standard in North America and northern Europe.[9]

The principle of autonomy must be seen in its historical context because it is not universally recognized. While references to the principle can be found throughout medical history,[10] physicians traditionally made decisions without explicit input from their patients. This parentalism continues to be the standard of practice in much of the Far East, Middle East, and southern Europe and in some subcultures in the United States.[11-16] The practice of shared decision making is not always possible in the emergency center when an emergency medical condition may have robbed the patient of decision-making capacity. Such circumstances negate the requirement that the physician obtain autonomous patient consent to treatment. Therefore, the emergency center (EC) physician must determine the patient's capacity.[17]

Beyond the four components stated above, emergency physicians must recognize that decisional capacity is task specific. That is, a patient may be able to demonstrate each of the components and thus possess sufficient capacity for making medical decisions, even while being unable to make other types of decisions.[18] When the primary physician is uncertain of whether a patient has sufficient capacity to make medical decisions, the opinion of a psychiatrist or other medical professional expert may be helpful in assessing capacity.

TABLE 3–1. Summary of an Algorithm for Ethical Medical Emergency Care

I. Determine whether emergent medical condition exists
  A. Yes, emergency condition exists
    1. Treat: go to II
    2. Transfer (avoid dumping)
    3. Follow reporting requirements
  B. No emergency condition exists: go to III

II. Proceed with treatment
  A. Determine patient's capacity
    1. Adults
    2. Minors
  B. Patient has capacity
    1. Patient consents to emergency treatment
    2. Patient refuses emergency treatment
    3. Patient leaves against medical advice
  C. Patient lacks capacity
    1. Determine existence of advance directives
    2. Identify surrogate decision maker
      a. Seeking telephone consent
      b. Challenging surrogate's decision
    3. Lacking advance directives or surrogate consent, provide appropriate medical care
  D. Patient or surrogate demands medically inappropriate or futile care

III. Ensure responsible discharge

IV. Meet responsibilities upon death of patient
  A. Request organ donation
  B. Meet inquest, autopsy, and reporting requirements

> Case 2: Jake, an 11-year-old boy, is brought to the EC by his parents. His leukemia has relapsed, and he needs immediate hospitalization. Jake agrees to the hospitalization but confides to the EC physician that he has decided that he will not agree to further chemotherapy; he has had enough. The EC physician now faces a dilemma: the boy is older than the age of assent, and he has indicated that he may refuse potentially life-prolonging treatment.

Society has traditionally judged children not to have the abilities necessary for capacity and entrusts appropriate surrogates to safeguard their autonomy. However, children who have lived with cancer are often mature beyond their years and have a sophisticated understanding of medical procedures. These children can sometimes participate in relatively complex discussions about treatment. The age of assent, the age when the child's assent to a procedure should be sought, is commonly considered to be 7 years.[19-21] A true ethical dilemma arises when a child older than 7 years does not assent to a procedure his or her parents choose. In the context of a stable physician-patient relationship and with the help of resources usually available in pediatric oncology settings (including child-life and social workers), these conflicts can usually be resolved. When there is no time to resolve the dilemma (as may often be the case in the emergency setting) the surrogate's consent is sufficient for treatment.

Patient Has Capacity and Consents to Emergency Treatment. If the patient has capacity and consents to emergency treatment, the physician should recommend the appropriate treatment and then abide by the patient's choice.

> Case 1 (continued): Mr. Slade's shortness of breath persists. The emergency physician explains that if prolongation of life is Mr. Slade's goal, he may need to be intubated. However, since future extubation is unlikely, the physician also explains that comfort measures are available if Mr. Slade wishes to avoid ventilator dependence. The patient manages to say that he wants everything possible done.

Every physician carries a "benefit/burden calculator" next to his beeper: Is a particular treatment likely to result in more benefits than burdens, and if so, will it yield more benefits than another treatment? This way of analyzing treatment options pervades medicine and is strongly rooted in the hippocratic bioethical principles of beneficence (striving to benefit the patient) and nonmaleficence (avoiding harm to the patient). These principles require the physician to weigh the benefits and burdens of treatment in light of the patient's overall treatment goals and to then recommend a course of action. Unless the options are medically equal, the physician should recommend the medically superior treatment, disclose the alternatives, and explain the reasons for the recommendation. Again, respect for patient autonomy requires that once the patient is informed, the patient be allowed to make the decision. In most circumstances, the patient's presentation to the EC reflects his or her desire for treatment, and consent for the recommended treatment is easily granted. However, a refusal or choice of an alternative treatment does not necessarily indicate that the patient lacks capacity.

Patient Refuses Emergency Treatment. There is now general agreement in the law and among bioethicists and the public that a competent patient has the right to refuse medical care.[22] This right to refuse care includes the right to refuse life-sustaining treatments such as cardiopulmonary resuscitation (CPR) and mechanical ventilation as well as the various forms of nutritional support.[23,24] One notable limitation of this right is a treatment refusal that would subject others to significant health risks. For example, a person with a highly communicable serious disease must either accept effective treatment or be placed in quarantine. When a physician judges a patient's treatment refusal to be irrational or to be threatening to others, noncoercive and nonmanipulative attempts to persuade such a patient to accept treatment do not violate the patient's autonomy and right of self-determination.[25]

When a patient refuses treatment, the physician must determine the factors that have contributed to the patient's refusal. This requires spending time talking with the patient, which may be difficult in emergency situations but which is necessary to enable the physician to evaluate whether the patient's refusal is informed according to the same criteria required for informed consent.[26] In the case of cancer patients, the physician must also consider whether the patient is in a state of denial. A patient who has not accepted the existence of his or her disease process might not understand the severity of the condition and might consequently make a choice he or she would not make if that understanding were clearer. Careful and sensitive information sharing is important in such circumstances.

Other factors may motivate cancer patients to refuse emergency medical care. Refusal of care may indicate the need for better symptom management. For example, since most patients with advanced cancer and up to 60% of patients at all stages of the disease experience significant pain,[27] physicians should ascertain whether the patient views refusal of care as a means of ending the pain. Patients also differ in the degree to which they are willing to tolerate painful treatments or conditions for the sake of others.[28] Only the patient can determine what burdens are worth enduring, and only the well-informed patient can make a decision that reflects his or her values and goals.

> Case 2 (continued): The EC physician probes Jake's reasons for refusing further chemotherapy and discovers that during Jake's last two courses of chemotherapy, symptoms were not well managed. She assures the boy that these symptoms are treatable and that he should not suffer in silence. She asks permission to contact Jake's attending physician to explain Jake's concerns.

A patient's religious beliefs may lead to a refusal of medical treatments. One well-known example is the competent patient who is a Jehovah's Witness and who explicitly states that because of long-standing religious beliefs, no blood or blood products are to be administered.[29] Although the physician may struggle with this decision, neither legal nor bioethical principles differentiate between a treatment refusal for religious reasons and a refusal for other reasons. Both require the physician to inform the patient of the benefits of the proposed treatment and the consequences of the treatment refusal. Competent individuals who reject lifesaving medical care may sue for battery if the treatment is administered against their wishes.[25]

Finally, the patient's refusal of medical treatment may reflect mismatched goals among the patient, family members, and medical team. While presentation to the EC presumes a patient's desire for life-prolonging treatment, some end-stage cancer patients wish to avoid aggressive interventions. Their treatment refusal may be an opportunity to discuss preferences for code status and to redirect treatment toward a palliative mode. Thus, treatment refusals may indicate the need for a more appropriate care plan.

Patient Leaves against Medical Advice.

Case 2 (continued): The EC physician leaves to invite Jake's parents back into the room. Alone with the nurse, Jake confides that he wants to be done with everything and that he is going home.

Patients with capacity who refuse treatment may wish to leave the EC against medical advice. Although the principle of autonomy ultimately supports a competent patient's right to leave, the principle of beneficence requires the emergency physician to try to prevent the patient's departure. Patients wish to leave for many reasons: fear of medical care, obligations to children at home or a demanding boss at work, or religious objections like those discussed above, among others. After exploring the patient's reasons for wanting to leave, the physician should try to persuade the patient to stay, perhaps enlisting other staff members with whom the patient has friendly relations and who may contact family members or other sources of social support to address the patient's concerns.

If all attempts fail, the physician should clearly inform the patient of the risks involved in leaving and suggest alternatives for obtaining care. Many institutions require patients to sign a form acknowledging departure against medical advice, or institutions may require other documentation under such circumstances.

Case 2 (concluded): At the prompting of the nurse, the EC physician returns to the room and again discusses Jake's fears and concerns. The parents tell the EC physician that their son trusts one of the child-life workers. The EC physician requests that the child-life worker come to the EC to be with the boy, but she also makes plans to admit the child against his wishes, with the consent of the parents, since hospitalization is medically necessary and because the boy will be at great risk if he goes home. The EC physician calls the attending physician; they agree that upon admission, a palliative-care consultation will be requested.

Patient Lacks Capacity.

Determine the Existence of Advance Directives.

Case 1 (continued): Mr. Slade continues to deteriorate, and he loses capacity as his hypoxia increases. His wife, who is present, reports that her husband's medical record, currently in the hospital's storage area, includes his handwritten living will. She emphasizes that the living will asks that everything possible be done. Retrieved from storage, Mr. Slade's nonstandard living will states, "Do everything possible in an emergency. I want full resuscitation—anything possible to keep me alive."

There are two basic types of advance directives: the living will, or directive to physicians, and the medical power of attorney. The living will is the patient's statement about his or her choice of treatment, usually near the end of life. Many state statutes recognize a standard living will stating that the patient refuses life-sustaining treatments for an irreversible and/or terminal condition.

The application of this type of living will is often ambiguous, particularly in the cancer setting. The emergency physician, who may have had little or no past contact with the patient and who has no time to explore options, may have difficulty determining whether or not the current crisis is a truly irreversible or terminal event. In case of reasonable doubt, a trial of therapy is appropriate and consistent with the language of most standard living wills.

Additionally, many people do not understand the meaning of the terms "irreversible" and "terminal" and assume that their living will covers all contingencies in which aggressive life-sustaining interventions may be offered. The emergency physician must be prepared to discuss the actual content of the living will with families, explaining, when appropriate, that the patient's current crisis cannot be definitively determined to be irreversible and that a trial of therapy is recommended.

Physicians can no longer assume that a living will reflects the previously typical refusal of aggressive life-sustaining interventions. Patients may write specific instructions that delete or add to language in living-will forms, or they may compose a new original document. Recent living-will legislation by several states allows the standard living-will form to offer the choice of receiving rather than refusing life-sustaining treatments.[30,31] To honor living wills, physicians must read them carefully and understand them since there are various forms of living wills.

The second kind of advance directive, the medical power of attorney, allows the patient to appoint an agent to express the patient's choices when the patient is unable to do so. The medical power of attorney gives the physician the opportunity to explain the details of the patient's condition to the agent, who can then interpret them in light of the patient's wishes.

If a physician determines that decisions made by the patient's agent do not represent the patient's wishes or do not reflect the patient's best interests, state statutes may direct the physician to seek judicial intervention to appoint an appropriate decision maker. State courts often have judges on call to adjudicate medically emergent issues.

In some jurisdictions, the prehospital or out-of-hospital do-not-resuscitate (OOH-DNR) order is a third type of advance directive. In most states, the OOH-DNR order is a medical order, acknowledged by the patient, that authorizes emergency personnel to forgo resuscitation.[32] The order may be considered an advance directive because, like the living will and medical power of attorney, it allows patients to express their wishes about the use of medical interventions when they cannot speak for themselves. The OOH-DNR order differs significantly from the living will or medical power of attorney in that in all but a few states, patients cannot obtain the document merely by their own request; a physician must complete and sign the document. Several states do permit a patient to create an OOH-DNR order without a physician's signature, by signing the document before witnesses. Instead of carrying the actual order, patients may hold or wear evidence of the OOH-DNR order in the form of an identifying bracelet or card. When a patient presents an OOH-DNR order or appropriate evidence of it, emergency personnel should stop or not begin resuscitation attempts.

The movement to recognize OOH-DNR orders originated with emergency response teams who faced legal penalties for failing to attempt resuscitation even of patients who did not wish to be resuscitated. Legislation enacted to address such concerns established the OOH-DNR order and provided civil and criminal immunity to health care providers who honor the order. Because the orders are largely a matter of state law, health care professionals should know the legal rules in their jurisdictions. In Ohio, for example, legislation created two types of OOH-DNR orders: (1) DNR comfort care, which prohibits aggressive life-sustaining and resuscitative measures both before and during a respiratory or cardiac arrest; and (2) DNR comfort care–arrest, which allows all life-sustaining interventions until the patient experiences cardiac or respiratory arrest.[33] Oregon created four specific optional orders: "comfort measures only," "limited interventions," "advanced interventions," and "full treatment/resuscitation." Each has particular treatment implications.[34]

As illustrated by the case narrative, the unavailability of advance directives is a significant limitation in the emergency setting. Unless the family or patient has the documents in hand, an advance directive may not be an available authority for decisions regarding emergency treatment. Barring an informed treatment refusal by a patient with capacity or by a surrogate, physicians should proceed with emergency treatment.

Identify a Surrogate Decision Maker. When a patient loses the ability to make an informed decision, someone else must make a decision based on what the patient would have wanted or, if this is unknown, on the patient's best interests. Ideally, the patient has a medical power of attorney naming a surrogate whom the patient trusts to make decisions in the event of the patient's incapacity. When such a designation does not exist, state law typically designates a surrogate decision maker. In typical order of priority, possible surrogates are the patient's legal guardian or medical power of attorney, the patient's spouse, an adult child or a majority of the patient's reasonably available adult children, the patient's parents, or the nearest living relative.[35] Reliance on family members reflects the assumption that families are usually most concerned about the patient's welfare and most likely to know the patient's preferences.

Communicating by telephone with the surrogate decision maker to obtain consent for medical or surgical treatment for an incapacitated patient or a patient who is a minor may be necessary in the emergency setting. To meet the legal and ethical requirements of informed consent, the physician should inform all parties on the telephone that a nurse or other health care provider will listen to the telephone conversation to witness it. The patient's record should clearly list the names of the individuals contacted for consent, the names of the physician and the witness, and the date and time of the conversation.

> Case 1 (continued): Based on both Mr. Slade's living-will note in the medical record and his surrogate's (ie, his wife's) instructions, he is intubated and sent to the intensive-care unit (ICU), where he continues to receive aggressive treatment. Growing increasingly uncomfortable with providing what it considers to be medically inappropriate care, the health care team questions whether the wife's surrogacy is to be trusted. Both the social worker and chaplain involved with the Slades affirm that Mrs. Slade believes she is upholding her husband's wishes as stated in his living will. She firmly believes that the current dismal medical prognosis would not change his mind. She states, "A day alive in the ICU is worth it." Facing strong family objection to withdrawing treatment, the physicians continue aggressive treatment.

Some ethicists argue that certain conditions need to be met before one can rely on surrogates.[36] First, the surrogate must be willing to participate in the decision. Second, the surrogate must know the patient well so that decisions reflect the patient's preferences. Third, decisions must be made without undue influence by financial factors, the emotional burdens of caregiving, or the behavior of dysfunctional families. Finally, reliance on surrogates must result in an outcome much like the one the patient would reasonably be expected to choose. Since decisions about a patient's welfare are usually made jointly by the physician and the surrogate, the physician must be sure that the path chosen is one of the medically sound alternatives. Although the emergency physician's ability to ascertain that these conditions are met may be limited, in most cases, the surrogate is best suited to promote the patient's best interests and goals.

Three circumstances, however, may justify challenging a surrogate's decision.[23] First, a surrogate's decisions should be challenged if he or she has been involved in the abuse or neglect of the patient. Second, the surrogate should be disqualified if the surrogate lacks decisional capacity. Third, the surrogate's decision should be discredited if a serious conflict of interest is likely to bias the decision against the patient's rights and interests. This last consideration includes instances when family members are in such disagreement that they cannot function as a decision-making unit. Unfortunately, neither the courts nor legislatures have provided significant guidance regarding what constitutes a conflict of interest serious enough to disqualify the surrogate or to require referral to the courts, and it is unclear how often such problems occur. Physicians must apply their judgment in these cases and use institutional resources to reach acceptable outcomes. Social workers are usually trained in guardianship procedures and can assist the physician who believes that a guardian is needed. If the need for a guardian is not clear, an ethics committee may be able to assist in principled decision making although the recommendations of an ethics committee are typically advisory only. When a member of the health care team questions a surrogate's decision, designated authorities within the institution (such as the chief medical officer, chief of nursing, legal counsel, or head of the institution's ethics committee) may assist the medical staff in assessing a surrogate's qualifications or in seeking judicial intervention.

In the Absence of Advance Directives or Surrogate Consent, Provide Appropriate Medical Care. The so-called emergency rule stipulates that appropriate medical care must be rendered in an emergency even when obtaining informed consent is not possible. According to one view, this rule is grounded in the notion of presumed consent,[37] according to which the physician presumes consent to treatments that a reasonable person would want in an emergency. Another rationale of the emergency rule is implied consent: the patient's help-seeking and cooperative actions (eg, coming to the EC and cooperating with physicians, if able) imply consent. Others argue that no consent, whether presumed, implied, or informed, is needed for such treatments. Since the patient cannot express an autonomous choice, the ethical principle of beneficence dictates that it is the physician's responsibility to initiate appropriate medical treatment immediately.[38]

To invoke the emergency rule, the emergency physician must determine (a) that the patient is incapable of consenting and (b) that harm from a failure to treat is imminent and outweighs any harm threatened by the proposed treatment.[39] As a corollary, the physician must also determine that delaying care in order to obtain consent from the patient's legal surrogate would increase the patient's risk. Simultaneously, the physician must direct a staff member not immediately involved in the patient's examination and treatment to attempt to contact the patient's relatives. While providing emergency care promotes the patient's well-being, the simultaneous attempt to inform relatives of the patient's condition and to obtain consent from the legal surrogate respects the patient's right of self-determination.

In strictly limited circumstances, both the US Department of Health and Human Services and the Food and Drug Administration permit emergency research (ie, the application of emergency interventions that are the subject of research) without the consent of participants. The criteria for the approval of such research proposals by an institutional review board (IRB) are that (1) potential participants face life-threatening situations for which available treatments are unproven or unsatisfactory; (2) obtaining informed consent from the participant or surrogate is precluded by the need to perform the intervention before consent can be obtained; (3) participation holds the prospect of direct benefit to the participant; (4) the research could not practicably be carried out without the waiver; (5) the investigator will attempt to reach a surrogate to request consent during a "potential therapeutic window"; and (6) the IRB has reviewed and approved an informed-consent procedure and document to be used when feasible.[40,41] Moreover, approval requires the inclusion of additional protections for research participants, including consultation with representatives of the communities in which the research will be done; public disclosure of the research plan and its risks, benefits, and anticipated results; review by a data-monitoring board; and (if consent was not obtained during the initial "window") the commitment of the investigator to find out whether a surrogate objects to the patient's participation.[41]

Patient Demands Medically Inappropriate or Futile Care.

> Case 1 (concluded): Mr. Slade is in the ICU for 6 weeks and dies during a code. Although the staff is tempted to believe that the conflict and the long ICU stay could have been avoided if the EC physician had refused resuscitation, respect for patient autonomy had made this course premature. This case and others like it prompt the hospital to join with other hospitals in the area to suggest community guidelines for responding to patient and surrogate requests for medically inappropriate interventions.[42]

The ethical standard of honoring a patient's autonomous choice does not require physicians to concede to patients' requests for medically inappropriate or futile care. Patient autonomy may be limited by physicians' professional integrity and duty of beneficence, which require physicians not to provide treatments that will bring more harm than benefit, even when a patient or surrogate demands such treatment.

These are complex issues. Some ethicists distinguish quantitatively or physiologically futile treatments (ie, treatments that will not have the intended physiologic effect), such as providing platelets to a platelet-refractory patient, from qualitatively futile treatments (ie, treatments that will prolong life without a minimum amount of quality), such as the cardiopulmonary resuscitation of a person in a persistent vegetative state.[43] Among ethicists, there is stronger support for the position that a physician may unilaterally refuse to provide a physiologically futile treatment than there is for the position that a physician may refuse to provide a qualitatively futile treatment.[44] For example, Youngner limits the physician's prerogative to the refusal of physiologically futile treatments[45] whereas Schneiderman and colleagues take a more expansive view that condones the refusal of qualitatively futile treatments.[46]

Others argue that medical futility cannot be defined and advocate a "due-process" approach to determining whether an intervention is medically inappropriate and therefore need not be offered or provided.[47] Several state legislatures[30,31] as well as the American Medical Association's Council on Ethical and Judicial Affairs[48] have endorsed this procedural approach, which authorizes an institutional committee to review a physician's decision not to honor a request for treatment the physician deems medically inappropriate. As enacted, the process is relatively unhelpful in the emergency setting because of mandated waiting periods before a physician can withhold or withdraw the demanded intervention. (These waiting periods are intended to allow patients the opportunity to transfer to another facility before an intervention is withdrawn.)

Process-based futility policies that may result in a directive from an institutional review committee not to provide life-sustaining care for a patient can create a difficult problem for emergency physicians. For example, if a review committee rules that CPR is futile for a particular patient and if institutional policy directs that no physician at that hospital may then provide CPR, the emergency physician may face a true ethical bind. If the patient presents to the hospital's EC in arrest, the physician, as an emergency physician subject to EMTALA, must provide CPR. However, as a physician governed by the policies of the hospital, he or she cannot do so. Emergency physicians at institutions with binding futility policies should address this potential conflict with hospital administration in advance of an actual case.

Physicians dealing with oncologic emergencies may particularly face two requests for inappropriate interventions. The first involves the end-stage cancer patient who requests CPR. Several studies have shown that following CPR, patients with metastatic cancer who are hospitalized[49] or in an ICU[50] do not survive to discharge. Most medical professional guidelines state that futile CPR need not be provided. For example, the American Heart Association's Guidelines for Cardiopulmonary Resuscitation and Emergency Cardiac Care allow unilateral DNR orders when "no survivors after CPR have been reported under the circumstances in well-designed studies."[51] Ethicists have also argued against futile CPR[46] although they often recommend such safeguards as a review mechanism[52] or referral to an ethics committee.[53] Some take the opposing stance and argue for providing CPR when the patient requests it.[54,55]

When the emergency physician determines that a patient's chance of survival to discharge following CPR is extremely small, the physician should explain to the patient and surrogates that appropriate palliative care will be provided but that interventions such as cardiac compression and intubation, which would not benefit the patient and would be invasive and even violent, will be withheld. If the patient or surrogate strongly objects to this forceful recommendation, the emergency physician should set in motion the review mechanism that is provided for his or her setting, even though the review and its attendant delay may result in the performance of CPR.

One response to the demand for CPR is to conduct a sham resuscitation attempt. Slow codes, Hollywood codes, or other sham codes are not appropriate.[56] Legitimate CPR and Advanced Cardiopulmonary Life Support (ACLS) should be performed with the intention of resuscitating the patient. Physicians have the prerogative to end a code when, in their medical judgment, the intervention will not restore spontaneous circulation.

The second frequent request for inappropriate treatment in the setting of an oncologic emergency involves hospital admission. Patients and families may request hospital admission for a number of reasons (eg, to relieve burned-out caregivers, to effect the patient's transition to hospice or nursing-home care, or to avoid caring for the patient at home during the last stages of illness). Admitting the patient to an acute-care setting may not be the appropriate course of action and may involve reimbursement difficulties. If no other options exist, however, a brief hospital stay may provide a transition to a more appropriate setting.[37]

In sum, there is no overriding ethical obligation to provide medically inappropriate interventions. When the balance of benefits over burdens of an intervention is uncertain, medical professionals should err on the side of honoring the patient's or surrogate's request for treatment.

Step III. Ensure Responsible Discharge

Having provided emergency treatment that enables the patient to leave in a stable condition, physicians must give the patient adequate information about follow-up care. They also must ensure a safe discharge, which may require having the patient's relatives or friends or social services take custody or assume responsibility for the patient's return home and for follow-up care.

Discharge of a patient who cannot reach home safely or who was not informed of necessary follow-up care may constitute negligence if the patient is injured as a result of the oversight. Moreover, discharging a patient prematurely, inappropriately, or without ascertaining the patient's safety leaves a physician vulnerable to charges of malpractice and patient abandonment.[57] Legal abandonment occurs when the physician terminates the physician-patient relationship without giving the patient due notice and an opportunity to secure other medical assistance.[58] To avoid such charges, many hospitals require documentation of (a) the instructions given to patients regarding home care, (b) the need for further medical treatment, or (c) the fact that the patient was discharged to the custody of a responsible family member.

Step IV: Meet Responsibilities upon Death of Patient

Organ Donation. Most oncology patients will not be eligible for organ donation. However, emergency personnel should be familiar with the rules of their local organ procurement organization for evaluating donors and requesting donation. In the cancer setting, some patients express a wish to donate organs or offer some use of their body after death, as a way of contributing to science and to the search for a cure. The emergency physician should be aware of opportunities to fulfill these patients' altruistic wishes, such as body donation or contributions to research.

Inquest, Autopsy, and Reporting Requirements. An inquest is a judicial investigation into the cause of a person's death, for the purposes of detecting a crime and gathering evidence when a crime may have been committed. An autopsy is the examination of a body by dissection and other medical tests, to ascertain the cause of death or to determine other medical facts about the body. Typically, state law defines the circumstances that require an inquest or autopsy and also regulates the specific inquiries and resulting documentation related to the necessary procedures. Who may consent to autopsy is usually legislated as well. Emergency room physicians should be aware of local requirements for an inquest or autopsy by the county coroner or medical examiner.

Entries in the cause-of-death section of a patient's death certificate provide epidemiologic information important for public health planning and other societal goals. Useful information includes the single disease or condition that began the sequence of events leading directly to the patient's death, the most important events or complications that occurred between the underlying and immediate causes of death, the final condition that directly caused death, and other significant conditions that contributed to death.[59] Emergency physicians should also be aware of specific cancer-related information required by the state.[60]

Physicians may encounter objections to autopsy that are based on patients' religious beliefs; prohibitions against the practice may be found in Orthodox Judaism and among some conservative Islamic sects.[61] Although the citizens who use ECs are subject to the civil laws governing autopsy in the particular jurisdiction, respect for autonomy and cultural differences requires both recognition of and sensitivity to patients' and families' objections based on these beliefs. For EC physicians, respect for autonomy might also mean *not* assuming that a patient of a particular religion or culture automatically adopts the doctrines associated with that group. However, familiarity with the beliefs of religious and cultural groups in the community will help an EC physician to manage requests for autopsy (as well as any other medical intervention) with sensitivity and professional skill.

OTHER ETHICAL ISSUES IN EMERGENCY CARE

Truth Telling

A corollary of respect for patient autonomy is the principle of truth telling. The accepted medical practice in the United States, Canada, and northern Europe is to inform patients of their diagnosis.[9] In the case of most cancer patients, who likely undergo a thorough examination before their diagnosis, this task is not usually the emergency physician's. The more common dilemma is posed by patients who arrive at the EC with no clear idea of their prognosis. When the prognosis is dismal, the emergency physician is thrust into the position of telling bad news to a patient and family whom the physician does not know. The task is complicated by the absence of consensus about how much information about prognosis should be shared.[62] While respect for autonomy generally entails the full disclosure of information, respect for patients also includes a regard for a patient's desire not to know certain things. Sharing bad news must therefore be done sensitively. One recommended protocol for breaking bad news is the SPIKES protocol: (1) create an appropriate, private **S**etting; (2) determine the patient's **P**erception of the problem; (3) obtain the patient's **I**nvitation to proceed and to disclose details, asking, for example, "Are you the type of person who likes to know everything?"; (4) provide the appropriate **K**nowledge and information in small chunks; (5) **E**mpathize and explore emotions; and (6) summarize and discuss **S**trategy for follow-up.[63,64]

The emergency physician can reasonably be expected to initiate the process of sharing bad news. Ascertaining the patient's understanding of the illness and how much the patient wants to know is a particularly important step. Although the EC may not be the most appropriate setting for such conversations, the emergency physician has a crucial role in initiating the conversation in an empathetic way, responding sensitively to patients' cues about how much they are ready to hear at that time, and (if nothing else) providing an initial warning that the disease is progressing.

Justice

Although there is no agreement on one principle of justice that governs the delivery of health care in the United States, principles of justice have been clearly defined by ECs. Anyone who comes to an emergency room has the right to receive stabilizing health care regardless of ability to pay or individual characteristics. In 1959, Darien Manlove, a 4-month-old child, died of bronchial pneumonia after being refused emergency care.[65] In a resulting suit, the Delaware Supreme Court ruled that even though hospitals are not required to have ECs, "liability on the part of the hospital may be predicated on the refusal of services to a patient in the case of an unmistakable emergency, if the patient has relied upon well-established custom of the hospital to render aid in such cases."[66] Cases such as *Wilmington General Hospital v. Manlove* established the common-law right to emergency care, a right that was given federal statutory enforcement with the passing of EMTALA. Although patients in the United States have not been granted a universal legal right to health care, they have the right to medical care in the emergency setting.

Scarcity of resources is one exception to the right to emergency care. Here again, the EC has an accepted procedure for allocating resources. Emergency triage stipulates that the sickest patient has the highest priority for treatment, as long as the emergency interventions have a possibility of benefiting the patient. Thus, triage divides patients into three categories of treatment priority: (1) those who are in dire need and can benefit from emergency intervention; (2) those who can benefit from emergency intervention but who can safely wait for medical intervention; and (3) those who cannot benefit from medical intervention. If there are more patients in a category than can be treated, ECs often adopt a policy of first-come, first-served. Emergency triage differs from a strictly utilitarian triage that gives priority to those who will be most useful in achieving some societal goal after treatment (such as soldiers returning to the front lines in war). The Seattle kidney triage, which allocated access to dialysis machines on the basis of "age, sex, marital status, number of dependents, education, occupation, past performance and future potential,"[67] was criticized for using an utilitarian form of triage. Emergency triage, on the other hand, is well accepted as respectful of human life.

Privacy of Patients

Emergency physicians may receive requests for information about patients under their care. Full disclosure to the patient's agent (under a medical power of attorney) or to another legal surrogate is necessary to enable informed consent, which makes the release of information to the patient's immediate family or caregiver seem noncontroversial. Yet, such requests may impinge on the health professional's ethical obligation to maintain patient confidentiality. Even when someone apparently close to the patient initiates a request for information, EC staff members should use discretion in disclosing a patient's medical information.

Requests for information may come from those outside the patient's family after a publicized accident or tragedy, during a community crisis, or when a well-known figure is admitted by way of the EC. Like all other patients, emergency patients have a right to privacy and to the confidentiality of their medical information. Providing certain information to police or other civil authorities may be required by law, but hospitals have no legal obligation to disclose medical-record information to news media.

Even when the release of medical information as public news is legal, discretion should be used in determining content. Publicizing shocking or embarrassing details or images or incorporating personal or moral judgments in the released information without the patient's consent is neither necessary nor ethical and may be actionable. Particularly sensitive information (such as a patient's intoxication, suicide, or criminal involvement related to the reason for the emergency visit) should not be disclosed. Emergency physicians should ascertain whether their institution maintains a policy for handling media requests. Such policies typically direct all communications with radio, newspaper, or television reporters to one hospital-designated person.

Attempted Suicide

Although some research shows that most oncology patients do not attempt suicide,[68–70] physicians in oncologic emergency settings may encounter suicide cases. Distinguishing a suicide attempt from disease progression or a treatment complication may be difficult. Even if the patient has clearly attempted suicide, emergency treatment raises many ethical concerns. When the precipitating event is an attempted suicide, some professionals may object to honoring advance directives refusing aggressive interventions. Ethicists who argue that patients should have the right to choose the time and means of their death through suicide predicate their arguments on a high esteem for patient autonomy. Yet, a primary cause of attempted suicide is clinical depression. This creates a catch-22 for respecting autonomy, because a clinically depressed person has diminished autonomy and may not be able to make truly autonomous choices. Others who support the right to commit suicide require safeguards such as repeated requests for nontreatment, proper treatment of pain, and consultation with family. In the emergency setting, these safeguards often cannot be met, nor will it be possible to rule out reversible clinical depression in most cases. Therefore, a patient suspected of attempted suicide should usually be given aggressive treatment, at least until evidence justifying a less aggressive approach accrues.

CONCLUSION

Basic ethical principles are the same in the EC as in all hospital departments. However, emergency health care providers face special challenges because of time pressures, patients' lack of capacity, the absence of therapeutic relationships, and the unavailability of advance directives and sometimes even of surrogates. In the emergency setting, the cancer patient may present additional concerns that reflect the nature of the disease and the aggressive interventions available to ECs. This chapter has provided an algorithm to guide oncologic emergency health professionals as they strive to provide ethical care.

REFERENCES

1. Beauchamp TL, Childress JF. Principles of biomedical ethics. 4th ed. New York: Oxford University Press; 1994.
2. Fletcher JC, Lombardo PA, Marshall MF, et al, editors. Introduction to Clinical Ethics. Frederick (MD): University Publishing Group; 1997.
3. 42 U.S.C. § 1395dd (a)–(e) (1999). http://uscode.house. gov/usc.html (accessed Feb 12, 2002).
4. Hyman DA. Patient dumping and EMTALA: past imperfect/future shock. Health Matrix 1998;8:29–56.
5. Texas Cancer Incidence Reporting Act, Health and Safety Code § 82.001 et seq., Texas Cancer Registry (1999), ii–iii.
6. *Scholoendorff v. New York Hospital*, 211 NY 125, 105 NE 92.
7. Rothman DJ. Strangers at the bedside: a history of how law and bioethics transformed medical decision making. New York: HarperCollins; 1991. p. 107.
8. Faden RR, Beauchamp TL. A history and theory of informed consent. New York: Oxford University Press; 1986. p. 87.
9. Holland JC, Geary N, Marchini A. An international survey of physician attitudes and practice in regard to revealing the diagnosis of cancer. Cancer Invest 1987;5:151–4.
10. Faden RR, Beauchamp TL. A history and theory of informed consent. New York: Oxford University Press; 1986. p. 53–110.
11. Blackhall L, Murphy ST, Frank G, et al. Ethnicity and attitudes toward patient autonomy. JAMA 1995;274:820–5.
12. Carrese J, Rhodes L. Western bioethics on the Navajo reservation: benefit or harm? JAMA 1995;274:826–9.
13. Harrison A, al-Saadi AM, al-Kaabi MR, et al. Should doctors inform terminally ill patients? The opinions of nationals and doctors in the United Arab Emirates. J Med Ethics 1997;23:101–7.
14. Torreccillas L. Communication of the cancer diagnosis to Mexican patients: attitudes of physicians and patients. Ann N Y Acad Sci 1997;809:188–96.
15. Elwyn TS, Fetters MD, Gorentlo W, et al. Cancer disclosure in Japan: historical comparisons, current practices. Soc Sci Med 1998;46(9):1151–63.
16. Gordon D, Paci E. Disclosure practices and cultural narratives: understanding concealment and silence around cancer in Tuscany, Italy. Soc Sci Med 1997;44:1433–52.
17. Appelbaum PS, Grisso T. Assessing patients' capacities to consent to treatment. N Engl J Med 1998;319:1635–8.
18. Grisso, T, Appelbaum PS. Assessing competence to consent to treatment: a guide for physicians and other health professionals. London: Oxford University Press; 1998.
19. American Academy of Pediatrics, Committee on Drugs. Guidelines for the ethical conduct of studies to evaluate drugs in pediatric populations. Pediatrics 1995;95:286–94.
20. American Academy of Pediatrics, Committee on Drugs. Informed consent, parental permission, and assent in pediatric practice. Pediatrics 1995;95:314–7.
21. Sigman G, O'Connor C. Exploration for physicians of the mature minor doctrine. J Pediatrics 1991;119(4):520–5.
22. President's Commission. Deciding to forego life-sustaining treatment. Washington (DC): US Government Printing Office; 1983. p. 89–90.
23. Buchanan AE, Brock D. Deciding for others: the ethics of surrogate decision making. New York: Cambridge University Press; 1989.
24. *Cruzan v. Director*, Missouri. Health Dept. 497 US 261 (1990).
25. Brock DW, Wartman SA. Sounding board. When competent patients make irrational choices. N Engl J Med 1990;322:1595–9.
26. Katz J. Why doctors don't disclose uncertainty. Hastings Cent Rep 1984;14(1):35–44.
27. Bonica JJ. Treatment of cancer pain: current status and future needs. In: Fields HL, Dubner R, Cervero F, et al, editors. Advances in pain research and therapy. Vol 9. New York: Raven Press; 1985. p. 589–616.
28. Cassell EJ. The relief of suffering. Arch Intern Med 1983;143:522–3.
29. Iserson KV. Bioethics. In: Rosen P, Barkin RM, Braen GR, et al, editors. Emergency medicine: concepts and clinical practice. 3rd ed. St. Louis: Mosby Year Books; 1992. p. 37–48.
30. Texas Health & Safety Code § 166.033 (1999).
31. Virginia Code § 54.1-2990 (2000).
32. Sabatino CP. Survey of state EMS-DNR laws and protocols. J Law Med Ethics 1999;27:297–315.
33. Ohio Rev. Code § 2133.21–.26 (Banks-Baldwin 1999).
34. Or. Admin. R. 847-035-0030(7) (1998). http://arcweb.sos. state.or.us/rules.
35. Texas Health & Safety Code § 166.039 (1999).

36. Sass HM, Veatch RM, Kimura R. Advance directives and surrogate decision making in health care. Baltimore (MD): Johns Hopkins University Press; 1998.

37. Iserson KV. Ethical dilemmas in hematologic/oncologic emergencies. Emerg Med Clin North Am 1993;11: 531–43.

38. Annas G. New York's do-not-resuscitate law: bad law, bad medicine, and bad ethics. In: Baker, Strosberg MA, editors. Legislating medical ethics: a study of the New York do-not-resuscitate law. The Netherlands: Kluwer Academic Publishers; 1995. p. 141–55.

39. *Canterbury v. Spence*, 464 F2d 772, 788–789 (DC Cir 1972).

40. 5 C.F.R. § 46.101(i) (1999). http://www.access.gpo.gov.nara/cfr.

41. 21 C.F.R. § 50.24 (2000). http://www.access.gpo.gov.nara/cfr.

42. Pentz RD. The need for a community-wide futility policy, or, how not to handle a case of medical futility. In: Misbin RI, editor. The search for answers. Frederick (MD): University Publishing Group; 1995. p. 41–8.

43. Brody B, Halevy A. Is futility a futile concept? J Med Philos 1995;20:123–44.

44. Rubin SB. When doctors say no: the battleground of medical futility. Bloomington (IN): Indiana University Press; 1998. p. 88.

45. Youngner S. Who defines futility? JAMA 1988;260:2094–5.

46. Schneiderman LJ, Jecker N, Jonsen A. Medical futility: its meaning and ethical implications. Ann Intern Med 1990;112:952–3.

47. Brody B, Halevy A, Atkinson G, et al. A multi-institution collaborative policy on medical futility. JAMA 1996; 276:571–4.

48. Council on Ethical and Judicial Affairs, American Medical Association. Medical futility in end-of-life care: report of the Council on Ethical and Judicial Affairs. JAMA 1999;281:937–41.

49. Faber-Lagendorf K. Resuscitation of patients with metastatic cancer: is transient benefit still futile? Arch Intern Med 1991;151:234–9.

50. Kish SK, Ewer MS, Price KJ, et al. Outcome of cardiopulmonary resuscitation in cancer patients admitted to an intensive care unit in a tertiary cancer center. Chest 1998;114:334S.

51. Emergency Cardiac Care Committee and Subcommittees of the American Heart Association. Guidelines for cardiopulmonary resuscitation and emergency cardiac care Ethical considerations in resuscitation. JAMA 1992;268:2282–8.

52. Alpers A, Lo B. When is CPR futile? JAMA 1995;273:156–8.

53. Lo B. Unanswered questions about DNR orders. JAMA 1991;265:1874–5.

54. Lantos JD, Singer PA, Walker PM, et al. The illusion of futility in clinical practice. Am J Med 1989;87:81–4.

55. Truog RD, Brett AS, Fradre J. The problem with futility. N Engl J Med 1992;326:1560–4.

56. Gazelle G. The slow code—should anyone rush to its defense? N Engl J Med 1998;338:467–9.

57. *Davis v. Weiskopf*, 439 NE2d 60 (Ill. App 1982).

58. *Payton v. Weaver*, 182 Cal. Rptr. 225 (1982).

59. Hutchins G, Berman J, Moore G, et al. Practice guidelines for autopsy pathology: autopsy reporting. Arch Pathol Lab Med 1999;123:1085–8.

60. California Health & Safety Code § 102860. http://caselaw.1p.findlaw.com/cacodes/ (accessed Feb 12, 2002).

61. Geller SA. Religious attitudes and the autopsy. Arch Pathol Lab Med 1984;108:494–6.

62. Anderlik MR, Pentz RD. Revisiting the truth-telling debate. J Clin Ethics 2000;11:251–9.

63. Buckman R, editor. How to break bad news: a guide for health care professionals. Baltimore: Johns Hopkins University Press; 1992.

64. Baile WF, Kudelka AP, Beale EA, et al. Communication skills training in oncology: description and preliminary outcomes of workshops on breaking bad news and managing patient reactions to illness. Cancer 1999;86:887–96.

65. Dougherty CJ. The right to health care: first aid in the emergency room. St Louis University Public Law Forum 1984;4:101–28.

66. *Wilmington General Hospital v. Manlove*, 54 DE 15, 174 A2d 135 (1961) at 140.

67. Baker R, Strosberg M. Triage and equality: an historical reassessment of utilitarian analyses of triage. Kennedy Inst Ethics J 1992;2:117.

68. Brown JH, Henteleff P, Barakat S, et al. Is it normal for terminally ill patients to desire death? Am J Psychiatry 1986;143:208–11.

69. Chochinov HM, Wilson KKG, Enns M, et al. Desire for death in the terminally ill. Am J Psychiatry 1995;152: 1185–91.

70. Emanuel EF, Fairclough DL, Daniels ER, et al. Euthanasia and physician-assisted suicide: attitudes and experiences of oncology patients, oncologists, and the public. Lancet 1996;347:1805–10.

CHAPTER 4

MAJOR PRESENTING SYMPTOMS

CARMEN P. ESCALANTE, MD

JESSICA P. HWANG, MD, MPH

TEJPAL S. GROVER, MD, MBA

ARUN RAJAGOPAL, MD

GARY E. DENG, MD, PHD

GUILLERMO LAZO-DIAZ, MD

ARTHUR D. FORMAN, MD

ELLEN F. MANZULLO, MD

SHUWEI GAO, MD

NARIN APISARNTHANARAX, MD

MADELEINE DUVIC, MD

This chapter gives an overview of common symptoms in cancer patients presenting to an acute-care facility. Symptoms are described with the development of a differential diagnosis and/or diagnostic algorithm. In addition, important points to remember, "clinical pearls," are included. (Please refer to Chapter 1, Figure 1–2, for chief complaints of patients at triage in a comprehensive cancer center's emergency center.)

FEVER AND HYPERTHERMIA

An elevation in body temperature can result from cytokine activation and subsequent changes in the thermoregulatory center of the hypothalamus, leading to fever, or from exogenous or endogenous reasons exclusive of hypothalamic input, otherwise known as hyperthermia. Hyperthermia is briefly discussed because this diagnosis should always be included in the differential diagnosis of an individual presenting to an emergency room with an elevation of temperature, regardless of disease status. However, the rest of this section emphasizes fever, particularly neutropenic fever, in the cancer patient.

Hyperthermia

Hyperthermia results from a failure of thermoregulation. Body temperature is maintained within a limited range, balanced between heat load and heat dissipation. Heat load is composed of endogenous factors such as metabolic processes and by exogenous factors such as ambient temperature.[1] Regardless of the reason, when the core body temperature rises, the hypothalamus stimulates the autonomic nervous system to initiate heat-dissipating mechanisms such as evaporation (ie, sweating and cutaneous vasodilation). In extreme heat and humidity, however, evaporation, as well as other heat dissipation methods such as conduction, convection, and radiation, cannot transfer heat efficiently when ambient temperatures exceed body core temperature. Heat stroke, one example of hyperthermia, is defined as a body temperature > 40.5°C (105°F) with associated central nervous system dysfunction (ie, seizure, coma, delirium) in the setting of a large environmental heat load that cannot be dissipated.[2] Patients with a history of cardiovascular disease, the very young and the very old, and those who exert themselves in high ambient temperatures and humidity are at higher risk for heat stroke.

Hyperthermia can also result from endogenous metabolic processes that do not alter the hypothalamic set point (see below). Neuroleptic malignant syndrome, one example, is an idiosyncratic reaction to antipsychotic agents such as piperazine, butyrophenones, and haloperidol.[3,4] Clinical manifestations include hyperthermia, altered mental status, tremors, autonomic dysfunction, and muscle rigidity. Neuroleptic malignant syndrome is thought to be secondary to central nervous system dopamine receptor blockade or withdrawal of exogenous dopaminergic agonists.[4] Another example is malignant hyperthermia, a rare condition thought to be genetically based, which may manifest after the administration of anesthetic agents such as succinylcholine and halothane.[5] Clinical features include marked hyperthermia up to 42.5°C (108.5°F), muscle rigidity, hypotension, arrythmias, and even disseminated intravascular coagulation.[6]

Serotonin syndrome is a constellation of symptoms affecting the autonomic nervous system (hyperthermia, shivering), cognition (disorientation, confusion), behavior (agitation, restlessness), and neuromuscular activity (ataxia, myoclonus). It can occur in the setting of a recent addition of a serotonergic agent. The most common drug combinations include selective serotonin reuptake inhibitors (SSRIs) and monoamine oxidase inhibitors (MAOIs). Serotonin syndrome has also been implicated in the combination of MAOIs with tricyclic antidepressants, tryptophan, or meperidine. The syndrome itself is caused by excess serotonin in the central nervous system (CNS) at the serotonin receptor ($5\text{-}HT_{1A}$) site.[7]

Thyroid storm is another example of an endogenous process causing hyperthermia. Other features include tachycardia, altered mental state (seizures, delirium, coma), as well as emesis and diarrhea. Thyroid storm is usually precipitated by an acute illness (infection, diabetic ketoacidosis, or trauma), surgery (usually on the thyroid), or iodine contamination in a patient with hyperthyroidism.[8,9] Exogenous thyroid hormone can also increase the body's metabolic rate and subsequently increase heat production (Table 4–1, Figure 4–1).[10]

TABLE 4–1. Differential Diagnosis of Elevated Temperature

Hyperthermia
    Heat stroke
    Drugs
        Neuroleptic malignant syndrome
        Malignant hyperthermia
        Serotonin syndrome
    Endocrine disease
        Thyroid storm
Fever
    Infection
        Neutropenic fever
        Non-neutropenic fever
    Transfusion reaction
    Tumor fever
    Drug reaction
    Jarisch-Herxheimer reaction
    Vaccines

Fever

Fever is regulated by the physiologic thermostat, the anterior hypothalamus. The release of cytokines shifts the set point of the hypothalamus upwards, thereby activating the CNS to initiate vasoconstriction, minimizing heat loss. Shivering, a method of heat production, may also occur at this time. When the set point is shifted downward (as a result of antipyretics, for example), the CNS is stimulated to commence vasodilation (ie, sweating or flushing), which continues until the set point is reached.[11]

Although fever can occur for a variety of reasons, between 48 and 60% of neutropenic patients with fever have an established or occult infection. The definitions of fever and neutropenia may differ, depending on the institution; however, according to the 1997 Guidelines from the Infectious Diseases Society of America, fever is defined as a single oral temperature of > 38.3°C (101.0°F) or a temperature of ≥ 38.0°C (100.4°F) for over 1 hour in the absence of obvious environmental causes. Neutropenia is defined as an absolute neutrophil count (ANC) of < 1,000 cells/mm^3.[12] Patients with neutrophil counts of ≤ 500 cells/mm^3 are at greater risk of infection than those patients with an ANC of 1,000 cells/mm^3, and patients with neutrophil counts of ≤ 100 cells/mm^3 are at greater risk of infection than those patients with an ANC of 500 cells/mm^3.[13]

Predisposition for Infection

The following are risk factors potentially predisposing the cancer patient to infection.

1. Neutropenia. Chemotherapy and radiation therapy may result in neutropenia, as does bone marrow replacement by hematologic or metastatic tumor. Treatment-related neutropenia may be associated with a breakdown of normal skin and mucosal barriers that thus provide a potential port of entry for microorganisms.

2. Humoral immunity. Abnormal immunoglobulin production and subsequently impaired function in states such as multiple myeloma, chronic lymphocytic leukemia, and Waldenström's macroglobulinemia predispose these patients to infections with encapsulated bacteria (ie, *Haemophilus influenzae*, *Neisseria meningitidis*, *Klebsiella pneumoniae*, and *Streptococcus pneumoniae*).

3. Cell-mediated immunity. Impaired cell-mediated immunity has been associated with Hodgkin's lymphoma, resulting in an increased risk of infection with intracellular pathogens such as *Listeria monocytogenes*, *Salmonella* species, *Cryptococcus neoformans*, and *Mycobacterium* species.

4. Hyposplenism. Neoplastic infiltration as well as surgical removal of the spleen for staging purposes can

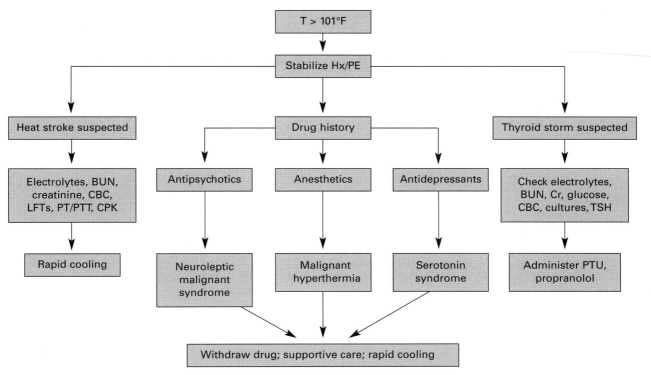

Figure 4–1. Management of hyperthermia. BUN = blood urea nitrogen; CBC = complete blood count; CPK = creatinine phosphokinase; Cr = creatinine; Hx = history; LFT = liver function test; PE = physical examination; PT = prothrombin time; PTT = partial prothrombin time; PTU = propylthiouracil; T = temperature; TSH = thyroid-stimulating hormone.

result in increased risk of infections with bacteria that use opsonization as a defense mechanism (ie, *Streptococcus pneumoniae*, *Neisseria meningitidis*, *Escherichia coli*, *Haemophilus influenzae*, and *Staphylococcus* species).

5. Tumor growth. The tumor can infiltrate and break down natural barriers of skin, head and neck, gastrointestinal tract, and genitourinary tracts, subsequently causing local infection and bacteremia. Tumor growth can cause compression and obstruction of (1) the bronchioles, leading to postobstructive pneumonia; (2) the gastrointestinal tract, causing perforation and sepsis; and (3) the urinary tract, contributing to urinary-tract infection.

6. Indwelling catheters. Central venous catheters and urinary catheters can contribute to an increased risk of infection.[14]

Fever in the cancer patient may be caused by drugs. Bleomycin and methotrexate are two chemotherapeutic drugs that have been found to elicit fever.[15,16] Common antibiotics such as trimethoprim/sulfamethoxazole, ciprofloxacin, and rifampin can cause fever.[17–19] Fever can occur shortly after antibiotic administration for certain infections; fever in such a setting is postulated to result from injured or dying bacteria that release products into the blood system,

thereby eliciting an exaggerated inflammatory response, the Jarisch-Herxheimer reaction.[20] Human immunodeficiency virus (HIV)–infected patients who are taking zidovudine (AZT) may have drug fever.[21] Sulfasalazine, used in the treatment of ulcerative colitis, has been implicated in causing fever.[22] Anticonvulsants can also cause fever; carbamazepine and phenytoin are two examples.[23,24]

The tumor itself may cause fever through rapid tumor growth or through tumor necrosis. Fever is a well-known phenomenon observed in lymphomas, leukemias, lung cancer, prostate cancer, and gastrointestinal tumors. In breast cancer patients, tumor fever has been described as a sign of metastases or the progression of disease.[25] Fever may play a role in the staging of some cancers. The Ann Arbor Staging System for Hodgkin's Disease includes B symptoms such as persistent or recurrent fever, weight loss, or night sweats. The fever may persist for days to weeks, followed by afebrile intervals and then recurrence of fever; this pattern is known as Pel-Ebstein fever. The presence of B symptoms, such as fever, weight loss, or night sweats, influences treatment modalities in that it may warrant a complete course of chemotherapy with doxorubicin, bleomycin, vinblastine, and dacarbazine (ABVD), mechlorethamine, vincristine, procarbazine, and prednisone (MOPP), or a combination of drugs in these regimens[26] (Figure 4–2).

Patients may demonstrate fever for still other reasons. Fever is the most common presenting symptom in delayed hemolytic transfusion reactions,[27] and this is clinically relevant for cancer patients who have a great need for blood products. Complications of radiation can cause fever in patients with postradiation pneumonitis. Fever is a common reaction in patients who have received tetanus toxoid.[28] Toxic reactions to insect bites have also been implicated in causing fever.[29]

Treatment

For patients with suspected hyperthermia, frequent, if not continuous, core temperature monitoring and rapid evaporative cooling methods are important. For neuroleptic or malignant hyperthermia, suspected antipsychotic or anesthetic medicines should be discontinued. Serotonin syndrome usually resolves within hours after drug withdrawal and supportive care. In patients with thyroid storm, large doses of propylthiouracil (PTU) are given orally, via nasogastric tube, or rectally; PTU inhibits the conversion of thyroxine (T_4) to tri-iodothyronine (T_3). β-Blockers such as propranolol should be given immediately to reduce tachycardia and other adrenergic manifestations. Propranolol has also been found to decrease the T_4-to-T_3 conversion.[9] Antipyretics do not help in cases of hyperthermia.

In cases in which infection is the cause of fever, particularly neutropenic fever, empiric as well as nonempiric antibiotics are the mainstay of treatment and should be given rapidly. Bodey and colleagues reported that among patients with acute leukemia who were found to have *Pseudomonas* infection, a 1- to 2-day delay in antibiotic therapy reduced the cure rate from 74 to 46%.[30] Combinations of β-lactams plus aminoglycosides had been the standard of care for neutropenic fever. However, data from the International Antimicrobial Therapy Group did show that monotherapy with meropenem had similar success rates when compared with combination

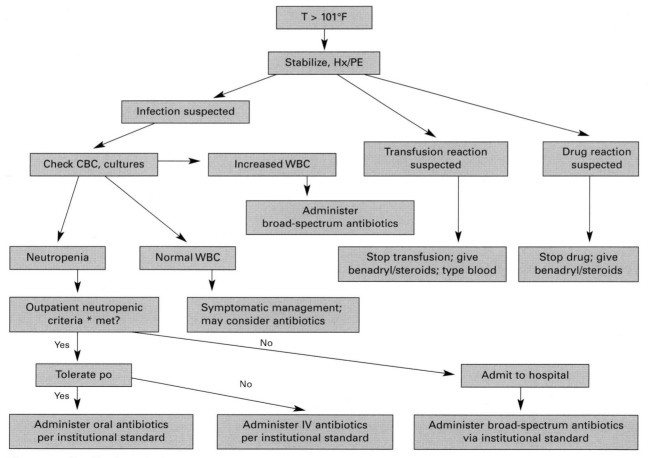

Figure 4–2. Algorithm for evaluation and treatment of fever. CBC = complete blood count; Hx = history; IV = intravenous; PE = physical examination; po = by mouth; WBC = white blood cell count. *Criteria for outpatient treatment of neutropenic fever: (1) less than 1 week anticipated neutropenia; (2) no unstable comorbid conditions; (3) normal renal and liver functions; (4) no history of hematologic cancer (lymphoma, leukemia) or status post bone marrow transplantation; (5) history of patient compliance; (6) 24-hour caregiver available; (7) telephone access; (8) lives within 30 miles; and (9) transportation available.

therapy with β-lactams plus aminoglycosides.[31]

For noninfectious causes of fever, it is prudent to avoid the instigating factors. If a drug reaction or transfusion reaction is suspected, it is necessary to stop the drug and to be ready to administer diphenhydramine, epinephrine, or steroids, depending on the severity of the reaction. In the case of transfusion reactions, the blood product must be evaluated for blood type.

Points to Remember

There are reasons other than neutropenic fever that can cause an elevated temperature in the cancer patient. If, however, neutropenic fever is identified as a possible suspect, start empiric antibiotics immediately.

A good history and a physical examination are paramount to the elucidation of the etiology of elevated temperature.

CANCER FATIGUE

Fatigue is the most widely experienced symptom in cancer patients. One recent survey showed that 73% of cancer patients experienced fatigue; this was even greater than the percentage of cancer patients who experienced pain.[32] Patients suffering from cancer fatigue also experience significant morbidity and decreased quality of life.

Given its prevalence, cancer fatigue has received relatively little attention in the literature until recently. It also appears to be undertreated clinically.[33] This may be due to conflicting perceptions by physicians and patients of the severity of the fatigue and its effects on quality of life. Also, the evaluation and management of cancer fatigue are both time and labor intensive, making them difficult to perform in a busy clinical setting.

Much of the information in this section is based on experiences in the Emergency Center and Fatigue Clinic at The University of Texas M. D. Anderson Cancer Center. In that experience, fatigue tends to be multifactorial, adding to the difficulty of evaluating and managing it.

Pathophysiology

Fatigue as a symptom of cancer may be the end point of one or many different pathophysiologic states (Table 4–2). The exact pharmacophysiologic pathway leading to fatigue remains unknown, which significantly limits the treatment of fatigue with pharmaceuticals.

Diagnostic Approach

A complete evaluation of the etiology of cancer fatigue is outside the scope of most emergency centers. Due to the nature of the processes that cause fatigue, the medical history and physical examination tend to be nondiagnostic. However, a number of etiologies can be evaluated via a directed medical history, physical examination and appropriate laboratory evaluation, allowing for proper follow-up and referral for further focused testing. Clinical indications and resources available in the emergency center or hospital should direct this testing.

History. There are many questions that should be asked during the patient's medical history.[33] They include the following:

- How severe is the fatigue?
- How significantly does the fatigue affect the patient's ability to function?
- When did the fatigue start?
- Is the fatigue getting better or worse?
- Is the fatigue worse at a particular time of day?
- Was the onset of the fatigue associated with therapy?
- What are the patient's expectations regarding the fatigue?
- How significant is the underlying malignancy?
- Is there any evidence of infection?
- Is there a sleep disturbance?
- How well is the patient eating and drinking?
- How much pain is the patient experiencing?
- How well controlled is the pain?
- What medications is the patient currently taking?
- Is there any evidence of depression or a psychological disorder?

Physical Examination. The physical examination should be directed toward any evidence supportive of an underlying disease process. Questions should include the following:

- Is the patient orthostatic?
- Is there any evidence of infection?
- Is there pallor? Is there jaundice?
- Is there any evidence of hypothyroidism?
- Is there any evidence of hypocalcemia?
- Is the patient's stool guaiac positive?

Tests. Cancer fatigue tests include the following:

- Check electrolyte levels for evidence of a metabolic disturbance.
- Check calcium, magnesium, and phosphorus levels

TABLE 4–2. Differential Diagnosis of Fatigue

Fluid and electrolyte imbalances
Hypothyroidism
Addison's disease
Infection
Drug side effects or toxicity
Cancer treatment side effects (chemotherapy, radiotherapy, immunotherapy)
Radiotherapy side effects
Sleep disorders
Anemia
Depression
Pain
Fatigue caused by the cancer itself

for deficiencies. Check blood urea nitrogen and creatinine levels for evidence of renal dysfunction.
- Check liver function tests for evidence of hepatic dysfunction.
- Check thyroid function tests for hypothyroidism.
- Check the complete blood count for anemia; if the patient is anemic, consider performing iron studies, checking the vitamin B_{12} and folate levels, and performing a hemolysis panel as clinically indicated.
- Consider a morning cortisol level or cosyntropin stimulation challenge if the patient is orthostatic or hypotensive for a reason other than fluid depletion.
- An overnight sleep study may be indicated if the medical history reveals disturbed sleep patterns.

Management

If evidence of a specific treatable problem (such as significant anemia) becomes apparent after the above evaluation, therapy for the underlying disease should begin in the emergency center. If the evaluation is nondiagnostic or if the problem is chronic, the initiation of symptom therapy should usually await further evaluation by the patient's oncologist or primary care provider to ensure appropriate long-term follow-up and management.

Fluid and electrolyte replacement should be started in the emergency center. Administration of appropriate antimicrobials should be started if there is evidence of infection. Uncontrolled pain should be treated by using the appropriate amount of analgesics. Severe anemia should be treated according to local guidelines for transfusion for symptomatic anemia. Mild to moderate anemia should be treated with epoetin alfa and iron supplements. Thyroid and corticosteroid replacement usually should be started in the follow-up setting unless the deficiency is significant.

Polypharmacy can usually be partially addressed in the emergency setting but also requires appropriate follow-up. Pharmacologic treatment options for symptoms include the use of psychostimulants (such as methylphenidate and dextroamphetamine), low-dose corticosteroids, antidepressants, and analgesics. Nonpharmacologic treatment options include energy conservation training, exercise programs, strength training, sleep hygiene training, stress management, cognitive therapy, counseling, and support groups.

EDEMA

Edema, whether generalized or localized, can result from a variety of causes; thus, a complete medical history and physical examination are essential for an effective diagnosis in the emergency center. Although the pathophysiology of edema may be multifactorial, an approach by region of presentation, generalized versus localized edema, and acute versus chronic edema can help determine the cause in most cases.

Generalized edema, or anasarca, is usually due to systemic causes. It is the excessive accumulation of interstitial fluid throughout the body, usually due to a change in plasma oncotic pressure or to increased fluid retention. Localized edema is usually related to local factors affecting blood and lymph flow from a limb.

Pathophysiology

Edema results from an imbalance in the Starling forces that control the amount of interstitial fluid in the body, resulting in an excess of sodium and water in the interstitial space.[34] Two basic opposing forces determine the quantity of interstitial fluid in the body. The first force is the filtration of plasma out of the vasculature and into the surrounding tissue. Factors that affect this include the hydrostatic and osmotic colloid pressure in the capillaries and surrounding tissue, the permeability of the vasculature, and obstruction of venous return. The filtration of plasma can be affected by the total circulatory volume and (therefore) by cardiac, hepatic, and renal function and sodium retention. The second force is the reabsorption of interstitial fluid back into the systemic circulation via the lymphatic system. Factors that affect this include obstruction of the lymphatic system, usually by metastatic disease or mass effect, and surgical removal of the lymphatic system, usually in the course of surgical resection of tumor.

Etiology

Generalized Edema. It is important to distinguish generalized edema from bilateral lower-extremity edema since generalized edema is almost always caused by systemic factors whereas bilateral edema may just be related to local causes. In the cancer patient population, hypoproteinemia due to malnutrition is probably the most common cause of newly diagnosed generalized edema. Additionally, hepatic dysfunction leading to hypoproteinemia can occur as a result of decreased liver function or liver failure. This failure can be a result of cirrhosis, invasion or infiltration by tumor, or hepatic vein or portal vein thrombosis. Hypoproteinemia may also be caused by gastrointestinal malabsorption due to damage to the endothelium from chemotherapy or, in the case of bone marrow transplant recipients, graft-versus-host disease. Occasionally, chemotherapy regimens may lead to significant nephrotic-level protein losses in the urine,[35] but such regimens usually cause nephrotoxicity. Also, increased vasculature permeability (usually due to the chemotherapeutic agent) may be seen. Other known but less frequent causes of increased vascular permeability include vasculitis and anoxia.

Systemic increased venous pressure is usually cardiac in nature and may be due to congestive heart failure, restrictive cardiac disease, tricuspid regurgitation, constrictive pericarditis from irradiation to the area, malignant pericardial tamponade, or even salt overloading and decompensation in the face of pre-existing cardiac disease.

Cardiac decompensation is usually due to previously recognized or unrecognized coronary artery disease or congestive heart failure. However, new presentations of cardiac decompensation should always be evaluated for other causes related to the underlying malignancy or treatment of the malignancy, such as malignant pericardial effusions or chemotherapy-induced cardiotoxicity. Usually, cardiac decompensation due to any of the reasons described above will initially present as bilateral lower-extremity edema, but this can quickly progress to generalized edema. Also, large amounts of edema can be missed in bedridden or hospitalized patients. Less frequent causes in this population include endocrine etiologies, such as Cushing's disease or thyroid disease, and increased loss of protein via the skin or feces. Physiologic causes such as pregnancy are rarely seen in this patient population (Table 4–3).[36]

Edema of the Arms or Legs. Unilateral edema of any extremity suggests a local mechanism, such as a mechanical or inflammatory cause.[37] The most emergent cause that should be considered is venous thrombosis, and this may be due to a variety of reasons. Previous or concurrent central venous catheter placement can often lead to clot formation in an upper extremity. In addition, decreased physical activity, chronic venous insufficiency, and compression of the venous vasculature by tumor all may contribute to the formation of deep venous thrombosis in the lower extremities. Invasion and destruction of the lymphatic system by gynecologic or prostate cancer can also lead to unilateral or bilateral lower-extremity edema. Furthermore, postsurgical changes may lead to lymphedema in an extremity. An example of a surgical procedure causing lymphedema would be mastectomy plus lymph node dissection. Usually, the timing of the development of the edema in relation to the surgical history is obvious. Unilateral edema caused by vasculitis has also been described.[38]

Bilateral lower-extremity edema usually suggests a systemic mechanism affecting the general circulation or chemical composition of the blood. This usually precedes a transition to generalized edema if the problem is not recognized or treated. These causes are the same as those of generalized edema. However, certain mechanical causes can present as bilateral lower-extremity edema, especially if they affect the inferior vena cava. Inferior vena cava syndrome due to obstruction by a clot or tumor can present as sudden bilateral lower-extremity edema. Worsening of unilateral lower-extremity edema or progression to bilateral edema after placement of an inferior vena cava filter may be a result of occlusion of the filter by a captured clot. Other local mechanical causes include compression or invasion of inguinal or retroaortic lymph nodes by a tumor. Rare causes include retroperitoneal fibrosis.

Additionally, rapidly developing isolated edema of both arms, with or without facial involvement, is rare. The possibility of superior vena cava syndrome needs to be considered in these cases.

Edema of the Face. Angioedema of the face is the most important emergent cause of facial edema and usually is easily recognizable. A history of exposure to new chemotherapeutic agents or medications must be elicited, but it should not hold up treatment, especially if airway involvement is of concern. For unclear reasons, patients may also develop angioedema due to medications that they have been receiving chronically. Previous surgery in the area, as in head and neck cancers, may also predispose a patient to facial edema.[39]

Edema of the face is often caused by thrombosis of a major vein. Typical causes include thrombosis after central venous catheter placement in the internal jugular or

TABLE 4–3. Differential Diagnosis of Edema

Impaired synthesis
    Malnutrition
    Malabsorption
    Hepatic dysfunction, such as cirrhosis
Increased loss
    Urinary losses due to nephrotic syndrome or glomerulonephritis
    Fecal losses due to malabsorption, protein-losing enteropathy, or graft-versus-host disease
Increased venous pressure
    Congestive heart failure
    Restrictive cardiac disease
    Tricuspid valve disease
    Constrictive pericarditis
    Pericardial tamponade
    Renal failure
    Compartment syndrome
    Secondary hyperaldosteronism
    Extrinsic compression or invasion by tumor
    Iatrogenic problems due to increased intravenous fluids and feedings
    Chemotherapy-induced cardiotoxicity
Local venous disease
    Venous thrombosis (including superior or inferior vena cava syndrome)
    Venous insufficiency
Increased capillary permeability
    Side effects of drugs*
    Histamine release
    Angioedema
    Infection
    Neuropathy
    Septic shock
    Vasculitis
    Postanoxic syndrome
    Thyroid dysfunction
Idiopathic edema

Adapted from Powell AA.[36]
*Antihypertensives, corticosteroids, androgenic and anabolic steroids, estrogens, and nonsteroidal anti-inflammatory drugs (including phenylbutazone, ibuprofen, and naproxen).

subclavian vein or superior vena cava syndrome. Also, it is important to examine the patient for any evidence of generalized edema. Edema of the face has also been described in cases of retro-orbital lymphoma.[40] Other possible localized causes include allergic reactions, cavernous sinus thrombosis, conjunctivitis, acne vulgaris, periorbital cellulitis, peritonsillar abscess, allergic rhinitis, and superior vena cava syndrome.

Diagnostic Approach

Although most cases of edema are slow in development, patients may present emergently if the edema becomes severe enough to affect breathing or if it develops suddenly. The severity of the edema should be judged quickly. The examiner should give particular attention to patency of the airway and should be especially alert for hypoxia, distension of the neck veins, and evidence of cardiac failure or pulmonary congestion. The physician should be prepared to administer oxygen, nitrates, narcotics, and intravenous diuretics. If the patient is stable, the medical history and physical examination can proceed, being tailored to the clinical situation at hand.[41]

Medical History. The medical history should include the following questions:

- When did the edema begin?
- Was the onset of edema sudden or gradual?
- Is the edema localized or general? Unilateral or bilateral?
- Is the edema position dependent?
- Is there any history of weight gain?
- Are there any changes in urine output?
- Is there a history of malnutrition?
- Have any new medications been taken?
- Is the edema more prominent upon awakening or arising?
- Is there any history of surgery on the arm or chest wall?
- Is there any history of intravenous line placement in the affected limb?
- Is there any history of recent surgery or illness that may have immobilized the patient?
- Is there any previous history of cardiac, renal, hepatic, endocrine, or gastrointestinal disorders?

Associated Symptoms Assessment. Assessment of associated symptoms may include the following inquiries:

- Is there any shortness of breath?
- Does any such shortness of breath occur at rest, with exertion, or both?
- Is there orthopnea or paroxysmal nocturnal dyspnea?
- Is there any history of pain (such as thrombophlebitis, compartment syndrome, thrombosis, ruptured Baker's cyst, or a ruptured gastrocnemius) that may localize the cause of the edema?

Physical Examination. Physical examinations for edema include the following:

- Examine the patient to determine if the edema is generalized or localized.
- If the latter, is it localized to the arms, legs, or face?
- Is it bilateral or unilateral?
- Examine the patient for cyanosis. Examine the heart and lungs for evidence of congestive heart failure.
- Examine the back and sacrum for dependent edema if the patient is bedridden.
- Examine the patient for pitting. Pitting of the skin with little resistance and a quick recovery time is usually considered to represent underlying hypoproteinemia. Long-standing edema may cause interstitial fibrosis, resulting in prolonged pitting recovery times even in the face of hypoproteinemia.
- Measure the girth of the affected and opposite limbs.
- Check and compare the pulse in the affected and opposite arms.
- Check for coolness or clamminess, acute injuries, gas crepitation, numbness, and loss of sensation. If there is any evidence of neurovascular compromise, as in compartment syndrome, elevate the extremity.
- Examine the skin for spider angiomas, palmar erythema, hepatomegaly, jaundice, and ascites, all of which may be signs of cirrhosis.
- Check for periorbital edema, which is associated with hypoproteinemic states such as nephrotic syndrome, especially after recumbency.

Tests. Edema tests include the following:
- Check the serum electrolyte levels.
- Check the blood urea nitrogen and creatinine levels for evidence of renal dysfunction.
- Check the complete blood count for evidence of infection.
- Check serum albumin and total protein levels for hypoproteinemia.
- Check liver function tests and clotting times for evidence of liver dysfunction.
- Check thyroid function tests for evidence of thyroid dysfunction.
- Check urinalysis results for evidence of protein wasting and renal dysfunction.
- Check a chest radiograph for evidence of congestive heart failure. Echocardiography may be necessary to rule out cardiac dysfunction.
- Perform duplex Doppler ultrasonography[42] of the affected extremities, or perform nuclear or contrast venography to rule out venous thrombosis. These tests are often necessary on an emergent basis. Computed tomography or magnetic resonance imaging[43] may be needed in some difficult cases to differentiate between fat deposition and fluid in the subcutaneous,

muscular, and interstitial spaces. Lymphangiography appears to be more and more difficult to perform in the clinical setting but remains the "gold standard" for evaluating lymphatic flow.

Emergent Management

In the case of severe generalized edema, management should address the ensuring of adequate oxygenation. This may require the administration of supplemental oxygen, intravenous diuretics, nitrates to assist with venous dilatation, and morphine for dyspnea. Once the patient is stable, the medical history and physical examination should help the physician select the appropriate tests to perform for further evaluation.[44]

Venous thrombosis requires anticoagulation using unfractionated or low-molecular-weight heparin followed by warfarin. If anticoagulation is contraindicated, vena cava filter placement should be considered. Furthermore, cardiac dysfunction should be evaluated for oncologic causes if this is a new presentation, as mentioned above. Further management requires discovering and responding to the underlying cause of the edema. Once the patient is stabilized and emergent causes have been treated or ruled out, appropriate follow-up for further evaluation and management of the edema is essential for the well-being of the patient.[44]

HEADACHE

In general, headaches can be classified into two groups: chronic headaches (migraines, cluster headaches, tension-type headaches, and cranial neuralgias) and acute headaches (exacerbation of chronic headache and headaches due to raised intracranial pressure, intracranial hemorrhage, infection, trauma, and withdrawal). Of all the causes of headaches, the two that require the most immediate attention, especially in the cancer pain setting, are raised intracranial pressure (whether from a mass, hemorrhage, or thrombosis) and infection.[45,46] A complete discussion of the infectious causes of headaches is beyond the scope of this chapter, but those causes that may relate to cancer are outlined in Table 4–4 and Figure 4–3.

There are some key points to remember in treating a headache in cancer patients. First, headache is a very common complaint in cancer patients. Second, the most important diagnostic assessment that must be made is differentiating between (a) a chronic or benign headache that has worsened and (b) a possibly impending catastrophe. Last, the clinician should maintain a high degree of suspicion if the patient has a malignancy that is known to metastasize to the head or brain.

BACKACHE

Back pain can be classified into two groups: chronic back pain and acute back pain. In some instances, acute back pain can be superimposed on long-standing back pain. In the cancer setting, the diagnosis of back pain and determining the etiology of the pain can be challenging. Back pain is one of the most common symptoms in the general population. It can be due to organic conditions such as chronic degenerative changes in the spine, chronic myofas-

TABLE 4–4. Differential Diagnosis of Headache*

Migraine
Tension-type headache
Cluster headache and chronic paroxysmal hemicrania
Miscellaneous headaches not associated with structural lesions
    Idiopathic "stabbing" headache
    External-compression headache
    Cold stimulus headache
    Benign cough headache
    Benign exertional headache
    Headache associated with sexual activity
Headache associated with head trauma
Headache associated with vascular disorders
    Acute ischemic cerebrovascular disorder
    Intracranial hematoma
    Subarachnoid hemorrhage
    Unruptured vascular malformation
    Arteritis
    Carotid or vertebral artery pain
    Venous thrombosis
    Arterial hypertension
    Other vascular disorder
Headache associated with nonvascular intracranial disorder
    High CSF pressure
    Low CSF pressure
    Intracranial infection
    Intracranial neoplasm
    Intrathecal injections
    Sarcoidosis
Headache associated with substance or substance withdrawal
    Induced by substance use, chronic or acute
    Induced from substance withdrawal, acute or chronic
Headache associated with noncephalic infection
    Viral or bacterial infection
Headache associated with metabolic disorder
    Hypoxia
    Hypercapnia
    Hypoglycemia
    Dialysis
Headache associated with disorder of facial or cranial structures
    Cranial bone
    Temporomandibular joint
    Eyes, ears, nose, sinuses
    Teeth, jaw, related structures
Cranial neuralgias, nerve trunk, or de-afferentation pain
    Persistent pain of cranial-nerve origin
    Trigeminal neuralgia
    Glossopharyngeal neuralgia
    Nervus intermedius neuralgia
    Superior laryngeal neuralgia
    Occipital neuralgia
    Central pain syndromes
Nonclassifiable headache

CSF = cerebrospinal fluid.
*International Headache Society classification.

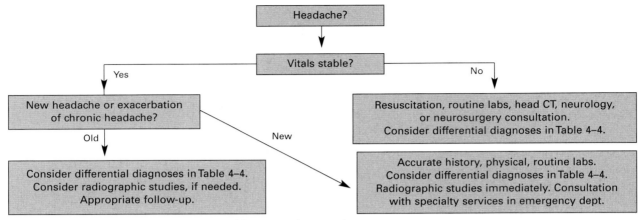

Figure 4–3. Algorithm for evaluation of headache. CT = computed tomography.

cial pain, herniated disks, or joint arthropathy. Chronic back pain is also the most common somatic complaint in many patients who have anxiety, unrelieved stress, and depression. All of these psychological issues may be magnified in the cancer patient. Unfortunately, in the cancer patient, the presence of malignant disease involving the neuraxis and the remote possibility of infection (eg, epidural abscess) are also possible and further confound the diagnosis[47] (Table 4–5;[48] Figure 4–4).

There are some key points to remember in treating cancer patients with a backache. The presentation of back pain can pose a challenge to the emergency-room clinician. Overall, the key point is the ruling out of potentially catastrophic conditions such as an epidural abscess or imminent cord compression. In a patient with a malignancy or a history of a malignancy known to metastasize to the vertebral column or associated soft tissues, a diagnosis of new-onset back pain should be thoroughly evaluated. Once all the relevant data have been obtained, the clinician must make a reasonable decision, based on risk versus relative benefit.

LIMB PAIN

Limb pain in the cancer setting can be caused directly by the presence of tumor in the affected limb or indirectly by the neurotoxic effects of chemotherapy. The presence of tumor in the neuraxis can also manifest as a radicular pain in the affected limb. The etiology of limb pain can usually be differentiated on the basis of a thorough history and physical examination[49,50] (Table 4–6; Figure 4–5).

As in other clinical conditions, the clinician must maintain a high index of suspicion regarding patients who present with isolated limb pain. Causes may be as mild as the occasional sprain or strain but may also be potentially far more serious, such as a pathologic fracture, a new metastasis, recent epidural disease manifesting as radicular pain, a vascular problem, or an infection.

The onset of diffuse bilateral pain, whether neuropathic or somatic, generally indicates a more benign condition, such as neuropathy from chemotherapy or joint or muscle pain from certain adjuvant agents.

ABDOMINAL PAIN

Patients presenting with acute abdominal pain may have etiologies ranging from benign self-limiting conditions to life-threatening illnesses. The practitioner must be able to quickly recognize serious conditions and initiate

TABLE 4–5. Differential Diagnosis of Backache

Vertebral and paravertebral causes of back pain (with or without radiculopathy)
    Herniated nucleus pulposus: cervical, thoracic, lumbar (most commonly)
    Degenerative joint disease: disk space narrowing, spinal stenosis, facet normality
    Arachnoiditis: after surgery or after intrathecal injection of contrast material
    Musculoskeletal disorder: strain, sprain, spasm, vertebral fracture
    Neoplasm: metastatic, multiple myeloma, other primary spinal tumors
    Infection: epidural abscess, vertebral osteomyelitis, Pott's disease, herpes zoster
    Rheumatic conditions: ankylosing spondylitis, Reiter's syndrome, fibromyalgia
Referred causes of back pain (usually without radiculopathy)
    Vascular origin: abdominal aortic aneurysm, arterial occlusive disease
    Biliary origin: obstructed bile ducts, distended gallbladder
    Gastrointestinal: perforated viscus
    Pancreatic origin: pancreatic carcinoma, pancreatitis
    Uterine origin: ovarian carcinoma, endometrial carcinoma
    Renal origin: renal carcinoma, kidney stones, ureteral stones, pyelonephritis, bladder carcinoma
Psychiatric causes of low back pain
    Chronic low back pain secondary to
        Somatization
        Compensation hysteria
        Malingering
        Substance abuse
        Anxiety states
        Depression

Reproduced with permission from Engstrom JW, Bradford DS.[48]

proper treatment, including surgical consultation, without delay. This is made more challenging by the atypical presentation frequently seen in cancer patients.

Common Causes of Abdominal Pain

A common cause of mild abdominal cramps is reaction to medications, frequently antibiotics. The onset of the pain coincides with recent medication changes. The patient generally looks well, the symptoms are mild, and the examination and diagnostic studies are unremarkable.

Another common reason for patients seeking acute treatment for abdominal pain is cancer pain that is not being controlled by the current medication regimen. These patients usually have abdominal or pelvic malignant lesions and are taking some form of analgesic. The patient usually states that there is no change in the nature of the pain; however, the current pain medication is not effective (Table 4–7).[51–57]

Diagnostic Approach

During the evaluation of any patient seeking acute care, the practitioner must first consider and exclude true emergencies that may cause catastrophic consequences in the absence of prompt intervention. One may then evaluate for the common causes that are the bases of the majority of the cases; this is followed by a more exhaustive search for less common etiologies to arrive at a final diagnosis.[58,59]

- Information regarding the onset, duration, timing, quality, and location of the abdominal pain must be obtained.
- Associated symptoms (such as nausea and vomiting, diarrhea, or fever) and aggravating or alleviating factors need to be elicited.
- Pay particular attention to peritoneal signs such as abdominal wall rigidity and rebound tenderness during the abdominal examination.
- Watch for alarming signs such as hypotension, altered mental status, tachypnea, and persistent tachycardia not responding to intravenous fluids.[51]
- A complete blood count, assessment of electrolytes, biochemical survey, urinalysis, liver function tests, analyses of amylase and lipase, are usually indicated.
- Stool should be tested for occult blood.
- Supine and erect abdominal radiography and upright chest radiography should be included as part of the evaluation in most patients.
- Perform electrocardiography if the pain is located in the upper abdomen of a patient at risk for myocardial ischemia.

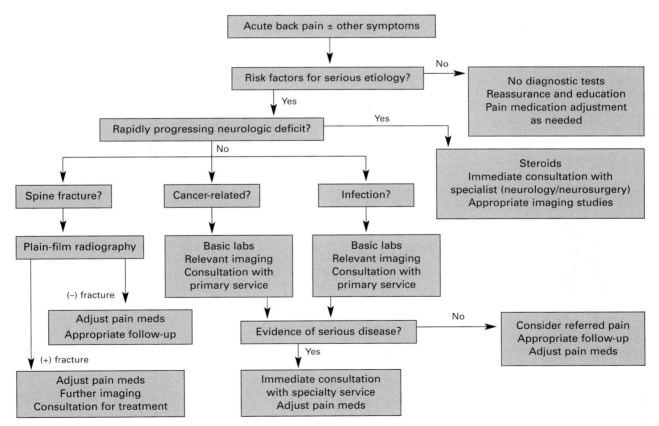

Figure 4–4. Algorithm for evaluation and treatment of back pain.

TABLE 4–6. Differential Diagnosis of Limb Pain

Musculoskeletal disorder
　Muscle sprain or strain
Neurologic disorders
　Sympathetically-mediated pain syndromes
　　Complex regional pain syndrome type I (CRPS I)
　　Complex regional pain syndrome type II (CRPS II)
　Neuropathic pain
　　Chemotherapy-induced: involvement is usually symmetrical, affects
　　　distal areas (hands/feet), and progresses proximally.
　　Neuraxial involvement: epidural disease can cause a radicular pain
　　　involving one (or both) extremities. Presentation is usually
　　　asymmetrical.
Somatic Pain
　Tumor involvement of the affected limb (usually affects only the limb
　　involved)
Vascular disease
Inflammatory disease
Infection
　Osteomyelitis
Psychiatric causes
　Exaggerated limb pain, rarely secondary to somatization, compensation
　　hysteria, malingering, substance abuse, anxiety states, depression

- Arterial blood gas analysis is indicated if acidosis is suspected in patients with tachypnea or when a significant anion gap is present.
- Coagulation panel and a type and screen of blood should be ordered if surgical intervention is anticipated.
- So that signs and symptoms are not masked, one may have to withhold analgesics until the patient is evaluated by a surgeon (Figure 4–6).[60,61]

True Emergencies

Perforated viscus is usually caused by invasion and weakening of the intestinal wall by cancer or peptic ulcer disease. The acute onset of pain, a rigid abdomen, unstable vital signs, and intra-abdominal free air on abdominal radiography are typically seen in these patients. Surgery consultation should be expedited.[62–65]

Acute intestinal obstruction usually presents as nausea and vomiting with or without abdominal pain. It is described in more detail in Nausea and Vomiting, below. The presence of air-fluid levels on abdominal series warrants consultation for possible surgical intervention.[66,67]

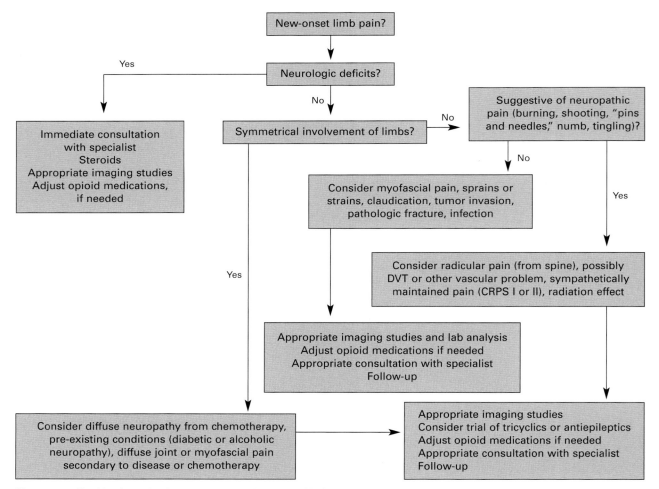

Figure 4–5. Algorithm for evaluation and treatment of limb pain. CRPS = complex regional pain syndrome; DVT = deep venous thrombosis.

Neutropenic enterocolitis is a necrotizing lesion of the bowel in leukemia or solid-tumor patients with chemotherapy-induced neutropenia. It should be considered in neutropenic patients with fever, severe abdominal pain, and evidence of sepsis. Blood culture should be obtained, and broad-spectrum antibiotics and aggressive fluid resuscitation must be started immediately.

Intra-abdominal or retroperitoneal hemorrhage is primarily associated with cancer invading local vascular structures or with spontaneous cancer bleeding in patients with thrombocytopenia or coagulopathy. Abdominal computerized tomography or ultrasonography is usually diagnostic. Serial hematocrits should be monitored. Transfusion of packed red cells and platelets may become necessary. Surgical intervention is indicated if the hemorrhage persists.

In patients with splenomegaly due to hematologic malignancy, splenic rupture may occur with mild trauma or even spontaneously. Left upper-quadrant pain, diaphoresis, and history of trauma are the usual presenting elements. Volume resuscitation and surgical consultation is mandatory.

Urinary outlet obstruction due to space-occupying pelvic lesions is not an uncommon reason for patients to seek acute care for abdominal pain. The pain is localized in the lower abdominal suprapubic area.[56] The patient almost always relays a history of inability to void. The distended bladder is palpable. The insertion of a urinary catheter immediately relieves the symptom.

Points to Remember

Cancer patients frequently have atypical presentations of their underlying pathology. For instance, patients on steroids, either as part of their chemotherapy or as treatment for a brain lesion or emesis, may have little or none of the symptoms of an acute abdomen during the early stage of a catastrophic abdominal event. Therefore, every patient seeking acute care must be evaluated thoroughly to exclude true abdominal emergencies.

Cancer patients also develop conditions seen in the general population. One needs to include conditions such as myocardial infarction, ruptured abdominal aortic aneurysm, mesenteric ischemia, ovarian torsion, ectopic pregnancy (rare), nephrolithiasis, diverticulitis, gallbladder diseases, and incarcerated hernia in the differential diagnosis.

Gastrointestinal involvement of graft-versus-host disease should be considered in bone marrow transplantation patients. These patients are also prone to opportunistic infections. Patients with hematologic malignancies may develop splenic rupture due to massive splenomegaly, intra-abdominal or retroperitoneal bleeding due to thrombocytopenia, and abdominal or pelvic infection or abscess due to neutropenia. Some patients with solid tumors may develop Budd-Chiari

TABLE 4–7. Differential Diagnosis of Abdominal Pain

Abdominal
  Hollow viscera (stomach, small bowel, large bowel, rectum, biliary tract)
    Perforation
    Obstruction
    Inflammation, infection, abscess
    Neoplasm
  Solid viscera (liver, spleen, pancreas)
    Rupture
    Distention
    Inflammation, infection, abscess
    Neoplasm
  Vascular
    Ischemia due to thrombosis, embolism, or spasm
    Rupture or dissection of abdominal aortic aneurysm
  Peritoneal
    Inflammation, infection, abscess
    Hemorrhage
    Neoplasm
  Retroperitoneal (kidney, ureter, lymph nodes)
    Inflammation, infection, abscess
    Hemorrhage
    Neoplasm
Extra-abdominal
  Thoracic
    Pulmonary
    Pneumonia
    Pneumothorax
    Pleuritis
    Primary or metastatic neoplasm
    Cardiac
      Myocardial ischemia
      Pericarditis
      Benign or malignant pericardial effusion
    Esophageal
      Esophagitis, infectious or radiation-induced
      Esophageal rupture
      Neoplasm
  Pelvic (ovary, uterus, cervix, prostate, bladder)
    Inflammation, infection, abscess
    Distention, torsion
    Neoplasm
  Spinal
    Herpes zoster
    Spinal-cord compression
    Leptomeningeal disease with nerve root involvement
    Spinal metastasis
  Systemic
    Leukemia
    Lymphoma
    Hemolytic anemia
    Sickle cell crisis
  Metabolic
    Addisonian crisis
    Uremia
    Diabetic ketoacidosis
    Porphyria
    Venom (black widow spider, snake)
  Other
    Depression
    Anxiety
    Psychiatric disorder
    Factitious

syndrome (hepatic vein obstruction) due to their hyper-coagulable state.

With a patient who has had a percutaneous endo-scopic gastrostomy (PEG) within 24 to 48 hours, free air may be seen on abdominal radiography and mild to mod-erate abdominal pain may be present. The patient can be safely observed and followed with repeated evaluations if the position of the PEG tube is confirmed and if the patient is stable. The symptoms usually resolve within a couple of days. Sometimes, a diagnosis cannot be achieved after the initial work-up. It is prudent to admit the patient for observation of evolving symptoms and signs until the true nature of the underlying process emerges.

Summary

Cancer patients presenting with abdominal pain have variable underlying etiologies. The practitioner must remain vigilant in identifying ominous signs and symp-toms in a patient with atypical presentations. Surgical consultation should be obtained without delay when sur-gical abdomen is suspected.

NAUSEA AND VOMITING

Nausea and vomiting is the second most common pre-senting symptom of cancer patients seeking acute or emergent care. Almost any acute or chronic illness can cause nausea and vomiting. Frequently, cancer patients present with nausea and vomiting due to emetogenic chemotherapeutic agents; however, etiologies with poten-tially devastating complications must be considered.

Common Causes of Nausea and Vomiting

The most common causes of nausea and vomiting in cancer patients result from complications of chemo-therapy. Common emetogenic agents include carbo-platin, cisplatin, cyclophosphamide, cytarabine, doxoru-bicin, etoposide, gemcitabine, ifosfamide, methotrexate, mitomycin, and topotecan, especially when used at a high dose.[68] Other chemotherapeutic agents may less frequently cause nausea and vomiting in some patients. The patient usually has few other associated symptoms besides evidence of dehydration. Control of symptoms and correction of dehydration and electrolyte abnor-malities remain the mainstays of treatment.[69,70] Occa-sionally, emesis becomes so debilitating that admission for intravenous fluid and symptom control is justified.

Another common cause of anorexia or nausea and vomiting in cancer patients (as well as in the general pop-ulation) is medication side effects. The medications in question include potassium supplements, morphine and its derivatives, and some antibiotics.

The etiologies that can cause nausea and vomiting are numerous. The more common causes are listed in Table 4–8.

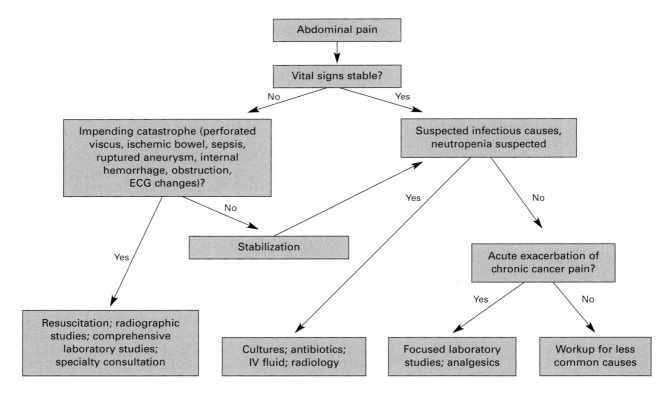

Figure 4–6. Algorithm for evaluation of abdominal pain. ECG = electrocardiogram; IV = intravenous.

TABLE 4–8. Differential Diagnosis of Nausea and Vomiting

Gastrointestinal
  Obstructive
    Mechanical
      Extraluminal
        Primary or metastatic neoplasm
        Peritoneal carcinomatosis
        Postsurgical adhesion
        Hematoma
        Abscess
      Intraluminal
        Neoplasm
        Bowel wall thickening by infiltration of malignant cells
        Surgical anastomosis
        Fecal impaction
        Radiation stenosis
        Intussusception, volvulus
    Nonmechanical, adynamic ileus
      Peritoneal irritation
        Peritonitis
        Perforated viscus
        Postoperative irritation
      Retroperitoneal irritation
        Hemorrhage
        Abscess
        Renal colic
        Pyelonephritis
        Pancreatitis
        Neoplasm (eg, lymphoma)
      Systemic and metabolic causes (see below)
  Non-obstructive
    Neoplasmic lesion (primary or metastatic)
    Graft-versus-host disease
    Gastroenteritis
    Gastroesophageal reflux disease (GERD)
    Diabetic gastroparesis
    Peptic ulcer disease
    Pancreatitis
    Cholecystitis
    Choledocholithiasis
    Hepatitis (viral or drug-induced)
    Ascites
    Ischemic bowel disease
    Food poisoning
Systemic
  Infection
  Severe pain
  Myocardial ischemia
  Congestive heart failure
  Radiation sickness
  Progression of cancer
Metabolic
  Electrolyte abnormalities, hypokalemia, hypercalcemia, hyponatremia
  Uremia
  Metabolic acidosis
  Adrenal insufficiency
  Hypothyroidism, hyperthyroidism
Neurologic
  Increased intracranial pressure
    Primary or metastatic brain lesion
    Hemorrhage into neoplasm
    Subarachnoid hemorrhage
    Trauma (eg, fall, thrombocytopenia)
    Leptomeningeal disease
    Hydrocephalus, obstruction of cerebrospinal-fluid flow
    Meningitis, encephalitis
  Disorders of the middle ear
    Neoplasm involvement
    Infection
  Migraine headache

TABLE 4–8. Continued

Pharmacologic
  Chemotherapeutic agents
  Morphine and derivatives
  Nonsteroidals (NSAIDs)
  Oral antibiotics
  Potassium supplement
  Digitalis
  Anticholinergics
Other
  Psychogenic
  Pregnancy
  Drug withdrawal
  Carbon monoxide poisoning

Diagnostic Approach

During the evaluation of any patient seeking acute care, the practitioner must first consider and exclude true emergencies that may cause catastrophic consequences in the absence of prompt intervention. One may then evaluate for the common causes that are the bases of the majority of cases; this is followed by a more exhaustive search for less common etiologies to arrive at a final diagnosis.

During the patient interview, the onset of nausea and vomiting and its temporal relationship with chemotherapy must be clarified.[71,72] Associated symptoms, such as abdominal distention, pain, or diarrhea, must be elicited. In general, most emesis due to chemotherapeutic agents regresses after the fifth day following the administration of the agent. The locations of the malignancies and metastases often shed light on the underlying etiology. The exact nature of prior abdominal surgery is also important.

Fever may indicate underlying infection. Evidence of neurologic involvement must be actively sought. Abdominal examination may or may not be helpful in narrowing the differential diagnosis in the absence of other associated symptoms and signs.[73,74]

The practitioner should have a low threshold in ordering supine and erect abdominal radiography looking for evidence of obstruction. A complete blood count, assessment of electrolytes, magnesium level, and urinalysis are almost always required. Biochemical surveys and analyses of amylase and lipase may be indicated. If a serious systemic or cardiopulmonary process is suspected, electrocardiography, chest radiography, and arterial blood gas analysis should also be performed (Figure 4–7).

True Emergencies

Increased intracranial pressure due to a brain lesion, hemorrhage, obstruction of the flow of cerebrospinal fluid (CSF), or central nervous system infection may manifest as nausea and vomiting. Look for neurologic changes, a known brain lesion or metastasis, thrombocy-

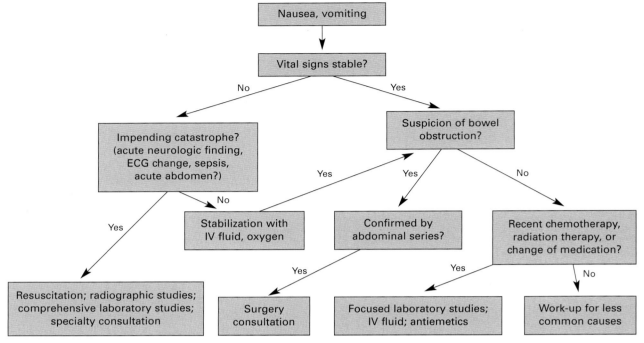

Figure 4–7. Algorithm for evaluation of nausea and vomiting. ECG = electrocardiogram; IV = intravenous.

topenia, coagulopathy, fever, meningeal signs, or a history of trauma. Prompt imaging studies by computed tomography (CT) or magnetic resonance imaging (MRI) followed by consultation with neurology or neurosurgery are warranted. Immediate intervention to lower the intracranial pressure should be initiated.

Serious infection or cardiopulmonary events causing tissue hypoperfusion may also cause nausea and vomiting. The patient usually has other associated symptoms and signs, such as fever, altered mental status, dyspnea, or diaphoresis. Look for unstable vital signs, neutropenia, and evidence of myocardial ischemia or pulmonary embolism. Results of the appropriate diagnostic studies should be obtained. Stabilization of the patient and proper treatment for the underlying processes should be started without delay.

Obstruction of the gastrointestinal tract is usually seen in patients with gastrointestinal involvement of either primary or metastatic neoplasms. Patients with gastrointestinal malignancies, gynecologic malignancies, peritoneal metastasis or carcinomatosis, and a history of prior abdominal surgery and patients developing intractable nausea and vomiting in the absence of recent chemotherapy have higher frequencies of bowel obstruction. Abdominal radiography to obtain supine, erect, and decubitus abdominal films is usually diagnostic. Adynamic ileus and partial bowel obstruction usually present a similar pattern. Timely surgical consultation should be obtained.

Points to Remember

A history of recent chemotherapy or radiation therapy and a temporal relationship with the onset of symptoms are extremely helpful in reaching a diagnosis. Radiation treatment may cause the sensation of nausea. Radiation esophagitis or gastritis occasionally presents with nausea and vomiting but more frequently presents with odynophagia.[73]

In hematologic patients, diffuse infiltration of the gastrointestinal wall can cause progressive nausea and vomiting. In bone marrow transplantation patients, graft-versus-host disease in the gastrointestinal tract must be considered.

Many cancer patients have atypical presentations of typical illness. This fact demands that the practitioner have a high level of suspicion for serious underlying diseases. One should exercise a low threshold for more extensive work-ups in this particular patient population.

Finally, severe cancer pain alone may induce nausea and vomiting. The progression of cancer and psychological factors such as depression may also cause anorexia and may occasionally cause nausea.

Summary

Nausea and vomiting is a very common complaint in cancer patients. Although it can be caused by almost any illness, the vast majority of cases fall into two groups: chemotherapy-induced emesis and bowel obstruction by underlying malignancy. The role of abdominal radiography should be emphasized.

CONSTIPATION

Constipation is usually a chronic problem among cancer patients. However, patients occasionally present to an emergency department, seeking relief. Constipation in these patients is usually due to impaired physical mobility caused by the disease or the treatment as well as by the narcotic analgesics that many cancer patients take.

Differential Diagnosis

The chronic use of morphine and its derivatives is among the most common cause of constipation in cancer patients.[75] Concurrent stool softeners should be given to the many cancer patients who are on narcotics for chronic pain. A medication history should be elicited, and a digital rectal examination should be done on those patients who are without contraindication (such as neutropenia). Chronic constipation may perpetuate into fecal impaction that requires digital disimpaction.

Physical inactivity is another common cause of constipation. Many cancer patients are debilitated by the disease or the complications of treatment. These patients should avoid chronic laxative use. Instead, increased physical activity, dietary adjustment, and adequate hydration should be encouraged[76–78] (Table 4–9).

Diagnostic Approach

The duration of the constipation and associated symptoms such as abdominal pain, distention, nausea, vomiting, and diarrhea must be elicited. A detailed medication history often helps in the diagnosis. During the examination, one must specifically look for signs of acute abdomen, neurologic compromises, and severe systemic illness. A rectal examination should be done on all patients who have no contraindication (such as neutropenia).

Laboratory studies and abdominal radiography help eliminate serious underlying conditions from the diagnosis. Abdominal CT with oral and rectal contrast may be needed if obstruction is suspected. More elaborate work-up procedures such as sigmoidoscopy or colonoscopy may be scheduled for difficult cases but are seldom required in the emergency department.[79–84]

True Emergencies

Spinal-cord compression at the level of lower sacral segments sometimes presents as constipation. It is usually associated with local pain, lower-extremity weakness, and loss of sphincter tone. It should be high on the differential diagnosis list for patients with known spinal metastasis or patients with neurologic findings in a lower extremity. Magnetic resonance imaging of the spine is the diagnostic test of choice. Neurology, neurosurgery, and radiation oncology services should be consulted for definitive treatment. Meanwhile, high-dose steroids such as dexamethasone (40 to 100 mg intravenously) should be started in the emergency department without delay if spinal-cord compression is highly suspected.

Extraluminal or luminal obstruction of the colon or rectum may be present in patients who complain only of having constipation and having no bowel movements for a number of days. Obstruction of the colon or rectum is seen in patients with gastrointestinal (GI)-tract involvement of primary or metastatic cancer, most commonly colon cancer, anorectal cancer, gynecological cancer, genitourinary cancer, lymphoma, and carcinoid. Evidence of GI-tract obstruction should be sought. Supine

TABLE 4–9. Differential Diagnosis of Constipation

Gastrointestinal
  Anorectal
    Primary anorectal neoplasm
    Pelvic neoplasm (prostatic, cervical, vaginal)
    Proctitis (radiation, infection)
    Hemorrhoids
    Anal fissures or fistula
    Perineal abscess
  Colonic
    Colon cancer
    Extraluminal primary or metastatic neoplasm
    Postoperative stricture, adhesion
    Ascites
    Fecal impaction
    Intussusception
    Inflammatory bowel disease (Crohn's disease)
    Granulomatous disease (tuberculosis)
    Irritable bowel syndrome
    Diverticular disease
Systemic
  Physical inactivity
  Low-residue diet
Metabolic
  Hypercalcemia
  Hypokalemia
  Hypothyroidism
  Diabetes mellitus
  Uremia
Neurologic
  Lower-spinal-cord compression by neoplasm or hematoma
  Autonomic neuropathy
Pharmacologic
  Morphine and derivatives
  Laxative or enema abuse
  Nonabsorbable antacids
  Calcium channel blockers
  Anticholinergics
  Antidepressants
  Diuretics
Other
  Psychiatric disorders
  Senile dementia

and erect plain-film radiography of the abdomen, supplemented by abdominal CT or barium enema, helps in reaching a diagnosis.

Points to Remember

Other medications that may cause decreased bowel mobility include anticholinergics, nonabsorbable antacids, and diuretics. Among chemotherapeutic agents, thalidomide is notorious for causing constipation. Recent changes of medications should always be queried as part of the interview.

Hypercalcemia is occasionally the etiology of constipation. The type of cancer and the site of metastasis should raise the suspicion for this condition. Assessments of serum calcium level, albumin level, and ionized calcium level (if indicated) should be ordered as a part of the work-up.

Fecal impaction may present as both constipation and overflow diarrhea. Severe anorectal pain due to hemorrhoid, fissure or cancer may prevent a patient from having regular bowel movements. A digital rectal examination usually establishes the diagnosis. Treatment with oral agents such as lactulose is preferred to treatment with rectal suppositories or enemas.[85] One must be careful in giving enemas in patients with abdominal pain. Rectal suppository or enema treatment is generally contraindicated in neutropenic patients.

Summary

True emergencies are few in patients who present with isolated constipation. Once true emergent conditions are eliminated, symptomatic treatment is usually all that is needed in the emergency department.

DIARRHEA

Acute diarrhea in cancer patients may result from de novo pathologic processes (as seen also in the general population) as well as from complications of the underlying neoplasm or the treatment received. Infectious etiologies that cause self-limiting diarrhea in healthy populations may cause protracted symptoms in cancer patients because of their weakened immune system.

Differential Diagnosis

Antibiotics are common culprits, causing gastrointestinal upset and diarrhea in patients seeking acute care. They are used more frequently as prophylaxis or treatment in cancer patients because of the patients' immunosuppressed state. Broad-spectrum antibiotics may induce pseudomembranous colitis. Stool samples should be submitted for testing of *Clostridium difficile* toxin.[86,87] Some chemotherapeutic agents (eg, irinotecan [CPT-11]) are also known to cause diarrhea (Table 4–10).

Diagnostic Approach

It is important to know the onset, frequency, and severity of the diarrhea. The amount and consistency of the stool, the presence of any blood or mucus, and any associated fever, abdominal pain, and nausea and vomiting must be part of the history obtained. Evidence of hemodynamic instability, such as tachycardia and orthostatic hypotension, indicates the severity of the problem. A careful abdominal and rectal examination is performed with attention to signs of acute abdomen.

Blood counts and analyses of electrolytes, magnesium, blood urea nitrogen, and creatinine are usually required for the evaluation of any significant diarrhea. Stool samples should be collected for testing for occult blood, fecal leukocytes, and *C. difficile* toxin as indicated. Abdominal series must be obtained if obstruction or perforation is suspected. Endoscopy should be considered for any patient with bloody diarrhea[88–93] (Figure 4–8).

TABLE 4–10. Differential Diagnosis of Diarrhea

Gastrointestinal
   Infectious
      Toxin-related (*Staphylococcus aureus, Escherichia coli*, etc)
      Viral (*Enterovirus, Cytomegalovirus*, herpes simplex, etc)
      Bacterial (*Escherichia coli, Salmonella, Clostridium difficile*, etc)
      Parasitic (amebiasis, giardiasis, etc)
      Fungal (*Candida, Cryptococcus*, etc)
   Noninfectious
      Gastrointestinal-tract hemorrhage (mistaken as diarrhea)
      Intestinal lymphoma
      Graft-versus-host disease
      Partial bowel obstruction by neoplasm
      Radiation enteritis
      Postoperative change (blind loop syndrome, short-bowel syndrome, etc)
      Ischemic bowel disease
      Inflammatory bowel disease
      Irritable bowel disease
      Malabsorption
Systemic
   Infection (eg, toxic shock syndrome)
   Stress
   Diabetic autonomic neuropathy
   Collagen/vascular disease
Metabolic
   Carcinoid syndrome
   Hyperthyroidism
   Addisonian crisis
   Uremia
Pharmacologic
   Laxatives
   Antibiotics
   Chemotherapeutic agents
   Opiates (withdrawal)
   Antacids containing magnesium
Other
   Psychiatric disorders
   Dietary factors
   Senile incontinence

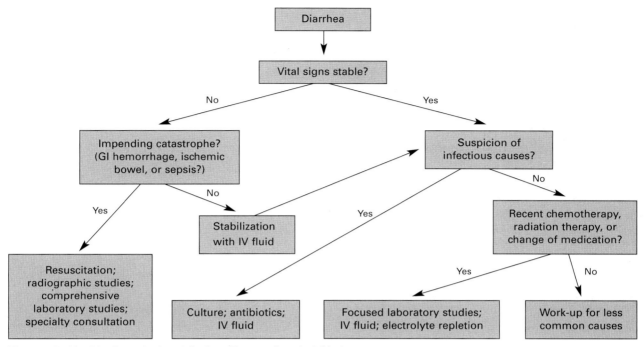

Figure 4–8. Algorithm for evaluation of diarrhea. GI = gastrointestinal; IV = intravenous.

True Emergencies

Gastrointestinal hemorrhage must be eliminated during evaluation. Occasionally, a patient may complain of diarrhea that, upon further questioning, is found to be actually melena. Melena usually becomes apparent after a thorough history and a rectal examination with tests for gross or occult blood.

Copious diarrhea in a short period of time from any etiology can result in severe intravascular depletion manifesting as hemodynamic collapse. In patients presenting with diarrhea and hypotension, fluid resuscitation must be initiated without delay while the cause of the diarrhea is being evaluated.

Points to Remember

Other infectious causes of diarrhea need to be considered, including those of bacterial, viral, and parasitic origin. Patients who have hematologic malignancies, who have had bone marrow transplantation, who are on immunosuppressants, or who are neutropenic are especially prone to opportunistic infections.

Radiation enterocolitis or proctitis should be considered in patients who have had recent abdominal or pelvic irradiation treatments. A history of bone marrow transplantation should remind the evaluator of the possibility that graft-versus-host disease with gastrointestinal involvement could be the cause of the patient's diarrhea.

One must pay particular attention to the patient's hemodynamic status and electrolyte levels. Aggressive fluid administration and correction of potassium and magnesium abnormalities are often required.

Summary

Most diarrheas are self-limiting upon the removal of the offending elements. However, patients with explosive diarrhea can lose significant amounts of fluid and electrolytes in a short period of time and develop hemodynamic instability. Fluid resuscitation should be aggressive in this situation. Stabilization of the patient is more important than reaching a definitive diagnosis in an emergency setting.

DYSPNEA

Dyspnea is a subjective awareness of difficulty in breathing. It is one of the symptoms most likely to cause patients with advanced cancer to seek medical attention in the acute setting.

Along with the overall performance status of the patient, dyspnea is considered to be a prognostic indicator of survival.[94] It may occur in 21 to 78% of all patients days to weeks before their deaths and is reported to be severe in as many as 63% of patients.[95]

In a study conducted at The University of Texas M. D. Anderson Cancer Center, Escalante and colleagues found that 37% of the patients with dyspnea in the study cohort who sought medical care from an emergency center had the diagnosis of lung cancer and that 30% had breast cancer. In this study, patients with dyspnea had an overall median survival duration of 12 weeks after the initial visit to the emergency center. Patients with lung cancer had the shortest survival (an average of only 4 weeks, compared with 22 weeks for patients with breast cancer).[96]

Dyspnea is usually the result of one of the three following abnormalities: (1) an inability to increase breathing effort to reach a certain respiratory workload, (2) respiratory muscle weakness, and (3) increasing ventilatory requirements.[97]

Differential Diagnosis

Dyspnea has several different etiologies, and in about half of the patients who have it, more than one factor contributes to the symptom. In one study of patients with breast cancer, pleural effusions and congestive heart failure were the leading causes of dyspnea whereas the primary tumor, chronic obstructive pulmonary disease, and pneumonia were the contributing factors in patients with lung cancer.[96]

Lung cancer is the primary malignancy that is most commonly associated with dyspnea although the genesis of the symptom may have an important patient-to-patient variation as the location and size of the tumor generally determine the severity and characteristics of dyspnea. Severity and characteristics differ according to whether the tumor is growing centrally (endobronchial) or in the periphery. Obstruction, dyspnea, and stridor mainly characterize central lesions; peripheral lesions lead to pain, coughing, and dyspnea, often as a consequence of a lung-restrictive pattern.[98]

It is important to keep in mind that patients with cancer may also have other pulmonary comorbidities, such as chronic bronchitis, asthma, or emphysema. Cardiac-related pathologies such as congestive heart failure and coronary insufficiency can contribute to dyspnea, as can other musculoskeletal, hematologic, or psychological abnormalities.[99]

In addition, in cancer patients with dyspnea cardiac tamponade or restrictive pericardial, conditions should also be considered. Interstitial lung disease, such as lymphangitic metastases and pulmonary embolism are also part of the differential diagnosis of dyspnea in the cancer patient. For more detailed discussions of these topics, refer to Chapters 10, 14 and 15. Therapeutic interventions such as bleomycin, doxorubicin, and mitomycin C can cause dyspnea, and other conditions, such as cachexia, ascites, anemia, respiratory muscle weakness, or even anxiety,[100] can contribute as well.

The role of anemia in the genesis of dyspnea deserves some discussion because the treatment of anemia is widely used to alleviate dyspnea along with other symptoms such as fatigue, weakness, and tachycardia. Nevertheless, only a small amount of contradictory data regarding the effectiveness of peripheral red blood cell transfusions on the subjective relief of the sensation of breathlessness can be found in the literature[97] (Figure 4–9).

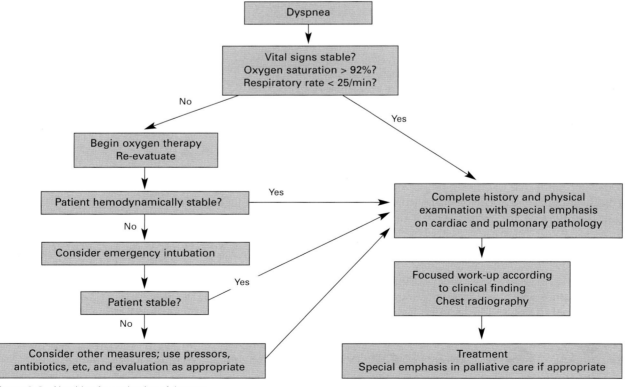

Figure 4–9. Algorithm for evaluation of dyspnea.

Points to Remember

Dyspnea is a very common symptom in patients with virtually every kind of advanced cancer. It is a subjective sensation that is unique to each individual although some scoring systems are available to "quantify" its magnitude.[101]

Breathlessness has been linked at presentation in as many as 60% of patients diagnosed with non-small-cell lung cancer in one study[102] and has been associated with a very short median survival duration (as brief as 2 weeks) in another series.[96] In the cancer population, therefore, this symptom ought to be considered an ominous sign in patients with advanced malignancies.

In the subset of patients with advanced cancer, a number of different drugs and treatments have been given for the palliation of dyspnea, depending on the severity and acuity of the symptom and on the clinical circumstances. The treatments and drugs most commonly used have been oxygen, opioids, benzodiazepines, bronchodilators, antibiotics (when clinically appropriate), and general support measures.[103,104]

Summary

Dyspnea has several different causes, including muscular weakness and hypoxia. It occurs frequently in patients with advanced cancer. It may present at diagnosis or during the terminal stages of disease, or it may precede an oncologic catastrophe. Potentially, dyspnea is at least partially correctable, usually with a palliative goal.

COUGH

Cough is one of the most common reasons patients seek medical attention. To them, a persistent cough means "something is wrong," and they may seek care for a variety of reasons, including a fear of cancer, tuberculosis, or aquired immunodeficiency syndrome (AIDS).[105] Cough can be a protective mechanism, triggered by foreign materials such as airway irritants (including smoke and dust) or aspirated materials (such as upper-airway secretions or gastric contents).

Differential Diagnosis

Any disorder that causes inflammation, constriction, infiltration, or compression of the airway can be associated with a cough. Airway infections, including viral and bacterial infections, commonly result in inflammation of the bronchial tree.[105] Also, any neoplasm (such as a bronchogenic malignancy or carcinoid tumor) that infiltrates or compresses the airway may result in a cough. Other comorbidities can cause a cough; these include a number of pulmonary conditions such as asthma, postnasal drip, pertussis, sarcoidosis, and interstitial lung disease and some nonpulmonary-related etiologies such as gastroe-sophageal reflux disease, congestive heart failure, and the use of angiotensin-converting enzyme inhibitor.[105]

Although there are no reports in the literature about the association between cough and malignancy, cough is a symptom of particular importance in oncology. The most common clinical circumstances that involve cough are infections in the general oncologic/hematologic population that can range from simple viral or bacterial infections to complicated fungal pulmonary infections. Even more important, these infections also occur in other immunocompromised patients. Also, intrinsic pulmonary malignancies and pulmonary metastases may present with bronchial-tree infiltration or external compression, both of which produce a cough.

In most patients, the cause of a cough can be determined by simple diagnostic tests, beginning with a general physical examination and including proper auscultation, chest radiography, microscopic sputum examination, and pulmonary function testing if clinically appropriate[105] (Figure 4–10).

Summary

The cause of a chronic cough can almost always be determined by appropriate patient evaluation, and it may be possible to prescribe a specific therapy that can be almost uniformly successful.

ALTERED MENTAL STATUS

Altered mental status is a common reason for neurologic consultation for the cancer patient presenting to the emergency center. The differential diagnosis runs the gamut from sepsis, metabolic disturbances, and drug intoxication to intracerebral hemorrhage. The initial evaluation must be expedient and thorough if appropriate therapy is to be undertaken. History is frequently limited, given the nature of the complaint, and the neurologic examination, coupled with appropriate studies, directs the direction and pace of management. An accurate assessment of the patient by the receiving physician will greatly aid diagnosis, and as with many emergencies, the evaluation is often concurrent with therapy. While clinicians worry about mass lesions as the cause of altered mental status, particularly in oncologic patients, toxic metabolic encephalopathy is the far more common etiology[106] (Table 4–11).

Initial Measures

Prior to performing a detailed examination, the clinician should be certain that the patient with altered mental status has an adequate airway and adequate blood pressure. Blood for glucose should be drawn as well as for blood cultures, tests for electrolytes, calcium and magnesium, and an arterial blood gas analysis (Table 4–12). The patient should then receive 100 mg of thiamine and 50 g

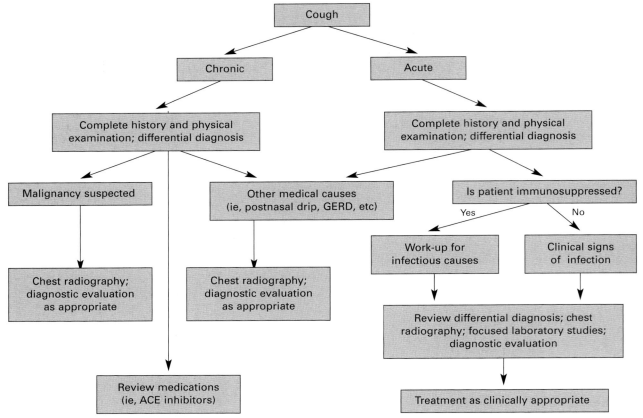

Figure 4–10. Algorithm for evaluation of cough. ACE = angiotensin-converting enzyme; GERD = gastroesophageal reflux disease.

of glucose.[107] A single bolus of glucose may prevent permanent neuronal damage should hypoglycemia be the cause of the altered mental state.

Thiamine deficiency will cause irreparable brain damage if uncorrected, and this deficiency has protean manifestations. A confusional state, nystagmus, ophthalmoplegia, and ataxia are central nervous system manifestations of acute thiamine deficiency although the clinical picture for any individual is highly variable. Thiamine deficiency is commonly thought of as a problem that chiefly affects alcoholics (hence the useful mnemonic DRUNK [Dullness of mentation, Rectus palsy, Unsteady gait, Nystagmus, Korsakoff's psychosis]), (P Gross, personal communication, March 1976) but thiamine is critical to carbohydrate metabolism. Thiamine deficiency is not uncommon in cancer patients, who often eat poorly and who, when they do eat, frequently consume mainly carbohydrates. Severe thiamine deficiency may produce lactic acidosis that is refractory to correction until thiamine is given parenterally.[108] A urine specimen should be sent for toxicology screen if there is a possibility that the patient may be intoxicated.

Hints of intoxication include miotic pupils (seen in narcotic intoxication), an unexplained anion gap that occurs with lactic acidosis, and unexplained hyperosmolality that may be present with high serum alcohol levels. Patients who are on narcotics other then meperidine will have miotic pupils, but these will be seen to constrict although a hand lens may be needed for this assessment. Unless the pupils are constricted, it is unlikely that narcotics are the sole reason for the patient's confusion. Widely dilatated but reactive pupils, particularly when associated with erythematous skin and dry mucous membranes, point to anticholinergic overdose, a common cause of confusional state in oncologic emergency patients who take a host of anticholinergic drugs for symptomatic relief of everything from nausea to bladder spasms. The saying "dry as a bone, red as a beet, mad as a hatter" reminds the clinician of the cardinal signs of anticholinergic overdose, but these signs may be seen only in extreme instances.

Anticholinergic and anxiolytic drugs contribute to many more encephalopathic states than those for which they are credited whereas narcotics seem to be blamed for a good deal more confusional states than they actually cause. Mixing medications often has a synergistic confusional effect. Narcotic or benzodiazepine antagonists (eg, nalorphine) should be used with caution[109] (seizures

TABLE 4–11. Differential Diagnosis of Altered Mental Status

Structural causes
    Primary brain tumor
    Metastatic brain lesion
    Cerebrovascular disease
    Leptomeningeal disease
Metabolic abnormalities
    Anemia
    Hyponatremia or hypernatremia
    Hypoglycemia or hyperglycemia
    Uremia
    Hypoxia
    Hypercalcemia
    Hepatic dysfunction
Infection
    Sepsis
    Meningitis
Toxic effects
    Medications
    Alcohol
    Drugs
Head trauma
Treatment side effects
    Chemotherapy
    Radiation therapy
    Bone marrow transplantation
Endocrine disorders
    Thyroid disorder
    Adrenal insufficiency
Psychiatric disorders
Nutritional deficiencies
    Thiamine
    B_{12}
    Folate
Seizures
Paraneoplastic syndromes

TABLE 4–12. Routine Laboratory Studies for Patients with Altered Mental Status

Blood cultures
Complete blood count
Electrolytes (Na, K, Cl, CO_2, Ca, Mg, PO_4)
Glucose
Blood urea nitrogen, creatinine
Aspartate transaminase, γ-glutamyltransferase
Osmolality
Arterial blood gases, ammonia
Thyroid function

Ca = calcium; Cl = chlorine; CO_2 = carbon dioxide; K = potassium; Mg = magnesium; Na = sodium; PO_4 = serum phosphate.

Sepsis

Sepsis occurs with great frequency in cancer patients. Septic patients will sometimes become encephalopathic even before mounting a fever. In the general critically ill population, sepsis is the most common cause of encephalopathy,[110,111] in the acutely ill oncologic patient, sepsis is the most frequent cause of encephalopathy, after drug intoxication.[106] Acute infectious meningitis is a relatively infrequent cause of acute confusion in oncologic patients; chronic meningitis associated with leptomeningeal malignancy or fungal infection may produce a confusional state. Chronic meningitis presents in a multitude of ways, and patients often will have had symptoms (sometimes dismissed by the patient or caregivers) for weeks prior to the diagnosis being made.[112] Diagnostic lumbar puncture should not be performed until imaging studies document the absence of mass lesions, which occur with a higher frequency in the cancer patient than in the general population.

Patients with advanced malignancy may develop perversions of coagulation, which manifest as nonbacterial

have been reported with their use, as well as aspiration pneumonia). Clinicians may gain a false sense of security in the belief that the sole cause of the altered mental status relates to the intoxication when intoxication may be only a contributing factor. As the agents mentioned above have a relatively short half-life, it is imperative that patients be monitored carefully following their use.

While these routine measures are being done and while any deficiencies found are being corrected, the clinician should proceed to a neurologic examination that is modified to evaluate altered mental status. The Glasgow Coma Scale (Table 4–13) is invaluable for assessing the progression of altered consciousness. The scale is simple to use, is accurate (particularly for advanced altered states), and takes but a few minutes to perform. Ideally, the Glasgow Coma Scale should be incorporated into the patient's record of vital signs, with the test done serially. The patient's clinical state at presentation is most important in assessing the temporal course of altered mental status (Figure 4–11).

TABLE 4–13. Glasgow Coma Scale

Eye opening
    4 Spontaneous
    3 To speech
    2 To pain
    1 None
Best motor response (arm)
    6 Obeying
    5 Localizing pain
    4 Withdrawal
    3 Abnormal flexing
    2 Extensor response
    1 None
Best verbal response
    5 Oriented
    4 Confused conversation
    3 Inappropriate words
    2 Incomprehensible sounds
    1 None

thrombotic endocarditis or disseminated intravascular coagulopathy, mimicking uncontrolled sepsis in many ways. These states may be seen with any malignancy but are most commonly encountered with mucin-producing carcinomas and with acute promyelocytic leukemia.

Focal Disturbances

Neuro-ophthalmologic examination yields the most information about the etiology of coma.[113] The assess-ment of pupillary function by examining the patient in a room with the lights dimmed and checking for symme-try of constriction to light should be carefully done, not-ing the speed as well as the completeness of constriction. Irregularly shaped pupils (corectopia) may be seen in cases of diencephalic lesions, and miotic pupils can be seen in cases of brain stem or diencephalic lesions, alert-ing the clinician that serious structural disease may be the cause of the patient's altered mental state. Vascular

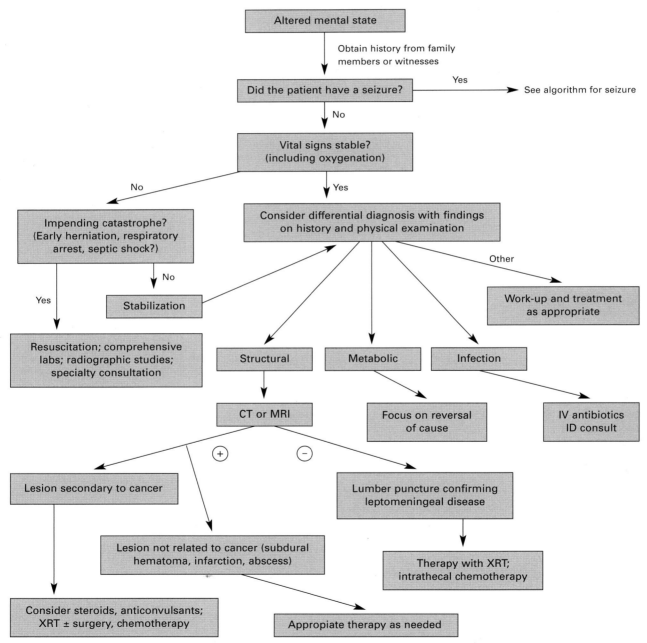

Figure 4–11. Algorithm for evaluation and treatment of altered mental status. CT = computed tomography; ID = infectious disease; IV = intravenous; MRI = magnetic resonance imaging; XRT = radiation therapy.

lesions such as hemorrhage or infarction are common in this location although some viruses and even *Listeria* have a predilection for midbrain involvement.

Asymmetry of pupillary reflexes raises the specter of an uncal herniation syndrome due to a supratentorial mass lesion. Masses in the posterior fossa are more treacherous as they do not produce third-nerve palsy but rather compress vasomotor and respiratory centers directly, with death often developing swiftly and with little warning. Unfortunately, posterior fossa masses produce nondescript symptoms such as lethargy, headache, giddiness, dizziness, or nausea and vomiting. These highly variable presentations are frequently misdiagnosed or dismissed by the evaluating physician with symptomatic management. As brain metastases from pelvic and gastrointestinal primaries have a predilection for the posterior fossa,[114] physicians caring for such patients should have a low threshold for ordering brain imaging studies as part of their acute evaluation. The inability to walk is a fairly constant finding in patients who harbor a significant cerebellar mass.[115] Starting oncologic patients on dexamethasone upon suspicion of a herniation syndrome is wise practice. A single corticosteroid dose has minimal toxicity. In instances of presumed herniation, intubation and hyperventilation as well as a bolus of mannitol should be considered since the dexamethasone may take hours to take full effect. Patients who do not respond to painful stimuli should be electively intubated for protection of their airway as well as for hyperventilation.[109]

As multifactorial etiologies are common, oncology patients with altered mental status should routinely undergo an imaging procedure. Noncontrast CT can be performed on a modern scanner in a matter of minutes and will reveal the vast majority of lesions responsible for altered mental status. Confused patients cannot cooperate for magnetic resonance scanning which takes 30 to 45 minutes to do and which is much more easily degraded by patient movement. Magnetic resonance scanning is also a closed system that does not permit close monitoring of these critically ill patients.

Mass Lesions

Mass lesions affecting cancer patients are metastasis, hemorrhage, and abscess. Alterations in mental status from mass lesions are caused by increased intracranial pressure, acute hydrocephalus, or disturbances of critical centers in the brain stem, midbrain, interior frontal lobe, or medial temporal lobe. Lesions of the dominant caudal superior temporal gyrus produce a fluent aphasia (Wernicke's aphasia) in which the patient appears to be confused and without any comprehension of language, not even their own. Such patients speak fluently, but their well-articulated speech consists of words strung together completely without meaning and often without grammar. These

patients have no awareness of their difficulties, which often prompts psychiatric evaluation for confusion.

Metastasis produces cerebral edema that often exceeds the size of the actual tumor and that is responsible for many of the symptoms. When a mass lesion is identified on imaging, administration of dexamethasone should begin (Table 4–14). Subsequent therapy with radiation, surgery, or systemic treatment depends on the tumor type. Prior to starting treatment, steroids should be administered for at least 48 hours; this avoids the transient and sometimes life-threatening worsening of edema seen at the initiation of central nervous system metastasis therapy.[116] Multiple small metastases may cause altered mental status, but noncontrast CT scan often misses small metastases. A contrast study or magnetic resonance scanning should be performed once the patient is stabilized and their renal function determined to be normal.

An abscess may be extremely difficult to distinguish from a tumor with a necrotic center.[117] Immunocompromised cancer patients, particularly those with pulmonary infections, are at risk for cerebral abscess. Stereotactic or open biopsy should be considered for patients whose diagnosis is questionable. If there is symptomatic brain edema, corticosteroid therapy is warranted, pending definitive diagnosis.

Hemorrhage

Hemorrhage is usually easily seen by CT. The exception is the subdural hematoma that may appear isodense with the adjacent brain early in its course. Unilateral loss of sulcal markings is an important sign of early subdural hematoma. While cerebral hemorrhage is generally not improved by corticosteroid therapy, bleeding may arise from a metastatic deposit in the cancer patient, justifying corticosteroid therapy during acute management, particularly if there is evidence of depressed sensorium. Measures to address increased intracranial pressure should be

TABLE 4–14. Emergency Measures for Patients with Intracranial Mass Lesions

Protect airway: intubate if patient does not localize pain
Correct hypoxemia
Reverse Trendelenburg's position to 30°
Correct coagulopathy with platelets supplemented with fresh frozen plasma, vitamin K if needed
Hyperventilation: increase respiratory rate to 20 breaths/min, aim at PCO_2 of 25–30 mm Hg
Administer mannitol, 20%, 1g/kg; if no effect, 2g/kg; aim at plasma osmolality of 310 mOsm/L
If medically appropriate:
    Administer dexamethasone
    Resect tumor
    Irradiate tumor
    Drain subdural hematoma

PCO_2 = carbon dioxide partial pressure.

started if there is shift of midline structures or effacement of cortical sulci. Neurosurgical consultation should be obtained, particularly for cerebellar hemorrhages, which have a more favorable prognosis, given the relative ease with which they can be approached and the devastating consequences of posterior fossa masses. Cerebellar hemorrhages generally have a more favorable outcome from neurosurgical evacuation than do supratentorial hemorrhages. Only if the volume of the hemorrhage is < 60 mL (4 cm by 4 cm by 4 cm), the hemorrhage is in an accessible location, and the patient has a Glasgow Coma Score of > 9 may neurosurgical evacuation offer some benefit for supratentorial hemorrhages.[118]

Acute Hydrocephalus

Acute hydrocephalus complicates many of the pathologic processes associated with altered mental status. Transudation of cerebrospinal fluid into the surrounding periventricular tissues is the hallmark of acute hydrocephalus and is easily recognized by CT or MRI. Corticosteroids and cytoreductive therapy may help relieve hydrocephalus when it is due to malignant meningitis or tumor obstruction, but neurosurgical placement of a draining catheter is usually required, especially if the patient is acutely symptomatic.

Seizures

Following a major seizure, the patient's neurologic function is suppressed due to the release of inhibitory endogenous neurotransmitters, chiefly γ-aminobutyric acid. Postictal cortical suppression may last for as long as 24 hours, but the patient usually has a gradual steady improvement. When the seizure is unwitnessed, the diagnosis can be difficult. Signs of bruises (particularly on the tongue), incontinence, and the presence of lactic acidosis with elevated muscle enzymes suggest that the patient may have had a seizure although these findings are nonspecific. Nonconvulsive status is usually caused by focal cerebral dysfunction and manifests itself much more as confusion than as coma. The state of bewilderment can last for days and is best diagnosed with electroencephalography; the characteristic spike activity clears with intravenous benzodiazepine administration[119] (Figure 4–12).

Distinguishing the tonic phase of a generalized seizure from posturing due to midbrain damage can be difficult even for experienced clinicians, especially if there is no clonic episode. Bilateral extension of the limbs, especially if sustained, strongly favors midbrain trouble that requires urgent imaging and measures to treat increased intracranial pressure.

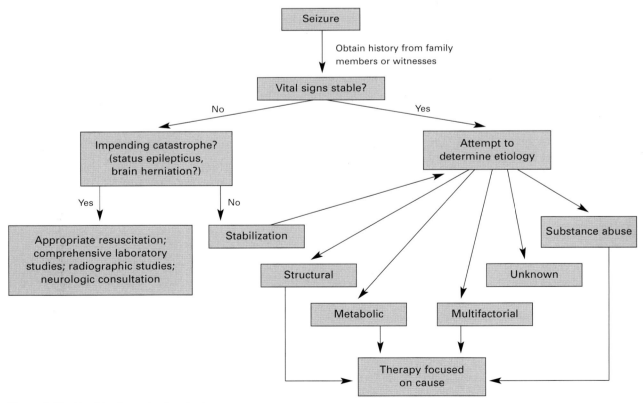

Figure 4–12. Algorithm for evaluation of seizure.

Summary

The management of altered mental status in a cancer patient requires diligent attention to detail and careful observation from both medical and nursing staff in the emergency center as these patients are unable to care or speak for themselves. How neurologic illness unfolds is critical to making a diagnosis as there are often few distinguishing characteristics at the onset; therefore, the initial assessment must be accurate. The speed and manner in which patients are treated in the emergency center often determines their chances for a good outcome.

SYNCOPE

Syncope is a sudden temporary non-epileptic loss of consciousness that has many potential etiologies in cancer patients. Any event or sequence of events that interferes with cerebral perfusion can impair consciousness. Depending on the rapidity and severity of the reduction of cerebral perfusion and on the patient's general condition, diminished cerebral perfusion can lead to weakness, light-headedness, disturbance of vision, and loss of consciousness and muscle tone. Brief myoclonic jerking and urinary incontinence occasionally occur, owing to cerebral hypoxia. Most patients rapidly and completely regain consciousness when normal cerebral perfusion resumes, usually after the patient assumes a supine position. When faced with a patient who has sustained a syncopal episode, it is important first to stabilize the patient and then to consider both the oncologic and non-oncologic etiologies for this symptom. Identifying the etiology of syncope will help the clinician to determine appropriate therapeutic measures (Table 4–15).

Diagnostic Approach

Identifying the cause of syncope is very important in determining both the prognosis and the management strategy. An accurate diagnosis of the underlying etiology of syncope can often be made on the basis of the medical history, the physical examination, simple laboratory tests, and an electrocardiogram (ECG).[120] Information obtained from these evaluations can also guide further analysis if the cause of syncope remains unknown.[121]

TABLE 4–15. Differential Diagnosis of Syncope

Hypoperfusion
  Volume loss
    Acute hemorrhage
    Dehydration
      Nausea/vomiting secondary to chemotherapy, or tumor
      Decreased oral intake secondary to oral/gastrointestinal mucositis
      Diarrhea
    Adrenal insufficiency
  Inadequate postural reflexes
    Central autonomic dysfunction
      Parkinson's disease
      Striatonigral degeneration
      Pure autonomic failure
    Peripheral autonomic dysfunction
      Baroreceptor dysfunction
      Spinal-cord disease
      Sympathectomy
      Guillain-Barré syndrome
      Neuropathies (secondary to diabetes, amyloidosis, or chemotherapy)
    Medications
      Antihypertensive medications
      Phenothiazine
      Tricyclic antidepressants
      Levodopa
  Increased vagal tone
    Emotional stimulus
    Carotid sinus hypersensitivity
    Glossopharyngeal neuralgia
    Valsalva's maneuver
    Micturition syncope
  Cardiac disorders
    Electrical disorders
      Conduction (sinoatrial or atrioventricular)
      Atrial arrhythmias
      Ventricular arrhythmias
      Valvular abnormalities (especially aortic stenosis, prosthetic valve malfunction)

TABLE 4–15. Continued

  Other obstructions
    Hypertrophic cardiomyopathies
    Congenital heart disease
    Atrial myxoma
    Pericardial tamponade
    Chest mass
    Impaired venous return
      Cough syncope
      Abdominal or thoracic masses
    Pulmonary hypertension
    Low-output cardiac failure
      Myocardial infarction
      Cardiomegalies (eg, cardiomyopathy secondary to doxorubicin use)
      Congenital diseases
Situational causes (combination of mechanisms)
  Micturition
  Cough
  Breath holding
  Hyperventilation or hypercarbia
  Valsalva's maneuver
Acute intracranial hypertension
  Mass (primary brain tumors or brain metastases)
  Hemorrhage
  Cerebrospinal-fluid obstruction
Metabolic impairment with adequate perfusion
  Inadequate oxygen delivery
    Hypoxia
    Carbon monoxide, other poisonings
    Anemia, hemoglobinopathies
  Impaired metabolism
    Hypoglycemia (insulin-secreting tumors)
    Poisons

Adapted from Drislane, FW. Transient events. In: Samuels MA, Feske S, editors. Office practice of neurology. New York: Churchill Livingstone Inc; 1996. p. 112.

Syncope is common in cancer patients. When faced with a patient with this symptom, it is important to evaluate the patient within the context of the malignancy. The clinician must quickly obtain the patient's cancer history, including details of the primary malignancy, presence of metastatic disease, and the type of cancer therapy the patient has received. It is important to learn the timing of the therapy with regard to the patient's syncopal episode. The clinician must also consider nononcologic causes for the syncope, focusing on any other major medical illnesses (such as cardiac disease) and the patient's medications for those diseases.

Once the clinician has obtained the above information on the patient, further details surrounding the event should be obtained. The clinical features associated with a syncopal episode are extremely important.[120,122] Witnesses to the syncopal episode are particularly helpful because they can provide details of possible precipitating events such as sudden changes in position, urination, and unpleasant sights. They can also describe the suddenness and duration of the loss of consciousness and how quickly the patient recovered; this may help to exclude the possibility of the patient having had a seizure. Finally, witnesses can provide information on any preceding symptoms the patient could have experienced, such as chest pain, palpitations, and dyspnea.

The clinician evaluating a cancer patient after a syncopal episode must also ascertain whether the patient experienced any other significant symptoms in the preceding days. For example, it is important to determine whether the patient had nausea, vomiting, or diarrhea prior to the syncopal episode; any of these could have resulted in dehydration.

A thorough physical examination must also be performed since several findings can help to identify some of the common causes of syncope.[120] Orthostatic vital signs should be measured because a drop of > 15 mm Hg in blood pressure or a pulse increase of > 20 bpm upon rising from a lying position to a standing position indicates hypovolemia or inadequate postural reflexes. Particular focus should also be placed on the cardiac and neurologic examinations, with all test results taken into consideration.

Finally, a careful diagnostic work-up is warranted. The laboratory, cardiac, and radiologic studies that are ordered should be guided by the history and physical examination, as outlined above (Figure 4–13).

True Emergencies

Cardiac Etiologies. There are a number of serious cardiac causes of syncope, so it is important to ascertain whether a patient has a history of cardiac disease. Patients who have had a syncopal episode require a thorough cardiac examination to detect signs of arrhythmia or valvular heart disease. The clinician must be particularly concerned about possible myocardial infarction, malignant ventricular arrhythmia, and cardiac tamponade. A pulsus paradoxus may indicate a pericardial effusion. If a cardiac etiology is of concern, patients will require continuous cardiac monitoring and electrocardiography. Electrocardiography will help in finding evidence of heart block, long QT syndrome, arrhythmias, or cardiac ischemia. Echocardiography can assist with the diagnosis of a pericardial effusion and valvular heart disease. Routine laboratory studies will be needed and cardiologic consultation should be contemplated.

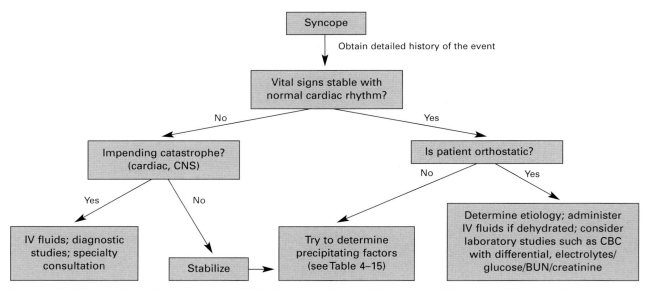

Figure 4–13. Algorithm for evaluation of syncope. BUN = blood urea nitrogen; CBC = complete blood count; CNS = central nervous system; IV = intravenous.

Neurologic Etiologies. Increased intracranial pressure due to intracerebral lesions, hemorrhage, or CSF obstruction can result in syncope. Computed tomography or MRI is typically required to determine the extent of the disorder in a patient. Consultation with a neurologist and possibly a neurosurgeon should be considered.

Hemorrhage. Cancer patients can be predisposed to acute hemorrhage for a variety of reasons, including thrombocytopenia and coagulopathy. Patients with hypoperfusion due to acute hemorrhage usually require aggressive therapy, such as blood product support.

Common Causes

A common cause of syncope in cancer patients is dehydration, which has a number of possible sources. Typically, dehydrated patients display orthostatic changes on physical examination. The patient's history will usually provide clues to the fact that the patient is dehydrated. For example, the patient might have had significant nausea or vomiting as a result of chemotherapy, or he or she may have had impaired oral intake as a result of radiation-induced mucositis. Patients may also have significant fluid losses from diarrhea, resulting in dehydration. Less commonly, patients will have a decreased oral intake as a result of the tumor itself. Another common cause of syncope is increased vagal tone due to an emotional stimulus, carotid sinus hypersensitivity, glossopharyngeal neuralgia, Valsalva's maneuver, or micturition.

Medication effects may cause syncope. Particular attention must be paid to medications that have an adverse effect on autonomic function, such as antidepressants. Also, certain chemotherapy agents can result in a peripheral neuropathy, which will have an effect on the patient's postural reflexes. Finally, patients who have been receiving steroid therapy may have adrenal insufficiency, which may result in hypoperfusion.

Points to Remember

When evaluating a patient who has had a syncopal episode, it is critical to obtain a detailed history of the event. Witnesses are invaluable for providing details. A possible cardiac etiology must always be considered in the differential diagnosis. The cause of syncope cannot always be determined, even though a thorough investigation has been performed. At times, the diagnosis may become apparent during follow-up.

RASH

Oncologic patients are susceptible to rashes that are commonly seen in the general population. The diagnosis of rash in oncologic patients is further complicated by their inherent history of underlying malignancy, by polypharmacy, and by the added risks of infection that are associated with immunosuppressive therapy and the constant exposure to the nosocomial environment. In the face of a cutaneous eruption in a patient with cancer, consideration must be given to primary dermatologic diseases, cutaneous manifestations of malignancy, infectious processes, and reactions to drugs and treatments. While some rashes are ultimately benign, many eruptions in the oncologic patient are potentially fatal and require emergent management and treatment (see Chapter 20, Dermatologic Emergencies). Thus, quick recognition and diagnosis of cutaneous eruptions in this group of patients is essential (Table 4–16).[123–126]

Chemotherapy-Induced Eruptions

A majority of emergent rashes in the oncologic patient are due to complications of chemotherapy (Figure 4–14). Although the dermatologic complications of chemotherapy are rarely fatal, it is important to recognize potential reactions because they may result in significant morbidity, cosmetic disfigurement, and psychological distress.[123] Eruptions that are falsely attributed to chemotherapy may also result in inappropriate dose reduction or the premature discontinuation of therapy. Chemotherapeutic reactions generally complicate the diagnosis of rash in the oncologic patient. For example, neutrophilic eccrine hidradenitis is a clinically variable eruption that may mimic septic emboli, vasculitis, metastatic infiltrates, erythema multiforme, and Sweet's syndrome. Usually, however, the relationship between the time of the onset of rash and the administration of chemotherapy is a helpful diagnostic clue. Cases of chemotherapy-induced irritant and vesicant reactions (Figure 4–15) are common and are easily traced to the causative therapy. Palmoplantar erythema presents a potential diagnostic dilemma in a patient undergoing stem cell transplantation after myeloablative chemotherapy, as acral erythema (Figure 4–16) may mimic early acute graft-versus-host disease.

Radiation-Induced Reactions

Many cancer patients also undergo radiation therapy and develop radiation dermatitis, which sometimes produces a more generalized id reaction (Figure 4–17). With the widespread use of combined-modality regimens that involve both chemotherapy and radiation therapy, radiation recall and radiation enhancement reactions have become more common. Radiation enhancement occurs as a result of the augmentation of radiation therapy effects when both chemotherapy and radiation therapy are given within 1 week of each other. Bleomycin, dactinomycin, doxorubicin, fluorouracil, hydroxyurea, and methotrexate are most commonly involved.[123] Radiation recall is an erythematous inflammatory reaction in areas of previously irradiated skin and usually occurs with the

TABLE 4–16. Differential Diagnosis of Rash in the Oncologic Patient.

Macules and papules	Petechiae/purpura
Erythema multiforme	Thrombocytopenia
Erythema marginatum	Disseminated intravascular
Systemic lupus erythematosus	coagulation
Dermatomyositis	Cryoglobulinemia/
Drug hypersensitivity	cryofibrinogenemia
Serum sickness	Anticoagulant-induced necrosis
Sweet's syndrome	Infectious emboli
Acute graft-versus-host disease	Ecthyma gangrenosum
Lymphoma/leukemia cutis	Henoch-Schönlein purpura
Cutaneous metastatic carcinoma	Hypersensitivity vasculitis
Eruption of lymphocyte recovery	Amyloidosis
Neutrophilic eccrine hidradenitis	Systemic lupus erythematosus
Acral erythema	Acute rheumatic fever
Radiation recall	Endocarditis
Toxic shock syndrome	Meningococcemia
Viral exanthems	Gonococcemia
Rocky Mountain spotted fever	Hepatitis B
	EBV infection
Papules and nodules	Enteroviral infection
Lymphoma cutis	Bacterial infections
Leukemia cutis	
Cutaneous metastatic carcinoma	Annular lesions
Lymphocytoma cutis	Tinea
Vasculitis	Urticaria
Kaposi's sarcoma	Granuloma annulare
Sweet's syndrome	Pustular psoriasis
Neuromas (MEN syndrome	Secondary syphilis
type 2b)	Sarcoidosis
Tricholemmomas (Cowden's	Subacute lupus erythematosus
disease)	Erythema migrans
Sebaceous adenomas	Erythema marginatum
(Torre's syndrome)	Erythema annular centrifugum
Neurofibromas (von	Erythema gyratum repens
Recklinghausen's disease)	Cutaneous T-cell lymphoma
Basal cell epitheliomas	Necrolytic migratory erythema
(basal cell nevus syndrome)	

TABLE 4–16. Continued

Erythroderma	Vesicles and bullae
Atopic dermatitis	Contact dermatitis
Chronic actinic dermatitis	Paraneoplastic pemphigus
Drug hypersensitivity reactions	Porphyria cutanea tarda
Pseudolymphoma	Toxic epidermal necrolysis
Lymphoma/carcinoma	Stevens-Johnson syndrome
Mycosis fungoides/	Acute graft-versus-host disease
Sézary syndrome	Varicella-zoster virus
Pityriasis rubra pilaris	Herpes simplex virus
Superficial pemphigus	*Candida*
Erythrodermic pemphigoid	Bullous impetigo
Erythrodermic psoriasis	
Erythrodermic dermatomyositis	Oral ulceration
	Apthous ulcers
Cutaneous ulceration	Gingivostomatitis
Pyoderma gangrenosum	Chemotherapy mucositis
Vasculitis	Lupus erythematosus
Viral, bacterial infections	Erythema multiforme
Antiphospholipid syndrome	Stevens-Johnson syndrome
Cryoglobulinemia/	Toxic epidermal necrolysis
cryofibrinogenemia	Acute graft-versus-host disease
Raynaud's phenomenon	
Lymphoma	
Cutaneous T-cell lymphoma	
Urticaria	
Allergic urticaria	
Angioedema	
Serum sickness	
Vasculitis	
Malignancy	
Hepatitis B	
Mycoplasma infection	
EBV infection	

Adapted from Apisarnthanarax N, Duvic M;[123] Robson KJ, Piette WW;[124] Schlossberg D;[125] Fitzpatrick et al.[126]
EBV = Epstein-Barr virus; MEN = multiple endocrine neoplasia.

administration of dactinomycin and doxorubicin from 8 days to 15 years after radiation therapy.

Metastatic Eruptions

Rashes in the oncologic patient are often due to cutaneous spread or extension of malignancy. Cutaneous metastases are common (with an incidence of approximately 2 to 10%), and may mimic other cutaneous diseases.[127] Rash may be the first presenting sign of malignancy, especially melanoma, breast cancer, and mucosal cancers of the head and neck. Lesions commonly appear as erythematous or skin-colored nodules that appear suddenly and grow rapidly. Breast cancer often manifests in the skin as erythema, edema, and warmth that mimics cellulitis. Alopecia neoplastica of the scalp may develop and is clinically similar to the scarring alopecia of discoid lupus erythematosus or morphea. The most common primary cancers that present with cutaneous metastases in males are lung cancers (22%), melanoma (18%), colo-rectal cancers (18%), and oral cancers (12%). In women, cutaneous metastases are predominantly from breast cancers (71%), followed by melanoma (9%) and colo-rectal cancers (5%). Metastasis of gastric adenocarcinoma to the periumbilical area results in Sister Mary Joseph's nodules. Lymphoma and leukemia cutis are relatively common, occurring in approximately 7% of lymphoma and leukemia patients, depending on the specific cancer.[128,129] Lymphoma cutis usually appears as firm violaceous to erythematous nodules or plaques whereas leukemia cutis appears with greater clinical variability, manifesting as macules, papules, plaques, nodules, ecchymoses, palpable purpura, or ulcerations. Acute monocytic, myelomonocytic, and T-cell leukemias have the highest incidence of leukemia cutis.[130]

Paraneoplastic Eruptions

Several skin diseases and conditions have been associated with malignancy (Table 4–17). Dermatomyositis is asso-

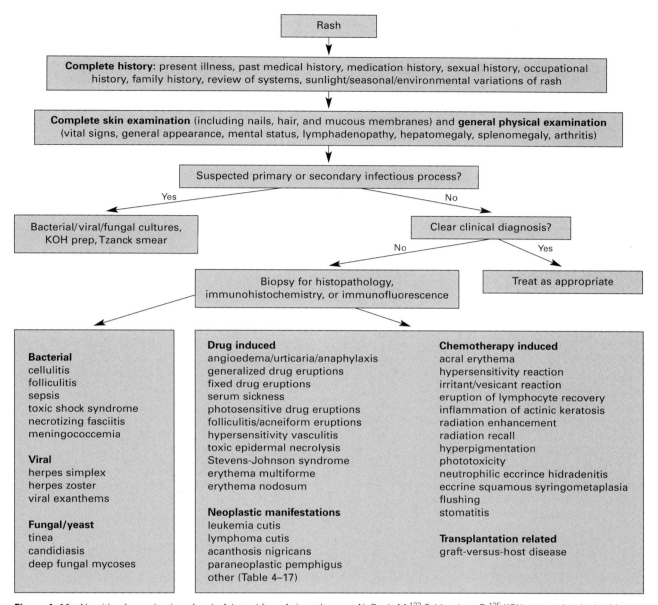

Figure 4–14. Algorithm for evaluation of rash. Adapted from Apisarnthanarax N, Duvic M;[123] Schlossberg D.[125] KOH = potassium hydroxide.

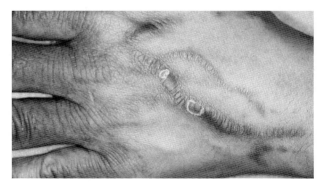

Figure 4–15. This chemotherapy-induced irritant is easily identified by following the venous system.

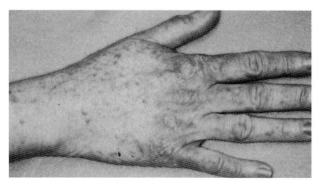

Figure 4–16. An example of acral erythema, which may mimic early graft-versus-host disease in patients undergoing stem cell transplantation.

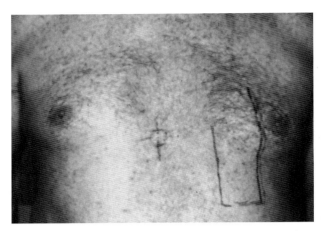

Figure 4–17. Radiation dermatitis in a patient undergoing chest irradiation.

ciated with a higher risk of malignancy and may mimic seborrheic dermatitis with a pattern of facial and scalp involvement of scaly erythematous patches and plaques.[124] However, dermatomyositis usually presents with Gottron's papules, a characteristic heliotrope rash, and proximal muscle weakness. Sweet's syndrome is often nodular, but it may also be mistaken for cellulitis that does not respond to antibiotics (Figure 4–18) Among ulcerative conditions, pyoderma gangrenosum is a chronic painful ulcerative condition that may be associated with systemic diseases, including lymphoproliferative disorders and monoclonal gammopathy. Erythema gyratum repens is a rapidly migrating serpiginous erythema with a wood-grained appearance; it is nearly always associated with malignancy. Paraneoplastic pemphigus is particularly associated with a high risk of mortality; it is discussed in depth in Chapter 20.

Erythroderma

Erythroderma (exfoliative dermatitis) is a distinct severe eruption that has a variety of causes, including various dermatoses, infections (especially with *Staphylococcus aureus*), drugs, and cancers[131] (see Table 4–16). A large percentage (9 to 47%) of erythrodermic cases are idiopathic. Although erythroderma usually evolves slowly, it may be associated with an acute and rapid onset in the setting of conditions such as drug hypersensitivity, superficial pemphigus, and pityriasis rubra pilaris. Fever, malaise, fatigue, and pruritus often accompany the eruption. Diffuse alopecia, keratoderma, nail dystrophy, and ectropion may occur, especially with chronic erythroderma. Lymphadenopathy and peripheral edema are also common. Laboratory findings include anemia, leukocytosis, eosinophilia, lymphocytopenia, elevated immunoglobulin E (IgE), elevated erythrocyte sedimentation rate, hypoalbuminemia, and increased uric acid. Circulating Sézary cells may be seen, but findings of < 10% are nonspecific whereas higher counts of > 20% are more specific for Sézary syndrome.[132] A positive T-cell receptor β gene rearrangement analysis of peripheral blood helps to differentiate Sézary syndrome from other causes of erythroderma.[133] Complications of erythroderma are related to fluid and electrolyte imbalance, hypoalbuminemia, capillary leak syndrome, thermoregulatory disturbance, high-output cardiac failure, and infection.[132] Immediate supportive and skin care is required.

Fever and Rash

Patients who present with fever and rash should raise the suspicion of infection. Infections may present as petechial, maculopapular, vesicbullous, erythrodermic, and urticarial rashes (see Table 4–16). Petechial rashes are generally the most life-threatening; their causes include endocarditis, meningococcemia, gonococcemia, other bacteremia, Rocky Mountain spotted fever, typhus, rat-bite fevers, dengue, and hepatitis B.[125] It is also important to consider noninfectious causes of rash and fever, such as allergic reactions, Henoch-Schönlein purpura, vasculitis, acute rheumatic fever, systemic lupus erythematosus, Sweet's syndrome, and malignancy.

TABLE 4–17. Dermatologic Disorders and Associated Malignancies

Disorder	Dermatologic Findings	Associated Malignancies
Hypertrichosis lanuginosa	Sudden development of fine, unpigmented hair	Lung carcinoma
Acquired ichthyosis	Large, polygonal white to brown scales	Hodgkin's lymphoma
Paget's disease of the breast	Eczematous red plaques around breast nipples	Ductal breast adenocarcinoma
Muir-Torre syndrome	Sebaceous tumors	Gastrointestinal carcinoma
Leser-Trélat sign	Sudden development of multiple seborrheic keratoses	Internal malignancies (especially intra-abdominal adenocarcinoma)
Acquired porphyria cutanea tarda	Photosensitive vesiculobullous eruption with skin fragility, facial hypertrichosis, and hyperpigmentation	Hepatocellular carcinoma
Cowden's disease	Facial trichilemmomas, "cobblestone" papules of oral mucosa and gums	Breast and thyroid carcinoma
Necrolytic migratory erythema	Centrally distributed erythema and erosions	Glucagon-producing tumors
Sweet's syndrome	Painful erythematous plaques, pustules, vesicles, or ulcerations, with fever, arthralgias, and leukocytosis	Acute myelogenous leukemia; genitourinary carcinoma

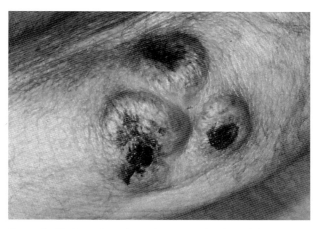

Figure 4–18. Sweet's syndrome is an example of a nodular paraneoplastic eruption and is often associated with acute myelogenous leukemia and genitourinary carcinoma.

Points to Remember

The following are recommendations for evaluating rashes in cancer patients:

1. Consider chemotherapy, other drugs, cancer, and infection as possible causes of rash.
2. Take a detailed medication history.
3. Consider disseminated viral, bacterial, and fungal infections in immunosuppressed patients.
4. Consider graft-versus-host disease in the transplantation patient.
5. Remember that the presentation of fever and rash is an emergency situation.

Summary

A high index of suspicion should be held when evaluating an oncologic patient with rash. In addition, manifestations may be related to drugs, malignancy, or infection. While most eruptions are a manifestation of a benign process, consideration must be given to life-threatening conditions. Quick recognition and diagnosis of emergent rashes will allow for more effective management and therapy and for the possibility of decreased morbidity and mortality.

REFERENCES

1. Khosla R, Guntupalli KK. Heat-related illnesses. Crit Care Clin 1999;15:251–63.
2. Bross MH, Nash BT Jr, Carlton FB Jr. Heat emergencies. Am Fam Physician 1994;50:389–96, 398.
3. Schneider SM. Neuroleptic malignant syndrome: controversies in treatment. Am J Emerg Med 1991;9:360–2.
4. Totten VY, Hirchenstein E, Hew P. Neuroleptic malignant syndrome presenting without initial fever: a case report. J Emerg Med 1994;12:43–7.
5. Denborough M. Malignant hyperthermia. Lancet 1998;352:1131–6.
6. Delaney KA, Vassallo SU, Goldfrank LR. Thermoregulatory principles. In: Goldfrank LR, Flomenbaum NE, Lewin NA, et al, editors. Toxicologic Emergencies. 5th ed. Norwalk (CT): Appleton and Lange; 1994. p. 151–70.
7. Sporer KA. The serotonin syndrome. Implicated drugs, pathophysiology and management. Drug Saf 1995; 13:94–104.
8. Burger AG, Philippe J. Thyroid emergencies. Baillieres Clin Endocrin Metab 1992;6:77–93.
9. Jameson JL, Weetman AP. Disorders of thyroid gland. In: Braunwald E, Fauci AS, Kasper DL, et al, editors. Harrison's principles of internal medicine. 15th ed. New York: McGraw-Hill Companies; 2001. p. 2073.
10. McDonald M, Sexton DJ. Drug fever. In: Rose BD, editor. Up to date. Wellesley: UpToDate;2001. Version 92.
11. Porat R, Dinarello CA. Pathophysiology and treatment of fever. In: Rose BD, editor. Up to date. Wellesley: UpToDate;2001. Version 92.
12. Hughes WT, Armstrong D, Bodey GP, et al. 1997 guidelines for the use of antimicrobial agents in neutropenic patients with unexplained fever. Clin Infect Dis 1997; 25:551–73.
13. Bodey GP, Buckley M, Sathe YS, et al. Quantitative relationships between circulating leukocytes and infection in patients with acute leukemia. Ann Intern Med 1966; 64:328–40.
14. Gucalp R, Dutcher JP. Fever and infection. In: Dutcher JP, Wiernik PH, editors. Handbook of hematologic and oncologic emergencies. New York: Plenum Publishing Corporation; 1987. p. 155–8.
15. Oken MM, Loch J. Corticosteroid and antihistamine modification of bleomycin-induced fever. Exp Biol Med 1979;161:594–6.
16. Blanco R, Martinez-Taboada VM, Gonzalez-Gay MA, et al. Acute febrile toxic reaction in patients with refractory rheumatoid arthritis who are receiving combined therapy with methotrexate and azathioprine. Arthritis Rheum 1996;39:1016–20.
17. Gluckstein D, Ruskin J. Rapid oral desensitization to trimethoprim-sulfamethoxazole (TMP-SMZ): use in prophylaxis for *Pneumocystis carinii* pneumonia in patients with AIDS who were previously intolerant to TMP-SMZ. Clin Infect Dise 1995;20:849–53.
18. Deamer RL, Prichard JG, Loman GJ. Hypersensitivity and anaphylactoid reactions to ciprofloxacin. Ann Pharmacother 1992;26:1081–4.
19. Martinez E, Collazos J, Mayo J. Hypersensitivity reactions to rifampin. Pathogenetic mechanisms, clinical manifestations, management strategies, and review of the anaphylactic-like reactions. Medicine 1999;78:361–9.
20. Beutler B, Munford RS. Tumor necrosis factor and the Jarisch-Herxheimer reaction. New Engl J Med 1996; 335:347–8.
21. Wassef M, Keiser P. Hypersensitivity of zidovudine: report of a case of anaphylaxis and review of the literature. Clin Infect Dis 1995;20:1387–9.
22. Nakajima H, Munakata A, Yoshida Y. Adverse effects of

sulfasalazine and treatment of ulcerative colitis with mesalazine. J Gastroenterol 1995;30(Suppl 8):115–7.

23. De Vriese AS, Phillippe J, Van Renterghem DM, et al. Carbamazepine hypersensitivity syndrome: report of 4 cases and review of the literature. Medicine (Baltimore) 1995;74:144–51.

24. Gennis MA, Vemuri R, Burns EA, et al. Familial occurrence of hypersensitivity to phenytoin. Am J Med 1991; 91:631–4.

25. Chawla SP, Buzdar AU, Hortobagyi GN, Blumenschein GR. Tumor-associated fever in breast cancer. Cancer 1984;53:1596–9.

26. Armitage JO, Longo DL. Malignancies of lymphoid cells. In: Braunwald E, Fauci AS, Kasper DL, et al, editors. Harrison's principles of internal medicine. 15th ed. New York: McGraw-Hill Companies; 2001. p. 720, 726.

27. Pineda AA, Taswell HF, Brzica SM. Transfusion reaction. An immunologic hazard of blood transfusion. Transfusion 1978;18:1–7.

28. Jacobs RL, Lowe RS, Lanier BQ. Adverse reactions to tetanus toxoid. JAMA 1982;247:40–2.

29. Gaunder BN. Insect bites and stings: managing allergic reactions. Nurse Pract 1986;11:16, 19–22, 27–8.

30. Bodey GP, Jadeja L, Elting L. Pseudomonas bacteremia. Retrospective analysis of 410 episodes. Arch Intern Med 1985;145:1621–9.

31. Cometta A, Calandra T, Gaya H, et al. Monotherapy with meropenem versus combination therapy with ceftazidime plus amikacin as empiric therapy for fever in granulocytopenic patients with cancer. The International Antimicrobial Therapy Cooperative Group of the European Organization for Research and Treatment of Cancer and the Gruppo Italiano Malattie Ematologiche Maligne dell'Adulto Infection Program. Antimicrob Agents Chemother 1996;40:1108–15.

32. Vogelzang NJ, Breitbart W, Cella D, et al. Patient, caregiver, and oncologist perceptions of cancer-related fatigue: results of a tripart assessment survey. Semin Hematol 1997;34:4–12.

33. Portenoy RK, Itri LM. Cancer-related fatigue: guidelines for evaluation and management. Oncologist 1999;4:1–9.

34. Bichet DG. Pathogenesis of edematous states. Clin Invest Med 1989;12:316–22.

35. Dhib M, Bakhace E, Postec E, et al. Nephrotic syndrome complicating treatment with interferon alpha. Presse Med 1996;25:1066–8.

36. Powell AA, Armstrong MA. Peripheral edema. Am Fam Physician 1997;55:1721–6.

37. Young JR. The swollen leg. Clinical significance and differential diagnosis. Cardiol Clin 1991;9:443–56.

38. Nash P, Fryer J, Webb J. Vasculitis presenting as chronic unilateral painful leg swelling. J Rheumatol 1988;15: 1022–5.

39. Laitinen K. Life-threatening laryngeal edema in a pregnant woman previously treated for thyroid carcinoma. Obstet Gynecol 1991;78:937–8.

40. Dragan LR, Baron JM, Stern S, Shaw JC. Solid facial edema preceding a diagnosis of retro-orbital B-cell lymphoma. J Am Acad Dermatol 2000;42:872–4.

41. Seller RH. Differential diagnosis of common complaints. Philadelphia: W.B. Saunders Company; 1996. p. 335–41.

42. Barloon TJ, Bergus GR, Seabold JE. Diagnostic imaging of lower limb deep venous thrombosis. Am Fam Physician 1997;56:791–802.

43. Meler JD, Solomon MA, Steele JR, et al. The MR appearance of volume overload in the lower extremities. J Comput Assist Tomogr 1997;21:969–73.

44. Weber R. Leg edema. In: Rakel R, editor. Saunders manual of medical practice. 1st ed. Philadelphia: W.B. Saunders Company; 1996. p. 287–9.

45. Raskin NH. Headache. In: Fauci AS, Braunwald E, Isselbacher KJ, Wilson JD, editors. Harrison's principles of internal medicine. New York: McGraw-Hill Publishers; 1998.

46. Biondi DM. Headache. In: Abram SE, Haddox JD, editors. The pain clinic manual. Philadelphia: Lippincott, Williams & Wilkins; 2000.

47. Calder TM, Rowlingson JC. Low back pain. In: Raj PP, editor. Pain medicine: a comprehensive review. St Louis: Mosby Publishing; 1996.

48. Engstrom JW, Bradford DS. Back and neck pain. In: Fauci AS, Braunwald E, Isselbacher KJ, Wilson JD, editors. Harrison's principles of internal medicine. New York: McGraw-Hill Publishers; 1998.

49. Sullivan JGB. The anesthesiologist's approach to back pain. In: Nothman RH, Simeone FA, editors. The spine. 3rd ed. Philadelphia: W.B. Saunders; 1992.

50. Burton RJ. Musculoskeletal pain. In: Raj PP, editor. Pain medicine: a comprehensive review. St. Louis: Mosby-Year Book, Inc.; 1996.

51. Stone R. Acute abdominal pain. Lippincotts Prim Care Pract 1998;2:341–57.

52. Roy S, Weimersheimer P. Nonoperative causes of abdominal pain. Surg Clin North Am 1997;77:1433–54.

53. Zackowski SW. Chronic recurrent abdominal pain. Emerg Med Clin North Am 1998;16:877–94.

54. Olden KW. Rational management of chronic abdominal pain. Compr Ther 1998;24:180–6.

55. Tarraza HM, Moore RD. Gynecologic causes of the acute abdomen and the acute abdomen in pregnancy. Surg Clin North Am 1997;77:1371–94.

56. Samm BJ, Dmochowski RR. Urologic emergencies. Conditions affecting the kidney, ureter, bladder, prostate, and urethra. Postgrad Med 1996;100:177–80, 183–4.

57. Ho K. Noncardiac chest pain and abdominal pain. Ann Emerg Med 1996;27:457–60.

58. Graff LG 4th, Robinson D. Abdominal pain and emergency department evaluation. Emerg Med Clin North Am 2001;19:123–36.

59. al-Musawi D, Thompson J. The important signs in acute abdominal pain. Practitioner 2000;244:312–4, 316–8, 320.

60. LoVecchio F, Oster N, Sturmann K, et al. The use of analgesics in patients with acute abdominal pain. J Emerg Med 1997;15:775–9.

61. Pace S, Burke TF. Intravenous morphine for early pain relief in patients with acute abdominal pain. Acad Emerg Med 1996;3:1086–92.

62. Martin RF, Rossi RL. The acute abdomen. An overview and algorithms. Surg Clin North Am 1997;77:1227–43.

63. Waterston T. A strategy for abdominal pain. Practitioner 1997;241:316–8, 320.

64. Gupta H, Dupuy DE. Advances in imaging of the acute abdomen. Surg Clin North Am 1997;77:1245–63.

65. Mindelzun RE, Jeffrey RB. The acute abdomen: current CT imaging techniques. Semin Ultrasound CT MR 1999;20:63–7.

66. Macari M, Megibow A. Imaging of suspected acute small bowel obstruction. Semin Roentgenol 2001;36:108–17.

67. Maglinte DD, Balthazar EJ, Kelvin FM, Megibow AJ. The role of radiology in the diagnosis of small-bowel obstruction. AJR Am J Roentgenol 1997;168:1171–80.

68. Fauser AA, Fellhauer M, Hoffmann M, et al. Guidelines for anti-emetic therapy: acute emesis. Eur J Cancer 1999;35:361–70.

69. Briscoe K. Optimal management of nausea and vomiting in clinical oncology. Oncology (Huntingt) 1989;3(8 Suppl):11–5.

70. Hesketh PJ. Defining the emetogenicity of cancer chemotherapy regimens: relevance to clinical practice. Oncologist 1999;4:191–6.

71. Morrow GR, Roscoe JA, Kirshner JJ, et al. Anticipatory nausea and vomiting in the era of 5-HT3 antiemetics. Support Care Cancer 1998;6:244–7.

72. Kris MG, Roila F, De Mulder PH, Marty M. Delayed emesis following anticancer chemotherapy. Support Care Cancer 1998;6:228–32.

73. Feyer PC, Stewart AL, Titlbach OJ. Aetiology and prevention of emesis induced by radiotherapy. Support Care Cancer 1998;6:253–60.

74. Donnelly S, Walsh D, Rybicki L. The symptoms of advanced cancer: identification of clinical and research priorities by assessment of prevalence and severity. J Palliat Care 1995;11:27–32.

75. Sykes NP. The relationship between opioid use and laxative use in terminally ill cancer patients. Palliat Med 1998;12:375–82.

76. Fielding JF, Badenoch J, Millward-Sadler GH. Dysphagia, vomiting and obdurate constipation as a metabolic manifestation of malignancy. J Ir Med Assoc 1973;66:384–5.

77. Portenoy RK. Constipation in the cancer patient: causes and management. Med Clin North Am 1987;71:303–11.

78. Mancini I, Bruera E. Constipation in advanced cancer patients. Support Care Cancer 1998;6:356–64.

79. Tramonte SM, Brand MB, Mulrow CD, et al. The treatment of chronic constipation in adults. A systematic review. J Gen Intern Med 1997;12:15–24.

80. Locke GR 3rd, Pemberton JH, Phillips SF. American Gastroenterological Association Medical Position Statement: guidelines on constipation. Gastroenterology 2000;119:1761–6.

81. Prather CM, Ortiz-Camacho CP. Evaluation and treatment of constipation and fecal impaction in adults. Mayo Clin Proc 1998;73:881–6.

82. Floch MH, Wald A. Clinical evaluation and treatment of constipation. Gastroenterologist 1994;2:50–60.

83. Barloon TJ, Lu CC. Diagnostic imaging in the evaluation of constipation in adults. Am Fam Physician 1997;56:513–20.

84. Camilleri M, Thompson WG, Fleshman JW, Pemberton JH. Clinical management of intractable constipation. Ann Intern Med 1994;121:520–8.

85. Kot TV, Pettit-Young NA. Lactulose in the management of constipation: a current review. Ann Pharmacother 1992;26:1277–82.

86. Yassin SF, Young-Fadok TM, Zein NN, Pardi DS. *Clostridium difficile*-associated diarrhea and colitis. Mayo Clin Proc 2001;76:725–30.

87. Anand A, Glatt AE. *Clostridium difficile* infection associated with antineoplastic chemotherapy: a review. Clin Infect Dis 1993;17:109–13.

88. DuPont HL. Guidelines on acute infectious diarrhea in adults. The Practice Parameters Committee of the American College of Gastroenterology. Am J Gastroenterol 1997;92:1962–75.

89. Scheidler MD, Giannella RA. Practical management of acute diarrhea. Hosp Pract (Off Ed) 2001;36:49–56.

90. Kroser JA, Metz DC. Evaluation of the adult patient with diarrhea. Prim Care 1996;23:629–47.

91. Matseshe JW, Phillips SF. Chronic diarrhea. A practical approach. Med Clin North Am 1978;62:141–54.

92. Cheney CP, Wong RK. Acute infectious diarrhea. Med Clin North Am 1993;77:1169–96.

93. Ilnyckyj A. Clinical evaluation and management of acute infectious diarrhea in adults. Gastroenterol Clin North Am 2001;30:599–609.

94. Ripamonti C, Fulfaro F, Bruera E. Dyspnea in patients with advanced cancer: incidence, causes and treatments. Cancer Treat Rev 1998;24:69–80.

95. Ripamonti C, Bruera E. Dyspnea: pathophysiology and assessment. J Pain Symptom Manage 1997;13:220–32.

96. Escalante CP, Martin CG, Elting LS, et al. Dyspnea in cancer patients. Etiology, resource utilization, and survival-implications in a managed care world. Cancer 1996;78:1314–9.

97. Ripamonti C. Management of dyspnea in advanced cancer patients. Support Care Cancer 1999;7:233–43.

98. Drings P. Dyspnea in cancer patients [editorial]. Support Care Cancer 1999;7:215–6.

99. Dudgeon DJ, Lertzman M. Dyspnea in the advanced cancer patient. J Pain Symptom Manage 1998;16:212–9.

100. Bruera E, Schmitz B, Pither J, et al. The frequency and correlates of dyspnea in patients with advanced cancer. J Pain Symptom Manage 2000;19:357–62.

101. Mancini I, Body JJ. Assessment of dyspnea in advanced cancer patients. Support Care Cancer 1999;7:229–32.

102. Muers M. Understanding breathlessness. Lancet 1993;342:1190–1.

103. Bruera E, Neumann CM. Management of specific symptom complexes in patients receiving palliative care. Can Med Assoc J 1998;158:1717–26.

104. LeGrand SB, Walsh D. Palliative management of dyspnea in advanced cancer. Curr Opin Oncol 1999;11:250–4.

105. Irwin RS, Curley FJ, Bennett FM. Appropriate use of antitussives and protussives. A practical review. Drugs 1993;46:80–91.

106. Tuma R, DeAngelis LM. Altered mental status in patients with cancer. Arch Neurol 2000:57:1727–31.

107. Plum F, Posner JB. The diagnosis of stupor and coma. 3rd ed. Philadelphia: F.A. Davis Company; 1982.

108. Kuba H, Inamura T, Ikezaki K, et al. Thiamine-deficient lactic acidosis with brain tumor treatment. Report of three cases. J Neurosurg 1998;89:1025–8.

109. Widjdicks EF. Altered arousal and coma. Neurologic catastrophes in the emergency department. Boston: Butterworth – Heinemann; 2000. p. 3–39.

110. Bleck TP, Smith MC, Pierre-Louis SJ, et al. Neurologic complications of critical medical illnesses. Crit Care Med 1993;21:98–103.

111. Sprung CL, Peduzzi PN, Shatney CH, et al. Impact of encephalopathy on mortality in the sepsis syndrome. The Veterans Administration Systemic Sepsis Cooperative Study Group. Crit Care Med 1990;18:801–6.

112. Wilhelm C, Ellner JJ. Chronic meningitis. Neurol Clin 1986;4:115–41.

113. Fisher CM. The neurological examination of the comatose patient. Acta Neurol Scand Suppl 1969;36:1–56.

114. Delattre JY, Krol G, Thaler HT, Posner JB. Distribution of brain metastases. Arch Neurol 1988;45:741–4.

115. Elting LS, Rubenstein EB, Martin CG, et al. Incidence, cost, and outcomes of bleeding and chemotherapy dose modification among solid tumor patients with chemotherapy-induced thrombocytopenia. J Clin Oncol 2001;19:1137–46.

116. Galicich JH, French LA, Melby JC. Use of dexamethasone in the treatment of cerebral edema associated with brain tumors. Lancet 1961;81:46–53.

117. Monabati A, Kumar PV, Kamlarpour A. Intraoperative cytodiagnosis of metastatic brain tumors confused clinically with brain abscess. A report of three cases. Acta Cytol 2000;44:437–41.

118. Qureshi AI, Tuhrim S, Broderick JP, et al. Spontaneous intracerebral hemorrhage. N Engl J Med 2001;344:1450–60.

119. Drislane FW. Nonconvulsive status epilepticus in patients with cancer. Clin Neurol Neurosurg 1994;96:314–8.

120. Linzer M, Yang EH, Estes NA, et al. Diagnosing syncope. Part 1: Value of history, physical examination and electrocardiography. Clinical efficacy assessment project of the American College of Physicians. Ann Intern Med 1997;126:989–96.

121. Linzer M, Yang EH, Estes NA, et al. Diagnosing syncope. Part 2: Unexplained syncope. Clinical efficacy assessment project of the American College of Physicians. Ann Intern Med 1997;127:76–86.

122. Calkins H, Shyr Y, Frumin H, et al. The value of the clinical history in the differentiation of syncope due to the ventricular tachycardia, atrioventricular block, and neurocardiogenic syncope. Am J Med 1995;98:365–75.

123. Apisarnthanarax N, Duvic M. Dermatologic complications of cancer chemotherapy. In: Holland JF, Frei E III, Bast RC Jr, et al, editors. Cancer Medicine. 5th ed. Hamilton: B.C. Decker; 2000. p. 2271–78.

124. Robson KJ, Piette WW. Cutaneous manifestations of systemic diseases. Med Clin North Am 1998;82:1359–79.

125. Schlossberg D. Fever and rash. Infect Dis Clin North Am 1996;10:101–10.

126. Fitzpatrick TB, Bernhard JD, Cropley TG. The structure of skin lesions and fundamentals of diagnosis. In: Freedberg IM, Eisen AZ, Wolff K, et al, editors. Fitzpatrick's dermatology in general medicine. 5th ed. New York: McGraw-Hill; 1999. p. 1642–53.

127. Lookingbill DP, Spangler N, Helm KF. Cutaneous metastases in patients with metastatic carcinoma: a retrospective study of 4020 patients. J Am Acad Dermatol 1993;29:228–36.

128. Schwartz RA. Cutaneous metastatic disease. Dermatol Clin 1996;33:161–82.

129. Spencer PS, Helm TN. Skin metastases in cancer patients. Cutis 1987;39:119–21.

130. Ratnam KV, Khor CJ, Su WP. Leukemia cutis. Dermatol Clin 1994;12:419–31.

131. Rothe MJ, Bialy TL, Grant-Kels JM. Erythroderma. Dermatol Clin 2000;18:405–15.

132. Sigurdsson V, Toonstra J, Hezemans-Boer M, et al. Erythroderma: a clinical and follow-up study of 102 patients, with special emphasis on survival. J Am Acad Dermatol 1996;35:53–7.

133. Bakels V, van Oostveen JW, Gordijn RLJ, et al. Diagnostic value of T-cell receptor beta gene rearrangement analysis on peripheral blood lymphocytes of patients with erythroderma. J Invest Dermatol 1991;97:782.

CHAPTER 5

PATHOPHYSIOLOGY OF EMERGENCY ILLNESS DUE TO CANCER

GIAMPAOLO TALAMO, MD

EMERGENCY ILLNESSES DUE TO ORGAN INFILTRATION OR METASTASIS TO ORGANS

The clonal proliferation of cancer cells can lead to contiguous invasion of adjacent tissues or to metastasis to distant sites. Gradually, the infiltrating or metastasizing tumor cells replace the normal parenchyma and compromise the function of involved tissues, leading to clinically relevant complications. Organ failure from tumor invasion is the most common cause of death in patients with metastatic cancer.[1] A progressively growing malignant tumor may spread by infiltration of surrounding tissue, by hematogenous or lymphatic routes, or by implantation in serous cavities.

The distribution of metastases varies widely, depending on the origin of the primary tumor and its histologic type. Malignant tumors frequently have predictable patterns of metastasis. The preferential spread of primary tumors to specific organs can be explained by three factors: (1) blood flow and anatomic relationships, (2) adhesive interactions between endothelium and cancer cells, and (3) soluble factors.[2]

When groups of cells detach from a primary tumor, they invade the blood stream and mechanically lodge in a capillary bed. Thus, in many types of invasive cancer, the organ most frequently invaded by distant metastases is the one that contains the first capillary bed encountered by the circulating cells. Examples of this phenomenon are liver metastases from colorectal cancer and brain metastases from lung cancer. On the other hand, some patterns of metastasis cannot be predicted on the basis of anatomic considerations alone (eg, ovarian metastases from breast cancer, or thyroid metastases from clear cell carcinoma of the kidney).

Another factor that affects the preferential spread of tumors to specific organs is the presence of specific surface antigens on the endothelial cells of the target organ; these surface antigens function as recognition signals and mediate the adhesion of circulating tumor cells.[3] E-selectin, an adhesion molecule expressed by endothelial cells, provides an example of this mechanism.[4]

The third and final mechanism that explains the preferential spread of tumors to specific organs is the target organ's production of local growth factors, growth inhibitors (eg, tumor necrosis factor alpha, transforming growth factor beta, and tissue-specific inhibitory molecules), hormones, and chemotactic factors that attract the tumor cells.[5]

The most important consequences of the invasion of organs by tumor cells are organ failure; hemorrhage; the obstruction of vessels, ducts, and hollow viscera; and malignant effusion. The first part of this chapter discusses the consequences of each of these complications and the mechansisms responsible for them.

Complications Due to Organ Invasion

In this section, the term "invasion" is used to refer to both the infiltration of organs by adjacent tumors and metastasis to organs from distant tumors. The following describes the pathologic consequences of the invasion of specific organs by tumor cells.

The Lungs. Because the lungs are richly vascularized and because they contain the first capillary bed encountered by cancer cells that detach from primary tumors at other sites (except for abdominal tumors that drain into the portal vein), the lungs are a common site for metastases. Metastatic disease in the lungs usually presents as nodular lesions. However, it can also present as diffuse lymphangitic carcinomatosis, especially in the case of some adenocarcinomas of the gastrointestinal tract, such as gastric cancer. In this case, cancer cells first metastasize to the mediastinal or hilar lymph nodes and then spread in a retrograde manner to the pulmonary lymphatics.[6] Although the flow of lymph in the pulmonary lymphatics is normally centripetal, lymphatic obstruction induces reversal of flow.

Pulmonary leukostasis, which occurs primarily with leukemias, is another form of direct damage to the lungs by cancer cells. If the white blood cell count exceeds $100,000/mm^3$, the plugging of small vessels by the leukemic blasts causes pulmonary dysfunction with hypoxia and diffuse infiltrates.

When tumors involve a great amount of lung tissue, hypoxia and respiratory failure ensue.

The Heart. Cancerous invasion of the heart can be caused by direct spread from tumors in the mediastinum or lungs or by metastasis from tumors at distant sites, through either lymphatic or hematogenous routes. The great majority of tumors involving the heart are noncardiac neoplasms (primarily melanoma, lung cancer, breast cancer, lymphomas, and leukemias) that involve the pericardium or the myocardium. Metastatic involvement of the heart valves or the endocardium is rare.[7] Involvement of the pericardium can lead to pericardial effusion or constrictive pericarditis. The latter condition is due to the encasement of the pericardium without an effusion and is often observed with mesotheliomas.[8] Although the finding of myocardial metastases is not uncommon at autopsy, most patients with such metastases never have symptoms.[9] However, when the conduction system is invaded, patients develop arrhythmias and various degrees of heart block,[10] and sudden death may occur.

Gastrointestinal Tract. Certain tumors, such as lymphomas of the gastrointestinal tract, can erode the walls of the stomach and intestine, leading to perforation in some cases. A rare but reported complication is the formation of an internal malignant fistula involving two or more loops of different bowel segments and genitourinary structures. The colon is frequently one of the involved loops.[11]

The Liver. The liver is a common site for metastatic lesions because the venous drainage of many abdominal organs enters the portal circulation. Liver metastases are of two types: nodular (most common) and diffuse. Diffuse liver metastases most frequently occur with lymphomas, small-cell lung cancer (SCLC), breast cancer, and poorly differentiated gastrointestinal tumors. Patients with SCLC and diffuse metastatic infiltration of the liver may have a very unusual presentation, namely, acute hepatic failure with normal findings on chest radiography and no evidence of a neoplastic process on abdominal imaging.[12] The liver has an enormous functional reserve and impressive regenerative properties; replacement of the normal hepatic parenchyma by liver metastases causes hepatic failure only when the hepatic reserve is less than 10%. However, when tumor growth cannot be controlled, hepatic coma and death are the inevitable consequences of liver invasion.

The Bones. Most skeletal neoplasms represent metastases from other sites rather than primary tumors of the bone. Skeletal metastases are more common in bones with more vascular supply. Thus, the thoracolumbar spine, which contains highly vascular bone marrow, is the most common site of bone metastases[13] whereas the bones below the elbows and knees, which contain less vascular bone marrow, are rarely involved by metastases. The high frequency of metastasis from pelvic tumors to the thoracolumbar spine is related to the presence of Batson's plexus, a network of deep pelvic veins with rich anastomoses to the vertebral plexus.[14]

The replacement of calcifies bone with tumor weakens the structure of the bone and alters its geometry. The application of bending, compressing, or rotational forces on a weakened bone can produce a pathologic fracture. The risk of fracture depends on the site of involvement, the extent of the lesion, and the type of metastases. The anatomic location is important because each bone has a specific architecture and is subjected to different stress forces. This explains why the proximal femur is the site of approximately 10% of bone metastases but is responsible for about 40% of all pathologic fractures.

Bone metastases are of two types: osteolytic (as in multiple myeloma and renal carcinoma), characterized predominantly by the destruction of bone, and osteoblastic (as in prostate carcinoma), in which the metastatic lesion induces sclerosis and bone formation.[15] Fractures are more common with lytic than with blastic bone metastases.[16] The mechanism of bone resorption and destruction is mediated by osteoclasts and involves the release of osteoclastic stimulating substances by tumor cells and inflammatory cells. Such substances include interleukin-1, tumor necrosis substance, transforming growth substances, and prostaglandins. After pathologic fractures, the healing response is inhibited by the tumoral growth; only 35% of pathologic fractures heal.[17] Healing rates vary according to cancer type. For example, healing rates are high in multiple myeloma and very low in lung cancer.

The infiltration of the bone marrow with consequent replacement of the hematopoietic cells by metastatic tumor leads to pancytopenia or to the isolated deficit of a cell lineage (granulocytopenia, anemia, or thrombocytopenia).

Nervous System. Neoplasms can invade the brain, the meninges, peripheral nerves, the spinal cord, and the autonomic nervous system.

The most common route by which neoplasms invade the brain is the arterial circulation. Most brain tumors are of metastatic origin, mainly from lung cancer. Eighty percent of intracranial metastases are located in the cerebral hemispheres, 15% are located in the cerebellum, and 5% are located in the brain stem. The boundary area between the cortex and the white matter is the most common location of supratentorial metastases because the narrowed arterial vessels at this level trap the tumor emboli. With brain tumors, edema develops in the adjacent normal tissues; sometimes, the edema is out of proportion to the size of the neoplasm. The clinical manifestations of brain tumors are those of any mass lesion in the brain: headache, focal neurologic deficits, cognitive dysfunction, and seizures. Metastases in the central nervous system can cause death by interfering with vital central nervous system structures, such as the respiratory centers in the brain stem.

Approximately 5% of tumors metastasize to the meninges. The most common sources of leptomeningeal metastases are leukemia, lymphoma, melanoma, SCLC, and breast cancer. Leptomeningeal metastases cause neurologic dysfunction by several mechanisms: (1) direct infiltration of the brain parenchyma, which produces cerebral symptoms (headache, seizures, altered mental status, lethargy, gait ataxia); (2) direct infiltration of the spinal cord, which causes spinal symptoms (radicular pain, weakness or numbness of extremities, bladder or bowel dysfunction); (3) encasement or infiltration of the portion of the cranial nerves and spinal roots that traverses the subarachnoid space, leading to cranial nerve symptoms (visual loss, diplopia, facial weakness or numbness, hearing loss, dysphagia) and spinal symptoms; (4) interruption of cerebrospinal fluid absorption, which results in an increase in intracranial pressure and hydrocephalic symptoms (headache, altered mental status, gait imbalance, urinary incontinence); and (5) brain ischemia and cerebral infarction.[18] The most commonly involved portions of the meninges are the inferior surface of the brain, the dorsal surface of the spinal cord, and the cauda equina.

Tumor infiltration may be macroscopically visible (either as a diffuse leptomeningeal involvement or as tumor nodules) or may be microscopic. The arachnoid membranes may be infiltrated by an inflammatory reaction or may be fibrotic. Cancer cells can gain entrance to the subarachnoid space by several routes. One route is directly from metastases to the capillaries of the leptomeninges;[19] another route is from metastatic lesions to the bone (skull or vertebrae). An experimental leukemia model in mice showed that neoplastic cells first infiltrated the bone marrow in the skull, then invaded the bridging veins, and finally entered the subarachnoid space.[20] Neoplastic lesions in the brain parenchyma can erode directly into the subarachnoid space or ventricles.[21] Two other mechanisms by which cancer cells can enter the subarachnoid space are infiltration from dural metastases [22] and infiltration along nerve roots. In the latter case, cancer cells first invade nerve roots and then grow along the nerve sheath.

Peripheral nerves may be involved individually or in combination (mononeuritis multiplex). Neural plexuses may be infiltrated as well; the invasion of the brachial plexus (usually by lung cancer arising in the superior sulcus) results in pain and Pancoast's syndrome. Cranial nerves may be affected by the neoplasm (a) at their origin near the brain stem, (b) along their course (eg, facial nerve paralysis is a common occurrence in parotid neoplasms), or (c) at the level of their end organ. Trigeminal neuropathy (with facial pain or paresthesias) can result from the perineural spread of head and neck carcinomas.[23]

Finally, even the autonomic system may be involved by cancerous spread. If a tumor or its metastases invade the subdiaphragmatic sympathetic plexus, the patient is at risk for acute colonic pseudo-obstruction (Ogilvie's syndrome), which is characterized by severe dilatation of the colon, without obstruction. This syndrome is due to damage of the parasympathetic nerves, which inhibits intestinal peristalsis and leads to colonic atony and functional obstruction.[24]

Endocrine Glands. In autopsy studies, thyroid metastases are present in approximately 15% of patients with metastatic carcinoma. However, most patients have microscopic metastases, and hypothyroidism secondary to organ failure is exceedingly rare. Conversely, hyperthyroidism has been reported in patients with thyroid metastases; the mechanism is believed to be similar to that of subacute thyroiditis, in which destruction of thyroid tissue leads to the release of high levels of thyroid hormone and thyroglobulin.[25]

Metastatic involvement of the adrenal glands is present in 10 to 20% of patients who die of cancer. Despite this relatively high prevalence of adrenal infiltration, clinically evident adrenal insufficiency (Addison's disease) is very rare.[26] This is due to the large functional reserve of the adrenal glands: more than 80% of adrenal tissue must be destroyed before hormonal production will be impaired; therefore, Addison's disease develops only in patients with bilateral metastases.[27] In cancer patients with adrenal insufficiency, the possibility of hypothalamic or pituitary metastases must always be considered.

Metastases to the pituitary gland can cause diabetes insipidus, anterior pituitary insufficiency, painful ophthalmoplegia, and visual-field deficits.[28]

The Skin. Tumor invasion of the skin occurs in about 25% of breast cancers, 7% of lung cancers, 5% of renal cancers, 3% of colorectal cancers, and 1% of other neoplasms. Tumor masses can erode through the skin and ulcerate. When such skin ulcers are large, they can become necrotic and malodorous.

Complications Due to Mechanical Pressure from Tumor Masses

Because of their tendency to grow and invade adjacent tissues, neoplasms can cause compressions and obstructions of vessels, ducts, and hollow viscera. If left untreated, these mechanical events will lead sooner or later to an oncologic emergency.

Obstruction of Airways. Obstruction of the upper airway (the hypopharynx, larynx, and high tracheal region) is a common complication of head and neck carcinomas (carcinomas of the base of the tongue, the hypopharynx, and the larynx), thyroid cancers, and mediastinal lymphomas.[29] Obstruction of the lower airway (the main stem bronchi, the lobar bronchi, and their derivatives) is a frequent complication of primary carcinoma of the lung but can also be caused by metastases from melanoma, breast cancer, colorectal cancer, or other carcinomas.[30] Obstruction of the lower airway leads to atelectasis and postobstructive pneumonias.

Obstruction of the Esophagus, Stomach, Small Intestine, or Colon. Esophageal obstruction is a common consequence of esophageal cancer but can be caused (in rare cases) by tumors arising in adjacent organs or by large nodal metastases. Obstruction of the esophageal lumen leads to serious complications such as malnutrition and aspiration pneumonia. In approximately 10% of patients with esophageal obstruction, erosion of the esophageal wall is complicated by the development of esophagopulmonary fistula.

Obstruction of the stomach can occur at the level of the pylorus or the duodenum. Before the availability of effective ulcer therapy with antacid medications (eg, H_2 blockers), the most common cause of gastric-outlet obstruction was peptic ulcers. Nowadays, in 60 to 75% of patients with gastric-outlet obstruction, the cause is malignancy. Pyloric stenosis in cancer patients is usually caused by a primary gastric cancer whereas occlusion at the duodenal level is usually a complication of pancreatic cancer. When the obstruction delays gastric emptying, patients develop gastric-outlet syndrome, a condition characterized by nausea, vomiting, epigastric fullness, anorexia, and early satiety. Vomiting starts 1 hour or more after eating and may contain undigested food but usually no bile. If severe and persistent, vomiting will lead to dehydration and electrolyte imbalance.

Occlusion of the small intestine (resulting from either direct invasion or metastasis from colorectal cancer, ovarian cancer, peritoneal carcinomatosis, or other neoplasms) leads to vomiting and abdominal pain.

Because the colon has a larger lumen, obstruction of the colon is less frequent than obstruction of the small intestine. Colonic obstruction occurs in approximately 10% of patients with colorectal adenocarcinomas. When the colon is completely obstructed, the severity of symptoms depends on the continence of the ileocecal valve. If this valve is not competent, the colonic distension will be transmitted to the small intestine; if the valve is competent, the colonic distension could lead to visceral rupture (usually at the level of the cecum), a life-threatening complication.

Obstruction of the Biliary Tract. Neoplasms arising from the head of the pancreas and cholangiocarcinomas are common causes of biliary tract obstruction. Biliary tract obstruction leads to liver insufficiency with a cholestatic pattern, and patients with this condition are at risk for sepsis secondary to cholangitis.

Acute Pancreatitis. In the cancer setting, obstruction of the pancreatic duct occurs mainly as a consequence of pancreatic cancer or lymph nodes enlarged by metastases.[31]

Obstruction of the Urinary Tract. Urinary tract obstruction can occur at the levels of the ureter, bladder, or urethra. Ureteral obstruction occurs when retroperitoneal lymph nodes become involved because of lymphomatous infiltration or metastases from cancers of the genitourinary tract, especially prostate, testicular, and cervical cancers. The periaortic lymph nodes in the retroperitoneal space are the drainage sites for many urologic and gynecologic cancers. The mechanism of urinary tract obstruction is almost always extrinsic compression of the ureteral lumen, without invasion of the wall of the ureter.

Bladder-outlet obstruction, seen primarily with prostate and cervical cancers, typically produces bilateral hydronephrosis and (in the case of long-standing obstructive uropathy) atrophic kidneys. Urethral obstruction can occur in patients with prostate cancer, bladder cancer, or primary urethral tumors.

Spinal-Cord Compression. The spinal cord is a nearly round structure that is contained in the spinal canal. The spinal cord is almost 1 cm in diameter, is 42 to 45 cm long, and ends at the level of the L1 or L2 lumbar vertebra. Five percent of patients with cancer experience spinal-cord compression, most commonly from metastases of breast cancer (25%), lung cancer (20%), and prostate cancer (15%). There are five main mechanisms of spinal-cord compression (Figure 5–1). The first and most common mechanism is direct epidural compression due to the extension of metastases located in the vertebrae. Cancer cells reach the vertebrae hematogenously, traveling by either arterial vessels or the paravertebral venous plexus system described by Batson.[14] The second mechanism of spinal-cord compression is vertebral compression associated with a pathologic fracture: when the vertebral body collapses, the bone and the tumor can invade the spinal canal and compress the anterior surface of the spinal cord.[32] The third mechanism is epidural extension resulting from direct spread of a paravertebral tumor mass. In this case, the tumor does not invade the bone but reaches the epidural space through the intervertebral foramina. This event accounts for approximately 10% of cases of spinal-cord compression and is especially common in cases of lymphoma and multiple myeloma.[33] Spinal-cord compression can also be caused by the direct metastasis of tumor into the spinal cord and by the metastasis of tumor into the epidural space.

Spinal-cord compression may occur at the level of the cervical spine (10%), thoracic spine (70%), or lumbar spine (20%); in 20% of cases, multiple sites are involved. The resulting neurologic deficits are determined by the level of involvement of the cord: a cervical compression can cause quadriplegia, a thoracic compression can cause paraplegia, and a compression at the upper lumbar level can cause bladder or bowel incontinence. Compression at the level of the cauda equina (below L1-L2) can cause bowel and bladder dysfunction, paraparesis, and sensory loss in a saddle distribution. In terms of clinical symptoms, the most important neural structures affected by spinal-cord compression are the anterior and lateral corticospinal tracts (descending pathways formed by upper motor neurons that control the skeletal muscle fibers), the spinocerebellar tracts (ascending pathways that convey spinal information to the cerebellum), and the posterior columns (ascending pathways involved in processing sensory information). Lateral compression of the cord can cause Brown-Séquard's syndrome, which is characterized by a loss of vibratory and position sensations on the side of the compression and by a contralateral loss of pain and temperature sensations.[34]

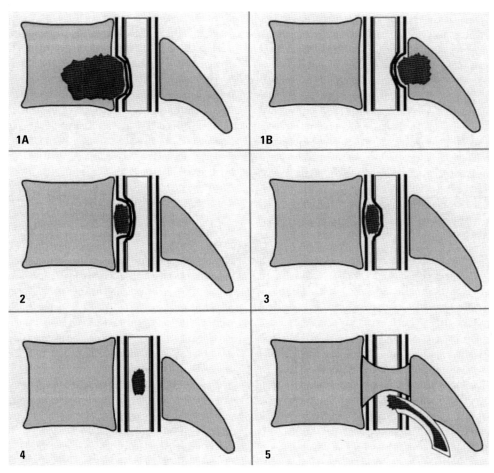

Figure 5–1. Mechanisms of spinal cord compression. 1A and 1B: Bony metastasis, either in the vertebral body (1A) or in the vertebral arch (1B). 2: Epidural metastasis. 3: Subdural metastasis. 4: Intramedullary metastasis. 5: Paraspinal tumor infiltrating through the vertebral foramen.

Histologic studies have shown demyelination, axonal swelling, and interstitial edema at the level of spinal-cord compression. The spinal-cord edema seen in patients with spinal-cord compression is believed to result from both the mechanical pressure on the cord and the compression of the epidural venous plexus. In an experiment in mice, all pathologic lesions observed in spinal-cord compression could be reproduced by occlusion of the venous outflow from the cord.[13] Cord edema plays an important role in the pathogenesis of the acute neurologic deficit, as is suggested by the frequent improvement of symptoms with the use of corticosteroids. Cord ischemia, which is caused by the obliteration of parenchymal vessels, is a late event in patients with spinal-cord compression.[35]

Compression of Nerves. The effects of nerve irritation or paralysis due to mechanical pressure caused by tumor depend on the specific functions of the involved nerves. When neoplasms of the anterior mediastinum compress the phrenic nerve, patients may develop chest pain and hiccups (in the case of nerve irritation) or paralysis of the homolateral hemidiaphragm (in the case of nerve paralysis). Compression of the vagus nerve, which may occur with intrathoracic neoplasms, can lead to cervical pain, coughing, tachycardia, gastric retention, and (occasionally) bronchospasm. Compression of the recurrent laryngeal nerve, which in cancer patients is usually a complication of thyroid neoplasms, can cause spasms of the glottis (in the case of nerve irritation) or vocal-cord paralysis with dysphonia (in the case of nerve paralysis). Apical tumors of the lung often cause Pancoast's syndrome (lower brachial plexopathy, shoulder pain, and Horner's syndrome) because they invade the stellate ganglion and the lower brachial plexus (C8–T1 nerve roots). Compression of the brachial plexus occurs in approximately 35% of patients with carcinoma of the superior pulmonary sulcus.

Increased Intracranial Pressure. Increased intracranial pressure can be caused by either a mass lesion or an obstruction of cerebrospinal fluid flow by tumor. Normal intracranial pressure is less than 10 mm Hg; clinical manifestations occur when intracranial pressure increases to > 20 mm Hg. Since the brain is surrounded by a rigid skull, the expansion of an intracranial tumor displaces brain tissue and structures and may lead to herniation. There are three types of herniation: central, uncal, and tonsillar. Central herniation is caused by hemispheric tumor masses. Uncal herniation is caused by tumors located above the tentorium (eg, tumors in the temporal lobe or the lateral fossa of the frontal lobe). The tentorium cerebelli separates the cerebral hemispheres above from the cerebellum and brain stem below. Supratentorial tumors can displace the uncus (the medial portion of the temporal lobe) beneath the tentorium. Tonsillar herniation is caused by infratentorial neoplasms. Neoplasms located in the posterior fossa can displace the cerebellar tonsils either upward through the tentorium or (more commonly) downward through the foramen magnum. Cerebellar tonsil–foramen magnum herniation can be aggravated by acute obstructive hydrocephalus. Herniation syndromes are highly lethal because the compression of the respiratory centers in the brain stem leads to respiratory arrest.[34] In patients with glioblastoma multiforme, herniation is the most frequent cause of death.

Superior Vena Cava Syndrome. Neoplasms account for 90% of cases of superior vena cava (SVC) syndrome. The most common neoplastic causes of SVC syndrome are lung cancer (80%) and lymphoma (10%). The SVC starts at the junction of the left and right innominate veins and ends at the right atrium. The SVC is responsible for the drainage of venous blood from the head, neck, upper thorax, and upper extremities. The SVC is approximately 8 cm long and has a diameter of 2 cm. Its thin wall is easily compressible by an adjacent tumor mass. Although a thrombotic process is present in 40% of cases of SVC syndrome,[36] the pathogenesis of this syndrome is mainly related to extrinsic compression of the SVC, which causes obstruction of the blood flow and diminished blood return to the heart. The venous pressure in the SVC can increase to levels as high as 200 to 500 cm H_2O.[37] The clinical manifestations of SVC syndrome (mainly dyspnea, coughing, facial edema, a sense of fullness in the head, and the distension of veins on the neck and upper thorax) are due to the increased venous pressures secondary to the obstructed drainage of the upper thorax and head. The compensatory redistribution of venous blood flow in SVC syndrome is shown in Figure 5–2.

Hemorrhage

Hemorrhage is one of the most common causes of death in patients with metastatic cancer. Hemorrhage may result either from direct tumor invasion and destruction of blood vessels or from neovascularization of the tumor. It is also important to note that many patients with cancer have concomitant pathologic conditions that precipitate or predispose to hemorrhage—for example, thrombocytopenia related to bone marrow involvement or chemotherapeutic drugs, or coagulopathy related to disseminated intravascular coagulation, which may be caused either directly by the cancer or by a supervening infection.

Hemorrhage in patients with cancer can range from minimal and clinically occult hemorrhages to massive hemorrhages that lead to cardiovascular shock and death. In determining the seriousness of a hemorrhage, the rapidity of blood loss is more important than the amount of blood lost; a very gradual loss of more than 70% of the total blood volume can be well tolerated whereas the sudden loss of 500 mL (approximately 10% of the normal total blood volume) can lead to cardiovascular collapse (hemorrhagic shock).

Epistaxis. Epistaxis occurs primarily with nasopharyngeal carcinoma. Epistaxis is rarely massive or life threatening.

Hemoptysis. Massive hemoptysis, defined as blood loss greater than 500 mL per 24 hours, can lead to death from hemorrhagic shock or from asphyxiation when the bronchial tree is flooded with blood. The most common causes of hemoptysis in cancer patients are neoplasms of the lung, followed by carcinoma of the larynx.[38]

Gastrointestinal Hemorrhage. The tumor most likely to directly cause massive gastrointestinal bleeding is a gastric lymphoma; however, gastrointestinal hemorrhage may also be seen in patients with cancer of the esophagus, stomach, and colon.[39] Among nongastrointestinal cancers, melanoma that has metastasized to the bowel wall is the most common cause of bleeding.

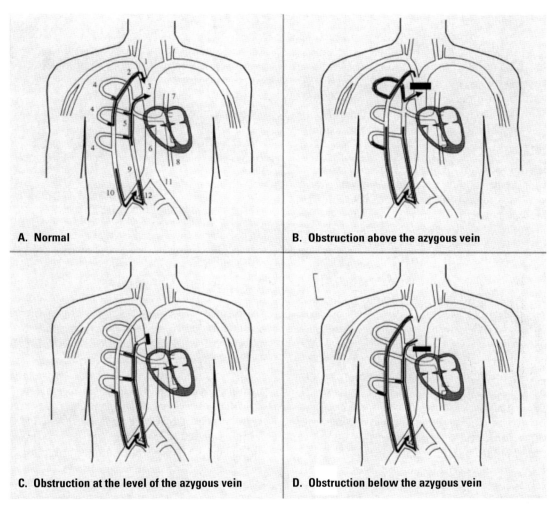

A. Normal

B. Obstruction above the azygous vein

C. Obstruction at the level of the azygous vein

D. Obstruction below the azygous vein

Figure 5–2. Compensatory redistribution of venous blood flow in superior vena cava (SVC) syndrome. A: Schematic representation of the normal venous circulation. 1 = right brachiocephalic vein; 2 = right internal mammary vein; 3 = superior vena cava; 4 = right intercostal veins (only three are shown); 5 = azygous vein; 6 = inferior vena cava; 7 = accessory hemiazygous vein; 8 = hemiazygous vein; 9 = right ascending lumbar vein; 10 = right inferior epigastric vein; 11 = right common iliac vein; 12 = right ileolumbar vein. The superior vena cava arises from the junction of the right and left brachiocephalic veins and enters the right atrium. It drains blood from the head, neck, upper extremities, and upper thorax. The superior and inferior vena cava are connected because the internal mammary veins form anastomoses with the inferior epigastric veins, and the azygous and hemiazygous veins form anastomoses with the right and left ascending lumbar veins, respectively. These join the ileolumbar veins, which enter the internal iliac vein. B, C, and D: The direction of the venous circulation when the superior vena cava is obstructed by a tumor above, at the level of, and below the azygous vein, respectively.

Hemoperitoneum. Bleeding from cancer is a rare cause of hemoperitoneum. One of the neoplasms most commonly associated with this life-threatening complication is uterine leiomyoma.[40]

Hematuria. The most common causes of tumor-related hematuria are (in order of decreasing frequency) bladder carcinoma and local infiltration by carcinoma of the prostate, uterine cervix, or rectum.

Intracranial Hemorrhage. Cerebral hemorrhage related to direct involvement of tumor of the brain can develop with any intracranial neoplasm, but it is primarily seen in patients with intracranial metastases from lung cancer, melanoma, or renal cell carcinoma.[41] In patients with leukemia, cerebral leukostasis may lead to intracranial hemorrhage, especially when the white cell count is greater than 100,000/mm^3. Although intracranial bleeding in cancer patients can occasionally result from a spontaneous intratumoral hemorrhage, intracranial bleeding in most cases is precipitated by thrombocytopenia secondary to chemotherapy or bone marrow infiltration by cancer.

Rupture of the Aorta or Major Artery. Carcinomas of the lung and esophagus can erode the aortic wall; rupture of the aorta leads to sudden death.[42,43] Head and neck tumors can erode into the carotid arteries, and so-called carotid blowout can also lead to sudden death.

Malignant Effusions

The pleural, pericardial, and peritoneal cavities are the three large serous cavities of the human body. The membranes that surround these cavities are formed by a parietal layer that covers the external surface of the cavity and a visceral layer that covers the organs. Normally, only a minimal amount of fluid is present inside the cavities. The function of the fluid is to facilitate the motion of the covered organs by reducing the friction between the membranes. When fluid accumulates in the closed space, the effusion may be clinically silent or may severely compromise organ function, depending on the amount of fluid and the rapidity of fluid accumulation.

Neoplasms produce malignant effusions by three main pathogenetic mechanisms: contiguity (ie, growth through the wall of an organ and infiltration of the serous membranes), hematogenous spread to the capillary vessels underlying the serous membranes and blockage of lymphatic drainage.

While pathologic processes such as congestive heart failure, nephrotic syndrome, and liver cirrhosis produce a transudate (a thin watery fluid with few blood cells and proteins), malignant effusions usually produce an exudate. By definition, a pleural fluid is an exudate if it has at least one of the following three features: a pleural protein/serum protein ratio > 0.5; a pleural lactate dehydrogenase (LDH)/serum LDH ratio > 0.6; or a pleural LDH level > two-thirds of the upper limit of the normal level for serum LDH. Malignancies can also produce chylous effusions, which are characterized by elevated levels of triglycerides (>110 mg/dL). When chylous effusions are seen, the most likely cause is lymphoma.

Malignant effusions are often serosanguineous or frankly hemorrhagic. The fluid is said to be hemorrhagic if the red blood cell count is > 100,000/mm^3. The white blood cell count is often elevated (> 3,000/mm^3), usually with a predominance of lymphocytes and mononuclear cells. The serosanguineous appearance of the effusion and the elevated blood counts are due to the direct invasion of blood vessels by cancer cells and to the inflammatory response to them. The latter results in the dilatation and increased permeability of the capillaries and in the infiltration of the pleura by lymphocytes. In some cases, the increased glucose use by cancer cells leads to reduced concentrations of glucose in the pleural fluid.[44]

Pleural Effusion. The accumulation of a pathologic fluid in the pleural space is a common complication of cancers, especially lymphomas and cancers of the lung and breast. Under normal conditions, 5 to 10 L of fluid are produced in the pleural space each day, but most of this fluid is reabsorbed, so that only 5 to 20 mL of fluid are present in the pleural cavity at any given time.[45] Factors influencing the dynamics of pleural fluid are hydrostatic pressure, oncotic pressure, capillary permeability, and lymphatic drainage (Figure 5–3). Accumulation of fluid in the pleural space can occur by several mechanisms: increased hydrostatic pressure (as in congestive heart failure), increased negative intrapleural pressure (as in pulmonary atelectasis), decreased oncotic pressure (as in hypoalbuminemia), and increased capillary permeability (as in pneumonia). The most important mechanism involved in the development of malignant pleural effusions is blockage of lymphatic drainage. Other factors that may be involved are increased capillary permeability (related to the disruption of the capillary endothelium by tumor and the resulting inflammatory response) and increased pleural fluid oncotic pressure (related to the proliferation of cancer cells).[46]

The amount of fluid that accumulates in the pleural space varies. When fluid accumulation is minimal, the effusion is asymptomatic and can be detected only with imaging studies. Blunting of a costophrenic angle seen on routine posteroanterior chest radiography means that approximately 500 mL of fluid is already present. Symptoms of respiratory insufficiency related to the compression of the lung parenchyma and to consequent reduced lung volume usually develop if the volume of accumulated fluid is > 2,000 mL.[47] Massive and uncon-

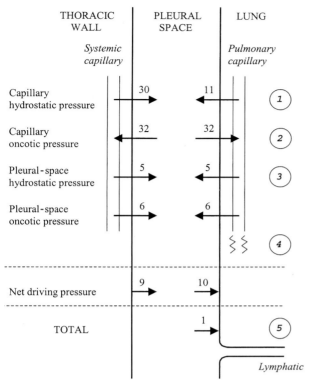

THORACIC WALL | PLEURAL SPACE | LUNG

Systemic capillary | *Pulmonary capillary*

Capillary hydrostatic pressure — 30 | 11 — (1)

Capillary oncotic pressure — 32 | 32 — (2)

Pleural-space hydrostatic pressure — 5 | 5 — (3)

Pleural-space oncotic pressure — 6 | 6 — (4)

Net driving pressure — 9 | 10 —

TOTAL | 1 — (5)

Lymphatic

Figure 5–3. Mechanisms for the production and absorption of pleural fluid. Numbers refer to pressure (in cm H$_2$O). The figure shows only mean pressures, and does not include variations due to gravitational forces or related to the respiratory cycle. The pleural-space hydrostatic pressure is negative because of the elastic recoil of the lungs. Circled numbers refer to the five mechanisms for the accumulation of pleural fluid: (1) increased plasma hydrostatic pressure (eg, congestive heart failure); (2) decreased plasma oncotic pressure (eg, hypoalbuminemic states); (3) increased negative intrapleural pressure (eg, lung atelectasis); (4) increased capillary permeability (eg, inflammatory processes); (5) block of lymphatic drainage (eg, cancer).

trolled pleural effusions lead to cardiopulmonary decompensation and death.

Pericardial Effusion. Metastatic pericardial effusions are the most common cause of cardiac tamponade. Cancers of the lung and breast account for 75% of cases of malignant pericardial effusion; other tumors that may be involved include carcinomas of the esophagus and stomach, melanoma, lymphoma, and leukemia. Primary tumors of the pericardium are very rare. Normally, only up to 50 mL of fluid is present in the pericardial space. The following factors can cause an accumulation of fluid in the pericardium of a patient with cancer: alteration of vascular permeability, obstruction of the efferent lymphatic vessels by tumor cells, and localized bleeding from tumor implants.[45] When mediastinal lymph nodes are infiltrated by tumor, as is often seen in patients with breast and lung cancers, the pericardial lymphatic drainage is impeded.[48]

Hemodynamic compromise occurs when there is a high level of intrapericardial pressure. This pressure depends not only on the amount of fluid but also on the distensibility of the parietal pericardial sac, the intravascular volume, and the rapidity of fluid accumulation. A rapid accumulation of as little as 200 mL of fluid in a scarcely elastic pericardial sac can induce hemodynamic instability whereas the slow accumulation of more than 1 L in a distensible sac can be accommodated without decompensation.[49] As intrapericardial pressure increases, compensatory mechanisms (increased heart rate, myocardial contractility, and systemic resistance) ensue. Cardiac tamponade results when the pressure of the fluid within the pericardial sac equals the right atrial and ventricular diastolic pressure, so that the cardiac output is compromised.

Malignant Ascites. Malignant ascites is usually related to the dissemination of cancer in the peritoneal cavity. In rare cases, however, malignant ascites is due to the presence of liver metastases. Widespread peritoneal seeding is common with gastrointestinal and ovarian tumors. The principal mechanism involved in the development of malignant ascites is the blockage of lymphatic drainage. However, it has been shown that when the concentration of cancer cells in the peritoneal fluid is elevated (> 4,000/mm^3), their presence alone can sustain the formation of the ascites because of the production of chemical mediators (cytokines, histamine, lactate) with irritative effect.[50] Some gynecologic tumors can produce hydrothorax and ascites simultaneously (Meigs' syndrome). This syndrome is possible because the peritoneal cavity communicates with the right pleural cavity through lymphatic vessels that are usually nonfunctional but that become permeable when peritoneal pressure increases significantly.

It is interesting that while spontaneous bacterial peritonitis occurs in 8% of patients with ascites secondary to liver cirrhosis, bacterial peritonitis usually does not develop in patients with malignant ascites.[51] It can be speculated that bacterial peritonitis in the course of cirrhosis is promoted by a decreased hepatic reticuloendothelial function and by portosystemic shunting.

PARANEOPLASTIC SYNDROMES

In addition to infiltrating organs and causing mechanical pressure due to masses, cancers are capable of producing paraneoplastic syndromes—combinations of signs and symptoms that occur at a distance from the primary tumor or its metastases (Table 5–1).

Many paraneoplastic syndromes are related to substances, such as hormones, that are produced by the abnormal activation of normal cellular genes. Every cell in the body has a complete genome, with approximately 40,000 genes. In a typical cell, however, only about 1% of these genes are expressed, and transcription of the remaining genes is repressed. For example, myocytes contain the gene for antidiuretic hormone (ADH) in their deoxyribonucleic acid (DNA), but unlike pituitary cells, myocytes do not produce ADH because that gene remains silent (ie, it is constitutively repressed). Cancer cells have the capacity to produce and secrete a wide array of substances by derepressing normal genes. The detailed molecular mechanisms underlying the activation of specific genes in transformed cells are generally unknown.

Many of the molecules (such as carcinoembryonic antigen and α-fetoprotein) produced by cancer cells do not produce clinical manifestations and can be used as tumor markers. Paraneoplastic syndromes occur only when the substances produced by cancer cells are biologically active (eg, as hormones, cytokines, or growth factors [Table 5–2]) and are secreted in amounts that are sufficient to induce clinical manifestations.

The following section describes paraneoplastic syndromes according to their pathogenesis. Paraneoplastic syndromes for which the underlying mechanism is obscure (such as acute necrotizing myopathy, hypertrophic osteoarthropathy, and many dermatologic disorders [eg, dermatomyositis, acanthosis nigricans, ichthyosis, necrolytic migratory erythema, and vasculitis]) are not discussed.

Syndromes Due to Hormones and Cytokines

Many non-endocrine cancer cells are able to produce hormones. Often, the secreted hormones are either nonfunctional or precursors that possess only a small portion of the biologic activity of the mature form of the hormone. The term "ectopic" is used to describe these hormones because they are not normally found in the tissue in which the neoplasm develops.

The production of specific hormones by certain cancers can often be explained by the development and differentiation of cell lineage that occurs during embryogenesis. For example, SCLC, a tumor often associated with the production of several hormones (eg, adrenocorticotropic hormone, ADH, and calcitonin), is a pulmonary neoplasm that arises from neuroendocrine cells that belong to the amine precursor uptake and decarboxylation (APUD) system. This system is anatomically disassociated and is bound together by several embryologic, biochemical, and ultrastructural features. Cells of the APUD system produce polypeptide hormones of low molecular weight by decarboxylating amine precursors, such as dopa. All APUD cells derive from the neuroectoderm.[52]

Syndrome of Inappropriate Secretion of Antidiuretic Hormone. The most common neoplasm associated with the syndrome of inappropriate ADH (SIADH) is SCLC, which accounts for 60% of cases. The physiologic role of ADH is to act on the renal tubule to increase the absorp-

TABLE 5–1. Paraneoplastic Syndromes and Commonly Associated Neoplasms

Paraneoplastic Syndrome	Associated Neoplasms
Intestinal pseudo-obstruction	SCLC
Glomerulonephritis	Lung, breast, and gastrointestinal cancers
Neurologic syndromes	
Eaton-Lambert syndrome	SCLC
Myasthenia gravis	Thymoma
Guillain-Barré syndrome	HD
Encephalopathy	SCLC, breast cancer
Cerebellar degeneration	SCLC, breast cancer, ovarian cancer, HD
Myelopathy	SCLC, breast cancer
Motor neuropathy	HD, NHL, SCLC, multiple myeloma
Sensory neuropathy	SCLC
Opsoclonus/myoclonus	Neuroblastoma; breast, lung, and ovarian cancers
Retinopathy	SCLC, NSCLC, melanoma, uterine cancer, breast cancer
Dermatologic syndromes	
Dermatomyositis	Lung cancer, cancers of the female genital tract
Pemphigus	Breast cancer, ovarian cancer, cancer of the thymus, lung cancer, gastrointestinal tract cancers, lymphomas
Acanthosis nigricans	Gastrointestinal cancers
Ichthyosis	Lymphomas
Keratosis palmaris or plantaris	Lung cancer, bladder carcinoma
Leser-Trélat sign	Adenocarcinomas of the gastrointestinal tract (stomach)
Necrolytic migratory erythema	Glucagonoma
Vasculitis	Leukemias, lymphomas
Hematologic syndromes	
Secondary polycythemia	Renal carcinoma, cerebellar hemangioblastoma, HCC
ITP	Lymphomas
Pure red cell aplasia	Thymoma
Aplastic anemia	Thymoma, lymphomas, lung cancer
DIC	APL, adenocarcinomas
Endocrinologic syndromes	
Hypercalcemia	Lung cancer (SCC), renal cancer, ovarian cancer, multiple myeloma
SIADH	SCLC
Cushing's syndrome	SCLC, cancer of the thymus, islet cell tumors, MCT
Hypoglycemia	Mesenchymal tumors, HCC, adrenal carcinoma
Acromegaly	Pancreatic islet cell tumors, bronchial carcinoid
Zollinger-Ellison syndrome	Gastrinoma
Fever	Renal cell carcinoma, HD
Polymyositis	SCLC, breast cancer, ovarian cancer, lymphomas

APL = acute promyelocytic leukemia; DIC = disseminated intravascular coagulation; HCC = hepatocellular carcinoma; HD = Hodgkin's disease; ITP = idiopathic thrombocytopenic purpura; MCT = medullary carcinoma of the thyroid; NHL = non-Hodgkin's lymphoma; NSCLC = non-small-cell lung cancer; SCC = squamous cell carcinoma; SCLC = small-cell lung cancer; SIADH = syndrome of inappropriate secretion of antidiuretic hormone.

tion of water during hypovolemia (eg, in case of dehydration). In the paraneoplastic syndrome, the secretion of ADH is "inappropriate" because it occurs in a normovolemic patient. The syndrome is characterized by hyponatremia, inappropriately concentrated urine (the urine osmolality is usually > 100 mOsm/L) in the presence of hypotonic plasma (the serum osmolality is usually < 260 mOsm/L), and high urinary sodium levels (> 20 mEq/L). It is notable that many patients with cancer have elevated levels of ADH in plasma but do not develop SIADH. These patients would most likely have SIADH if they were subjected to a water load. Whether or not symptoms (eg, anorexia, nausea, vomiting, and signs of cerebral edema, such as confusion, seizures, and coma) develop depends not only on the severity of hyponatremia but also on the rapidity with which hyponatremia occurs. Many patients with SIADH have increased levels of atrial natriuretic factor (ANF), a peptide hormone that is normally secreted by the cardiac atria and that promotes the renal excretion of sodium. This can be a compensatory mechanism that antagonizes the water

TABLE 5–2. Biologically Active Substances Produced by Cancer Cells

Hormones and hormone precursors
    Antidiuretic hormone
    Corticotropin-releasing hormone
    Pro-opiomelanocortin, lipocortin
    Melanocyte-stimulating hormone
    Adrenocorticotropic hormone
    Chorionic gonadotropin and its subunits (alpha and beta)
    Growth hormone (GH), GH-releasing hormone
    Prolactin
    Parathyroid hormone
    Parathyroid hormone–related protein
    Calcitonin
    Somatostatin
    Serotonin
    Gastrin
    Gastrin-releasing peptide
    Bombesin
    Vasoactive intestinal peptide
    Glucagon
    Insulin
    Prohormone form of insulin-like growth factor II
    Renin, prorenin
    Atrial natriuretic factor
    Erythropoietin
Cytokines
    Interleukin-1
    Tumor necrosis factors
Growth factors
    Transforming growth factor beta
    Epidermal growth factor
Enzymes
    Alkaline phosphatase
    Thymidine kinase

retention associated with the inappropriately high levels of ADH. However, cancer cells can ectopically secrete ANF, as seen in many cases of SCLC. The relative contribution of ADH and ANF to the hyponatremia associated with SIADH is unclear.[53]

Cushing's Syndrome. Paraneoplastic Cushing's syndrome is usually caused by adrenocorticotropic hormone (ACTH) and ACTH precursors.[54] Very rarely, Cushing's syndrome results from the production of corticotropin-releasing factor. Tumors that produce ACTH include lung cancer, particularly SCLC (50% of cases); carcinoma of the thymus (10%); islet cell tumors of the pancreas (10%); and medullary carcinoma of the thyroid (5%). The precursor molecule of ACTH is pro-opiomelanocortin (POMC). The gene that encodes for POMC is a very large gene that also codes for lipotropin, melanocyte-stimulating hormone, ACTH, endorphins, and enkephalins. Experimental evidence suggests that many carcinomas synthesize large amounts of POMC, but only a few of them metabolize it to mature ACTH and produce Cushing's syndrome. Whereas pituitary cells contain all the enzymes required for processing POMC, cancer cells have variable amounts of these enzymes, and therefore, they often cannot process POMC.[55] Clinical manifestations of neoplastic Cushing's syndrome include weakness, weight loss, hypertension, hyperglycemia, hypokalemia, and metabolic alkalosis. Clinicians must remember that because of the short duration of paraneoplastic Cushing's syndrome, the full spectrum of manifestations typical of adrenal or pituitary Cushing's syndrome is often absent.

Hypoglycemia. Approximately 45% of cases of hypoglycemia that is associated with malignancy are caused by mesenchymal tumors (sarcomas, mesotheliomas, neurofibromas, and spindle cell carcinomas); the remaining cases are caused by hepatocellular carcinoma (23%), adrenocortical carcinoma (10%), and other cancers (< 10% each). These neoplasms induce hypoglycemia through the production of insulin-like growth factors (IGFs). The IGF family includes three peptide hormones—insulin, IGF-I (formerly called somatomedin C), and IGF-II—that have approximately 50% of their amino acids in common. Whereas insulin is synthesized in the pancreas as proinsulin, which is cleaved to form insulin and C peptide, IGFs are synthesized primarily in the liver, and they retain the C peptide.

The IGF usually produced by the above-mentioned neoplasms is a prohormone form of IGF-II termed "big IGF-II" because of its higher-than-normal molecular weight. Big IGF-II causes hypoglycemia by stimulating the uptake of glucose by the tumor, by inhibiting hepatic glucose uptake, and by enhancing the disposal of glucose into insulin-responsive tissues such as muscle and fat. Big

IGF-II has a reduced ability to interact with the IGF-binding protein complex; this leads to an increase in the bioavailability of big IGF-II.[56]

Acromegaly. Paraneoplastic acromegaly, seen especially with pancreatic islet cell tumors and bronchial carcinoids, is usually due to the secretion of growth hormone–releasing hormone.[57] Paraneoplastic acromegaly can also be caused by ectopic production of growth hormone, but this is extremely rare.[58]

Secondary Erythrocytosis. Some tumors cause polycythemia by producing an excess of erythropoietin, the hormone that stimulates the production of erythrocytes in the bone marrow. Since erythropoietin is normally secreted by the kidney, it is not surprising that the most common types of neoplasms associated with its production are renal carcinomas.[59]

Hypocalcemia. Medullary carcinoma of the thyroid can secrete calcitonin, a hormone normally synthesized by the C cells of the thyroid that induces hypocalcemia by inhibiting bone reabsorption and by increasing the renal excretion of calcium. Paraneoplastic hypocalcemia is usually asymptomatic, but tetany and seizures have been reported.[60]

Hypertension and Hypokalemia. Cancer cells can secrete renin and induce hypertension and hypokalemia. In some patients, inactive renin (prorenin) constitutes 90% of the total plasma renin concentration.[61] Paraneoplastic hypertension may also result from overproduction of angiotensin I.[62]

Humoral Hypercalcemia of Malignancy. Hypercalcemia is a common metabolic problem in patients with cancer; it is seen in approximately 15% of patients with metastatic disease. Normally, the serum calcium concentration is regulated by three hormones: parathyroid hormone (PTH), calcitonin, and vitamin D. Parathyroid hormone promotes calcium reabsorption in the distal nephron and enhances the conversion of 25-hydroxycholecalciferol to 1,25-dihydroxycholecalciferol (also called 1,25-dihydroxyvitamin D). Parathyroid hormone also activates both osteoblasts and osteoclasts, enhancing the rate of bony calcium turnover. Calcitonin counters these effects by suppressing osteoclast activity and stimulating the deposition of calcium in the skeleton. 1,25-dihydroxycholecalciferol, which is the active form of vitamin D, increases the intestinal absorption of calcium. It should be remembered that "vitamin D" is actually a misnomer because 1,25-dihydroxycholecalciferol is a hormone, not a vitamin (ie, a coenzyme).

Hypercalcemia of malignancy can be mediated by the following substances: (1) 1,25-dihydroxyvitamin D, produced mainly by lymphomas;[63] (2) cytokines that activate osteoclasts and promote bone resorption, such as interleukin-1, transforming growth factor alpha, and prostaglandins of the E family[64] (the previously described "osteoclast-activating factor" produced by multiple myeloma cells is actually a mixture of these cytokines); (3) PTH (which is produced by cancer cells very rarely);[65] and (4) PTH-related protein (PTH-RP), which is the most common cause of humoral hypercalcemia of malignancy.[66]

Like PTH, PTH-RP increases calcium resorption from bone and decreases the renal excretion of calcium, inducing hypercalcemia, hypercalciuria, hypophosphatemia, and hyperphosphaturia. The pathogenesis of humoral hypercalcemia of malignancy resembles that of Jansen's metaphyseal chondrodysplasia, a rare genetic disease characterized by short-limbed dwarfism, hypercalcemia, and hypophosphatemia. However, whereas humoral hypercalcemia of malignancy is related to an increased level of PTH-RP, the hypercalcemia associated with Jansen's metaphyseal chondrodysplasia is due to a DNA mutation that results in a constitutively activated PTH-RP receptor.[67]

The *PTH-RP* gene is able to generate three proteins because of alternative splicing of the messenger ribonucleic acids (mRNAs). The proteins contain 139, 141, and 173 amino acids, and the first 139 amino acids are common to all three proteins (Figure 5–4). Parathyroid hormone–related protein is produced not only by cancer cells but also (at low levels) by many normal tissues such as bone, skin, stomach, brain, vascular endothelium, placenta, and lactating breast tissue.[68] In contrast, PTH is produced only in the parathyroid glands. Parathyroid hormone and PTH-RP share a sequence homology (eight amino acids in the aminoterminal portion) and bind to a common receptor (PTH/PTH-RP receptor) with equal affinity. Thus, some of the biologic effects of PTH-RP are PTH-like; both PTH and PTH-RP promote bone resorption and reduce the renal excretion of calcium, thereby increasing serum levels of calcium. However, other effects of PTH-RP are different from those of PTH; PTH-RP is involved in the normal lactation process, in placental calcium transport, and in keratinocyte differentiation in the skin.[66,69] Thus, other receptors must be involved.

In the plasma of usual subjects, PTH-RP is not detectable; PTH-RP is detectable only in lactating women, fetuses, and most patients with humoral hypercalcemia of malignancy. This suggests that PTH-RP is not a hormone but a cytokine because it exerts paracrine or autocrine actions in the tissues in which it is normally produced. To clarify the physiologic role of PTH-RP, experiments of ablation and overexpression of the *PTH-RP* gene have been performed in mice. Knockout mice that are homozygous for the deletion of the *PTH-RP* gene show accelerated differentiation of the endochondral bone, which results in the development of short limbs.[70] On the other hand,

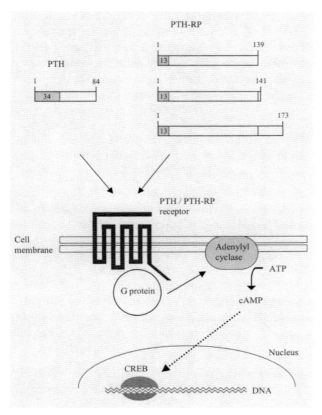

Figure 5–4. Mechanism of action of parathyroid hormone–related protein (PTH-RP). The shaded portion in the PTH molecule corresponds to the amino terminal 34 amino acids possessing full biologic activity. The shaded portion in the PTH-RP molecules corresponds to the region homologous with PTH. The PTH/PTH-RP receptor is a protein containing seven transmembrane-spanning domains and linked to G protein. Binding of PTH or PTH-RP to the extracellular portion of the receptor activates the G protein, and this initates the production of two "second messengers": (1) cAMP, that binds to and activates CREB, a DNA-binding protein that controls the transcription of specific genes; and (2) inositol 1,4,5-triphosphate, induces the release of calcium stores within the cytoplasm (not shown here). ATP = adenosine triphosphate; cAMP = cyclic adenosine monophosphate; CREB = cAMP response element-binding protein; DNA = deoxyribonucleic acid.

transgenic mice in which the *PTH-RP* gene is overexpressed show delayed differentiation of the endochondral bone and delayed osteogenesis.[71] Of interest, the pathologic findings in the latter mice resemble those of Jansen's metaphyseal chondrodysplasia. The mechanism by which cancer cells activate the *PTH-RP* gene is unknown, but a study has shown that the transcription of this gene is activated by the oncogenes *src* and *ras*.[68]

Syndromes Due to Antibodies

Tumor antigens stimulate the formation of antibodies that sometimes cross-react with normal tissues and damage them. In recent years, intense research has led to

important advances in the understanding of the pathophysiology of several neurologic syndromes that occur in patients with cancer. It is now known that many of these syndromes are mediated by autoantibodies that react against neuronlike components of the tumor cells.[72]

Eaton-Lambert Syndrome. Eaton-Lambert syndrome is a paraneoplastic neurologic disorder characterized by myasthenia (proximal muscle weakness, especially of the pelvic girdle) and most often associated with SCLC. The central pathogenic role of antibodies in Eaton-Lambert syndrome has been demonstrated by elegant experiments in animals; in mice injected with the immunoglobulin G (IgG) fraction of serum from a patient with Eaton-Lambert syndrome, a profound neuromuscular transmission defect developed (Figure 5–5).[73] Normally, acetylcholine is released from storage vesicles in response to an action potential; this mechanism requires the regulated influx of calcium through voltage-gated channels in nerve terminals. Patients with Eaton-Lambert syndrome have autoantibodies in their serum that are directed against voltage-gated calcium channels of the anti-P/Q type,[74] which regulate the influx of calcium and induce the release of acetylcholine from the storage vesicle (see Figure 5–5). In patients with Eaton-Lambert syndrome, the presence of anti–calcium channel antibodies impairs the presynaptic release of acetylcholine at the neuromuscular junction.[73,75] It is interesting that Eaton-Lambert syndrome is also seen in patients without cancer, in which case it is an autoimmune disease.

Myasthenia Gravis. Paraneoplastic myasthenia gravis, which develops in about 40% of patients with thymomas, is associated with the presence of helper T cell–dependent autoantibodies directed against the postsynaptic acetylcholine receptor (AChR) of the neuromuscular junction. These autoantibodies block the interaction of acetylcholine with AChR and thus impair neuromuscular transmission (see Figure 5–5). It has been shown that thymoma cells express subunits of AChR and sensitize developing thymocytes or recirculating peripheral T cells against AChR epitopes.[76]

Encephalopathy. Paraneoplastic encephalopathy is characterized by cognitive dysfunction (dementia) and myelopathy and occurs mainly in patients with SCLC (most commonly) and breast cancer. Paraneoplastic encephalopathy is associated with the presence of anti-neuronal nuclear autoantibodies type 1 (ANNA-1, or anti-Hu) and type 2 (ANNA-2, or anti-Ri), which are so named because they react with a group of proteins contained in the nuclei of neurons.[72] It has been shown that Hu, the protein recognized by the anti-Hu antibody, is responsible for the synthesis of a nuclear protein involved in neuronal development in *Drosophila*.[77] In patients with breast cancer, the involved antibodies are ANNA-2.

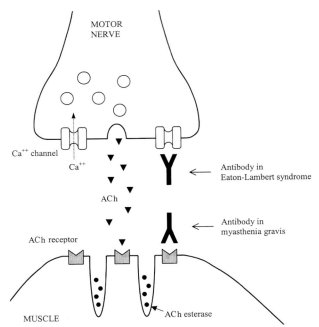

Figure 5–5. Schematic representation of the neuromuscular junction. Normally, when the nerve action potential invades the nerve terminal, the release of acetylcholine (ACh) activates muscle contraction. In paraneoplastic Eaton-Lambert syndrome and myasthenia gravis, the presence of antibodies disrupts the normal communication between the nerve and muscle (see text for details). Ca = calcium.

(labels in figure: MOTOR NERVE; Ca⁺⁺ channel — Ca^{++} channel; Ca^{++}; ACh; ACh receptor; MUSCLE; ACh esterase; Antibody in Eaton-Lambert syndrome; Antibody in myasthenia gravis)

Cerebellar Degeneration. Paraneoplastic cerebellar degeneration is a very disabling syndrome; most affected patients are unable to walk without assistance. The pathologic change characteristic of this syndrome is the diffuse or patchy loss of Purkinje's cells in the cerebellum. Affected patients have been found to have autoantibodies in their serum and cerebrospinal fluid that react with both the neoplastic cells and the cerebellar tissue.[72,78] Many patients with cerebellar degeneration in the course of breast and gynecologic cancers have an antibody called anti-Yo in their serum; this antibody has been shown to react with Purkinje's cells of the cerebellum. The ANNA-1 and ANNA-2 antibodies are involved as well; ANNA-1 has been found primarily in patients with SCLC, and ANNA-2 has been found primarily in patients with breast cancer.

Motor Neuropathy. Paraneoplastic motor neuropathy is characterized by the loss of anterior horn cells in the spinal cord, which results in an impairment of motor function and in sensory sparing. Paraneoplastic motor neuropathy is associated with SCLC and with lymphomas. Type-1 antineuronal nuclear autoantibodies have been detected in the serum of patients with SCLC and motor neuropathy.[72]

Subacute Sensory Neuropathy. Paraneoplastic subacute sensory neuropathy is characterized by the loss of sensory

function, proprioception, and vibration sensation. Pain, temperature, and touch sensation are affected to a lesser degree. The sensory ataxia can leave patients in a bedridden state. Paraneoplastic subacute sensory neuropathy is associated primarily with SCLC. Pathologically, this syndrome is characterized by neuronal loss, degeneration of axons, and demyelination in dorsal and posterior roots of the spinal cord. The damage seems to be mediated by the ANNA-1 antibody, which reacts with both the neoplastic cells and the neurons of the dorsal root ganglia.[79]

Opsoclonus/Myoclonus. The term "opsoclonus" refers to irregular multidirectional eye movements that persist after eye closure. The term "myoclonus" refers to brief jerking contractions of muscles. Approximately 20% of adults and 50% of children who present with opsoclonus/myoclonus are found to have an underlying neoplasm, usually a neuroblastoma (in children) or a carcinoma of the lung or breast (in adults). Paraneoplastic opsoclonus/myoclonus occurs in approximately 2% of children with neuroblastoma, and it is often the presenting symptom. The ANNA-2 antibody has been found in the serum of patients with this syndrome in the course of breast cancer.[80]

Autonomic Neuropathy. Paraneoplastic autonomic neuropathy is a severe subacute disorder characterized mainly by postural tachycardia and gastrointestinal dysmotility. Recently, the pathogenesis of this syndrome has been attributed to the presence of autoantibodies against ganglionic AChRs.[81] Intestinal pseudo-obstruction, usually associated with SCLC, is a form of autonomic neuropathy. The serum of affected patients contains IgG antibodies that react with neurons of the myenteric and submucosal plexus of the gastrointestinal tract.[82]

Glomerulonephritis. The most common form of glomerulonephritis seen in patients with cancer is membranous glomerulonephritis. It is caused by the deposition of immune complexes in the glomerular membrane. The involved tumor antigens may be fetal proteins.[83] Patients with paraneoplastic immunoglobulin A (IgA) nephropathy have an immune injury of the glomeruli due to a tumor-induced antigen-antibody response.[84]

Retinopathy. Paraneoplastic retinopathy is characterized by the rapid onset of blindness secondary to degeneration of photoreceptors. Several studies in patients with paraneoplastic retinopathy have documented the presence of antibodies reacting with both cancer and retinal cells (either the retinal ganglion cells or the photoreceptors).[85,86] The involved antigen has been identified as a recoverin-like protein.[87] Recoverin is a calcium-binding protein that is present in retinal rods and cones and that is involved in the transduction of light by photoreceptors.

Pemphigus. Patients with paraneoplastic pemphigus have been found to have serum autoantibodies that react with desmoplakin I, a protein found in desmosomes of epithelial cells.[88] This finding indicates that the appearance of bullae in the skin and mucosae of affected patients is due to the loss of normal cell-to-cell adhesion in the epidermis.

Autoimmune Hemolytic Anemia. Autoimmune hemolytic anemia can be mediated by two types of autoantibodies: warm antibodies and cold antibodies. The anemia mediated by warm antibodies (IgG) is seen mainly in patients with B-cell lymphomas and leukemias. In these cases, the hemolysis is extravascular (ie, it involves phagocytosis by the spleen). The anemia mediated by cold antibodies is associated with intravascular hemolysis. A cold antibody is a complement-fixing immunoglobulin M (IgM) that leaves the surface of red blood cells in the warm visceral circulation but attacks red blood cell membranes at cold temperatures. The clinical manifestations of autoimmune hemolytic anemia are related to small-vessel occlusion and include acrocyanosis of the ears, the tip of the nose, the fingers, and the toes.

Autoimmune anemia in patients with cancer is not always characterized by hemolysis in the peripheral blood; pure red cell aplasia, a paraneoplastic syndrome seen in about 5% of patients with thymoma, is characterized by decreased reticulocytes in the peripheral blood and the absence of erythroblasts in the bone marrow. Immunoglobulin G autoantibodies that destroy the erythroblasts have been found in the serum of affected patients.

Idiopathic Thrombocytopenic Purpura. Idiopathic thrombocytopenic purpura, which is associated with the production of antiplatelet antibodies, can complicate the course of lymphomas and several types of carcinomas.[89]

REFERENCES

1. Klastersky J, Daneau D, Verhest A. Causes of death in patients with cancer. Eur J Cancer 1972;8:149–54.
2. Zetter BR. The cellular basis of site-specific tumor metastasis. N Engl J Med 1990;332:605–12.
3. Nicolson GL. Differential organ tissue adhesion, invasion and growth properties of metastatic rat mammary adenocarcinoma cells. Breast Cancer Res Treat 1988;12:167–76.
4. Takada A, Ohmori K, Yoneda T, et al. Contribution of carbohydrate antigens sialyl Lewis A and sialyl Lewis X to adhesion of human cancer cells to vascular endothelium. Cancer Res 1993;53:345–61.
5. Kohn EC, Francis EA, Liotta LA, et al. Heterogeneity of the motility responses in malignant tumor cells: a biological basis for the diversity and homing of metastatic cells. Int J Cancer 1990;46:287–92.
6. Heitzman ER, Markarian B, Raasch BN, et al. Pathways of tumor spread through the lung: radiologic correlations with anatomy and pathology. Radiology 1982;144:3–14.
7. Schoen FJ, Berger BM, Guerina NG. Cardiac effects of noncardiac neoplasms. Cardiol Clin 1984;2:657–70.
8. Agatston AS, Robinson ML, Trigo L, et al. Echocardiographic findings in primary pericardial mesothelioma. Am Heart J 1986;111:986–8.
9. Cates C, Virmani R, Vaughn W, et al. Electrocardiographic markers of cardiac metastasis. Am Heart J 1986;112:1297–303.
10. Koiwaya Y, Nakamura M, Yamamoto K. Progressive ECG alterations in metastatic cardiac mural tumor. Am Heart J 1983;105:339–41.
11. Jeon HM, Kim JS, Oh ST, et al. Ileo-rectal fistula complicating advanced ovarian carcinoma. Oncol Rep 1999;6:1243–7.
12. McGuire BM, Cherwitz DL, Rabe KM, et al. Small-cell carcinoma of the lung manifesting as acute hepatic failure. Mayo Clin Proc 1997;72:133–9.
13. Arguello F, Baggs RB, Duerst RE, et al. Pathogenesis of vertebral metastases and epidural spinal cord compression. Cancer 1990;65:98–106.
14. Geldof AA. Models for cancer skeletal metastasis: a reappraisal of Batson's plexus. Anticancer Res 1997;17:1535–9.
15. Galasko CSB. Mechanism of lytic and blastic metastatic disease of bone. Clin Orthop 1982;169:120–7.
16. Hipp JA, Rosenberg AE, Hayes WC. Mechanical properties of trabecular bone within and adjacent to osseous metastases. J Bone Miner Res 1992;7:1165–71.
17. Gainor BJ, Buchert P. Fracture healing in metastatic bone disease. Clin Orthop 1983;178:297–302.
18. Klein P, Haley EC, Wooten GF, et al. Focal cerebral infarctions associated with perivascular tumor infiltrates in carcinomatous leptomeningeal metastases. Arch Neurol 1989;46:1149–52.
19. Nicolson GL, Kawaguchi T, Kawaguchi M, et al. Brain surface invasion and metastasis of murine malignant melanoma variants. J Neurooncol 1986;4:209–18.
20. Varakis JN, Kase CS, Wilborn WH, et al. Pathogenesis of an experimental meningeal leukemia model. Clin Immunol Immunopathol 1982;23:400–7.
21. Rosen ST, Aisner J, Makuch RW, et al. Carcinomatous leptomeningitis in small cell lung cancer: a clinicopathologic review of the National Cancer Institute experience. Medicine 1982;61:45–53.
22. Redman BG, Tapazoglou E, Al-Sarraf M. Meningeal carcinomatosis in head and neck cancer: report of six cases and review of the literature. Cancer 1986;58:2656–61.
23. Boerman RH, Maassen EM, Joosten J, et al. Trigeminal neuropathy secondary to perineural invasion of head and neck carcinomas. Neurology 1999;13:213–6.
24. Vanek VW, Al-Salti M. Acute pseudo-obstruction of the colon (Ogilvie's syndrome): an analysis of 400 cases. Dis Colon Rectum 1986;29:203–10.
25. Shimaoka K, Vanherle AJ, Dindogru A. Thyrotoxicosis secondary to involvement of the thyroid with malignant lymphoma. J Clin Endocrinol Metab 1976;43:64–8.
26. Redman BG, Pazdur R, Zingas AP, et al. Prospective evaluation of adrenal insufficiency in patients with adrenal masses. Cancer 1987;60:103–7.
27. Lutz A, Stojkovic M, Schmidt M, et al. Adrenocortical function in patients with macrometastases of the adrenal gland. Eur J Endocrinol 2000;143:91–7.

28. Morita A, Meyer FB, Laws ER Jr. Symptomatic pituitary metastases. J Neurosurg 1998;89:69–73.

29. Sise JG, Crichlow RW. Obstruction due to malignant tumors. Semin Oncol 1978;5:213–24.

30. Baumgartner WA, Mark JB. Metastatic malignancies from distant sites to the tracheobronchial tree. J Thorac Cardiovasc Surg 1980;79:499–503.

31. Gutman M, Inbar M, Klausner JM. Metastases-induced acute pancreatitis: a rare manifestation of cancer. Eur J Surg Oncol 1993;19:302–4.

32. Kakulas BA, Harper CG, Shibasaki K, et al. Vertebral metastases and spinal cord compression. Clin Exp Neurol 1978;15:98–113.

33. Markman M. Common complications and emergencies associated with cancer and its therapy. Cleve Clin J Med 1994;61:105–14.

34. Willson JKV, Masaryl TJ. Neurologic emergencies in the cancer patient. Semin Oncol 1989;16:490–503.

35. Kato A, Ushio Y, Hayakawa T, et al. Circulatory disturbance of the spinal cord with epidural neoplasm in rats. J Neurosurg 1985;63:260–5.

36. Goodman R. Superior vena cava syndrome. Clinical management. JAMA 1975;231:58–61.

37. Dombernowsky P, Hansen HH. Combination chemotherapy in the management of superior vena caval obstruction in small-cell anaplastic carcinoma of the lung. Acta Med Scand 1978;204:513–6.

38. Miller RR, McGregor DH. Hemorrhage from carcinoma of the lung. Cancer 1980;46:200–5.

39. Allum WH, Brearley S, Wheatley KE, et al. Acute hemorrhage from gastric malignancy. Br J Surg 1990;77:19–20.

40. Danikas D, Theodorou SJ, Kotrotsios J, et al. Hemoperitoneum from spontaneous bleeding of a uterine leiomyoma: a case report. Am Surg 1999;65:1180–2.

41. Graus F, Rogers LR, Posner JB. Cerebrovascular complications in patients with cancer. Medicine 1985;64:16–35.

42. Sapone FM, Reyes CV. Unusual faces of lung cancer. J Surg Oncol 1985;30:1–5.

43. Cilley RE, Strodel WF, Peterson RO. Causes of death in carcinomas of the esophagus. Am J Gastroenterol 1989;84:147–9.

44. Rodriguez-Panadero F, Lopez-Mejias J. Low glucose and pH levels in malignant pleural effusions. Am Rev Respir Dis 1989;139:663–7.

45. McKenna RJ, Ali MK, Ewer MS, et al. Pleural and pericardial effusions in cancer patients. Curr Probl Cancer 1985;9:1–44.

46. Leff A, Hopewell PC, Costello J. Pleural effusion from malignancy. Ann Intern Med 1978;88:532–7.

47. Maher GG, Berger HW. Massive pleural effusion: malignant and nonmalignant causes in 46 patients. Am Rev Respir Dis 1972;105:458–60.

48. Onuigbo WI. The spread of lung cancer to the heart, pericardium, and great vessels. Jpn Heart J 1974;15:234–8.

49. Shabetai R, Mangiardi L, Bhargava V, et al. The pericardium and cardiac function. Prog Cardiovasc Dis 1979;22:107–34.

50. Nagy JA, Herzberg KT, Dvorak JM, et al. Pathogenesis of malignant ascites formation: initiating events that lead to fluid accumulation. Cancer Res 1993;53:2631–43.

51. Kurtz RC, Bronzo RL. Does spontaneous bacterial peritonitis occur in malignant ascites? Am J Gastroenterol 1982;77:146–8.

52. Pearse AG. Common cytochemical and ultrastructural characteristics of cells producing polypeptide hormones (the APUD series) and their relevance to thyroid and ultimobranchial C cells and calcitonin. Proc R Soc London Biol Sci 1968;170:71–80.

53. Pierce ST. Paraendocrine syndromes. Curr Opin Oncol 1993;5:639–45.

54. Stewart PM, Gibson S, Crosby SR, et al. ACTH precursors characterize the ectopic ACTH syndrome. Clin Endocrinol 1994;40:199–204.

55. Wolfsen AR, Odell WD. ProACTH: use for early detection of lung cancer. Am J Med 1979;66:765–72.

56. Baxter RC. The role of insulin-like growth factors and their binding proteins in tumor hypoglycemia. Horm Res 1996;46:195–201.

57. Barkan AL, Shenker Y, Grekin RJ, et al. Acromegaly due to ectopic growth hormone (GH)-releasing hormone (GHRH) production: dynamic studies of GH and ectopic GHRH secretion. J Clin Endocrinol Metab 1986;63:1057–64.

58. Melmed S, Ezrin C, Kovacs K, et al. Acromegaly due to secretion of growth hormone by an ectopic pancreatic islet-cell tumor. N Engl J Med 1985;312:9–17.

59. Thorling EB. Paraneoplastic erythrocytosis and inappropriate erythropoietin production. Scand J Haematol Suppl 1972;17:1–166.

60. Tashjian AH, Wolfe HJ, Voelkel EF. Human calcitonin: immunologic assay, cytologic localization and studies of medullary thyroid carcinoma. Am J Med 1974;56:840–9.

61. Kew MC, Leckie BJ, Greeff MC. Arterial hypertension as a paraneoplastic phenomenon in hepatocellular carcinoma. Arch Intern Med 1989;149:2111–3.

62. Arai H, Saitoh S, Matsumoto T, et al. Hypertension as a paraneoplastic syndrome in hepatocellular carcinoma. J Gastroenterol 1999;34:530–4.

63. Rosenthal N, Insogna KL, Godsall JW, et al. Elevations in circulating 1,25-dihydroxyvitamin D in three patients with lymphoma-associated hypercalcemia. J Clin Endocrinol Metab 1985;60:29–33.

64. Rosol TJ, Capen CC. Mechanisms of cancer-induced hypercalcemia. Lab Invest 1992;67:680–702.

65. Rizzoli R, Pache JC, Didierjean L, et al. A thymoma as a cause of true ectopic hyperparathyroidism. J Clin Endocrinol Metab 1994;79:912–5.

66. De Papp A, Stewart AF. Parathyroid hormone-related protein: a peptide of diverse physiologic functions. Trends Endocrinol Metab 1993;4:181–7.

67. Schipani E, Kruse K, Juppner H. A constitutively active mutant PTH-PTHrP receptor in Jansen-type metaphyseal chondrodysplasia. Science 1995;268:98–100.

68. Li X, Drucker DJ. Parathyroid hormone-related peptide is a downstream target for ras and src activation. J Biol Chem 1994;269:6263–6.

69. Thiede MA, Rodan GA. Expression of a calcium-mobilizing parathyroid hormone-like peptide in lactating mammary tissue. Science 1988;242:278–80.

70. Karaplis AC, Luz A, Glovacki J, et al. Lethal skeletal dysplasia from targeted disruption of the parathyroid hormone-related peptide gene. Genes Dev 1994;8:277–89.

71. Herderson JE, Amizuka N, Warshawsky H, et al. Nucleolar localization of parathyroid hormone-related peptide enhances survival of chondrocytes under conditions that promote apoptotic cell death. Mol Cell Biol 1995;15:4064–75.

72. Lennon VA. Paraneoplastic autoantibodies: the case for a descriptive generic nomenclature. Neurology 1994;44:2236–40.

73. Lambert EH, Lennon VA. Selected IgG rapidly induces Lambert-Eaton myasthenic syndrome in mice: complement independence and EMG abnormalities. Muscle Nerve 1988;11:1133–45.

74. Lennon VA, Kryzer TJ, Griesmann GE, et al. Calcium-channel antibodies in the Lambert-Eaton syndrome and other paraneoplastic syndromes. N Engl J Med 1995;332:1467–74.

75. Roberts A, Perera S, Lang B, et al. Paraneoplastic myasthenic syndrome IgG inhibits 45Ca2+flux in a human small cell carcinoma line. Nature 1985;317:737–9.

76. Nagvekar N, Moody AM, Moss P, et al. A pathogenetic role for the thymoma in myasthenia gravis. Autosensitization of IL-4-producing T cell clones recognizing extracellular acetylcholine receptor epitopes presented by minority class II isotypes. J Clin Invest 1998;101:2268–77.

77. Sekido Y, Bader SA, Carbone DP, et al. Molecular analysis of the HuD gene encoding a paraneoplastic encephalomyelitis antigen in human lung cancer cell lines. Cancer Res 1994;54:4988–92.

78. Furneaux HM, Rosenblum MK, Dalmau J, et al. Selective expression of Purkinje-cell antigens in tumor tissue from patients with paraneoplastic cerebellar degeneration. N Engl J Med 1990;322:1844–51.

79. Graus F, Elkon KB, Cordon-Cardo C, et al. Sensory neuronopathy and small cell lung cancer. Antineuronal antibody that also reacts with the tumor. Am J Med 1986;80:45–52.

80. Buckanovich RJ, Posner JB, Darnell RB. Nova, the paraneoplastic Ri antigen, is homologous to an RNA-binding protein and is specifically expressed in the developing motor system. Neuron 1993;11:657–72.

81. Vernino S, Low PA, Fealey RD, et al. Autoantibodies to ganglionic acetylcholine receptors in autoimmune autonomic neuropathies. N Engl J Med 2000;343:847–55.

82. Lennon VA, Sas DF, Busk MF, et al. Enteric neuronal autoantibodies in pseudoobstruction with small-cell lung carcinoma. Gastroenterology 1991;100:137–42.

83. Kaplan BS, Klassen J, Gault MH, et al. Glomerular injury in patients with neoplasia. Annu Rev Med 1977;27:117–25.

84. Magyarlaki T, Kiss B, Buzogany I, et al. Renal cell carcinoma and paraneoplastic IgA nephropathy. Nephron 1999;82:127–30.

85. Grunwald GB, Klein R, Simmonds MA, et al. Autoimmune basis for visual paraneoplastic syndrome in patients with small-cell lung carcinoma. Lancet 1985;1:658–61.

86. Kornguth SE, Klein R, Appen R, et al. Occurrence of anti-retinal ganglion cell antibodies in patients with small cell carcinoma of the lung. Cancer 1982;50:1289–93.

87. Polans AS, Witkowska D, Haley TL, et al. Recoverin, a photoreceptor-specific calcium-binding protein, is expressed by the tumor of a patient with cancer-associated retinopathy. Proc Natl Acad Sci U S A 1995;92:9176–80.

88. Anhalt GJ, Kim SC, Stanley JR, et al. Paraneoplastic pemphigus. An autoimmune mucocutaneous disease associated with neoplasia. N Engl J Med 1990;323:1729–35.

89. Kim HD, Boggs DR. A syndrome resembling idiopathic thrombocytopenic purpura in 10 patients with diverse forms of cancer. Am J Med 1979;67:371–7.

CHAPTER 6

PATHOPHYSIOLOGY OF EMERGENCY ILLNESS DUE TO TREATMENT OF CANCER

GIAMPAOLO TALAMO, MD

COMPLICATIONS OF SURGERY

Surgery has many applications in the management of cancer; it is the treatment of choice for most localized solid neoplasms and often represents the only chance for cure. Surgical procedures are also performed for diagnostic purposes (eg, for biopsy or staging), cancer prevention, hormonal ablation, disease palliation, reconstruction, and the insertion of vascular devices.

For a variety of reasons, oncologic surgery is often more difficult than surgery performed for other diseases. First, the organ resection in most cases must be wider than usual because it is impossible to define macroscopically the precise boundary between normal tissue and cancerous infiltration. Often, tumor extends to a greater area than was expected on the basis of imaging studies, and surgical procedures may take longer than anticipated. Second, cancers may present with related conditions (such as hemorrhage, obstruction, or perforation of hollow viscera) that require emergent surgical procedures that increase the risk of perioperative mortality.[1] Third, cancer patients are often debilitated and subject to complications due to their disease or its treatment. For example, patients may be neutropenic or thrombocytopenic as a result of chemotherapy-induced myelosuppression.[2] Finally, many patients with cancer who undergo surgery also undergo preoperative or postoperative chemotherapy or radiotherapy, and the toxicities induced by these modalities can add to the morbidity due to surgery alone.

Factors Influencing the Occurrence of Surgical Complications

Factors Related to the Patient. Patients with severe compromise in pulmonary, renal, hepatic, or cardiovascular function may be unable to undergo major surgical procedures. Therefore, a tumor that is considered resectable on the basis of technical considerations may be inoperable in light of the patient's general medical condition. Age alone is not a contraindication to major surgery. However, the preoperative assessment of elderly patients should take into account that advanced age is often associated with decreased organ function (eg, decreased myocardial reserve) and comorbid conditions.[3,4]

The cardiovascular system should always be assessed before a surgical intervention because cardiac events, including arrhythmias, myocardial infarction, unstable angina, and congestive heart failure, are the factors most responsible for perioperative mortality (ie, deaths occurring within 30 days after a surgical procedure). Criteria that indicate a high risk of cardiac events during surgery include myocardial infarction in the previous 6 months, angina, hemodynamically significant valvular heart disease, atrial fibrillation, and a left-ventricle ejection fraction < 50%. Arrhythmias are often precipitated by hypoxemia, medications, fever, and electrolyte abnormalities. Surgery in a patient with ischemic heart disease puts the patient at risk for myocardial infarction and death, especially if the patient has had a recent ischemic event; a major operation performed within 3 months after a myocardial infarction results in a re-infarction in 27% of patients, but this percentage falls to 6% for patients who have surgery performed more than 6 months after the myocardial infarction.[5] It is important to note that 60% of perioperative myocardial infarctions are silent. Among valvular heart diseases, significant aortic stenosis poses a particular surgical risk because it causes a fixed cardiac output that cannot increase in response to surgical stress.

Factors Related to the Affected Organ. The reserve of the affected organ varies, depending on a patient's lifestyle and diseases. In some cases, the organ may be so severely compromised that resection of a primary tumor in the organ is risky or even lethal. For example, severe liver cirrhosis, a common finding in patients with hepatocellular carcinoma, often prohibits any resection more extensive than a segmentectomy. Likewise, chronic lung disease, a common finding in patients with lung cancer, contributes to the increased complication rates observed in patients with surgically resected lung cancer, compared to patients without lung cancer who require pulmonary resection.[6] The risk of hypoventilation or lung atelectasis is increased by any condition that decreases the pulmonary reserve (eg, chronic obstructive pulmonary disease, obesity, and cigarette smoking). Arterial blood gases are often measured and pulmonary function tests are often performed before surgery, to obtain a functional assessment of the lung. If the forced expiratory volume in 1 second (FEV_1) is > 2 L, the patient can safely undergo the surgical procedure whereas if FEV_1 is < 1 L, the risk of postoperative pulmonary complications is particularly high.

Factors Related to the Cancer. A tumor's location and size will influence the technical approach to surgery and the complexity of the procedure. In addition, a neoplasm can have a profound influence on the perioperative management of a patient because the presence of the tumor produces both anatomic and physiologic effects.[7] Examples of anatomic effects are airway obstruction due to head and neck cancer, respiratory compromise due to mediastinal masses, and cardiac tamponade due to malignant pericardial effusions. Examples of physiologic effects are the hormonal syndromes induced by endocrine tumors. These syndromes include wide swings in blood glucose concentrations in patients with insulinoma; hypokalemia and hypertension in patients with adrenocortical neoplasms; dangerous elevations in blood pressure, caused by the release of catecholamines following the surgical removal of pheochromocytomas; and severe hypotension, hypertension, tachycardia, or bronchospasm due to the surgical manipulation of carcinoid tumors.[8] All of these endocrine effects pose special risks for the anesthetic management of patients with cancer.

Factors Related to the Surgery. The type, length, and technical complexity of a surgical procedure are major determinants of perioperative risk. Any operation that requires general anesthesia can be complicated by hypotension, which can precipitate a vascular event in the brain or cause renal failure. The longer the period of anesthesia, the higher the risk of hypotension. Although it is generally believed that spinal anesthesia is safer than general anesthesia, this is not true from a cardiopulmonary standpoint because spinal anesthesia can also cause vasodilation and cardiovascular collapse. The risk of surgical complications is also affected by the experience of the anesthesiologist and surgeon.

The following complications can occur with any type of major surgery, regardless of the specific procedure: hemorrhage; cardiopulmonary, renal, or liver dysfunction; nutritional deficiencies; fluid, electrolyte, and metabolic abnormalities; and thromboembolic events (ie, deep venous thrombosis and pulmonary embolism). The risk of deep venous thrombosis and pulmonary embolism is particularly important in oncologic surgery because 70% of cancer patients have a hypercoagulable state.

Selected Surgical Procedures and Specific Associated Complications

Thoracic Surgery. The most common complications of thoracic surgery are pulmonary: respiratory failure, pneumonia, pleural effusion, bronchopleural fistula with empyema, and pulmonary embolism.[9] Respiratory failure is occasionally related to phrenic-nerve damage. Unilateral paralysis of a recurrent laryngeal nerve caused by damage during thoracic surgery causes dysphonia, hoarseness, and symptomatic aspiration.[10]

Esophagectomy. Esophagectomy can cause tracheal lacerations, chylothorax, strictures, and esophagovisceral anastomotic leaks. Anastomoses are more likely to leak if they are hand-sewn or single-layer anastomoses as opposed to stapled or double-layer anastomoses.[11] Extensive lymphadenectomy performed during surgical removal of the abdominal esophagus can cause ascites and massive pleural effusion due to disruption of the lymphatic drainage system.[12]

Gastric Resection. Gastric resection can be complicated by anastomotic failure, hemorrhage, cholecystitis, pancreatitis, and pulmonary problems. Ileus can occur secondary to adhesions. Gastric resection can also cause pernicious anemia (due to reduced absorption of vitamin B_{12}) and dumping syndrome (due to dysfunctional emptying of food). Anastomotic leaks account for about one-half of surgery-related deaths after total gastrectomy.[13]

Intestinal Resection. Intestinal resection and abdominal surgery in general can be complicated by the development of fistulae, adhesions, mechanical obstruction, and problems related to anastomoses.

Pancreatoduodenectomy. Pancreatoduodenectomy (Whipple's operation) for pancreatic cancer can be complicated by pancreatic fistulae, biliary leakage, and stomal ulcerations. This operation involves the invagination of the pancreas into the jejunum. The required ligation of arterial vessels may lead to necrosis and sloughing of the pancreatic side of the surgical anastomosis, resulting in a pancreatic leak. Although most leaks are not clinically relevant, they occasionally require surgical repair or drainage.[14] Biliary leakage occurs when surgical mobilization disrupts the vascularization of the common bile duct (mainly the retroportal artery). This leads to necrosis and stenosis of the duct.[15] Ulcers of the surgical stoma (the gastrojejunal margin) are a frequent complication of Whipple's operation. The formation of these ulcers is promoted by the decrease in secretin, enterogastrone, and other hormones that are secreted by the pancreas and duodenum and that normally inhibit gastric acid secretion. Vagotomy during pancreatoduodenectomy protects against stomal ulcers,[16] which indicates that vagal stimuli contribute to the pathogenesis of such ulcers.

The removal of pancreatic tissue also leads to deterioration of both the endocrine and exocrine functions of the pancreas. A complete lack of insulin induces secondary diabetes mellitus. Postoperative glucose metabolism is dependent not only on the amount of pancreatic tissue resected but also on the degree of pre-existing endocrine function. Hemipancreatectomy leads to impaired glucose tolerance in 25% of healthy humans. With the insufficiency of the exocrine pancreas, the lack of digestive enzymes (eg, lipase) induces malabsorption and diarrhea.[17]

Hepatic Resection. The major complications associated with hepatic resection are hemorrhage, liver insufficiency, bile leak, biliary fistulae, perihepatic abscess, and sepsis. In addition, liver failure can occur in the case of technical errors in the manipulation of hepatic ducts or when there is insufficient hepatic reserve. Because of the regenerative capability of the liver, as much as 85% of the liver can be safely removed. Liver regeneration starts within the first few weeks after surgical resection and is complete in 4 to 12 months. During regeneration, the liver increases the number of hepatocytes. This hyperplasia is mediated by hepatocyte growth factor, transforming growth factor alpha, epidermal growth factor, fibroblast growth factor, and several other growth factors.[18]

Splenectomy. Patients who have undergone splenectomy (eg, patients with Hodgkin's disease) are at risk for the development of serious infections. The loss of the spleen's phagocytic function and the decreased production of opsonizing antibodies predispose patients who have undergone splenectomy to fulminant and life-threatening sepsis, usually caused by *Streptococcus pneumoniae, Haemophilus influenzae, Neisseria meningitidis, Babesia* species, or *Capnocytophaga* species.[19]

Nephrectomy. Classic radical nephrectomy involves the removal of the entire kidney and Gerota's fascia, the ipsilateral adrenal gland, and regional lymph nodes. The most common complications are injuries to the spleen and large vessels.[20]

Prostatectomy. Radical prostatectomy involves the excision of the prostate gland, the attached seminal vesicles, and a layer of the surrounding connective tissue. The most common complications are hemorrhage, impotence, and urinary incontinence. These complications may be reduced by nerve-sparing techniques.[21]

Craniotomy. The major complications of craniotomy are herniation (due to edema), hemorrhage in the operative site, thromboembolic events, wound infection, pseudomeningocele (a collection of cerebrospinal fluid due to a dural leak), and various neurologic deficits, depending on the site and function of the excised brain tissue.

Placement of Access Devices. Patients with cancer often need surgical placement of access devices. Central venous catheters (eg, Broviac, Hickman, and Groshong catheters) and subcutaneously implanted venous access ports (eg, Port-A-Cath and Infus-A-Port systems) are inserted to provide long-term access for intravenous fluids, parenteral nutrition, blood products, and medication, including chemotherapy and antibiotics. The insertion of these devices may be complicated by pneumothorax or hemothorax. Arterial catheters or ports, primarily used for the infusion of regional intra-arterial chemotherapy agents, may be complicated by arterial thrombosis, arterial damage, and hemorrhage uncontrolled by pressure.[22] Intraperitoneal catheters or ports, used to deliver antineoplastic agents directly into the peritoneal cavity of patients with intra-abdominal tumors, may be associated with fluid leakage around the catheter, abdominal pain, bacterial peritonitis, and bowel perforation.[23] Intraventricular reservoirs (often referred to as Ommaya reservoirs, after the neurosurgeon A. K. Ommaya, who in 1963 devised the first intraventricular implanted reservoir) are used to deliver antineoplastic agents directly into the cerebrospinal fluid. The presence of the reservoirs may be complicated by displacement or migration of the catheter and infection (meningitis).[24]

In summary, two types of complications are associated with catheters and ports: mechanical and infectious. The most frequent mechanical complications are thrombosis around the catheter and displacement of the catheter's tip. With central venous access devices, thrombosis around the catheter is present in 80% or more of patients, but it is clinically silent in most cases. However, if an incomplete vascular occlusion progresses to a complete occlusion, patients can develop superior vena cava syndrome or pulmonary embolism.[25,26] Infectious complications of catheters and ports are either localized or disseminated; local contamination causes infection in the implantation site of the catheter, and dissemination of the infection may cause septic shock. The three most frequently isolated organisms responsible for catheter-related sepsis are *Staphylococcus aureus, Staphylococcus epidermidis,* and *Candida* species.[27,28]

COMPLICATIONS OF CHEMOTHERAPY

Since most antineoplastic drugs are simply antiproliferative agents, they lack the ability to differentiate malignant cells from normal cells. Thus, tumor selectivity is often the result of kinetic differences between cancer cells and normal cells. On the basis of their effect on the cell cycle (Figure 6–1), antineoplastic agents can be divided into three groups: (1) cell cycle–nonspecific agents; (2) cell cycle–specific/phase-nonspecific agents; and (3) cell cycle–specific/phase-specific agents. Cell cycle–nonspecific agents are toxic to both dividing and quiescent (cell-cycle phase G_0) cells; examples are alkylating agents. Cell cycle–specific/phase-nonspecific agents kill dividing cells regardless of the cells' phase; examples are anthracyclines and mitoxantrone. Cell cycle–specific/phase-specific agents kill dividing cells at specific phases of the cell cycle; examples are antimetabolites, epipodophyllotoxins, vinca alkaloids, and bleomycin. Chemotherapeutic drugs are most cytotoxic for rapidly proliferating tissues; a given dose of drug administered for a given period will have a bigger effect on cell populations with a large percentage of cycling cells than on cell populations with a large percentage of cells in the G_0 (resting) phase. This explains why some tumor selectivity is obtained by administering antineoplastic agents in high intermittent pulses; this strategy has a relatively small effect on the gastrointestinal tract and the bone marrow because these organs contain many stem cells that are in the G_0 phase.

More than 50 different chemotherapeutic agents are currently approved by the US Food and Drug Administration for the treatment of cancer (Table 6–1). Their mechanism if action is shown in Figure 6–2. Because of their different reactivity, distribution, and metabolism (Table 6–2), each of these agents—even those that have mechanisms of action in common with other agents—produces a characteristic set of toxic effects (Tables 6–3 and 6–4). The pattern of toxic effects may also differ, depending on the schedule. For example, when doxorubicin is administered in boluses, the main toxic effect is myelosuppression whereas when doxorubicin is administered with a 96-hour infusion, the main toxic effect is mucositis. The patient's metabolism may also affect a drug's toxicity. For example, in patients with liver insufficiency, the toxicity of vinca alkaloids is increased because these drugs are excreted primarily by the hepatobiliary system whereas the toxicity of cyclophosphamide is reduced because its conversion to active metabolites is impaired. Finally, it must be considered that chemotherapeutic drugs are often administered in combination (polychemotherapy), in which case the observed toxic effects may be the result of additive or synergistic effects of the single agents.

Mechanism of Action and Toxicity of Chemotherapeutic Agents

Alkylating Agents. Alkylating agents are compounds that form reactive intermediates that are capable of promoting the transfer of alkyl groups to several molecules, including deoxyribonucleic acid (DNA), ribonucleic acid (RNA), and proteins. The cytotoxic effect of alkylating agents is due to the interaction with DNA; after binding to the nitrogens in the DNA bases, alkylating agents induce cross-links in the DNA helix and break its strands, leading to inhibition of DNA replication and cell division. Since alkylating agents kill a fixed percentage of cells at a given dose, they have a linear dose-response curve: the greater the amount of drug administered, the greater the fraction of cells killed. There are four classes of alkylating agents: (1) bischloroethylamines, (2) platinum compounds, (3) nitrosoureas, and (4) other alkylating agents.

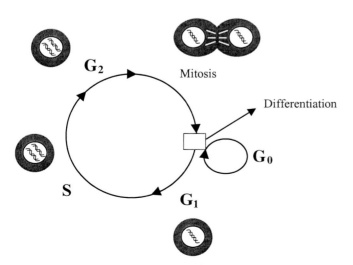

Figure 6–1. The cell cycle. G_1 = gap 1: production of all cellular components (proteins, enzymes, ribonucleic acid [RNA]) that are necessary for the synthesis of deoxyribonucleic acid (DNA). S = synthesis: new DNA is synthesized, and the genome is duplicated. G_2 = gap 2: the newly duplicated chromosomes condense, and all cellular components necessary for the mitosis are synthesized. M = mitosis: chromosomes are segregated, and the cell divides into two daughter cells. After mitosis, cells may enter (a) a G_1 phase, starting a new cell cycle; (b) a quiescent phase, called G_0; or (c) differentiation, with loss of the replicating capabilities.

TABLE 6–1. Commonly Used Chemotherapeutic Drugs

Drugs	Indications*	Dose†
Alkylating agents		
Bischloroethylamines		
Cyclophosphamide	Various neoplasms	50–100 mg/m² PO × 10–14 days or 50–1,000 mg/m² IV q2–3 weeks
Ifosfamide	Various neoplasms	1.2 g/m² IV × 5 days q 3 weeks
Melphalan	MM, ovarian cancer	6 mg PO qd × 2–3 weeks or 0.2 mg/kg PO × 5 days q4–5 weeks
Chlorambucil	CLL, lymphomas	4–10 mg/day PO daily
Mechlorethamine	HD, other neoplasms	0.4 mg/kg either as single dose or in divided doses of 0.1–0.2 mg/kg/day
Platinum compounds		
Cisplatin	Various neoplasms	30–120 mg/m² IV q3–4 weeks
Carboplatin	Various neoplasms	240–450 mg/m² IV q4 weeks
Nitrosoureas		
Carmustine	Brain tumors, MM, HD, NHL	30–200 mg/m² IV q6 weeks
Lomustine	Brain tumors, HD	75–130 mg/m² PO q6–8 weeks
Streptozocin	Pancreatic islet cell cancers	500 mg/m² × 5 days IV q6 weeks
Other		
Thiotepa	Bladder carcinoma	0.3–0.4 mg/kg IV q1–4 weeks
Busulfan	CML, ET, PV	1.8 mg/m² PO daily
Mitomycin C	GI cancers	10–20 mg/m² IV q6–8 weeks
Procarbazine	HD	100 mg/m² PO × 14 days q4 weeks
Dacarbazine	HD, melanoma	150 mg/m² IV × 5 days q4 weeks or 2.0–4.5 mg/kg IV × 10 days q4 weeks
Antimetabolites		
Pyrimidine antagonists		
5-Fluorouracil	Various neoplasms	400–1,000 mg/m² IV × 5 days q4 weeks
Floxuridine	GI cancers	0.2–0.3 mg/kg IV × 14 days q4 weeks via hepatic artery
Cytarabine	Leukemias, lymphomas	100 mg/m²/day or q12h IV × 7 days
Gemcitabine	Pancreatic cancer	1,000 mg/m² weekly × 7 doses
Purine antagonists		
Thioguanine	AML, ALL, CML	75–200 mg/m²/day PO × 5–7 days
Mercaptopurine	AML, ALL, CML	1.5–2.5 mg/kg PO qd × several weeks
Pentostatin	Leukemias, lymphomas	4 mg/m² IV q2 weeks
Fludarabine	CLL, lymphomas	25 mg/m² IV × 5 days q4 weeks
Cladribine	Leukemias, lymphomas	0.09 mg/kg IV × 7 days
Antifolates		
Methotrexate	Various neoplasms	30–40 mg/m² IV q1 week or 3–12 g/m² IV q1 week with LV rescue
Hydroxyurea	CML, AML, PV, other	800–1,200 mg/m² PO daily or 2,000–3,200 mg/m² q3d
Topoisomerase inhibitors		
Type I		
Irinotecan	Colorectal cancer	125 mg/m² IV weekly × 4 doses
Topotecan	Ovarian cancer	1.5 mg/m² IV × 5 days q3 weeks
Type II		
Doxorubicin	Various neoplasms	60–75 mg/m² IV q3 weeks
Daunorubicin	Leukemias	45 mg/m² IV × 3 days
Idarubicin	AML	12 mg/m² IV × 3 days
Mitoxantrone	Leukemias	14 mg/m² IV q3 weeks
Dactinomycin	Various neoplasms	500 μg IV × 5 days q4–6 weeks
Etoposide	SCLC, testicular cancer	35–100 mg/m² IV × 3–5 days q 3–4 weeks
Teniposide	ALL, AML	165 mg/m² IV twice weekly × 8–9 doses or 250 mg/m² IV weekly × 4–8 doses
Antimicrotubule agents		
Vinca alkaloids		
Vincristine	Various neoplasms	1.4 mg/m² IV weekly
Vinblastine	HD, testicular cancer	6 mg/m² IV q2 weeks
Vinorelbine	NSCLC	25–30 mg/m² IV weekly
Taxoids		
Paclitaxel	Breast cancer, ovarian cancer	135–175 mg/m² IV q3 weeks
Docetaxel	Breast cancer	60–100 mg/m² IV q3 weeks
Other		
Bleomycin	Various neoplasms	0.25–0.50 U/kg IV/IM/SC × once or twice weekly
Asparaginase	ALL	200 IU/kg IV × 28 days

*Only the most common and Food and Drug Administration (FDA)-approved indications are shown.
†Doses refer to standard or most commonly used regimens, and they are intended to have a mere orientative purpose. Route of administration is intravenous unless otherwise specified.

ALL = acute lymphoblastic leukemia; AML = acute myeloblastic leukemia; CLL = chronic lymphocytic leukemia; CML = chronic myelogenous leukemia; ET = essential thrombocythemia; GI = gastrointestinal; HD = Hodgkin's disease; LV = leucovorin; MM = multiple myeloma; NHL = non-Hodgkin's lymphoma; NSCLC = non-small-cell lung cancer; PV = polycythemia vera; SCLC = small-cell lung cancer.

Bischloroethylamines. Bischloroethylamines include cyclophosphamide, ifosfamide, chlorambucil, melphalan, and mechlorethamine. Cyclophosphamide is a nonreactive compound that is converted by the hepatic microsomal system to the active metabolites 4-hydroxycyclophosphamide and aldophosphamide. Ifosfamide is a structural isomer of cyclophosphamide and undergoes metabolic reactions similar to those of cyclophosphamide. Both drugs can cause myelosuppression, hemorrhagic cystitis, and pulmonary and cardiac damage. The development of hemorrhagic cystitis is principally due to acrolein, an inactive metabolite that is toxic to the urothelial mucosa; however, other metabolites, such as chlorethylazeridine and chloracetaldehyde, may also contribute to hemorrhagic cystitis.[29,30] The efficacy of the sulfhydryl compound mesna (2-mercaptoethanesulfonate sodium) in the prevention of hemorrhagic cystitis is actually related to the compound's neutralizing activity toward acrolein.[31] With cyclophosphamide, pulmonary damage is not dose or time dependent; cases of such damage have been reported after administration of as little as 150 mg, and the delay from the initiation of treatment to the development of symptoms has varied from 2 weeks to 13 years.[32] In contrast, cyclophosphamide produces cardiac damage only with high doses (200 mg/kg or more), such as those used in the setting of bone marrow transplantation. The course of illness is fulminant, and congestive heart failure and pericarditis develop in 10 to 14 days.[33–35] Cyclophosphamide can exert an antidiuretic effect on the distal renal tubules. The syndrome of inappropriate secretion of antidiuretic hormone (SIADH) induced by this drug may cause severe hyponatremia, seizures, and even death.[36]

Chlorambucil and melphalan produce interstitial pneumonitis and fibrosis in addition to myelosuppression.

With the bischloroethylamines, myelosuppression may be prolonged and cumulative. The destruction of stem cells and progenitor cells leads to a reduction of components in all three hematopoietic lineages, which results in leukopenia, anemia, and thrombocytopenia. Since the half-life of neutrophils is 6 to 8 hours, the half-life of platelets is 5 to 7 days, and the half-life of erythrocytes is

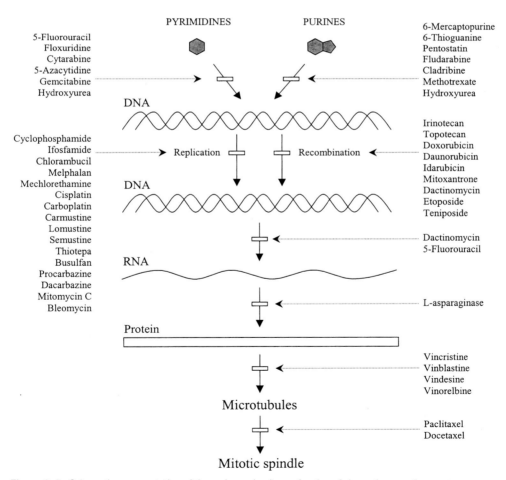

Figure 6–2. Schematic representation of the main mechanisms of action of chemotherapeutic agents. DNA = deoxyriboncleic acid; RNA = ribonucleic acid.

TABLE 6–2. Pharmacokinetics of Chemotherapeutic Drugs

Agents	Absorption	Metabolism	Elimination	Half-Life*
Asparaginase	Not absorbed from the GI tract	Degraded by proteolytic enzymes	Metabolic	8–30 h
Bleomycin	45% absorbed after IP or intrapleural administration	Enzyme degradation in tissues	Urine (65%)	2 h
Busulfan	Completely absorbed from the GI tract	Rapidly metabolized in the liver	Urine	2.5 h
Carboplatin	20% absorbed systemically after IP administration	Transformed to diamine metabolites	Urine	3–6 h
Carmustine	Low oral bioavailability	Rapidly transformed in the liver to active metabolites	Urine (70%); metabolic	20 min
Chlorambucil	Rapidly and completely absorbed from the GI tract	Transformed in the liver to the active metabolite bischloroethylphenylacetic acid	Urine	145 min
Cisplatin	75% absorbed systemically after IP administration	Nonenzymatic conversion to inactive metabolites	Urine	58–73 h
Cladribine	Low oral bioavailability	Metabolized to 2-chloro-2′-deoxyadenosine-5′-triphosphate	Urine	7 h
Cyclophosphamide	85% absorbed from the GI tract	Transformed in the liver to active alkylating metabolites	Urine (70%)	6 h
Cytarabine	< 20% absorbed from the GI tract	Deaminated to the inactive metabolite arabinosyluracil (ara-U)	Metabolic	1–3 h
Dacarbazine	Low oral bioavailability	Metabolized in the liver	Urine	5 h
Dactinomycin	Low oral bioavailability	Minimally metabolized; concentrated in nucleated cells	Bile (50%); urine (10%)	36 h
Daunorubicin	Low oral bioavailability	Transformed in the liver to the active metabolite daunorubicinol	Bile (40%); urine (25%)	20 h
Docetaxel	Low oral bioavailability	Metabolized by hepatic cytochrome P-450 isoenzymes in the CYP3A subfamily to one major and three minor metabolites	Bile (75%); urine (5%)	11 h
Doxorubicin	Low oral bioavailability	Transformed in the liver to the active metabolite doxorubicinol	Bile (50%); urine (10%)	20–48 h
Etoposide	Oral bioavailability variable (25–75%)	Transformed in the liver to inactive metabolites	Urine (40%); bile (10%)	4–11 h
Floxuridine	Low oral bioavailability	Metabolized in the liver and tissues to the monophosphate derivative and fluorouracil	Metabolic	20 min
Fludarabine	Low oral bioavailability	Dephosphorylated in serum to the active metabolite 2-fluoro-ara-A, then phosphorylated intracellularly to 2-fluoro-ara-ATP, the main active metabolite	Urine	10 h
5-Fluorouracil	Low oral bioavailability (10–25%)	Rapidly transformed in the tissues to the active metabolite floxuridine monophosphate	Metabolic; urine (15%)	8–15 min
Gemcitabine	Low oral bioavailability	Transformed to two active metabolites (gemcitabine diphosphate and gemcitabine triphosphate) and an inactive metabolite (dFdU)	Urine	32–94 min
Hydroxyurea	Well absorbed from the GI tract	Metabolized in the liver	Urine	4 h
Idarubicin	Well absorbed from the GI tract	Hepatic and extrahepatic transformation to the metabolite idarubicinol, which is equipotent with idarubicin	Bile (15%); urine (10%)	22 h
Ifosfamide	Well absorbed from the GI tract	Requires metabolic activation by microsomal liver enzymes to produce active metabolites	Urine (80%)	15 h
Irinotecan	Low oral bioavailability	Converted to the active metabolite SN-38 by carboxylesterases in plasma, intestinal mucosa, and liver	Bile (60%); urine (30%)	13 h
Lomustine	80% absorbed from the GI tract	Rapidly transformed in the liver to active metabolites	Urine	16–48 h
Mechlorethamine	Low oral bioavailability	Rapidly deactivated in body fluids and tissues	Urine	Few min
Melphalan	Oral bioavailability erratic, average ~50%	Hydrolysis to monohydroxy- and dihydroxymelphalan	Metabolic	90 min
Mercaptopurine	Oral bioavailability erratic, average ~50%	Enters the anabolic and catabolic pathways for purines	Metabolic	10 h
Methotrexate	Oral absorption highly variable and dose dependent	Metabolized in the liver; converted intracellularly to active polyglutamated forms	Urine (85%); bile (< 10%)	3–15 h
Mitomycin C	Low oral bioavailability	Metabolized in the liver (primarily) and other tissues	Urine (20%)	1 hr
Mitoxantrone	Low oral bioavailability	Transformed in the liver to inactive metabolites	Bile (40%); urine (10%)	6 d
Paclitaxel	Low oral bioavailability; detected in ascitic fluid but not CSF	Metabolized primarily to 6-alpha-hydroxypaclitaxel by the hepatic cytochrome P-450 isoenzyme CYP2C8	Bile (70%); urine (5%)	29 h
Pentostatin	Low oral bioavailability	Only small amounts are metabolized (liver)	Urine	6 h
Procarbazine	Rapidly and completely absorbed from the GI tract	Metabolized primarily in the liver and kidneys	Urine (70%)	10 min

(continued)

TABLE 6–2. *Continued*

Agents	Absorption	Metabolism	Elimination	Half-Life*
Streptozocin	< 20% absorbed from the GI tract	Metabolized in the liver and kidneys	Urine (65%); metabolic	35 min
Teniposide	Low oral bioavailability	Transformed in the liver to various metabolites	Urine (10%); bile (< 10%)	6–10 h
Thioguanine	Variable and limited oral bioavailability (~30%)	Enters the anabolic and catabolic pathways for purines	Metabolic	80 min
Thiotepa	Low oral bioavailability	Transformed in the liver to TEPA, a less active metabolite	Urine (85%)	2 h
Topotecan	Low oral bioavailability	Hydrolyzed to an active lactone form and an inactive hydroxyacid form	Urine (30%)	2–3 h
Vinblastine	Erratic absorption from the GI tract	Metabolized by hepatic cytochrome P-450 isoenzymes in the CYP3A subfamily	Bile; urine (< 10%)	25 h
Vincristine	Low oral bioavailability	Metabolized by hepatic cytochrome P-450 isoenzymes in the CYP3A subfamily	Bile (80%); urine (15%)	85 h
Vinorelbine	Well absorbed from the GI tract	Metabolized in the liver to deacetylvinorelrelbine, which possesses antitumor activity	Bile (46%); urine (< 10%)	27–44 h

*Refers to the terminal elimination half-life of active metabolites.
CSF = cerebrospinal fluid; dFdU = difluorodeoxyuridine; GI = gastrointestinal; IP = intraperitoneal; TEPA = triethylenephosphramide.

50 to 65 days, the first manifestation of myelosuppression is often leukopenia, and the last is usually anemia. As is the case for many other chemotherapeutic agents, the nadir occurs at about day 10, and recovery takes 3 to 4 weeks.

Platinum Compounds. Platinum compounds (cisplatin, carboplatin, and oxaliplatin) bind covalently to DNA and produce intrastrand and interstrand cross-links in the DNA helix. Cisplatin (*cis*-diamminedichloroplatinum, or CDDP) is the most commonly used platinum compound. It can cause renal failure, peripheral neuropathy, myelosuppression, and vomiting.

The most serious toxic effect of cisplatin is renal. Cisplatin is generally contraindicated when the creatinine clearance is < 40 mL/min. The renal damage caused by cisplatin is characterized by focal acute tubular necrosis, dilatation of convoluted tubules, formation of casts, and epithelial atypia of the collecting ducts.[37] The primary lesion in the kidneys appears to be necrosis of the proximal convoluted tubules. Because the *trans* isomer of cisplatin is not nephrotoxic, cisplatin-induced kidney damage is not related to the tubular damage associated with the administration of heavy metals.

Cisplatin-induced neuropathy appears as the result of a total cumulative dose > 300 mg/m^2 and is usually reversible. It is a peripheral neuropathy, characterized mainly by sensory loss in a "stocking-and-glove" distribution. Other symptoms are a loss of proprioception, reduced vibratory perception, hyporeflexia, and damage to hearing and balance.

Cisplatin-induced myelosuppression may be prolonged and cumulative. The primary cause of cisplatin-induced anemia is not myelosuppression but a decrease in erythropoietin production, which results from the renal tubular damage induced by cisplatin.[38]

Cisplatin can also cause episodes of myocardial ischemia, manifested as angina pectoris or even myocardial infarction.[39] Angiographic studies in patients with cisplatin-induced ischemia showed patent coronary arteries and significant ergonovine-induced vasospasm, indicating that the most likely mechanism of cisplatin-induced ischemia is coronary artery vasospasm.[40] Cerebral vasospasm may occur as well, with transient ischemia and seizures.[41]

Cisplatin is one of the most emetic drugs. As is the case with many other chemotherapeutic agents, the pathophysiology of cisplatin-induced nausea and vomiting involves the direct stimulation of the chemoreceptor trigger zone, a chemosensor center located on the area postrema (ie, the caudal margin of the fourth ventricle). The main neurotransmitters that activate the chemoreceptor trigger zone (in order from greatest to least importance in terms of activity) are serotonin (5-hydroxytryptamine, or 5-HT), dopamine, histamine, acetylcholine, and apomorphine. In cats, surgical ablation of the area postrema eliminates cisplatin-induced vomiting.[42] As do other antineoplastic agents, cisplatin induces emesis not only by acting centrally but also by acting peripherally via the afferent nerves from the gastrointestinal tract.[43] When chemotherapy damages the intestinal mucosa, the injured mucosal enterochromaffin cells release serotonin; the high levels of serotonin activate the 5-HT$_3$ receptors on the vagal primary afferent neurons, which in turn stimulate the chemoreceptor trigger zone (Figure 6–3).

Carboplatin is better tolerated than cisplatin because it is much less nephro- and neurotoxic.

Nitrosoureas. The nitrosoureas include carmustine, lomustine, semustine, and streptozocin. Carmustine,

TABLE 6–3. Toxic Effects of Chemotherapeutic Drugs

Organ System and/or Type of Toxic Effect	Commonly Associated Agents*
Eye	
Conjunctivitis	Cytarabine, doxorubicin, 5-fluorouracil, methotrexate
Necrotizing uveitis	Mechlorethamine
Retinopathy	IA nitrosoureas
Papilledema, optic neuropathy	Cisplatin
Ear	
Ototoxicity	Cisplatin
Lung	
Acute hypersensitivity pneumonitis	Bleomycin, methotrexate, procarbazine
Chronic pneumonitis/fibrosis	Bleomycin, busulfan, chlorambucil, cyclophosphamide, melphalan, mitomycin C, nitrosoureas
Acute pulmonary edema	Cyclophosphamide, cytarabine, methotrexate, mitomycin C, teniposide
Pleural effusion	Bleomycin, busulfan, cyclophosphamide, docetaxel, methotrexate, mitomycin C, procarbazine
Heart	
Arrhythmias	Cyclophosphamide, paclitaxel
Congestive heart failure	Anthracyclines, cyclophosphamide, ifosfamide, mitoxantrone, mitomycin C
Myocardial ischemia	Anthracyclines, cisplatin, etoposide, 5-fluorouracil, vinca alkaloids
Acute myocarditis-pericarditis	Anthracyclines, cyclophosphamide
GI system	
Nausea, vomiting	Variety of agents
Mucositis	Anthracyclines, cisplatin, cytarabine, etoposide, 5-fluorouracil, methotrexate
Diarrhea	Cytarabine, 5-fluorouracil, irinotecan, methotrexate
Paralytic ileus	Vinca alkaloids
Hepatocellular injury	Variety of agents
Cholestasis	IA floxuridine, 6-mercaptopurine, busulfan
Fibrosis, cirrhosis	Methotrexate
Sclerosing cholangitis	IA floxuridine
Veno-occlusive disease	Variety of agents
Pancreatitis	Asparaginase
Genitourinary system	
Renal failure	Cisplatin, methotrexate, mitomycin C, nitrosoureas
Hemorrhagic cystitis	Cyclophosphamide, ifosfamide
Azoospermia	Alkylating agents
Nervous system	
Acute encephalopathy	Cytarabine, IT/IV methotrexate
Chronic encephalopathy	Carmustine, cytarabine, fludarabine, methotrexate
Cerebellar dysfunction	Cytarabine, 5-fluorouracil, procarbazine
Cranial neuropathy	IA cisplatin, vincristine
Aseptic meningitis	IT cytarabine, IT methotrexate
Myelopathy	IT ara-C, cisplatin, IT methotrexate
Peripheral neuropathy	Cisplatin, paclitaxel, vincristine, vindesine
Seizures	Asparaginase, busulfan, carmustine, cisplatin, cyclophosphamide, etoposide, methotrexate, paclitaxel, teniposide, vinca alkaloids
Skin	
Local vesicants	Anthracyclines, mechlorethamine, methotrexate, vinca alkaloids
Urticaria/angioedema	Asparaginase, cisplatin, cyclophosphamide, thiotepa, mechlorethamine, melphalan, methotrexate
Macular or papular eruptions	Busulfan, dacarbazine, hydroxyurea, methotrexate
Photosensitivity	Dacarbazine, 5-fluorouracil, methotrexate, vinblastine
Radiation recall reaction	Anthracyclines, dactinomycin, hydroxyurea, methotrexate
Vasculitis	Cytarabine, hydroxyurea, methotrexate
Hematopoietic system	
Myelosuppression	Most agents
Microangiopathic hemolytic anemia	Mitomycin C
Coagulopathy	Asparaginase
Systemic reactions	
Fever	Bleomycin, dacarbazine, gemcitabine
Hypersensitivity reactions	Asparaginase, paclitaxel
Metabolic disturbances	
Hyperuricemia	Alkylating agents
Tumor lysis syndrome	Cytarabine
SIADH	Cyclophosphamide, vincristine

*Route of administration is intravenous unless otherwise specified.
ara-C = cytosine arabinoside; GI = gastrointestinal; IA = intra-arterial; IT = intrathecal; IV = intravenous; SIADH = syndrome of inappropriate secretion of antidiuretic hormone.

lomustine, and semustine have limited clinical use because they produce marked and prolonged hematopoietic suppression. They can also cause severe renal failure and pulmonary fibrosis.[44] The kidney damage caused by nitrosoureas is associated with the development of interstitial nephritis. Years after the completion of therapy, the observed pathologic lesions are interstitial fibrosis and glomerular sclerosis.[45]

Other Alkylating Agents. Alkylating agents that do not fit into the previously discussed categories include thiotepa, busulfan, procarbazine, dacarbazine, and mitomycin C.

The main side effect of thiotepa is mucositis.

Busulfan is an alkyl alkane sulfonate. It produces severe myelosuppression and lung injury. Clinically apparent lung injury occurs in approximately 4% of patients, but up to 46% of patients treated with busulfan have subclinical lung damage, as determined at autopsy.[32] The interval between the initiation of treatment and the onset of symptoms is generally longer for busulfan than for other cytotoxic agents and can be as much as 10 years.[32] Although a strict dose-toxicity relationship does not exist for busulfan, there appears to be a threshold cumulative dose of 500 mg, above which pulmonary fibrosis may occur and below which the risk is minimal.

A flulike syndrome occurs in up to 50% of patients who receive high-dose dacarbazine. A rare but serious hypersensitivity-type hepatocellular injury has also been described in patients treated with dacarbazine. The clinical picture includes the acute onset of upper abdominal pain, ascites, jaundice, and elevated transaminase levels. The pathogenesis of this toxic reaction is most likely a hypersensitivity reaction to the drug as most patients develop this complication in the second cycle of treatment and as the tissue findings are characterized by an eosinophilic infiltration of the hepatic vessels.

Mitomycin C is an antitumoral antibiotic that functions as an alkylating agent. Mitomycin C can produce myelosuppression (dose-limiting), thrombotic microangiopathy, pneumonitis or pulmonary fibrosis, and extravasation injury. Administration of mitomycin C is associated with congestive heart failure in approximately 5% of patients, and the incidence of congestive heart failure increases with cumulative doses > 300 mg/m^2.[46] Thrombotic microangiopathy includes clinical entities such as microangiopathic hemolytic anemia, thrombotic

TABLE 6–4. Toxic Doses of Selected Chemotherapeutic Drugs

Agent	Toxic Dose*				
	Pulmonary Toxicity[†]	Cardiotoxicity[‡]	Hepatic Toxicity[§]	Renal Toxicity[¶]	Neurotoxicity[#]
Asparaginase	—	—	Conventional dose	—	Conventional dose [j]
Bleomycin	> 400 U total dose [a]	—	—	—	—
Busulfan	Conventional dose PO [a]	Conventional dose PO [f]	—	—	—
Carmustine	> 1,500 mg/m^2 total dose [a]	—	Conventional dose	> 1,200 mg/m^2 total dose [g]	—
Chlorambucil	Conventional dose [a]	—	—	—	—
Cisplatin	—	Conventional dose [e]	—	> 100 mg/m^2 [g]	> 300 mg/m^2 total dose [i]
Cyclophosphamide	Conventional doses [a]	> 200 mg/kg total dose [c]	—	> 50 mg/kg [h]	—
Cytarabine	Conventional dose [b]	—	Conventional dose	—	> 2 g/m^2 IV [j]
					>100 mg/m^2 IT [jk]
Dacarbazine	—	—	Conventional dose	—	—
Daunorubicin	—	> 550 mg/m^2 total dose [c]	—	—	—
Doxorubicin	—	> 550 mg/m^2 total dose [c]	—	—	—
Fludarabine	Conventional dose [a]	—	—	—	Low dose [i]; high dose [j]
5-Fluorouracil	—	Conventional dose [e]	—	—	Conventional dose [k]
Hydroxyurea	—	—	Conventional dose	—	—
Ifosfamide	—	> 6 g/m^2 [f]	—	1.2 g/m^2/d × 5 d [h]	High dose [j]
Melphalan	High dose [a]	—	—	—	—
Methotrexate	Conventional dose [a]	—	Conventional dose	> 1 g/m^2 [g]	>12 mg/m^2 IT [j]
Mitomycin C	Conventional dose [a]	Conventional dose [c]	—	> 50 mg/m^2 total dose [g]	—
Mitoxantrone	—	> 120 mg/m^2 total dose [c]	—	—	—
Paclitaxel	—	Conventional dose [f]	—	—	Conventional dose [i]
Streptozocin	—	—	Conventional dose	Conventional dose [g]	—
Vincristine	—	Conventional dose [e]	—	—	Conventional dose [i]

*For each agent, only the most frequent toxic effects are shown. Route of administration is intravenous unless otherwise specified.
[†]a = interstitial pneumonitis/fibrosis; b = pulmonary edema.
[‡]c = congestive heart failure; d = endocardial fibrosis; e = myocardial ischemia; f = arrhythmias.
[§]Elevation of transaminases/alkaline phosphatase levels.
[¶]g = renal insufficiency; h = hemorrhagic cystitis.
[#]i = peripheral neuropathy; j = central nervous system neuropathy; k = cerebellar dysfunction.
IT = intrathecal; PO = oral.

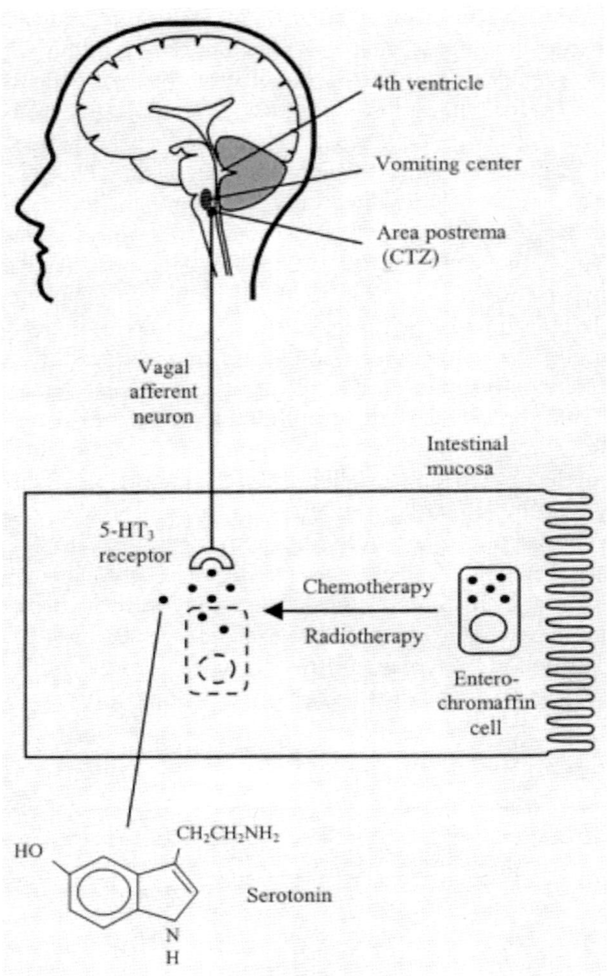

Figure 6–3. Peripheral mechanism of emesis in patients treated with chemotherapy or radiotherapy (see text). CTZ = chemoreceptor trigger zone; 5-HT3 = 5-hydroxytryptamine3.

thrombocytopenic purpura, and hemolytic-uremic syndrome.[47] The hemolysis is caused by mechanical damage: the red blood cells stick to deposited fibrin and break off. The initiating factor in the development of thrombotic microangiopathy is direct endothelial cell injury, but the pathogenesis of this syndrome is unknown. Autoimmune mechanisms have been proposed on the basis of two clinical observations: (1) red blood cell transfusions may aggravate the syndrome, and (2) the therapeutic use of staphylococcal protein A immunoperfusion column, which removes plasma immunoglobulin G (IgG), ameliorates the thrombotic microangiopathy. Immune complexes that aggregate platelets have been observed after the administration of mitomycin C.

Antimetabolites. Antimetabolites are compounds with a chemical structure that is similar to that of normal metabolites. They act by inhibiting DNA synthesis.

Because their activity is greatest in the S phase of the cell cycle, these agents are most effective when cell proliferation is rapid. The dose-response curve for antimetabolites is nonlinear; above a certain dose, further increases in drug dose (with the exception of 5-fluorouracil [5-FU]) do not result in greater cell killing.

Pyrimidine Antagonists. Pyrimidine antagonists include 5-FU, floxuridine, cytarabine, 5-azacytidine, and gemcitabine.

5-Fluorouracil acts on cells in the S phase and in other phases of the cell cycle. The target sites for the biologic action of 5-FU are DNA, RNA, and the enzyme thymidylate synthetase. 5-Fluorouracil can be directly incorporated into DNA in the place of thymine, leading to errors during DNA transcription or repair. The 5-FU metabolite uridine triphosphate can incorporate into RNA, leading to the miscoding of protein synthesis, the inhibition of RNA polyadenylation, and the altered maturation of ribosomal RNA. Finally, the 5-FU metabolite uridine monophosphate can bind to and inhibit thymidylate synthetase, an enzyme involved in the conversion of deoxyuridylic acid to thymidylic acid. The inhibition of this enzyme leads to intracellular depletion of thymidine and the consequent impairment of DNA synthesis. In chemotherapy protocols, 5-FU is often administered together with leucovorin, which enhances the binding of 5-FU to thymidylate synthetase and therefore increases both the antitumoral activity and toxicity of 5-FU. Adverse reactions to 5-FU include mucositis (dose-limiting), myelosuppression, hand-foot-and-mouth syndrome, conjunctivitis, dermatitis, myocardial ischemia (1%),[48] and cerebellar dysfunction (1%). Mucositis includes inflammation of the tongue (glossitis) and mouth (stomatitis), esophagitis, and enteritis, with diarrhea. Mucositis generally begins 3 to 8 days after the administration of 5-FU and lasts approximately 7 to 12 days. Its mechanism is a direct cytotoxic effect on the rapidly growing basal epithelium of the gastrointestinal tract. Lesions due to mucositis may range from mild erythema to severe erosions and diffuse ulcerations. Besides causing local pain, mucositis may lead to superinfections; the protective barrier of the oral epithelium is disrupted, and the ulcerations that accompany mucositis are frequent portals of entry for indigenous oral microorganisms. Infection and sepsis are often caused by *Candida* species, herpes simplex virus type 1, and bacteria. Moreover, odynophagia and dysphagia caused by mucositis may compromise the patient's hydration and nutritional status.

Floxuridine is often administered via the hepatic intra-arterial route; its main toxic effects are hepatitis and sclerosing cholangitis.

Cytarabine (ara-C) is a nucleoside analogue of deoxycytidine. Its cytotoxic effect is related to its incorporation into DNA, which terminates the DNA-chain elongation catalyzed by DNA polymerase. The toxic effects of cytarabine are myelosuppression (dose-limiting), mucositis (dose-limiting), and nausea and vomiting. At high doses (> 500 mg/m^2), cytarabine can lead to severe central nervous system (CNS) and cerebellar damage.[49] Cerebellar damage results from specific damage to cerebellar Purkinje's cells; pathologic studies have correlated the clinical manifestations of cytarabine-related cerebellar toxicity (dysmetria, ataxic gait, dysarthria, and nystagmus) to the loss of Purkinje's cells in the deep cerebellar nuclei.[50] "Cytarabine syndrome" consists of diffuse rash, conjunctivitis, malaise, fever, and arthralgias that occur in 2% of treated patients, usually 6 to 12 hours after administration; its mechanism is unclear.

5-Azacytidine is a cytidine analogue primarily used in the treatment of myelodysplastic syndromes and acute myeloblastic leukemia. Its dose-limiting toxic effect is myelosuppression.

Gemcitabine is a deoxycytidine analogue used for the treatment of pancreatic cancer. Its cytotoxicity is related to the DNA and RNA incorporation of its triphosphate and diphosphate metabolites. Important side effects are myelosuppression (dose-limiting), fever (seen in 30% of patients), nausea and vomiting, and skin rash.

Purine Antagonists. Purine antagonists include 6-mercaptopurine, 6-thioguanine, pentostatin, fludarabine, and cladribine.

6-Mercaptopurine and 6-thioguanine inhibit purine synthesis and purine interconversion. Myelosuppression is the dose-limiting toxic effect.

Pentostatin, fludarabine, and cladribine (2-CdA) are synthetic analogues of adenosine. They are especially useful in the treatment of lymphoproliferative disorders. The development of these drugs resulted from the search for compounds that could inhibit adenosine deaminase (ADA) activity. Adenosine deaminase normally serves to degrade purine and deoxypurine nucleotides through the irreversible deamination of adenosine to inosine. This enzyme became a target in the research for antiproliferative drugs because it was known that the lymphopenia observed in patients with congenital ADA deficiency, a form of severe combined immunodeficiency, was caused by the intracellular accumulation of deoxypurine nucleotides. Researchers believed that drugs capable of inhibiting ADA and increasing deoxynucleotide levels in lymphocytes could prove useful in the treatment of diseases with abnormal lymphocyte proliferation. The dose-limiting toxic effect of pentostatin, fludarabine, and cladribine is myelosuppression. Because of their potent lymphotoxic effect, these agents induce a profound and prolonged immunosuppression, predisposing patients to a broad spectrum of infections.

Folate Antagonists. Folate antagonists include methotrexate (MTX) and trimetrexate.

Methotrexate binds to and blocks dihydrofolate reductase, the enzyme that converts dihydrofolate to tetrahydrofolate. Tetrahydrofolate is a coenzyme that mediates the transfer of carbon units in various reactions. When cells are depleted of tetrahydrofolate, the formation of thymidylate from deoxyuridylate is impaired; consequently, the biosynthesis of purines (and thus, DNA) is impaired. Patients with pleural or peritoneal effusions are at increased risk for the toxic effects of MTX because the drug accumulates in the effusion, from which it is slowly released, leading to sustained elevated MTX concentrations in the serum.[51]

Adverse effects of MTX include myelosuppression, mucositis, liver damage, pulmonary damage, skin rash, nervous system damage, and renal failure. Patients in whom pulmonary damage occurs usually present with the clinical picture of hypersensitivity pneumonitis, pulmonary fibrosis, or (less commonly) acute pleuritis or noncardiogenic pulmonary edema. Intrathecal administration of MTX can induce acute aseptic meningitis and chronic encephalopathy or myelopathy.[52] This is thought to be caused by either direct chemical arachnoiditis or the release of adenosine (a potent CNS depressant) in the CNS. (Since it inhibits purine synthesis, MTX leads to increased adenosine levels, including elevated adenosine concentrations in the cerebrospinal fluid.) This hypothesis appears to be confirmed by the clinical improvement of MTX-induced nervous system damage produced by the administration of methylxanthines (ie, aminophyllin and theophylline), which act by displacing adenosine from its receptors.[53] Methotrexate-related kidney damage involves two mechanisms: (1) a direct effect on renal tubular cells and (2) the crystallization and precipitation of MTX and its less soluble metabolite, 7-hydroxy-MTX, in the renal tubules, possibly leading to obstructive nephropathy.[54] The use of vigorous hydration and urine alkalinization for the prevention of this complication has the effect of increasing the solubility of MTX and 7-hydroxy-MTX.

Trimetrexate inhibits dihydrofolate reductase. Whereas MTX requires a folate transport carrier, trimetrexate enters cells by passive or facilitative diffusion. Thus, trimetrexate is cytotoxic in MTX-resistant cells when the mechanism of resistance is impaired MTX uptake.

Hydroxyurea. Hydroxyurea inhibits DNA synthesis by blocking ribonucleotide reductase, the enzyme that converts ribonucleosides to deoxyribonucleosides (the DNA bases). The main side effects of hydroxyurea are myelosuppression (dose-limiting) and gastrointestinal side effects.

Topoisomerase Inhibitors. Topoisomerase I inhibitors include irinotecan and topotecan. Topoisomerase I is an enzyme that untwists supercoiled DNA by producing and resealing single-strand breaks. The action of this enzyme is important in DNA recombination and repair. Topoisomerase I inhibitors stabilize the enzyme/DNA complexes so that the DNA replication fork collides with the topoisomerase I/DNA complex, resulting in an accumulation of DNA breaks. The final effect is cell cycle arrest in the G_2 phase (because the M phase [ie, mitosis] cannot take place) and cell death. Irinotecan (CPT-11) is a semisynthetic drug derived from the tree *Camptotheca acuminata,* which grows in Asia. The main side effects of irinotecan are diarrhea (seen in 88% of treated patients), nausea and vomiting (in 86%), and myelosuppression (in 63%). The dose-limiting toxic effect of topotecan is myelosuppression.

Topoisomerase II inhibitors can be divided into four groups: anthracyclines, the anthracenedione mitoxantrone, dactinomycin, and epipodophyllotoxins.

Anthracyclines. Anthracyclines include doxorubicin, daunorubicin, epirubicin, and idarubicin. Anthracyclines act by several mechanisms. They are DNA intercalators because their planar aromatic ring structure is capable of inserting itself between DNA base pairs. The DNA intercalation alters the supercoiling of the DNA strands and the DNA topology. Anthracyclines also inhibit topoisomerase II, a nuclear enzyme that catalyzes the breaking and resealing of double-stranded DNA, thereby allowing strand passing (ie, the exchange of one segment of double-stranded DNA with another). Strand passing is essential for the separation of daughter DNA strands just prior to mitosis. Anthracyclines stabilize the topoisomerase II/DNA complex, interfering with the reunion of DNA and resulting in double-strand DNA breakage. The major side effects of anthracyclines are myelosuppression (dose-limiting), heart damage (dose-limiting), mucositis, skin rash, conjunctivitis, urine discoloration (red color), and extravasation injury. Cardiac damage manifests as an acute myocarditis-pericarditis syndrome,[55] arrhythmia, or chronic cardiomyopathy. Congestive heart failure is dose dependent; it develops in approximately 1% of patients who receive a cumulative doxorubicin dose of 450 mg/m^2, in 5% who receive a cumulative dose of 550 mg/m^2, in 15% who receive 600 mg/m^2, and in 20% who receive 700 mg/m^2.[56] The cardiotoxicity of doxorubicin is significantly lower if the drug is infused over 24 to 96 hours, which suggests that high peak concentrations are an important factor in doxorubicin's cardiotoxicity. The pathophysiology of anthracycline-induced cardiotoxicity involves the chelation of iron and the generation of free radicals, such as hydrogen peroxide, superoxide, and the hydroxyl radical (Figure 6–4).[57,58] After entering the cell, doxorubicin binds ferric iron (Fe^{+++}). Then, the anthracycline/Fe^{+++} complex binds to cell membranes and DNA and acts as a redox

catalyst, generating highly reactive hydroxyl radical species. These attack phospholipids (lipid peroxidation) in the mitochondrial membrane and sarcoplasmic reticulum. The sarcoplasmic reticulum is essential in the physiology of the normal cardiac contractile cycle; after the wave of electrical depolarization occurs, the calcium bound to the sarcoplasmic reticulum is released and activates a calcium-dependent adenosinetriphosphatase (ATPase) that triggers the contraction. The oxidative damage to the sarcoplasmic reticulum results in defective calcium binding. The final effect is myocyte degeneration, loss of muscle fibers, and the replacement of normal tissue by fibrotic tissue. The use of the ethylenediaminetetraacetic acid (EDTA) derivative dexrazoxane in the prevention of anthracycline-induced cardiac damage appears to confirm this pathophysiologic mechanism: after entering the cell, dexrazoxane is hydrolized to form a potent metal chelating agent that accepts the iron from the anthracycline/Fe^{+++} complex and removes it from the myocytes, thereby protecting these cells from free-radical generation and oxidative injury. The most frequent electrocardiographic abnormalities observed during anthracycline treatment are nonspecific ST changes, T-wave changes, decreased QRS voltages,

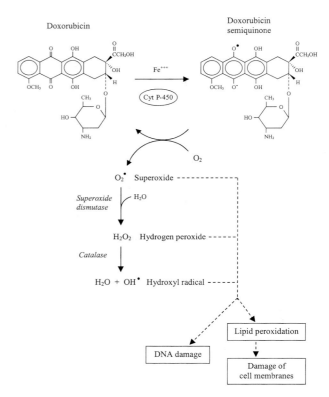

Figure 6–4. Mechanism of free radical–dependent doxorubicin toxicity. "Lipid peroxidation" is the destruction of double bonds in unsaturated fatty acids contained in membrane phospholipids. The oxidative damage to the sarcoplasmic reticulum of myocytes contributes to the cardiotoxicity induced by anthracyclines. Cyt = cytochrome; DNA = deoxyribonucleic acid.

sinus tachycardia, supraventricular tachycardias, premature atrial contractions, premature ventricular contractions, and a prolonged Q–T interval.[56] These changes are usually self-limited, resolve within 1 week, and are often asymptomatic. Although acute arrhythmias have been reported in up to 40% of patients treated with doxorubicin, life-threatening arrhythmias such as ventricular tachycardia rarely develop.[59]

The immunomodulator, trastuzumab, has recently been associated with an increased risk of cardiac dysfunction, especially in patients receiving concurrent anthracyclines. The incidence was highest in patients receiving trastuzumab and anthracycline plus cyclophosphamide concurrently (27%). Patients receiving paclitaxel and trastuzumab (13%) or trastuzumab alone (3 to 7%) had lower risk of cardiac dysfunction.[60,61]

Mitoxantrone. Like anthracyclines, the anthracenedione mitoxantrone is a DNA intercalator and topoisomerase II inhibitor. It was developed in the search for anthracycline analogues with a better tolerability. Compared with anthracyclines, mitoxantrone causes less nausea and vomiting and is less cardiotoxic (cardiomyopathy occurs in less than 5% of patients); an additional benefit is that mitoxantrone does not produce extravasation injury. It is less cardiotoxic than anthracyclines because of its minor ability to generate free radicals. The main side effects of mitoxantrone are myelosuppression (dose-limiting) and bluish discoloration of urine, sclerae, fingernails, and the site of injection.

Dactinomycin. Dactinomycin is another DNA intercalator. The main adverse reactions associated with this drug are myelosuppression (dose-limiting) and extravasation injury.

Epipodophyllotoxins. The epipodophyllotoxins etoposide and teniposide are semisynthetic derivatives of podophyllotoxin, a compound derived from the American mandrake *(Podophyllum peltatum)*. The major side effects of the epipodophyllotoxins are myelosuppression (dose-limiting), gastrointestinal side effects (nausea, vomiting, and diarrhea), hepatic dysfunction, and hypersensitivity reactions.

Antimicrotubule Agents. *Vinca Alkaloids.* The vinca alkaloids (vincristine, vinblastine, vindesine, and vinorelbine) are specific for cells in the M phase of the cell cycle. Unlike most chemotherapeutic agents, they do not target DNA but rather bind to tubulin, the subunit protein of microtubules, blocking microtubule assembly (Figure 6–5). Since microtubules are required for the formation of the mitotic spindle, vinca alkaloids lead to a mitotic arrest of cells in metaphases and ultimately to cell death. Despite their chemical similarity, the various vinca alkaloids have significantly different toxic effects. For example, whereas vincristine is profoundly neurotoxic and is rarely myelosuppressive, the opposite is true for vinorelbine.

The most common neurologic side effect of vincristine is peripheral neuropathy, with paresthesias in the fingers and toes and a decrease or loss of deep tendon reflexes. In severe cases, motor function is impaired, and the patient suffers from muscle weakness, gait abnormalities, wrist or foot drop, and quadriparesis. Vincristine can also cause autonomic neuropathy, with constipation, paralytic ileus, abdominal pain, urinary retention, and orthostatic hypotension. Finally, vincristine can cause cranial neuropathy in rare cases. Extraocular eye movement abnormalities are most commonly seen, but ptosis, facial and laryngeal paralysis, and optic-nerve neuropathy have also been observed.[62] The mechanism of action of the vinca alkaloids explains their neurotoxicity; microtubules are required not only for the formation of the mitotic spindles but also for the cytoskeleton, which is essential for the movement of mitochondria and secretory granules along neural processes.[63,64] Severe local extravasation injury is common to the use of all vinca alkaloids. Vincristine exerts an antidiuretic effect on the distal renal tubules and occasionally induces the syndrome of inappropriate secretion of antidiuretic hormone (SIADH).

Taxoids. Unlike the vinca alkaloids, which cause the disassembly of microtubules, taxoids (ie, paclitaxel and docetaxel) promote microtubule assembly; they form tubulin dimers and stabilize the microtubules against depolymerization, thereby impeding cellular mitosis (see Figure 6–5).[65] The taxoid-binding site is on the β-tubulin and is distinct from the binding site for the vinca alkaloids. Paclitaxel was first isolated from the western yew tree *(Taxus brevifolia)*. Its important toxic effects are myelosuppression (dose-limiting), peripheral neuropathy (dose-limiting), type I hypersensitivity reactions (an incidence of 2% in patients who receive the premedication with dexamethasone, diphenhydramine, and an H_2 antagonist), and cardiac arrhythmias. Paclitaxel can induce asymptomatic bradycardia, premature ventricular contractions, ventricular tachycardia, and varying degrees of heart block. In one trial, transient asymptomatic bradycardia occurred in 29% of patients.[66] Paclitaxel causes a peripheral neuropathy very similar to that seen with the administration of vincristine; this is not surprising, given that the taxoids have an action that is opposite to that of the vinca alkaloids (taxoids promote microtubule assembly) but that produces the same effect (ie, disruption of cytoskeleton). Docetaxel is a semisynthetic taxoid whose toxic effects are similar to those of paclitaxel. One toxic effect seen with docetaxel but not paclitaxel is fluid retention, which manifests as weight gain, peripheral edema, and pleural effusions.

Other Antineoplastic Agents. *Bleomycin.* Bleomycin is a mixture of several polypeptides, all of which contain a component called bleomycinic acid. Like anthracyclines,

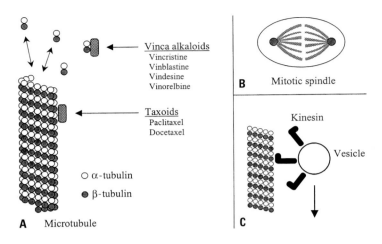

Figure 6–5. Drugs that disrupt microtubules. A: Vinca alkaloids bind tubulin and block microtubule assembly whereas taxoids bind to a polymer and induce microtubule stabilization. B and C: The opposite mechanism of action of these two classes of compounds leads to the same effects: mitotic arrest of cells in metaphase (because microtubules are required for the formation of the mitotic spindles) (B) and neurotoxicity (because microtubules are required for the movement of vesicles and secretory granules along neural processes) (C).

bleomycin binds to iron and induces the formation of highly reactive free-radical species, particularly superoxide. Moreover, bleomycin binds to DNA and induces single-strand and chromosomal breaks, and it prevents DNA repair by inhibiting DNA ligase. The main side effects of bleomycin are fever, hypersensitivity reactions, and pulmonary damage (dose-limiting). Fever and shaking chills occur in 25% of patients after the first few treatments, often within 4 to 10 hours of injection. Interstitial pneumonitis, which can progress to pulmonary fibrosis, appears in 1% of patients who receive a total cumulative dose of < 200 U/m^2 and in 10% of patients who receive a total cumulative dose of > 200 U/m^2. Interstitial pneumonitis can occur even several months after the last dose of bleomycin.[67] The sensitivity of the lung to bleomycin is explained by the fact that this drug is inactivated by a hydrolase enzyme that is relatively deficient in the lung, compared with its presence in other tissues, such as liver tissue.[32] The cells most vulnerable to the effects of bleomycin are type I pneumocytes and vascular endothelial cells. Type I pneumocytes are the alveolar-lining cells whereas type II pneumocytes are the progenitor cells that proliferate in response to damage to type I pneumocytes. Damage of vascular endothelial cells leads to exudation of fluid into interstitial and intra-alveolar spaces, but the extent to which this contributes to the final fibrosis is unknown.[68] The damage appears to be mediated by three main mechanisms: (1) the generation of free radicals, which damage capillary endothelium and pneumocytes;[69] (2) the induction of an immune response in the lungs;[69] and (3) the stimulation of collagen synthesis. It has been shown that bleomycin is able to directly stimulate fibroblast growth.[70]

L-Asparaginase. L-Asparaginase is an enzyme derived from two bacterial species, *Escherichia coli* and *Erwinia* species. L-Asparaginase hydrolyzes L-asparagine into L-aspartic acid and ammonia, thereby causing a depletion of L-asparagine in the plasma. Neoplastic lymphoblasts and other tumor cells are unable to synthesize asparagine de novo because they lack the enzyme L-asparagine synthetase; therefore, their protein synthesis and their survival ultimately depends on the presence of L-asparagine in the serum. Unlike many chemotherapeutic agents, L-asparaginase is generally not myelosuppressive and does not cause gastrointestinal toxic effects. The most important side effects are hypersensitivity reactions, which include urticaria (most common), chills, fever, laryngospasm, asthma, and life-threatening anaphylactic shock. Side effects develop within 1 hour of administration and may occur at any time during treatment although they are more likely to occur after several doses have been given. The organs frequently affected by L-asparaginase are those with high rates of protein synthesis in their cells, such as the liver and pancreas. Damage to the liver manifests as elevated transaminases and decreased levels of albumin and other serum proteins synthesized by the hepatocytes. Damage to the exocrine pancreas manifests as malabsorption, and damage to the endocrine pancreas manifests as hyperglycemia and secondary diabetes mellitus. Acute pancreatitis occurs in 15% of treated patients. By inhibiting protein synthesis, asparaginase reduces the hepatic production of several coagulation factors, both procoagulant proteins (including prothrombin; factors XI, X, IX, VIII, VII, and V; and fibrinogen) and anticoagulant proteins (antithrombin III, protein C, and protein S). As a consequence, 1% of patients develop coagulopathy, manifested either as thrombotic events (eg, deep venous thrombosis and pulmonary embolism) or as hemorrhages (eg, stroke).[71] Two mechanisms have been proposed to explain the development of acute encephalopathy in patients treated with L-asparaginase. The first is the production of glutamic acid, which is known to be neurotoxic. In fact, L-asparaginase hydrolyzes not only L-asparagine to aspartic acid but also L-glutamine to glutamic acid. Second, by hydrolyzing asparagine to aspartic acid and ammonia, L-asparaginase elevates the ammonia levels in the blood, as seen in patients with hepatic encephalopathy.

COMPLICATIONS OF
EXTERNAL-BEAM RADIOTHERAPY

External-beam radiotherapy (referred to as simply "radiotherapy" in the remainder of this section) involves the use of a radiation beam that is focused on a target region. Radiotherapy is an important component of the management of cancer because it can cure or control the primary tumor and the involved regional lymph nodes. Radiotherapy also has an important role in the setting of metastatic disease, where it is employed in the palliation of cancer symptoms. The term "radiation" normally refers to ionizing radiation that is either electromagnetic (roentgen and gamma radiation) or particulate (electrons, protons, alpha particles, and neutrons). When interacting with matter, ionizing radiation causes the ejection of an orbital electron, with the absorption of energy. The unit of absorbed dose of radiation is the gray (Gy). One gray is equivalent to 1 joule of energy absorbed per kilogram of tissue exposed to radioactive emissions (J/kg). Grays have replaced rads, the older units for reporting absorbed dose of radiation. One centigray is equivalent to 1 rad.

Radiation is cytotoxic because it damages DNA. The radiation particles produce scattered electrons that can either interact directly with the DNA or collide with water molecules to form superoxide, hydrogen peroxide, or hydroxyl radicals that are capable of covalently binding to DNA, damaging and breaking it. Radiotherapy induces DNA lesions in the forms of single- or double-strand breaks, alteration or loss of nucleotide bases, and cross-links between DNA strands. The lesion most responsible for radiation-induced cell death is the double-strand break.[72] Besides cell death due to DNA damage, radiotherapy can produce other biologic effects: the stimulation of the production of growth factors, such as fibroblast growth factor and transforming growth factor beta;[73] the activation of oncogenes, such as c-*jun*, c-*fos*, and c-*abl*;[74] the production of cytokines, (eg, interleukin-1 [IL-1], one of the mediators of tissue inflammation);[75] the stimulation of prostaglandin synthesis; and apoptosis.[76] Radiotherapy initiates apoptosis through several mechanisms, both genetic and nongenetic; experiments involving membrane preparations devoid of nuclei have shown that the interaction between radiotherapy and cellular membranes induces sphingomyelin hydrolysis and that this event generates ceramide, which in turn activates certain serine/threonine protein kinases and causes DNA degradation.[77] Thus, radiation-induced cell killing does not necessarily require direct DNA damage.

The susceptibility of cells to radiotherapy, like the susceptibility of cells to chemotherapy, depends on the phase in the cell cycle; the most sensitive cells are those in the M phase (mitosis) and the G_1/S interphase whereas the most resistant cells are those in the G_0 (resting) phase.

The development and the severity of side effects related to radiotherapy depend on several factors, including the dose of radiation, the volume of the exposed area, the functional reserve of the organ, and the concomitant use of other treatment modalities. The higher the doses of radiation delivered, the higher the clinical efficacy (ie, the better the tumor control). However, the dose of radiotherapy that can be delivered to a tumor is limited by the occurrence of serious complications in the normal tissues (Table 6–5). To reduce the toxicity of radiotherapy, the total dose is "fractionated" into repeated small doses. Fractionation causes less damage to normal tissues because it allows them to repair sublethal damage. The toxicity of radiation increases with increasing volume of the exposed area. A dose of radiation as low as a few hundred rads may lead to hematopoietic failure and death within a few weeks if the dose is delivered to the whole body. In recent years, the therapeutic index of radiotherapy has been improved by new developments in three-dimensional treatment planning, which involves control of the radiation beam by a computer system and which may involve customized "beam-shaping blocks." With such techniques, the radiotherapist can tailor the radiation fields to the shape of the tumor, maximizing the exclusion of the adjacent normal tissues. The functional reserve of an organ also affects the toxicity of radiotherapy. For example, a certain dose to the liver might be without consequences because of the liver's regenerative capacity whereas the same dose of radiotherapy delivered to the spinal cord could be catastrophic. Neural cells have minimal or no regenerative capabilities; thus, damage to a few neurons can result in severe dysfunction. The functional reserve of an organ may also be compromised by underlying diseases that play a role in determining individual patient susceptibility to radiotherapy. The toxicity associated with radiotherapy can be increased by the concomitant use of chemotherapeutic agents because they

TABLE 6–5. Limiting Doses of External-Beam Radiotherapy

Tissue	Toxic Effects	Limiting Dose* (cGy)
Eye	Blindness, corneal ulcers	5,000
Heart	Pericarditis, myocarditis	4,500
Lung	Pneumonitis, fibrosis	1,500
GI tract	Ulcerations, fibrosis	5,000
Liver	Hepatitis	2,500
Kidney	Nephrosclerosis	2,000
Brain	Necrosis	5,500
Spinal cord	Necrosis	4,500
Bone marrow	Aplasia	250
Skin	Dermatitis, sclerosis	5,500
Thyroid gland	Hypothyroidism	4,500

*Defined as the dose that produces toxic effects in 5% of patients within 5 years after irradiation.
GI = gastrointestinal.

often have a spectrum of side effects that overlap with those induced by radiation. Many chemotherapeutic drugs, such as hydroxyurea, 5-FU, and paclitaxel, are used as "radiation sensitizers" (ie, they sensitize cells to the cytotoxic effect of radiation). Some radiation sensitizers enhance the DNA damage induced by radiation. Other radiation sensitizers alter the cell cycle; for example, paclitaxel arrests cells in mitosis by stabilizing microtubules whereas hydroxyurea and 5-FU arrest cells at the G_1/S interphase.[78] As mentioned above, these are the phases of the cell cycle in which cells are most sensitive to radiation.

Radiation-induced toxic effects can be divided into acute sequelae and late tissue injury. Acute reactions occur hours to days after irradiation. They involve tissues with rapidly proliferating cells, such as bone marrow, intestine, mucosae, and skin. Acute reactions in these tissues consist of myelosuppression, enteritis, mucositis, and cutaneous inflammation, respectively. Less commonly, the brain, lung, and pericardium are involved. Acute sequelae resemble an inflammatory response. In fact, their pathogenesis involves the release of pro-inflammatory cytokines (such as tumor necrosis factor and IL-1), the expression of the endothelial leukocyte adhesion molecule E-selectin, and the extravasation of neutrophils into the irradiated tissues.[79] The pathogenesis of chronic radiation injury to normal tissues is multifactorial. The main mechanisms are the killing of tissue stem cells and damage to vascular endothelial cells.[80,81] Vascular injury and leukocyte infiltration always precede the onset of late tissue damage related to radiotherapy. Depletion of the microvasculature leads to organ ischemia, parenchymal atrophy, fibrosis, and necrosis. If vital organs such as the heart or the brain are involved, the organ dysfunction leads to life-threatening complications.

Radiation-Induced Toxic Effects, by Organ System

Eyes. Radiation-induced conjunctivitis is an acute inflammatory reaction that is usually reversible and is without complications if infections do not supervene. Irradiation of the lacrimal gland can have serious consequences (such as corneal ulcerations) if the tissue becomes entirely atrophic. Epiphora (the overflow of tears, due to inadequate tear drainage) is a consequence of late sclerosis and stenotic obstruction of the lacrimal duct. Loss of visual acuity is usually related to cataract secondary to irradiation of the lens.

The Mouth. The severity of radiation-induced mucositis ranges from mild erythema to large ulcerative lesions and depends primarily on the total dose delivered. Mucosal damage starts when the total dose reaches 2,000 cGy. Lesions usually resolve within 2 to 3 weeks after completion of the radiotherapy course. Stomatitis is caused by inhibition of cellular proliferation in the basal layer of the oral epithelium. Damage to the submucosa increases the vascular permeability and leads to tissue edema.[82] Irradiation of the salivary glands can cause xerostomia.

Lungs. *Acute Pneumonitis.* Radiation pneumonitis occurs when the total dose of irradiation is high (> 5,000 cGy). The mechanism appears to be an immunologically mediated reaction secondary to direct lung injury in the treatment field. This mechanism has been suggested by the observation that although acute lung injury is limited to the irradiated field in most patients, it can also be seen outside this area, even in the contralateral lung. This implies that circulating factors, probably autoantibodies, contribute to the radiation injury.[83] Histopathologic studies show that the injured cells are both the alveolar-lining cells (type I and type II pneumocytes) and vascular endothelial cells. The lesions cannot be distinguished from those induced by chemotherapeutic agents, which suggests that similar pathogenetic mechanisms are involved. Since type I pneumocytes are unable to regenerate, the alveolar epithelium is repopulated by type II pneumocytes, the surfactant-producing cells; some of them differentiate into type I pneumocytes. Even if regeneration occurs, however, the damage to the extracellular matrix components alters the precise reconstruction of the three-dimensional structure of the alveolocapillary unit, resulting in functional impairment. Together with the exudation of fluid into the alveolar space, this leads to abnormal gas exchange and respiratory failure.[84]

Chronic Pulmonary Fibrosis. Late radiation fibrosis occurs approximately 6 months to 2 years after the delivery of radiation. Late radiation fibrosis is the result of both direct damage to pneumocytes and indirect damage resulting from microvascular injury. The destruction of type II pneumocytes leads to the loss of alveolar surfactant, which results in alveolitis and progressive interstitial fibrosis. Histopathologic studies show that after approximately 3 months, alveolar cells slough, and the permeability of the vascular endothelium increases, leading to the accumulation of protein-rich fluid in the interstitium and alveoli. After approximately 6 months, sclerosis of the alveolar walls and diffuse interstitial fibrosis ensue. This process leads to a progressive loss of lung volume and to pleural thickening.[85]

The Heart. Cardiac irradiation delivered during the treatment of thoracic neoplasms can have several serious consequences, among which are arrhythmias and electrocardiographic changes (T-wave abnormalities, prolonged P–R interval). The most clinically relevant arrhythmia induced by radiotherapy is complete atrioventricular block, which is caused by fibrosis of the conduction system, as demonstrated in autopsy studies.[86] Cardiac irradiation can also cause acute pericarditis or constrictive pericarditis, which appears months or even many years after the completion of radiotherapy and which results from pericardial fibrosis.[87] Chronic pericardial effusion may develop after cardiac irradiation; this condition is thought to derive from increased capillary permeability. If cardiac tamponade develops, the hemodynamic effects are similar to those of constrictive pericarditis because both conditions are associated with increased venous pressure and decreased cardiac output. Cardiac irradiation may also cause congestive heart failure secondary to radiation-induced myocardial fibrosis,[88] and myocardial ischemia, manifested as angina pectoris or myocardial infarction.[89] Irradiation of the heart induces coronary artery disease even in the absence of cardiovascular risk factors. Stenosis of the coronary arteries preferentially affects their proximal portion. The pathologic lesions induced by radiotherapy include intimal proliferation, medial fibrosis, and accelerated atherosclerosis. The mechanism responsible for damage to the coronary arteries seems to be apoptosis of the vascular endothelial cells.[90] The process is regulated by several cytokines, including basic fibroblast growth factor; experimental treatment with basic fibroblast growth factor in animals that have been subjected to chest irradiation decreases radiation-induced coronary artery stenosis.[91] Besides injuring the pericardium, myocardium, and coronary arteries, radiotherapy can also affect the endocardium; cardiac valves frequently show endocardial thickening, resembling fibroelastosis. However, this is usually a finding on autopsy studies and is without clinical consequences.[92]

Gastrointestinal Tract. *Nausea and Vomiting.* The development and severity of radiation-induced emesis depend on the dose per fraction, the size of the field, and the site irradiated. Total body irradiation and radiotherapy to the upper abdomen are commonly associated with vomiting. The pathogenesis of radiation-induced emesis seems to be the same as that seen with the use of chemotherapeutic drugs: a central mechanism of stimulation of the chemoreceptor trigger zone and a peripheral mechanism whereby the release of serotonin from the enterochromaffin cells of the gastrointestinal tract stimulates the chemoreceptor trigger zone by visceral afferent nerves.[93]

Mucositis and Diarrhea. Inflammation in the mouth (stomatitis) and esophagitis can be serious events because they can compromise the patient's hydration and nutritional status. Esophagitis is a frequent complication of chest irradiation and can cause severe chest pain. The mucosal damage induced by radiation may lead to the development of opportunistic infections, often with *Candida albicans,* herpes simplex virus type 1, varicella-zoster virus, and *Cytomegalovirus.* Irradiation of the lower gastrointestinal tract can lead to diarrhea and abdominal cramping. Radiotherapy inhibits the proliferation of stem cells, essential for the maintenance of villous height and function, in the intestinal crypts. The resultant flattening of the villi leads to the loss of surface area, decreased absorption, and diarrhea.

Liver Injury. Since the liver is an organ with an elevated functional reserve, excluding as little as 15% of the normal liver from the radiation field is sufficient to prevent the development of liver failure. Radiation doses to the liver that are > 3,500 cGy can produce radiation hepatitis, which is characterized histologically by a veno-occlusive disease, with central vein fibrosis and fibrous bridging.[94]

Other Events. Gastrointestinal bleeding, intestinal infarction, fistula formation, and small-bowel obstruction are other serious late events caused by radiotherapy. Lower gastrointestinal hemorrhage, occasionally massive, can complicate radiotherapy used for treatment of gastrointestinal or genitourinary cancers.[95,96] Chronic changes secondary to radiotherapy are hypertrophy and hyalinization of the intima and media, which lead to arterial narrowing. The resultant ischemia may lead to edema, necrosis, and ulcerations of intestinal segments, either in the small intestine or colon. When necrosis has involved the full thickness of the bowel wall, perforation occurs. With progression of collagenization and hyalinization, even the submucosa and serosa of the bowel thicken. Then, the inflammatory exudate covering the serosa promotes adherence to adjacent bowel segments and fibrous strictures, which predispose to bowel obstruction.

Genitourinary Tract. *Radiation Nephropathy.* Radiation damage to the kidneys is usually seen in the treatment of large abdominal and retroperitoneal neoplasms when both kidneys are included in the radiotherapy port. When 400 cGy or a higher dose is delivered to both kidneys, radiation damage occurs in the form of a reduction in the glomerular filtration rate and a decrease in tubular excretory capacity. The most important lesions in acute radiotherapy-induced nephropathy are located in the glomerular arterioles; tubular damage appears to be secondary to the glomerular injury. Chronic radiation nephropathy may occur as late as 10 years following radiotherapy and is often accompanied by severe hypertension.

Radiation Cystitis. Pelvic radiotherapy, often given for cancers of the bladder, rectum, cervix, or prostate, may result in severe hematuria (in 15% of patients) secondary to acute cystitis.[97] Acute cystitis is an irritative process, with edema, erythema, and increased vascularity of the mucosa. Ulcerations may develop, and superinfections are common. Chronically, the bladder damage is characterized by interstitial fibrosis and by the occasional formation of fistulae. The small-vessel injury leads to fragile telangiectatic blood vessels that can spontaneously rupture.

Vulvovaginitis. Pelvic radiotherapy can be complicated by vulvovaginitis, which is a form of mucositis. Vaginitis can cause severe pain, superinfection, and late complications such as vaginal atrophy and stenosis.

Neurologic System. *Encephalopathy.* Acute radiation-induced encephalopathy occurs immediately or several weeks after a radiotherapy course and is characterized by headache, nausea, vomiting, somnolence, worsening of neurologic symptoms, and (occasionally) cerebral herniation and death. It affects predominantly the white matter. Administration of corticosteroids can prevent radiation-induced encephalopathy; this indicates that cerebral edema and increased intracranial pressure may be involved. Chronic radiation encephalopathy occurs several months or many years after radiotherapy and is characterized by amnesia, cognitive dysfunction, learning disabilities in children, and gait abnormalities. It is associated with atrophy of the brain and is believed to be the result of cerebral demyelination related to radiation-induced damage of the oligodendrocytes.[98] Radionecrosis is manifested by a focal mass lesion; like any other mass lesion in the brain, it can manifest as headache, focal neurologic deficits, and seizures. Cerebral infarctions may occur several years after the completion of radiotherapy to the brain or cervical area, as a consequence of accelerated atherosclerosis induced by radiation. After cranial irradiation, stenosis of carotid and intracranial arteries is a common finding.[99]

Myelopathy. Acute radiation-induced myelopathy is the cause of Lhermitte's sign, a sensation of electric shock in the arms and legs that is precipitated by flexion of the neck. Lhermitte's sign is an uncommon complication of irradiation to the cervical and upper thoracic spinal cord. A study showed that in 1,112 patients who had at least 3,000 cGy to the cervical spinal cord, 40 (3.6%) had Lhermitte's sign.[100] The symptom is due to a temporary demyelination. Much more serious is transverse myelitis, a late and often nonreversible radiotherapy complication that manifests as paraplegia or tetraplegia. The involved pathogenetic mechanism is necrotic degeneration of the cord white substance secondary to microvascular injury.

The Bones. *Skeletal Complications.* Radiotherapy can cause osteonecrosis, which puts the involved bone at risk for pathologic fracture.[101] The pathogenesis of osteoradionecrosis involves cellular injury and vascular damage, which lead to inhibition of osteoblastic activity and to fibrosis. The irradiated bone becomes hypocellular, hypovascular, and hypoxic, thereby losing its metabolic and homeostatic properties; it becomes unable to replace normal collagen and cellular components lost through routine wear.[102]

Myelosuppression. Because of its high proliferative index, the bone marrow is one of the most radiosensitive organs in the body. The severity of radiation-induced myelosuppression is determined by the total radiation dose, the volume of the irradiated area, and the anatomic location irradiated. Total body irradiation, as used in conditioning regimens for bone marrow transplantation, can destroy all hematopoietic cells (including stem cells), even at low doses; patients who undergo this treatment would die if they did not receive transplants of hematopoietic cells. The anatomic location of the irradiated bones is important as well; major effects are seen when radiation is delivered to the pelvic bones and to the thoracolumbar spine because these sites account for approximately 45% and 25% of the proliferating bone marrow, respectively. However, in children up to 5 years of age, severe myelosuppression can be encountered even when the long bones of the extremities are irradiated because at that age, those bones contain almost half of the actively proliferating bone marrow.

The Skin. The clinical relevance of radiation-induced effects on the skin is limited because such effects are usually limited to temporary erythema. If severe necrosis occurs, the use of improper techniques or inappropriately high doses should be suspected.

Endocrine Glands. *Pituitary Insufficiency.* Hypopituitarism is a common complication of cranial irradiation. The hormone deficiency becomes clinically evident several years after irradiation. Hormonal studies have clarified that the pituitary dysfunction is actually secondary to hypothalamic insufficiency and that the hormone secretion most frequently compromised is that of growth hormone, follicle-stimulating hormone, luteinizing hormone, thyrotropin, and adrenocorticotropic hormone.[103] Consequently, patients with radiation-induced hypopituitarism may experience hypothyroidism, Addison's disease, infertility, and (in children) growth retardation.

Hypothyroidism. The main potential consequences of thyroid irradiation are the development of thyroid carcinoma, hypothyroidism, and thyroiditis. Hypothyroidism is the result of thyroid cell destruction, vascular damage, and immune-mediated phenomena.[104] Interestingly, patients may develop exophthalmos without hyperthyroidism. The pathogenesis of this event resembles the pathogenesis of Graves' disease: radiation induces thyroidal cell injury followed by an immunologically mediated process.[105]

COMPLICATIONS OF RADIOISOTOPES

Radioisotopes for the treatment of cancer can be delivered by several methods: (1) they can be sealed in needles, seeds, capsules, tubes, or wires (brachytherapy; examples

sis of complications associated with their use is often unknown. Antiestrogens (tamoxifen, toremifene, droloxifene) are mainly used in the treatment of breast carcinoma. Their most serious side effect is thromboembolism in the form of deep venous thrombosis or pulmonary embolism.[122] Vaginal bleeding, another side effect, may be related to the development of an endometrial cancer; it has been calculated that one endometrial cancer develops for approximately every 1,000 patients with breast cancer treated with tamoxifen.[123] Antiandrogens (flutamide and finasteride) are used to effect total androgen blockade in the treatment of prostate cancer. Flutamide can cause liver damage, anemia, and leukopenia. Important side effects of finasteride are diarrhea, vomiting, and hepatic dysfunction, which is potentially lethal if treatment is not stopped. Osteoporosis is a significant and debilitating side effect of androgen suppression therapy due to anti-testosterone effect. Bone mineral density loss is approximately 3 to 5% annually in the initial years of androgen suppression therapy with an increase risk for skeletal fracture and an increase risk with longer durations of therapy. Slender white men are at greatest risk of fracture.[120,121] Luteinizing hormone–releasing hormone (LH-RH) agonists (leuprolide, goserelin acetate, and buserelin) decrease the testosterone level by decreasing serum levels of luteinizing hormone (LH) and follicle-stimulating hormone. These agents are used in the treatment of prostate cancer and are administered as monthly injections of a depot preparation. Since LH-RH agonists initially stimulate LH release and thus cause a transient rise in testosterone level, they may cause a temporary "flare" of prostate cancer when therapy is first started. The flare usually manifests as an increase in bone pain, but it may have more serious consequences in patients with impending spinal-cord compression or urinary obstruction. This explains why antiandrogens should be started before the administration of LH-RH agonists in clinical practice. Progestins (megestrol acetate and medroxyprogesterone acetate), used mainly in the treatment of endometrial carcinoma and breast cancer, can cause gastrointestinal side effects (anorexia, vomiting, change in bowel habits), uterine bleeding, fluid retention, and thromboembolism. Aromatase inhibitors (anastrozole, letrozole, and vorozole) are indicated for breast cancer in postmenopausal women with disease progression following tamoxifen therapy. The enzyme aromatase is responsible for the conversion of androstenedione to estrone and the conversion of testosterone to estradiol. Side effects include gastrointestinal events (anorexia, vomiting, change in bowel habits), edema, and thromboembolism (which occurs in 1% of treated patients). Important side effects of the use of glucocorticoids (prednisone and dexamethasone) are hyperglycemia, psychosis, gastric hemorrhage, myopathy, and ischemic necrosis of the bone.

Questionable Cancer Therapies

Treatments for which there is no real evidence of value attract a large following; approximately one-third of cancer patients use unproven healing methods.[126] These include herbal treatment, dietary supplements, psychological approaches, electroacupuncture devices, homeopathy, and shark cartilage. Although erroneously regarded as generally safe by many patients (and physicians), questionable cancer drugs and herbs can be responsible for oncologic emergencies, as shown by the following examples. (a) Laetrile is the trade name for a synthetic relative of amygdalin, a chemical contained in some fruits and nuts (eg, apricots and almonds). When subjected to enzymatic breakdown, Laetrile can form cyanide. Some cancer patients who were treated with Laetrile on the basis of the erroneous belief that amygdalin could kill cancer cells experienced nausea, vomiting, and death from cyanide poisoning.[127] (b) "Fresh cell therapy," which involves the injection of fresh embryonic animal cells, has caused serious infections, immunologic reactions, and occasionally death.[128] (c) The "Gerson method" is a type of "nutritional therapy" that consists of "detoxifying" the body with frequent coffee enemas and a low-sodium diet rich in juices made from fruits, vegetables, and raw calf's liver. Some patients who were treated developed *Campylobacter fetus* sepsis and severe hyponatremia.[129] (d) "Hyperoxygenation" is a method of treatment based on the erroneous concept that cancer is caused by oxygen deficiency and can be cured by exposing cancer cells to more oxygen than they can tolerate. Germanium sesquioxide, a hyperoxygenating agent, has caused irreversible renal failure and death. Histologic examination showed tubular degeneration and interstitial fibrosis of the kidneys.[130]

REFERENCES

1. Greenburg AG, Saik RP, Pridham D. Influence of age on mortality of colon surgery. Am J Surg 1985;150:65–70.
2. Wade DS, Douglass H Jr, Nava HR, et al. Abdominal pain in neutropenic patients. Arch Surg 1990;125:1119–27.
3. Nishi M, Hiramatsu Y, Hioki K, et al. Risk factors in relation to postoperative complications in patients undergoing esophagectomy or gastrectomy for cancer. Ann Surg 1988;207:148–54.
4. Kemeny MM, Busch-Devereaux E, Merriam LT, et al. Cancer surgery in the elderly. Hematol Oncol Clin North Am 2000;14:169–92.
5. Steen PA, Tinker JH, Tarhan S. Myocardial infarction after anesthesia and surgery. JAMA 1978;239:2566–70.
6. Fowler WC, Langer CJ, Curran WJ Jr, et al. Postoperative complications after combined neoadjuvant treatment of lung cancer. Ann Thorac Surg 1993;55:986–9.
7. Lefor AT. Perioperative management of the patient with cancer. Chest 1999;115(Suppl):165S–71S.

8. Dougherty TB, Cronan LH Jr. Anesthetic implications for surgical patients with endocrine tumors. Int Anesthesiol Clin 1998;36:31–44.

9. Kohman LJ, Meyer JA, Ikins PM, et al. Random versus predictable risks of mortality after thoracotomy for lung cancer. J Thorac Cardiovasc Surg 1986;91:551–4.

10. Perie S, Laccourreye O, Bou-Malhab F, et al. Aspiration in unilateral recurrent laryngeal nerve paralysis after surgery. Am J Otolaryngol 1998;19:18–23.

11. Peracchia A, Bardini R, Ruol A, et al. Esophagovisceral anastomotic leak. A prospective statistical study of predisposing factors. J Thorac Cardiovasc Surg 1988;95:685–91.

12. Fujiwara Y, Nakagawa K, Kusunoki M, et al. Massive pleural effusion and ascites resulting from esophagectomy with extensive lymphadenectomy for cancer of the abdominal esophagus. Hepatogastroenterology 1999;46:290–4.

13. Paolini A, Tosato F, Cassese M, et al. Total gastrectomy in the treatment of adenocarcinoma of the cardia. Review of the results in 73 resected patients. Am J Surg 1986; 151:238–43.

14. Cullen JJ, Sarr MG, Ilstrup DM. Pancreatic anastomotic leak after pancreatoduodenectomy: incidence, significance, and management. Am J Surg 1994;168:295–8.

15. Northover JM, Terblanche J. A new look at the arterial supply of the bile ducts in man and its surgical implications. Br J Surg 1979;66:379–84.

16. Scott HW Jr, Dean RH, Parker T, et al. The role of vagotomy in pancreatoduodenectomy. Ann Surg 1980;191:688–96.

17. Sato N, Yamaguchi K, Yokohata K, et al. Changes in pancreatic function after pancreatoduodenectomy. Am J Surg 1998;176:59–61.

18. Michalopoulos GK. Liver regeneration: molecular mechanisms of growth control. FASEB J 1990;4:176–87.

19. Eraklis AJ, Kevy SV, Diamond LK, et al. Hazard of overwhelming infection after splenectomy in childhood. N Engl J Med 1967;276:1225–9.

20. Swanson DA, Borges PM. Complications of transabdominal radical nephrectomy for renal cell carcinoma. J Urol 1983;129: 704–7.

21. Walsh PC. Radical retropubic prostatectomy with reduced morbidity: an anatomic approach. J Natl Cancer Inst Monogr 1988;7:133–7.

22. Oberfield RA. Intraarterial hepatic infusion chemotherapy in metastatic liver cancer. Semin Oncol 1983;10:206–13.

23. Davidson SA, Rubin SC, Markman M, et al. Intraperitoneal chemotherapy: analysis of complications with an implanted subcutaneous port and catheter system. Gynecol Oncol 1991;41:101–6.

24. Obbens E, Leavens ME, Beal JW, et al. Ommaya reservoirs in 387 cancer patients: a 15 years experience. Neurology 1985;35:1274–8.

25. Bertrand M, Presant CA, Klein L, et al. Iatrogenic superior vena cava syndrome. A new entity. Cancer 1984;54: 376–8.

26. Lindbled B. Thromboembolic complications of central venous catheters. Lancet 1982;2:936–7.

27. Brothers TE, Von Moll LK, Niederhuber JE, et al. Experience with subcutaneous infusion ports in three hundred patients. Surg Gynecol Obstet 1988;166:295–301.

28. Raaf JH. Results from use of 826 vascular access devices in cancer patients. Cancer 1985;55:1312–21.

29. Cox PJ. Cyclophosphamide cystitis—identification of acrolein as the causative agent. Biochem Pharmacol 1979;28:2045–9.

30. Rubin JS, Rubin RT. Cyclophosphamide hemorrhagic cystitis. J Urol 1966;96:313–6.

31. Andriole GL, Sandlund JT, Miser JS, et al. The efficacy of mesna (2-mercaptoethane sodium sulfonate) as a uroprotectant in patients with hemorrhagic cystitis receiving oxazaphosphorine chemotherapy. J Clin Oncol 1987;5:799–803.

32. Cooper JA Jr, White DA, Matthay RA. Drug-induced pulmonary disease: part 1. Cytotoxic drugs. Am Rev Respir Dis 1986;133:321–40.

33. Baverman AC, Antin JH, Plappert MT, et al. Cyclophosphamide cardiotoxicity in bone marrow transplantation. J Clin Oncol 1991;9:1215–23.

34. Mills BA, Roberts RW. Cyclophosphamide induced cardiomyopathy: a report of two cases and a review of the English literature. Cancer 1979;43:2223–6.

35. Gottdiener JS, Appelbaum FR, Ferrans VJ, et al. Cardiotoxicity associated with high dose cyclophosphamide therapy. Arch Intern Med 1981;141:758–63.

36. Harlow PJ, DeClerck YA, Shore NA, et al. A fatal case of inappropriate ADH secretion induced by cyclophosphamide therapy. Cancer 1979;44:896–8.

37. Madias NE, Harrington JT. Platinum nephrotoxicity. Am J Med 1978;65:307–14.

38. Wood PA, Hrushesky WJ. Cisplatin-associated anemia: an erythropoietin deficiency syndrome. J Clin Invest 1995;95:1650–9.

39. Talcott J, Herman TS. Acute ischemic vascular events and cisplatin. Ann Intern Med 1987;107:121–2.

40. Doll DC, List AF, Greco A, et al. Acute vascular ischemic events after cisplatin-based combination chemotherapy for germ cell tumors of the testis. Ann Intern Med 1986;105:48–51.

41. Doll DC, Yarbro JW. Vascular toxicity associated with antineoplastic agents. Semin Oncol 1992;19:580–96.

42. McCarthy LE, Borison HL. Cisplatin-induced vomiting eliminated by ablation of the area postrema in cats. Cancer Treat Rep 1984;68:401–4.

43. Hawthorn J, Ostler KJ, Andrews PL. The role of the abdominal visceral innervation and 5-hydroxytryptamine M-receptors in vomiting induced by the cytotoxic drugs cyclophosphamide and cis-platin in the ferret. Q J Exp Physiol 1988;73:7–21.

44. Twohig KJ, Matthay RA. Pulmonary effects of cytotoxic agents other than bleomycin. Clin Chest Med 1990; 11:31–54.

45. Harmon WE, Cohen HT, Schneeberger E, et al. Chronic renal failure in children treated with methyl CCNU. N Engl J Med 1979;300:1200–3.

46. Verweij J, Funke-Kupper AJ, Teule GJ, et al. A prospective study on the dose dependency of cardiotoxicity induced by mitomycin C. Med Oncol Tumor Pharmacother 1988;5:159–63.

47. Cantrell JE, Phillips TM, Schein PS. Carcinoma-associated hemolytic-uremic syndrome: a complication of mitomycin C chemotherapy. J Clin Oncol 1985;3:723–34.

48. Freeman NJ, Costanza ME. 5-Fluorouracil-associated cardiotoxicity. Cancer 1988;61:36–45.

49. Barnett MJ, Richards MA, Ganesan TS, et al. Central nervous system toxicity of high-dose cytosine arabinoside. Semin Oncol 1985;12:227–32.

50. Dworkin LA, Goldman RD, Zivin LS, et al. Cerebellar tox-

icity following high-dose cytosine arabinoside. J Clin Oncol 1985;3:613–6.

51. Wan SH, Huffman DH, Azarnoff DL, et al. Effect of route of administration and effusion on methotrexate pharmacokinetics. Cancer Res 1974;34:3487–91.

52. Suzuki K, Takemura T, Okeda R, et al. Vascular changes of methotrexate-related disseminated necrotizing leukoencephalopathy. Acta Neuropathol 1984;65:145–9.

53. Bernini JC, Fort DW, Griener JC, et al. Aminophylline for methotrexate-induced neurotoxicity. Lancet 1995;345:544–7.

54. Jacobs SA, Stoller RG, Chabner BA, et al. 7-Hydroxymethotrexate as a urinary metabolite in human subjects and rhesus monkeys receiving high dose methotrexate. J Clin Invest 1976;57:534–8.

55. Bristow MR, Thompson PD, Martin RP, et al. Early anthracycline cardiotoxicity. Am J Med 1978;65:823–32.

56. Praga C, Beretta G, Vigo PL, et al. Adriamycin cardiotoxicity: a survey of 1273 patients. Cancer Treat Rep 1979;62:931–4.

57. Myers CE, McGuire WP, Liss RH, et al. Adriamycin: the role of lipid peroxidation in cardiac toxicity and tumor response. Science 1977;197:165–7.

58. Doroshow JH, Locker GY, Myers CE. Enzymatic defenses of the mouse heart against reactive metabolites: alterations produced by doxorubicin. J Clin Invest 1980;65:128–35.

59. Ali MK, Soto A, Maroongroge D, et al. Electrocardiographic changes after Adriamycin chemotherapy. Cancer 1979;43:465–71.

60. Seidman A, Hudis, Pierri MK, et al. Cardiac dysfunction in the trastuzumab clinical trials experience. J Clin Onco 2002;20:1215–21.

61. Speyer J. Cardiac dysfunction in the trastuzumab clinical experience. J Clin Oncol 2002;20:1156–7.

62. Sandler SG, Tobin W, Henderson ES. Vincristine-induced neuropathy: a clinical study of fifty leukemia patients. Neurology 1969;19:367–74.

63. Chan SY, Worth R, Ochs S. Block of axoplasmic transport in vitro by *Vinca* alkaloids. J Neurobiol 1980;11:251–64.

64. Topp KS, Tanner KD, Levine JD. Damage to the cytoskeleton of large diameter sensory neurons and myelinated axons in vincristine-induced painful peripheral neuropathy in the rat. J Comp Neurol 2000;424:563–76.

65. Schiff PB, Fant J, Horwitz SB. Promotion of microtubule assembly in vitro by taxol. Nature 1979;277:665–7.

66. McGuire WP, Rowinsky EK, Rosenshein NB, et al. Taxol: a unique antineoplastic agent with significant activity in advanced ovarian epithelial neoplasms. Ann Intern Med 1989;111:273–9.

67. Jules-Elysee K, White DA. Bleomycin-induced pulmonary toxicity. Clin Chest Med 1990;11:1–20.

68. Jordana M, Richards C, Irving LB, et al. Spontaneous in vitro release of alveolar macrophages cytokines after intrathecal instillation of bleomycin in rats: characterization and kinetic studies. Am Rev Respir Dis 1988;137:1135–40.

69. Chandler DB. Possible mechanisms of bleomycin-induced fibrosis. Clin Chest Med 1990;11:21–30.

70. Muggia FM. Pulmonary toxicity of antitumoral agents. Cancer Treat Rev 1983;10:221–43.

71. Feinberg WM, Swenson MR. Cerebrovascular complications of L-asparaginase therapy. Neurology 1988;38:127–33.

72. Elkind MM. DNA damage and cell killing: cause and effect? Cancer 1985;56:2351–63.

73. Haimovitz-Friedman A, Vlodavsky I, Chandhuri A, et al. Autocrine effects of fibroblast growth factor in repair of radiation damage in endothelial cells. Cancer Res 1991;51:2552–8.

74. Fornace AJ Jr. Mammalian genes induced by radiation; activation of genes associated with growth control. Annu Rev Genet 1992;26:507–26.

75. Rubin P, Johnston CJ, Williams JP, et al. A perpetual cascade of cytokines postirradiation leads to pulmonary fibrosis. Int J Radiat Oncol Biol Phys 1995;33:99–109.

76. Allan DJ. Radiation-induced apoptosis: its role in a MADCaT (mitosis-apoptosis-differentiation-calcium toxicity) scheme of cytotoxicity mechanisms. Int J Radiat Biol 1992;62:145–52.

77. Haimovitz-Friedman A, Kan CC, Ehleiter D, et al. Ionizing radiation acts on cellular membranes to generate ceramide and initiate apoptosis. J Exp Med 1994;180:525–35.

78. Schilsky RL. Biochemical pharmacology of chemotherapeutic drugs used as radiation enhancers. Semin Oncol 1992;19 Suppl:2–7.

79. Dunn MM, Drab EA, Rubin DB. Effects of irradiation on endothelial cell-polymorphonuclear leukocyte interactions. J Appl Physiol 1986;60:1932–7.

80. Hopewell JW, Calvo W, Jaenke R, et al. Microvasculature and radiation damage. Recent Results Cancer Res 1993;130:1–16.

81. Law MP. Radiation-induced vascular injury and its relation to late effects in normal tissue. Adv Radiat Biol 1981;9:37–73.

82. Baker DG. The radiobiological basis for tissue reactions in the oral cavity following therapeutic x-irradiation. Arch Otolaryngol 1982;108:21–4.

83. Gibson PG, Bryant DH, Morgan GW, et al. Radiation-induced lung injury: a hypersensitivity pneumonitis? Ann Intern Med 1988;109:288–91.

84. Gross NJ. The pathogenesis of radiation-induced lung damage. Lung 1981;159:115–25.

85. Rosiello RA, Merrill WW. Radiation-induced lung injury. Clin Chest Med 1990;11:65–71.

86. Slama MS, Le Guludec D, Sebag C, et al. Complete atrioventricular block following mediastinal irradiation: a report of six cases. Pacing Clin Electrophysiol 1991;14:1112–8.

87. Applefeld MM, Slawson RG, Hall-Craigs M, et al. Delayed pericardial disease after radiotherapy. Am J Cardiol 1981;47:210–3.

88. Fajardo L, Stewart J. Pathogenesis of radiation-induced myocardial fibrosis. Lab Invest 1973;29:244–57.

89. Cohn KE, Stewart JR, Fajardo LF, et al. Heart disease following radiation. Medicine 1967;46:281–98.

90. Om A, Ellahham S, Vetrovec GW. Radiation-induced coronary artery disease. Am Heart J 1992;124:1598–602.

91. Fuks Z, Persaud RS, Alfieri A, et al. Basic fibroblast growth factor protects endothelial cells against radiation-induced programmed cell death in vitro and in vivo. Cancer Res 1994;54:2582–90.

92. Brosius F III, Waller B, Roberts W. Radiation heart disease: analysis of 16 young (aged 15–33 years) necropsy patients who received over 3,500 rads to the heart. Am J Med 1981;70:519–30.

93. Bodis S, Alexander E, Kooy H, et al. The prevention of radiosurgery-induced nausea and vomiting by ondansetron: evidence of a direct effect on the central nervous system chemoreceptor trigger zone. Surg Neurol 1994;42:249–52.

94. Rollins BJ. Hepatic veno-occlusive disease. Am J Med 1986;81:297–306.

95. Benk VA, Adams JA, Shipley WU, et al. Late rectal bleeding following combined x-ray and proton high-dose irradiation for patients with stages T3–T4 prostate carcinoma. Int J Radiat Oncol Biol Phys 1993;26:551–7.

96. Calvo FA, Aristu JJ, Azinovic I, et al. Intraoperative and external radiotherapy in resected gastric cancer: an updated report of a phase II trial. Int J Radiat Oncol Biol Phys 1992;24:729–36.

97. Dean RJ, Lytton B. Urologic complications of pelvic irradiation. J Urol 1978;119:64–7.

98. Lampert PW, Davis RL. Delayed effects of radiation on the human central nervous system: "early" and "late" delayed reactions. Neurology 1964;14:912–7.

99. Murros KE, Toole JF. The effect of radiation on carotid arteries: a review article. Arch Neurol 1989;46:449–55.

100. Fein DA, Marcus RB Jr, Parsons JT, et al. Lhermitte's sign: incidence and treatment variables influencing risks after irradiation of the cervical spinal cord. Int J Radiat Oncol Biol Phys 1993;27:1029–33.

101. Blumke DA, Fishman EK, Scott WW Jr. Skeletal complications of radiation therapy. Radiographics 1994;14:111–21.

102. Lim AA, Karakla DW, Watkins DV. Osteoradionecrosis of the cervical vertebrae and occipital bone: a case report and brief review of the literature. Am J Otolaryngol 1999;20:408–11.

103. Constine LS, Woolf PD, Cann D, et al. Hypothalamic-pituitary dysfunction after radiation for brain tumors. N Engl J Med 1993;328:87–94.

104. DeGroot LJ. Effects of irradiation on the thyroid gland. Endocrinol Metab Clin North Am 1993;22:607–15.

105. Wasnich RD, Grumet FC, Payne RO, et al. Graves' ophthalmopathy following external neck irradiation for non-thyroidal neoplastic disease. J Clin Endocrinol Metab 1973;37:703–13.

106. Roach M, Leidholdt EM Jr, Tatera BS, et al. Endobronchial radiation therapy (EBRT) in the management of lung cancer. Int J Radiat Oncol Biol Phys 1990;18:1449–54.

107. Kucera H, Vavra N, Weghaupt K. Benefit of external irradiation in pathologic stage I endometrial carcinoma: a prospective clinical trial of 605 patients who received postoperative vaginal irradiation and additional pelvic irradiation in the presence of unfavorable prognostic factors. Gynecol Oncol 1990;38:99–104.

108. Wallner K, Roy J, Harrison L. Tumor control and morbidity following transperineal iodine 125 implantation for stage T1/T2 prostatic carcinoma. J Clin Oncol 1996;14:449–53.

109. Ankem MK, Decarvalho VS, Harangozo AM, et al. Implications of radioactive seed migration to the lungs after prostate brachytherapy. Urology 2002;59:555–9.

110. Older RA, Synder B, Krupski TL, et al. Radioactive implant migration in patients treated for localized prostate cancer with interstitial brachytherapy. J Urol 2001;165:1590–2.

111. Tharp M, Hornback NB. Complications associated with intraperitoneal 32P. Gynecol Oncol 1994;53:170–5.

112. Alexander C, Bader JB, Schaefer A, et al. Intermediate and long-term side effects of high-dose radioiodine therapy for thyroid carcinoma. J Nucl Med 1998;39:1551–4.

113. Van Nostrun D, Neutze J, Atkins F. Side effects of "rational dose" iodine-131 therapy for metastatic well-differentiated thyroid carcinoma. J Nucl Med 1986;27:1519–27.

114. Edmonds CJ, Smith T. The long-term hazards of the treatment of thyroid cancer with radioiodine. Br J Radiol 1986;59:45–51.

115. Nair N, Mahadeo DS, Patel R. Does renal damage occur after the administration of 32P for palliation of pain from skeletal metastases? Nucl Med Commun 1998;19:689–93.

116. Vriesendorp HM, Herpst JM, Germack MA, et al. Phase I-II studies of yttrium-labeled antiferritin treatment for end-stage Hodgkin's disease, including Radiation Therapy Oncology Group 87-01. J Clin Oncol 1991;9:918–28.

117. Maraveyas A, Snook D, Hird V, et al. Pharmacokinetics and toxicity of an yttrium-90-CITC-DTPA-HMFG1 radioimmunoconjugate for intraperitoneal radioimmunotherapy of ovarian cancer. Cancer 1994;73:1067–75.

118. Quesada JR, Talpaz M, Rios A, et al. Clinical toxicity of interferons in cancer patients: a review. J Clin Oncol 1988;4:234–43.

119. Conlon KC, Urba WJ, Smith JW II, et al. Exacerbation of symptoms of autoimmune disease in patients receiving alpha-interferon therapy. Cancer 1990;65:2237–42.

120. Ochoa JB, Curti B, Peitzman AB, et al. Increased circulating nitrogen oxides after human tumor immunotherapy: correlation with toxic hemodynamic changes. J Natl Cancer Inst 1992;84:864–7.

121. Lee RE, Lotze MT, Skibber JM, et al. Cardiorespiratory effects of immunotherapy with interleukin-2. J Clin Oncol 1989;7:7–20.

122. Lipton A, Harvey HA, Hamilton RW. Venous thrombosis as a side effect of tamoxifen treatment. Cancer Treat Rep 1984;68:887–9.

123. Fisher B, Costantino JP, Redmond CK, et al. Endometrial cancer in tamoxifen-treated breast cancer patients: findings from the National Surgical Adjuvant Breast and Bowel Project (NSABP) B-14. J Natl Cancer Inst 1994;86:527–37.

124. Ross RW, Small EJ, Osteoporosis in men treated with androgen deprivation therapy for prostate cancer. J Urol 2002;167:1952–6.

125. Oefelein MG, Ricchuiti V, Conrad W, et al. Skeletal fracture associatd with androgen suppression induced osteoporosis: the clinical incidence and risk factors for patients with prostate cancer. J Urol 2001;166:1724–8.

126. Eisenberg DM, Kessler RC, Foster C, et al. Unconventional medicine in the United States. Prevalence, costs, and patterns of use. N Engl J Med 1993;328:246–52.

127. American Cancer Society. Unproven methods of cancer management: laetrile. CA Cancer J Clin 1991;1:187–92.

128. American Cancer Society. Unproven methods of cancer management: fresh cell therapy. CA Cancer J Clin 1991;41:126–8.

129. Ginsberg MM, Thompson MA, Peter CR, et al. *Campylobacter* sepsis associated with "nutritional therapy"— California. Morb Mortal Wkly Rep 1981;30:294–5.

130. Obara K, Saito T, Sato H, et al. Germanium poisoning: clinical symptoms and renal damage caused by long-term intake of germanium. Jpn J Med 1991;30:67–72.

CHAPTER 7

METABOLIC AND ENDOCRINE EMERGENCIES

SAI-CHING JIM YEUNG, MD, PHD, RPH
GUILLERMO LAZO-DIAZ, MD
ROBERT F. GAGEL, MD

Cancer and its treatment can lead to endocrine and metabolic dysfunction. Oncologists and emergency physicians should have an appropriate level of suspicion for endocrine and metabolic sequelae so that prompt and appropriate treatment can be given to improve the patient's quality of life and to avoid serious morbidity or mortality. This chapter focuses on pituitary, thyroid, and adrenal dysfunction; imbalance in electrolytes; water; and glucose metabolism; and neuroendocrine crises caused by tumors.

TUMOR LYSIS SYNDROME

Acute tumor lysis syndrome (TLS) is caused by the death of a large number of neoplastic cells and is a complication of cancer therapy.[1–4] Hyperkalemia and renal failure usually are responsible for patients' deaths in TLS cases. Early recognition of metabolic perturbations and prompt appropriate treatment can prevent fatal outcomes.

Clinical Manifestations

Tumor lysis syndrome was first described in patients with Burkitt's lymphoma who suddenly died after chemotherapy. Chemotherapy usually precedes TLS by less than 72 hours in patients with leukemia and lymphoma, but new therapeutic methods may alter the time frame. Recently, more effective treatments have caused TLS in patients with even indolent and chronic diseases, such as chronic lymphocytic leukemia.[5,6] Tumor lysis syndrome has also been reported in nonhematologic malignancies, including small-cell carcinomas,[7] non-small-cell lung cancer,[8] breast cancer,[9] and ovarian adenocarcinomas.[10]

The symptomatology is nonspecific, but common symptoms include nausea, vomiting, weakness, fatigue, lethargy, cloudy urine, and arthralgia. Other signs and symptoms related to metabolic and electrolyte abnormalities include arrhythmias, neuromuscular irritability, muscle weakness, and seizures. Sudden death in patients with TLS may result from arrhythmia.[11]

Pathophysiologic Mechanisms

Several factors contribute to the development of TLS, including type of malignancy, responsiveness of the malignancy to therapy, rapidity of cell turnover, and tumor burden. Other risk factors include pre-existing renal insufficiency, acute renal failure developing shortly after the treatment has been initiated, and poor response to hydration. Pretreatment lactate dehydrogenase levels, which tend to correlate with tumor bulk in patients with stage C or D lymphoma, can predict the development of posttreatment azotemia. Although pretreatment hyperuricemia is often considered a problem, the serum uric acid level is not predictive of the development of azotemia.

The metabolic abnormalities associated with TLS are due to the massive release of the contents and degradation products of dead tumor cells in the blood stream. These abnormalities include hyperkalemia, hyperphosphatemia and secondary hypocalcemia, hyperuricemia, azotemia, and (sometimes) profound metabolic acidosis that is out of proportion to the degree of renal insufficiency. Hyperuricemia, hyperkalemia, and hypocalcemia may contribute to the development of cardiac arrhythmia, tetany, and sudden death.

Acute renal failure is caused by the precipitation of uric acid and/or calcium phosphate in the renal tubules. Initiation of allopurinol prior to chemotherapy has decreased the incidence of acute renal failure due to uric acid nephropathy, but severe hyperphosphatemia is now the usual cause of acute renal failure in TLS.

Etiology

Tumor lysis syndrome can occur spontaneously,[12] or (most commonly) it may be related to chemotherapy (including steroid use alone, in some very sensitive lymphomas),[13] immunotherapy,[6] or radiation therapy.[14] The specific chemotherapy agents or regimens involved are fludarabine, mitoxantrone, 6-mercaptopurine, methotrexate, chemotherapeutic conditioning or total-body irradiation for bone marrow transplantation, and various combination chemotherapy regimens.

Diagnosis

The diagnosis of TLS requires a high level of suspicion as the condition can have few or no clinical manifestations in the early stages. The diagnosis is primarily biochemical, and routine uric acid and electrolyte screening (including calcium and phosphorus) is indicated in patients with a high tumor bulk or with hematologic malignancies.

Prevention and Treatment

Prevention is the most important approach to TLS management and should be the initial concern. Special attention should be paid to identifying the patients at risk for TLS so that preventive measures can be started early. Aggressive hydration with normal saline (up to 3 L/m^2/d) may be required to promote a urine output of at least 100 mL/h with or without the addition of loop or osmotic diuretics. Prophylactic treatment with the xanthine oxidase inhibitor allopurinol should be started at doses of between 100 and 300 mg/d.

The patient with severe TLS should be under intensive care to continuously monitor hemodynamic and electrocardiographic parameters, increase allopurinol up to 900 mg/d, increase hydration, and promote diuresis with loop diuretics (eg, furosemide, 20 to 200 mg intravenously [IV] every 4 to 6 hours) and acetazolamide (250 to 500 mg IV daily). If aciduria is present, sodium bicarbonate or acetate infusion may be used to keep urine pH between 7.1 and 7.5. Urate oxidase (uricozyme, an enzyme of nonhuman origin that is capable of oxidizing human uric acid to allantoin) may soon be available for treating urate nephropathy.[15,16] Electrolyte measurements may be required every 4 to 6 hours. Hyperkalemia should be treated with insulin, calcium, and bicarbonate infusions along with oral potassium exchange resins (sodium polystyrene sulfonate [Kayexalate]). In a hyperphosphatemic patient with hypocalcemia, the addition of an oral calcium-based compound will reduce phosphate and enhance calcium absorption. Intravenous calcium administration can potentially cause calcium phosphate precipitation in the presence of severe hyperphosphatemia and should be used cautiously. Dialysis may be required for patients with symptomatic hypocalcemia and a serum phosphorus level > 3.3 mmol/L (> 10.2 mg/dL). Other indications for dialysis include persistent azotemia, hyperuricemia, decreased urine output despite diuretic use, refractory acidemia, and volume overload. Prompt dialysis should be instituted, with continued careful monitoring until biochemical abnormalities resolve. Hemodialysis is the most common mode of dialysis. Continuous arteriovenous hemodialysis with a high dialysate flow rate[17] and continuous venovenous hemofiltration[18] are also effective.

HYPONATREMIA

Hyponatremia (defined as a plasma sodium concentration < 135 mEq/dL) may be seen in up to 25% of all hospitalized patients and is one of the most common electrolyte abnormalities found in cancer patients.[19–21] Hyponatremia may be present as a chronic asymptomatic condition, but it becomes an emergency when the patient is symptomatic. Hyponatremia can be classified clinically as hypovolemic, euvolemic, or hypervolemic; each has a different etiology. Treatments should be based on the etiology.

Clinical Manifestations

The signs and symptoms of hyponatremia depend mainly on the severity and rapidity of the development of the hypo-osmotic state. In patients with chronic hyponatremia, adaptive mechanisms can protect against brain swelling, and the patient can be asymptomatic even with serum sodium at about 120 mEq/L. The symptoms of hyponatremia are primarily neurologic (hyponatremic encephalopathy) and consist of hyperexcitability, irritability, psychotic behavior, nausea, and vomiting. Seizures may occur. The symptoms may progress with lethargy and confusion. If hyponatremia is not treated appropriately, coma, permanent brain damage, brain stem herniation, respiratory failure, and death may occur.

Pathophysiologic Mechanisms

Normotonic hyponatremia, or pseudohyponatremia, is a laboratory artifact and is mainly seen with hyperlipidemia (sodium [Na] corrected = Na + 0.2 × triglyceride (TG) [grams per liter]) or hyperproteinemia (Na corrected = Na + 0.025 × protein [if protein > 8 g/dL]). This laboratory artifact is being avoided as more laboratories are measuring sodium concentration with a selective electrode that is not affected by the proportion of the nonaqueous phase of plasma.

Hypertonic hyponatremia occurs when active solutes shift intracellular water to the extracellular fluid, diluting the sodium concentration in plasma. This mainly occurs with extreme hyperglycemia. Other solutes, such as sorbitol and mannitol, have similar effects.

Hypovolemic hypotonic hyponatremia is associated with true volume depletion. Intravascular volume depletion can occur after acute bleeding or massive draining of ascites or pleural effusion or can be caused by diuretics, diarrhea, vomiting, severe hypoalbuminemia, and fluid third-spacing in ileus, peritonitis, or other serious infections. Such patients usually present with hypotension, tachycardia, orthostasis, oliguria, and low spot urine sodium (< 30 mEq/L). Renal sodium wasting due to platinum compounds, cyclophosphamide, or ifosfamide may cause a similar picture except that urine sodium may be higher.

Normal adults can excrete more than 10 L of water per day, and hyponatremia would not occur unless there were a combination of non-osmotic stimulation of antidiuretic hormone secretion and an excessive intake of water. Normovolemic hyponatremia is associated with increased vasopressin secretion. The causes of non-osmotic stimulation of vasopressin secretion include nausea and vomiting, liver disease, and congestive heart failure. Other causes are thiazide-associated hyponatremia, adrenal deficiency, severe hypothyroidism, and the syndrome of inappropriate antidiuretic hormone (SIADH).

The syndrome of inappropriate antidiuretic hormone was first described in the 1950s and is characterized by inappropriately concentrated urine (> 100 mOsm/kg) in the presence of hypotonic hyponatremia, euvolemia, and normal thyroid, adrenal, cardiac, hepatic, and renal functions. Antidiuretic hormone level (vasopressin) is elevated, particularly in relation to plasma osmolality. Hyponatremia in these patients is dilutional in origin. However, the hyponatremia may be exacerbated by the activation of natriuretic mechanisms, including the suppression of rennin and aldosterone secretion and a decrease in proximal tubular sodium reabsorption. Because of the increased natriuresis from these secondary mechanisms, normal saline administration may fail to correct the hyponatremia unless free water restriction is also instituted.

Hypervolemic hypotonic hyponatremia is manifested mainly by peripheral edema or ascites and is commonly found in cancer patients. Any condition that leads to a decrease in the effective circulating volume, such as hepatic tumoral infiltration, infection, veno-occlusive disease, ascites, Budd-Chiari syndrome, or congestive heart failure, can lead to water retention. These patients are seldom oliguric and have a low spot urine sodium level (15 mEq/L), low (< 1) fractional excretion of sodium (FENa), and increased total body water along with normal to increased total body sodium.

Etiology

Etiologic factors for hyponatremia include free water retention, renal sodium wasting, and disturbances in the intake of water and sodium (including intravenous fluids). In cancer patients, hypovolemic hypotonic hypona-

tremia is quite common. Intravascular volume depletion can be caused by diarrhea, vomiting, or acute bleeding or by massive draining of ascites or pleural effusion, severe hypoalbuminemia, fluid third-spacing in ileus, peritonitis, or other serious infections.

Renal sodium wasting due to platinum compounds, cyclophosphamide, or ifosfamide also is commonly seen.[22] Drug-induced renal salt wasting or tumor-induced salt wasting (mediated by atrial natriuretic peptide) also can cause hyponatremia, hypo-osmolality, elevated urinary sodium, and urinary osmolality. Damage to the renal tubules and resultant defects in salt and water transport may be the major cause of hyponatremia associated with low-dose cyclophosphamide therapy. The mechanism of cisplatin-induced hyponatremia is unclear, but the renal toxic effects of cisplatin, which decrease papillary solute content and decrease maximal urinary osmolarity, are perhaps the major factor in vasopressin secretion rather than a direct effect on the hypothalamus.

Ectopic vasopressin secreted by tumors, abnormal secretory stimuli, or cytotoxicity affecting paraventricular and supraoptic neurons may cause SIADH. It is also possible that chemotherapy-induced lysis of vasopressin-containing cancer cells leads to or worsens SIADH. Malignant diseases are the most common clinical disorders associated with nonpituitary SIADH. Small-cell carcinoma of the lung is the common tumor most often associated with ectopic vasopressin production. Less commonly, ectopic vasopressin production accompanies pancreatic cancer, prostate cancer, lymphoma, or extrapulmonary small-cell carcinoma. Although as many as two-thirds of patients with small-cell lung cancer may have impaired water excretion, less than 10% have clinically evident hyponatremia. The degree of water excretion impairment is not always related to the extent of disease or tumor burden. In certain cases, SIADH has presented prior to clinical recognition of small-cell lung cancer.

Primary or metastatic brain tumors also may cause SIADH, as may pituitary adenoma. The post-traumatic development of SIADH in patients is well known. The syndrome may also be caused by viral, tuberculous, or bacterial encephalitis or meningitis, as well as by meningitis of neoplastic origin.

Nonmalignant pulmonary tissue also is capable of synthesizing antidiuretic hormone. Such synthesis may occur primarily in the presence of inflammatory or infectious disorders as vasopressin appears to be synthesized in granulomatous lung tissue. SIADH also may be seen in patients with lung abscess, bacterial and viral pneumonia, and aspergillosis. These conditions may be seen as presenting signs of lung cancer or as infections in immunocompromised cancer patients. Impaired water excretion may also be seen in cases of chronic obstructive pulmonary disease.

Medications such as indomethacin, acetaminophen, carbamazepine, serotonin reuptake inhibitors, barbiturates, and opiates have been reported to cause SIADH. Diabetes in cancer patients may be treated with the hypoglycemic agents chlorpropamide and tolbutamide, which have been reported to cause SIADH. Chemotherapeutic agents such as vincristine, vinblastine, cyclophosphamide, melphalan, and cisplatin also have been reported to cause SIADH.[22] The vigorous hydration given to prevent hemorrhagic cystitis in patients who are taking high-dose cyclophosphamide or to prevent nephrotoxicity in patients who are taking cisplatin may contribute to the rapid development of potentially fatal hyponatremia. Nausea, being an important stimulus of vasopressin release, also contributes to the development of hyponatremia in these emetogenic chemotherapeutic agents.

Diagnosis

The first step in properly evaluating a hyponatremic patient is to measure serum osmolality to confirm the hypotonicity (Figure 7–1).[23] If the osmolality is found to be high, the presence of solutes such as glucose or mannitol must be investigated.

If hypotonicity is confirmed, the volume status of the patient should be clinically evaluated. Edema, ascites, congestive heart failure, cirrhosis, and nephrotic syndrome are readily identified through history, physical examination, and basic laboratory studies. Hypovolemic patients can be identified by tachycardia, oliguria, orthostasis (upon change of position from supine to upright, blood pressure decreases > 20/10 mm Hg, and pulse increases > 20/min), hypotension, and poor skin turgor. Many cancer patients who are actively undergoing therapy may have central venous lines, and the measurement of central venous pressure may be helpful in assessing intravascular volume status.

If the patient is thought to be euvolemic, urine osmolality and urine electrolytes should be measured, with special attention paid to serum uric acid and blood urea nitrogen (BUN). Low uric acid, low BUN, and inappropriately concentrated urine (> 100 mOsm/kg) characterize SIADH. In a recent study of patients with small-cell carcinoma of the lung, the presence of hyponatremia and hypouricemia (serum urate < 3.5 mg/dL) had a positive predictive value of 100% in identifying SIADH. A patient with these laboratory findings (in the absence of hypothyroidism, renal malfunction, or adrenal malfunction) might be considered to have SIADH. Plasma vasopressin concentration may be important for the diagnosis as SIADH causes an abnormal relationship between osmolality and vasopressin concentration. For the purpose of rapid diagnosis, a water load excretion test may be performed, but this test may be harmful to patients with a serum sodium concentration of < 125 mEq/L.

Treatment

Factors to consider in the treatment of a hyponatremic cancer patient include symptoms, comorbidities, and the etiology, severity, and duration of the hyponatremia. Patients with hypovolemic hyponatremia are treated primarily with intravenous isotonic crystalloid fluids (normal saline, lactated Ringer's solution, etc) to correct the intravascular volume. In patients with SIADH secondary to malignancy, treatment of the underlying disease (whether by resection, radiation, or chemotherapy) has proved successful in correcting water excretion abnormalities. Even if the tumor is deemed to be incurable, these treatments may be undertaken to relieve or prevent potentially life-threatening water intoxication. Nonmalignant pulmonary diseases or infections that cause SIADH may be treated with antimicrobial therapy, which will normalize serum sodium concentration. Any drugs that can cause water retention should be discontinued and replaced with medications that do not have this undesirable side effect. Stimuli for vasopressin secretion, such as nausea and pain, should be controlled with medications.

If the patient with SIADH is asymptomatic and has some features of hypervolemia or is euvolemic, the primary treatment is fluid restriction to 500 to 800 mL of free water per day. Such elective fluid restriction requires a compliant patient. The effect should be seen as a steady increase in serum sodium concentration as body weight steadily decreases. If hyponatremia persists (usually in refractory or relapsed malignant disease), demeclocycline, lithium, or fludrocortisone can be used. Demeclocycline produces a reversible form of nephrogenic diabetes insipidus, inhibiting antidiuretic hormone (ADH)-induced cyclic adenosine monophosphate (cAMP) formation. In the usual dose range of 600 to 1200 mg/d, demeclocycline usually is well tolerated although it can have some side effects, such as skin photosensitivity and retention of urea. Lithium has a 20% efficacy rate, but nontoxic serum concentrations of lithium are difficult to maintain in the presence of hyponatremia. Fludrocortisone is not as effective as demeclocycline and will usually raise sodium levels by 4 to 8 mEq/L.

If the patient is having clinical signs of hyponatremic encephalopathy syndrome and if the symptoms have developed in an acute period (< 48 hours), a more aggressive approach should be used. The sodium concentration should be raised by no more than 1 to 2 mEq/L/h by using either normal saline (0.9% sodium chloride [NaCl]) or hypertonic saline (3% NaCl), at a rate of 1 mL/kg/h. Serum and the overall clinical picture must be closely monitored in an intensive-care environment, and intravenous furosemide should be added to enhance the free water clearance. About 200 to 300 mL of 3% NaCl is generally adequate to increase serum sodium to a level at which symptoms improve. Fluid restriction must be continued. The acute treatment can be interrupted when any of the following end points is reached: (1) symptoms are reversed, (2) a sodium level of ≥ 125 mEq/L is reached, or (3) a total correction of 20 mEq/L in a 24-hour period is achieved.

The correction of hyponatremia may be complicated by central pontine myelinolysis (CPM), a syndrome characterized by spastic quadriparesis, pseudobulbar palsy, swallowing dysfunction, and mutism. The histologic findings in this syndrome are demyelinations in the central pons and extrapontine sites. The exact etiology of CPM is not known, but CPM is related primarily to the duration of the hyponatremia and the rapid correction of the hypotonic state.

HYPERNATREMIA

Hypernatremia is defined as a sodium concentration of > 145 mEq/L, and it is always accompanied by a hyperosmolar state and by cellular dehydration.[24,25] Hyper-

natremia is seen in about 1% of hospitalized patients.[26] Young, old, and chronically ill patients are particularly vulnerable.[27]

Clinical Manifestations

The clinical manifestations of hypernatremia are primarily related to cellular dehydration leading to central nervous system dysfunction and are more pronounced with a high level or an acute rise of sodium.[28] In young children, symptoms include restlessness, weakness, and lethargy that may progress to coma. In older children and adults, thirst is the first symptom unless there is hypodipsia due to hypothalamic dysfunction. Muscle weakness and central nervous system changes usually are not manifested until serum sodium is > 160 mEq/L.

Diabetes insipidus (DI) is characterized by polyuria (> 3L), with the excretion of large quantities of diluted urine (< 100 mOsm/kg), and compensatory polydipsia. If water loss exceeds water ingestion, then the patient will

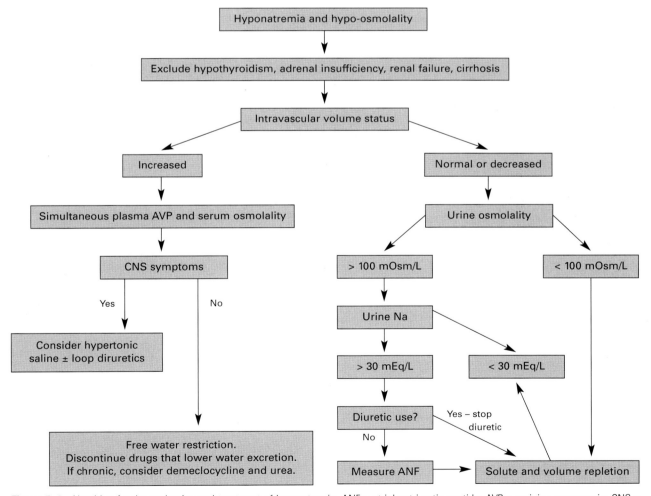

Figure 7–1. Algorithm for the evaluation and treatment of hyponatremia. ANF = atrial natriuretic peptide; AVP = arginine vasopressin; CNS = central nervous system.

have signs and symptoms of intravascular volume depletion and hypernatremia.

Pathophysiologic Mechanisms

Water makes up about 60% of the human body, and the balance of water and sodium is regulated by the renin-angiotensin system, by antidiuretic hormone, and by atrial natriuretic peptides. The serum sodium concentration is determined by the intake and loss of sodium relative to the intake and loss of water. Hypernatremia results from excess sodium intake, excess renal reabsorption of sodium, reduced water intake, or increased water loss.

Etiology

The causes of hypernatremia are listed in Table 7–1. Central DI is most frequently caused by events that affect the anterior pituitary or the related hypothalamic nuclei (eg, surgery, destruction by tumors, hemorrhage, head injury, infarction, or infection).[29]

TABLE 7–1. Causes of Hypernatremia in Cancer Patients

Decreased water intake
  Hypodipsia: loss of hypothalamic thirst center due to tumor or treatment
  Inability to take in water:
    Depressed mentation
    Intubated or paralyzed patient
    Inaccessibility of water; failure to provide care
    Nausea and vomiting
    Upper-GI obstruction
Increased water loss
  Gastrointestinal
    Vomiting, diarrhea
    Nasogastric suctioning
    Third-spacing
  Renal
    Tubular concentrating defects; nephrotoxicity of some
      chemotherapeutic drugs
    Acquired nephrogenic diabetes insipidus
    Osmotic diuresis (diabetes mellitus, mannitol)
    Postobstructive diuresis
  Respiratory
    Hyperventilation
  Dermatologic
    Excessive sweating: fever, night sweat
    Loss of barrier: graft-versus-host disease, cutaneous T-cell leukemia
Increased sodium intake
  Iatrogenic: improper IV fluid or TPN, improper dialysate (peritoneal or
    hemodialysis)
  Excess oral sodium intake
Increased sodium reabsorption
  Hypercortisolism
    Ectopic Cushing's syndrome
    Exogenous corticosteroids or mineralocorticoid
  Hyperaldosteronism

GI = gastrointestinal; IV = intravenous; TPN = total parenteral nutrition.
Adapted from Bibbs MA, Wolfson AB, Tayal VS. Electrolyte disturbances. In: Rosen P, Barkin R, editors. Emergency medicine: concepts and clinical practice. 4th ed. St. Louis: Mosby; 1998. p. 2432–2456.

Most cases of familial or congenital nephrogenic DI are caused by vasopressin (V_2) receptor mutations and aquaphorin-2 water channel mutations.[30,31] However, these causes are rare in cancer patients. Acquired nephrogenic DI can result from the nephrotoxicity of drugs. The most common cause of drug-induced nephrogenic DI is lithium, followed by foscarnet and clozapine.[32] Distal tubular defects develop in about half of patients treated with ifosfamide. However, frank nephrogenic DI leading to hypernatremia is uncommon.[33,34] Streptozocin (also known as streptozotocin) also is nephrotoxic. In addition to glomerular (proteinuria) and tubular (Fanconi's syndrome) defects, two cases of nephrogenic DI following streptozocin therapy have been reported.[35]

Other than disorders in free water metabolism, the most important factor in the development of hypernatremia is inadequate water intake in the setting of increased water loss. Elderly persons and debilitated patients are at risk. In cancer patients, there are many reasons for inadequate water intake, including obstruction of the gastrointestinal tract, chemotherapy-induced nausea and vomiting, and chemotherapy- or radiotherapy-induced mucositis. Primary hypodipsia can result from the destruction of the thirst center in the supraoptic nucleus of the hypothalamus. The possible causes of hypodipsia include primary or metastatic malignancy (eg, breast cancer and lung cancer), granulomatous disease, trauma, vasculitis, and treatment of central nervous system tumors by surgical resection and/or radiation. The causes of increased water loss include diuretics, high fever, burn injury, and diarrhea. Iatrogenic causes of hypernatremia include inappropriate intravenous-fluid administration, total parenteral nutrition,[36] and hemodialysis.[37]

Drugs that decrease the effect of antidiuretic hormone include demeclocycline, lithium, amphotericin, vinblastine, glyburide, propoxyphene, colchicine, acetohexamide, tolazamide, and methoxyflurane.

Diagnosis

The cause of hypernatremia usually is obvious from the history of illness (see Table 7–1). Urine osmolality, urine sodium, and serum sodium concentration are useful in diagnosing the cause of hypernatremia[38] (Table 7–2). A total body water deficit is associated with low urinary sodium and highly concentrated urine (> 700 mOsm/kg). With osmotic diuresis, renal salt wasting, and diuretics, urine osmolality tends to be isotonic.

To differentiate between central and nephrogenic DI, a water deprivation test may be performed (no fluid intake, with continuous measurements of weight and urine output). When two urine samples differ by less than 10% in osmolality or when the patient's weight has been reduced by at least 2%, the plasma vasopressin level

TABLE 7–2. Diagnosis and Treatment of Hypernatremia

Causes	Orthostasis	Spot Urine Sodium	Urine Osmolality	Treatment
Renal sodium and water loss	Yes	> 20	Decreased or unchanged	Hypotonic saline
Nonrenal sodium and water loss	Yes	< 10	Increased	Hypotonic saline
Sodium excess	No	> 20	Decreased or unchanged	Diuretics and water
Renal water loss	No	Variable	Variable	Water
Nonrenal water loss	No	Variable	Increased	Water

Adapted from Sanders LR. Disorders of water metabolism. In: McDermott MT, editor. Endocrine secrets. Philadelphia: Hanley and Belfus Inc; 1995. p. 122–134.

is measured, and the patient is given desmopressin (DDAVP). This should increase urine osmolality by more than 150 mOsm/kg in patients with central DI but not in patients with nephrogenic DI. Patients with partial central DI and nephrogenic DI may not be correctly identified because they may have only modest responses. The presence of a serum uric acid concentration of > 5 mg/dL in polyuric polydipsic patients is highly suggestive of central DI.[39]

Treatment

The treatment of hypernatremia is the administration of free water. This can be achieved enterally or intravenously with solutions low in electrolytes (ie, 5% dextrose or 0.2% NaCl). The total body water deficit can be estimated by 0.6 body weight (kg) × [(serum Na/140)−1]. Prolonged hypernatremia with protracted hypotension suggests a very poor prognosis.[40] In severe cases, hemodialysis to correct hypernatremia has been attempted.[41]

In acute hypernatremia, free water can be replaced rapidly. In chronic hypernatremia, serum sodium should be decreased by 1 to 2 mEq/L/h until the symptoms resolve. Correction of the remaining water deficit can be completed in 48 hours. Patients with hypodipsia should receive prescribed water on a regular basis.[42]

Central DI is usually treated with DDAVP at a typical dose of 5 to 20 μg every 12 hours intranasally, 1 to 2 μg daily SQ, or 0.1 to 0.2 mg orally twice daily.[43] Side effects are uncommon but are dose related and include rhinitis, abdominal cramping, headache, and nausea. Partial central DI usually requires close follow-up but no medical intervention.

A low-salt diet, along with thiazide diuretics that induce natriuresis is the treatment of choice for nephrogenic DI. Indomethacin has been used to treat drug-induced nephrogenic DI.[35,44] Clearly, any drugs (such as lithium)[45] that contribute to nephrogenic DI should be withheld if clinically appropriate.

HYPOKALEMIA

Hypokalemia may be defined as a serum potassium concentration of < 3.5 mEq/L. This is a common electrolyte abnormality in cancer patients.[46]

Clinical Manifestations

With mild hypokalemia (3.0 to 3.5 mEq/L), patients usually are asymptomatic. With severe hypokalemia (< 3.0 mEq/L), symptoms may range from mild to severe to potentially fatal. Cardiac manifestations may range from flat T waves, T-wave depression, and prominent U waves to serious arrhythmias. The neurologic manifestations may be muscle weakness, paresthesias, and paralysis.

Pathophysiologic Mechanisms

Potassium is one of the major ions that determines the resting membrane potential. Disturbances in potassium level affect tissues with excitable membranes, such as those in the nervous system and muscles. Disturbances in the level of potassium in the extracellular fluid lead to changes in the membrane potentials of excitable tissue and to clinical manifestations.

Etiology

Hypokalemia can be caused by low intake, by the shift of potassium into cells, by potassium losses from the gastrointestinal tract, skin, or kidneys, and by drug-related side effects.

Low potassium intake is rare in the general population because potassium is abundant in most foods. However, potassium intake in cancer patients may be decreased for various reasons (such as nausea, vomiting, anorexia, and gastrointestinal obstruction).

Alkalosis, either respiratory or, on a larger scale, metabolic, may precipitate hypokalemia through a transcellular shift of potassium. Hydrogen ions are actively transported out of cells to buffer the high-pH environment, and potassium ions are transported into cells to maintain the electrical potential across the cell membrane. Drugs that cause potassium redistribution include insulin, vitamin B_{12}, β-adrenergic agonists, theophylline, and chloroquine.

Potassium may be lost (1) from the gastrointestinal tract through vomiting or diarrhea, (2) from the skin during profuse sweating or severe burns, or (3) from the kidneys as a result of intrinsic tubular defects, type 1 renal tubular acidosis, or drug-related effects. Common examples of potassium-wasting drugs are loop diuretics, aminoglycosides, cyclophosphamide, ifosfamide, carboplatin, cisplatin, and amphotericin B.[46] Hypokalemia due to excess mineralocorticoid activity may result from the pharmacologic administration of corticosteroids or from ectopic Cushing's syndrome associated with some cancers.[47]

Diganosis

Hypokalemia is diagnosed by potassium measurement. Medication and dietary histories are helpful in determining the cause of hypokalemia. Physical examination will give clues to Cushing's syndrome. Measurement of serum electrolytes (including magnesium, BUN, and creatinine), urinalysis, and urine electrolyte measurement will help diagnose renal potassium losses.

Treatment

The rate of correction for hypokalemia and the route of administration will vary from patient to patient. The oral route is preferred if tolerated. The intravenous route may be used in patients with profound hypokalemia or an inability to tolerate oral intake. The rate of intravenous administration should not exceed 20 mEq/h diluted in intravenous fluid through a peripheral vein, and should not exceed 40 mEq/h through a central venous catheter. In general, the relation between the degree of hypokalemia and the total body deficit is linear. For each 1-mEq/L fall in serum, the total body deficit would be around 300 mEq, and this total body deficit may be corrected over days.

About 40 to 50% of patients with hypokalemia will also have hypomagnesemia. To fully correct the potassium-depleted state, hypomagnesemia must be corrected.

Potassium-sparing diuretics such as amiloride or spironolactone inhibit potassium excretion and may have a role in preventing hypokalemia, particularly when renal potassium wasting is involved.

HYPERKALEMIA

Primarily because a number of medications can interfere with potassium equilibrium, hyperkalemia is a common electrolyte disorder in patients with cancer.

Clinical Manifestations

Severe clinical manifestations usually are absent until serum potassium becomes > 7.5 mEq/L. However, some patients (eg, those in chronic renal failure) can tolerate high serum levels without evidencing clinical signs or symptoms. At a serum potassium level of > 7.5 mEq/L, patients may develop nonspecific symptoms, such as muscle weakness that can progress to complete paralysis of several different muscle groups, including the respiratory muscles. Muscle cramping is a frequent complaint.

Specific electrocardiographic changes may be present and can potentially lead to fatal arrhythmias, but no direct correlation exists between serum potassium level and a particular pattern on an electrocardiogram (ECG). Early electrocardiographic abnormalities associated with hyperkalemia are peak T waves, followed by a progressive widening in the QRS complex (Figure 7–2) and progression to a "sinusoidal" ECG pattern. If the hyperkalemia worsens or is left untreated, ventricular tachycardia, fibrillation, and asystole will occur.

Pathophysiologic Mechanisms

Hyperkalemia may cause depolarization. Membrane depolarization leads to excitability of nerves and muscles, causing cramps, muscle weakness, and paralysis. The most vital organ with excitable membranes is the heart. Hyperkalemia affects cardiac membrane potential, resulting in conduction disturbances and dysrhythmias. Ventricular fibrillation and asystole are the ultimate results of uncorrected hyperkalemia.

Etiology

Several mechanisms can lead to hyperkalemia in cancer patients, including increased intake, increased release from cells, and decreased excretion of potassium, and drug side effects.

Increased intake following an oral or intravenous load of potassium may lead to hyperkalemia. If the intake occurs over a long period of time, renal excretion will be increased, and the potassium elevation may be minimal. In contrast, with a rapid intake of a large dose, the elevation in serum level may be severe and life threatening. Inappropriate potassium content in intravenous fluid or total parenteral nutrition is a common iatrogenic cause of hyperkalemia.[48]

Significant release of intracellular potassium will cause hyperkalemia. Insulin deficiency, β-blocker therapy, and serum acidemia can elevate serum potassium. Massive cell breakdown, as in tumor lysis syndrome or rhabdomyolysis, also causes hyperkalemia.

Drug-induced hyperkalemia most often occurs in patients whose renal excretion of potassium is impaired.[49] Several drugs used by oncologists may contribute to hyperkalemia; the most common of these agents are cyclosporin A, tacrolimus, heparin,[49] mitomycin C,[50] and pentamidine.[51]

Diminished renal excretion is another mechanism of hyperkalemia. This primarily occurs in acute or chronic renal failure, renal hypoperfusion, or type 4 renal tubular acidosis. Drugs that can lead to decreased potassium excretion include the potassium-sparing diuretics and angiotensin-converting enzyme inhibitors.

Treatment

Treatment depends on the severity and rate of development of hyperkalemia. Medical intervention usually is

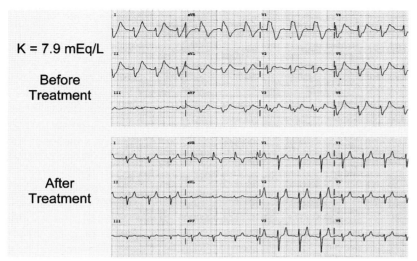

Figure 7–2. Electrocardiographic changes in hyperkalemia. This patient had acute renal failure after chemotherapy. The top electrocardiogram (ECG) was obtained when the serum potassium was 7.9 mEq/L. Note the widening of QRS complexes. The patient was immediately treated with sodium bicarbonate (50 mEq intravenously [IV]), calcium gluconate (1 g IV), and D50W (50 mL IV) with regular insulin (10 U IV). The bottom ECG was obtained about 15 minutes after infusing the medications. Note the normal QRS complexes and the peaked T waves.

not necessary unless the potassium level is > 6.0 mEq/L. In a patient with chronic hyperkalemia, attention should be focused on offending medications such as β-adrenergic blockers, nonsteroidal anti-inflammatory drugs, angiotensin-converting enzyme inhibitors, potassium supplements, and other drugs mentioned above.

In the acute setting, primarily in patients with electrocardiographic changes, the first step is the intravenous infusion of calcium (calcium gluconate, 1 to 2 g, or chloride, 0.5 to 1 g) with continuous electrocardiographic monitoring. Sodium bicarbonate, glucose (usually 25 g) plus 6 to 8 U of regular insulin, and β-adrenergic agonists promote potassium entry into the cells. These interventions usually last for less than 60 minutes. Increasing the renal excretion of potassium can be attempted by administering loop diuretics. An attempt should be made to remove potassium from the body by using ion exchange resins such as sodium polystyrene sulfonate (Kayexalate), which can be administered orally (15 to 30 g per dose) or per rectum (30 to 60 g per dose) as retention enemas. Emergent hemodialysis also may be used in refractory cases.

HYPOCALCEMIA

Calcium is required for the proper functioning of many intracellular and extracellular processes, such as muscle contraction, nerve conduction, and blood coagulation. Among hospitalized cancer patients, the frequency of hypocalcemia is about 13.4%.[52]

Clinical Manifestations

Hypocalcemia may be asymptomatic or may be associated with signs and symptoms that range from mild to serious and life threatening. The neuromuscular manifestations are muscle weakness, spasm, tetany, paresthe-sia, hyper-reflexia, Chvostek's sign, Trousseau's sign, and seizures. Involvement of the muscles in the respiratory system may lead to bronchospasm, laryngeal spasm, or respiratory arrest. The cardiovascular manifestations of hypocalcemia are bradycardia, hypotension, QT–interval prolongation, and cardiac arrest. The neuropsychiatric symptoms include anxiety, irritability, psychosis, depression, and confusion. Other chronic abnormalities include dry skin, frail nails, and coarse hair.

Pathophysiologic Mechanisms

About 99% of total body calcium is located in bones, leaving only 1% available in the extracellular fluid. Of this extracellular calcium, 40% is bound to albumin, and the remainder is ionized and physiologically active.

Bone, the gastrointestinal tract, the kidneys, the liver, the skin, the parathyroid glands, and the thyroid gland affect serum calcium. The serum calcium level is regulated by parathyroid hormone, 1,25-dihydroxyvitamin D, calcitonin, phosphate, and calcium itself. The parathyroid glands secrete parathyroid hormone (PTH), and the thyroid gland secretes calcitonin. Diet, skin, liver, and kidneys control the synthesis and metabolism of vitamin D. Vitamin D_2 is ingested in the diet, and vitamin D_3 is synthesized in the skin. In the liver, 25-hydroxylase hydroxylates vitamin D. In the proximal renal tubule, 1α-hydroxylase converts 25-hydroxyvitamin D to 1,25-dihydroxyvitamin D. Calcitonin inhibits osteoclastic bone resorption, decreases renal tubular reabsorption of calcium, and may also enhance osteoblast activity. Parathyroid hormone and 1,25-dihydroxyvitamin D_3 provide the main control of calcium. Calcitonin may play a role, but its significance is not well defined.

Excluding decreased serum calcium level due to low albumin and low serum proteins, the major causes of hypocalcemia are hypoparathyroidism and hypomagnesemia. Hypocalcemia may be one of the features of TLS, as discussed above. In cancer patients, osteoblastic bone metastases (especially from prostate carcinoma) are often associated with hypocalcemia. The toxicity of certain chemotherapeutic agents may also lead to hypocalcemia in cancer patients.[53]

Etiology

Many different mechanisms precipitate hypocalcemia (Table 7–3). Hypoparathyroidism (PTH deficiency) is one of the most prevalent. Secondary hypoparathyroidism is most often iatrogenic, resulting from the removal of the parathyroid glands or from disruption of the vascular supply during neck surgery. Excision of a functional parathyroid adenoma, leaving the chronically suppressed but otherwise unaffected parathyroid tissue, causes hypocalcemia that usually resolves over several days. Severe hypo- and hypermagnesemia may impair the release of PTH. Other mechanisms include vitamin D deficiency, renal failure with decreased formation of vitamin D metabolites, phosphorus excess, acute pancreatitis, citrate (in blood products or through apheresis),[54] and septic shock.

Elderly persons and chronically ill or debilitated patients may have limited exposure to sunlight. Vitamin D insufficiency can result from intestinal malabsorption in patients with small-bowel, biliary, or exocrine pancreatic diseases.

Drugs linked with hypocalcemia include anticonvulsants (mainly phenytoin) and rifampin. Bisphosphonates that are used to treat bone metastasis (especially from myeloma, breast cancer, and prostate cancer),

pamidronate,[55–57] and (perhaps) zoledronic acid also may cause hypocalcemia.

Platinum compounds are major chemotherapeutic drugs that can cause hypocalcemia. Hypocalcemia has been reported in 6 to 20% of cisplatin-treated patients. Cisplatin's effects on renal tubular function, magnesium metabolism, bone resorption, and vitamin D metabolism may explain this hypocalcemia. Hypomagnesemia may cause a decrease in PTH secretion and a reduction in the calcium-mobilizing effects of PTH. Hypomagnesemia also inhibits the formation of 1,25-dihydroxyvitamin D. Cisplatin may inhibit mitochondrial function in the kidney, thereby inhibiting the conversion of 25-hydroxyvitamin D to 1,25-dihydroxyvitamin D. Another mechanism of cisplatin-induced hypocalcemia may be hypomagnesemia, which causes hypoparathyroidism.[58] In addition, cisplatin may have a direct inhibitory effect on bone resorption. Similar to cisplatin, carboplatin therapy is associated with a 16 to 31% incidence of hypocalcemia.

Other chemotherapeutic drugs that can cause hypocalcemia include 5-fluorouracil with leucovorin,[59] plicamycin (mithramycin),[60–62] dactinomycin,[63] and the combination of doxorubicin and cytarabine.[64]

Diagnosis

The evaluation of hypocalcemia involves confirmation by measuring ionized calcium. Measurements of magnesium, phosphate, 25-hydroxyvitamin D_3, 1,25-dihydroxyvitamin D_3, PTH, and 24-hour urinary calcium are helpful in determining the source of hypocalcemia (Table 7–4).

Treatment

Chronic hypocalcemia can be treated orally with one of the available forms of calcium (eg, gluconate or carbonate) to provide 1 to 2 g of elemental calcium per day. Vitamin D supplements can be given in the 1-hydroxylated form or in calcitriol. Calcitriol is preferred in cases of renal insufficiency or failure because of decreased 1α-hydroxylase in the kidneys. Special attention should be paid to magnesium replacement and phosphate binding.

Acute severe hypocalcemia is treated parenterally with intravenous calcium chloride (0.5 to 1.0 g) or gluconate (1 to 2 g) over 5 to 10 minutes. Because the half-life is short, continuous infusion of calcium or proper oral replacement may be needed for complete replacement. Proper magnesium and potassium replacement also is required to completely restore the calcium level.

HYPERCALCEMIA

Hypercalcemia affects 0.5 to 1.0% of the general population. Hypercalcemia in the context of cancer is a poor prognostic sign that is associated with a short survival. Hypercalcemia of malignancy is observed in 10 to 15% of patients

TABLE 7–3. Major Causes of Hypocalcemia in Cancer Patients

Parathyroid hormone insufficiency
  Secondary hypoparathyroidism
    Neck surgery
    Drugs (cisplatin, carboplatin, cyclophosphamide, ifosfamide, amphotericin, dactinomycin, mithramycin, ethanol, cimetidine)
    Hypomagnesemia
    Sepsis
    Pancreatitis
Vitamin D deficiency
  Malnutrition and low sun exposure
  Malabsorption (eg, after small-bowel surgery)
  Liver disease
  Renal disease
    Acute and chronic renal failure
    Nephrotic syndrome
  Anticonvulsants (phenytoin, primidone)
Calcium chelation
  Hyperphosphatemia
  Citrate
  Alkalosis

Adapted from Bibbs MA, Wolfson AB, Tayal VS. Electrolyte disturbances. In: Rosen P, Barkin R, editors. Emergency medicine: concepts and clinical practice. 4th ed. St. Louis: Mosby; 1998. p. 2432–2456.

TABLE 7–4. Laboratory Evaluation of Hypocalcemia

	Phosphate	Parathyroid hormone	25-(OH)VitD	1,25-(OH)$_2$VitD
Hypoparathyroidism	High	Low	Normal	Low
Pseudohypoparathyroidism	High	High	Normal	Low or normal
Liver disease	Low	High	Low	Low or normal
Renal disease	High	Low	Normal	Low or normal

25-(OH)VitD = 25-hydroxyvitamin D; 1,25-(OH)$_2$ VitD = 1,25-dihydroxyvitamin D.
Adapted from Christensen RS. Hypocalcemia. In: McDermott MT, editor. Endocrine secrets. Philadelphia: Hanley and Belfus Inc; 1995. p. 81–84.

with any type of cancer and can be observed throughout the course of their disease. It is an ominous sign because it is a manifestation of advanced disease and is associated with a median survival as short as 30 to 90 days.[65]

Clinical Manifestations

Mild hypercalcemia (< 12 mg/dL) usually has no symptoms. However, patients with moderate or severe hypercalcemia are frequently symptomatic. Central nervous system symptoms are lethargy, ataxia, stupor, coma, mental status changes, and psychosis. Gastrointestinal tract symptoms are anorexia, nausea, constipation, ileus, dyspepsia, and pancreatitis. Renal symptoms or signs are polyuria, nephrolithiasis, and nephrocalcinosis. Musculoskeletal system symptoms are myalgias, arthralgias, and weakness. Electrocardiographic changes associated with hypercalcemia are a short Q–T interval, depression of the ST segment, sinus arrest, and atrioventricular blocks.

Pathophysiologic Mechanisms

The regulation of the calcium level has been discussed. Hypercalcemia results from increased bone resorption, renal tubular reabsorption, and the gastrointestinal absorption of calcium. Hyperparathyroidism, humoral hypercalcemia of malignancy, thyrotoxicosis, pheochromocytoma, excessive vitamin A, and immobilization all increase bone resorption. Milk-alkali syndrome, thiazide diuretics, and familial hypocalciuric hypercalcemia involve increased renal reabsorption or decreased excretion of calcium. Excessive vitamin D, sarcoidosis, and other inflammatory disorders increase gastrointestinal absorption of calcium.

Hypercalcemia associated with malignancy may have different pathophysiologic mechanisms. The most common humoral factor secreted by cancers causing hypercalcemia is PTH-related peptide (PTHrP).[66,67] This hormone is homologous to PTH and is released by many different tumors. It activates the PTH receptor, promoting renal reabsorption of calcium and stimulating bone resorption. In general, patients with PTHrP have advanced malignant disease and a poor prognosis. Other humoral mediators, such as interleukins-1 and -6, prostaglandins, and tumor necrosis factor (TNF), can mediate hypercalcemia in cancer patients.

A second mechanism of hypercalcemia in cancer patients is the induction of local bone destruction and subsequent lytic lesions by a mixture of different paracrine substances, such as transforming growth factors (TGFs) and prostaglandins. This phenomenon is seen primarily in breast cancer and multiple myeloma.

The third mechanism is a syndrome of increased levels of 1,25-dihydroxyvitamin D$_3$ that promotes calcium reabsorption and bone resorption. This mechanism is seen in patients with Hodgkin's disease and non-Hodgkin's lymphoma.

Etiology

The various causes of hypercalcemia in cancer patients are listed in Table 7–5.

Hypercalcemia of malignancy usually is seen in non-small-cell lung cancer, breast cancer, head and neck

TABLE 7–5. Common Causes of Hypercalcemia in Cancer Patients

Malignant disease
    Parathyroid hormone–related protein
    Ectopic production of 1,25-dihydroxyvitamin D
    Other bone-resorbing substance
    Osteolytic bone metastasis
Medications
    Thiazide diuretics
    Lithium
    Estrogens
    Tamoxifen
    Vitamin D toxicity
    Excess calcium ingestion
Granulomatous disorders
    Sarcoidosis
    Tuberculosis
    Coccidioidomycosis
    Histoplasmosis
Endocrine disorders
    Hyperparathyroidism
    Hyperthyroidism
    Adrenal insufficiency
    Pheochromocytoma
    Acromegaly
    Vasoactive intestinal polypeptide–producing tumor
Miscellaneous
    Milk-alkali syndrome
    Immobilization

Adapted from Bibbs MA, Wolfson AB, Tayal VS. Electrolyte disturbances. In: Rosen P, Barkin R, editors. Emergency medicine: concepts and clinical practice. 4th ed. St. Louis: Mosby; 1998. p. 2432–2456.

(squamous cell) cancer, multiple myeloma, hypernephroma, and some types of T-cell lymphomas. No chemotherapy has been found to cause hypercalcemia.

Radiation-induced hyperparathyroidism may be seen in long-term cancer survivors.[68,69] Among study patients who developed primary hyperparathyroidism, 14 to 30% had prior exposure to radiation.[70,71] The median time interval from irradiation to the development of hyperparathyroidism is about 30 years.[71] Concurrent thyroid cancer may be seen in more than 30% of patients with radiation-induced hyperparathyroidism.[72]

Diagnosis

Serum calcium should be interpreted in the context of protein binding. Serum albumin should be measured simultaneously. Formulas for the correction of calcium based on albumin level may be useful. However, accurate measurement of ionized calcium is indicated to confirm hypercalcemia. Unless the cancer patient already has an established diagnosis of the cause of hypercalcemia, laboratory studies are indicated for the following: intact PTH, PTH-related protein, 25-hydroxyvitamin D_3, and 1,25-dihydroxyvitamin D_3 (Table 7–6).

Despite ample reviews of the topic in the literature,[2,67,73–75] hypercalcemia of malignancy remains underdiagnosed.[76] The syndrome can be a late manifestation of advanced cancer or the first sign of an undiagnosed one.

Treatment

Primary hyperparathyroidism is amenable to cure by parathyroidectomy. Medications causing or contributing to hypercalcemia (eg, thiazides, lithium,[77] and vitamin supplements) should be discontinued. For hypercalcemia of malignancy, direct antitumoral therapy improves hypercalcemia, at least transiently.

The majority of patients with hypercalcemia present with severe intravascular volume depletion secondary to vomiting, decreased oral intake, or renal losses. Thus, immediate volume replacement with crystalloid intravenous fluid (eg, lactated Ringer's solution, 0.9% NaCl) to correct extracellular volume deficits is the first and emergent treatment for increasing the glomerular filtration rate and renal calcium excretion. Once volume depletion has been corrected, the addition of a loop diuretic that promotes calciuresis is indicated. (Note that thiazide diuretics are contraindicated because they decrease the excretion of calcium.)

Although rehydration often is the initial therapy for hypercalcemia, the cornerstone of therapy is the inhibition of bone resorption by osteoclasts.[78] The bisphosphonates, plicamycin, gallium nitrate, and calcitonin all inhibit bone resorption by osteoclasts. The use of bisphosphonates (etidronate, clodronate, pamidronate, and zoledronic acid) to treat hypercalcemia is clearly established.[79,80] Pamidronate is more widely used and is given at a dose of 60 to 90 mg as a single intravenous infusion over 4 to 24 hours;[81] the maximal effect is seen within 48 hours. Side effects include low-grade fever and mild hypocalcemia and hypomagnesemia. Zoledronic acid (4 mg IV) is a new bisphosphonate that can be administered more rapidly and that has fewer systemic side effects than pamidronate. Second-line agents include gallium nitrate (200 mg/m^2 IV)[82] and calcitonin (salmon calcitonin, 4 IU/kg subcutaneously [SQ] every 12 hours). Calcitonin has a rapid onset of action although its action decreases rapidly within 2 to 3 days. Other less widely used agents include plicamycin (25 μg/kg IV over 4 hours)[61] and corticosteroids.

HYPOMAGNESEMIA

In one series, the incidence of hypomagnesemia among hospitalized cancer patients was 17.1%.[52] Hypomagnesemia is a common electrolyte deficiency in clinical practice. Hypomagnesemia is defined as a plasma serum concentration of < 1.4 mEq/L.

Clinical Manifestations

The clinical manifestations of hypomagnesemia may be nonspecific and include anorexia, nausea, vomiting, lethargy, dizziness, muscle weakness, tremor, muscle fasciculation, tetany, and tonic-clonic seizures.

Pathophysiologic Mechanisms

Magnesium is a major cation of the body. It is needed for a wide variety of enzymatic reactions within the body, including those involving adenosine triphosphate (ATP) and nucleic acid metabolism. Magnesium also is directly related to calcium and potassium metabolism.

TABLE 7–6. Differential Diagnosis of Hypercalcemia in Cancer Patients

Etiology	Intact PTH	PTHrP	1,25-(OH)$_2$VitD
Primary hyperparathyroidism	High	Low	High
Malignancy secreting PTHrP	Low	High	Low
Non-PTHrP-mediated	Low	Low	Low

PTH = parathyroid hormone; PTHrP = PTH-related peptide; 1,25-(OH)$_2$ VitD = 1,25-dihydroxyvitamin D.
Adapted from Sanders LR. Hypocalcemia. In: McDermott MT, editor. Endocrine secrets. Philadelphia: Hanley and Belfus Inc; 1995. p. 71–80.

The kidney normally conserves magnesium efficiently. Significant hypomagnesemia occurs only when renal excretion and intestinal loss exceeds dietary intake and absorption.

Etiology

Hypomagnesemia is related usually to low intake and to impaired renal reabsorption or intestinal absorption (Table 7–7). It also has been related to prolonged intravenous feeding, nasogastric suction, chronic alcoholism, intestinal malabsorption, and diarrhea. The renal toxicity of chemotherapeutic drugs (platinum-based drugs,[83] cyclophosphamide, and ifosfamide) or antifungal medications (eg, amphotericin) is a major cause of magnesium deficiency in cancer patients. Diuretics used in patients with hypertension and congestive heart failure also increase renal magnesium loss. Hypomagnesemia also is commonly associated with certain aminoglycosides.[84]

Cisplatin causes morphologic changes and necrosis in the proximal tubule, an important site of magnesium reabsorption. Hypomagnesemia occurs in more than 90% of patients treated with cisplatin,[83,85] and 10% of these patients are symptomatic with muscle weakness, tremulousness, and dizziness. Vigorous hydration and the use of osmotic diuretics such as mannitol may prevent renal failure but have little effect on renal magnesium wasting. Hypomagnesemia may persist long after cisplatin therapy.[86] No large series in the literature have addressed the incidence, but information from the pharmaceutical manufacturer indicates that 60% of those taking cisplatin may be affected.

Diagnosis

Only 1 to 2% of total body magnesium is present in the extracellular space. As a result, serum magnesium values and erythrocyte magnesium concentrations are poor indicators of total body magnesium content. A single measurement of serum magnesium may not accurately reflect the true extent of magnesium deficiency in the body because most of the magnesium is intracellular and because transient redistribution of magnesium can occur between the extracellular space and intracellular stores. However, continual subnormal magnesium levels do suggest a deficiency in the whole body.

Hypomagnesemia is often associated with other electrolyte abnormalities, such as hypokalemia and hypocalcemia.[87] The concurrent measurement of other electrolytes (such as calcium, phosphate, and potassium) should be considered.

Treatment

Magnesium replacement is indicated when the deficiency state is symptomatic or is associated with persistent and severe hypomagnesemia (< 1 mEq/L) with deficits approaching 10 to 20 mg/kg of body weight.

Oral replacement is preferred over parenteral replacement when feasible. However, diarrhea may become a dose-limiting side effect. When intravenous replacement is needed, the usual practice is to replace half of the estimated dose over 24 hours and the remaining half over the next 3 to 4 days.

Recently, some clinicians have advocated "prophylactic" magnesium replacement in patients undergoing cisplatin-based chemotherapy[88] and the use of amifostine to ameliorate nephrotoxicity and to prevent hypomagnesemia.[89]

HYPERMAGNESEMIA

Hypermagnesemia is much more uncommon than hypomagnesemia. Hypermagnesemia is usually caused by an increased intake of magnesium in the presence of renal insufficiency.

Clinical Manifestations

The clinical manifestations of hypermagnesemia correlate well with the serum level. Early signs include nausea, vomiting, weakness, and cutaneous flushing, which can occur when the magnesium level is > 3 mg/dL. As the level goes above 4 mg/dL, hyporeflexia and loss of deep tendon reflexes may occur. At serum levels of 5 to

TABLE 7–7. Common Causes of Hypomagnesemia in Cancer Patients

Alcohol abuse or protein-calorie malnutrition
Renal loss
   Acute and chronic renal failure
   Postobstructive diuresis
   Acute tubular necrosis
   Chronic glomerulonephritis
   Interstitial nephropathy
Gastrointestinal loss
   Chronic diarrhea
   Nasogastric suctioning
   Short-bowel syndrome
   Bowel fistula
   Total parenteral nutrition
   Acute pancreatitis
Endocrine
   Diabetes mellitus
   Hyperaldosteronism
   Hyperthyroidism
   Hyperparathyroidism
Drug
   Amphotericin
   Pentamidine
   Theophylline
   Foscarnet
   Diuretics
   Cyclosporine
   Cisplatin
   β-Agonists
   Aminoglycosides

Adapted from Bibbs MA, Wolfson AB, Tayal VS. Electrolyte disturbances. In: Rosen P, Barkin R, editors. Emergency medicine: concepts and clinical practice. 4th ed. St. Louis: Mosby; 1998. p. 2432–2456.

6 mg/dL, hypotension and electrocardiographic changes (QRS widening, Q–T and P–R interval prolongation, and conduction abnormalities) may occur. Respiratory depression, coma, and complete heart block may occur at levels > 9 mg/dL. Asystole and cardiac arrest can occur at levels > 10 mg/dL.

Pathophysiologic Mechanisms

Supraphysiologic concentrations of magnesium suppress PTH secretion. Acute suppression of PTH may lead to hypocalcemia.

Etiology

The major causes of hypermagnesemia are renal failure and excessive ingestion of magnesium-containing medications in the presence of renal insufficiency (Table 7–8). In the absence of renal insufficiency, hypermagnesemia due to excessive oral intake of magnesium is very rare because excess magnesium in the gastrointestinal tract leads to diarrhea. Over-replacement in intravenous fluid or in hyperalimentation also can cause hypermagnesemia. Less common causes include TLS, rhabdomyolysis, adrenal insufficiency, hyperparathyroidism, hypothyroidism, and lithium therapy.

Diagnosis

Hypermagnesemia is diagnosed by direct measurement of serum magnesium. Excessive magnesium intake usually is evident from the dietary and medication history. Renal function should be assessed by measuring BUN and creatinine.

Treatment

Discontinuation of magnesium intake is the first step. Patients with mild symptoms and normal renal function can simply be observed to ensure that the magnesium level returns to normal. If symptoms are significant, hydration with crystalloid fluid and an intravenous loop diuretic will accelerate magnesium excretion. In cases of severe hypermagnesemia, intravenous calcium should be administered. Calcium directly reverses the effects of hypermagnesemia on excitable membranes and reverses respiratory depression, hypotension, and cardiac arrhythmia. Emergent dialysis should be considered for patients with coma, respiratory failure, hemodynamic instability, and severe hypermagnesemia with renal failure.

HYPOPHOSPHATEMIA

Hypophosphatemia is quite prevalent; it is found in about 2 to 3% of all hospitalized patients[90] and in about 30% of cancer patients.[87]

Clinical Manifestations

Muscle weakness is the most common complaint. Acute severe hypophosphatemia may lead to generalized neu-rologic findings, such as lethargy, confusion, disorientation, hallucinations, and to focal neurologic findings, including dysarthria, dysphagia, oculomotor palsies, anisocoria, nystagmus, ataxia, cerebellar tremor, ballismus, hyporeflexia, distal sensory deficits, paresthesia, and hyperesthesia. Severe neurologic symptoms, such as muscle paralysis, seizure, or coma, are observed only when the serum phosphate level is < 0.8 mg/dL. Cardiac muscle also can be affected by severe hypophosphatemia, and reversible left ventricular dysfunction can occur. Severe hypophosphatemia can lead to death.[91]

Bone pain is another prominent complaint of phosphate-depleted patients. Prolonged hypophosphatemia leads to rickets.[92] Growing children are particularly vulnerable. Hypophosphatemic rickets can result from ifosfamide nephrotoxicity.[33,93] Osteomalacia, waddling gait, bone tenderness, and pseudofractures can occur in adult patients with chronic hypophosphatemia. A severe loss of bone mass may lead to fractures.

Pathophysiologic Mechanisms

Acute hypophosphatemia occurs primarily in hospitalized patients with serious illnesses and pre-existing phosphate depletion due to unusual urinary losses, severe malabsorption, malnutrition, or antacid abuse. Chronic hypophosphatemia is largely limited to disorders of mineral and bone metabolism.

The risk factors for hypophosphatemia include malnutrition, diuretic or antacid therapy, sepsis, and alcoholism. Short-term fasting does not induce hypophosphatemia because the release of endogenous bone and intracellular phosphate is more than enough to compen-

TABLE 7–8. Common Causes of Hypermagnesemia in Cancer Patients

Impaired renal magnesium excretion
Exogenous magnesium administration
Antacids
Laxatives, cathartics (milk of magnesia, magnesium citrate)
Dialysate
Parenteral nutrition or intravenous fluid
Impaired gastrointestinal magnesium elimination
Anticholinergics
Narcotics
Chronic constipation
Bowel obstruction
Colitis
Miscellaneous
Rhabdomyolysis
Tumor lysis syndrome
Adrenal insufficiency
Hyperparathyroidism
Hypothyroidism
Lithium therapy

Adapted from Bibbs MA, Wolfson AB, Tayal VS. Electrolyte disturbances. In: Rosen P, Barkin R, editors. Emergency medicine: concepts and clinical practice. 4th ed. St. Louis: Mosby; 1998. p. 2432–2456.

Metabolic and Endocrine Emergencies / **117**

sate for the obligate phosphate loss in the kidneys. In the absence of elevated PTH or PTHrP, consumption of oral phosphate binders, or accelerated bone formation, chronic hypophosphatemia is due either to increased humoral factors suppressing renal reabsorption of phosphate or to an intrinsic renal tubular defect in phosphate reabsorption.

Tumor-induced (oncogenic) osteomalacia is a rare syndrome that is characterized by hypophosphatemia, excessive urinary phosphate loss, reduced 1,25-dihydroxy-vitamin D concentrations, and osteomalacia. Normalization of serum 1,25-dihydroxyvitamin D in this syndrome reverses secondary hyperparathyroidism but is associated with persistent hypophosphatemia and phosphaturia. Conditioned media derived from cultures of tumors causing oncogenic osteomalacia contain humoral factors that specifically inhibit sodium-dependent phosphate transport in cultured renal proximal tubular epithelia.[94] Candidate phosphate-wasting factors are FGF23,[95,96] the gene that is mutated in autosomal dominant hypophosphatemic rickets, and matrix extracellular phosphoglyco-protein (MEPE).[97]

Etiology

The causes of hypophosphatemia are listed in Table 7–9. The frequency of severe hypophosphatemia (< 1 mg/dL) is less than 0.1%. Acute severe hypophosphatemia usually results from the translocation of phosphate into cells. Respiratory alkalosis, intravenous glucose administration (including hyperalimentation), Gram-negative sepsis, or insulin therapy can induce the transcellular shift of phosphate.

Hypophosphatemia in malnourished patients (especially alcoholic patients) is due to a combination of magnesium deficiency, vitamin D deficiency, and malabsorption. Refeeding of high-calorie diets in severely malnourished patients can lead to a refeeding syndrome with hypophosphatemia.[98]

Rapid cell proliferation in ill patients with nutritional deprivation or catabolism may cause hypophosphatemia. Chronic hypophosphatemia, together with hypocalcemia, is occasionally associated with extensive osteoblastic metastasis due to prostate, breast, lung, or other malignancies. Patients with rapidly progressing leukemia or lymphoma (eg, Burkitt's lymphoma) may experience hypophosphatemia that coincides with tumor growth. The redistribution of body phosphorus with increased uptake by the rapidly replicating tumor cells is the likely cause (leading to the coining of the term "tumor genesis syndrome").[99] As with the use of granulocyte colony-stimulating factors or erythropoietin in severely ill patients, hematopoietic reconstitution after bone marrow transplantation[100] or stem cell harvesting in preparation for bone marrow transplantation[91] has also been reported to cause hypophosphatemia.

The liver also plays a significant role in phosphate homeostasis. Severe symptomatic dose-limiting hypophosphatemia can be induced by hepatic arterial infusion of recombinant TNF in patients with liver metastases.[101] In a retrospective study, the postoperative serum phosphate level dropped in all 44 patients who underwent right or extended right hepatic lobectomy.[102] Hypophosphatemia has been reported in a patient with hepatocellular carcinoma complicating liver cirrhosis.[103]

Intrinsic renal tubular defects in phosphate reabsorption may occur in Fanconi's syndrome, Wilson's disease, hereditary hypophosphatemic rickets, hypophosphatemic bone disease, osteomalacia, myeloma,[104] and amyloidosis. A proximal tubular dysfunction responsible for a reduced transport maximum of phosphate ($TmPO_4$) glomerular filtration rate (GFR) may be involved in the pathogenesis of hypophosphatemia in alcoholics, and liver function impairment is not required for the expression of this tubular dysfunction.[105] Hypophosphatemia may be associated with chemotherapeutic drugs such as platinum compounds[106,107] and alkylating agents.[93] Ifosfamide is a common agent that is associated with a 16% incidence of hypophosphatemia because of nephrotoxicity.[108] Hypophosphatemia occurs in 42% of patients with advanced prostate cancer treated with weekly paclitaxel in combination with estramustine and carboplatin (TEC).[107]

Several neoplastic processes, including mesenchymal tumors,[109] prostatic carcinoma,[110] and endodermal malig-

TABLE 7–9. Causes of Hypophosphatemia in Cancer Patients

Renal loss
    Diuretic therapy or osmotic diuresis due to hyperglycemia
    Renal tubular dysfunction (drug induced Fonconi syndrome)
    Oncogenic osteomalacia
    Hyperparathyroidism
    Hyperaldosteronism
    Glucocorticoid administration
Insufficient intestinal absorption
    Starvation/malnutrition
    Phosphate-binding antacids
    Vitamin D deficiency
    Chronic diarrhea
    Nasogastric suctioning
Transcellular shift
    Respiratory alkalosis
    Sepsis
    Heatstroke/hyperpyrexia
    Salicylate poisoning
    Neuroleptic malignant syndrome
    Hepatic encephalopathy
    Alcohol withdrawal
    Hyperglycemia
    Insulin administration

Adapted from Bibbs MA, Wolfson AB, Tayal VS. Electrolyte disturbances. In: Rosen P, Barkin R, editors. Emergency medicine: concepts and clinical practice. 4th ed. St. Louis: Mosby; 1998. p. 2432–2456.

nancy, cause oncogenic osteomalacia. In a review of 72 cases,[111] more than one-third of the tumors were classified as vascular tumors, and half of these were hemangiopericytomas. Other common pathologic diagnoses were nonossifying fibromas and "mesenchymal" and giant cell tumors. Subsequent reports have emphasized that this syndrome may be associated not only with mesenchymal tumors but also with prostate carcinoma.[103,112] Oncogenic osteomalacia is distinct from hypophosphatemia associated with hematogenous malignancies in which light-chain nephropathy causes phosphate wasting.[113]

Pseudohypophosphatemia due to interference in the laboratory assay of phosphate by a large amount of immunoglobulin G (IgG) secreted by a myeloma has been reported.[114]

Diagnosis

Hypophosphatemia is demonstrated by the direct measurement of serum phosphate level. Measurements of renal function, potassium, magnesium and calcium levels, vitamin D metabolites, and PTH level are helpful in determining the cause of hypophosphatemia. If urinary loss of phosphate is suspected, urine should be collected to measure $TmPO_4/GFR$ to confirm phosphaturia. It is necessary to monitor electrolytes and vitamin levels closely during the early stages of instituting enteral or parenteral nutrition.[98] In chronic hypophosphatemia, when bone metabolism is likely to be affected, measurements of bone mineral density and alkaline phosphatase may be indicated.

Treatment

Significant hypophosphatemia (< 2 mg/dL), especially in the context of underlying phosphate depletion, constitutes a potentially dangerous electrolyte abnormality and should be corrected promptly. Pharmaceutical preparations of phosphates are a combination of monobasic and dibasic phosphate salts. Therefore, it is general practice to prescribe phosphate in terms of millimoles to avoid confusion and errors in dosage.[90]

On the basis of studies from patients with diabetic ketoacidosis, phosphate can be safely administered intravenously at initial doses of 0.2 to 0.8 mmol/kg over 6 hours (ie, 10 to 50 mmol over 6 hours). Higher doses (1.5 to 3.0 mmol/kg over 12 hours) should be reserved for patients with a phosphate level of < 1.5 mg/dL and normal renal function. Serum phosphate and calcium must be monitored closely throughout the treatment. Because of potentially serious complications (such as severe hypocalcemia, calcified right ventricular thrombi, and nephrocalcinosis) long-term intravenous phosphate infusion should be reserved for patients who cannot tolerate adequate doses of oral phosphate and for whom the benefits outweigh the risks.[115]

Mild hypophosphatemia can be treated with oral phosphate in divided doses of 750 to 2,000 mg/d. In general, oral phosphate therapy is well tolerated although 5 to 10% of patients develop gastrointestinal symptoms such as nausea, vomiting, diarrhea, or abdominal pain. These side effects are generally dose related. The alternatives to oral phosphate therapy are few, and an inadequate oral dose may result in suboptimal treatment.

In oncogenic osteomalacia, complete resection of the tumor will reverse all the biochemical abnormalities, but complete resection is not possible in certain clinical situations. The management of this clinical syndrome in such patients is challenging. Reversal of 1,25-dihydroxyvitamin D deficiency (by administering calcitriol) and correction of hypophosphatemia are effective palliative therapies.[115]

HYPERPHOSPHATEMIA

Hyperphosphatemia is found in 2.5% of cancer patients.[87]

Clinical Manifestations

The clinical manifestations of acute hyperphosphatemia are similar to those of associated hypocalcemia. Paresthesia, muscle cramps, tetany, and prolongation of Q–T interval may be induced directly by severe hyperphosphatemia. Chronic hyperphosphatemia, especially associated with hypercalcemia, may lead to a diffuse visceral deposition of calcium phosphate. Soft-tissue deposition of calcium phosphate complexes may lead to renal failure.

Pathophysiologic Mechanisms

Eighty percent of the phosphate in the human body is in bone. The phosphate balance is maintained primarily by the intestine, the kidneys, and bone. Vitamin D and PTH are the major regulators of the serum phosphate level although they are released in response to changes in ionized calcium rather than in response to changes in phosphate. Vitamin D enhances the gastrointestinal absorption of both phosphate and calcium. Ninety percent of the phosphorus in the glomerular filtrate is reabsorbed in the proximal renal tubule. Parathyroid hormone inhibits renal reabsorption of phosphate. The release and uptake of phosphate by bone are determined by the mechanism that governs calcium metabolism. When the serum calcium level falls, both calcium and phosphate are released from bone by the action of PTH on osteoclasts.

Etiology

The causes of hyperphosphatemia are listed in Table 7–10. Pseudohyperphosphatemia can result from the presence of immunoglobulin in some patients with multiple myeloma, which interferes with the biochemical assay for phosphate.[116–118] In the absence of renal failure, the fasting serum phosphate level is determined primarily by the rate of renal tubular reabsorption.

A massive amount of phosphate can be released into the extracellular fluid by extensive cellular injury. Tumor lysis syndrome was discussed earlier. Rhabdomyolysis and hemolysis may cause hyperphosphatemia in the same way.

The translocation of phosphate from cells in response to metabolic or respiratory alkalosis also can lead to hyperphosphatemia, as can hypoparathyroidism. Excess phosphate intake (including that caused by the use of phosphate-containing laxatives)[119] is yet another potential cause of hyperphosphatemia.

Diagnosis

In patients with hyperglobulinemia, hyperphosphatemia probably needs to be confirmed by a specimen that is free of protein (removed by precipitation with sulfosalicylic acid).[120] In cases of true hyperphosphatemia, renal function must be assessed. In addition, measurements of lactic dehydrogenase, uric acid, potassium, and calcium are necessary for the detection and management of hyperphosphatemia due to cellular breakdown.

Treatment

The emergency treatment of hyperphosphatemia involves supportive care and the treatment of symptomatic hypocalcemia. In patients with normal renal function, the infusion of isotonic saline increases phosphate excretion. The administration of dextrose and insulin drives phosphate into cells, temporarily lowering the serum level. When hyperphosphatemia poses a life-threatening condition, hemodialysis or peritoneal dialysis should be considered.

Although it is an important factor in the control of serum phosphorus in the chronic setting, the dietary restriction of phosphorus has practical problems that

TABLE 7–10. Causes of Hyperphosphatemia in Cancer Patients

Pseudohyperphosphatemia
    Paraproteinemia (myeloma)
    Hyperlipidemia
    Hyperbilirubinemia
Renal dysfunction
    Renal failure
    Increased renal tubular reabsorption
        Hypoparathyroidism
        Thyrotoxicosis
        Excess vitamin D administration
Cellular breakdown
    Rhabdomyolysis
    Tumor lysis syndrome
    Hemolysis
Increased intake
    Phosphate enemas or laxatives (eg, Fleet's Phosphosoda)
    Intravenous or oral phosphate administration

Adapted from Bibbs MA, Wolfson AB, Tayal VS. Electrolyte disturbances. In: Rosen P, Barkin R, editors. Emergency medicine: concepts and clinical practice. 4th ed. St. Louis: Mosby; 1998. p. 2432–2456.

limit its success in most patients. Aluminum-containing antacids are used to inhibit phosphorus absorption in the gastrointestinal tract, but the accumulation of aluminum has serious long-term toxic effects in patients with impaired renal function. Calcium-based phosphate binders have largely replaced aluminum compounds. However, excessive amounts of absorbed calcium present a different problem. New strategies for managing hyperphosphatemia may include the use of nonabsorbed phosphate binders that are aluminum free and calcium free (sevelamer, 800 to 1,600 mg with each meal)[121,122] and the development of vitamin D analogues that control PTH activity with fewer calcemic effects.[123]

HYPOGLYCEMIA

Hypoglycemia is defined as a blood glucose level of < 50 mg/dL. The timing of symptoms relative to a fasting or postprandial state can distinguish the various etiologies.

Clinical Manifestations

A progressive pattern of responses to hypoglycemia is determined by the availability of glucose to the brain. At a plasma glucose level of about 70 mg/dL, the brain's glucose uptake can be reduced, and counter-regulatory hormone responses are triggered. At 60 mg/dL, autonomic symptoms such as hunger, anxiety, palpitations, sweating, and nausea are prevalent. When glucose drops to < 50 mg/dL, the neuroglycopenic symptoms of blurry vision, slurred speech, confusion, and difficulty with mental concentration will appear. When glucose decreases to < 40 mg/dL, the patient may become drowsy, confused, or combative. A further prolonged decrease to < 30 mg/dL can cause seizures, permanent neurologic deficits, and death.

Pathophysiologic Mechanisms

Glucagon and epinephrine are the two major counter-regulatory hormones. Other hormones that respond to hypoglycemia are norepinephrine, cortisol, and growth hormone, but their effects are delayed. Glucagon and epinephrine immediately stimulate hepatic glycogenolysis followed by gluconeogenesis. Primary adrenal insufficiency and primary hypothyroidism may be associated with fasting or reactive hypoglycemia. Hypoglycemia also may be seen in hypopituitarism, in which the secretion of growth hormone, adrenocorticotropic hormone, or thyroid-stimulating hormone is deficient.

The kidneys contribute about one-third of the overall gluconeogenesis during hypoglycemia stress, and the kidneys also are an important extrahepatic site of insulin degradation. Moreover, a number of oral hypoglycemic drugs are excreted by the kidneys. Therefore, a decline in renal function often leads to hypoglycemic episodes in diabetic patients.

In many cancer patients, hypoglycemia is associated with tumor-related malnutrition, weight loss, and muscle wasting that impairs gluconeogenesis. Non-islet cell tumors also may secrete hypoglycemia factors, such as insulin-like growth factor-II (IGF-II) which causes hypoglycemia by binding to insulin receptors in the liver. Hypoglycemia may occur with pheochromocytoma, carcinoid tumors, and hematologic malignancies (leukemia, lymphoma, and myeloma). Excessive glucose consumption by large tumors may cause hypoglycemia.

Etiology

The causes of hypoglycemia in cancer patients are listed in Table 7–11, and the precipitating factors for hypoglycemia in diabetic cancer patients are listed in Table 7–12. For diabetic patients who are on sulfonylurea or insulin, the most common cause of hypoglycemia is perhaps delayed or decreased food intake.

Cancer patients who have received radiation to the head and neck area are at risk of developing hypopituitarism. Hypoadrenalism, growth hormone deficiency, and hypothyroidism can cause hypoglycemia or can precipitate hypoglycemia in a diabetic patient who is taking insulin or oral antidiabetic agents. Metastatic or primary tumors that affect the hypothalamic-pituitary area can

TABLE 7–11. Causes of Hypoglycemia in Cancer Patients

Postprandial
    Alimentary hyperinsulinism
        Partial or total gastrectomy
        Pyloroplasty
        Gastrojejunostomy
        Peptic ulcer disease
        Early type 2 diabetes mellitus
Fasting
    Overuse of glucose
        Hyperinsulinism
            Insulinoma
            Exogenous insulin
            Sulfonylureas and meglitinide class of drugs
            Shock
        Tumors
            bulky mesenchymal tumor
            IGF-II–secreting tumors, (hepatoma, mesotheliomas, etc)
    Underproduction of glucose
        Hormone deficiencies
            Adrenal insufficiency
            Hypothyroidism
            Catecholamine deficiency
            Glucagon deficiency
        Malnutrition
        Severe liver dysfunction (acute toxic necrosis, viral hepatitis, cirrhosis, congestive heart failure)
        Drugs (β-blockers, ethanol, pentamidine, sulfonamides, etc)

Adapted from Aydulka R. Biabetes mellitus and disorders of glucose hemeostasis. In: Rosen P, Barkin R, editors. Emergency medicine: concepts and clinical practice. 4th ed. St. Louis: Mosby; 1998. p. 2456–2478.
IGF-II = insulin-like growth factor II.

TABLE 7–12. Precipitating Factors for Hypoglycemia in Diabetic Patients

Hypoadrenalism
Overaggressive treatment of diabetic ketoacidosis and hyperglycemic hyperosmolar nonketotic coma
Recent change of dose, type of insulin, or oral hypoglycemic agent
Decrease in usual food intake or malnutrition
Ethanol
Factitious hypoglycemia
Hepatic impairment
Hyperthyroidism
Increase in exercise
Sepsis
Worsening renal insufficiency
Malfunctioning, improperly adjusted, or incorrectly used insulin pump
Drugs (oral hypoglycemics, insulin, β-blockers, salicylates, pentamidine, phenylbutazone, antimalarials, some antibacterial sulfonamides)

Adapted from Aydulka R. Biabetes mellitus and disorders of glucose hemeostasis. In: Rosen P, Barkin R, editors. Emergency medicine: concepts and clinical practice. 4th ed. St. Louis: Mosby; 1998. p. 2456–2478.

cause problems similar to those caused by therapeutic radiation to the head and neck areas.[124]

Various mesenchymal tumors (mesothelioma,[125,126] fibrosarcoma,[127] leiomyosarcoma,[128] and hemangiopericytoma[129,130]) and organ-specific carcinomas (hepatic[131,132] pancreatic,[133] adrenocortical,[134] renal,[135] and mammary[136]) may be associated with non-islet cell tumor–induced hypoglycemia, which is often caused by the tumor's secretion of IGF-II. In a series of 44 patients, about 70% had large amounts of IGF-II.[137]

Diagnosis

Simultaneous measurements of fasting blood glucose and fasting insulin levels are helpful in investigating the cause of hypoglycemia. Hypoglycemia with an inappropriately elevated level of insulin suggests autonomous insulin secretion and factitious use of insulin or hypoglycemia agents. When the hypoglycemia occurs with a correspondingly suppressed level of insulin, non-insulin-mediated causes of fasting hypoglycemia need to be explored. The normal insulin-to-fasting plasma glucose ratio is less than 0.33. This ratio is increased in patients with insulinomas.

For many years, the demonstration of Whipple's triad in a 72-hour fast has been the standard method of diagnosing fasting hypoglycemia and insulinoma. A 72-hour fast with measurements of glucose and insulin every 6 hours will diagnose hypoglycemia in most patients with insulinomas. Recently, it was demonstrated that the current insulin and proinsulin assays allow insulinoma to be diagnosed within 48 hours of fasting.[138] The measurement of C peptide helps to distinguish between endogenous insulin secretion and exogenous insulin. Among patients who take oral sulfonylurea, levels of both C peptide and insulin are elevated, but the proinsulin level is normal. Measurements of IGF-II and the ratio of

IGF-II to IGF-I are useful in screening patients with hypoglycaemia induced by non-islet cell tumors that produce IGF-II.

Treatment

For mild hypoglycemia (glucose level of 50 to 60 mg/dL), 15 g of simple carbohydrates (such as 4 fl oz of unsweetened fruit juice or non-diet soft drink) is sufficient. For more severe hypoglycemia without loss of consciousness, 15 to 20 g of simple carbohydrates should be ingested quickly, followed by 15 to 20 g of a complex carbohydrate (such as crackers or bread).

In non-islet cell tumor–induced hypoglycemia, the most effective therapeutic approach is to resect or debulk the tumor. For unresectable tumors, reducing the bulk by external-beam radiation,[139] arterial chemoembolization, or percutaneous alcohol injection may be attempted. Otherwise, counter-regulatory hormones such as growth hormone,[140] glucocorticoids,[140,141] or glucagon may be tried as a means of raising the blood glucose level.

The treatment of postprandial hypoglycemia is primarily dietary. The diet should have a low carbohydrate content, and α-glucosidase inhibitors (acarbose or miglitol) may be helpful.[142]

The management of diabetes mellitus in a cancer patient is complicated by anorexia and by nausea or vomiting, which make caloric intake erratic.[143] Blood sugar swings and (especially) hypoglycemia should be avoided whenever possible. The degree of tight glycemic control should be viewed in the light of the patient's life expectancy. Aggressive blood sugar monitoring impairs quality of life, and intensive insulin therapy may not be appropriate because the long-term diabetic complications may not be relevant for a cancer patient with a short life expectancy.

HYPERGLYCEMIA

Diabetes mellitus is a common disease, and a large number of cancer patients have coexisting diabetes. Glucocorticoids are often used in cancer patients for various conditions, and steroid-induced diabetes mellitus is common. Since diabetes mellitus is an extensive subject, this section focuses on the acute complications of diabetes mellitus in cancer patients.

Clinical Manifestations

Most patients with significant hyperglycemia have polydipsia, polyuria, and polyphagia as symptoms. An extended period of unrecognized glycosuria may lead to weight loss. The dehydration of the lenses due to hyperglycemia leads to blurry vision.

In nonketotic hyperosmolar coma, the patient experiences mental status changes, hypotension, and severe dehydration. Nausea, vomiting, and abdominal pain are present in almost half of patients with diabetic ketoacidosis. Tachypnea (Kussmaul's respiration), tachycardia, hypotension, orthostatic blood pressure changes, acetone breaths, and other signs of severe dehydration are present in patients with diabetic ketoacidosis.

Pathophysiologic Mechanisms

Serum glucose is regulated by absorption, cellular uptake, gluconeogenesis, and glycogenolysis, which are processes regulated by the pancreas, intestine, liver, kidneys, and muscles. Hyperglycemia can result from perturbation of the hormones involved in glucose regulation (such as insulin or glucagon), or from dysfunction of the organs involved in glucose homeostasis.

The maintenance of normal glucose levels requires the matching of glucose absorption and production with glucose catabolism. Hormones that regulate glucose include insulin, glucagon, epinephrine, norepinephrine, cortisol, and growth hormone. When glucose is not transported inside the cells because of a lack of food and/or insulin, the body senses a fasting state and releases glucagon. Glucagon is secreted from the alpha-cells of the pancreatic islets into the hepatic portal circulation. Glucagon decreases glycolysis and increases gluconeogenesis. Epinephrine both stimulates hepatic glucose production and limits the glucose use through direct and indirect actions mediated through both α-adrenergic and β-adrenergic receptors. Epinephrine increases gluconeogenesis and glycogenolysis. Growth hormone release is not critical for rapid glucose counter-regulation, but growth hormone increases glucose production over a longer time frame.

Diabetic ketoacidosis is decompensated catabolism triggered by a relative or absolute deficiency of insulin secretion. A deficiency of insulin relative to glucagon inhibits glycolysis and increases glycogenolysis and gluconeogenesis in the liver. Levels of malonyl coenzyme A (CoA) decrease because acetyl CoA carboxylase and glycolysis are inhibited. As a result, the oxidation of fatty acids and the formation of ketone bodies are increased. The pathophysiology of hyperglycemic hyperosmolar nonketotic coma is similar to diabetic ketoacidosis except that ketone bodies are not formed and that the extremely high glucose level results from a diminished urine output.

Etiology

The factors that precipitate diabetic ketoacidosis and hyperosmotic hyperglycemic coma are listed in Table 7–13.

Glucocorticoid administration (in combination chemotherapy regimens or for treatment or prevention of edema of brain metastasis, transplant rejection, graft-versus-host disease, and nausea and vomiting) is the most common cause of diabetes mellitus in cancer patients, and it necessitates periodic screening for diabetes with fasting

TABLE 7–13. Precipitating Factors for Diabetic Ketoacidosis or Hyperglycemic Hyperosmolar Nonketotic Coma

External insult
   Trauma
   Burns
   Dialysis
   Hyperalimentation
Disease process
   Cushing's syndrome and other endocrinopathies
   Hemorrhage
   Myocardial infarction
   Renal disease
   Subdural hematoma
   Cerebrovascular accident
   Infection/sepsis
Drugs
   Antimetabolites
   L-Asparaginase
   Chlorpromazine
   Diazoxide
   Didanosine
   Glucocorticoids
   Immunosuppressives (FK506, cyclosporin A)
   Phenytoin
   Propranolol
   Thiazides

Adapted from Aydulka R. Biabetes mellitus and disorders of glucose hemeostasis. In: Rosen P, Barkin R, editors. Emergency medicine: concepts and clinical practice. 4th ed. St. Louis: Mosby; 1998. p. 2456–2478.

glucose levels during therapy. Treatment with streptozocin or L-asparaginase[144,145] may result in insulin-deficient diabetes mellitus. Although there is no evidence of a delayed onset of diabetes mellitus following treatment with streptozocin, follow-up has been limited and of a short term. Diabetes mellitus also may develop as a consequence of serious pancreatitis secondary to L-asparaginase treatment.[146–148] Tacrolimus (FK506) also has been shown to increase the incidence of diabetes,[149] perhaps by damaging islet beta cells and inhibiting insulin synthesis.[150] Patients who have received an allogeneic bone marrow transplant are likely to be on both glucocorticoid and tacrolimus and are particularly at risk of developing diabetes mellitus. Homoharringtonine is reported to increase insulin resistance and to cause hyperglycemia.[151] Anticancer cytokine drugs, such as interleukin-2,[152] interferon-α,[153–155] and interferon-γ,[156] also can cause diabetes.

Diagnosis

Some antineoplastic drugs affect the renal excretion of glucose without actually affecting glucose metabolism. Drugs such as ifosfamide[33] and mercaptopurine[157] can damage the renal tubules and cause glycosuria or Fanconi's syndrome. A false-positive reaction with the testing agent for urinary ketones can be caused by mesna (2-mercaptoethane sulfonate sodium),[158] an agent usually given together with ifosfamide to decrease the incidence of hemorrhagic cystitis.

As a general rule, a random glucose level of > 200 mg/dL or a fasting plasma glucose level of > 126 mg/dL on more than one occasion can establish the diagnosis of diabetes mellitus. A glucose tolerance test (2-hour oral glucose tolerance test: glucose measurements ≥ 200 mg/dL) usually is not necessary except in borderline cases. Glycosylated hemoglobin (Hgb A_{1C}) reflects the level of glucose in the preceding 1.5 months. The use of Hgb A_{1C} to monitor therapy is well established, but its use for diagnosing diabetes mellitus is controversial.[159,160]

Diabetic ketoacidosis is diagnosed by the triad of metabolic acidosis, hyperglycemia, and the presence of ketone bodies in the urine or blood. Increased gluconeogenesis and lipolysis lead to uncontrolled production of ketones by the liver and to metabolic acidosis. Hypertriglyceridemia and severe hyperglycemia can cause pseudohyponatremia. Arterial blood gas analysis will show acidemia and respiratory compensation of metabolic acidosis by hyperventilation. The anion gap will be elevated and serum ketone will be positive. A urine dipstick test for ketone can provide timely information for a quick bedside diagnosis. An absence of ketone in the urine practically excludes diabetic ketoacidosis. Leukocytosis may be associated with ketosis, but an infection must be considered as a precipitating factor for diabetic ketoacidosis. Serum creatinine can be falsely elevated because of ketosis. Abnormalities of potassium, phosphate, and magnesium are due to transcellular shifts caused by acidosis.

The differential diagnosis of diabetic ketoacidosis includes alcoholic ketoacidosis, cerebrovascular accident, trauma, sepsis, hyperosmolar hyperglycemic nonketotic coma, postictal states, lactic acidosis (possibly induced by malignancy),[161–163] uremic acidosis, and intoxication or poisoning by ethanol, methanol, isopropyl alcohol, salicylates, chloral hydrate, or cyanide.

In hyperglycemic hyperosmolar nonketotic coma, the plasma glucose level may be > 800 mg/dL, and the serum osmolality may be more than 100 mOsm higher than normal. Mild ketosis may be present because of starvation, but ketoacidosis is not present. In severe cases, when volume depletion causes circulatory collapse, lactic acidosis will develop.

Treatment

Management of the blood glucose level depends on the severity of the blood glucose abnormality and on the underlying pathophysiologic mechanism of the increase in blood sugar. In general, oral agents are less likely to be effective in patients who are deficient in insulin.

The treatment of diabetic ketoacidosis focuses on supplemental insulin, rehydration, correction of elec-

TABLE 7–14. Treatment of Diabetic Ketoacidosis

1st hour (which may very often take place in an emergency center)
1. Normal saline IV at 15 mL/kg/h.
2. Regular insulin: 10–20 U IV bolus, followed by continuous infusion, 0.1 U/kg/h. Monitor glucose at bedside every hour.
3. ECG: look for evidence of myocardial infarction as precipitating factor; look for peaked T waves or U waves as signs of severe abnormality in potassium level.
4. Arterial blood gases: confirm metabolic acidosis; if pH < 7.00, consider administration of small amount of sodium bicarbonate (about 1 mEq/kg).
5. Look for precipitating factors.

2nd hour
1. Continue normal saline IV at 15 mL/kg/h.
2. Regular insulin: continue insulin drip. If glucose < 250 mg/dL, change IV fluid to D5NS. If glucose does not decrease, double the insulin infusion rate.
3. Continue cardiac monitoring.

Subsequent hours
1. Adjust infusion rate of normal saline, based on hydration status. If serum sodium > 145 mEq/L, consider changing the fluid to 0.45% NaCl.
2. Anticipate potential need for potassium replacement. Monitor electrolytes closely.
3. Consider replacing phosphate if serum phosphorus < 1 mg/dL.
4. Continue insulin drip until anion gap becomes normal, serum bicarbonate becomes > 18 mEq/L, and urine ketone becomes negative. Patient may be fed or given D5W (if unable to eat) and subcutaneous regular insulin or fast-acting insulin analogues to control the blood sugar, using a sliding scale.

D5NS = dextrose 5% in normal saline; D5W = dextrose 5% in water; ECG = electrocardiogram; IV = intravenous; NaCl = sodium chloride.

trolyte abnormalities, correction of severe acidosis, and identification of the precipitating factors (Table 7–14). Regular insulin usually is given as an intravenous bolus of 0.1 U/kg followed by a maintenance intravenous infusion of 0.1 U/kg/hr.

The treatment of hyperglycemic hyperosmolar non-ketotic coma also focuses on intravenous fluid hydration and supplemental insulin although the amount of insulin required may be less than that required to treat diabetic ketoacidosis.

ADRENAL CRISIS

The adrenal gland is a common site of hematogenous metastasis, exceeded in frequency only by the lungs, the liver, and bone.[164] Despite the relatively high prevalence of adrenal infiltration by many common cancers, clinically evident primary adrenal insufficiency occurs infrequently. The hypothalamic-pituitary area may be damaged by tumor or by the treatment of tumor (radiation or surgery), and secondary adrenal insufficiency may result.

Clinical Manifestations

The symptoms of adrenal insufficiency include weakness, fatigue, nausea, vomiting, and weight loss. In cases of chronic primary adrenal failure, hyperpigmentation may occur. Acute adrenal crisis will involve hypoglycemia and hypotension.

The cachexia and weakness seen in patients with adrenal insufficiency can mimic the general wasting of extensive metastatic disease. Electrolyte abnormalities can easily be explained by poor intake, malnutrition, side effects of chemotherapy, or paraneoplastic syndromes. Adrenal insufficiency may develop so gradually that it goes unnoticed. Because the clinical manifestations of adrenal insufficiency are nonspecific and overlap other findings in cancer patients, a high index of suspicion is required to detect this treatable condition.

Pathophysiologic Mechanisms

Inadequate production of glucocorticoids needed to meet the metabolic requirements of the body leads to a potentially life-threatening adrenal crisis. In primary adrenal insufficiency, the adrenal glands are incapable of producing an adequate amount of cortisol and/or aldosterone. A lack of negative feedback leads to an elevation of adrenocorticotropic hormone (ACTH) levels. In secondary adrenal failure, the malfunction is in the hypothalamic-pituitary axis. Secondary adrenal insufficiency is characterized by (a) an inappropriately low level of ACTH in the context of low cortisol, (b) an appropriate level of aldosterone, controlled by the renin-angiotensin axis, and (c) hyperkalemia. Functional adrenal insufficiency may occur after the withdrawal of pharmacologic doses of glucocorticoids that suppressed the hypothalamic-pituitary-ACTH axis.

Etiology

The causes of adrenal insufficiency are listed in Table 7–15. Factors that precipitate adrenal crisis are listed in Table 7–16. In large autopsy studies, the prevalence of adrenal metastasis ranged from 9 to 27% among patients who died from malignant illness, and the involvement was bilateral in one-half to two-thirds of the patients with adrenal metastasis.[164] Research suggests that more than 80% of adrenal tissue must be destroyed before corticosteroid production (under both basal and stress conditions) is impaired.[165]

Other causes of primary adrenal insufficiency in cancer patients include autoimmune adrenalitis, adrenal hemorrhage, and granulomatous diseases. Many cancer patients are immunocompromised, particularly those with leukemia or lymphoma and those who have undergone bone marrow transplantation. In these patients, infection of the adrenal glands by *Cytomegalovirus* (CMV), mycobacteria, or fungus may lead to adrenal insufficiency. Adrenal insufficiency also may occur as a result of bilateral adrenalectomy; for instance, renal cell carcinoma often metastasizes to both adrenals, and radical nephrectomy is quite often performed along with contralateral adrenalectomy. Adrenal insufficiency may also be induced by drugs. Etomidate,[166] a common intravenous anesthetic, may inhibit cortisol synthesis, but its

TABLE 7–15. Causes of Adrenocortical Insufficiency in Cancer Patients

Primary adrenal failure
  Infectious causes
    Granulomatous
      Tuberculosis
    Fungal
      Histoplasmosis
      Blastomycosis
      Coccidiomycosis
      Candidiasis
      Cryptococcosis
    Viral
      Cytomegalovirus
      Herpes simplex virus
  Infiltration
    Sarcoidosis
    Neoplastic (metastatic)
    Lymphoma/leukemia
    Hemochromatosis
    Adrenoleukodystrophy
    Amyloidosis
  Post adrenalectomy
    Bilateral adrenal hemorrhage (eg, trauma, thrombocytopenia,
      coagulopathy, disseminated intravascular coagulation)
Secondary adrenal failure
  Pituitary insufficiency
    Apoplexy (hemorrhage)
    Pituitary or suprasellar tumor
    Isolated ACTH deficiency
    Infiltration disease
      Sarcoidosis
      Histiocytosis X
      Hemachromatosis
  Hypothalamic insufficiency
  Head trauma
  Status post surgical resection of brain tumor/metastasis
  Functional
      Glucocorticoid administration

ACTH = adrenocorticotropic hormone.
Adapted from Wogan JM. Endocrine disorders. In: Rosen P, Bartin R, editors. Emergency medicine: concepts and clinical practice. 4th ed. St. Louis: Mosby; 1998. p. 2488–2503.

short-term use (as in rapid-sequence intubation) does not create any clinically significant problems.[167] Imidazole antifungal drugs, ketoconazole,[168,169] and also fluconazole[170] and itraconazole[171] at high doses inhibit cytochrome P-450–dependent enzymes in the glucocorticoid synthetic pathway. Aminoglutethimide was originally used as an inhibitor of the synthesis of adrenocortical steroids, but now it is also used in endocrine therapy for breast cancer because of its inhibition of aromatase.[172] Patients with advanced breast cancer who are treated with megestrol acetate (60 mg/d) may develop symptomatic adrenal insufficiency.[173] Mitotane, structurally related to the insecticide dichorodiphenyltrichoroethane (DTT), has selective toxicity for normal and neoplastic adrenocortical cells. The biochemical mechanism of action for mitotane is unclear. Adrenal insufficiency is commonly observed at the doses used to treat adrenocortical cancer, making glucocorticoid replacement therapy mandatory. Serum levels of steroid-binding protein also have been reported to increase twofold to threefold during mitotane therapy.[174] Increased protein binding and increased clearance of steroid may lead to an increased daily requirement for glucocorticoid replacement during mitotane therapy.[175]

Secondary adrenal insufficiency because of metastasis to the pituitary and hypothalamus may also occur. The most common cause of secondary adrenal hypofunction, however, is the suppression of the hypothalamic-pituitary-adrenal-axis caused by exogenous glucocorticoid therapy. A prolonged course of therapy may lead to hypothalamic-pituitary-axis suppression that lasts for many months. It also has been demonstrated that short periods of steroid therapy (ie, 1, 2, or 4 weeks) suppress adrenal function for about 1 week in most patients.[176] In cancer patients who have received dexamethasone (12 mg/d for 4 days) together with paclitaxel and cisplatin, the hypothalamic-pituitary-adrenal axis may be suppressed for 8 to 14 days.[177] A 6-week course of high-dose dexamethasone as part of the induction chemotherapy for leukemia can suppress the hypothalamic-adrenal axis for more than 2 weeks,[178] and a 4-week course can suppress it for up to 4 weeks.[179] Therefore, these patients and those patients treated with a longer glucocorticoid course within the past year should receive stress dosages of glucocorticoid if an acute medical or surgical compli-

TABLE 7–16. Precipitating Factors for Adrenal Insufficiency

Surgery
Anesthesia
Volume loss, acute hemorrhage
Trauma
Asthma
Hypothermia
Alcohol
Myocardial infarction
Pyrogens
Sepsis
Hypoglycemia
Pain (severe)
Psychotic breakdown
Drugs
  Imidazole antifungals
  Etomidate
  Mitotane
  Megestrol
  Metyrapone
  Aminoglutethimide
  Morphine
  Reserpine
  Chlorpromazine
  Barbiturates

Adapted from Wogan JM. Endocrine disorders. In: Rosen P, Bartin R, editors. Emergency medicine: concepts and clinical practice. 4th ed. St. Louis: Mosby; 1998. p. 2488–2503.

cation occurs (eg, neutropenic fever with hypotension). Irradiation of the hypothalamic-pituitary region causes an ACTH deficiency and secondary adrenal insufficiency.[180–186] This may occur as early as the first 2 years after radiotherapy although the median time for occurrence is 5 years (see Figure 7–2).

Diagnosis

Cortisol has been measured primarily in the plasma to assess adrenal function, but measuring the cortisol concentration in the saliva may be an alternative.[187]

About 20 to 30% of patients with bilateral adrenal metastasis will develop adrenal insufficiency.[188] All of these patients should be evaluated by the ACTH stimulation test (cosyntropin [synthetic ACTH, amino acids 1 to 24], 250 µg). Recent advances in imaging techniques have allowed patients with adrenal lesions to be identified ante mortem as part of the tumor-staging evaluation. The location of the adrenal glands in the perinephric fat allows almost all normal glands and contour-deforming masses smaller than 5 to 10 mm to be detected. Computed tomography (CT) has a sensitivity of 86%, a specificity of 97%, and an accuracy of 93% in the detection of adrenal masses.[189] Adrenal cysts and myelolipomas usually can be definitely diagnosed, based on CT appearance. The characteristics on CT that suggest adrenal metastasis rather than primary adrenal disease include heterogeneity, contrast enhancement, bilaterality, and a size > 3cm.[190] Patients with metastatic cancer and bilateral adrenal involvement as shown by CT should be screened for adrenal insufficiency.[188]

Several diagnostic approaches have been used to evaluate secondary adrenal insufficiency. Screening tests include basal (8:00 am) serum cortisol measurements.[191] Further dynamic tests include stimulation with 1 µg of cosyntropin,[192] metyrapone (30 mg/kg orally overnight),[193] corticotropin-releasing hormone (CRH), and insulin-induced hypoglycemia (insulin tolerance test).

Treatment

If a cancer patient presents to an emergency center in a state of hemodynamic shock, there may be no time to confirm a diagnosis of adrenal insufficiency. In these instances, empiric treatment with a stress dose of hydrocortisone should be considered, especially if the patient has received high-dose glucocorticoid treatment within the past year. Moreover, in patients who are vasopressor dependent because of septic shock, replacement therapy with hydrocortisone may alleviate systemic inflammatory responses, shorten the duration of shock, and improve survival.[194] In unstable patients (those with circulatory instability, sepsis, prior emergency surgery, or other major complications), hydrocortisone (300 mg/d) or other glucocorticoids (in equipotent doses) may be administered intravenously in divided doses. For

instance, dexamethasone would not interfere with the assay for serum cortisol and thus would not hamper further diagnostic testing by cosyntropin stimulation.

The usual adult dose of glucocorticoid replacement is about 20 to 30 mg/d of hydrocortisone (eg, 10 to 20 mg in the morning and 10 mg in the early afternoon).[195] Other glucocorticoids at equipotent doses may be used. In the event of severe stress or febrile illness, the glucocorticoid dosage must be increased to prevent an "adrenal crisis." Fludrocortisone (9-α-fluor-hydrocortisone, 0.05 to 0.2 mg/d) may replace mineralocorticoids. Younger adult women with adrenal insufficiency may benefit, with regard to sexual function and a sense of well-being, from dehydroepiandrosterone (DHEA, 50 mg/d).[196]

Addisonian patients often are up to 20% volume depleted. Correction of hypovolemia should be aggressive, with intravenous boluses of normal saline or other crystalloid fluids such as lactated Ringer's solution. Up to a total of 3 L may be required in the first 8 hours. Treatment of hypoglycemia should be immediate if the patient is symptomatic. Dextrose (50% in water, 50 to 100 mL) may be given by intravenous push and should be followed by dextrose 5% in water (D5W). If intravenous access is not promptly available, 2 mg of glucagon may be given SQ or intramuscularly (IM), but the effect may be delayed by about 10 to 20 minutes.

CUSHING'S SYNDROME

Glucocorticoid increases glucose production, inhibits protein synthesis, promotes protein breakdown, stimulates lipolysis, and modulates immunologic and inflammatory responses. It is important in the maintenance of blood pressure and is part of the body's response to stress.

Clinical Manifestations

The signs and symptoms of glucocorticoid excess include central obesity (truncal obesity, moon face, supraclavicular fat pads, and buffalo hump), skin changes (thinning, facial plethora, easy bruising, and violaceous striae), muscle weakness with proximal myopathy, hypertension, atherosclerosis, edema, menstrual irregularities, depression, emotional lability, irritability, osteoporosis, infection, and poor wound healing. Patients with ectopic Cushing's syndrome experience weight loss, hypertension, hypokalemia, and hyperpigmentation.

Pathophysiologic Mechanisms

The synthesis of glucocorticoids in the adrenal cortex is regulated by ACTH, which is synthesized and secreted by corticotrophic cells in the anterior pituitary. The hypothalamus secretes corticotropin-releasing hormone (CRH), which stimulates the anterior pituitary to secrete ACTH. The secretion of ACTH is also inhibited by negative feedback from glucocorticoid levels.

Excess glucocorticoids may arise from exogenous sources, excess secretion of glucocorticoid by benign or malignant adrenal tumors, and excess production of ACTH by pituitary tumors or (ectopically) by carcinomas. Overall, exogenous Cushing's syndrome is the most common form. Among the endogenous causes of Cushing's syndrome, pituitary disease is the most common.

Etiology

Cancer patients receive glucocorticoids frequently and for various reasons. For instance, glucocorticoids may be given as part of the chemotherapy regimen or as premedication to prevent adverse reactions to the chemotherapeutic agent. In patients with brain metastasis or spinal-cord compression, high-dose glucocorticoids are required to decrease edema in the neural tissue. Prolonged use of supraphysiologic doses of glucocorticoids will lead to Cushing's syndrome.

Carney's complex is an inherited autosomal dominant disease with multiple tumors, including cardiac myxomas, pigmented skin lesions, pigmented nodular adrenal dysplasia, myxoid fibroadenoma of the breast, testicular tumors, acromegaly, and peripheral-nerve lesions. The tumor suppressor gene PRKAR1A, which codes for the type 1 α-regulatory subunit of protein kinase A (PKA), is mutated in about half of Carney's complex kindreds.[197]

Pituitary Cushing's syndrome is due to a benign pituitary adenoma that secretes ACTH inappropriately. Both benign and malignant adrenal tumors can cause Cushing's syndrome. Malignant adrenal carcinoma usually presents with widespread disease in the abdomen and has a poor prognosis. Both ACTH-secreting pituitary tumors and adrenocortical tumors are part of the multiple endocrine neoplasia type I, in which menin is mutated.[198]

Ectopic Cushing's syndrome may result from the ectopic production of ACTH or CRH.[47] In a Mayo Clinic series of ectopic Cushing's syndrome cases due to ectopic ACTH production, the frequency of the various causative tumors were as follows: bronchial carcinoid, 25%; islet cell cancer, 16%; small-cell lung carcinoma, 11%; medullary thyroid cancer, 8%; disseminated neuroendocrine tumor of unknown primary, 7%; thymic carcinoid, 5%; pheochromocytoma, 3%; disseminated gastrointestinal carcinoid, 1%; and other tumors, 8%.[199] Ectopic secretion of CRH has been reported in cases of small-cell lung cancer.[200]

Diagnosis

The single best screening test for diagnosing hypercortisolism is 24-hour urine collection for urinary free cortisol and creatinine. An overnight low-dose dexamethasone suppression test and a midnight cortisol saliva test are sensitive screening tests.[201] The next step is to determine whether the hypercortisolism is dependent on ACTH, by measuring plasma levels of ACTH on multiple occasions. Dexamethasone-CRH or desmopressin may distinguish between Cushing's disease and pseudo-Cushing's syrdrome.[201] The test for distinguishing a pituitary source from an ectopic source of ACTH is bilateral simultaneous inferior petrosal sinus sampling (IPSS) for ACTH levels. The adequacy of IPSS is further increased by measuring ACTH responses to CRH injection.[201] Magnetic resonance imaging (MRI) of the sella and CT of the abdomen will provide radiologic evidence of tumor locations.

Treatment

Cushing's disease may be amenable to resection by transsphenoidal resection of the pituitary adenoma. Surgical adrenalectomy may be performed for adrenocortical tumors. Hypercortisolism increases the likelihood of adrenalectomy, and patients may experience significant postoperative surgical morbidity (or even mortality), such as problems with wound healing, infection, coronary artery disease, and pulmonary embolism. Biochemical adrenalectomy with medications such as mitotane, ketoconazole (titrated up to 1,200 mg/d),[169,202] or metyrapone (750 to 6,000 mg/d)[203] may be performed preoperatively or if the patient is not a candidate for surgery.

HYPOTHYROIDISM

Hypothyroidism is a common disease, with a prevalence of 2 to 3% in the general population. Hypothyroidism is much more common in women, with a female-to-male ratio of 10:1. As a result, it is quite common to find a female cancer patient with pre-existing or coexisting hypothyroidism. Moreover, hypothyroidism may arise as a complication of cancer or cancer treatment.

Clinical Manifestations

Hypothyroidism is often associated with nonspecific symptoms, such as fatigue, general weakness, cold intolerance, depression, weight gain, joint aches, constipation, dry skin, and menstrual irregularities. With mild or subclinical hypothyroidism, physical examination may be normal. Signs of moderate to severe hypothyroidism include hypertension, bradycardia, coarse hair, periorbital edema, carpal tunnel syndrome, and delayed relaxation of the tendon reflexes. Unusual signs of severe hypothyroidism include megacolon, cardiomegaly, and congestive heart failure.

Myxedema coma is a life-threatening condition characterized by exaggerated signs and symptoms of hypothyroidism. Hypothermia, bradycardia, and hypoventilation are common in cases of myxedema coma, and pericardial, pleural, and peritoneal effusions are often present. An ileus is present in about two-thirds of patients. Central nervous system changes include seizures, stupor, and coma.

Pathophysiologic Mechanisms

Thyroid hormone synthesis depends on iodine uptake, the synthesis of thyroglobulin, the oxidative binding of iodide to thyroglobulin, and the oxidative coupling of two iodotyrosines into iodothyronines. These processes are regulated by thyroid-stimulating hormone (TSH). The secretion of TSH from the pituitary is under the negative feedback control of thyroid hormones in the hypothalamus, which release thyrotropin-releasing hormone (TRH) to stimulate the release of TSH from the pituitary.

The effects of thyroid hormones can be divided into two categories: (1) effects on cellular differentiation and development and (2) effects on metabolism. In adults, the primary effects of thyroid hormones are metabolic. Thyroid hormones have effects on essentially all metabolic pathways and organs. Thyroid hormones modulate the metabolic rate and affect oxygen consumption and the metabolism of lipids, proteins, and carbohydrates.

Etiology

The most common cause of hypothyroidism in the general population is chronic lymphocytic thyroiditis (Hashimoto's disease). Iodine deficiency is an important cause of hypothyroidism in some other parts of the world but is rare in the United States and Western Europe. Other causes include surgery, radioactive iodine, acute thyroiditis, postpartum thyroiditis, subacute thyroiditis, external-beam irradiation to the neck, amyloidosis, sarcoidosis, hemochromatosis, medications (antithyroid drugs, amiodarone, lithium, excess iodine, interferons, and interleukin-2), and congenital defects. Insults to the pituitary and hypothalamus lead to secondary and tertiary hypothyroidism, respectively (see discussion of hypopituitarism, below, for the causes of central hypothyroidism).

Irradiation is an important cause of hypothyroidism (primary, secondary, and tertiary) in cancer patients (see Figure 7–2). Radiation-induced primary hypothyroidism is caused by thyroid cell destruction, inhibition of cell division, vascular damage, and (possibly) immune-mediated phenomena. Factors that increase the risk of developing primary hypothyroidism include a high radiation dose to the vicinity of the thyroid gland, time since therapy, lack of shielding to the thyroid during radiotherapy, and combined irradiation and surgical treatments.[204] Other factors include hemithyroidectomy during laryngectomy and damage to the thyroid vascular supply during surgery.[204] The incidence of hypothyroidism after radiation therapy for various cancers and conditions is shown in Table 7–17.

Except for L-asparaginase, thyroid dysfunction from cytotoxic chemotherapeutic agents is uncommon. In addition to blocking synthesis of thyroid-hormone binding proteins, L-asparaginase may also inhibit TSH synthesis reversibly and lead to temporary hypothyroidism.[205,206] Several noncytotoxic anticancer drugs can cause hypothyroidism. In one study, targretin (a retinoid X-receptor selective ligand) caused secondary hypothyroidism in patients treated for cutaneous T-cell lymphoma, in a dose-related manner.[207] Thyroid dysfunction is a recognized side effect of cytokine treatments. Treatment with interleukin-2 produces thyroid dysfunction in approximately 20 to 35% of patients.[208,209] These patients have hypothyroidism, hyperthyroidism, or hyperthyroidism followed by hypothyroidism.[210,211] About 10% of interferon-treated patients develop primary hypothyroidism (mostly subclinical).[212,213] Patients with pre-existing thyroid autoimmunity are at a higher risk of cytokine-induced thyroid dysfunction.

It has been suggested that immunosuppression by chemotherapeutic agents may prevent the development of chronic autoimmune lymphocytic thyroiditis and subsequent hypothyroidism. However, a protective effect of chemotherapy could not be demonstrated in patients who received higher doses of radiation (< 30 Gy) or in long-term survivors of bone marrow transplantation (BMT), 43% of whom were hypothyroid after a 13-month follow-up period.[214] On the contrary, about 14% of BMT patients who did not receive radiation were hypothyroid.[215] This suggests a relationship between hypothyroidism and high-dose chemotherapy. This notion is further supported by several studies in which hypothyroidism occurred more frequently in a patient group treated with chemotherapy plus surgery or radiation than in a control group treated without chemotherapy.[216–218]

The potential contribution of lymphangiography to thyroid dysfunction has been controversial. Ethiodol is a fat-soluble organic iodide, and its slow release from lymph 4 months after lymphangiography carries the theoretic risk that the iodide excess can inhibit thyroid hormone biosynthesis and secretion, thereby producing

TABLE 7–17. Incidence of Hypothyroidism* after Radiation Therapy

Type of Malignancy	Radiation Dose (Gy)	Hypothyroidism (%)
Hodgkin's disease	30–60	30–50
Head and neck cancer	40–72	25–50
Lymphoma	20–40 (median, 36)	30–42
Breast carcinoma	?	15–21
Bone marrow transplantation (total-body irradiation)	13.75–15	15–43

*Adapted from Samaan NA, et al;[185] Tami TA, et al;[204] Sklar CA, et al;[214] Tamura K, et al;[221] Schimpff SC, et al;[228] Hancock SL, et al;[229] Constine LS, et al;[317] Devney RB, et al;[318] Grande C;[319] Vrabek DP and Heffron TJ;[320] Posner MR, et al;[321] Cannon CR;[322] Shafer RB, et al;[323] Fuks Z, et al;[324] Joensuu H and Viikari J;[325] Boulad F, et al.[326]
*Including compensated hypothyroidism.

hypothyroidism.[219] Lymphangiography also may increase the risk of radiation-associated thyroid dysfunction.[220] The risk appears to be highest for patients who have an interval of more than 30 days between lymphangiography and radiotherapy.[221]

Hypothyroidism secondary to metastatic infiltration and replacement of the thyroid by cancer is extremely rare.

Myxedema coma occurs most often in elderly hypothyroid patients with a superimposed precipitating event. The precipitating factors for myxedema coma are listed in Table 7–18.

Diagnosis

The diagnosis of hypothyroidism is confirmed by thyroid function tests. However, the interpretation of thyroid function tests can be complicated and challenging.

The level of thyroid hormone–binding proteins (thyroxine-binding globulin [TBG] and albumin) can be modified by sex hormones and nutritional factors, abnormalities of which are encountered frequently in cancer patients. Several chemotherapeutic drugs are known to affect thyroid function tests. L-Asparaginase appears to reversibly inhibit the synthesis of albumin and TBG, resulting in a low total thyroxine level but normal free thyroxine level.[222,223] Podophyllin combined with alkylating agents has also been reported to decrease TBG.[224] 5-Fluorouracil[225] and mitotane[174] both increase total thyroxine and triiodothyronine (T_3) levels without suppressing TSH, suggesting that these drugs increase thyroid hormone–binding capacity in the serum.

Alterations in thyroid hormone metabolism will occur in cancer and other serious nonthyroidal systemic illnesses.[226,227] Low serum T_3 levels, which may be found in up to 17% of moderately to seriously ill patients, are due to reduced extrathyroidal conversion of thyroxine (T_4) to T_3. Serum concentrations of free T_4 usually are normal or high whereas free T_3 concentrations are below normal or low. These patients are clinically euthyroid, and serum TSH level and TRH stimulation test results are normal. Thyroid hormone therapy is not indicated. As nonthyroidal illness progresses, the low-T_3 syndrome may evolve into the low-T_3 low-T_4 syndrome, in which the low total T_4 is caused by (a) decreased binding of T_4 to serum proteins; (b) decreased serum TBG, prealbumin, and/or albumin; or (c) an increase in T_4 clearance. In most of these patients, T_3, T_4, and TSH levels are normal. The clinical manifestations of hypothyroidism are usually absent, but assessment may be compounded by the obtundation, edema, and hypothermia that may accompany severe illness. Low free-T_4 levels usually indicate a grave prognosis, with a mortality rate in the range of 60%. Thyroid hormone replacement therapy has no benefit in these patients.

In cancer patients or long-term cancer survivors, a history of radiotherapy is particularly important. Long-term follow-up of patients suggests that there is a threshold of about 10 Gy for the development of hypothyroidism.[228,229] Almost 60% of patients who receive mantle irradiation for Hodgkin's disease have hypothyroidism 10 to 18 years later,[230] and the high risk of developing hypothyroidism persists for more than 25 years after radiotherapy for Hodgkin's disease.[229] These findings reinforce the importance of clinical vigilance in the detection of hypothyroidism in cancer survivors. In adults, neck irradiation for a variety of head and neck tumors and lymphoma is associated with a high incidence of primary hypothyroidism. Children who have received either head and neck or cranial irradiation should be routinely screened. Early detection will permit intervention before hypothyroidism causes adverse effects on physical and intellectual development and growth.

In patients with myxedema coma, serum thyroid hormones usually are low, and the TSH level is significantly elevated (except in cases of secondary hypothyroidism). Anemia, hyponatremia, hypoglycemia, hypothermia, and hypotension can be found. Analysis of arterial blood gases usually reveals retention of carbon dioxide and hypoxemia. Electrocardiography often shows sinus bradycardia, various types and degrees of heart block, low voltage, and T-wave flattening.

Recognizing hypothyroidism may be difficult in the emergency care setting. Thyroid function tests typically are not performed on a 24-hour basis, and it may take more than 1 day for results to become available. The emergency physician's responsibility is to consider the diagnosis of hypothyroidism and to order the appropriate thyroid function tests in the laboratory evaluation to ensure adequate patient care and follow-up.[231]

Treatment

Once hypothyroidism (frank or subclinical) is diagnosed, the patient should receive thyroid hormone replacement therapy.

TABLE 7–18. Factors That May Precipitate Myxedema Coma

Exposure to cold
Infection (usually pneumonia)
Congestive heart failure
Trauma
Drugs
    Phenothiazine, phenobarbital, narcotics, anesthetics, benzodiazepines, lithium, iodides
Cerebrovascular accident
Hemorrhage (especially gastrointestinal)

Adapted from Wogan JM. Endocrine disorders. In: Rosen P, Bartin R, editors. Emergency medicine: concepts and clinical practice. 4th ed. St. Louis: Mosby; 1998. p. 2488–2503.

The management of myxedema coma in the critical-care setting has been reviewed.[232] Rapid clinical diagnosis and early therapy may be lifesaving. Treatment may be emergent and is usually given prior to laboratory confirmation.[231] For critical patients, if myxedema coma is highly suspected, levothyroxine should be given (0.5 mg IV,[233] followed by 0.025 to 0.1 mg/d). Since the conversion of thyroxine to triiodothyronine is decreased in severe nonthyroidal illness, patients who require pressor support and who are unresponsive to 1 to 2 days of thyroxine therapy should be given triiodothyronine (12.5 µg IV every 6 hours). In one study, advanced age, cardiac problems, and high-dose thyroid hormone replacement (levothyroxine [≥ 0.5 mg/d] or triiodothyronine [≥ 75 µg/d]) were associated with death within 1 month of treatment.[233] Other supportive measures, such as the correction of hypothermia by slow rewarming and such as ventilatory and circulatory support, are critical.

THYROTOXICOSIS

Thyroid disorders and abnormalities of thyroid function are commonly associated with cancer and its therapy. Although less common than hypothyroidism, thyrotoxicosis is a common disease and has a prevalence of 20 to 25 per 100,000 in the general population. Again, as with hypothyroidism, there is a female dominance, with a female-to-male ratio of 5:1. Therefore, it is quite common to find a female cancer patient with pre-existing or coexisting hypothyroidism. Moreover, thyrotoxicosis may arise as a complication of cancer or its treatment.

Clinical Manifestations

Thyrotoxicosis is characterized by a hyperadrenergic state. A fine tremor can be seen in the hands. Sinus tachycardia, systolic flow murmur, and water-hammer pulse are commonly seen. Atrial dysrhythmias (atrial fibrillation, atrial flutter, and premature atrial contractions) and congestive heart failure are often observed. Eye signs include Graves' ophthalmopathy, exophthalmos, extraocular-muscle palsies, staring, lid lag, and upper-eyelid retraction. Neuropsychiatric symptoms (ie, agitation, anxiety, restlessness, fear, paranoia, and mood swings) are observed. Dyspnea on exertion and proximal myopathy are particularly common in elderly patients. Thyrotoxic hypokalemic paralysis has been observed mostly in Asians but has also been reported in Caucasians.[234,235] Acute thyrotoxic polyneuropathy also has been reported.[236] Gastrointestinal symptoms include hyperphagia, diarrhea, nausea, vomiting, and abdominal pain. Dermatologic symptoms include flushed skin, moist arms, fine and straight hair, alopecia, and pretibial myxedema. Apathetic hyperthyroidism is seen (primarily in elderly persons), and congestive heart failure, atrial fibrillation, and weight loss are prominent features. Depressed mental function may range from a placid demeanor to frank confusion.

Pathophysiologic Mechanisms

Thyrotoxicosis can result from the unregulated release of thyroid hormones and thyroglobulins. This may be caused by direct injury to the thyroid gland, destructive infiltrative processes, or autoimmune-mediated destruction of thyroid follicular cells. In these cases, radioiodine scanning will show decreased uptake of iodine. Iodine-induced hyperthyroidism also may show low radioiodine uptake. Amiodarone-induced hyperthyroidism may result from subacute thyroiditis or excess iodine.[237]

Hyperthyroidism can result from the unregulated or stimulated synthesis and release of thyroid hormones and from the unregulated growth of thyroid tissues. Toxic goiters, toxic adenomas, and thyroid carcinomas are examples of unregulated autonomous thyroid tissue. The inappropriate stimuli causing hyperfunction of the thyroid may be TSH, human chorionic gonadotropin, thyroid-stimulating immunoglobulins, and mutations in TSH receptors, or they may arise from faulty intracellular signal transduction mechanisms. Central hyperthyroidism results from the overproduction of TSH by the pituitary gland, which leads to thyroid enlargement and hyperfunction.[238] In these cases, radioiodine scanning will show increased uptake of iodine.

Etiology

Large quantities of iodide are present in many drugs (eg, approximately 9 mg of iodine, following a daily dose of 300 mg of amiodarone), antiseptics (eg, povidone-iodine), and contrast media for radiology. Cancer patients are frequently exposed to these iodide sources, especially to contrast media for radiologic studies. Iodine-induced hyperthyroidism usually occurs in euthyroid patients with previous thyroid diseases, active Graves' disease or recombinant interferon-α–induced destructive thyrotoxicosis.[239]

Thyrotoxicosis can result from autoimmune thyroiditis precipitated by bioimmunotherapy of cancer with cytokines.[209,211,240] Besides being the mechanism for excess iodine, as mentioned above, amiodarone also induces thyroiditis. Patients with amiodarone-induced thyroiditis may later develop permanent hypothyroidism.[239]

Radiation-induced painless thyrotoxic thyroiditis occurs infrequently after external-beam radiotherapy to the head and neck area. Transient hyperthyroidism may occur as a result of inflammation and destruction of thyroid tissue and is often followed by hypothyroidism. Transient hyperthyroidism has been reported after mantle radiotherapy in patients with Hodgkin's disease, typically within 18 months of treatment.[241] Low uptake of radioiodine in most of these cases suggests a diagnosis of silent thyroiditis.

Graves' disease, toxic multinodular goiter, and the solitary toxic nodule are the three forms of primary hyperthyroidism that account for most cases of hyperthyroidism in the general population. Graves' disease is an autoimmune disorder characterized by the production of antibodies to the TSH receptor. Hyperthyroidism results when thyroid-stimulating immunoglobulins stimulate the TSH receptor, leading to the enlargement of the thyroid gland and to increased thyroid hormone synthesis. Radiation-induced thyroidal dysfunction may be associated with the autoimmune processes directed against the thyroid and can cause either hypo- or hyperthyroidism.[242] A small percentage of patients develop Graves' disease after radiotherapy for Hodgkin's disease.[229,243] The risk of Graves' disease in these patients was estimated to be at least 7.2 times that found in the general population.

Ophthalmopathy similar to Graves' disease has been reported within 18 to 84 months of high-dose radiotherapy to the neck for lymphoma, breast cancer, or nasopharyngeal/laryngeal cancer. Ophthalmopathy may occur without hyperthyroidism and in the absence of human leukocyte antigen-B8 (HLA-B8).[244] This suggests that radiation-induced thyroid injury may induce an autoimmune process that is similar to Graves' disease.

Autopsy series demonstrated thyroid metastasis in 1.25 to 24% of patients with metastatic carcinoma.[245,246] The common primary tumor sites are the kidneys, lungs, breasts, esophagus, and stomach.[245] Thyrotoxicosis has been reported in patients with thyroid metastases[247] from lymphoma[248] and pancreatic cancers.[249] In these cases, the etiology of hyperthyroidism is similar to that seen in cases of subacute thyroiditis, with follicular destruction resulting in unregulated release of thyroid hormone and thyroglobulin.

Central hyperthyroidism is rare. Overproduction of TSH by the pituitary gland causes thyroid enlargement and hyperfunction. The two causes of central hyperthyroidism are TSH-producing pituitary tumors and the syndrome of pituitary resistance of thyroid hormone.[238]

Structural homology in human chorionic gonadotropin and TSH molecules, as well as in receptors, provides the biochemical basis for the ability of human chorionic gonadotropin to stimulate the TSH receptor.[250] Trophoblastic tumors, hydatidiform mole, and choriocarcinoma secrete large amounts of human chorionic gonadotropin and often cause hyperthyroidism. When serum human chorionic gonadotropin rises to > 200 IU/mL, hyperthyroidism is likely to occur. Surgical removal of the disease or effective chemotherapy can cure the hyperthyroidism.[251]

Other rare causes of hyperthyroidism include hormone-producing malignant struma ovarii,[252] destruction of normal thyroid tissue by anaplastic thyroid cancer,[253] McCune-Albright syndrome,[254,255] and an activating TSH receptor mutation in a Hürthle cell carcinoma.[256]

Thyroid storm, an acute severe decompensation of severe or untreated thyrotoxicosis, is a life-threatening complication with a high mortality.[257] The precipitating factors for thyroid storm are listed in Table 7–19.

Diagnosis

The diagnosis of thyrotoxicosis is achieved by measuring thyroid hormones (thyroxine and triiodothyronine) and thyroid-stimulating hormone. Pituitary and hypothalamic causes of thyrotoxicosis are unusual. Measuring free thyroid hormones instead of total serum hormone levels avoids changes introduced by variations of TBG. Radioiodine scanning is helpful in distinguishing hyperfunction of the thyroid gland from thyroiditis.

Thyroid storm should be considered in the differential diagnosis of hyperpyrexia in the emergency-care setting,[258] particularly in cancer patients with risk factors for Graves' disease (bioimmunotherapy or a history of radiotherapy to the neck or chest area) or who have tumors that may secrete human chorionic gonadotropin. A set of diagnostic criteria (fever, tachycardia, tachyarrhythmia, mental status change, etc) and a scoring system have been proposed by Burch and Wartofsky.[257]

Treatment

Treatment of Graves' disease includes antithyroid medication, radioactive iodine, and surgery. Treatment of thyroiditis primarily involves the removal of the causative factors and the control of hyperadrenergic symptoms with β-blockers. If the diagnosis of thyroid storm is highly likely on the basis of clinical criteria, diagnostic studies should be obtained, and therapy should be initiated immediately. The management of severe thyrotoxicosis or thyroid storm consists of treatments directed at inhibiting thyroid hormone synthesis, blocking thy-

TABLE 7–19. Precipitating Factors for Thyroid Storm

Infection
Iodine therapy
Contrast radiographic studies
Premature withdrawal of antithyroid therapy
Pulmonary embolism
Visceral infarction
Ingestion of thyroid hormone
Surgery
Trauma
Severe emotional stress
Hypoglycemia
Diabetic ketoacidosis
Hyperosmolar nonketotic coma

Adapted from Wogan JM. Endocrine disorders. In: Rosen P, Bartin R, editors. Emergency medicine: concepts and clinical practice. 4th ed. St. Louis: Mosby; 1998. p. 2488–2503.

roid hormone release, inhibiting the conversion of thyroxine to triiodothyronine, supporting systemic decompensation, and correcting the precipitating factors.[257] Rapid inhibition of thyroid hormone synthesis with thionamide drugs followed within hours by blockade of the release of preformed thyroid hormone by iodides is the cornerstone of acute management.

Thionamides function as antithyroids primarily by preventing the synthesis of thyroid hormones. The half-life of thyroxine (T_4) is 7 days in euthyroid individuals and somewhat shorter in thyrotoxic patients. This accounts for the delay of several weeks in the onset of clinical improvement in most patients. Doses range from 100 to 600 mg of propylthiouracil per day or 10 to 60 mg of methimazole per day. For patients who cannot receive medication orally or through nasogastric, gastrostomy, or jejunostomy tubes, rectal administration of propylthiouracil[259–261] or methimazole[262] has been described.

β-Blockers, both cardioselective and noncardioselective, are important adjuncts in treating hyperthyroidism. β-Blockade provides rapid relief of hyperadrenergic symptoms and signs of thyrotoxicosis, such as palpitations, tremors, anxiety, heat intolerance, and various eyelid signs, before any decrease in thyroid hormone levels. β-blockers are useful in preventing episodes of hypokalemic periodic paralysis in susceptible individuals, and they are the drugs of choice for thyroiditis, which is self-limiting. Higher doses of propranolol (> 160 mg/d) also can inhibit peripheral T_4-to-T_3 conversion.

Saturated potassium iodide solution (3 to 5 drops) is administered orally every 8 hours to block the release of thyroid hormones. In pharmacologic concentrations (100 times the normal plasma level), iodides decrease thyroid gland activity. This action involves decreasing thyroid iodide uptake, iodide oxidation, and organification and blocking the release of thyroid hormones (Wolff-Chaikoff effect). Iodide has substantial benefits in treating thyroid storm.[257] However, the administration of iodide may be problematic in thyrotoxic patients with severe dysfunction of the upper gastrointestinal tract. Rectal delivery of potassium iodide is an effective alternative to parenteral sodium iodide in treating a severely thyrotoxic patient with a small-bowel obstruction.[259]

The oral contrast agents ipodate or iopanoic acid also are potent inhibitors of T_4-to-T_3 conversion, making them ideal for treating severe or decompensated thyrotoxicosis. They are generally given after starting the patient on thioamide. Although intravenous iodinated radiographic contrast medium has been used to treat a case of thyroid storm,[263] this approach has significant nephrotoxicity, and its efficacy has not been firmly established.

The enterohepatic circulation of thyroid hormones is higher in thyrotoxicosis. Bile salt sequestrants bind thyroid hormones and thereby increase their fecal excretion. Colestipol has been shown to be an effective and well-tolerated adjunctive agent in the treatment of hyperthyroidism.[264]

Other treatment options include corticosteroids (such as dexamethasone, which inhibits peripheral thyroxine conversion), lithium, amiodarone, and potassium perchlorate. Plasmapheresis[265,266] and hemoperfusion[267,268] are effective ways to remove excess thyroid hormone. Emergent thyroidectomy is hazardous in the presence of severe thyrotoxicosis, and radioactive iodine does not offer rapid control of thyroid function.[257]

HYPOPITUITARISM

Hypopituitarism results from processes that affect the pituitary, hypothalamic, or parasellar areas and disrupt the normal function of the hypothalamic-pituitary axis by displacement, infiltration, or destruction.

Clinical Manifestations

The major clinical signs and symptoms of anterior pituitary dysfunction are those associated with hypothyroidism, hypoadrenalism, and hypogonadism. The clinical signs and symptoms of posterior pituitary dysfunction are those of diabetes insipidus (see specific sections above for more details about the clinical manifestations of each of these conditions). The major sign of hyposomatotropism in children is stunted growth, but the signs and symptoms in adults are subtle. Increased fat mass, reduced muscle and bone mass, impaired exercise capacity, decreased physical strength, fatigue, and a decreased sense of well-being (quality of life) are common in adults with growth hormone deficiency.[269]

Pathophysiologic Mechanisms

The hypothalamus links many other areas of the brain and integrates the signals that control the secretory function of the pituitary gland. Four major hormonal axes with negative-feedback control loops involve the anterior pituitary: the somatotropic, adrenocorticotropic, gonadotropic, and thyrotropic axes. Prolactin is primarily under the inhibitory control of dopamine. The regulatory hormones reach the anterior pituitary from the hypothalamus via the portal circulation. In contrast, the posterior pituitary consists of neurons extending from the hypothalamus, secreting vasopressin and oxytocin.

Many hormonal functions are crowded into a small anatomic area, making this an area of utmost endocrine importance. Any insult or injury to this anatomic area will lead to hormonal dysfunction (most often involving multiple hormones).

Etiology

The various causes of hypopituitarism in cancer patients are listed in Table 7–20.

TABLE 7–20. Causes of Hypothalamic-Pituitary Dysfunction in Cancer Patients

Invasive
    Craniopharyngioma
    Pituitary tumors
    Metastatic cancer
    Meningioma
    Optic glioma
    Leukemia/chordoma
    Lymphoma
Compressive
    Cyst
    Aneurysm
Iatrogenic
    Surgery
    Radiotherapy
Ischemic
    Poorly controlled diabetes mellitus
    Sickle cell anemia
    Arteritis and vasculitis
Infiltrative
    Hemochromatosis
    Sarcoidosis
    Amyloidosis
    Histiocytosis
    Wegener's granulomatosis
    Lymphocytic hypophysitis
Infectious
    Meningitis (bacterial, fungal, viral)
    Brain abscess (bacterial, fungal)
    Encephalitis (bacterial, viral)
    Tuberculosis
    Syphilis
    Brucellosis

Radiotherapy is the most common etiologic factor for hypothalamic-pituitary dysfunction in cancer patients.[270] No strong direct evidence has implicated chemotherapy as a cause of permanent dysfunction of the anterior pituitary. The development of radiation-induced hypothalamic dysfunction is insidious, and any clinical manifestation of hormone deficiency can occur years after radiation exposure. In general, the rapidity of onset and the severity of dysfunction depend on the total dose of radiation and on the rate of delivery. The sequence and frequency of hormonal dysfunction among the several axes varies considerably. The somatotropic axis appears to be the most sensitive[18,184–186] (Figure 7–3). Severe growth hormone deficiency is correlated with a high number of pituitary hormone deficits.[271]

Surgical intervention for pituitary tumors[272] or craniopharyngiomas[273] often leads to endocrine dysfunction within the hypothalamic-pituitary axes.

Pituitary apoplexy is an acute life-threatening event characterized by severe headache and circulatory collapse caused by intrapituitary hemorrhage.[274] The expanding hemorrhagic mass may compress parasellar structures, including cranial nerves.

Metastasic disease to the hypothalamic region or to the pituitary gland is uncommon,[275] and clinical manifestation of endocrine dysfunction due to displacement, infiltration, or destruction by metastatic disease in this region is rare. The most prevalent primary malignancies associated with pituitary metastases are breast cancer and lung cancer.[276] However, benign tumors, such as pituitary tumors and craniopharyngioma,[277] often arise in this anatomic region and cause endocrine dysfunction.

Diagnosis

The evaluation should include the assessment of anterior pituitary hormones and MRI. Nocturia, polyuria, and polydipsia suggest the need to test for diabetes insipidus.

The diagnosis of pituitary dysfunction requires vigilance because most of the presenting symptoms are nonspecific and can be easily discounted; for example, fatigue and weakness are common among cancer patients. A history of cranial or head and neck irradiation should prompt a serious consideration of hypopituitarism in the differential diagnosis. Diagnostic screening for hypothalamic and pituitary dysfunction should entail the measurement of growth hormone (GH) and an evaluation for gonadal failure. Other signs of overt hypopituitarism include hypoglycemia, hypotension, and hypothermia. The evaluation of sexual development should include Tanner staging, examination of pubic and axillary hair, review of menstrual history in girls, and notation of penile and testicular size in boys. Decreased insulin-like growth factor (IGF) I and IGF-binding protein 3 (IGF-BP3) levels *per se* do not establish growth hormone deficiency. If initial evaluation results are abnormal, stimulation of GH secretion by insulin-induced hypoglycemia, using the insulin tolerance test (ITT), should be performed unless contraindicated by cardiac disease or seizure disorders[278] (Table 7–21). Alternative provocative tests of the somatotropic axis include those for L-dopa, and growth hormone–releasing hormone (GHRH) and L-arginine.[278] The L-arginine stimulation test may be less sensitive than the ITT.[279] If screening tests with thyrotropin (TSH) and free thyroxine levels, cortisol (8:00 am), 24-hour urinary free cortisol, luteinizing hormone, follicle-stimulating hormone, estradiol, and testosterone are abnormal, then detailed dynamic testing should be performed.

Treatment

Although the classic sequence of loss of pituitary secretion is GH, gonadotropins, TSH, and, ACTH, the order of replacement therapy for deficient hormone(s) is cortisol, thyroxine, androgens/estrogens, and GH.[280] In emergent situations, cortisol and thyroxine replacements are most relevant. Depending on the patient's level of stress and severity of illness, stress doses of corticosteroid, up to 300

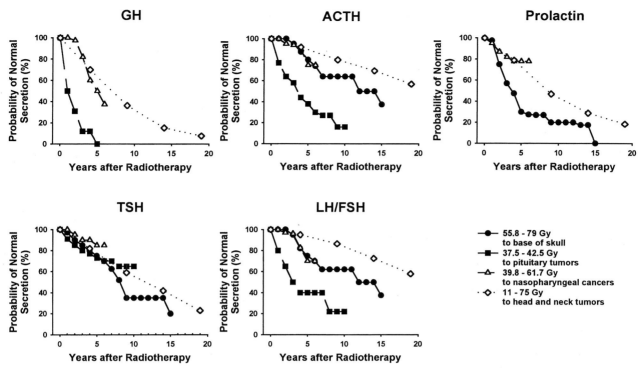

Figure 7–3. Probability of normal pituitary hormone secretion over time after radiation exposure to the hypothalamic-pituitary areas. Data from four studies were replotted on this single figure. The first set of values (*closed circles*) are from the study of Pai and colleagues, in which the patients received 55.8 to 79 Gy to the base of the skull. The second set of values (*solid squares*) are from the study of Shalet and colleagues, in which patients with pituitary tumors were treated with 37.5 to 42.5 Gy. The third set (*open triangles*), from the study by Lam and colleagues, shows the effect of radiation treatment for nasopharyngeal carcinoma with 39.8 to 61.7 Gy. The final set (*open diamonds*) represents data from the study of Samaan and colleagues, in which 11 to 75 Gy was administered to treat head and neck tumors. Adapted from Pai HH, et al;[182] Shalet SM, et al;[184] Samaan SM, et al;[185] Lam KS, et al.[186] ACTH = adrenocorticotropic hormones; FSH = follicle-stimulating hormone; GH = growth hormone; LH = luteinizing hormone; TSH = thyroid-stimulating hormone.

mg of hydrocortisone per day (or other glucocorticoids in equipotent doses), may be administered (see Hypothyroidism, above, and Hypoadrenalism, above).

Long-term experience with GH replacement in otherwise healthy adults seems to justify GH replacement therapy for patients with a clear-cut diagnosis of GH deficiency and continuation of long-term therapy for those who demonstrate beneficial effects, especially improvements in exercise performance and quality of life.[269,281] However, there is legitimate concern that GH may promote cancer growth. The safety of "physiologic"

replacement doses of growth hormone in cancer patients has not been established.

HYPERTENSIVE CRISIS DUE TO PHEOCHROMOCYTOMA OR PARAGANGLIOMAS

Pheochromocytomas and paragangliomas are catecholamine-producing tumors arising from chromaffin cells. These are rare tumors that cause hypertension in about 0.2% of all hypertensive patients. Pheochromocy-

TABLE 7–21. Dynamic Testing of the Growth Hormone Axis for the Diagnosis of Growth Hormone Deficiency

Test	Dose/Sampling	Contraindications
Insulin hypoglycemia	0.075–0.1 U regular insulin/kg IV to achieve glucose ≤ 40 mg/dL; sample for glucose and GH at 0, 30, 45, 60, and 90 min	Coronary heart disease; seizures
Arginine	0.5 g/kg (up to 30 g) IV over 30 min; sample for GH at 0, 30, 60, 90, and 120 min	Liver disease; renal disease
Arginine and GHRH	Arginine dose as above. GHRH 1 µg/kg IV push; sample for GH at 0, 30, 60, 90, and 120 min.	Liver disease; renal disease
L-Dopa	500 mg by mouth; sample for GH at 0, 30, 60, 90, and 120 min	Systolic blood pressure < 100 mm Hg; age > 60 yr

GH = growth hormone; GHRH = growth hormone–releasing hormone; IV = intravenously.

tomas arise from the adrenal medulla, and paragangliomas arise from the sympathetic ganglia. The tumors' release of large quantities of catecholamine can lead to a life-threatening crisis.

Clinical Manifestations

Hypertensive crises are life-threatening situations and may be defined as a sudden increase in systolic and diastolic blood pressure that causes dysfunction of the brain, heart, or kidneys. These crises require immediate treatment with antihypertensive drugs. Associated emergent conditions include dissecting aneurysms, acute left ventricular heart failure, intracranial bleeding, malignant hypertension resistant to treatment, hypertensive encephalopathy, and serious blood pressure elevations after vascular surgery.[282]

Pathophysiologic Mechanisms

Catecholamine synthesis begins with L-tyrosine. Dopamine, norepinephrine, and epinephrine are formed through the action of dopamine β-hydroxylase and phenylethanolamine-N-methyltransferase. These secreted catecholamines are metabolized by monoamine oxidase and catechol O-methyltransferase. The adrenergic receptors are classified into α_1, α_2, β_1, β_2, and β_3, with different organ distribution and functions.

The colocalization of various substances with catecholamines in the tumor (such as neuropeptide Y and opioid peptides) is recognized. The significance of these cosecreted substances in the clinical features of pheochromocytomas is not fully understood,[283] but immunoreactive neuropeptide-Y levels have been correlated with systemic vascular resistance.[284]

Etiology

Most pheochromocytomas arise sporadically, but about 10% are hereditary and are most often associated with the following familial tumor syndromes: multiple endocrine neoplasia type II (MEN II), von Hippel-Lindau (VHL) disease, and neurofibromatosis 1 (NF1).[285] Germline mutations of the VHL tumor suppressor gene are responsible for VHL disease, and germline RET proto-oncogene mutations are associated with MEN II.[286]

Factors that precipitate a hypertensive crisis in a pheochromocytoma patient include anesthesia, surgical resection of the tumor, and fine-needle biopsy of the tumor. The induction of a hypertensive crisis by chemotherapy for a malignant pheochromocytoma has been reported.[287] Drugs such as glucagon and metoclopramide also can provoke the release of catecholamines and cause a hypertensive crisis.

Diagnosis

Biochemical diagnosis is confirmed primarily by elevated urine vanillylmandelic acid (VMA) and/or catecholamine levels. Plasma metanephrines offer less variability in response to external factors and may be favored as a screening test for pheochromocytomas.[288,289] A high sensitivity of plasma levels of metanephrines supports a role for this test in a diagnostic algorithm.[290] Chromogranin-A levels may be a useful follow-up marker. The serum α-subunit of the glycoprotein hormone level may differentiate pheochromocytoma from other endoderm-derived neuroendocrine tumors (from which it is frequently secreted).[291]

Diagnostic testing has changed over the years.[292] Since the 1980s, CT has replaced venous sampling as the primary localizing procedure. Radionuclide-labeled metaiodobenzylguanidine (MIBG) scanning was used for almost all patients between 1984 and 1987 but was used only selectively after that period.[292] Iodine 123 (^{123}I), MIBG scintigraphy and 6-[^{18}F]-fluorodopamine positron emission tomography enhance diagnosis and tumor localization.[290] For tumor localization, MIBG scintigraphy is superior to CT in specificity, but CT has a higher sensitivity. After biochemical diagnosis, CT will detect most pheochromocytomas.[293]

All patients with incidental adrenal tumors should be biochemically screened for pheochromocytoma (especially before resection or needle biopsy) to avoid precipitating a lethal hypertensive crisis.[294]

The diagnosis of a hypertensive crisis is primarily clinical; a sudden increase in systolic and diastolic blood pressure that causes dysfunction of the brain, heart, or kidneys qualifies for one. Precipitating factors include surgery, needle biopsy, sudden withdrawal of antihypertensive medication, chemotherapy, and other drugs (saralasin, hydralazine, morphine, fentanyl, glucagon, metoclopramide, droperidol, amphetamine, tricyclic antidepressants, guanethidine, and monoamine oxidase inhibitors).

Treatment

Laparoscopic adrenalectomy (LA) has become a safe, efficient, and preferred method for removing most adrenal neoplasms. It has few major complications, and its clinical and biochemical cure rates are comparable to those of open adrenalectomy.[295,296] Laparoscopic excision of paragangliomas also is technically feasible.[297]

The combination of α-metyrosine and α-adrenergic blockade results in better blood pressure control during surgery, compared to the classic method of single-agent adrenergic blockade. Preoperative treatment with metyrosine along with an α-blocker is a useful strategy for decreasing surgical complications in patients with pheochromocytoma.[298]

In patients with hypertensive crisis, treatment should be started with an α-adrenergic receptor blocking agent if pheochromocytoma has not been excluded.[282] Antihypertensive agents with a rapid onset of action are used at present. These include nifedipine (10 mg sublingual (SL) every

15 to 30 min, for a total of 30 mg), clonidine (0.1 mg orally every 30 to 60 min, for a total of 0.3 mg), phentolamine (5 to 10 mg IV every 5 to 15 min), diazoxide (50 to 100 mg IV every 15 min up to 300 mg, then titration of the continuous infusion from 0.75 mg/min to a maximum of 30 mg/min), nitroglycerin (5 μg/min IV initially and titrated with close monitoring), and sodium nitroprusside (0.5 μg/kg/min IV initially and titrated with close monitoring). Generally, β-blockers such as propranolol, metoprolol, and atenolol will worsen the increase in blood pressure.

CARCINOID CRISIS

Carcinoid tumors secrete a variety of polypeptides, biogenic amines, and prostaglandins. The humoral factors and perhaps some other unknown factors cause a constellation of symptoms collectively known as carcinoid syndrome. Severe and life-threatening manifestations of carcinoid syndrome are called carcinoid crises.

Clinical Manifestations

Carcinoid syndrome includes the following symptoms: skin flushing, telangiectasia, cyanosis, diarrhea, intestinal cramping, bronchoconstriction, and valvular heart disease. In many patients, the primary complaints are severe flushing, nausea, and faintness. In a crisis situation, seizure, hypotension, severe bronchoconstriction, and cardiopulmonary arrest can occur.

Ectopic Cushing's syndrome may be caused by carcinoid tumors.[299,300] Bronchial carcinoid is the most common cause of Cushing's syndrome due to ectopic ACTH production.[301] (See Cushing's Syndrome, above, for a descripton of the signs and symptoms of Cushing's syndrome.)

Pathophysiologic Mechanisms

The provocation of 5-hydroxytryptamine (5-HT) and other humoral mediator release in carcinoid patients may be mediated through the release of catecholamines from the adrenals, which activates adrenergic receptors on tumor cells. Somatostatin receptors on the tumor cells exhibit a primarily inhibitory effect. Treatment with a somatostatin analogue can reduce these reactions and thus minimize the risk of carcinoid crisis.[302]

Etiology

Typical carcinoid syndrome is usually associated with midgut carcinoid tumors. Foregut carcinoid tumors may be associated with carcinoid syndrome with atypical symptoms. Hindgut carcinoid tumors are rarely associated with carcinoid syndrome. Ninety percent of patients with carcinoid syndrome have metastatic disease.

Foregut carcinoid tumors may be part of MEN I syndrome,[303] an autosomal dominant disease caused by mutation of the *MEN* I gene (menin).[303] Investigations to rule out other tumors of the MEN I syndrome should be carried out in these patients.

In one study, the presence of carcinoid heart disease or a high urinary output of 5-hydroxyindoleacetic acid (5-HIAA) preoperatively were statistically significant risk factors for perioperative complications.[304] Fatal carcinoid crisis has been reported immediately after a fine-needle aspiration biopsy was performed on a carcinoid tumor.[305,306] Carcinoid crisis also can be precipitated by chemotherapy[307] and laser bronchoscopy.[308]

Diagnosis

Typically, symptoms of diarrhea and skin flushing prompt an investigation into possible carcinoid syndrome. A 24-hour urine collection for 5-HIAA, the product of 5-HT metabolism, is a very specific test for carcinoid syndrome. However, this test may not be helpful in cases of foregut carcinoids and bronchial carcinoids, which often lack aromatic amino acid decarboxylase. Chromogranin A is released by neuroendocrine tumors. As a general rule, the serum concentration of chromogranin A correlates well with the urinary excretion of 5-HIAA. Knowing the fasting blood serotonin level is helpful, especially when the 24-hour urinary 5-HIAA excretion is borderline. Provocative testing with epinephrine or pentagastrin to bring out symptoms of flushing, hypotension, and tachycardia also can be performed. Scintigraphy using indium 111 (^{111}In)–labeled octreotide is the examination of choice for diagnosing and localizing carcinoid tumors as it is more sensitive than morphologic imaging techniques such as CT.[309]

Treatment

Symptomatic treatments usually target bronchoconstriction, flushing, and diarrhea. Mild bronchoconstriction may respond to inhaled anticholinergic and/or β-adrenergic agonists. Mild diarrhea usually responds to codeine and its derivatives or to cholestyramine. To block the effects of histamine, H_1 blockers (diphenhydramine, dimenhydrinate, and hydroxyzine) can be used in combination with H_2 blockers (ranitidine, famotidine, and cimetidine). Cyproheptadine also can block 5-HT receptors and may be helpful in controlling symptoms caused by 5-HT.

Patients with flushing and/or diarrhea not responsive to standard symptomatic measures may benefit from chemotherapy or hormonal therapy. Chemotherapy with either doxorubicin alone or streptozocin plus 5-fluorouracil (5-FU) achieves a response rate of about 23 to 33%.[310] Hepatic artery ligation or embolization are effective means of inducing rapid tumor shrinkage in patients who have hepatic-dominant metastases. Adding chemotherapy after the induction of a partial remission with hepatic artery embolization may prolong the response.[311] Chemoembolization infrequently causes cholecystitis or gallbladder infarction. Other complications include carcinoid crisis, pseudocirrhosis, liver infarction, abscess formation, hepatorenal syndrome, and liver rupture.[312]

Octreotide acetate, a somatostatin analogue, is effective in controlling and markedly reducing the symptoms of carcinoid crisis. Dose escalation of up to 5,950 μg/d has been reported.[313] Lanreotide is a somatostatin analogue whose activity persists for 10 to 14 days. Unlike octreotide, lanreotide can be administered once every 10 to 14 days instead of 2 or 3 times daily.[314] Slow-release octreotide preparations (eg, Sandostatin LAR), which can be injected monthly, are now available.

Both hypertensive and hypotensive carcinoid crises respond to octreotide, and octreotide or lanreotide should be considered for prophylactic and emergency use for all carcinoid syndrome patients prior to and during anesthesia, surgery, and biopsy or chemoembolization of liver lesions.[315]

Treatment with octreotide or dexamethasone decreases extracellular levels of tryptophan metabolites, but the mechanisms are partly different. In some tumors, octreotide decreases the synthesis of 5-HT whereas dexamethasone markedly increases intracellular 5-HIAA levels.[316] When a carcinoid crisis occurs, octreotide and dexamethasone should be administered quickly in addition to supportive measures such as oxygen administration, intubation (if necessary), intravenous fluid, and H_1 and H_2 blockers. Administration of catecholamine should be avoided.

REFERENCES

1. Arrambide K, Toto RD. Tumor lysis syndrome. Semin Nephrol 1993;13:273–80.
2. Flombaum CD. Metabolic emergencies in the cancer patient. Semin Oncol 2000;27:322–34.
3. Jones DP, Mahmoud H, Chesney RW. Tumor lysis syndrome: pathogenesis and management. Pediatr Nephrol 1995;9:206–12.
4. Markman M. Common complications and emergencies associated with cancer and its therapy. Clev Clin J Med 1994;61:105–14.
5. Jensen M, Winkler U, Manzke O, et al. Rapid tumor lysis in a patient with B-cell chronic lymphocytic leukemia and lymphocytosis treated with an anti-CD20 monoclonal antibody (IDEC-C2B8, rituximab). Ann Hematol 1998;77:89–91.
6. Yang H, Rosove MH, Figlin RA. Tumor lysis syndrome occurring after the administration of rituximab in lymphoproliferative disorders: high-grade non-Hodgkin's lymphoma and chronic lymphocytic leukemia. Am J Hematol 1999;62:247–50.
7. Kalemkerian GP, Darwish B, Varterasian ML. Tumor lysis syndrome in small-cell carcinoma and other solid tumors. Am J Med 1997;103:363–7.
8. Persons DA, Garst J, Vollmer R, Crawford J. Tumor lysis syndrome and acute renal failure after treatment of non-small-cell lung carcinoma with combination irinotecan and cisplatin. Am J Clin Oncol 1998;21:426–9.
9. Drakos P, Bar-Ziv J, Catane R. Tumor lysis syndrome in nonhematologic malignancies. Report of a case and review of the literature. Am J Clin Oncol 1994;17:502–5.
10. Bilgrami SF, Fallon BG. Tumor lysis syndrome after combination chemotherapy for ovarian cancer. Med Pediatr Oncol 1993;21:521–4.
11. Van Der Klooster JM, Van Der Wiel HE, Van Saase JL, Grootendorst AF. Asystole during combination chemotherapy for non-Hodgkin's lymphoma: the acute tumor lysis syndrome. Neth J Med 2000;56:147–52.
12. Jasek AM, Day HJ. Acute spontaneous tumor lysis syndrome. Am J Hematol 1994;47:129–31.
13. Loosveld OJ, Schouten HC, Gaillard CA, Blijham GH. Acute tumour lysis syndrome in a patient with acute lymphoblastic leukemia after a single dose of prednisone. Br J Haematol 1991;77:122–3.
14. Schifter T, Cohen A, Lewinski UH. Severe tumor lysis syndrome following splenic irradiation. Am J Hematol 1999;60:75–6.
15. Leach M, Parsons RM, Reilly JT, Winfield DA. Efficacy of urate oxidase (uricozyme) in tumour lysis induced urate nephropathy. Clin Lab Haematol 1998;20:169–72.
16. Mahmoud HH, Leverger G, Patte C, et al. Advances in the management of malignancy-associated hyperuricaemia. Br J Cancer 1998;77:18–20.
17. Agha-Razii M, Amyot SL, Pichette V, et al. Continuous veno-venous hemodiafiltration for the treatment of spontaneous tumor lysis syndrome complicated by acute renal failure and severe hyperuricemia. Clin Nephrol 2000;54:59–63.
18. Sakarcan A, Quigley R. Hyperphosphatemia in tumor lysis syndrome: the role of hemodialysis and continuous veno-venous hemofiltration. Pediatr Nephrol 1994;8:351–3.
19. Adrogue HJ, Madias NE. Hyponatremia. N Engl J Med 2000;342:1581–9.
20. The Merck Manual Editorial Panel. Water, electrolyte, mineral, and acid-base metabolism. In: Beers MH, Berkow R, editors. The Merck manual of diagnosis and therapy. 17th ed. Whitehouse Station: Merck Research Laboratories; 1999. p. 120–155.
21. McDonald GA, Dubose TD Jr. Hyponatremia in the cancer patient. Oncology (Huntington) 1993;7:55–64, 67–8, 70–1.
22. Berghmans T. Hyponatremia related to medical anticancer treatment. Support Care Cancer 1996;4:341–50.
23. Fall PJ. Hyponatremia and hypernatremia. A systematic approach to causes and their correction. Postgrad Med 2000;107:75–82.
24. Adrogue HJ, Madias NE. Hypernatremia. N Engl J Med 2000;342:1493–9.
25. Fried LF, Palevsky PM. Hyponatremia and hypernatremia. Med Clin North Am 1997;81:585–609.
26. Palevsky PM, Bhagrath R, Greenberg A. Hypernatremia in hospitalized patients. Ann Intern Med 1996;124:197–203.

27. Palevsky PM. Hypernatremia. Semin Nephrol 1998;18: 20–30.

28. DeVita MV, Michelis MF. Perturbations in sodium balance. Hyponatremia and hypernatremia. Clin Lab Med 1993;13:135–48.

29. Wong MF, Chin NM, Lew TW. Diabetes insipidus in neurosurgical patients. Ann Acad Med Singapore 1998;27: 340–3.

30. Deen PM, Knoers NV. Vasopressin type-2 receptor and aquaporin-2 water channel mutants in nephrogenic diabetes insipidus. Am J Med Sci 1998;316:300–9.

31. Morello JP, Bichet DG. Nephrogenic diabetes insipidus. Ann Rev Physiol 2001;63:607–30.

32. Bendz H, Aurell M. Drug-induced diabetes insipidus: incidence, prevention and management. Drug Saf 1999;21:449–56.

33. Skinner R, Pearson AD, Price L, et al. Nephrotoxicity after ifosfamide. Arch Dis Child 1990;65:732–8.

34. Negro A, Regolisti G, Perazzoli F, et al. Ifosfamide-induced renal Fanconi syndrome with associated nephrogenic diabetes insipidus in an adult patient. Nephrol Dial Transplant 1998;13:1547–9.

35. Delaney V, de Pertuz Y, Nixon D, Bourke E. Indomethacin in streptozocin-induced nephrogenic diabetes insipidus. Am J Kidney Dis 1987;9:79–83.

36. Sunyecz L, Mirtallo JM. Sodium imbalance in a patient receiving total parenteral nutrition. Clin Pharm 1993; 12:138–49.

37. Williams DJ, Jugurnauth J, Harding K, et al. Acute hypernatraemia during bicarbonate-buffered haemodialysis. Nephrol Dial Transplant 1994;9:1170–3.

38. Buonocore CM, Robinson AG. The diagnosis and management of diabetes insipidus during medical emergencies. Endocrinol Metab Clin North Am 1993;22: 411–23.

39. Decaux G, Prospert F, Namias B, Soupart A. Hyperuricemia as a clue for central diabetes insipidus (lack of V1 effect) in the differential diagnosis of polydipsia. Am J Med 1997;103:376–82.

40. Mandal AK, Saklayen MG, Hillman NM, Markert RJ. Predictive factors for high mortality in hypernatremic patients. Am J Emerg Med 1997;15:130–2.

41. Pazmino PA, Pazmino BP. Treatment of acute hypernatremia with hemodialysis. Am J Nephrol 1993;13:260–5.

42. Yeung SJ, Chui AC, Balasubramanyam A. Diagnostic challenge: a young woman with no thirst for life. Cortlandt Forum 2000;13:42–43.

43. Singer I, Oster JR, Fishman LM. The management of diabetes insipidus in adults. Arch Intern Med 1997;157: 1293–301.

44. Hohler T, Teuber G, Wanitschke R, Meyer zum Buschenfeld KH. Indomethacin treatment in amphotericin B induced nephrogenic diabetes insipidus. Clin Invest 1994;72:769–71.

45. Stone KA. Lithium-induced nephrogenic diabetes insipidus. J Am Board Fam Pract 1999;12:43–7.

46. Milionis HJ, Bourantas CL, Siamopoulos KC, Elisaf MS. Acid-base and electrolyte abnormalities in patients with acute leukemia. Am J Hematol 1999;62:201–7.

47. Becker M, Aron DC. Ectopic ACTH syndrome and CRH-mediated Cushing's syndrome. Endocrinol Metab Clin North Am 1994;23:585–606.

48. Trujillo EB, Young LS, Chertow GM, et al. Metabolic and monetary costs of avoidable parenteral nutrition use. JPEN J Parenter Enteral Nutr 1999;23:109–13.

49. Perazella SO. Drug-induced hyperkalemia: old culprits and new offenders. Am J Med 2000;109:307–14.

50. Wu DC, Liu JM, Chen YM, et al. Mitomycin-C induced hemolytic uremic syndrome: a case report and literature review. Jpn J Clin Oncol 1997;27:115–8.

51. Kumura T, Yamane T, Ohta K, et al. [Acute myelogenous leukemia with hyperkalemia induced by pentamidine administration]. Rinsho Ketsueki 1998;39:398–401.

52. D'Erasmo E, Celi FS, Acca M, et al. Hypocalcemia and hypomagnesemia in cancer patients. Biomed Pharmacother 1991;45:315–7.

53. Abramson EC, Gajardo H, Kukreja SC. Hypocalcemia in cancer. Bone Miner 1990;10:161–9.

54. Uhl L, Maillet S, King S, Kruskall MS. Unexpected citrate toxicity and severe hypocalcemia during apheresis. Transfusion 1997;37:1063–5.

55. Comlekci A, Biberoglu S, Hekimsoy Z, et al. Symptomatic hypocalcemia in a patient with latent hypoparathyroidism and breast carcinoma with bone metastasis following administration of pamidronate. Intern Med 1998;37:396–7.

56. Sims EC, Rogers PB, Besser GM, Plowman PN. Severe prolonged hypocalcaemia following pamidronate for malignant hypercalcaemia. Clin Oncol (R Coll Radiol) 1998;10:407–9.

57. McIntyre E, Bruera E. Symptomatic hypocalcemia after intravenous pamidronate. J Palliat Care 1996;12:46–7.

58. Mune T, Yasuda K, Ishii M, et al. Tetany due to hypomagnesemia induced by cisplatin and doxorubicin treatment for synovial sarcoma. Intern Med 1993;32:434–7.

59. Kido Y, Okamura T, Tomikawa M, et al. Hypocalcemia associated with 5-fluorouracil and low dose leucovorin in patients with advanced colorectal or gastric carcinomas. Cancer 1996;78:1794–7.

60. Caro JF, Besarab A, Glennon JA. Symptomatic hypocalcemia following combined calcitonin and mithramycin therapy for hypercalcemia due to malignancy. Cancer Treat Rep 1978;62:1561–3.

61. Slayton RE, Shnider BI, Elias E, et al. New approach to the treatment of hypercalcemia. The effect of short-term treatment with mithramycin. Clin Pharmacol Therapeut 1971;12:833–7.

62. Dube WJ, Oberfield RA. Hypocalcemia from mithramycin therapy in malignant disease. Lahey Clin Found Bull 1970;19:85–91.

63. Khoo EC, Kowalewski K. Effect of actinomycin-D on calcium homeostasis. Proc Soc Exp Biol Med 1965;119: 946–8.

64. Freedman DB, Shannon M, Dandona P, et al. Hypoparathyroidism and hypocalcaemia during treatment for acute leukaemia. Br Med J (Clin Res Ed) 1982;284:700–2.

65. Vassilopoulou-Sellin R, Newman BM, Taylor SH, Guinee VF. Incidence of hypercalcemia in patients with malignancy referred to a comprehensive cancer center. Cancer 1993;71:1309–12.

66. Strewler GJ. The parathyroid hormone-related protein. Endocrinol Metab Clin North Am 2000;29:629–45.

67. Esbrit P. Hypercalcemia of malignancy—new insights into an old syndrome. Clin Lab 2001;47:67–71.

68. Tezelman S, Rodriguez JM, Shen W, et al. Primary hyperparathyroidism in patients who have received radiation therapy and in patients who have not received radiation therapy. J Am Coll Surg 1995;180:81–7.

69. Cohen J, Gierlowski TC, Schneider AB. A prospective study of hyperparathyroidism in individuals exposed to radiation in childhood. JAMA 1990;264:581–4.

70. Christensson T. Hyperparathyroidism and radiation therapy. Ann Intern Med 1978;89:216–7.

71. Russ JE, Scanlon EF, Sener SF. Parathyroid adenomas following irradiation. Cancer 1979;43:1078–83.

72. De Jong SA, Demeter JG, Jarosz H, et al. Thyroid carcinoma and hyperparathyroidism after radiation therapy for adolescent acne vulgaris. Surgery 1991;110:691–5.

73. Barri YM, Knochel JP. Hypercalcemia and electrolyte disturbances in malignancy. Hematol Oncol Clin North Am 1996;10:775–90.

74. Kelly KM, Lange B. Oncologic emergencies. Pediatr Clin North Am 1997;44:809–30.

75. Pimentel L. Medical complications of oncologic disease. Emerg Med Clin North Am 1993;11:407–19.

76. Lamy O, Jenzer-Closuit A, Burckhardt P. Hypercalcaemia of malignancy: an undiagnosed and undertreated disease. J Intern Med 2001;250:73–9.

77. Rifai MA, Moles JK, Harrington DP. Lithium-induced hypercalcemia and parathyroid dysfunction. Psychosomatics 2001;42:359–61.

78. Nussbaum SR. Pathophysiology and management of severe hypercalcemia. Endocrinol Metab Clin North Am 1993;22:343–62.

79. Theriault RL, Hortobagyi GN. The evolving role of bisphosphonates. Semin Oncol 2001;28:284–90.

80. Body JJ. Current and future directions in medical therapy: hypercalcemia. Cancer 2000;88:3054–8.

81. Nussbaum SR, Younger J, Vandepol CJ, et al. Single-dose intravenous therapy with pamidronate for the treatment of hypercalcemia of malignancy: comparison of 30-, 60-, 90-mg dosages. Am J Med 1993;95:297–304.

82. Warrell RP Jr, Murphy WK, Schulman P, et al. A randomized double-blind study of gallium nitrate compared with etidronate for acute control of cancer-related hypercalcemia. J Clin Oncol 1991;9:1467–75.

83. Lajer H, Daugaard G. Cisplatin and hypomagnesemia. Cancer Treat Rev 1999;25:47–58.

84. Wu B, Atkinson SA, Halton JM, Barr RD. Hypermagnesiuria and hypercalciuria in childhood leukemia: an effect of amikacin therapy. J Pediatr Hematol Oncol 1996;18:86–9.

85. Stewart AF, Keating T, Schwartz PE. Magnesium homeostasis following chemotherapy with cisplatin: a prospective study. Am J Obstet Gynecol 1985;153:660–5.

86. Markmann M, Rothman R, Reichman B, et al. Persistent hypomagnesemia following cisplatin chemotherapy in patients with ovarian cancer. J Cancer Res Clin Oncol 1991;117:89–90.

87. D'Erasmo E, Acca M, Celi FS, et al. A hospital survey of hypocalcemia and hypophosphatemia in malignancy. Tumori 1991;77:311–4.

88. Martin M, Diaz-Rubio E, Casado A, et al. Intravenous and oral magnesium supplementations in the prophylaxis of cisplatin-induced hypomagnesemia. Results of a controlled trial. Am J Clin Oncol 1992;15:348–51.

89. Hartmann JT, Knop S, Fels LM, et al. The use of reduced doses of amifostine to ameliorate nephrotoxicity of cisplatin/ifosfamide-based chemotherapy in patients with solid tumors. Anticancer Drugs 2000;11:1–6.

90. Lloyd CW, Johnson CE. Management of hypophosphatemia. Clin Pharm 1988;7:123–8.

91. Clark RE, Lee ES. Severe hypophosphataemia during stem cell harvesting in chronic myeloid leukaemia. Br J Haematol 1995;90:450–2.

92. Ashraf MS, Skinner R, English MW, et al. Late reversibility of chronic ifosfamide-associated nephrotoxicity in a child. Med Pediatr Oncol 1997;28:62–4.

93. Ho PT, Zimmerman K, Wexler LH, et al. A prospective evaluation of ifosfamide-related nephrotoxicity in children and young adults. Cancer 1995;76:2557–64.

94. Kumar R. Tumor-induced osteomalacia and the regulation of phosphate homeostasis. Bone 2000;27:333–8.

95. White KE, Jonsson KB, Carn G, et al. The autosomal dominant hypophosphatemic rickets (ADHR) gene is a secreted polypeptide overexpressed by tumors that cause phosphate wasting. J Clin Endocrinol Metab 2001;86:497–500.

96. Shimada T, Mizutani S, Muto T, et al. Cloning and characterization of FGF23 as a causative factor of tumor-induced osteomalacia. Proc Natl Acad Sci U S A 2001; 98:6500–5.

97. Rowe PS, de Zoysa PA, Dong R, et al. MEPE, a new gene expressed in bone marrow and tumors causing osteomalacia. Genomics 2000;67:54–68.

98. Shadaba A, Paine J, Adlard R, Dilkes M. Re-feeding syndrome. J Laryngol Otol 2001;115:755–6.

99. Wollner A, Shalit M, Brezis M. Tumor genesis syndrome. Hypophosphatemia accompanying Burkitt's lymphoma cell leukemia. Miner Electrolyte Metab 1986;12:173–5.

100. Steiner M, Steiner B, Wilhelm S, et al. Severe hypophosphatemia during hematopoietic reconstitution after allogeneic peripheral blood stem cell transplantation. Bone Marrow Transplant 2000;25:1015–6.

101. del Giglio A, Zukiwski AA, Ali MK, Mavligit GM. Severe, symptomatic, dose-limiting hypophosphatemia induced by hepatic arterial infusion of recombinant tumor necrosis factor in patients with liver metastases. Cancer 1991;67:2459–61.

102. George R, Shiu MH. Hypophosphatemia after major hepatic resection. Surgery 1992;111:281–6.

103. Mizuno Y, Masaki N, Hashimoto H, et al. Marked hypophosphatemia with decreased serum 1,25-dihydroxyvitamin D in a patient with hepatocellular carcinoma complicating liver cirrhosis. Jpn J Med 1991;30:81–6.

104. Dash T, Parker MG, Lafayette RA. Profound hypophosphatemia and isolated hyperphosphaturia in two cases of multiple myeloma. Am J Kidney Dis 1997;29:445–8.

105. Angeli P, Gatta A, Caregaro L, et al. Hypophosphatemia and renal tubular dysfunction in alcoholics. Are they

related to liver function impairment? Gastroenterology 1991;100:502–12.

106. Davis S, Kessler W, Haddad BM, Maesaka JK. Acute renal tubular dysfunction following cis-dichlorodiammine platinum therapy. J Med 1980;11:133–41.

107. Kelly WK, Curley T, Slovin S, et al. Paclitaxel, estramustine phosphate, and carboplatin in patients with advanced prostate cancer. J Clin Oncol 2001;19:44–53.

108. Lee BS, Lee JH, Kang HG, et al. Ifosfamide nephrotoxicity in pediatric cancer patients. Pediatr Nephrol 2001;16: 796–9.

109. Reyes-Mugica M, Arnsmeier SL, Backeljauw PF, et al. Phosphaturic mesenchymal tumor-induced rickets. Pediatr Dev Pathol 2000;3:61–9.

110. Nakahama H, Nakanishi T, Uno H, et al. Prostate cancer-induced oncogenic hypophosphatemic osteomalacia. Urol Int 1995;55:38–40.

111. Nuovo MA, Dorfman HD, Sun CC, Chalew SA. Tumor-induced osteomalacia and rickets. Am J Surg Pathol 1989;13:588–99.

112. Lyles KW, Berry WR, Haussler M, et al. Hypophosphatemic osteomalacia: association with prostatic carcinoma. Ann Intern Med 1980;93:275–8.

113. Rao DS, Parfitt AM, Villanueva AR, et al. Hypophosphatemic osteomalacia and adult Fanconi syndrome due to light-chain nephropathy. Another form of oncogenous osteomalacia. Am J Med 1987;82:333–8.

114. Loghman-Adham M, Walton D, Iverius PH, et al. Spurious hypophosphatemia in a patient with multiple myeloma. Am J Kidney Dis 1997;30:571–5.

115. Yeung SJ, McCutcheon IE, Schultz P, Gagel RF. Use of long-term intravenous phosphate infusion in the palliative treatment of tumor-induced osteomalacia. J Clin Endocrinol Metab 2000;85:549–55.

116. Busse JC, Gelbard MA, Byrnes JJ, et al. Pseudohyperphosphatemia and dysproteinemia. Arch Intern Med 1987; 147:2045–6.

117. Sonnenblick M, Eylath U, Brisk R, et al. Paraprotein interference with colorimetry of phosphate in serum of some patients with multiple myeloma. Clin Chem 1986;32:1537–9.

118. Oren S, Feldman A, Turkot S, Lugassy G. Hyperphosphatemia in multiple myeloma. Ann Hematol 1994;69: 41–3.

119. Vukasin P, Weston LA, Beart RW. Oral Fleet Phospho-Soda laxative-induced hyperphosphatemia and hypocalcemic tetany in an adult: report of a case. Dis Colon Rectum 1997;40:497–9.

120. Adler SG, Laidlaw SA, Lubran MM, Kopple JD. Hyperglobulinemia may spuriously elevate measured serum inorganic phosphate levels. Am J Kidney Dis 1988;11:260–3.

121. Ramsdell R. Renagel: a new and different phosphate binder. ANNA J 1999;26:346–7.

122. Burke SK. Renagel: reducing serum phosphorus in haemodialysis patients. Hosp Med 2000;61:622–7.

123. Malluche HH, Monier-Faugere MC. Hyperphosphatemia: pharmacologic intervention yesterday, today and tomorrow. Clin Nephrol 2000;54:309–17.

124. Lebl J, Snajderova M, Kolouskova S. Severe hypoglycemia

and reduction of insulin requirement in a girl with insulin-dependent diabetes mellitus: first sign of a craniopharyngioma. J Pediatr Endocrinol Metab 1999; 12:695–7.

125. Schweichm M, Hennessey JV, Cole P, et al. Hypoglycemia in pregnancy secondary to a non-islet cell tumor of the pleura and ectopic insulin-like growth factor II hormone production. Obstet Gynecol 1995;85:810–3.

126. Sakamoto T, Kaneshige H, Takeshi A, et al. Localized pleural mesothelioma with elevation of high molecular weight insulin-like growth factor II and hypoglycemia. Chest 1994;106:965–7.

127. Kotani K, Tsuji M, Oki A, et al. IGF-II producing hepatic fibrosarcoma associated with hypoglycemia. Intern Med 1993;32:897–901.

128. Strauss G, Christensen L, Zapf J. Tumour-induced hypoglycaemia due to "big" IGF-II. J Intern Med 1994;236:97–9.

129. Hoekman K, van Doorn J, Gloudemans T, et al. Hypoglycaemia associated with the production of insulin-like growth factor II and insulin-like growth factor binding protein 6 by a haemangiopericytoma. Clin Endocrinol (Oxf) 1999;51:247–53.

130. Pavelic K, Spaventi S, Gluncic V, et al. The expression and role of insulin-like growth factor II in malignant hemangiopericytomas. J Mol Med 1999;77:865–9.

131. Yamaguchi M, Kamimura S, Takada J, et al. Case report: insulin-like growth factor II expression in hepatocellular carcinoma with alcoholic liver fibrosis accompanied by hypoglycaemia. J Gastroenterol Hepatol 1998;13:47–51.

132. Tietge UJ, Schofl C, Ocran KW, et al. Hepatoma with severe non-islet cell tumor hypoglycemia. Am J Gastroenterol 1998;93:997–1000.

133. Mizuta Y, Isomoto H, Futuki Y, et al. Acinar cell carcinoma of the pancreas associated with hypoglycemia: involvement of "big" insulin-like growth factor-II. J Gastroenterol 1998;33:761–5.

134. Eguchi T, Tokuyama A, Tanaka Y, et al. Hypoglycemia associated with the production of insulin-like growth factor II in adrenocortical carcinoma. Intern Med 2001;40:759–63.

135. Holt RI, Teale JD, Jones JS, et al. Gene expression and serum levels of insulin-like growth factors (IGFs) and IGF-binding proteins in a case of non-islet cell tumour hypoglycaemia. Growth Horm IGF Res 1998;8:447–54.

136. Bessell EM, Selby C, Ellis IO. Severe hypoglycaemia caused by raised insulin-like growth factor II in disseminated breast cancer. J Clin Pathol 1999;52:780–1.

137. Hizuka N, Fukuda I, Takano K, et al. Serum insulin-like growth factor II in 44 patients with non-islet cell tumor hypoglycemia. Endocr J 1998;45:S61–5.

138. Hirshberg B, Livi A, Bartlett DL, et al. Forty-eight-hour fast: the diagnostic test for insulinoma. J Clin Endocrinol Metab 2000;85:3222–6.

139. Kishi K, Sonomura T, Sato M. Radiotherapy for hypoglycaemia associated with large leiomyosarcomas. Br J Radiol 1997;70:306–8.

140. Gullo D, Sciacca L, Parrinello G, et al. Treatment of hemangiopericytoma-induced hypoglycemia with growth hormone and corticosteroids. J Clin Endocrinol Metab 1999;84:1758–9.

141. Teale JD, Marks V. Glucocorticoid therapy suppresses abnormal secretion of big IGF-II by non-islet cell tumours inducing hypoglycaemia (NICTH). Clin Endocrinol (Oxf) 1998;49:491–8.

142. Brun JF, Fedou C, Mercier J. Postprandial reactive hypoglycemia. Diabetes Metab 2000;26:337–51.

143. Poulson J. The management of diabetes in patients with advanced cancer. J Pain Symptom Manage 1997;13:339–46.

144. Cetin M, Yetgin S, Kara A, et al. Hyperglycemia, ketoacidosis and other complications of L-asparaginase in children with acute lymphoblastic leukemia. J Med 1994;25:219–29.

145. Whitecar JP Jr, Bodey GP, Hill CS Jr, Samaan NA. Effect of L-asparaginase on carbohydrate metabolism. Metabolism 1970;19:581–6.

146. Sahu S, Saika S, Pai SK, Advani SH. L-asparaginase (Leunase) induced pancreatitis in childhood acute lymphoblastic leukemia. Pediatr Hematol Oncol 1998;15:533–8.

147. Alvarez OA, Zimmerman G. Pegaspargase-induced pancreatitis. Med Pediatr Oncol 2000;34:200–5.

148. Weetman RM, Baehner RL. Latent onset of clinical pancreatitis in children receiving L-asparaginase therapy. Cancer 1974;34:780–5.

149. Przepiorka D, Khouri I, Ippoliti C, et al. Tacrolimus and minidose methotrexate for prevention of acute graft-versus-host disease after HLA-mismatched marrow or blood stem cell transplantation. Bone Marrow Transplant 1999;24:763–8.

150. Drachenberg CB, Klassen DK, Weir MR, et al. Islet cell damage associated with tacrolimus and cyclosporine: morphological features in pancreas allograft biopsies and clinical correlation. Transplantation 1999;68:396–402.

151. Sylvester RK, Lobell M, Ogden W, Stewart JA. Homoharringtonine-induced hyperglycemia. J Clin Oncol 1989;7:392–5.

152. Sievers EL, Lange BJ, Sondel PM, et al. Feasibility, toxicity, and biologic response of interleukin-2 after consolidation chemotherapy for acute myelogenous leukemia: a report from the Children's Cancer Group. J Clin Oncol 1998;16:914–9.

153. Gori A, Caredda F, Franzetti F, et al. Reversible diabetes in patient with AIDS-related Kaposi's sarcoma treated with interferon alpha-2a. Lancet 1995;345:1438–9.

154. Whitehead RP, Hauschild A, Christophers E, Figlin R. Diabetes mellitus in cancer patients treated with combination interleukin 2 and alpha-interferon. Cancer Biother 1995;10:45–51.

155. Guerci AP, Guerci B, Levy-Marchal C, et al. Onset of insulin-dependent diabetes mellitus after interferon-alfa therapy for hairy cell leukaemia. Lancet 1994;343:1167–8.

156. Shiba T, Higashi N, Nishimura Y. Hyperglycaemia due to insulin resistance caused by interferon-gamma. Diabet Med 1998;15:435–6.

157. Butler HE Jr, Morgan JM, Smythe CM. Mercaptopurine and acquired tubular dysfunction in adult nephrosis. Arch Intern Med 1965;116:853–6.

158. Cantwell BM, Pooley J, Harris AL. False-positive ketonuria during ifosfamide and mesna therapy. Eur J Cancer Clin Oncol 1986;22:229–30.

159. Perry RC, Shankar RR, Fineberg N, et al. HbA1c measurement improves the detection of type 2 diabetes in high-risk individuals with nondiagnositc levels of fasting plasma glucose: the Early Diabetes Intervention Program (EDIP). Diabetes Care 2001;24:465–71.

160. Ko GT, Chan JC, Tsang LW, Cockram CS. Combined use of fasting plasma glucose and HbA1c predicts the progression to diabetes in Chinese subjects. Diabetes Care 2000;23:1770–3.

161. Sculier JP, Nicaise C, Klastersky J. Lactic acidosis: a metabolic complication of extensive metastatic cancer. Eur J Cancer Clin Oncol 1983;19:597–601.

162. Sillos EM, Shenep JL, Burghen GA, et al. Lactic acidosis: a metabolic complication of hematologic malignancies. Cancer 2001;92:2237–46.

163. Doolittle GC, Wurster MW, Rosenfeld CS, Bodensteiner DC. Malignancy-induced lactic acidosis. South Med J 1988;81:533–6.

164. Abrams H, Spiro R, Goldstein N. Metastasis in carcinoma—one thousand autopsied cases. Cancer 1950;3:74.

165. Cedermark BJ, Sjoberg HE. The clinical significance of metastases to the adrenal glands. Surg Gynecol Obstet 1981;152:607–10.

166. Fellows IW, Bastow MD, Byrne AJ, Allison SP. Adrenocortical suppression in multiply injured patients: a complication of etomidate treatment. Br Med J (Clin Res Ed) 1983;287:1835–7.

167. Sokolove PE, Price DD, Okada P. The safety of etomidate for emergency rapid sequence intubation of pediatric patients. Pediatr Emerg Care 2000;16:18–21.

168. Khosla S, Wolfson JS, Demerjian Z, Godine JE. Adrenal crisis in the setting of high-dose ketoconazole therapy. Arch Intern Med 1989;149:802–4.

169. Sonino N, Boscaro M, Paoletta A, et al. Ketoconazole treatment in Cushing's syndrome: experience in 34 patients. Clin Endocrinol (Oxf) 1991;35:347–52.

170. Albert SG, DeLeon MJ, Silverberg AB. Possible association between high-dose fluconazole and adrenal insufficiency in critically ill patients. Crit Care Med 2001;29:668–70.

171. Sharkey PK, Rinaldi MG, Dunn JF, et al. High-dose itraconazole in the treatment of severe mycoses. Antimicrob Agents Chemother 1991;35:707–13.

172. Lonning PE, Kvinnsland S. Mechanisms of action of aminoglutethimide as endocrine therapy of breast cancer. Drugs 1988;35:685–710.

173. Subramanian S, Goker H, Kanji A, Sweeney H. Clinical adrenal insufficiency in patients receiving megestrol therapy. Arch Intern Med 1997;157:1008–11.

174. van Seters AP, Moolenaar AJ. Mitotane increases the blood levels of hormone-binding proteins. Acta Endocrinol (Copenh) 1991;124:526–33.

175. Robinson BG, Hales IB, Henniker AJ, et al. The effect of o,p'-DDD on adrenal steroid replacement therapy requirements. Clin Endocrinol (Oxf) 1987;27:437–44.

176. Carella MJ, Srivastava LS, Gossain VV, Rovner DR. Hypothalamic-pituitary-adrenal function one week after a short burst of steroid therapy. J Clin Endocrinol Metab 1993;76:1188–91.

177. Del Priore G, Gurski KJ, Warshal DP, et al. Adrenal function following high-dose steroids in ovarian cancer patients. Gynecol Oncol 1995;59:102–4.

178. Kuperman H, Damiani D, Chrousos GP, et al. Evaluation of the hypothalamic-pituitary-adrenal axis in children with leukemia before and after 6 weeks of high-dose glucocorticoid therapy. J Clin Endocrinol Metab 2001;86:2993–6.

179. Felner EI, Thompson MT, Ratliff AF, et al. Time course of recovery of adrenal function in children treated for leukemia. J Pediatr 2000;137:21–4.

180. Constine LS, Woolf PD, Cann D, et al. Hypothalamic-pituitary dysfunction after radiation for brain tumors. N Engl J Med 1993;328:87–94.

181. Oberfield SE, Garvin JH Jr. Thalamic and hypothalamic tumors of childhood: endocrine late effects. Pediatr Neurosurg 2000;32:264–71.

182. Pai HH, Thornton A, Katznelson L, et al. Hypothalamic/pituitary function following high-dose conformal radiotherapy to the base of skull: demonstration of a dose-effect relationship using dose-volume histogram analysis. Int J Radiat Oncol Biol Phys 2001;49:1079–92.

183. Littley MD, Shalet SM, Beardwell CG, et al. Hypopituitarism following external radiotherapy for pituitary tumours in adults. QJM 1989;70:145–60.

184. Shalet SM, Clayton PE, Price DA. Growth and pituitary function in children treated for brain tumours or acute lymphoblastic leukaemia. Horm Res 1988;30:53–61.

185. Samaan NA, Schultz PN, Yang KP, et al. Endocrine complications after radiotherapy for tumors of the head and neck. J Lab Clin Med 1987;109:364–72.

186. Lam KS, Tse VK, Wang C, et al. Effects of cranial irradiation on hypothalamic-pituitary function—a 5-year longitudinal study in patients with nasopharyngeal carcinoma. QJM 1991;78:165–76.

187. Laudat MH, Cerdas S, Fournier C, et al. Salivary cortisol measurement: a practical approach to assess pituitary-adrenal function. J Clin Endocrinol Metab 1988;66:343–8.

188. Redman BG, Pazdur R, Zingas AP, Loredo R. Prospective evaluation of adrenal insufficiency in patients with adrenal metastasis. Cancer 1987;60:103–7.

189. Abrams HL, Siegelman SS, Adams DF, et al. Computed tomography versus ultrasound of the adrenal gland: a prospective study. Radiology 1982;143:121–8.

190. Hussain S, Belldegrun A, Seltzer SE, et al. CT diagnosis of adrenal abnormalities in patients with primary non-adrenal malignancies. Eur J Radiol 1986;6:127–31.

191. Shankar RR, Jakacki RI, Haider A, et al. Testing the hypothalamic-pituitary-adrenal axis in survivors of childhood brain and skull-based tumors. J Clin Endocrinol Metab 1997;82:1995–8.

192. Rasmuson S, Olsson T, Hagg E. A low dose ACTH test to assess the function of the hypothalamic-pituitary-adrenal axis. Clin Endocrinol (Oxf) 1996;44:151–6.

193. Fiad TM, Kirby JM, Cunningham SK, McKenna TJ. The overnight single-dose metyrapone test is a simple and reliable index of the hypothalamic-pituitary-adrenal axis. Clin Endocrinol (Oxf) 1994;40:603–9.

194. Annane D. Corticosteroids for septic shock. Crit Care Med 2001;29:S117–20.

195. Oelkers W, Diederich S, Bahr V. Therapeutic strategies in adrenal insufficiency. Ann Endocrinol (Paris) 2001;62:212–6.

196. Arlt W, Callies F, van Vlijmen JC, et al. Dehydroepiandrosterone replacement in women with adrenal insufficiency. N Engl J Med 1999;341:1013–20.

197. Stratakis CA, Kirschner LS, Carney JA. Clinical and molecular features of the Carney complex: diagnostic criteria and recommendations for patient evaluation. J Clin Endocrinol Metab 2001;86:4041–6.

198. Stratakis CA. Clinical genetics of multiple endocrine neoplasias, Carney complex and related syndromes. J Endocrinol Invest 2001;24:370–83.

199. Aniszewski JP, Young WF Jr, Thompson GB, et al. Cushing syndrome due to ectopic adrenocorticotropic hormone secretion. World J Surg 2001;25:934–40.

200. Auchus RJ, Mastorakos G, Friedman TC, Chrousos GP. Corticotropin-releasing hormone production by a small-cell carcinoma in a patient with ACTH-dependent Cushing's syndrome. J Endocrinol Invest 1994;17:447–52.

201. Cavagnini F, Pecori Giraldi F. Epidemiology and follow-up of Cushing's disease. Ann Endocrinol (Paris) 2001;62:168–72.

202. Winquist EW, Laskey J, Crump M, et al. Ketoconazole in the management of paraneoplastic Cushing's syndrome secondary to ectopic adrenocorticotropin production. J Clin Oncol 1995;13:157–64.

203. Verhelst JA, Trainer PJ, Howlett TA, et al. Short and long-term responses to metyrapone in the medical management of 91 patients with Cushing's syndrome. Clin Endocrinol (Oxf) 1991;35:169–78.

204. Tami TA, Gomez P, Parker GS, et al. Thyroid dysfunction after radiation therapy in head and neck cancer patients. Am J Otolaryngol 1992;13:357–62.

205. Heidemann PH, Stubbe P, Beck W. Transient secondary hypothyroidism and thyroxine binding globulin deficiency in leukemic children during polychemotherapy: an effect of L-asparaginase. Eur J Pediatr 1981;136:291–5.

206. Ferster A, Glinoer D, Van Vliet G, Otten J. Thyroid function during L-asparaginase therapy in children with acute lymphoblastic leukemia: difference between induction and late intensification. Am J Pediatr Hematol Oncol 1992;14:192–6.

207. Sherman SI, Gopal J, Haugen BR, et al. Central hypothyroidism associated with retinoid X receptor-selective ligands. N Engl J Med 1999;340:1075–9.

208. Atkins MB, Mier JW, Parkinson DR, et al. Hypothyroidism after treatment with interleukin-2 and lymphokine-activated killer cells. N Engl J Med 1988;318:1557–63.

209. Krouse RS, Royal RE, Heywood G, et al. Thyroid dysfunction in 281 patients with metastatic melanoma or renal carcinoma treated with interleukin-2 alone. J Immunother Emphasis Tumor Immunol 1995;18:272–8.

210. Sauter NP, Atkins MB, Mier JW, Lechan RM. Transient thyrotoxicosis and persistent hypothyroidism due to acute autoimmune thyroiditis after interleukin-2 and interferon-alpha therapy for metastatic carcinoma: a case report. Am J Med 1992;92:441–4.

211. Vassilopoulou-Sellin R, Sella A, Dexeus FH, et al. Acute

thyroid dysfunction (thyroiditis) after therapy with interleukin-2. Horm Metab Res 1992;24:434–8.

212. Carella C, Mazziotti G, Morisco F, et al. Long-term outcome of interferon-alpha-induced thyroid autoimmunity and prognostic influence of thyroid autoantibody pattern at the end of treatment. J Clin Endocrinol Metab 2001;86:1925–9.

213. Jones TH, Wadler S, Hupart KH. Endocrine-mediated mechanisms of fatigue during treatment with interferon-alpha. Semin Oncol 1998;25:54–63.

214. Sklar CA, Kim TH, Ramsay NK. Thyroid dysfunction among long-term survivors of bone marrow transplantation. Am J Med 1982;73:688–94.

215. Toubert ME, Socie G, Gluckman E, et al. Short- and long-term follow-up of thyroid dysfunction after allogeneic bone marrow transplantation without the use of preparative total body irradiation. Br J Haematol 1997;98:453–7.

216. Sutcliffe SB, Chapman R, Wrigley PF. Cyclical combination chemotherapy and thyroid function in patients with advanced Hodgkin's disease. Med Pediatr Oncol 1981;9:439–48.

217. Ogilvy-Stuart AL, Shalet SM, Gattamaneni HR. Thyroid function after treatment of brain tumors in children. J Pediatr 1991;119:733–7.

218. Stuart NS, Woodroffe CM, Grundy R, Cullen MH. Long-term toxicity of chemotherapy for testicular cancer—the cost of cure. Br J Cancer 1990;61:479–84.

219. Markou K, Georgopoulos N, Kyriazopoulou V, Vagenakis AG. Iodine-induced hypothyroidism. Thyroid 2001;11:501–10.

220. Kaplan MM, Garnick MB, Gelber R, et al. Risk factors for thyroid abnormalities after neck irradiation for childhood cancer. Am J Med 1983;74:272–80.

221. Tamura K, Shimaoka K, Friedman M. Thyroid abnormalities associated with treatment of malignant lymphoma. Cancer 1981;47:2704–11.

222. Garnick MB, Larsen PR. Acute deficiency of thyroxine-binding globulin during L-asparaginase therapy. N Engl J Med 1979;301:252–3.

223. Bartalena L, Martino E, Antonelli A, et al. Effect of the antileukemic agent L-asparaginase on thyroxine-binding globulin and albumin synthesis in cultured human hepatoma (HEP G2) cells. Endocrinology 1986;119:1185–8.

224. Djurica SN, Plecas V, Milojevic Z, et al. Direct effects of cytostatic therapy on the functional state of the thyroid gland and TBG in serum of patients. Exp Clin Endocrinol 1990;96:57–63.

225. Beex L, Ross A, Smals A, Kloppenborg P. 5-Fluorouracil-induced increase of total serum thyroxine and triiodothyronine. Cancer Treat Rep 1977;61:1291–5.

226. McIver B, Gorman CA. Euthyroid sick syndrome: an overview. Thyroid 1997;7:125–32.

227. Chopra IJ. Clinical review 86: euthyroid sick syndrome: is it a misnomer? J Clin Endocrinol Metab 1997;82:329–34.

228. Schimpff SC, Diggs CH, Wiswell JG, et al. Radiation-related thyroid dysfunction: implications for the treatment of Hodgkin's disease. Ann Intern Med 1980;92:91–8.

229. Hancock SL, Cox RS, McDougall IR. Thyroid diseases after treatment of Hodgkin's disease. N Engl J Med 1991;325:599–605.

230. Peerboom PF, Hassink EA, Melkert R, et al. Thyroid function 10–18 years after mantle field irradiation for Hodgkin's disease. Eur J Cancer 1992;28A:1716–8.

231. Mitchell JM. Thyroid disease in the emergency department. Thyroid function tests and hypothyroidism and myxedema coma. Emerg Med Clin North Am 1989;7:885–902.

232. Ringel MD. Management of hypothyroidism and hyperthyroidism in the intensive care unit. Crit Care Clin 2001;17:59–74.

233. Yamamoto T, Fukuyama J, Fujiyoshi A. Factors associated with mortality of myxedema coma: report of eight cases and literature survey. Thyroid 1999;9:1167–74.

234. Bazzani M, Benati L, Bosi M, et al. Hypokalemic thyrotoxic paralysis: a rare cause of tetraparesis with acute onset in Europeans. Ital J Neurol Sci 1998;19:307–9.

235. Berwaerts J, Verhelst J, Vandenbroucke M, et al. Thyrotoxic periodic paralysis, an unusual cause of hypokalemic periodic paralysis. Acta Neurol Belg 1996;96:301–6.

236. Pandit L, Shankar SK, Gayathri N, Pandit A. Acute thyrotoxic neuropathy—Basedow's paraplegia revisited. J Neurol Sci 1998;155:211–4.

237. Ross DS. Syndromes of thyrotoxicosis with low radioactive iodine uptake. Endocrinol Metab Clin North Am 1998;27:169–85.

238. McDermott MT, Ridgway EC. Central hyperthyroidism. Endocrinol Metab Clin North Am 1998;27:187–203.

239. Roti E, Uberti ED. Iodine excess and hyperthyroidism. Thyroid 2001;11:493–500.

240. Csaki AC, Blum M. Thyrotoxicosis after interferon-alpha therapy. Thyroid 2000;10:101.

241. Petersen M, Keeling CA, McDougall IR. Hyperthyroidism with low radioiodine uptake after head and neck irradiation for Hodgkin's disease. J Nucl Med 1989;30:255–7.

242. Katayama S, Shimaoka K, Osman G. Radiation-associated thyrotoxicosis. J Surg Oncol 1986;33:84–7.

243. Hancock SL, McDougall IR, Constine LS. Thyroid abnormalities after therapeutic external radiation. Int J Radiat Oncol Biol Phys 1995;31:1165–70.

244. Wasnich RD, Grumet FC, Payne RO, Kriss JP. Graves' ophthalmopathy following external neck irradiation for nonthyroidal neoplastic disease. J Clin Endocrinol Metab 1973;37:703–13.

245. Nakhjavani MK, Gharib H, Goellner JR, van Heerden JA. Metastasis to the thyroid gland. A report of 43 cases. Cancer 1997;79:574–8.

246. Lam KY, Lo CY. Metastatic tumors of the thyroid gland: a study of 79 cases in Chinese patients. Arch Pathol Lab Med 1998;122:37–41.

247. Shimaoka K. Thyrotoxicosis due to metastatic involvement of the thyroid. Arch Intern Med 1980;140:284–5.

248. Shimaoka K, VanHerle AJ, Dindogru A. Thyrotoxicosis secondary to involvement of the thyroid with malignant lymphoma. J Clin Endocrinol Metab 1976;43:64–8.

249. Eriksson M, Ajmani SK, Mallette LE. Hyperthyroidism from thyroid metastasis of pancreatic adenocarcinoma. JAMA 1977;238:1276–8.

250. Yoshimura M, Hershman JM. Thyrotropic action of human chorionic gonadotropin. Thyroid 1995;5:425–34.

251. Hershman JM. Human chorionic gonadotropin and the thyroid: hyperemesis gravidarum and trophoblastic tumors. Thyroid 1999;9:653–7.

252. Matsuda K, Maehama T, Kanazawa K. Malignant struma ovarii with thyrotoxicosis. Gynecol Oncol 2001;82:575–7.

253. Alagol F, Tanakol R, Boztepe H, et al. Anaplastic thyroid cancer with transient thyrotoxicosis: case report and literature review. Thyroid 1999;9:1029–32.

254. Lawless ST, Reeves G, Bowen JR. The development of thyroid storm in a child with McCune-Albright syndrome after orthopedic surgery. Am J Dis Child 1992;146:1099–102.

255. Isotani H, Sanda K, Kameoka K, Takamatsu J. McCune-Albright syndrome associated with non-autoimmune type of hyperthyroidism with development of thyrotoxic crisis. Horm Res 2000;53:256–9.

256. Russo D, Wong MG, Costante G, et al. A Val 677 activating mutation of the thyrotropin receptor in a Hurthle cell thyroid carcinoma associated with thyrotoxicosis. Thyroid 1999;9:13–7.

257. Burch HB, Wartofsky L. Life-threatening thyrotoxicosis. Thyroid storm. Endocrinol Metab Clin North Am 1993;22:263–77.

258. McGugan EA. Hyperpyrexia in the emergency department. Emerg Med (Fremantle) 2001;13:116–20.

259. Yeung SC, Go R, Balasubramanyam A. Rectal administration of iodide and propylthiouracil in the treatment of thyroid storm. Thyroid 1995;5:403–5.

260. Walter RM Jr, Bartle WR. Rectal administration of propylthiouracil in the treatment of Graves' disease. Am J Med 1990;88:69–70.

261. Bartle WR, Walker SE, Silverberg JD. Rectal absorption of propylthiouracil. Int J Clin Pharmacol Ther Toxicol 1988;26:285–7.

262. Nabil N, Miner DJ, Amatruda JM. Methimazole: an alternative route of administration. J Clin Endocrinol Metab 1982;54:180–1.

263. Koguchi T, Yoshizawa S, Iguchi T, et al. [Case of thyroid crisis effectively treated with a urinary tract angiographic medium]. Nippon Naika Gakkai Zasshi 1992;81:262–3.

264. Hagag P, Nissenbaum H, Weiss M. Role of colestipol in the treatment of hyperthyroidism. J Endocrinol Invest 1998;21:725–31.

265. Tajiri J, Katsuya H, Kiyokawa T, et al. Successful treatment of thyrotoxic crisis with plasma exchange. Crit Care Med 1984;12:536–7.

266. Derksen RH, van de Wiel A, Poortman J, et al. Plasma-exchange in the treatment of severe thyrotoxicosis in pregnancy. Eur J Obstet Gynecol Reprod Biol 1984;18:139–48.

267. Candrina R, Di Stefano O, Spandrio S, Giustina G. Treatment of thyrotoxic storm by charcoal plasmaperfusion. J Endocrinol Invest 1989;12:133–4.

268. Burman KD, Yeager HC, Briggs WA, et al. Resin hemoperfusion: a method of removing circulating thyroid hormones. J Clin Endocrinol Metab 1976;42:70–8.

269. ter Maaten JC. Should we start and continue growth hormone (GH) replacement therapy in adults with GH deficiency? Ann Med 2000;32:452–61.

270. Littley MD, Shalet SM, Beardwell CG. Radiation and hypothalamic–pituitary function. Baillieres Clin Endocrinol Metab 1990;4:147–75.

271. Toogood AA, Beardwell CG, Shalet SM. The severity of growth hormone deficiency in adults with pituitary disease is related to the degree of hypopituitarism. Clin Endocrinol (Oxf) 1994;41:511–6.

272. Webb SM, Rigla M, Wagner A, et al. Recovery of hypopituitarism after neurosurgical treatment of pituitary adenomas. J Clin Endocrinol Metab 1999;84:3696–700.

273. Sklar CA. Craniopharyngioma: endocrine sequelae of treatment. Pediatr Neurosurg 1994;21:120–3.

274. Fernandez-Real JM, Villabona C, Acebes JJ, et al. Pituitary apoplexy into nonadenomatous tissue: case report and review. Am J Med Sci 1995;310:68–70.

275. Sioutos P, Yen V, Arbit E. Pituitary gland metastases. Ann Surg Oncol 1996;3:94–9.

276. Morita A, Meyer FB, Laws ER Jr. Symptomatic pituitary metastases. J Neurosurg 1998;89:69–73.

277. Sklar CA. Craniopharyngioma: endocrine abnormalities at presentation. Pediatr Neurosurg 1994;21:18–20.

278. Ghigo E, Aimaretti G, Corneli G, et al. Diagnosis of GH deficiency in adults. Growth Horm IGF Res 1998;8:55–8.

279. Lissett CA, Saleem S, Rahim A, et al. The impact of irradiation on growth hormone responsiveness to provocative agents is stimulus dependent: results in 161 individuals with radiation damage to the somatotropic axis. J Clin Endocrinol Metab 2001;86:663–8.

280. Orrego JJ, Barkan AL. Pituitary disorders. Drug treatment options. Drugs 2000;59:93–106.

281. Abs R, Bengtsson BA, Hernberg-Stahl E, et al. GH replacement in 1034 growth hormone deficient hypopituitary adults: demographic and clinical characteristics, dosing and safety. Clin Endocrinol (Oxf) 1999;50:703–13.

282. Rahn KH. How should we treat a hypertensive emergency? Am J Cardiol 1989;63:48C–50C.

283. Nakao K, Itoh H, Takaya K. Current topics in pheochromocytoma. Biomed Pharmacother 2000;54:124s–8s.

284. Eurin J, Barthelemy C, Masson F, et al. Release of neuropeptide Y and hemodynamic changes during surgical removal of human pheochromocytomas. Regul Pept 2000;86:95–102.

285. Koch CA, Vortmeyer AO, Huang SC, et al. Genetic aspects of pheochromocytoma. Endocr Regul 2001;35:43–52.

286. Bender BU, Gutsche M, Glasker S, et al. Differential genetic alterations in von Hippel-Lindau syndrome-associated and sporadic pheochromocytomas. J Clin Endocrinol Metab 2000;85:4568–74.

287. Wu LT, Dicpinigaitis P, Bruckner H, et al. Hypertensive crises induced by treatment of malignant pheochromocytoma with a combination of cyclophosphamide, vincristine, dacarbazine. Med Pediatr Oncol 1994;22:389–92.

288. Raber W, Raffesberg W, Bischof M, et al. Diagnostic efficacy of unconjugated plasma metanephrines for the detection of pheochromocytoma. Arch Intern Med 2000;160:2957–63.

289. Eisenhofer G, Lenders JW, Linehan WM, et al. Plasma normetanephrine and metanephrine for detecting

pheochromocytoma in von Hippel-Lindau disease and multiple endocrine neoplasia type 2. N Engl J Med 1999;340:1872–9.

290. Pacak K, Linehan WM, Eisenhofer G, et al. Recent advances in genetics, diagnosis, localization, and treatment of pheochromocytoma. Ann Intern Med 2001;134:315–29.

291. Guignat L, Bidart JM, Nocera M, et al. Chromogranin A and the alpha-subunit of glycoprotein hormones in medullary thyroid carcinoma and phaeochromocytoma. Br J Cancer 2001;84:808–12.

292. Geoghegan JG, Emberton M, Bloom SR, Lynn JA. Changing trends in the management of phaeochromocytoma. Br J Surg 1998;85:117–20.

293. Berglund AS, Hulthen UL, Manhem P, et al. Metaiodobenzylguanidine (MIBG) scintigraphy and computed tomography (CT) in clinical practice. Primary and secondary evaluation for localization of phaeochromocytomas. J Intern Med 2001;249:247–51.

294. Hanna NN, Kenady DE. Hypertension in patients with pheochromocytoma. Curr Hypertens Rep 1999;1:540–5.

295. Brunt LM, Moley JF, Doherty GM, et al. Outcomes analysis in patients undergoing laparoscopic adrenalectomy for hormonally active adrenal tumors. Surgery 2001;130:629–35.

296. Col V, de Canniere L, Collard E, et al. Laparoscopic adrenalectomy for phaeochromocytoma: endocrinological and surgical aspects of a new therapeutic approach. Clin Endocrinol (Oxf) 1999;50:121–5.

297. Janetschek G, Neumann HP. Laparoscopic surgery for pheochromocytoma. Urol Clin North Am 2001;28:97–105.

298. Steinsapir J, Carr AA, Prisant LM, Bransome ED Jr. Metyrosine and pheochromocytoma. Arch Intern Med 1997;157:901–6.

299. Amer KM, Ibrahim NB, Forrester-Wood CP, et al. Lung carcinoid related Cushing's syndrome: report of three cases and review of the literature. Postgrad Med J 2001;77:464–7.

300. Chabot V, de Keyzer Y, Gebhard S, et al. Ectopic ACTH Cushing's syndrome: V3 vasopressin receptor but not CRH receptor gene expression in a pulmonary carcinoid tumor. Horm Res 1998;50:226–31.

301. Oliaro A, Filosso PL, Casadio C, et al. Bronchial carcinoid associated with Cushing's syndrome. J Cardiovasc Surg (Torino) 1995;36:511–4.

302. Ahlman H, Nilsson O, Wangberg B, Dahlstrom A. Neuroendocrine insights from the laboratory to the clinic. Am J Surg 1996;172:61–7.

303. Schussheim DH, Skarulis MC, Agarwal SK, et al. Multiple endocrine neoplasia type 1: new clinical and basic findings. Trends Endocrinol Metab 2001;12:173–8.

304. Kinney MA, Warner ME, Nagorney DM, et al. Perianaesthetic risks and outcomes of abdominal surgery for metastatic carcinoid tumours. Br J Anaesth 2001;87:447–52.

305. Karmy-Jones R, Vallieres E. Carcinoid crisis after biopsy of a bronchial carcinoid. Ann Thorac Surg 1993;56:1403–5.

306. Bissonnette RT, Gibney RG, Berry BR, Buckley AR. Fatal carcinoid crisis after percutaneous fine-needle biopsy of hepatic metastasis: case report and literature review. Radiology 1990;174:751–2.

307. Bonomi P, Hovey C, Dainauskas JR, et al. Management of carcinoid syndrome. Med Pediatr Oncol 1979;6:77–83.

308. Mehta AC, Rafanan AL, Bulkley R, et al. Coronary spasm and cardiac arrest from carcinoid crisis during laser bronchoscopy. Chest 1999;115:598–600.

309. Chatal JF, Le Bodic MF, Kraeber-Bodere F, et al. Nuclear medicine applications for neuroendocrine tumors. World J Surg 2000;24:1285–9.

310. Kvols LK. The carcinoid syndrome: a treatable malignant disease. Oncology (Huntingt) 1988;2:33–41.

311. Kvols LK. Metastatic carcinoid tumors and the carcinoid syndrome. A selective review of chemotherapy and hormonal therapy. Am J Med 1986;81:49–55.

312. Gates J, Hartnell GG, Stuart KE, Clouse ME. Chemoembolization of hepatic neoplasms: safety, complications, and when to worry. Radiographics 1999;19:399–414.

313. Deguchi H, Deguchi K, Tsukada T, et al. Long-term survival in a patient with malignant carcinoid treated with high-dose octreotide. Intern Med 1994;33:100–2.

314. Tomassetti P, Migliori M, Gullo L. Slow-release lanreotide treatment in endocrine gastrointestinal tumors. Am J Gastroenterol 1998;93:1468–71.

315. Warner RR, Mani S, Profeta J, Grunstein E. Octreotide treatment of carcinoid hypertensive crisis. Mt Sinai J Med 1994;61:349–55.

316. Westberg G, Ahlman H, Nilsson O, et al. Secretory patterns of tryptophan metabolites in midgut carcinoid tumor cells. Neurochem Res 1997;22:977–83.

317. Constine LS, Donaldson SS, McDougall IR, et al. Thyroid dysfunction after radiotherapy in children with Hodgkin's disease. Cancer 1984;53:878–83.

318. Devney RB, Sklar CA, Nesbit ME Jr, et al. Serial thyroid function measurements in children with Hodgkin disease. J Pediatr 1984;105:223–7.

319. Grande C. Hypothyroidism following radiotherapy for head and neck cancer: multivariate analysis of risk factors. Radiother Oncol 1992;25:31–6.

320. Vrabec DP, Heffron TJ. Hypothyroidism following treatment for head and neck cancer. Ann Otol Rhinol Laryngol 1981;90:449–53.

321. Posner MR, Ervin TJ, Miller D, et al. Incidence of hypothyroidism following multimodality treatment for advanced squamous cell cancer of the head and neck. Laryngoscope 1984;94:451–4.

322. Cannon CR. Hypothyroidism in head and neck cancer patients: experimental and clinical observations. Laryngoscope 1994;104:1–21.

323. Shafer RB, Nuttall FQ, Pollak K, Kuisk H. Thyroid function after radiation and surgery for head and neck cancer. Arch Intern Med 1975;135:843–6.

324. Fuks Z, Glatstein E, Marsa GW, et al. Long-term effects on external radiation on the pituitary and thyroid glands. Cancer 1976;37:1152–61.

325. Joensuu H, Viikari J. Thyroid function after postoperative radiation therapy in patients with breast cancer. Acta Radiol Oncol 1986;25:167–70.

326. Boulad F, Bromley M, Black P, et al. Thyroid dysfunction following bone marrow transplantation using hyperfractionated radiation. Bone Marrow Transplant 1995;15:71–6.

EMERGENT AND SERIOUS INFECTIONS IN CANCER PATIENTS

ROLA HUSNI, MD
ISSAM I. RAAD, MD

NEUTROPENIC FEVER

Neutropenic fever is the most common presenting diagnosis in the emergency room at The University of Texas M. D. Anderson Cancer Center. Infection remains the leading cause of morbidity and mortality in neutropenic patients.[1,2] Of cancer patients, 5 to 10% succumb to infectious complications associated with neutropenia.[3–5] As neutropenic fever is a true medical emergency, the timely administration of antibiotics can never be overemphasized. This section discusses the general approach to neutropenic patients in the emergency room.

Pathophysiology and Etiology

The most common granulocyte defect is a reduction in the number of circulating neutrophils. Neutrophils are phagocytic cells that defend against bacterial and fungal infections.[6–15] Neutropenia is defined as a neutrophil count of ≤ 1,000 cells per microliter, absolute neutropenia is a neutrophil count of ≤ 500 cells per microliter, and profound neutropenia is defined as a neutrophil count of ≤ 100 cells per microliter.[6] It has become clear that neutropenic febrile patients are a heterogeneous group. The risk of infection varies with the duration of neutropenia.[16] Associated changes in lymphocytes and mechanical-barrier defense (eg, mucositis, skin disease, central line), colonization, environmental exposure, and the use of prophylaxis add to the heterogeneity of this group.[8,17] Inpatients on prophylaxis and the masking of the source of infection are two main concerns. The most recently introduced concept in the evaluation of fever in neutropenic patients is risk assessment during the initial phase of a febrile episode.[18–20] It is now possible to identify patients with neutropenic fever who are at low risk

and who can thus be treated as outpatients. The model of Talcott and colleagues explains this concept in detail (Table 8–1). The most important risk factor for developing fever after chemotherapy appears to be the degree and duration of neutropenia.[21] In the 1970s and 1980s, 50 to 80% of febrile episodes were associated with clinical or microbiologic documentation of infection.[22] The type of infection depends on the underlying disease, the type of chemotherapy, the history of exposure, iatrogenic manipulation, prior use of antibacterial agents, and the use of respiratory equipment. Up to the mid-1980s, aerobic Gram-negative bacteria were the most common agents, but Gram-positive cocci (especially *Staphylococcus aureus*, *Staphylococcus epidermidis*, and *Streptococcus* species) have recently emerged as important pathogens in neutropenic patients. The reasons for the recent predominance of Gram-positive bacterial infections are the increased use of chemotherapeutic agents that cause mucositis, the use of central venous catheters (CVCs), and the use of anti-Gram-negative prophylactic antibiotics. In addition, *Candida albicans* and (more recently) non–*Candida albicans* species have emerged because of the use of fluconazole in leukemia and bone marrow transplantation (BMT) patients. Finally, *Aspergillus*

TABLE 8–1. Risk Categories in Febrile Neutropenic Patients

Risk Category	Criteria
High	Hematologic maligancy, bone marrow transplantation, or comorbidity (eg, hypotension, organ dysfunction, uncontrolled bleeding, altered mentation)
Medium	Progressive malignancy but no comorbidity
Low	Responding malignancy and no comorbidity

remains a significant pathogen in patients with prolonged and profound neutropenia, as well as emerging fungi such as *Fusarium*, *Trichosporon*, and *Alteranansis*.

Clinical Manifestations

The most important clinical clue in neutropenic patients is the inability to have a complete inflammatory reaction to infections. Any symptom or sign that the patient has should be investigated fully. A thorough daily physical examination is important in febrile neutropenic patients. Mucous-membrane and skin lesions can be viral (eg, herpes simplex virus [HSV] and varicella zoster virus [VZV]), bacterial (eg, ecthyma gangrenosum), or fungal (eg, disseminated *Candida*, *Aspergillus*, and *Fusarium*). Sinus symptoms can be secondary to bacterial or fungal infections. Abdominal pain, distention, and bloody diarrhea with nausea and vomiting are classic findings in neutropenic enterocolitis. Right-upper-quadrant pain in a patient recovering from neutropenia may suggest hepatosplenic candidiasis. Perianal symptoms, even if minimal, can hint of perianal abscess.

Pulmonary symptoms and findings on chest x-ray (CXR) films are a clinical challenge in the neutropenic patient. The differential diagnosis of pulmonary disease in this setting includes infection (viral, bacterial, fungal, and parasitic), radiation-induced pathology, chemotherapy toxicity, pulmonary hemorrhage, and pulmonary infarct. Physical findings in the chest are present in 30% of neutropenic patients with a normal chest radiograph.[23] A clinical correlation of pulmonary and extrapulmonary findings (skin; central nervous system [CNS]; and ear, nose, and throat) can help in establishing the etiologic agents.[24,25] In neutropenic patients, bacteremia occurs secondary to the translocation of organisms from their gastrointestinal tract. Thus, the organism cultured is usually whatever the patient is colonized by.

Diagnosis

Blood cultures may be helpful in diagnosing neutropenic patients because the cultures, when positive, can provide a definite diagnosis of the type of infection.[26] However, in persistently febrile patients on broad-spectrum antimicrobials, less than 1% of blood cultures yield organisms.[21] Sputum cultures should be obtained when the patient is expectorating. However, many neutropenic patients will not produce sputum even when there is a documented pulmonary infection. A positive sputum culture may provide the diagnosis of the etiologic agent causing the pulmonary infection. For example, *Aspergillus*, which can be a colonizer in normal hosts, is a significant pathogen in the neutropenic patient. If the patient is already on broad-spectrum antibiotics, a bronchoalveolar-lavage culture might not add to the yield of a sputum culture. A transbronchial biopsy specimen is also of limited use in this setting.[21] Any site with a localized sign of infection should be aggressively pursued with aspiration and/or a biopsy specimen culture (since it may lead to the definite diagnosis), but the presence of a low platelet count in the neutropenic patient can be a limiting factor in obtaining biopsy specimens from some sites. Chest x-ray films are abnormal in 17 to 25% of patients with neutropenic fever, in spite of negative symptoms or signs;[23,27] that is why chest radiography should be included in the workup of all febrile neutropenic patients. The degree of overlap in the findings of all infections on chest radiography limits its use in differentiating the type of infection. Computed tomography (CT) can be helpful in identifying pulmonary infections in the neutropenic patient in special situations such as the persence of the halo sign (an area of attenuation around a pulmonary infiltrate) or an air crescent within an infiltrate or nodule, both highly suggestive of *Aspergillus* infection. Serologic tests have been helpful in identifying infections in neutropenic patients. Polymerase chain reaction (PCR) tests and antigen detection techniques for mycobacterial infections, *Aspergillus* infection, and some viral infections can help in the early identification of a suspected infection.

Management

In 1971, it was shown that empiric use of a two-drug combination leads to significant improvement in the survival of febrile neutropenic patients.[22] Monotherapy with β-lactam including carbopenems (eg, imipenem or meropenem) or fourth-generation cephalosporin (eg, cefepime) agents has also been established.[28] All of these regimens have a success rate of 60 to 80%.[21] The Infectious Diseases Society of America recommendations for therapy are shown in Figure 8–1. Gram-negative bacilli coverage is mandatory since these infections carry a high mortality. Dual therapy and monotherapy as shown in Figure 8–1 are acceptable. Vancomycin as empiric therapy is acceptable if there is a suspected or documented infection with a Gram-positive organism (eg, cellulitis, a catheter-related infection, or severe mucositis); if the patient does not respond to the initial therapy, then vancomycin can be added as the isolation of Gram-positive organisms in these patients has been documented.[29–31] Antifungal therapy is recommended for patients with persistent fever after 4 to 7 days of broad-spectrum antibiotics. Amphotericin B has shown an improved response in patients who are not receiving antifungal prophylaxis, in patients with persistent neutropenia for more than 15 days, and in patients with a documented fungal infection. More data are available now about the use of fluconazole as initial empiric therapy in patients who have not received prior antifungal prophylaxis. In some studies, adjunctive use of hematopoietic growth

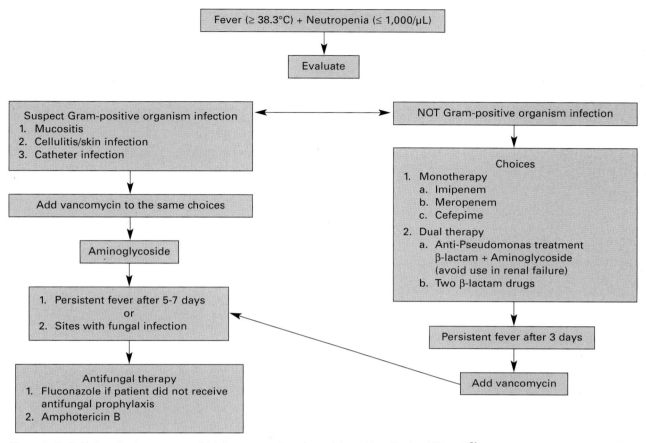

Figure 8–1. Guidelines for the treatment of febrile neutropenic patients. Adapted from Hughes WT, et al.[31]

factors was found to decrease hospital stay and to decrease the duration of neutropenia, but no reduction in the duration of fever or the rate of infectious mortality was documented.[32–34] Granulocyte transfusion is still being evaluated in the setting of fungal infections in the neutropenic patient.

Summary

Infection in neutropenic patients causes significant morbidity and mortality. Evaluation should include blood cultures and CRX. Empiric coverage for Gram-negative bacilli is recommended; coverage for Gram-positive organisms is indicated when infection with such pathogens is suspected. Antifungal therapy can be delayed until there have been 4 to 7 days of persistent fever. Outpatient therapy in low-risk neutropenic patients is considered acceptable management.

FEVER IN THE IMMUNOCOMPROMISED CANCER PATIENT

Over the past decade, there has been an increase in the number of immunocompromised patients. The most

important causes include the advances in chemotherapeutic agents, the increase in the number of patients infected with human immunodeficiency virus (HIV), and the increase in transplantations. Infections in the immunocompromised patient are numerous, but following the specific immune defect is helpful in evaluating and managing these patients.[35] The five main immune defect categories are summarized in Figure 8–2, which shows an algorithm for evaluating fever in the immunocompromised patient. (Neutropenia and its related infections in leukemic and BMT patients were discussed in the prior section.)

Pathophysiology and Etiology

The first category of immune deficiency is a defect in the mucosal and skin barriers. This predisposes to infection with bacteria or to fungus colonizing the affected area. In splenectomized patients (the second category), the main defect is in the clearing of the organisms by the use of receptors for the crystallizable fragment (Fc) portion of the immunoglobulin present on splenic macrophages. The spleen is also a major site for antibody synthesis. These patients are predisposed to infections with encapsulated organisms (*Streptococcus pneumoniae, Neisseria meningi-*

tidis, Haemophilus influenzae, Capnocytophaga canimorsus, and *Babesia microti),* especially if not immunized. Immunoglobulin and complement deficiency is the third category. Immunoglobulins G and M (IgG and IgM) play an important role in the opsonization and killing of encapsulated organisms. Deficiency of IgG seems to be the most serious deficiency. On the other hand, when antibodies are bound to the surface of the microbes, the complement system is activated, causing phagocytosis, a major process in the host immune defense system. Thus, immunoglobulin and complement deficiency predispose to bacterial infections, including infection with *Streptococcus pneumoniae, Haemophilus influenzae,* and *Staphylococcus aureus.* In the hereditary deficiency of IgG, *Mycoplasma hominis, Giardia, Campylobacter jejunii,* and enteroviral infections are common.[36–38] Multiple myeloma and chronic lymphocytic leukemia are examples of immunoglobulin deficiency in adults. Immunoglobulin levels fall with disease progression, rendering the patient more susceptible to bacterial infections.[39]

Finally, cell-mediated immunity is a complex process. Infections in patients with impaired cellular immunity (eg, transplantation and lymphoma patients) and in patients who are on certain chemotherapeutic agents such as fludarabine are caused by a wide variety of bacterial (*Salmonella, Streptococcus, Pseudomonas*), mycobacterial, viral (herpes viruses, respiratory viruses), and other opportunistic (*Pneumocystis carinii, Toxoplasma, Cryptococcus*) organisms. It should be noted that cancer patients and transplantation patients could have more than one defect in the immune system. A good example is BMT patients. They are predisposed to neutropenia-related and mucositis-related infections in the month after transplantation. They then develop a cellular immune defect secondary to graft-versus-host disease (GVHD) and the immunosuppressive therapy used to treat it. Bacteria, *Cytomegalovirus* (CMV), *Candida,* and *Aspergillus* are important pathogens in the first 100 days after transplantation. After that, varicella virus and *Streptococcus pneumoniae* infections become more important.[40]

Clinical Manifestations

Immunocompromised patients in general have minimal symptoms and signs of infection but can succumb quickly. Detailed and frequent examination is helpful in evaluating these patients. Bacteremia is common in patients with skin and mucosal-barrier defects. Meningi-

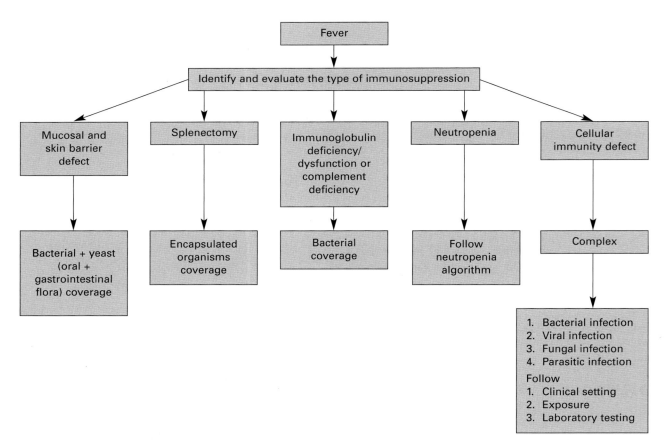

Figure 8–2. Algorithm for evaluating fever in cancer patients.

tis and pneumonia, in addition to bacteremia, are common in splenectomized as well as immunoglobulin- and complement-deficient patients.[35] In lymphoma and BMT patients whose main defect is cell-mediated immunodeficiency, all organ systems can be affected with the different types of infections to which they are predisposed. The most serious infection in the latter group is lung infection, in which diagnosis and management are difficult.

Diagnosis

To establish a quick diagnosis, advanced laboratory techniques should be considered in addition to the detailed history and examination when evaluating the immunocompromised patient. For example, CMV antigen testing or PCR (as well as PCR to detect other organisms such as *Mycobacterium tuberculosis*, herpesviruses, and hepatitis C virus) can be very useful in making an early diagnosis to help direct appropriate therapy.[35] A low threshold for performing advanced tests and radiologic examinations (CT, or magnetic resonance imaging) should be adopted when evaluating these patients.

Management

The management of fever and infection in immunocompromised patients should be guided by the specific immune defect, the type of infection, the site of infection, and the severity of infection. Empiric antimicrobial therapy directed against the specific pathogen to which the patient is predisposed should be initiated.[41–45] Patients with prolonged immunosuppression and multiple febrile episodes and infections or who have a persistent or relapsing fever may need frequent modification of their antimicrobial therapy, guided by detailed evaluation and follow-up. Prolonged antimicrobial therapy is also a consideration in those patients. Outpatient therapy should be limited to the small group of immunosuppressed patients who are considered to be at low risk and compliant and who can be easily followed up.[46–48]

Summary

The evaluation of fever in the immunocompromised patient should be guided by the specific immune defect. Diagnosis of the type of infection can be difficult.[49] Empiric antimicrobial therapy should be started, and careful follow-up is needed to help adjust therapy for these fragile patients.

INFECTIONS IN HIV-INFECTED PATIENTS WITH CANCER

Malignancies related to human immunodeficiency virus include Kaposi's sarcoma (KS), non-Hodgkin's lymphoma (NHL), squamous cell carcinoma, Hodgkin's disease (HD), plasmacytoma, and leiomyosarcoma in children. The acquired immunodeficiency syndrome (AIDS)–defining malignancies are KS, high-grade B-cell lymphoma, primary CNS NHL, and invasive cervical cancer. With the advent of highly active antiretroviral therapy, the incidence of some of these malignancies (eg, KS and NHL) has decreased.[50] Still, these patients are vulnerable to opportunistic infections and are the most difficult to manage.

Pathophysiology and Etiology

The risk factors for infection in HIV patients with malignancies, as detailed by Brown and Nadler, are neutropenia secondary to decreased production; increased destruction and sequestration; chemotherapy effect; impaired granulocyte function; disruption of the mechanical barriers secondary to infections such as Candida, HSV, and CMV or to cancer induced (eg, in KS),[51,52] and malnutrition (wasting disease).[53] Opportunistic infections and their relationship to progressive immune dysfunction are well documented in AIDS patients. At a CD4 count of > 200 cells per microliter, the main pathogens are *Pneumococcus*, HSV, VZV, *Mycobacterium tuberculosis*, *Salmonella*, and *Bartonella*. At a CD4 count of < 200 cells per microliter, *Candida* and *Pneumocystis carinii* are the main concern. At a CD4 count of < 100 cells per microliter, *Cryptococcus* and *Toxoplasma* play a major role. In a patient who is severely immunosuppressed at a CD4 count of < 50 cells per microliter, *Mycobacterium avium* complex (MAC) and CMV become the pathogens in play.[53,54] In AIDS patients with cancer, the difficulty is in trying to evaluate whether the infection is related to HIV, to cancer, or to both. For example, in AIDS patients with KS, oral *Cryptococcus* has been reported.[55] Bacillary angiomatosis and histoplasmosis have also been reported in KS lesions.[56,57] Pulmonary CMV infection is seen in AIDS patients with NHL and KS.[58]

Clinical Manifestations

Depending on the type of organism and the system affected, the clinical symptoms and signs in HIV-infected patients with cancer are extremely variable. For example, in patients with *Pneumocystis carinii* pneumonia (PCP) and AIDS without cancer, the presentation is rather indolent, with exacerbation by effort or exercise; but if the same patient has lymphoma and is undergoing chemotherapy, the presentation can be acute and fulminant. Infection or cancer or chemotherapy toxicity can be in the differential diagnosis of fever and organ abnormality (especially in the respiratory system). A poor outcome is associated with sepsis pneumonia and bacteremia.[59] Even minimal respiratory symptoms should be investigated in AIDS patients with cancer.

Diagnosis

Patients with HIV infection are difficult to evaluate. Detailed history and examination are helpful. The disease status of the HIV infection is important in establishing which opportunistic infections the patient is predisposed to. Thus, a recent CD4 count and viral load are necessary. Knowledge of the stage of the cancer and the chemotherapy received helps in evaluating the immune status. Knowledge of the prophylaxis the patient is receiving also helps in narrowing the differential diagnosis of the infection. A patient's being on trimethoprim/sulfamethoxazole makes PCP and *Toxoplasma* infection less likely. Early diagnosis is important, and advanced laboratory and radiologic tests may be helpful in establishing a diagnosis. Bronchoscopy and CT can help in diagnosing the type of pulmonary infection the HIV-infected patient with malignancy has. It is worth noting that more than one organ system and more than one type of infection can coexist in this subgroup of patients.

Management

It is compulsory to continue antiretroviral therapy and to maximize it if possible in HIV-infected patients with malignancy. Less myelotoxic antiretroviral therapy can be used safely with chemotherapy for treating the malignancy.[60,61] Empiric antimicrobial therapy for suspected infection should be the rule. The use of cytokines like erythropoietin and granulocyte colony-stimulating factor may help in reducing myelotoxicity in HIV-infected patients who are receiving chemotherapy.[62,63]

Summary

Malignancy in HIV-infected patients can worsen their immunosuppression. The clinical presentation of any infection is variable and can be difficult to diagnose. Thus, empirical antimicrobial therapy is recommended while continuing to administer effective and safe antiretroviral therapy.

INFECTIONS RELATED TO CENTRAL VENOUS CATHETERS

Central venous catheters (CVCs) are widely used for both hospital and home care of cancer patients. With prolonged CVC use, CVC-related infections eventually occur in nearly 25% of such patients.[64] Sepsis is the most serious life-threatening complication associated with CVC use.[65] The rate of infection for short-term CVC use is 3 to 7% whereas the rate for long-term CVC use (Hickman or Broviac catheters) is 1 to 2%.[66]

Infections related to CVC use can be divided into the following four categories:

1. Exit site infections, defined as < 2 cm of inflammation around the exit site
2. Tunnel infections, defined as > 2 cm of inflammation around the exit and tunnel site
3. Pocket space abscess or cellulitis with inflammation around the subcutaneously implanted catheter hub
4. Catheter-related bacteremia and sepsis.

Pathophysiology and Etiology

The two most common sources of catheter colonization and infection are the catheter insertion site and the hub.[64] Catheter colonization can occur 1 hour after insertion.[67] Contamination is the most likely cause of tunnel infection.[68,69] The usual organisms are the skin flora from the patient's insertion site or from the hands of medical personnel. In long-term CVC use, internal-surface colonization becomes a significant source of infection and sepsis.[66] The other route of CVC-related infection is hematogenous, commonly of gastrointestinal origin, as seen with *Candida* and Gram-negative bacilli infections.[66,70] The main organism cultured in catheter-related infection remains *Staphylococcus*. However, all types of bacteria, mycobacteria, and fungi can cause catheter infection in the immunocompromised cancer patient.

It is important to note that the location of the CVC plays a role in its infection. A femoral-line catheter has a higher rate of infection and related bacteremia than jugular and subclavian catheters have.[71] The question of whether the number of lumens (more than one) increases the risk of infection remains controversial.[72–74]

Clinical Manifestations

A CVC site–related infection causes local inflammation (redness, swelling, pain, and tenderness). If the area involved is < 2 cm, it is considered a simple site infection. If > 2 cm in a tunneled catheter is involved, then it is a tunnel infection. If there is pocket fluctulance, then abscess formation is suspected. Site infection may not cause much fever.[66] Catheter-related bacteremia or fungemia usually presents with fever and chills, which can only be present after use of an infusate. Complications of catheter-related infections include septic thrombophlebitis and (uncommonly) right-sided endocarditis. Finally, sepsis syndrome with fever and hypotension can result from a catheter infection, especially in the severely immunocompromised patient.

Diagnosis

For site or tunnel infection, physical examination is diagnostic. Site culture findings often correlate with the pathogen that is causing the infection.[75] Mostly, organisms are *Staphylococcus* species. A positive blood culture drawn from the catheter, showing clinical manifestations of sepsis having no apparent other source, is suggestive of a CVC-related infection. A fivefold or greater increase in colony-forming units (CFUs) in blood drawn through the CVC versus a peripheral blood culture, in the absence of a positive peripheral blood culture, is diagnostic of catheter-related bacteremia or fungemia, as is a catheter tip culture that is positive for > 15 CFUs.[74,76–78] The "gold standard" test for CVC-related infection is catheter culture. The most commonly used technique is the roll-plate method, in which the catheter tip is rolled directly on a plate. A CFU count of ≥ 15 is diagnostic of catheter colonization. Other techniques used are catheter flushing and sonication. Sonication might be superior since it captures organisms inside and outside the lumen. The disadvantage of all these techniques is that they are always retrospective. Quantitative blood culture offers a better method of assessing catheter-related blood stream infections.

Management

Exit site infections can generally be cured with appropriate antibiotics. Tunnel infection requires catheter removal.[79] Peripheral septic thrombophlebitis requires surgical removal and thrombectomy.[80] The role of anticoagulation in septic thrombophlebitis is not known. Appropriate antibiotics should be used for catheter-related bacteremia. Treatment of catheter-related infection can be attempted in the case of avirulent organisms such as coagulase-negative *Corynebacterium* species (not group JK). Catheter removal is recommended in cases of persistent bacteremia with any organism after 48 hours of appropriate antimicrobial therapy, relapse of bacteremia after an adequate course of antibiotics, infection with "sticky" virulent organisms (*Staphylococcus aureus*, *Corynebacterium* [group JK], *Bacillus*, *Lactobacillus*, *Mycobacterium*, vancomycin-resistant enterococci [VRE], *Pseudomonas aeruginosa*, polymicrobial-bacteremia organisms, *Candida*, and *Fusarium* and other fungi).[66,81] For *Staphylococcus aureus* or *Candida* blood stream infection after CVC removal, an average of 2 weeks of antimicrobial therapy is needed. If catheter-related bacteremia is associated with septic thrombosis or endocarditis, it is to be treated for 4 to 6 weeks. Using a guidewire to exchange a catheter, a quantitative tip culture should be obtained. If the tip culture shows > 15 CFUs, a new site is recommended.[72] Antibiotic lock therapy has not been adequately studied so far and is not recommended as part of therapy for infected catheters.[82] Antibiotic-impregnated and -coated catheters are now being used, to prevent catheter-related infections.[83–87]

Summary

Catheter-related infection is a common complication in cancer patients. Different types of infection exist. Catheter-related bacteremia can cause serious morbidity in the immunocompromised cancer patient. Although antibiotic therapy is easy to manage, removal of the catheter should be considered in certain situations, as discussed above.

INFECTIONS IN NONVASCULAR CATHETERS

Nonvascular catheters are commonly used to relieve obstruction or to install chemotherapy in cancer patients. Infections related to these catheters are the most common complications seen. This section focuses on infections in biliary and CNS catheters in cancer patients. Percutaneous drainage of the biliary system and ventriculostomies are usually used temporarily; they can become infected, but they are easier to treat. The infection rate associated with Ommaya reservoirs is reported to be between 5 and 50%,[88] whereas that associated with ventriculoperitoneal (VP) shunts is 5.9 to 9.3%.[89]

Pathophysiology and Etiology

The source of infection in CNS catheters is contamination at the time of surgery, from the skin of the patient or the hands of surgical personnel, from the environment, or from later manipulation and use of the catheter. The organisms involved are skin flora, most commonly *Staphylococcus* or nosocomial organisms such as *Pseudomonas aeruginosa*. *Staphylococcus* and *Corynebacterium* are more common with the Ommaya reservoir and ventriculostomy, whereas Gram-negative bacilli play a more important role in VP-shunt infection since the catheter is inserted in the peritoneum. In biliary catheters, gastrointestinal organisms are the most common. *Candida* infection is less common but can be seen with prolonged antibiotic use and in patients colonized with *Candida*.

Clinical Manifestations

Fever, chills, headache, nausea, vomiting, decreased mental status, and catheter obstruction are the most common findings with CNS catheter infections. Examination may find signs of meningitis and/or encephalitis. With VP-shunt infections, abdominal pain and signs of peritonitis can be present. Fever, chills, jaundice, abdominal pain, and sepsis are the most common symptoms of biliary-catheter infection. Septic shock can occur in these patients.

Diagnosis

Blood and fluid cultures should be obtained from these patients. Cerebrospinal fluid often shows pleocytosis and left shift, low to normal sugar levels, and high protein levels unless the patient is profoundly neutropenic. Any cultured organism is considered a pathogen. Bacterial antigen detection is not useful for CNS catheter infections. On the other hand, external biliary stents are usually colonized with one or more organisms; thus, a positive culture does not necessarily mean infection. A positive blood culture (in the right clinical setting) and signs of biliary-stent obstruction is a definite diagnosis of stent infection.

Management

Appropriate intravenous antimicrobial therapy should be started in patients with this type of infection. Vancomycin and ceftazidime are proper therapy for CNS catheter infection since they cover the pathogens involved and concentrate well in the cerebrospinal fluid (CSF). Antibiotics covering Gram-negative bacilli, enterococci, and anaerobes should be used in biliary-catheter infections. Many infections in Ommaya reservoirs can be treated with antimicrobial therapy without catheter removal.[90] The instillation of vancomycin into an Ommaya reservoir has been tried successfully in some studies.[90–92] Uncommonly, antibiotic therapy alone may fail, and then reservoir removal is needed. Infection in a VP shunt more frequently requires catheter removal to clear the infection, especially when Gram-negative bacilli are the pathogens cultured.[93] Temporary ventriculostomy is needed until the infection is clear, and another VP shunt can then be inserted.[93] Infections in internal and external biliary catheters should be treated with antibiotics and catheter exchange to relieve obstruction. A 2-week course of antimicrobial therapy can be used after the relief of obstruction.[94]

Summary

Infections in nonvascular catheters in cancer patients can be serious. Cancer patients with these catheter infections can present with meningitis or sepsis and can be very sick. They require immediate antimicrobial therapy and catheter removal, except in the case of infection in an Ommaya reservoir, for which intravenous and (sometimes) intrathecal antibiotics may be sufficient.

WOUND AND TUMOR INFECTION

Immunosuppression is the major factor predisposing cancer patients to surgical-wound infection.[95] However, solid tumors can get infected without surgical intervention. This usually occurs after chemotherapy or when the tumor increases in size, thus causing necrosis, where infection can occur. Both wound and tumor site infection are discussed in this section.

Pathophysiology and Etiology

Surgical-wound infection results from the interaction between the host factor (immunity, nutrition, and type of cancer), wound factor (magnitude of tissue devitalization, hematoma, and dead space), and microbial factor (virulence, adherence, and invasive ability). In cancer patients, the first factor is augmented secondary to decreased immunity from primary disease, from chemotherapy, or from both. The second factor becomes significant. When major surgery such as debulking is performed, with its increased risk of bleeding and hematoma formation, cancer patients are exposed to nosocomial pathogens and may be colonized with resistant organisms. The tumor site itself can become infected, especially when necrosis occurs and provides the proper medium for bacterial growth (especially anaerobes) and a hideout from host defense mechanisms.[96–98]

Organisms causing wound infections in cancer patients are skin flora or organisms that are colonizing the patients or contaminating the environment. Recently, more cases of wound infections from VRE have been reported in cancer patients who are colonized with those organisms.

Clinical Manifestations

Fever, wound pain, and erythema are the main clinical presentations of wound infection in the cancer patient. Drainage and inflammation, as in the normal host, can be present in the immunocompromised patient but can be minimal if the patient is severely immunosuppressed.[99,100] Complications of wound infection, such as abscess formation and sepsis, can be seen. Leukocytosis is usually present. With tumor site infection, fever is the most common clinical finding. No other cause of infection is present. CT scanning or ultrasonography shows a large tumor with necrosis. This presentation can occur after chemotherapy or in the setting of a fast growing tumor.

Diagnosis

Fever and wound inflammation (with or without drainage) and leukocytosis are the most common symptoms and signs seen with wound infection. However, in cancer patients, especially after chemotherapy or during neutropenia or steroid treatment, these signs can be minimal. Wound culture is important to guiding therapy. Gram's stains of wound drainage can help identify the category of pathogen responsible. Sepsis can occur secondary to wound infection, and blood cultures may be positive then. The preoperative prophylaxis used should be known since the organism causing wound infection is usually resistant to it. If the patient is colonized with certain organisms, they should be considered as possible pathogens in wound infection. Computed tomography or ultrasonography may show a fluid collection in the center of an infected tumor. The aspirate of this fluid can be cultured to confirm the infection.

Management

Antimicrobial therapy should be guided by findings from Gram's staining of the discharge if available. Empiric coverage should be started, especially if the patient is neutropenic or in unstable condition. The antimicrobials used should be effective against *Staphylococcus* in the case of most wound infections and against Gram-negative organisms in the case of abdominal wounds. Anaerobic coverage is needed in necrotic tumor infection or abscess formation. To guide therapy, preoperative prophylaxis should be known because the pathogen involved can be resistant to those antibiotics.[101,102] If the patient is colonized with VRE, empiric coverage for VRE should be considered in the wound or tumor infection with either quinupristin/dalfopristin or linezolid. The final culture result will help tailor the antibiotic therapy used. Managing wound infection in these patients can be difficult, and controlling other diseases (such as diabetes and chronic obstructive lung disease) is important.[103]

Summary

The management of wound infection in cancer patients should be similar to the management of wound infection in a normal host, keeping in mind that cancer patients can be colonized with resistant organisms. Tumor infection can be treated when suspected. Antibiotic therapy should include anaerobe coverage.

VIRAL INFECTIONS

Viral infections can cause serious disease in cancer patients, especially leukemia, lymphoma, and BMT patients. Herpesviruses (mainly CMV and VZV) and respiratory viruses such as influenza virus, respiratory syncytial virus (RSV), and parainfluenza virus (PIV) are the most important viruses causing disease in this group of patients. In both types of infection, the immunosuppression significantly increases the risk for severe disease.[104,105] This section focuses on all aspects of infections caused by the viruses mentioned above.

Pathophysiology and Etiology

In CMV and VZV infection, re-activation of latent virus often occurs; however, primary infection may also occur. The initial site of entry could be the respiratory system, the skin, or the conjunctiva. With herpesviruses, the most common cause of re-activation is allogeneic activation and iatrogenic immunosuppression. On the other hand, CMV is an immunomodulatory virus that can suppress T-cell function as well as increase the risk of rejection and GVHD in transplantation patients.[105] Respiratory

viruses differ from herpesviruses in their seasonality. They can be community or hospital acquired through the respiratory system.[104]

Clinical Manifestations

Infection with VZV can present as primary infection, localized zoster, or disseminated zoster.[106–112] Because of the more intensive chemotherapy now used, the frequency of zoster has increased. The infection occurs more frequently in areas of regionalized tumors or localized radiation. Patients receiving combined chemotherapy and radiation are at a higher risk of zoster than patients who are receiving radiation alone. The infection usually occurs within the first 12 months after radiation.[92] Visceral dissemination is associated with a higher mortality rate. Second cases of chickenpox in immunosuppressed patients are not uncommon.[106,110,112,113]

Cytomegalovirus can cause a variety of conditions in cancer and transplantation patients. Excretion of CMV in urine is well described in the transplantation patients. Infection with CMV is defined by fever, malaise, myalgias, arthralgias, night sweats, and viremia. On the other hand, CMV disease is more serious and is defined as end-organ damage related to CMV. *Cytomegalovirus* pneumonitis is the most common CMV disease in transplantation patients.[114] Colitis and bone marrow suppression are also common. Unlike in AIDS patients, CMV retinitis is rare in transplantation patients. The patients who are at highest risk for CMV disease are bone marrow transplant recipients who are CMV IgG positive and those who are IgG negative while their donor is CMV IgG positive. In spite of therapy, CMV pneumonia carries a high mortality. In infections with the respiratory viruses, the initial presentation of fever and upper-respiratory symptoms may be similar, but severe pneumonia varies with the type of virus and the degree of immunosuppression. In bone marrow transplant recipients, influenzal pneumonia occurs in 50% of patients with influenza virus infection, RSV pneumonia occurs in 60%, and PIV pneumonia occurs in 78%.[115–118] However, it is clear that these infections carry a high mortality with lower-respiratory-tract infection (13 to 41%).[104]

Diagnosis

Cytomegalovirus viremia can be detected by culture in 2 to 3 weeks, CMV antigen detection takes 1 to 3 days, and the PCR technique takes 24 hours. Serologic testing is not helpful in transplantation patients because of their inability to mount a proper humoral immunologic response, and the infection is most commonly secondary to the re-activation of the virus. Immunohistochemistry analysis done on tissue biopsy specimens gives a definite diagnosis, but biopsy may carry a risk of bleeding in patients with low platelet counts.

Infection with VZV is clinically diagnosed, but a Tzanck test and culture of a vesicle scraping can be done. Serologic testing for VZV and PCR tests can be performed on CSF when VZV CNS infection is suspected. In the case of respiratory viruses, diagnosis can be established for RSV and for influenza virus by rapid antigen detection tests done on nasal washings and a throat swab, respectively. Culture of respiratory viruses is rather slow but is the most sensitive test.

Management

For VZV infection, the drug of choice is acyclovir at a dose of 10 mg/kg every 8 hours. Varicella immunoglobulin is recommended in cases of dissemination or for chicken pox with pneumonia; foscarnet is an alternative therapy. *Cytomegalovirus* infection and disease can be treated with ganciclovir at a dose of 5 mg/kg every 12 hours; foscarnet is an alternative therapy. Pre-emptive therapy for CMV infection by using ganciclovir along with antigen detection or PCR testing to detect the period of maximal immunosuppression reduces the frequency and severity of CMV disease.[119,120] For infection with respiratory viruses, treatment is limited. Aerosolized ribavirin with intravenous immunoglobulins is recommended in cases of pneumonia secondary to infection with RSV and PIV.[121,122] For infection with influenza A virus, amantadine or rimantadine is available although resistance to these drugs has been recognized.[123] A new medication is available for infection with influenza A and B viruses and is effective in normal hosts,[124] but its use in the immunocompromised patient is not yet established. It is clear that delayed therapy in sick cancer patients infected with respiratory viral infection is not effective.

Summary

The most common types of viruses causing serious infections in cancer patients are herpesviruses and respiratory viruses. The diagnosis might be difficult in some cases, but rapid tests are available now. In spite of therapy, these infections carry a high mortality in the immunocompromised patient.

MYCOBACTERIAL INFECTIONS

Mycobacterial disease results from the interaction between virulent mycobacteria and the host immune defense response. Mycobacterial disease can be divided into tuberculous (ie, tuberculosis and leprosy) and nontuberculous forms. Although most mycobacteria cause disease in the normal host, some mycobacteria (such as MAC) cause serious infection in the immunocompromised patient. Mycobacterial disease occurs in cancer patients at a rate of 65 in 100,000 patients. At M. D. Anderson Cancer Center, about one-half of 59 patients with mycobacterial infection

had tuberculosis, and 64% of the nontuberculous infections were with *Mycobacterium kansasii* and *Mycobacterium fortuitum*.[125] In one study, 6% of patients with a hematologic malignancy had active tuberculosis while only 2% of patients who were admitted to hospital during the same time had tuberculosis.[126]

Pathophysiology and Etiology

Mycobacterial tuberculosis is spread from person to person via the respiratory route whereas *Mycobacterium leprae* is spread via contact. The other mycobacteria spread from animals and the environment to humans by the respiratory route, by ingestion of contaminated water or food, or by direct inoculation into the skin. The factors that predispose cancer patients to mycobacterial infection include poor nutritional status, a disruption of the normal mucosal barrier, and impaired cellular immunity due to underlying disease or due to chemotherapy.[127] Patients with lung cancer or hematologic malignancy or who chronically use high-dose steroids or muromonab-CD3 (OKT3) are at higher risk for active tuberculosis.[126,128–130]

Clinical Manifestations

Tuberculosis most commonly affects the lung. It usually has an indolent presentation but can present a fulminating and disseminated picture in the immunocompromised patient. Extrapulmonary tuberculosis can present with fever only. *Mycobacterium leprae* causes a skin disease that results in the destruction of peripheral nerves. Most nontuberculous mycobacteria present with pulmonary disease; a few (such as *Mycobacterium marinum, Mycobacterium ulcerans*, and *Mycobacterium hemophilum*) can cause skin disease (nodule, ulcer) after percutaneous inoculation.[131–133] Patients with mycobacterial infection can present with fever, night sweats, and weight loss. Disseminated disease can occur in severely immunocompromised patients; such patients are harder to treat, and disseminated disease is usually associated with a fatal outcome.

Diagnosis

Skin testing in patients with cellular immune deficiency is not helpful. A purified protein derivative (PPD) test in the immunosuppressed patient is considered positive if the test result is ≥ 5 mm. Culture remains the gold standard for diagnosing this disease. Special smears are done on fluid or tissue from the affected sites to help arrive at an early diagnosis, but a more sensitive and specific method for tuberculosis is PCR. The most important factor in establishing a diagnosis of mycobacterial disease remains a high index of suspicion in the right clinical setting.

Management

The main principle of treating the immunosuppressed patient who has a mycobacterial infection is choosing a regimen that has good efficacy without major toxicity. Multiple drugs are used in the early phase, and a longer course is recommended (8 to 20 months).[127] For tuberculosis, the first-line drugs are isoniazid, rifampin, ethambutol, pyrazinamide, and streptomycin. A four-drug regimen is used in the first 2 months. If resistance is suspected or documented, the second-line drugs should be used. Susceptibility testing should be done to help guide therapy. Sterilization of cultures should be documented. For nontuberculous mycobacterial infections, combination therapy should be used (consisting of doxycycline, macrolides [particularly clarithromycin], imipenem, amikacin, the quinolones, trimethoprim/sulfamethoxazole, ethionamide, rifabutin, etc).

Summary

Mycobacterial infection is seen more frequently in patients with cellular immunodeficiency. Mycobacterial infection is harder to diagnose without obtaining tissue cultures and special smears. Therapy is more difficult in such patients since an efficient but minimally toxic regimen is needed. A longer duration of treatment is recommended.

FUNGAL INFECTIONS

Invasive fungal infection is a serious infection in cancer patients and has high morbidity and mortality. *Candida* and *Aspergillus* infections are the most common types of fungal infection in the neutropenic patient whereas *Cryptococcus* and *Histoplasma* infections are more common in the patient with cellular immune deficiency. Emerging fungi such as *Fusarium*, *Trichosporon*, and *Pseudoallescheria* are becoming more frequent as organisms of fungal infection.

Pathophysiology and Etiology

The main defense mechanisms against fungal infection are mechanical barriers, phagocytes (neutrophils, monocytes, and macrophages), and T cell–mediated immunity. Chemotherapy used in cancer patients can affect the integrity of mucosal barriers, predisposing to *Candida* infection. Also, central venous access disrupts the skin barrier, resulting in a portal of entry for yeastlike fungi. Corticosteroid therapy used in cancer or BMT patients affects neutrophil, monocyte, macrophage, and T-lymphocyte function, thus predisposing to all types of fungal infection. Cyclosporine and tacrolimus used in transplantation patients affect mostly T-cell function, thus increasing the risk for fungal infection.[134] *Candida* and *Aspergillus* remain the most common fungi causing infection in the immunocompromised patient. Environmental factors play a role in exposing patients to fungi such as *Fusarium*, *Trichosporon*, *Zygomycetes*, and *Pseudoallescheria*.

Clinical Manifestations

Candida infection has a spectrum of presentation in cancer patients.[135] It can be divided into mucosal infection and deep tissue infection. Mucosal infection includes oropharyngeal, esophageal, vaginal, and bladder infections. Deep tissue infection includes fungemia,[136,137] disseminated candidiasis, and single-organ candidiasis. Disseminated candidiasis can be acute in presentation, or it can be chronic, with an indolent course.[138,139] A typical presentation is fever in a neutropenic patient, recurring after an initial antibiotic response, or skin nodules with fever, abdominal pain, nausea and vomiting, and elevated alkaline phosphatase in a patient recovering from neutropenia.

Invasive aspergillosis (IA) usually occurs in neutropenic patients who are on steroids. It affects many organ systems but mainly affects the respiratory tract,[140] sinuses, and CNS. Other mold infections affect the respiratory system and sinuses mostly.

Diagnosis

Candida mucosal infections are diagnosed by history and physical examination, together with endoscopic findings in esophageal candidiasis. Culture and susceptibility testing should be considered in cancer patients because of the increase in the rate of resistant and non-albicans *Candida*.[141–143] Clinical presentation and CT of the abdomen can help establish the diagnosis of hepatosplenic candidiasis. The diagnosis of IA is difficult, and biopsy with special stains remains the gold standard for diagnosis. However, antigen detection and PCR in serum and alveolar-lavage specimens are being evaluated and used in some laboratories.[144–149]

Management

Mucosal candidiasis can be treated with a topical antifungal (such as nystatin and clotrimazole) or with oral fluconazole. Deep tissue candidiasis, if not disseminated, can be treated with fluconazole if it is from *Candida albicans* or a fluconazole-sensitive non-*C. albicans*. For *Candida kruseii* or *Candida glabrata* infection, amphotericin B remains the drug of choice. Such infection should be treated with high-dose liposomal amphotericin B (7.5 to 5.0 mg/kg/d)[150,151] with or without caspofungin (Cancidas). Empiric therapy should be started if *Aspergillus* is suspected since delayed therapy carries a high mortality. Even with therapy, IA has a mortality rate of 80 to 90% unless neutropenia resolves. The main problem with amphotericin B is its renal and infusion-related toxicity, which can be diminished by the use of the new lipid formulation.[152–154] The combination of rifampin with flucytosine is controversial. Itraconazole is another drug that has a role in treating IA, especially with the advent of the intravenous formulation, which has overcome the oral formulation's bioavailability problem. Several new antifungals are being studied, such as voriconazole, posaconazole, caspofungin (an echinocandin).[155,156] The future of the management of fungal infection might be a combination antifungal regimen. Other aspects of managing fungal infection in the cancer patient include decreasing immunosuppressive therapy, the use of granulocyte colony-stimulating factors to reverse neutropenia, and granulocyte transfusion, which is still being evaluated.[157,158]

Summary

Invasive fungal infection in cancer patients can be fatal. *Candida* infection is easier to treat than a mold infection. Antifungal therapy is an evolving field with promising aspects, but the fact remains that for now, reversal of suppression (especially neutropenia) remains the best solution.

REFERENCES

1. Pizzo PA. Granulocytopenia and cancer therapy: past problems, current solutions, future challenges. Cancer 1984;54:2649–61.
2. Schimpff S. Overview of empiric antibiotic therapy for the febrile, neutropenic patient. Rev Infect Dis 1985;7:734–40.
3. De Pauw B, Deresinski SC, Feld R, et al. Ceftazidime compared with piperacillin and tobramycin for the empiric treatment of fever in neutropenic patients with cancer. Am J Med 1994;120:834–44.
4. Freifeld A, Walsh T, Marshall D, et al. Monotherapy for fever and neutropenia in cancer patients. A randomized comparison of ceftazidime versus imipenem. J Clin Oncol 1995;13:165–76.
5. Pizzo PA, Hathorn JW, Hiemenz J, et al. A randomized trial comparing ceftazidime alone with combination antibiotic therapy in cancer patients with fever and neutropenia. N Engl J Med 1986;315:552–8.
6. Bodey GP, Buckley M, Sathe YS, et al. Quantitative relationships between circulating leukocytes and infections in patients with acute leukemia. Ann Intern Med 1966; 64:328–40.
7. Boogaerts M, Cavalli F, Cortes-Funes H, et al. Granulocyte growth factors: achieving a consensus. Ann Oncol 1995;6:237–44.
8. Bow EJ, Raynor E, Louie T. Comparison of norfloxacin with clotrimazole for infection prophylaxis in acute leukemia. Am J Med 1988;84:847–54.
9. Christensen R, Rothstein G. Exhaustion of mature marrow neutrophils in neonates with sepsis. J Pediatr 1980; 96:316–8.
10. Berenguer J, Allende M, Lee J, et al. Pathogenesis of pulmonary aspergillosis: granulocytopenia versus cyclosporine and methylprednisolonone-induced immunosuppression. Am J Respir Crit Care Med 1995;152: 1079–86.
11. Chen S-M, Dumler J, Bakken J, et al. Identification of a granulocytotropic *Ehrlichia* species as the etiologic agent of human disease. J Clin Microbiol 1994;32:589–95.
12. Buchanan GR. Approach of the treatment of the febrile cancer patient with low-risk neutropenia. Hematol Oncol Clin North Am 1993;7:919–35.
13. Chanock S. Evolving risk factors for infectious complications of cancer therapy. Hematol Oncol Clin North Am 1993;7:771–93.
14. Chow JW, Fine MJ, Shlaes DM, et al. *Enterobacter* bacteremia: clinical features and emergence of antibiotic resistance during therapy. Ann Intern Med 1991;115: 585–90.
15. Centers for Disease Control and Prevention. Recommendations for prevention of the spread of vancomycin resistance. Morb Mortal Weekly Rep 1993;44 (RR-12):1.
16. Rubin M, Hathorn JW, Pizzo PA, et al. Controversies in the management of febrile neutropenic cancer patients. Cancer Invest 1988;6:167–84.
17. Archimbaud E, Guyotat D, Maupas J, et al. Perfloxacin and vancomycin vs gentamicin, colistin sulphate, and vancomycin for prevention of infections in granulocytopenic patients: a randomized double-blind study. Eur J Cancer 1991;27:174–8.
18. Talcott JA, Finberg R, Mayer RJ, et al. The medical course of patients with fever and neutropenia. Arch Intern Med 1988;148:2561–8.
19. Talcott JA, Siegel RD, Finberg R, et al. Risk assessment in patients with cancer and neutropenia: a prospective two-center validation of a prediction rule. J Clin Oncol 1992;10:316–22.
20. Talcott JA, Whalen A, Clark J, et al. Home antibiotic therapy for low-risk cancer patients with fever and neutropenia: a pilot study of 30 patients based on a validated prediction rule. J Clin Oncol 1994;12:107–14.
21. Donowitz GR. Fever in the compromised host. Infect Dis Clin North Am 1996;10:129–48.
22. Schimpff SL, Satterlee W, Young VM, Serpick A. Empirical therapy with carbenicillin and gentamicin for febrile patients with cancer and granulocytopenia. N Engl J Med 1971;284:1061–5.
23. Donowitz GR, Harman C, Pope T, et al. The role of the chest roentgenogram in febrile neutropenic patients. Arch Intern Med 1991;151:701–4.
24. Fishman J. Diagnostic approach to pneumonia in the immunocompromised host. Semin Respir Infect 1986; 1:133–44.
25. Wilson W, Cockerill FR, Rosenow EC. Pulmonary disease in the immunocompromised host. Mayo Clin Proc 1985;60:473–87, 610–31.
26. Washington JA III. Blood cultures—principles and techniques. Mayo Clin Proc 1975;59:91–8.
27. Jochelson MS, Altschaton J, Stomper PC. The yield of chest radiology in febrile and neutropenic patients. Ann Intern Med 1986;105:708–9.

28. Biron P, Furhmann C, Cure H, et al. Cefepime versus imipenem-cilastatin as empirical monotherapy in 400 febrile patients with short duration neutropenia. CEMIC (Study Group of Infectious Diseases in Cancer). J Antimicrob Chemother 1998;42:511–8.

29. Hughes WT, Armstrong D, Bodey GP, et al. 2002 IDSA guidelines for the use of antimicrobial agents in neutropenic patients with cancer. Clin Infect Dis 2002; 34:730–751.

30. EORTC International Antimicrobial Therapy Cooperative Group and the National Cancer Institute of Canada—Clinical Trials Group: Vancomycin added to empirical combination antibiotic therapy for fever in granulocytopenic cancer patients. J Infect Dis 1991;163:951–8.

31. Hughes WT, Armstrong D, Bodey GP, et al. Guidelines for the use of antimicrobial agents in neutropenic patients with unexplained fever. J Infect Dis 1990;161:381–96.

32. Wingard JR, Elfenbein GJ. Host immunologic augmentation for the control of infection. Infect Dis Clin North Am 1996;10:245–64.

33. Papadimitris C, Dimopoulos MA, Kostis E, et al. Outpatient treatment of neutropenic fever with oral antibiotics and granulocyte colony-stimulating factor. Oncology 1999;57:127–30.

34. Nemunaitis J, Buckner CD, Dorsey KS, et al. Retrospective analysis of infectious disease in patients who received recombinant human granulocyte-macrophage colony-stimulating factor versus patients not receiving a cytokine who underwent autologous bone marrow transplantation for treatment of lymphoid cancer. Am J Clin Oncol 1998;21:341–6.

35. Pizzo PA. Fever in immunocompromised patients. N Engl J Med 1999;341:893–9.

36. McKinney RE Jr, Karz SL, Wilfert CM. Chronic enteroviral meningoencephalitis in agammaglobulinemia patients. Rev Infect Dis 1987;9:334–56.

37. Roifman CM, Rao CP, Lederman HM, et al. Increased susceptibility to *Mycoplasma* infection in patients with hypogammaglobulinemia. Am J Med 1986;80:590–4.

38. LoGalbo PR, Sampson HA, Buckley RH. Symptomatic giardiasis in three patients with X-linked agammaglobulinemia. J Pediatr 1982;101:78–80.

39. Robertson TI. Complications and causes of death in B cell chronic lymphocytic leukaemia: a long term study of 105 patients. Aust N Z J Med 1990;20:44–50.

40. Walter EA, Bowden RA. Infection in the bone marrow transplant recipient. Infect Dis Clin North Am 1995; 9:823–47.

41. Hughes WT, Armstrong D, Bodey GP, et al. 1997 guidelines for the use of antimicrobial agents in neutropenic patients with unexplained fever. Clin Infect Dis 1997; 25:551–73.

42. Pizzo PA, Hathorn JW, Hiemenz J, et al. A randomized trial comparing ceftazidime alone with combination antibiotic therapy in cancer patients with fever and neutropenia. N Engl J Med 1986;315:552–8.

43. Sanders JW, Powe NR, Moore RD. Ceftazidime monotherapy for empiric treatment of febrile neutropenic patients: a meta-analysis. J Infect Dis 1991;164:907–16.

44. De Pauw BE, Deresinski SC, Feld R, et al. Ceftazidime compared with piperacillin and tobramycin for the empiric treatment of fever in neutropenic patients with cancer. Ann Intern Med 1994;120:834–44.

45. Freifeld AG, Walsh T, Marshall D, et al. Monotherapy for fever and neutropenia in cancer patients: a randomized comparison of ceftazidime versus imipenem. J Clin Oncol 1995;13:165–76.

46. Rubenstein EB, Rolston K, Benjamin RS, et al. Outpatient treatment of febrile episodes in low-risk neutropenic patients with cancer. Cancer 1993;71:3640–6.

47. Malik IA, Khan WA, Karim M, et al. Feasibility of outpatient management of fever in cancer patients with low-risk neutropenia: results of a prospective randomized trial. Am J Med 1995;98:224–31.

48. Freifeld A, Marchigiani D, Walsh T, et al. A double blind comparison of empirical oral and intravenous antibiotic therapy for low-risk febrile patients with neutropenia during cancer chemotherapy. N Engl J Med 1999;341:305–11.

49. Ouari TL, Brown AE. Infectious complications in the critically ill patient with cancer. Semin Oncol 2000;27:335–46.

50. O'Connor PG, Scandden DS. AIDS oncology. Infect Dis Clin North Am 2000;14:945–65.

51. Aboulafia D, Mathisen G, Mitsuyasu R. Case-report aggressive Kaposi sarcoma and *Campylobacter* bacteremia in a female with transfusion associated AIDS. Am J Med Sci 1991;301:256–8.

52. Kemper CA, Mickelson P, Morton A, et al. *Campylobacter fennelliae*-like organism as an important but occult cause of bacteremia in a patient with AIDS. J Infect 1993;26:97–101.

53. Katz MH, Hessol NA, Buchbinder SP, et al. Temporal trends of opportunistic infections and malignancies in homosexual men with AIDS. J Infect Dis 1994;170:198–202.

54. Woraphot T, William GP. Prophylaxis of opportunistic infections. Infect Dis Clin North Am 2000;14:929–44.

55. Kuruvilla A, Humphrey MD, Emko P. Coexistent oral cryptococcosis and Kaposi sarcoma in acquired immune deficiency syndrome. Cutis 1992;49:206–4.

56. Cole MC, Cohen PR, Satra KH, et al. The concurrent presence of systemic disease pathogens and cutaneous Kaposi sarcoma in the same lesion: *Histoplasma capsulatum* and Kaposi sarcoma coexisting in a single skin lesion in a patient with AIDS. J Am Acad Dermatol 1992;26:285–7.

57. Steeper TA, Rosenstein H, Weiser J, et al. Bacillary epithelioid angiomatosis involving the liver, spleen and skin in an AIDS patient with concurrent Kaposi's sarcoma. Am J Clin Pathol 1992;97:713–8.

58. Northfelt DW, Sollitto RA, Miller TR, et al. *Cytomegalovirus* pneumonitis: an unusual cause of pulmonary nodules in a patient with AIDS. Chest 1993;103:1918–20.

59. Hambelton J, Aragon T, Modin G, et al. Outcome for hospitalized patients with fever and neutropenia who are infected with the human immunodeficiency virus. Clin Infect Dis 1995;20:363–71.

60. Ho DD. Time to hit HIV, early and hard. N Engl J Med 1995;333:450–1.

61. Ho DD, Neumann AU, Perelson AS, et al. Rapid turnover

of plasma virus and CD4 lymphocytes in HIV-1 infection. Nature 1995;373:123–6.

62. Levine JD, Allan JD, Tessitore JH, et al. Recombinant human granulocyte-macrophage stimulating factor ameliorates zidovudine-induced neutropenia in patients with acquired immune deficiency syndrome. Blood 1991;78:3148–54.

63. Miles SS, Mitsuyasu RT, Baldwin G. Combined therapy with recombinant granulocyte colony stimulating factor and erythropoietin decreases hematologic toxicity from zidovudin. Blood 1991;77:2109–17.

64. Pizzo PA. Anticipated treatment is the best guide to catheter choice. Oncology Times 1992;14:2.

65. Raad II, Bodey GP. Infectious complications of indwelling vascular catheters. Clin Infect Dis 1992;15:197–208.

66. Greene JN. Catheter-related complications of cancer therapy. Infect Dis Clin North Am 1996;10:255–95.

67. Raad II, Hohn DC, Gilbreath BJ, et al. Prevention of central venous catheter-related infections caused using maximal sterile barrier precautions during insertion. Infect Control Hosp Epidemiol 1994;15:231–8.

68. Banerjee C, Bustamente CI, Wharton R, et al. *Bacillus* infections in patients with cancer. Arch Intern Med 1998;148:1769.

69. Raad I, Costerton W, Sabharwal U, et al. Ultrastructural analysis of indwelling vascular catheters: a quantitative relationship between luminal colonization and duration of placement. J Infect Dis 1993;168:400–7.

70. Kurkchubasche AG, Smith SD, Rowe MI. Catheter sepsis in short-bowel syndrome. Arch Surg 1992;127:21–4.

71. Goetz AM, Muder RR, Wagener MM, et al. Risk of infection due to femoral placement of central venous catheters [abstract J6]. In: Programs and Abstracts of the 35th Interscience Conference on Antimicrobial Agents and Chemotherapy, San Francisco, California. Washington (DC): American Society for Microbiology; 1995.

72. Circeo L, McGee W, Brown RB. Management of infections in adult intensive care unit patients: Part II. Infect Dis Clin Pract 1995;3:254.

73. Early TF, Gregory RT, Wheeler JR, et al. Increased infection rate in double-lumen versus single-lumen Hickman catheters in cancer patients. South Med J 1990;83:34–60.

74. Henrique HF 3rd, Karmy-Jones R, Knoll SM, et al. Avoiding complications of long term venous access. Am Surg 1993;59:555–8.

75. Maki DG. Infection caused by intravascular devices: pathogenesis, strategies for prevention. Royal Society of Medicine Services International Congress and Symposium 1991;179:3.

76. Maki DG, Weise CE, Sarafin HW. A semiquantitative culture method for identifying catheter-related infection. N Engl J Med 1977;296:1305–9.

77. Rello J, Coll P, Prats G. Laboratory diagnosis of catheter-related bacteremia. Scand J Infect Dis 1991;23:583–8.

78. Raad II, Sabbagh MF, Rand KH, et al. Quantitative tip culture methods and the diagnosis of catheter-related infections. Diagn Microbiol Infect Dis 1992;15:13–20.

79. Press OW, Ramsey PG, Larson EB, et al. Hickman catheter infection in patients with malignancies. Medicine 1984;63:189–200.

80. Horn CK, Conway SP. Candidemia: risk factors in patients with cystic fibrosis who have totally implantable venous access systems. J Infect 1993;26:127–32.

81. Raad II, Vartivarian S, Khan A, et al. Catheter-related infections caused by *Mycobacterium fortuitum* complex: 15 cases and review. Rev Infect Dis 1991;13:1120–5.

82. Kryzwda EA, Gotoff RA, Andris DA, et al. Antibiotic lock treatment (ALT): impact on catheter salvage and cost savings (abstract J4). In: Programs and Abstracts of the 35th Interscience Conference on Antimicrobial Agents and Chemotherapy, San Francisco, California. Washington (DC): American Society for Microbiology; 1992.

83. Groeger JS, Lucas AB, Coit D, et al. A prospective, randomized evaluation of the effect of silver impregnated subcutaneous cuffs for preventing tunneled chronic venous access catheter infections in cancer patients. Ann Surg 1993;218:206–10.

84. Jansen B, Jansen S, Peters G, Pluverer G. In vitro efficacy of a central venous catheter (hydrocath) loaded with teicoplanin to prevent bacterial colonization. J Hosp Infect 1992;22:92–107.

85. Raad I, Darouiche R, Hachem R, et al. The broad-spectrum activity and efficacy of catheters coated with minocycline and rifampin. J Infect Dis 1996;173:418–24.

86. Raad I, Hanna H. Intravascular catheters impregnated with antimicrobial agents: a milestone in the prevention of bloodstream infections. Support Care Cancer 1999;7:386–90.

87. Darouiche RO, Raad II, Heard SO, et al. A comparison of two antimicrobial-impregnated central venous catheters. Catheter study group. N Engl J Med 1999;340:1–8.

88. Lishner M, Scheinbaum R, Messner HA. Intrathecal vancomycin in the treatment of Ommaya reservoir infection by *Staphylococcus epidermidis*. Scand J Infect Dis 1991;23:101–4.

89. Borgbjerg BM, Gjerris F, Albeck MJ, Boresen SE. Risk of infection after cerebrospinal fluid shunt: an analysis of 884 first-time shunts. Acta Neurochir (Wien) 1995; 136:1–7.

90. Siegal T, Pfeffer MR, Steiner I. Antibiotic therapy for infected Ommaya reservoir systems. Neurosurgery 1998;22:97–100.

91. Hirsch BE, Amodio M, Einzig AI, et al. Instillation of vancomycin into a cerebrospinal fluid reservoir to clear infection: pharmacokinetic considerations. J Infect Dis 1991;163:197–200.

92. Morissette I, Gourdeau M, Francoeur J. CSF shunt infection: a fifteen-year experience with emphasis on management and outcome. Can J Neurol Sci 1993;20:118–22.

93. Stamos JK, Kaufman BA, Yogev R. Ventriculoperitoneal shunt infections with Gram-negative bacteria. Neurosurgery 1993;33:858–62.

94. Khardori N, Wong E, Carrasco CH, et al. Infections associated with biliary drainage procedures in patients with cancer. Rev Infect Dis 1991;13:587–91.

95. Kernodle DS, Kaiser AB. Postoperative infections and antimicrobial prophylaxis. In: Mandell GL, Benett JE, Dolin R, editors. Principles and practice of infectious diseases. New York: Churchill Livingstone; 1995. p. 2743–56.

96. Arbeit RD, Dunn RM. Expression of capsular polysaccha-

ride during experimental focal infection with *Staphylococcus aureus*. J Infect Dis 1987;156:947–52.

97. Kaiser AB, Kernodle DS, Parker RA. A low-inoculum animal model of subcutaneous abscess formation and antimicrobial prophylaxis. J Infect Dis 1992;166:393–9.

98. Elek SD, Conen PE. The virulence of *Staphylococcus pyogenes* for man. A study of the problems of wound infection. Br J Exp Pathol 1958;38:573–86.

99. Velasco ED, Martins CA, Vidal E, et al. Hospital infections at an oncology hospital. Rev Paul Med 1990;108:61–70.

100. Barber GR, Miransky J, Brown AE, et al. Direct observations of surgical wound infections at a comprehensive cancer center. Arch Surg 1995;130:1042–7.

101. Fong IW, Engelking ER, Kirby WMM. Relative inactivation by *Staphylococcus aureus* of eight cephalosporin antibiotics. Antimicrob Agents Chemother 1976;9:939–44.

102. Kernodle DS, Stratton CW, McMurray LW, et al. Differentiation of B-lactamase variants of *Staphylococcus aureus* by substrate hydrolysis profiles. J Infect Dis 1989;159:103–8.

103. Rodrigo Tapia JP, Alvarez Mendez JC, Martinez G, Suarez Nieto C. Risk factors in surgical wound infection in oncological surgery of the head and neck. Acta Otorrinolaringol Esp 1998;49:221–4.

104. Sable CA, Hayden FG. Orthomyxoviral and paramyxoviral infections in transplant patients. Infection in transplantation. Infect Dis Clin North Am 1995;9:987–1003.

105. Hirsch MS. Herpes group virus infection in the compromised host. In: Rubin RH, Young LS, editors. Clinical approach to infection in the compromised host. New York: Plenum Medical Book Company; 1994. p. 379–96.

106. Sokal JE, Firat D. Varicella-zoster infection in Hodgkin's disease. Am J Med 1965;39:452–63.

107. Goffinett DR, Glatstein EJ, Merigan TC. Herpes zoster-varicella infections and lymphoma. Ann Intern Med 1972;76:235–40.

108. Monfardini S, Bajetta E, Arnold CA, et al. Herpes zoster-varicella in malignant lymphomas. Eur J Cancer 1975; 11:51–7.

109. Ruckdeschel JS, Schimpff SC, Smyth AC, et al. Herpes zoster and impaired cell-associated immunity to the varicella-zoster virus in patients with Hodgkin's disease. Am J Med 1977;62:77–85.

110. Schimpff S, Serpick A, Stoler B, et al. Varicella-zoster infection in patients with cancer. Ann Intern Med 1972;76:241–54.

111. Wilson JF, Marsa GW, Johnson RE. Herpes zoster in Hodgkin's disease. Cancer 1972;29:461–5.

112. Mazur MH, Dolin R. Herpes zoster at the NIH: a 20 year experience. Am J Med 1978;65:738–44.

113. Dolin R, Reichman RC, Mazur MH, et al. Herpes zoster-varicella infections in immunosuppressed patients. Ann Intern Med 1978;89:375–88.

114. Meyers JD. *Cytomegalovirus* infection following marrow transplantation: risk, treatment and prevention. In: Plotkin SA, Michelson S, Pagano JS, et al, editors. CMV: pathogenesis and prevention of human infection. New York: Liss; 1984. p. 101–17.

115. Reusser P. Current concepts and challenges in the prevention and treatment of viral infections in immunocompromised cancer patients. Support Care Cancer 1998; 6:39–45.

116. Whimbey E, Couch RB, Englund JA, et al. Respiratory syncytial virus pneumonia hospitalized adult patients with leukemia. Clin Infect Dis 1995;21:376–9.

117. Elting LS, Whimbey E, Lo W, et al. Epidemiology of influenza A virus infection in patients with acute or chronic leukemia. Support Care Cancer 1995;3:198–202.

118. Lewis VA, Champlin R , Englund J, et al. Respiratory disease due to parainfluenza virus adult bone marrow transplant recipients. Clin Infect Dis 1996;23:1033–7.

119. Hibberd PL, Tolkoff-Rubin NE, Conti D, et al. Preemptive ganciclovir therapy to prevent cytomegalovirus disease in cytomegalovirus antibody-positive renal transplant recipients. Arandomized controlled trial. Ann Intern Med 1995;123:18–26.

120. Merigan TC, Renlund DG, Keay S, et al. A controlled trial of ganciclovir to prevent *Cytomegalovirus* disease after heart transplantation. N Engl J Med 1992;26:1182–6.

121. Whimbey E, Champlin RE, Couch RB, et al. Community respiratory virus infections among hospitalized adult bone marrow transplant recipients. Clin Infect Dis 1996;22:778–82.

122. Ghosn S, Champlin RE, Englund J, et al. Respiratory syncytial virus upper respiratory tract infection in adult bone marrow transplant recipients: combination therapy with aerosolized ribavirin and intravenous immunoglobulin. Bone Marrow Transplant 2000;25:751–5.

123. Douglas RJ Jr. Prophylaxis and treatment of influenza. N Engl J Med 1990;322:443–50.

124. Hayden FA, Treanor JJ, Fritz RS. Use of the oral neuraminidase inhibitor oseltamivir in experimental human influenza: randomized controlled trials for prevention and treatment. JAMA 1999;282:1240–6.

125. Feld R, Bodey GP, Groschel D. Mycobacteriosis in patients with malignant disease. Arch Intern Med 1976;136: 67–70.

126. Morrow LB, Anderson RE. Active tuberculosis in leukemia, malignant lymphoma and myelofibrosis. Arch Pathol 1965;79:484–93.

127. Barber T, Sugar AM. Mycobacteriosis and nocardiosis in the immunocompromised host. In: Rubin RH, Young LS, editors. Clinical approach to infection in the compromised host. New York: Plenum; 1994. p. 239–73.

128. Kaplan MH, Armstrong D, Rosen P. Tuberculosis complicating neoplastic disease: A review of 201 cases. Cancer 1974;33:850–8.

129. Ortbals DW, Marr JJ. A comparative study of tuberculous and other mycobacterial infections and their associations with malignancy. Am Rev Respir Dis 1978;117:39–45.

130. Oh C-S, Stratta RJ, Fox BC, et al. Increased infections associated with the use of OKT3 for treatment of steroid-resistant rejection in renal transplantation. Transplantation 1988;45:68–73.

131. Wolinsky E. Nontuberculous mycobacteria and associated diseases. Am Rev Respir Dis 1979;119:107–59.

132. Woods GL, Washington JA. Mycobacteria other than *Mycobacterium* tuberculosis: review of microbiologic and clinical aspects. Rev Infect Dis 1987;9:275–94.

133. Roberts GD , Koneman EW, Kim YK. *Mycobacterium.* In:

Hausler WJ, Kerrmann KL, Isenberg HD, et al, editors. Manual of clinical microbiology. Washington (DC): American Society for Microbiolgy; 1991, p. 304–39.

134. Walsh TJ, Hiemenz JW, Aniaissie E. Recent progress and current problems in the treatment of invasive fungal infections in neutropenic patients. Infect Dis Clin North Am 1996;10:365–400.

135. Kroschinsky F, Naumann R, Ehninger G. Candidiasis in cancer patients: epidemiology, diagnosis prophylaxis and therapy. Mycoses 1999;42:53–9.

136. Verduyn Lunel FM, Meis JF, Voss A. Nosocomial fungal infections: candidemia. Diagn Microbiol Infect Dis 1999;34:213–20.

137. Viscoli C, Girmenia C, Marinus A, et al. Candidemia in cancer patients: a prospective, multicenter surveillance study by the Invasive Fungal Infection Group (IFIG) of the European Organization for Research and Treatment of Cancer (EORTC). Clin Infect Dis 1999;28:1071–9.

138. Bodey GP, Anaissie EJ. Chronic systemic candidiasis. Eur J Clin Microbiol Infect Dis 1989;8:855–7.

139. Thaler M, Pastakia B, Shawker TH, et al. Hepatic candidiasis in cancer patients: the evolving picture of the syndrome. Ann Intern Med 1988;108:88–100.

140. Gentile G, Micozzi A, Girmenia C, et al. Pneumonia in allogeneic and autologous bone marrow recipients. A retrospective study. Chest 1993;104:371–5.

141. Anaissie EJ, Karyotakis NC, Hachem R, et al. Correlation between in vitro and in vivo activity of antifungal agents against Candida species. J Infect Dis 1994;170:384–9.

142. Karyotakis NC, Anaissie EJ, Hachem R, et el. Comparison of the efficacy of polyenes and triazoles against hematogenous Candida krusei infection in neutropenic mice. J Infect Dis 1993;168:1311–3.

143. Wingard JR, Merz WG, Rinaldi MG, et al. Increase in Candida krusei infections in bone marrow transplant recipients given fluconasole prophylaxis. N Engl J Med 1991;325:1274–7.

144. Dupont B, Huber M, Kim SJ, et al. Galactomannan antigenemia and antigenuria in aspergillosis: studies in patients with experimentally infected rabbits. J Infect Dis 1987;155:1–11.

145. EORTC International Antimicrobial Therapy Cooperative Group. Empiric antifungal therapy in febrile granulocytopenic patients. Am J Med 1989;86:668–72.

146. Melchers WJ, Verweij PE, Van den Hurk P, et al. General primer-mediated PCR for detection of Aspergillus species. J Clin Microbiol 1994;32:1710–7.

147. Talbot GH, Weiner MH, Gerson SL, et al. Serodiagnosis of invasive aspergillosis in patients with hematologic malignancy: validation of the Aspergillus fumigatus antigen radioimmunoassay. J Infect Dis 1987;155:12–27.

148. Verweij PE, Stynen D, Rijs AJ, et al. Sandwich enzyme-linked immunosorbent assay compared with pastorex latex agglutination test for diagnosing invasive aspergillosis in immunocompromised patients. J Clin Microbiol 1995;33:1912–4.

149. Walsh TJ, Wyman CA, Pizzo PA. Laboratory diagnosis of invasive fungal infections in patients with neoplastic diseases. Baillieres Clin Infect Dis 1995;2:25.

150. Burch PA, Karp JE, Merz WG, et al. Favorable outcome of invasive aspergillosis in patients with acute leukemia. J Clin Oncol 1987;5:1985–93.

151. Karp JE, Burch PA, Merz WG. An approach to intensive antileukemia therapy in patients with previous invasive aspergillosis. Am J Med 1988;85:203–6.

152. Hiemenz JW, Walsh TJ. Lipid formulations of amphotericin B: recent progress and future directions. Clin Infect Dis 1996;22:133–44.

153. Hiemenz JW, Greene JN. Special considerations for the patient undergoing allogeneic or autologous bone marrow transplantation. Hematol Oncol Clin North Am 1993;7:961–1002.

154. Viscoli C , Castagnola E. Emerging fungal pathogens, drug resistance and the role of lipid formulations of amphotericin B in the treatment of fungal infections in cancer patients; a review. Int J Infect Dis 1998–99;3:109–18.

155. Chiou CC, Groll AH, Walsh TJ. New drugs and novel targets for treatment of invasive fungal infections in patients with cancer. Oncologist 2000;5:120–35.

156. Anaissie EJ, Kontoyiannis DP, Vartivarian S, et al. Effectiveness of an oral triazole for opportunistic mold infections in partients with cancer experience with SCH 39304. Clin Infect Dis 1993;17:1022–31.

157. Rodriguez-Adrian LJ, Grazziutti ML, Rex JH, Anaissie EJ. The potential role of cytokine therapy for fungal infections in patients with cancer: is recovery from neutropenia all that is needed? Clin Infect Dis 1998;26:1270–8.

158. Chanock SJ, Gorlin JB. Granulocyte transfusion: time for a second look. Infect Dis Clin North Am 1996;10:327–43.

CHAPTER 9

GASTROINTESTINAL EMERGENCIES

HARISH K. GAGNEJA, MD
FRANK A. SINICROPE, MD

NAUSEA AND VOMITING

Nausea and vomiting are common occurrences in cancer patients. Nausea can be difficult to define, extremely unpleasant, and painless or associated with discomfort. It may precede vomiting. Nausea can be associated with autonomic symptoms, including pallor, cold sweats, and tachycardia. Some patients experience retching, which is a spasmodic movement of the diaphragm and abdominal musculature and which may be associated with vomiting. Vomiting (also called emesis) is the forceful expulsion of gastric contents from the mouth due to the contraction of the abdominal musculature and the diaphragm.[1,2] Cancer patients identify nausea and vomiting as two of the most distressing and feared side effects of their illness and therapy. Nausea and vomiting are common symptoms in cancer patients and have a number of underlying causes. These symptoms may be due to the cancer itself or may occur as a consequence of chemotherapy and/or radiation.[2]

Almost 75% of cancer patients undergoing chemotherapy experience nausea and vomiting during the course of chemotherapy. The appropriate management of nausea and vomiting in cancer patients is important for maintaining patient comfort and quality of life and also is economically beneficial.

In the majority of patients, vomiting can be controlled with antiemetic agents, particularly serotonin type 3 (5-HT$_3$) receptor antagonists. Nausea, particularly as a chronic symptom, can be more challenging to treat and to resolve. Nearly two decades ago, vomiting was regarded as the most severe adverse effect of chemotherapy. In a study of 155 patients done nearly one decade ago, nausea was the most severe side effect while vomiting ranked fifth.[3] Risk of nausea and vomiting can be classified according to the specific chemotherapeutic

agent administered. A prophylactic antiemetic regimen is then developed, depending upon the anticipated risk.

All advanced cancers can be associated with nausea and vomiting, and such symptoms are relatively common during the terminal phase of the illness. Nausea contributes to cachexia of advanced cancer, and vomiting exacerbates the pain associated with the metastatic disease. These symptoms may therefore negatively impact the patient's quality of life, and their effective treatment is an important goal of palliation.[4] Nausea and vomiting are frequently associated with primary gastrointestinal cancers (including those of the stomach, esophagus, and colon and rectum) but may also occur due to involvement of the gastrointestinal tract, either by direct extension or by metastasis. Metastasis to the brain from any cancer may elicit nausea and vomiting and should be excluded if the index of suspicion for metastatic disease is sufficiently high.

The complications of nausea and vomiting include a number of important clinical and metabolic events. Protracted vomiting may result in dehydration and metabolic alterations, including hypochloremic alkalosis, hypokalemia, and hyponatremia. Other consequences of protracted nausea and vomiting include Mallory-Weiss tears at the gastroesophageal junction, Boerhaave's syndrome (esophageal rupture), and thinned or damaged tooth enamel secondary to chronic acid injury. Another important complication is malnutrition due to decreased oral intake.

Chemotherapy-Induced Nausea and Vomiting

Conditioned, Acute, and Delayed Onset. Chemotherapy-induced nausea and vomiting can be classified as anticipatory, acute, or delayed, based on the time of occurrence relative to chemotherapy administration. Anticipatory nausea and vomiting is a conditioned response seen in

10 to 44% of patients receiving chemotherapy.[5] It occurs before or during the administration of chemotherapy but earlier than expected for the particular regimen being administered.

The onset of anticipatory vomiting before chemotherapy varies, but vomiting is prominent after the first few courses of chemotherapy.[6] Young adults (women, in particular) are at higher risk for this type of nausea and vomiting. Anticipatory nausea and/or vomiting can be triggered by certain sights or odors, including those experienced while traveling to or arriving at the hospital or chemotherapy administration area. Anxiety plays an important role in precipitating this condition.[5] Behavioral modification and biofeedback techniques may be helpful, and antianxiolytic agents (including lorazepam) are often used for treatment. Lorazepam (1 mg orally at bedtime the night before chemotherapy and 1 mg the morning of chemotherapy) may be beneficial.[7]

Acute nausea and vomiting occurs within 24 hours of chemotherapy administration. The onset can vary from a few minutes to several hours, according to the specific drug administered. Serotonin release and activation of 5-HT$_3$ receptor appear to be most important in the pathogenesis of this symptom when it occurs acutely.[5] The suggested therapy for this symptom is outlined below, and guidelines for antiemetic therapy are presented. Delayed nausea and vomiting is seen 24 hours or later after the administration of chemotherapeutic agents and may last for several days. The mechanism of this type of nausea and vomiting is less well understood, and the therapeutic approach is often more challenging.[5] In many cases, no etiology other than recent chemotherapy is found. However, in patients receiving intensive chemotherapy alone or combined with radiation, esophageal and/or gastric mucosal injury may be present and may be responsible for the nausea and vomiting. In immunocompromised patients, infectious etiologies with fungal or bacterial esophagitis are considerations.

Categories of Risk. The four categories of risk of emesis range from very low risk to severe risk. Antiemetic therapy is directed at the agent with the highest emetic potential. Cisplatin is the only agent in the severe-risk category and is the most emetogenic anticancer drug. Without antiemetic agents, the risk of nausea and vomiting is nearly 100%, and it is against cisplatin-induced emesis that antiemetic agents are tested.[8] Chemotherapeutic drugs that are in the high- and moderate-risk categories are shown in Table 9–1; the treatment approaches are similar and often include a combination of antiemetic agents. The low-risk category, as defined, has a lower emetic risk, and the use of a single antiemetic agent is usually sufficient therapy. Chemotherapeutic agents with a very low emetic potential do not require the

prophylactic use of antiemetics. Patients who are receiving such drugs can generally take oral antiemetics on an as-needed basis.

Affective Factors. Controlling emesis in older patients is generally easier than in younger patients. Younger patients are more prone to dystonic reactions with antiemetics that block dopamine receptors.[9] A 27% incidence of dystonia was reported in 500 patients under 30 years of age, as compared to only a 2% incidence of trismus or torticollis in older patients (> 30 years of age). Patients over 70 years of age who are treated with metoclopramide or ondansetron generally tolerate these agents at the same doses given to younger patients, and efficacy is preserved. Furthermore, full doses of serotonin receptor antagonists are appropriate for elderly persons.[10] Women are more prone to emesis, and this may be due to the fact they often receive highly emetogenic drug combinations, including cisplatin/cyclophos-

TABLE 9–1. Emetic Risks of Commonly Used Chemotherapeutic Agents

Severe emetic risk
    Cisplatin
Moderate to high emetic risk
    Dacarbazine
    Actinomycin D
    Nitrogen mustard
    Carboplatin
    Cyclophosphamide
    Lomustine
    Carmustine
    Daunorubicin
    Doxorubicin
    Epirubicin
    Idarubicin
    Cytarabine
    Ifosfamide
Low emetic risk
    Mitoxantrone
    Paclitaxel
    Docetaxel
    Mitomycin
    Irinotecan
    Topotecan
    Gemcitabine
    Etoposide
    Vinorelbine
Very low emetic risk
    Methotrexate
    Bleomycin
    Vindesine
    Vinblastine
    Vincristine
    Busulfan
    Chorambucil
    Alkeran
    Melphalan
    Hydroxyurea

phamide for cancer of the ovary. If emesis is not well controlled with previous courses of chemotherapy, it predisposes the patient to emesis with subsequent chemotherapy, even with the use of antiemetics.

Nausea and vomiting is a frequent side effect of high-dose chemotherapy, particularly in the setting of myeloablative conditioning regimens employed in hematopoietic cell transplantation.[11] It can also occur in relation to conditioning total body irradiation (TBI), as discussed below. In these patients, nausea and vomiting can also occur due to upper-gastrointestinal mucosal erosion or ulceration. In immunocompromised patients infectious etiologies, including fungal or bacterial esophagitis, must be considered as a cause of persistent nausea and vomiting. With varying degrees of efficacy, serotonin antagonists are frequently used to treat nausea and vomiting following high-dose chemotherapy with or without TBI.[12] Nausea and vomiting is a frequent side effect of acute or chronic graft-versus-host disease (GVHD); protracted symptoms are associated with chronic GVHD and may be a presenting symptom. (For further discussion of this topic, please refer to an oncology textbook.)

Nausea and vomiting following irradiation is often a complex multifactorial symptom. The intensity and severity of emesis are related to the site treated, the dose and the size of the field, and clinical considerations, including prior surgery, cytotoxic drugs, and the metabolic status of the patient. In patients receiving radiation to the upper abdomen, radiation-induced emesis will occur within 2 to 3 weeks of therapy in approximately 50% of patients after conventional fractionated radiotherapy (200 cGy per fraction). It will occur acutely in more than 90% of patients receiving fractionated TBI for hematopoietic cell transplantation. Furthermore, more than 80% of patients will develop an acute onset of nausea and vomiting following single-dose (> 500 cGy per large field) hemibody irradiation.[13]

Pathophysiologic Mechanisms. Vomiting is under central neurologic control by the "vomiting center" in the dorsal aspect of the lateral reticular formation in the medulla of the brain.[14] The vomiting center coordinates input from other medullary centers to produce a preprogrammed emetic response. Vomiting can be caused by emetogenic stimuli activating afferent vagal and sympathetic neural pathways within the gastrointestinal tract that act directly on the vomiting center.[5] Additionally, the vomiting center can be activated by afferent impulses from the vestibular system, the pharynx, the heart, the peritoneum, and other parts of the brain (ie, thalamus, hypothalamus, and cortex). A second site that controls emesis is located outside of the blood-brain barrier in the area postrema in the floor of the fourth ventricle and is called the chemoreceptor trigger zone (CTZ).[15] This zone is responsive to chemical stimuli in the circulation but not to electrical stimulation. Emetogenic stimuli that act on the CTZ include uremia, hypoxia, diabetic ketoacidosis, radiation sickness, motion sickness, and drugs (eg, digitalis, opiates, ergot derivatives, syrup of ipecac, salicylate, emetine, dopamine agonists, and bacterial enterotoxin).

The discovery of serotonin (5-HT) and its receptors, specifically the 5-HT$_3$ receptor, in the area postrema and CTZ as well as in the gastrointestinal (GI) tract led to the development of 5-HT$_3$ receptor antagonists like ondansetron and granisetron, which are extremely effective in preventing nausea and vomiting induced by chemotherapeutic agents.[5] Chemotherapy may induce vomiting by damaging enterochromaffin cells, thereby releasing serotonin in the GI tract, or by acting directly on medullary centers in the brain. The released serotonin binds to 5-HT$_3$ receptors in the gut, triggering impulses that travel up the vagus nerve to 5-HT$_3$ receptors in the brain. A number of brain neurotransmitters (including dopamine, histamine, acetylcholine, endogenous opiates, serotonin, γ-aminobutyric acid, and substance P) are important to the emetic response. Pharmacologic manipulation of these final common mediators and their receptors forms the basis for current and future therapies for nausea and vomiting.

Antiemetic Agents. *Serotonin Antagonists.* Serotonin type 3 receptor antagonists have significantly reduced nausea and vomiting within the 1st 24 hours of chemotherapy administration (Table 9–2). These agents are also effective in controlling nausea associated with radiation, bowel obstruction, renal failure, and brain injury.[16] There are currently five serotonin receptor antagonists commercially available, including azasetron, granisetron, ondansetron, and tropisetron. All are highly selective, with a high affinity to the 5-HT receptor, and all share the same low incidence of side effects, which include mild headache, elevated transient transaminase, and constipation or diarrhea.[17] Delayed nausea in response to cisplatin is likely unrelated to 5-HT release from gut enterochromaffin cells and remains poorly controlled.[2] Nausea in advanced cancer patients responds to 5-HT$_3$ antagonists used either alone or in combination with other agents. A well-known synergistic effect occurs with 5-HT antagonists used in combination with corticosteroids.[4] Overall, the introduction of 5-HT antagonists into clinical practice resulted in a dramatic improvement in the management of nausea and vomiting. Despite these drugs, chemotherapy-induced emesis remains a significant problem in many patients even when a combination of antiemetic drugs is used.

Corticosteroids. Corticosteroids have a high therapeutic index when used for chemotherapy-induced emesis. They

TABLE 9–2. Antiemetic Agents, Doses, and Administration Schedules

Antiemetic Agent	Dose Range	Schedule*
Serotonin receptor antagonists		
Dolasetron	100 mg or 1.8 mg/kg IV;	Once, before chemo
	100 mg PO	Once, before chemo
Granisetron	1 mg or 0.010 mg/kg IV;	Once, before chemo
	1 mg or 2 mg PO	Once, before chemo
Ondansetron	8 mg or 0.15 mg/kg IV[†]	Once, before chemo
Tropisetron	5 mg IV;	Once, before chemo
	5 mg PO	Once, before chemo
Corticosteroids		
Dexamethasone	8–20 mg IV;	Once, before chemo
	4–20 mg PO	Once, before chemo
Methylprednisolone	40–100 mg IV	Once, before chemo

chemo = chemotherapy; IV = intravenously; PO = orally.

*For acute chemotherapy-induced emesis.

[†]Oral doses have not been well studied for acute emesis. Usual dose is 8 mg two to three times daily for delayed or radiation emesis.

are among the most frequently used antiemetic agents, and single-agent use is appropriate in some settings. They are especially effective when given in combination with 5-HT receptor antagonists in patients receiving moderate to highly emetogenic chemotherapeutic agents.

Phenothiazines and Butyrophenones. Phenothiazines and butyrophenones are type 2 dopaminergic antagonists. Chlorpromazine, prochlorperazine, and promethazine serve as dopaminergic, cholinergic, and histamine receptor antagonists.[2] Prochlorperazine given in typical oral and intramuscular doses in random-assignment trials was found to be less active than metoclopramide or dexamethasone.[8] The butyrophenones haloperidol and droperidol are active antiemetic agents. A formal study comparing haloperidol with metoclopramide in patients receiving cisplatin reported that both antiemetics were effective although greater activity was seen with metoclopramide.[18]

Substituted Benzamides. Metoclopramide is a substituted benzamide and is both a dopaminergic antagonist and a serotonin type 4 (5-HT$_4$) agonist.[19] At doses greater than 120 mg per 24 hours, it becomes a 5-HT$_3$ antagonist.[20] Its side effects include restlessness and extrapyramidal reactions, which may not necessarily be dosage dependent.[21] Dexamethasone may add to its antiemetic properties and may salvage those patients resistant to metoclopramide who are receiving chemotherapy.[22] Metoclopramide is effective in delayed-onset emesis and is also used for the treatment of gastroparesis.

Anticholinergic and Antihistaminics. These agents are antimuscarinic, and their use for nausea and vomiting is limited.[2] Atropine has been shown to be effective in man-

aging the acute onset of cholinergic symptoms with diarrhea during the intravenous administration of irinotecan. Cyclizine and meclizine are effective for nausea associated with increased intracranial pressure, pharyngeal stimulation, and mechanical bowel obstruction.[2] Drowsiness and antimuscarinic effects are the main adverse effects of antihistamines.

Octreotide. Octreotide may reduce nausea and vomiting as well as abdominal cramps associated with malignant bowel obstruction. This is due to the inhibition of both motilin and vasoactive intestinal peptide release.[23]

Tachykinin/Neurokinin Receptor Antagonists. New agents include the neurokinin receptor antagonists. There are three well described neurokinin receptors; neuorkinin type 1 (NK-1) receptor is stimulated by substance P. Neurokinin type 1 receptor antagonists have cross-species antiemetic activity induced by radiation, cisplatin, cyclophosphamide, and morphine.[24] These agents are given orally and may provide better control of delayed emesis associated with cisplatin. These drugs also ameliorate acute nausea and vomiting when added to 5-HT$_3$ receptor antagonists and dexamethasone.[25]

Management

Treatment of the patient with nausea and vomiting is directed at the suppression of this symptom in addition to the thorough medical evaluation and correction of fluid, electrolyte, or nutritional deficiencies, especially in the setting of persistent or protracted vomiting. Fluid resuscitation includes normal saline solution and electrolyte supplementation as needed. In some cases, a nasogastric tube is placed to relieve gastric distension.

Antiemetic guidelines (Table 9–3) have been established and reported by investigators at the Mayo Clinic.[6] These guidelines pertain to all risk categories of emesis (see Table 9–1) and are useful for the management of adult patients receiving cytotoxic chemotherapy.

High-Risk Settings. Chemotherapeutic agents with the highest emetic potential (including development of grade 4 nausea and vomiting), per National Cancer Institute (NCI) common toxicity criteria can be managed by the following:

- Dexamethasone, 20 mg orally (PO) pretreatment.
- Granisetron, 1 mg PO pretreatment. (This is as effective as intravenous administration.)
- Dexamethasone, 8 mg PO twice a day (bid) for 2 days, and then 4 mg PO bid for 2 days. (This is for prevention of delayed-onset nausea and vomiting.)
- Prochlorperazine, 10 mg PO every 6 hours as needed.
- Lorazepam, 1 mg PO every hour (not used if the patient experiences excessive drowsiness).

The use of serotonin receptor antagonist together with the following corticosteroids represents the antiemetic combination most commonly used in the setting of grade 3 emisis potential:

- Dexamethasone, 20 mg PO pretreatment
- Ondansetron, 16 mg PO pretreatment
- Dexamethasone, 4 mg PO bid for 2 days (optional)
- Prochlorperazine, 10 mg PO every 6 hours prn
- Lorazepam, 1 mg PO every hour (not given if patient has excessive drowsiness)

Low-Risk Emetogenic Potential. Without antiemetic medications, some but not all patients may experience vomiting. Accordingly, emesis in this group is easier to control than in the higher-risk groups. Management is as follows:

- Dexamethasone, 20 mg PO (optional)
- Prochlorperazine, 10 mg PO pretreatment (optional)
- Prochlorperazine, 10 mg every 6 hours

Very-Low-Risk Emetogenic Potential. Prophylactic antiemetics are not recommended, but patients are provided with an oral antiemetic such as metoclopramide (10 to 20 mg in an oral dose) or prochlorperazine (10 to 20 mg in an oral dose) for use on an as-needed basis.

Acute-Onset Emesis after Chemotherapy. Several standard treatments for nausea and vomiting are used when 5-HT$_3$ receptor antagonists are not effective. One of the following medications can be selected for prompt management in the acute setting: (1) prochlorperazine, 10 mg PO every 6 hours, or 15 mg in time-release capsules every 12 hours, or 25 mg per rectum every 12 hours for nausea, vomiting, or both; (2) haloperidol, 1 mg PO every 4 hours; or (3) promethazine, 25 to 50 mg every 6 hours.

In addition, the following medications can be combined as necessary:

- Lorazepam, 1 mg PO every 1 to 2 hours (not given in drowsy patients)
- Diphenhydramine, 50 mg PO every 4 to 6 hours
- Dexamethasone, 4 to 8 mg PO bid (for maximum of 4 days)
- Promethazine, 25 to 50 mg every 6 hours
- Dronabinol, 2.5 to 7.5 mg PO every 4 hours

Chemotherapy-Induced Delayed Emesis. As shown in Table 9–4, several agents are used in the management of delayed-onset nausea and vomiting.

Corticosteroids are the most consistently useful drugs for the prevention of delayed emesis (eg, dexamethasone, 4 to 8 mg PO bid, for a maximum of 4 days).

Several trials have reported on metoclopramide given in combination with corticosteroids. Doses are typically 20 to 40 mg given two to four times per day for 3 to

TABLE 9–3. Antiemetic Guideline Summaries for Patients Receiving Chemotherapy

Emesis Potential	Antiemetics and Dosages*
Grade 4[†]	Dexamethasone, 20 mg PO Granisetron, 1 mg PO Dexamethasone, 8 mg PO bid for 4 days, then 4 mg PO bid for 2 days Prochlorperazine, 10 mg PO q6h prn Lorazepam, 1 mg PO qh prn (Metoclopramide no longer used)[‡]
Grade 3	Dexamethasone, 20 mg PO Ondansetron, 16 mg PO Dexamethasone, 4 mg PO bid for 2 days[§] Prochlorperazine, 10 mg PO q6h prn Lorazepam, 1 mg PO qh prn
Grade 1 or 2	Dexamethasone, 20 mg PO[§] Prochlorperazine, 10 mg PO[§] Prochlorperazine, 10 mg PO q6h prn

bid = twice daily; PO = by mouth; prn = as circumstances require; qh = every hour; q6h = every 6 hours.
*December 1998 guidelines (these guidelines also provided recommendations for the treatment of nausea and vomiting that occur despite standard prophylactic therapy).[6]
[†]With or without cisplatin.
[‡]Changed from previous guidelines.
[§]For inpatients, ondansetron could be given as an 8-mg IV bolus followed by continuous infusion of 1 mg/h.

4 days.[26] Studies have shown conflicting results concerning the use of serotonin antagonists for delayed emesis. These agents are used either as single agents or in combination with corticosteroids.

Recommendations for the subsequent cycle of the same chemotherapeutic regimen are given according to the patient's experience with the previous cycle of chemotherapy. When the patient is experiencing severe nausea or vomiting, the next level of antiemetogenic treatment should be applied (see Table 9–4).

If the patient is receiving grade 4 emetogenic chemotherapy and if treatment for acute-onset and delayed-onset nausea and vomiting is not effective, consider changing the patient to a different chemotherapeutic regimen.

ILEUS, OBSTIPATION, AND BOWEL OBSTRUCTION

The term "intestinal obstruction" refers to the interference of the normal passage of gastrointestinal contents through the gastrointestinal tract, caused by an intraluminal process or extrinsic compression. The obstruction can be partial (the passage continues but is difficult) or complete (intestinal contents are completely unable to pass through the gastrointestinal tract). Ileus is a failure of normal intestinal motility in the absence of obstruction. Idiopathic dilatation of the colon in the absence of mechanical

TABLE 9–4. Chemotherapeutic Agents and Regimens for Delayed Emesis

Emetic Category	Antiemetic Regimen	Doses and Schedules
Severe risk	Oral corticosteroid + oral metoclopramide (or + oral 5-HT$_3$ antagonist)	Dexamethasone, 8 mg bid daily for 3 to 4 days + Metoclopramide, 30 mg or 0.5 mg/kg 2 to 4 times per day for 2 to 4 days or 5-HT$_3$ antagonists at doses in Table 9–2, twice daily for 2 to 3 days
Moderate to high risk	Oral corticosteroid ± oral metoclopramide (or ± oral 5-HT$_3$ antagonist)	Same doses for agents, as above; agents given at the same schedule, but for 2 to 3 days
Low risk	No regular preventive use of antiemetics	—
Very low risk	No regular preventive use of antiemetics	—

5-HT3 antagonist = serotonin receptor type 3 antagonist.

obstruction is referred to as acute colonic pseudo-obstruction or Ogilvie's syndrome. Toxic megacolon is a type of ileus that can occur in patients with ulcerative colitis and in which there is transmural inflammation and colonic dilatation. "Obstipation" refers to flatus, acute abdominal pain, and cessation of bowel movements. Obstipation is associated with both mechanical obstruction and functional ileus. The term "strangulated obstruction" is used if the blood supply of the involved bowel is compromised.

Clinical Manifestations of Intestinal Obstruction

Whenever a patient presents with crampy abdominal pain, vomiting, abdominal distension, and obstipation, intestinal obstruction is the first diagnostic consideration. The clinical features of bowel obstruction and ileus are dependent on the site of obstruction. Proximal obstructions (gastric outlet, duodenum) are associated with persistent and copious vomiting, significant abdominal pain, and minimal abdominal distension. Distal small-bowel obstruction (SBO) is associated with vomiting that can be malodorous, abdominal distension, and pain. Vomiting is uncommon in colonic obstruction, but pain and distension are pronounced. In cases of ileus, vomiting is usually infrequent; pain is mild, and distension is moderate to severe. Typically, the pain in SBO is crampy, with paroxysms occuring at 4- to 5-minute intervals for proximal obstruction and less frequently for more distal obstruction. The development of continuous, localized, and very severe pain suggests the possibility of strangulated obstruction.

Pathophysiologic Mechanisms

Changes in blood flow, bowel flora, intestinal contents, and motility are important in the pathophysiology of SBO. The consequences of intestinal obstruction are determined by the duration of the obstruction and the presence or absence of ischemia. The intestinal vascular supply can be compromised by external compression of the bowel or its mesentery by adhesions, tumors, torsions, hernial orifices, or intussusception. Pressures reach only 8 to 10 cm H$_2$O in simple obstruction and are not high enough to produce ischemia.[26] Under special conditions, intraluminal pressure may reach a level that compromises blood flow.[26] The mucosal layer of the intestine is the first to become ischemic.[27] Muscosal ischemia results in the extravasation of protein-rich fluid into the bowel wall and lumen. A variety of inflammatory and vasoactive mediators have been incriminated in the pathogenesis of this injury.

Experimental and clinical evidence suggests that bacterial overgrowth is involved in the pathophysiology of SBO. Obstruction of the ileum in germ-free dogs induces intestinal distension without hypersecretion, suggesting that hypersecretion may be related to bacterial overgrowth and not intestinal distension per se.[28] In partial obstruction or with impaired motility, intestinal stasis promotes bacterial overgrowth and malabsorption. Small-bowel obstruction results in the accumulation of fluid proximal to the obstruction as water and electrolyte absorption is impaired, and secretion is increased, resulting in the net movement of isotonic fluid from the intravascular space into the intestinal lumen.[29] Intestinal distension also results from the accumulation of gas in the obstructed lumen. This gas originates from swallowed air and from bacterial overgrowth. The competency of the ileocecal valve is very important in the pathophysiology of colonic obstruction. With a competent ileocecal valve, the cecum cannot decompress fluid and gas into the small bowel, resulting in a closed-loop obstruction. Cecal diameters ≥ 13 cm carry a risk of perforation, particularly when the obstruction is relatively acute in onset. Ileus is thought to result from an imbalance between sympathetic and parasympathetic motor activity, resulting in intestinal atony and pseudo-obstruction.

Etiology

Although there are many causes of SBO (Table 9–5), three etiologies are most common and include adhesions resulting from prior abdominal surgery, hernias, and neoplasms. Obstruction may occur anytime after the initial abdominal surgery, but the average interval between the initial operation and development of adhesive obstruction reported in one study was 6 years.[30] Hernias are the second leading cause of obstruction. Neoplasms cause obstruction of the small intestine as well as the colon. Malignant etiology should be one's first impression in a large-bowel obstruction. Obstruction can be caused by primary tumors or by metastatic cancer, including metastases to the mesentary, serosa of the intestine, or peritoneal carcinomatosis.

Ileus and pseudo-obstruction. The underlying cause of mechanical obstruction is usually apparent whereas in cases of ileus or pseudo-obstruction, it is usually occult and multifactorial. In cancer patients, the most common causes include opioid use, electrolyte imbalance, certain chemotherapeutic agents (such as vincristine), and metabolic disturbances. Table 9–6 lists the causes of ileus and pseudo-obstruction.

TABLE 9–5. Causes of Mechanical Obstruction

Extrinsic
    Adhesions
    Hernias
    Volvulus
    Endometriosis
    Abscess
    Carcinomatosis
    Vascular
Intrinsic (intramural)
    Strictures
        Inflammation
        Crohn's disease
        NSAIDs
        Radiation
        Caustic ingestion
        Post-trauma
        Postanastomosis
        Neoplastim
        Ischemia
    Intussusception
    Congenital
        Atresias
        Annular pancreas
        Duplication cysts
        Hirschsprung's disease
    Hematomas
Intraluminal
    Fecal impaction
    Barium impaction
    Gallstone
    Bezoar
    Foreign body
    Worms
    Polypoid neoplasms

NSAIDs = nonsteroidal anti-inflammatory drugs.

Diagnosis

History. A detailed history is one of the key elements in pinpointing the site of obstruction. It is also important to ascertain the duration of symptoms to distinguish acute from chronic conditions. A history of previous abdominal surgery, previous episodes of obstruction, inflammatory bowel disease, herniation in the abdominal wall or previous incisions, prior abdominal or pelvic radiation, or previous cancers or polyps provide important clues as to cause of obstruction. A careful medication review that includes narcotic history is important in discovering the underlying cause of ileus.

Physical Examination. Inspection of the abdomen may reveal distension, previous surgical scars, and hernias. The degree of distension varies depending on the level of obstruction. Distension is marked in distal SBO and long-standing colonic obstruction. In cases of ileus, the degree of distension is quite variable. An area of erythematous or bluish skin may indicate the site of a strangulated hernia as the cause of obstruction. Palpation of the abdomen may reveal areas of marked tenderness, rebound guarding, or rigidity, indicating a strangulated hernia or a localized perforation requiring immediate surgical attention. Palpation of the abdomen may also reveal a mass, indicating tumor. Auscultation of the abdomen may reveal periods of increasing bowel sounds with periods of relative quiet. With obstruction, the bowel sounds are usually high-pitched or musical. In cases of prolonged obstruction and ileus, bowel sounds may disappear due to decreased motility. The patient's vital signs provide clues to the systemic response to the underlying obstruction.

Laboratory Studies. Laboratory studies have limited usefulness in the diagnosis of obstruction but are useful in the diagnosis of ileus, which can be caused by an electrolyte imbalance. Leukocytosis with left shift is common in cases of inflammation and infection. Metabolic abnormalities and electrolyte derangements are commonly associated with, and are a consequence of, prolonged and intestinal obstruction. The monitoring of electrolytes, blood urea nitrogen, and creatinine is helpful in assessing the fluid balance. In severe cases, measuring arterial blood gas is helpful in assessing the acid-base balance. Proximal obstruction produces more acid-base derangements, and distal obstruction produces more electrolyte disturbances.

Abdominal Radiography. Abdominal radiography is extremely helpful in confirming the diagnosis of obstruction, differentiating ileus from obstruction, and localizing the level of obstruction. A complete abdominal series that includes an upright chest film, an upright and supine abdominal film, and a lateral decubitus abdominal film

TABLE 9–6. Causes of Ileus

Postlaparotomy effects
Intra-abdominal conditions
    Acute appendicitis
    Acute diverticulitis
    Perforated viscus
    Acute cholecystitis
    Acute pancreatitis
    Pyelonephritis
    Bacterial peritonitis
    Chemical peritonitis
    Inflammatory bowel disease
Drugs
    Opioids
    Anticholinergics
    Calcium channel blockers (diltiazem, verapamil)
    Phenothiazines
    Chemotherapeutic agents
    Tricyclic antidepressants
Electrolyte imbalance
    Hypokalemia
    Hyponatremia
    Hypomagnesemia
Retroperitoneal hemorrhage
    Ruptured abdominal aortic aneurysm
    Lumbar compression fracture
Thoracic processes
    Pneumonia
    Lower-rib fractures
    Pulmonary embolus
    Myocardial infarction
    Open heart surgery
Metabolic disturbances
    Uremia
    Diabetic ketoacidosis
Systemic sepsis

should be obtained. Patients with a complete SBO generally have dilated intestinal loops proximal to the obstruction and no gas in the colon or rectum. Abdominal radiography may also show multiple air-fluid levels with distended loops of bowel. The rectum will be devoid of any gas in cases of colonic obstruction, but the proximal colon may or may not have gas. Abdominal radiography may also show free air, indicating perforation, or air in the intestinal wall, indicating pneumatosis or bowel ischemia. About 20 to 30% of patients with SBO produce equivocal or normal abdominal radiographs.[31,32] In cases of ileus, gas is generally present throughout the intestinal tract, including the rectum, but it is sometimes difficult to distinguish obstruction from ileus on the basis of abdominal plain radiography alone.

Contrast Studies. Contrast studies are helpful in differentiating between obstruction and ileus, identifying the site of obstruction, and differentiating between partial and complete obstruction. If colonic obstruction has been ruled out or is deemed very unlikely, barium sulfate can be given orally for an antegrade contrast study since net secretion in the intestinal lumen keeps the barium in solution. Water-soluble contrast agents such as diatrizoate meglumine (Gastrograffin) usually get diluted (because of the large amount of fluid present within the obstructed bowel) and prevent the definition of distal obstruction. If colonic obstruction is suspected, a Gastrograffin or barium enema should be done as the first test. Care is taken to avoid getting a large amount of barium above the obstruction, which can become inspissated due to net absorption of fluid in the colon and which can be removed only at the time of operation and can be hazardous due to the risk of spillage.

Computed Tomography. Computed tomography may be helpful in establishing the diagnosis if other studies are inconclusive. The demonstration of a transition zone with dilated fluid-, air-, or air-fluid-filled loops above collapsed loops of bowel distally suggests the presence of SBO. Computed tomography (CT) is very sensitive (90%) for high-grade obstruction, but sensitivity is low (50%) for low-grade obstruction.[33] It is also very useful in cases of suspected tumor involvement or recurrence, bowel strangulation, inflammatory mass, and extrinsic obstruction by masses. Computed tomography also detects air in the bowel wall or in the peritoneal cavity in cases of perforation.

Treatment

Obstruction. After diagnosis, patients should be resuscitated with intravenous fluids, and any electrolyte derangements should be corrected. A Foley catheter is suggested to measure intake and output and also to assess the immediate effects of fluid resuscitation on urine output. A nasogastric tube should be placed to decompress the stomach and intestine and to avoid further abdominal distension. Acid-base abnormalities should be sought and corrected. A surgical consultation should be obtained to determine whether operative treatment or expectant management should be employed. This decision depends on the patient's clinical condition, the degree of obstruction, the rapidity with which the obstruction developed, the presence of strangulation or perforation, and any signs of peritonitis. Intravenous antibiotics covering Gram-negative and anaerobic bacteria should be started in cases of suspected strangulation, inflammatory mass, or perforation. A cautious emergency endoscopy may be attempted in cases of distal obstructions that require further diagnostic evaluation or in cases of pseudo-obstruction with a very dilated bowel segment, for placement of a decompression tube. Recently, the use of self-expanding metal stents for acute colonic obstruction before elective surgery has been reported as having a 90% success rate. The mean time between stent placement and surgery was 8.6 days.[34]

Ileus. The most important principle for the treatment of ileus is to treat the underlying cause. Other important steps to take are (1) limiting oral intake, (2) maintaining intravascular volume, (3) correcting electrolyte abnormalities (especially hypokalemia), (4) stopping the administration of the offending drugs if possible, (5) using nasogastric suction, (6) decompressing the rectal tube, and (7) frequently changing the position of the patient. These conservative measures are successful in the majority (85%) of patients in a mean of 3 days.[35] In the case of a patient with colonic pseudo-obstruction, the decision to intervene with medical therapy, colonoscopy, or (rarely) surgery should be dictated by the patient's clinical status. In a recent double-blind placebo-controlled trial, neostigmine proved efficacious in patients with colonic pseudo-obstruction after the failure of conservative management.[36] Colonic decompression may be required in patients with persistent marked colonic distension that has failed to respond to conservative medical management or when neostigmine is contraindicated. The contraindications to neostigmine include mechanical colonic obstruction, pregnancy, renal insufficiency, cardiac arrhythmias, active bronchospasm, and signs of ischemia or perforation. Surgical intervention is reserved for cases with signs of colonic ischemia and perforation.

Summary

Ileus, obstipation, and bowel obstruction are encountered frequently in emergency-room settings. It is important to establish the correct diagnosis so as to institute appropriate treatment in a timely fashion. With available diagnostic studies, diagnosis can be made accurately and promptly in most cases. In addition to the time-honored treatments, the successful use of self-expanding metal stents for colonic obstruction and of neostigmine for ileus has been recently reported.

PERFORATED VISCUS

The perforation of a viscus along the GI tract is a serious emergency. Perforation can occur at any level in the GI tract, including that of the esophagus, the stomach, the duodenum, the small intestine, and the colon. The clinical presentation, cause, treatment, and outcome vary, depending on the level of the GI tract at which the perforation occurred.

Clinical Manifestations

Cervical esophageal perforation can present with neck pain, dysphonia, dysphagia, hoarseness, and subcutaneous emphysema. Upper-abdominal rigidity, severe retrosternal chest pain, odynophagia, and hematemesis are some of the common presentations of thoracic esophageal perforation. Acute onset of severe abdominal pain is usually the first symptom of gastric perforation. The pain is occasionally associated with nausea and vomiting, and significant bleeding may be present in about 15% of patients.[37] The pain usually becomes more diffuse, it may be felt in the lower abdomen, or it may radiate to the shoulders because of irritation of the diaphragm.

Accompanying abdominal distension and signs of peritonitis may occur in cases of free perforation into the peritoneal cavity. Subcutaneous emphysema is an important clue in cases of perforation. Patients may present with the tetralogy of a distended abdomen, shock, subcutaneous emphysema, and physical findings consistent with diffuse peritoneal irritation.[38] Fever and leukocytosis may eventually develop with any of these varieties of perforation.

Pathophysiologic Mechanisms

Perforation of the esophagus results in the entry of air, food, esophageal secretions, refluxed gastric contents, and bacteria into periesophageal space, with subsequent mixed bacterial infection and chemical destruction. The clinical course depends on the location and duration of the perforation. As infection progresses, signs of systemic sepsis are noted, including shock and sequestration of extravascular fluid. In diverticular disease of the colon, the degree of inflammatory reaction plays an important part in determining whether there is free perforation or whether there is a contained perforation resulting in abscess formation. If the inflammatory reaction is minimal at the time of loss of nutrient flow, the thin-walled diverticulum is likely to undergo necrosis and perforation. In contrast, if the inflammatory reaction has involved the diverticulum sufficiently to produce thickening of the wall, the infection is also likely to produce thickening of the wall, involving more diverticula and colonic wall and ultimately resulting in abscess formation. In patients with severe ulcerative colitis or ischemic injury to the bowel wall, perforation occurs in an area of transmural involvement.

Etiology

The most common causes of perforation in cancer patients are spontaneous perforation secondary to tumor and iatrogenic perforation secondary to instrumentation (endoscopy). Table 9–7 lists the different causes of perforation along the GI tract.

Diagnosis

Physical Examination. The patient with a perforated viscus may be asymptomatic or have very overt signs and symptoms. The physical examination begins with the assessment of the patient's vital signs, appearance, breathing pattern, ability to converse, posture, position in bed, and degree of discomfort. Facial expressions add to

TABLE 9–7. Etiology of Gastrointestinal-Tract Perforation

Esophagus
    Iatrogenic causes
        Endoscopy
        Bougie and balloon dilation
        Sclerotherapy
        Surgery in the mediastinal region
        Anastomotic leak
    Boerhaave's syndrome
    Foreign body
    Caustic ingestion
    Trauma
    Esophageal cancer
    Bronchogenic cancer
    Esophageal ulcer
    Gastric
    Peptic ulcer disease
    Malignancy
    Endoscopy
    Nasogastric tube
    Gastric syphilis
    Gastric volvulus
    Foreign body ingestion
    Metastatic carcinoma
    Severe forceful vomiting
    Spontaneous rupture
    Trauma
Duodenum and small intestine
    Endoscopy including ERCP
    Surgery
    Trauma
    Malignacy
    Lymphoma
    Diverticular disease
    Ischemic enteritis
    Infectious enteritis
    Inflammatory bowel disease
    NSAID ulcers
    Chronic ulcerative jejunoileitis
    Small-bowel obstruction
Colon
    Endoscopy
    Malignancy
    Diverticulitis
    Ischemic bowel disease
    Inflammatory bowel disease
    Colonic obstruction
    Barium enema
    Foreign body
    Stercoral ulcer

ERCP = endoscopic retrograde cholangiopancreatography; NSAID = non-steroidal anti-inflammatory drug.

the overall picture. A patient who lies still in bed with his or her extremities flexed and who is reluctant to move or speak is likely to have peritonitis. The abdominal examination should include inspection, palpation, percussion, and auscultation. On inspection, the abdomen may be distended. Palpation should begin at the point of least tenderness and proceed to the point of greatest tender-ness. Abdominal rigidity and rebound tenderness are present in cases of peritonitis. Gentle percussion is often superior to deep palpation for eliciting these signs. Percussion may also yield a tympanitic note due to air in the peritoneal cavity. Auscultation of the abdomen may yield few or no bowel sounds in cases of diffuse peritonitis. Bowel sounds can be normal or hyperperistaltic (in patients who have not developed diffuse peritonitis). Examination of the extremities may provide evidence for inadequate perfusion, as occurs in shock.

Laboratory Studies. The initial laboratory studies should include a complete blood count with differential, chemistry and liver function tests, and amylase and lipase assessments. Leukocytosis with bandemia may be present in patients with peritonitis or abscess formation. Amylase levels may be high in cases of intestinal, esophageal, or gastric perforation, and lipase levels may be high in cases of gastric perforation.

Radiology. Plain-film radiography can provide the first evidence for the diagnosis of perforation. In cervical perforation, a radiograph of the neck in lateral projection may show air in the deep cervical tissues before it is felt clinically or seen by chest radiography.[39] A plain-film radiograph of the chest is abnormal in 60 to 80% of cases; after instrumentation, the usual findings are pneumomediastinum and loss of contour of descending aorta at the level of the left diaphragm. A pleural effusion may be seen, especially with Boerhaave's syndrome. Subcutaneous air signifying subcutaneous emphysema may also be present. After 10 minutes of position maintenance, an upright and left-decubitus radiograph can demonstrate as little as 1 to 2 mL of free air.[40] When evaluating for free air, one should never request only a supine radiograph. Plain-film radiography may show air in the retroperitoneal space or retroperitoneal contrast collection in cases of duodenal perforation. Other signs of perforation include visualization of the hepatic ligament and prominence and visualization of both sides of the bowel wall.

Contrast studies are used when doubt exists. Water-soluble contrast is used initially and is followed by barium when no perforation is seen on the initial study. Water-soluble contrast is used initially because barium causes a severe inflammatory reaction in the peritoneum.

Computed tomography is very accurate in establishing the diagnosis of perforation. It can provide information about subcutaneous air, retroperitoneal air, pneumomediastinum, and free peritoneal air with a great deal of accuracy.

Treatment

Treatment of a perforated viscus can be expectant, expectant followed by surgery, or immediate surgery, depending on a number of factors, including the size and location of the defect, the type of defect (free or contained), and the patient's clinical course. Nonoperative treatment includes nothing by mouth, nasogastric-tube suction, broad-spectrum antibiotics, intravenous hydration, hyperalimentation, and close monitoring of the patient. If any signs of clinical deterioration develop while the patient is receiving expectant treatment, a decision to operate can be made. Perforations caused by peptic ulcer disease usually require emergent surgery, as do colonic perforations caused by megacolon. Factors predictive of mortality after ulcer perforation include major medical illness, preoperative shock, and perforation lasting longer than 24 hours.[41]

Summary

A perforated viscus in the GI tract is a serious emergency that requires prompt diagnosis and treatment. The clinical presentation varies, depending on the site of perforation. A careful history and careful physical examination are of utmost importance in establishing an early diagnosis of perforation, which will result in a better outcome. Laboratory tests and radiologic studies should be used judiciously when required. The treatment of perforation can be nonoperative or operative, depending on the size of the defect and the patient's clinical course.

ENTEROCOLITIS

Esophagitis

In addition to mucositis, esophageal injury and infection are frequently recognized in patients who are undergoing cancer treatment and in the immunocompromised host. Esophagitis can be caused by cytotoxic chemotherapy and irradiation as well as by viral, bacterial, and fungal organisms.[42] Other causes include acid-peptic esophagitis, pill-induced injury, trauma caused by nasogastric tubes, and GVHD in hematopoietic cell transplant recipients.[43,44] In nontransplantation patients, *Candida albicans* and herpes simplex virus (HSV) are the most common pathogens, but bacterial organisms and other viruses (including *Cytomegalovirus* [CMV]) are also responsible.[43] In severely immunocompromised patients, infections with multiple organisms may coexist, and these organisms can become invasive due to mucosal disruption. Other predisposing factors include corticosteroids, diabetes mellitus, and acquired immune deficiency states. In patients receiving bone marrow or stem cell transplants, prophylaxis with antifungal and antiviral drugs has substantially reduced the incidence of esophageal infections.[45,46] When esophagitis is suspected, endoscopy is the preferred diagnostic procedure and allows the early administration of appropriate therapy. In addition to visual inspection, endoscopic brushings and biopsy specimens can be obtained for microscopic examination, special stains, and culture.[43] Double-contrast esophagraphy will reveal evidence of esophagitis in severe cases, but its sensitivity and specificity are limited.

Infectious Esophagitis

***Candida* Esophagitis.** Many *Candida* species normally colonize the oropharynx and can become pathogenic and produce esophagitis in immunocompromised patients.[43,45] Patients may be asymptomatic or may complain of odynophagia (painful swallowing) and/or dysphagia (difficulty in swallowing). Oral thrush may be absent. Endoscopy reveals slightly raised, adherent whitish plaques or linear streaks with surrounding erythema.[47] In more severe cases, these plaques may be confluent; in thrombocytopenic patients, bleeding may occur. In granulocytopenic patients, exudative material is usually absent. In either setting, the diagnosis is made at endosopy by the finding of yeast or hyphal forms on cytologic smears of exudative material from esophageal brushings; mucosal biopsy is frequently nondiagnostic. Drugs that suppress acid production (H_2 blockers and proton pump inhibitors) contribute to fungal and bacterial colonization of the upper gastrointestinal tract that can predispose to infectious esophagitis.[43] Fluconazole is an effective treatment of esophageal candidiasis in immunocompromised patients.[43,45] Unlike ketoconazole, its absorption is not affected by the gastric hydrogen ion concentration (pH). Treatment-refractory patients, those with granulocytopenia, or those with suspected disseminated infection should be treated with amphotericin B. In nonimmunocompromised patients, oral nystatin or clotrimazole troches are often successfully used for initial therapy. In patients with acquired immunodeficiency syndrome (AIDS) and suspected esophageal candidiasis, empiric treatment with fluconazole is frequently administered.[48]

Viral Esophagitis. Viral infections of the esophagus are caused by HSV, CMV, and (rarely) varicella-zoster virus (VZV).[43,49] Symptoms include odynophagia, dysphagia, retrosternal chest pain, and nausea and vomiting. In transplant recipients, nausea and vomiting appears to be the most frequent presenting symptom.[48,50] A history of an oral herpetic lesion or the presence of vesicles on the lips or buccal mucosa can be an important clue to the diagnosis of herpetic esophagitis. Mucosal cells from a biopsy sample taken at the edge of an ulcer or from a cytologic smear show intranuclear inclusions in normal epithelial cells; multinucleated giant cells may also be observed.[51] Using monoclonal antibodies to HSV, inclusion can be detected by immunohistochemistry.[43,51] Culture for HSV becomes positive within days and can be helpful in diagnosis; acyclovir is used for both prophylaxis and treatment. Either type 1 or type 2 HSV may afflict patients who are immunosuppressed.

Varicella-zoster virus can produce esophagitis in adults with herpes zoster, usually in the setting of disseminated infection.[43,50] In some cases, esophageal VZV infection can be the source of disseminated VZV infection in the absence of skin involvement. In the immunocompromised host, VZV esophagitis causes vesicles and confluent ulcers and usually resolves spontaneously. On histologic examination of biopsy specimens or cytologic material, the distinction of VZV from HSV requires immunohistochemistry or culture.

Esophageal infection by CMV occurs only in immunocompromised patients and is usually activated from a latent stage or acquired from blood product transfusions.[43,52] *Cytomegalovirus* infects endothelial cells and fibroblasts but not epithelial cells as do HSV and VZV. *Cytomegalovirus* infection produces esophageal ulcerations that are often serpiginous and that can coalesce to form very large ulcers, particularly in the midesophagus and distal esophagus.[47] Diagnosis requires endoscopy and biopsy of the center of the ulcer crater. Routine histology demonstrates intranuclear inclusions in fibroblasts and endothelial cells. Immunohistochemistry with anti-CMV antibodies is more sensitive than routine histology but is less so than viral culture for establishing the diagnosis.[53] In contrast to routine viral culture, the shell vial culture method provides a rapid (24-hour) result. Gancyclovir is the treatment of choice,[54] and foscarnet is an effective alternative treatment.[55] Human immunodeficiency virus (HIV) may be associated with esophageal ulceration, oral ulcers and a maculopapular skin rash that occurs at the time of HIV seroconversion.[43,48] Persistent deep esophageal ulcers may occur in chronically infected individuals and in those with AIDS.

Bacterial esophagitis occurs in the immunocompromised host, is usually polymicrobial, and derives from oral flora.[50,56] This entity is underdiagnosed in severely granulocytopenic patients, given that the bacteria are difficult to identify on routine histologic examination. In such patients, bacterial infection often coexists with viral or fungal organisms that are more readily detected. The diagnosis is made by endoscopic biopsy and in these specimens, clusters of bacteria are mixed with necrotic epithelial cells.[56] Treatment consists of broad-spectrum antimicrobial therapy.

Radiation esophagitis commonly occurs during the treatment of intrathoracic malignancies, particularly lung and esophageal cancers. The frequency and severity of esophagitis increases with radiation dose and with the use of certain chemotherapeutic agents, including doxorubicin, bleomycin, cyclophosphamide, and cisplatin.[43,57–59] Endoscopy findings include erythema, edema, and friabililty of the esophageal mucosa, as well as ulceration

with eventual stricture formation.[47] Strictures result from submucosal fibrosis and degenerative changes involving blood vessels.[60] Symptomatic strictures can be managed with esophageal dilation. Treatment includes the relief of odynophagia with viscous lidocaine during the acute phase and the use of H_2 blockers or proton pump inhibitors to prevent further acid-related injury.

Pill-induced esophagitis can occur in patients who take medications at bedtime or in the recumbent position and with too little liquid.[43] Some of the medications associated with esophageal injury are potassium chloride, tetracycline, and phenytoin. Acid-peptic injury to the esophagus can result in patients who are undergoing cancer treatment.[43] Predisposing factors include delayed gastric emptying, esophageal dysmotility, impaired acid clearance, and a history of gastroesophageal reflux disease.

Esophageal involvement by GVHD is uncommon in patients with chronic GVHD.[44,61] Affected patients have desquamation of the esophageal mucosa and may also develop submucosal fibrosis and stricture formation.[62] Patients usually complain of dysphagia but may also have retrosternal discomfort and reflux-related symptoms due to reduced esophageal peristalsis. Salivary gland destruction secondary to GVHD also impairs swallowing and reduces acid neutralization and clearance. Treating chronic GVHD at its early stages may prevent esophageal involvement.

GASTROINTESTINAL BLEEDING

Etiology and Diagnosis

The diagnosis and management of acute GI bleeding is well covered in standard textbooks on gastroenterology. The goal of this section is to focus on aspects of intestinal mucosal injury and infection that can lead to significant bleeding in cancer patients who are undergoing therapy. In patients receiving chemotherapy, retching and nausea and vomiting are better controlled with antiemetics, including serotonin antagonists.[63] However, emetogenic injury to the gastric mucosa and the gastroesophageal junction (ie, Mallory-Weiss tear) commonly occurs and produces upper-gastrointestinal bleeding.[64] These injuries can produce very significant bleeding in the setting of thrombocytopenia. The etiology of bleeding in the upper GI tract in patients with cancer is commonly due to benign causes. In a series that included 122 cancer patients with upper-gastrointestinal bleeding, 95 (78%) had gastritis, peptic ulcer disease, or severe esophagitis as the cause of their hemorrhage.[65] Importantly, the development of thrombocytopenia and/or coagulopathy can unmask focal pathology and lead to the development of GI bleeding. Patients with cancer and patients undergoing cancer treatment are at risk for stress-related mucosal injury.

Stress-related mucosal injury is a common problem that is frequently seen in critically ill patients, including those with cancer. Many terms have been associated with this entity, including "stress-related mucosal damage," "stress ulceration," "erosive gastritis," and "stress ulcer syndrome." Such patients develop painless, occult, or overt upper-gastrointestinal bleeding in up to 20% of patients in the setting of an intensive care unit (ICU).[66] Significant hemorrhage was reported to occur in approximately 6% of patients. The likelihood of significant bleeding from stress-related mucosal lesions depends on risk factors such as thrombocytopenia, coagulopathy, sepsis, major surgical procedures, and the presence of organ failure.[67] The use of nonsteroidal anti-inflammatory drugs (NSAIDs) is also a relevant factor. Endoscopic findings include multiple superficial erosions or ulcers that arise most often in the gastric antrum. Most deaths are due to underlying illness; however, up to 30% of patients with clinically significant hemorrhage die as a direct result of bleeding.[68] The pathophysiology of stress-related mucosal injury involves an imbalance between injurious and defensive mucosal factors. In addition, a low gastric-luminal pH and reflex of acid and bile into the esophagus and stomach may serve as exacerbating factors; the role of *Helicobacter pylori* infection remains to be determined. While most patients do not have acid hypersecretion, it appears that acid is an essential permissive factor since the reduction of gastric acidity with antacids, H_2 receptor antagonists, and proton pump inhibitors can prevent these lesions.[69]

Primary tumors of the GI tract and mucosal metastatic tumor or chloroma are causes of occult bleeding but can also produce acute hemorrhage. With intestinal primary cancers, bleeding often ceases spontaneously and with conservative therapy. Endoscopic therapy is frequently not helpful due to diffuse oozing from the tumor surface and therefore, lack of a discreet focus amenable to electrocautery or other endoscopic modalities. Patients with hemodynamically significant bleeding can be referred for angiography with possible embolization; in some cases, surgery is required.

In bone marrow transplant recipients, gross intestinal bleeding occurs in fewer than 10% of patients within the first 100 days,[70] and its frequency in this population has fallen significantly over the past decade. This drop is attributed to effective prophylaxis against viral and fungal infection and acute GVHD. Of note, acute GVHD with diffuse small-intestinal ulceration is the most common cause of bleeding in these patients.[70] In transplantation patients, transfusion of platelets to achieve counts of ≥ 60,000/μL will generally control bleeding such that endoscopic control is often unneeded. Pre-existing ulcers may bleed profusely post transplantation, particularly those lesions with an exposed submucosal vessel. Importantly, endoscopic therapies are unsuccessful in the thrombocytopenic patient but can be attempted if the platelet count is > 50,000/μL and stable. Otherwise, embolization or surgery are usually urgently needed. Ulcers of the esophagus, stomach, or duodenum in the post-transplantation patient may be caused by GVHD or by CMV and HSV (esophageal) infection, particularly in patients not receiving antiviral prophylaxis,[43] and such ulcers can bleed profusely.

The goals of management include hemodynamic stabilization, the establishment of an accurate diagnosis, and the initiation of medical therapy with the objective of preventing further bleeding. Endoscopy is the preferred diagnostic procedure and should be performed in all patients with gross bleeding and in patients with ongoing occult blood loss. Treatment-related anemia also decreases reserves, and GI hemorrhage can therefore be life threatening in cancer patients.

Treatment

Cook and colleagues[66] reviewed 63 relevant randomized studies regarding stress ulcer prophylaxis in critically ill patients and concluded that there is strong evidence of reduced clinically important GI bleeding with H_2 antagonists versus no therapy. However, no evidence exists that prophylactic therapy decreases mortality rates. Fluid resuscitation and blood transfusion are important for re-establishing and maintaining hemodynamic stability. Attempts to correct coagulopathy with fresh frozen plasma are made in patients with active bleeding. In thrombocytopenic patients, platelet transfusions are used to maintain a platelet count of > 60,000/μL and preferably > 100,00/μL. Intravenous H_2 blockers are used in severely thrombocytopenic patients; the authors generally recommended removing nasogastric tubes due to their ability to produce erosion and bleeding in such patients. Endoscopic therapies used to achieve hemostasis include bicap electrocoagulation, heater probe, and the argon plasma laser coagulator.[71] Epinephrine injections are also used for the treatment of actively bleeding lesions.[71] Other therapies include the use of intravenous vasopressin or somatostatin although these drugs have not shown benefit in patients with ulcer-related bleeding, in contrast to patients with bleeding esophageal varices.[72] Other alternatives include surgical therapy or arteriography with embolization.

DIARRHEA

Pseudomembranous Colitis

Clostridium difficile is the most common bacterial cause of infectious diarrhea in antibiotic-treated patients[73] and in those undergoing cancer chemotherapy.[74–76] Essentially, any antibiotic can cause this syndrome; however, those drugs that are prescribed most frequently (ie, cephalosporins, followed by the penicillins) are most commonly implicated. Cancer patients receiving chemotherapy appear to be predisoposed to *C. difficile*–induced diarrhea even in the absence of antibiotics.[74–76] In a study of such patients, methotrexate, doxorubicin, and cyclophosphamide were the drugs most frequently associated with *C. difficile* infection.[76] It is speculated that anticancer-drug-mediated mucosal injury may produce the anaerobic environment conducive to *C. difficile* colonization.

Diarrhea is the key feature and is usually watery, voluminous, and without gross blood. Most patients have abdominal pain and tenderness, fever, and leukocytosis although symptoms vary.[73,77] Symptoms generally begin at 5 to 10 days of antibiotic therapy; however, they may occur as late as 3 to 4 weeks after the discontinuation of therapy.[78] Diarrheal volumes in *C. difficile*–infected patients are generally lower than those found in patients with acute GVHD. Diarrheal disease due to *C. difficile* is toxin mediated.[79,80] Diagnosis requires the detection of *C. difficile* toxin in the diarrheal fluid or by culture.[80] Nearly all patients who are found to have pseudomembranes of the colo-rectal mucosa at endoscopy will have stool assays that are positive for *C. difficile* toxin. Examination of the stool frequently reveals leukocytes. The left colon, including the rectum, is most commonly involved, but a predominantly right-sided colitis is also possible. Therefore, a normal flexible sigmoidoscopic examination does not exclude the infection but will detect approximately 80% of cases. Endoscopic evaluation reveals a spectrum from mild colitis to classic pseudomembranous colitis.[77] Importantly, typical pseudomembranes on the colo-rectal mucosa may be absent in granulocytopenic patients. Pseudomembranes appear as distinct adherent raised yellow-white plaques that are usually 2 to 5 mm in diameter but can be confluent, covering several centimeters of colonic mucosa.[47,77] Pseudomembranes are composed of polymorphonuclear leukocytes, chronic inflammatory cells, epithelial debris, and fibrin.

Clostridium difficile is a large, spore-forming, and Gram-positive anaerobic rod that is rarely detected in the feces of healthy adults who have not received antimicrobial therapy.[80,81] Isolation of the organism does not in itself imply active disease. Rather, in the proper clinical context, identification of the toxin in stool is consistent with infection and remains the best diagnostic test for pseudomembranous colitis.[73,77] After the organism is acquired, a change in intestinal flora due to antibiotics appears to permit *C. difficile* to overpopulate the intestine.[80] Infection is noninvasive, and blood cultures are therefore negative. At least three potential virulence factors have been described: an enterotoxin (toxin A), a cytotoxin (toxin B), and a distinct motility-altering factor.[79] Toxin A mediates alterations in fluid secretion and enhances inflammation; toxin B is more active than A in causing damage and exfoliation of intestinal epithelial cells. Laboratory diagnosis depends on examination of the feces for the presence of *C. difficile* toxin A. A rapid latex agglutination test for the detection of toxin A is available. Since immunospecific cross-reactions have been documented with certain other organisms, the latex test should be used only as a screening procedure.[82] Positive latex tests should be confirmed by another assay when clinically indicated.

The treatment of antibiotic-associated pseudomembranous colitis requires the discontinuation of the implicated antibiotic.[73] Many patients improve spontaneously with only this measure; however, specific therapy shortens the duration of symptoms. The most widely used agent is oral vancomycin, which (like metronidazole) is poorly absorbed and which reaches high concentrations in the stool.[73,77] Both oral vancomycin and metronidazole are effective treatments of pseudomembranous colitis, and comparison of these agents in a randomized trial demonstrated equal efficacy and relapse rates of 8 to 9% respectively.[83] Metronidazole is much more economical than vancomycin and is therefore recommended for initial therapy.[73,76] The usual initial dosage is 250 mg four times daily; 500 mg three times daily is also appropriate. Vancomycin is often reserved for patients who fail to respond to metronidazole therapy. A randomized trial found that vancomycin at a dosage of 125 mg orally four times daily for an average of 10 days was as active as the 500-mg dose given four times daily.[84] A relapse of symptoms and a repeat positive toxin assay is not uncommon after a patient responds to and completes initial therapy. Most relapsing patients will respond to a second course of treatment, but some patients suffer multiple relapses.[73,74] One can use vancomycin if metronidazole was used initially, and vice versa. Cholestyramine is an anion exchange resin that binds to the enterotoxin of *C. difficile* (ie, aborts its cytotoxic activity in vitro) and has been used with success in refractory cases.[77] Cholestyramine also binds vancomycin, and these agents should therefore not be used in combination. In the rare patient with a severe complication such as toxic megacolon or perforation, surgical management may be required.[73,85]

TYPHLITIS

Typhlitis is a clinical syndrome of fever and right-lower-quadrant tenderness in a neutropenic patient after cytotoxic chemotherapy. Typhlitis (from the Greek word "typhlon," meaning cecum) is also referred to as neutropenic colitis,[86,87] necrotizing colitis,[88] ileocecal syndrome, or cecitis.[89] This syndrome is seen in patients treated with cytotoxic drugs, usually for hematologic malignancies (especially acute myelogenous leukemia and acute lymphoblastic leukemia).[90] Typhlitis appears to be more common among children than among adults.[89,91–94] Typhlitis may also complicate the treatment of patients with solid tumors[95] and with granulocytopenia from other causes.[96,97] Although the cecum is most commonly affected, other potential areas of involvement include the ileum and ascending colon.[88,89,94,98] In our experience, patients with typhlitis have been granulocytopenic for 1 or more weeks before the onset of symptoms. Typhlitis is a consequence of an overgrowth of clostridia (particularly *Clostridium septicum*) in granulocytopenic patients.[99] The process appears to begin with mucosal disruption and leads to secondary intramural infection and subsequent edema, induration, and wall thickening.[88,98,100] Chemotherapeutic agents may themselves alter mucosal integrity.[101] To date, a predictor of this syndrome has not been identified; chemotherapy, neutropenia, fever, and antibiotic use are found with equal frequency in patients with and without typhlitis.[88,98,102]

Clinical Presentation and Diagnosis

Typhlitis should be suspected when a neutropenic patient presents with fever and abdominal pain, particularly in the right lower quadrant, with or without rebound tenderness. Associated diarrhea, often bloody, is common. Abdominal distention and nausea and vomiting are also common symptoms.[88,93,98] Given that the clinical presentation can be subtle and that there are no pathognomonic clinical findings, one must consider other entities in the differential diagnosis, such as pseudomembranous colitis, colonic pseudo-obstruction, acute appendicitis, ischemic colitis, inflammatory bowel disease, and infectious colitis. Imaging studies can be useful in supporting a diagnosis of typhlitis. Computed tomography and ultrasonography can demonstrate bowel wall thickening and can exclude other intra-abdominal processes. Computed tomography and magnetic resonance imaging (MRI) are more sensitive for diagnosis than are other imaging modalities, and they are noninvasive.[100,103] Plain-film radiography is nonspecific but may show any of the following features: (a) a relative paucity of bowel gas in the right lower quadrant, with a slight distention of surrounding small bowel; (b) a soft-tissue density secondary to an atonic fluid-filled right colon that may be dilated and exhibit thumbprinting of the mucosa; or (c) a small-bowel obstruction.[94,104] Findings at colonoscopy include mucosal erythema, edema, friability, and ulcerations. In some cases, a nodular tumorlike mass is seen.[105] Colonoscopy should be done cautiously to minimize the risk for perforation. Alternatively, flexible sigmoidoscopy can be performed to exclude pseudomembranous colitis, inflammatory bowel disease, and infectious colitis. Barium enema should also be done with caution; findings

will include cecal distortion, with edema and effacement of the mucosa; rigidity; loss of haustral markings; and thumbprinting.[89,106] At pathology, the bowel is dilated and edematous, and the mucosa is frequently hemorrhagic and may contain multiple ulcerations.[98] Transmural involvement may be present, and there is usually a sparse inflammatory infiltrate, edema (so-called phlegmonous colitis), intramural hemorrhage, necrosis, and evidence of either bacterial or fungal infection. Leukemic infiltration is not routinely found.[102]

Management

Patients with typhlitis are often very ill and have an increased mortality rate.[93] The treatment is conservative medical management while awaiting the recovery of granulocytes. At diagnosis, patients should receive broad-spectrum antibiotics with anaerobic coverage.[68,70] In some cases, patients have been found to have positive blood cultures for aerobic Gram-negative bacilli. Marrow-stimulating growth factors may be considered. There are anecdotal reports of successful treatment with oral vancomycin; antiperistaltic agents should be avoided.[102] Recurrence is rare, and most patients recover uneventfully. Surgical therapy has been successful in rare patients who failed medical treatment.[87,90,93,95] Proposed criteria for surgical intervention include (a) persistent GI bleeding after the resolution of neutropenia and thrombocytopenia and the correction of clotting abnormalities; (b) evidence of free intraperitoneal perforation; (c) clinical deterioration requiring support with vasopressors or large volumes of fluid, suggesting uncontrolled sepsis; and (d) development of symptoms of an intra-abdominal process, which would normally require surgery in the absence of neutropenia.[87,93] A review of the published literature suggests that surgical versus medical management is associated with a better outcome. However, these results must be cautiously interpreted as the two groups are not comparable. It is likely that the medically treated patients had a greater severity of illness and may have been unfit for surgery.[87]

CHEMOTHERAPY-RELATED ILEUS

Vincristine treatment is associated with adynamic ileus and has been implicated in some cases of cecal perforation.[107] Although the etiology of vincristine-induced ileus is not known, improvement has been reported with the use of metoclopramide.[108] Patients with vincristine-induced ileus often have obstipation, and aggressive use of cathartics may be needed.

Acute Colonic Pseudo-obstruction

Acute colonic pseudo-obstruction was first described in 1948 by Sir Ogilvie when he reported two patients with nonobstructive abdominal distention who were ultimately found to have metastases invading the subdiaphragm sympathetic plexus.[109] This condition is characterized by massive dilatation of the colon without apparent mechanical obstruction.[110]

Pathogenesis. The pathogenesis of acute colonic pseudo-obstruction is unknown. Autonomic nervous system imbalance has been suggested. The predilection towards massive cecal distention may be related to poor intestinal motility, prolonged recumbency in the supine position, or a mobile cecum on a loose mesentery.[111]

Clinical Presentation and Diagnosis. Patients with acute colonic pseudo-obstruction are generally quite ill and may have any of a wide range of underlying medical or surgical problems, including underlying malignancy and cancer treatment. Patients typically present with moderate to marked abdominal distention. Symptoms may include nausea, vomiting, abdominal pain, constipation, diarrhea, and (occasionally) fever.[112] The physical examination reveals abdominal distention, and bowel sounds may be diminished, normal, or hyperactive. Mild abdominal tenderness may be present; however, peritoneal signs suggest complications of ischemia or perforation.[113] Mild leukocytosis and electrolyte imbalances (particularly hypokalemia) are common.

Plain-film abdominal radiography provides the most useful diagnostic information. All patients have marked dilatation of the colon, usually most severe in the cecum and transverse colon. Increased cecal diameter and the absence of differential air-fluid levels are evident on an upright abdominal film. The absence of mechanical colonic obstruction is demonstrated by using views and other maneuvers to allow gas to move freely into the left colon and the rectum. The differential diagnosis includes true colonic obstruction, ischemic colitis, and toxic megacolon. Sigmoidoscopy, colonoscopy, or barium contrast studies can help to rule out distal mechanical obstruction but must be done with caution due to the risk of cecal perforation. A diatrizoate meglumine (Gastrograffin) enema should be performed if colonic perforation is suspected.

Treatment. Acute colonic pseudo-obstruction is a transient reversible condition whose most feared complication is perforation of the cecum or right colon. The cecum is most vulnerable to perforation due to Laplace's law, which states that the pressure required to stretch the wall of a hollow viscus decreases in proportion to the radius of the curative of the viscus. Although perforation is relatively unusual, the goal of treatment is to avoid its occurence. Neither the national history nor the specific factors that may predict perforation are known with certainty. However, the variables most often cited are the maximal cecal diameter and the duration of colonic dilatation. Various authors have recommended some form of intervention when the cecum reaches a diameter of from 9 to 14 cm.[114,115] Others have considered the duration of cecal enlargement to be more important. In one series, 75% of patients who suffered a perforation had documented cecal dilatation for at least 5 days.[111] Therapeutic modalities include conservative measures, colonoscopic decompression, and surgery.

Conservative measures include correction of fluid and electrolyte abnormalities; intravenous fluids; restriction of oral intake; nasogastric suction to minimize swallowing; discontinuation or (at least) decrease of any medications that may interfere with bowel motility (especially narcotics); and serial physical examination and abdominal radiography to assess improvement, worsening, or the development of perforation.[112,116] Frequent turning of the patient to the prone position allows redistribution of colonic gas into the descending colon and easier evacuation. In one study of 25 cancer patients with acute colonic pseudo-obstruction, 23 of 24 patients treated conservatively improved (according to clinical and radiologic criteria) in a mean of 3 days.[116]

Colonoscopic decompression should be considered when conservative management is unsuccessful or when the cecal diameter is deemed to be dangerously dilatated.[117] The success rate is very high, and an indwelling decompression tube (over a guidewire) is often placed. This decompression catheter may need to remain in place for longer-term benefit.

Surgical intervention is required when the therapeutic options mentioned above fail or when there is evidence of colonic perforation.[118] Tube cecostomy has been recommended for the patient with perforation.[114] Perforations should be exteriorized and there should be adequate decompression; some patients may require colectomy.[119]

DIARRHEA

Chemotherapy and Radiation-Related Diarrhea

A common complication of cytotoxic therapy, diarrhea can result in fluid and electrolyte imbalance and can compromise nutritional status. Cytotoxic agents target metabolically active tissues, including the small-intestinal and colonic epithelium of the GI tract.[120] Mucosal damage by these agents produces net fluid secretion by the intestine, and damage to intestinal villi results in a loss of absorptive capacity.[121] The net effect is a secretory diarrhea; however, such patients often have a reduced capacity to handle an osmotic load, and diarrhea is thus worsened by oral intake. Some anticancer drugs, including 5-fluorouracil (5-FU),[122–124] cisplatin,[125] and irinotecan (CPT-11),[126–128] have a greater propensity than others to produce diarrhea. The incidence of diarrhea with 5-FU is increased by the addition of leucovorin.[122,123] In a phase III study comparing different regimens for the treatment of colo-rectal cancer, the frequency of severe diarrhea was highest in the group receiving weekly 5-FU plus high-dose leucovorin (25%, compared with 13% for the group receiving 5-FU plus low-dose leucovorin).[129] When 5-FU alone was given for 5 consecutive days every 4 weeks, the frequency of severe diarrhea was 9%.[129] The toxic effects of 5-FU also depend on age and sex, being more common in women than in men and being worse in women over the age of 70 years.[124]

The type I topoisomerase inhibitor irinotecan (CPT-11) can cause diarrhea by two separate mechanisms. A hyperacute diarrhea with abdominal cramping appears to be mediated by a cholinergic effect and can be effectively treated with atropine as well as loperamide.[126,130] The delayed (ie, more than 24 hours post infusion) type of diarrhea induced by this agent correlates with the peak plasma concentration of the metabolite 7-ethyl-10-hydroxycamptothecin (SN-38).[131] The exact mechanism of this type of diarrhea remains unknown. Irinotecan-induced diarrhea can be severe, and more than 18% of patients treated with this agent require hospitalization for management of diarrhea alone or combined with other GI symptoms.[132] Early and aggressive antidiarrheal therapy with loperamide and/or diphenoxylate can significantly reduce the proportion of patients developing uncontrolled diarrhea and its complications of dehydration and electrolyte imbalance.[126] Gastrointestinal toxicities of irinotecan can lead to, or contribute to, premature deaths of cancer patients, and close monitoring, early detection, and aggressive intervention of the GI toxicities are recommended.[133,134]

Radiation therapy produces GI mucosal injury that peaks at 1 to 2 weeks after irradiation, with the subsequent resolution of symptoms. Worsening of diarrhea is seen with combined-modality therapy and also with the neoadjuvant treatment of rectal cancer.[135] When combined with radiation, continuous infusion of 5-FU produced a significant increase in the incidence and severity of diarrhea than was seen with intravenous boluses of 5-FU.[135]

Diarrhea in Patients Undergoing Hematopoietic Stem Cell Transplantation

In patients who are undergoing bone marrow or stem cell transplantation, diarrhea may be secondary to the conditioning regimen or to GVHD, or it may be due to infections related to immunosuppressive therapy. Diarrhea in the immediate post-transplantation period is generally due to injury to the intestinal mucosa caused by the conditioning regimen. This regimen includes total body irradiation (TBI) and/or a combination of chemothera-

peutic agents. Regimens that contain cytarabine and the combination of busulfan, melphalan, and thiotepa[136–138] have been associated with more severe and prolonged diarrhea. The severity of enteritis can vary and may reflect variability in the metabolism and concentration of toxic metabolites.[139,140] In general, diarrhea related to the conditioning regimen resolves by the 3rd week after treatment. Histologically, this injury is characterized by crypt abnormalities including nuclear atypia, mucosal flattening, and crypt cell degeneration and crypt obliteration due to apoptosis.[141,142] Mucosal injury results in net fluid secretion by the intestine (ie, secretory diarrhea) and resolves with mucosal restitution. After day 20, acute GVHD is the most common cause of diarrhea in these patients.[138] Therefore, persistent diarrhea should raise the suspicion of acute GVHD and/or infectious etiologies although the latter occur less frequently in this population. In patients with persistent diarrhea, a colo-rectal mucosal biopsy can be performed to assess for mucosal regeneration and to evaluate for GVHD.[141,142]

Graft-versus-Host Disease

Graft-versus-host disease is the most common cause of diarrhea in hematopoietic cell transplant recipients[143] and is more frequent in recipients of allogeneic transplants than in those with autologous transplants.[138,144] In a prospective study of 296 consecutive patients undergoing bone marrow transplantation, 43% developed diarrhea after day 20 and during the first 10 months of follow-up; of these cases, 48% were attributed to acute GVHD.[143] Patients with GVHD-related diarrhea pass large volumes of watery fluid that often contains some mucoid material.[145] Diarrhea related to GVHD is secretory and occurs in the absence of oral intake although such intake usually exacerbates the diarrhea. The suspicion of GVHD is supported by the presence of GVHD-associated skin and liver abnormalities that are nearly diagnostic of intestinal GVHD when present. Graft-versus-host disease as the cause of diarrhea is supported by stool studies that are negative for *C. difficile* toxin and enteric pathogens and by falling serum albumin secondary to intestinal protein loss.[143] Patients with intestinal GVHD usually complain of anorexia and crampy abdominal pain and may also have nausea and vomiting and fever. In more severe cases, patients can develop intestinal ileus or pseudo-obstruction. When the diagnosis is in question, endoscopic examination and biopsy are useful for a definitive diagnosis and for excluding *Cytomegalovirus* (CMV) enteritis. The latter is important in CMV-seropositive patients who have not received prophylactic gancyclovir when endoscopic biopsy will differentiate the two conditions.[145]

The yield from mucosal biopsy specimens for establishing the diagnosis of GVHD is higher from gastric specimens than from duodenal or rectal specimens.[143,146] However, a rectal biopsy is easier to perform (using a flexible sigmoidoscope) and is less costly than upper-GI biopsy. A recent report emphasizes the complementary nature of endoscopic and histologic examination and demonstrates that histologic findings in the upper GI tract, unless severe, can underestimate the severity of GVHD elsewhere in the GI tract.[142] For patients with significant nausea and/or vomiting, upper endoscopy with biopsy is the preferred diagnostic test. In mild GVHD, the intestinal mucosa may appear grossly normal or may have a mild granular appearance. Moderate to severe GVHD is associated with granular, erythematous, and edematous mucosa, and mucosal ulceration or large areas of mucosal sloughing may be present in severe cases.[147–149] Patients with severe cases will often pass bloody stools, and this is worsened by concurrent thrombocytopenia. Abdominal radiography and CT reveal edema of the intestinal wall.[150,151] Although not specific for GVHD, these studies can sometimes reveal the extent of intestinal involvement. Barium studies of the small bowel reveal bowel wall thickening, with effacement of folds and excess luminal fluid.[152]

The mechanisms of diarrhea in GVHD include epithelial cell loss, impaired absorption, and increased vascular permeability due to cytokine release.[138,153] The histologic hallmark of GVHD is apoptosis of intestinal crypt epithelial cells.[148,154] This mechanism of epithelial cell loss is mediated by cytotoxic T lymphocytes[153] and is detected by microscopic examination of biopsy specimens.[141,155,156] Acute GVHD is treated with immunosuppressive drugs, which can dramatically reduce stool volume and accompanying GI symptoms. Evidence indicates that approximately one-half of patients with acute GVHD respond to initial therapy.[144] The somatostatin analogue octreotide can also reduce stool volume in patients with mild to moderate GVHD.[157,158] The antidiarrheal effects of octreotide are due to enhanced electrolyte absorption, decreased motility and inhibition of fluid secretion. Octreotide, however, was shown to be ineffective in steroid-resistant cases of intestinal GVHD.[159] Opioids can also be used to treat GVHD-related diarrhea; the patient should be observed carefully for abdominal distention.

Enteric Infections in Bone Marrow Transplantation Patients

Infectious diarrhea is relatively uncommon in the period after bone marrow transplantation (BMT). In a prospective study of patients after BMT, 43% of 296 patients developed diarrhea, and only 13% of these had a documented enteric infection.[143] The pathogens that were identified in this study included *Astrovirus*, adenovirus, *Rotavirus*, and CMV; the bacteria included C. *difficile* and *Aeromonas* species. As a cause of diarrhea, viral infection was more common than bacterial infection. The incidence of CMV infection has decreased markedly with the use of gancyclovir prophylaxis. *Cytomegalovirus* frequently produces diarrhea and bleeding due to mucosal ulceration.[147,160] The presence of discreet or large serpiginous ulcers is highly suggestive of CMV infection.[161,162] The diagnosis of CMV infection is made by endoscopic biopsy, the specimen of which should be sent for immunohistochemistry to detect CMV antigen, and viral culture.[163] Herpes simplex virus infection rarely causes intestinal disease, except for esophageal infection.[164] Although *Astrovirus* was the most frequently detected enteric virus in a recent study,[143] commercial tests are not yet available for detecting this virus (which does not appear to produce serious infection). Of note, *Rotavirus*, adenovirus, and coxsackievirus are causes of sporadic diarrhea that are detectable by enzyme-linked immunosorbent assay (ELISA) or by stool culture.[165–167] Infectious diarrhea related to *Salmonella*, *Shigella*, and *Campylobacter* species is very rare in hospitalized BMT patients. Diarrhea related to parasites (*Cryptosporidium*, *Giardia lamblia*, and *Entamoeba histolytica*) is also rare, and most of these patients are infected prior to transplantation.[168–170] Another treatable cause of diarrhea is an overgrowth of *Candida albicans*.[171,172]

Other Causes

Diarrhea occurs in up to 20% of patients who receive antibiotics and is usually a self-limited process.[173] Most patients with antibiotic-associated diarrhea have normal-appearing or minimally erythematous colo-rectal mucosa at endoscopy. Carbohydrates that are incompletely absorbed by the small intestine reach the colon, where anaerobic flora normally converts them to short-chain fatty acids. In patients who are receiving broad-spectrum antibiotics, the colonic flora are unable to perform this function, and diarrhea results. Similarly, patients with GVHD or enteric infections that involve the small intestine often malabsorb carbohydrate due to loss of mucosal brush border disaccharidases, resulting in diarrhea after oral intake.[174] Other causes of diarrhea in cancer patients include surgery (postresection diarrhea) and neuroendocrine tumors that produce hormones that stimulate net fluid secretion (eg, carcinoid, vipoma, and somatostatinoma). Iatrogenic forms of diarrhea are frequently encountered in clinical practice. Diarrhea can occur secondary to the oral intake of magnesium salts or magnesium-containing antacids. In addition, prokinetic agents such as metoclopramide can produce or contribute to diarrhea. In cases of unexplained diarrhea, a careful review of the patient's medication list is warranted. In the inpatient setting, orders for laxatives or stool softeners may not have been canceled despite the onset of diarrhea.

Treatment

The objective of antidiarrheal therapy is to reduce fluid loss from the gut by inhibiting intestinal secretion, promoting absorption, and decreasing intestinal motility. Opioid agonists are the most commonly used agents. Noninfectious diarrhea, including that induced by the conditioning regimen, can be treated with opioid agonists (including loperamide at doses up to 4 mg taken every 6 hours orally) or with diphenoxylate atropine,[175] an opioid-anticholinergic combination that can be given at doses of up to 2 tablets every 6 hours. Careful observation of patients receiving these drugs is warranted due to their impaired intestinal motility. In patients with diarrhea that is refractory to opioid agonists and to other conventional treatments, octreotide therapy should be considered. Octreotide has been shown to be effective therapy.[176–179] A consensus panel has put forth guidelines for octreotide therapy for secretory diarrhea related to chemotherapy, radiation, or GVHD which is refractory to conventional therapy.[180] Patients should receive fluid and electrolyte replacement and be kept in a nil per os (NPO) status until symptoms are improved. Prompt and aggressive antidiarrheal therapy can significantly enhance the quality of life of cancer patients and can reduce hospital admissions, thereby reducing health care expenditures.

CHOLESTASIS (OBSTRUCTIVE JAUNDICE)

Jaundice is the abnormal accumulation of bilirubin in body tissues and is marked by the yellow discoloration of sclerae, skin, and mucous membranes. This can be due to a pathologic process that extends anywhere between the hepatocyte and the ampulla of Vater. The term "cholestasis" is preferred to "obstructive jaundice" as no mechanical block can be detected in the biliary tract in many instances. If a mechanical obstruction exists, it is desirable to relieve the obstruction to prevent cholangitis. Chronic biliary obstruction can lead to biliary cirrhosis, which may take months to years to develop.

Clinical Manifestations

A thorough history and physical examination directed toward the cause of jaundice are valuable tools for a correct diagnosis. Patients present with a yellow discoloration of the sclerae, skin (a patient with yellow skin due to hypercarotenemia can be recognized by the white sclerae), or mucous membranes, usually noticed by a third person. Patients may present with dark urine and acholic stools in cases of extrahepatic cholestasis. A history of shaking chills, fever, and abdominal pain in the setting of jaundice is strongly suggestive of ascending cholangitis. Presenting symptoms of malaise, anorexia, and myalgias point toward viral hepatitis as cause of the jaundice. When evaluating the patient with jaundice, clinicians should look carefully for hepatomegaly, hepatic tenderness, and stigmata of chronic liver disease (eg, spider angiomata, palmar erythema, Dupuytren's contracture, parotid enlargement, xanthelasma, gynecomastia, and testicular atrophy). Patients may present with increasing abdominal girth or with signs and symptoms of GI bleeding. Encephalopathy with jaundice is another presentation of fulminant hepatic failure or the deterioration of chronic liver disease. Patients may present with severe itching associated with cholestatic jaundice.

Pathophysiologic Mechanisms

Bilirubin is an organic anion formed from the breakdown of hemoglobin. The liver plays a major role in the metabolism and excretion of bilirubin. Approximately 80% of the total 250 mg of bilirubin that is produced daily comes from dying red blood cells; the rest of it comes from heme moieties of other hemoproteins such as myoglobin and tissue cytochromes. Normal serum bilirubin level usually ranges from 0.2 to 1.0 mg/dL. An increased serum bilirubin level is due to one or both of the following events: (a) increased production (due to hemolysis) or (b) decreased hepatic clearance (due to either hepatocyte dysfunction or obstruction of the intrahepatic or extrahepatic biliary system). Bilirubin is transported to the liver as unconjugated bilirubin bound reversibly to albumin. Unconjugated bilirubin separates from albumin on reaching the hepatocyte. It is then transported across the cell membrane and reaches the microsomal enzyme oxidizing system, where glucuronyl transferase converts it to conjugated bilirubin. Conjugated bilirubin is actively secreted into the biliary ductal system.

Etiology

Pathophysiologically, jaundice can be classified as unconjugated or conjugated hyperbilirubinemia. Hyperbilirubinemia associated with malignant disease is almost always of the conjugated type. Hepatic bilirubin uptake and conjugation are preserved in most liver diseases. Canalicular excretion represents the rate-limiting step in overall bilirubin metabolism. Conjugated hyperbilirubinemia occurs in a wide spectrum of hepatic diseases, including disorders associated with hepatocellular and cholestatic injury, extrahepatic biliary obstruction, familial abnormalities of bilirubin excretion, Dubin-Johnson and Rotor's syndromes (Table 9–8), and space-occupying hepatic mass lesions that directly impede the excretion of bile. Such lesions are either primary tumors, as with hepatocellular carcinoma, or metastatic tumors. A common cause of extrahepatic obstruction is tumor metastasis to lymph nodes in the porta hepatis. Increased bilirubin production, impaired hepatic uptake, or impaired conjugation results in unconjugated

TABLE 9–8. Differential Diagnosis of Jaundice

Disorders of bilirubin metabolism
    Gilbert syndrome
    Crigler-Najjar syndrome
    Dubin-Johnson syndrome
    Rotor's syndrome
    Hemolysis
    Ineffective erythropoiesis
    Resorption of hematomas
Hepatocellular dysfunction
    Viral hepatitis (A,B, and C)
    Hepatotoxins
    Drugs
    Alcohol
    Ischemia
    Wilson's disease
    Acute fatty liver of pregnancy
    Autoimmune hepatitis
    Hemochromatosis
    α_1 Antitrypsin deficiency
Intrahepatic cholestasis
    Drugs
    Primary biliary cirrhosis
    Sarcoidosis
    Amyloidosis
    Lymphoma
    Mycobacterial infections
    Total parenteral nutrition
    Malignancy
    Hepatic metastasis
    Graft-versus-host disease
    Postoperative cholestasis
    Primary sclerosing cholangitis
Extrahepatic cholestasis
    Choledocholithiasis
    Cholangiocarcinoma
    Pancreatic malignancy
    Metastatic tumor
    Extrinsic compression of biliary tree
    Hepatic arterial chemotherapy
    Primary sclerosing cholangitis
    Postsurgical strictures
    AIDS cholangiopathy
    Parasites

AIDS = acquired immunodeficiency syndrome.

hyperbilirubinemia. Impaired hepatic uptake at the sinusoidal membrane occurs in Gilbert syndrome. Reduced activity of uridine diphosphate (UDP) glucuronyl transferase leads to impaired bilirubin conjugation and is seen in patients with Gilbert and Crigler-Najjar (types I and II) syndromes.

Diagnosis

History and Physical Examination. A thorough medical history and a physical examination directed toward signs, symptoms, and the identifying of risk factors for liver disease remain very important tools for reaching an accurate diagnosis of jaundice. Age, history of alcohol use, family history of liver disease; history of blood transfusions, intravenous drug use, tattoos, travel, body piercing; medication history, surgical history, history of exposure to others with liver disease; and history of pain, fever, anorexia, weight loss, and pruritis are all items of information that should be sought. The physical findings to look for are outlined in the above section on the clinical manifestations. Clinical evaluation in conjunction with routine laboratory tests can correctly distinguish between intra- and extrahepatic causes of liver disease with an 85 to 90% accuracy.[181,182]

Laboratory Tests. Essential laboratory studies include measurements of serum total and fractionated bilirubin, aspartate and alanine transaminases (AST and ALT), alkaline phosphatase, albumin, and prothrombin time. Patients are considered to have conjugated bilirubinemia if > 50% of the total bilirubin is conjugated. Transminase levels > 400 IU generally indicate hepatocellular injury; levels > 1,000 IU usually indicate ischemic liver injury or acute hepatitis. A pattern of increased alkaline phosphatase that is 2 to 3 times normal and transaminase levels of < 300 IU usually indicate extrahepatic cholestasis. Conversely, if alkaline phosphatase is normal, extrahepatic obstruction is unlikely.[183] In infiltrative diseases such as sarcoidosis, amyloidosis, and tumor metastases, alkaline phosphatase is generally elevated out of proportion to serum bilirubin.

Abdominal Ultrasonography. Ultrasonography is a very useful modality for the evaluation of hepatobiliary disease. It determines the caliber of the ductal system and reveals intra- and extrahepatic mass lesions. The major advantages of ultrasonography are that it is noninvasive, portable, and relatively inexpensive. Its major disadvantages are that it is operator dependent and that its images are difficult to interpret in obese patients and in patients with overlying bowel gas. Ultrasonography has a sensitivity of 71% for delineating the level of obstruction and a sensitivity of 57% for delineating the level of obstruction. It detects choledocholithiasis in 32% of patients with that condition.[184] Ultrasonography should be the initial radiologic test in the evaluation of otherwise healthy patients with suspected biliary obstruction and should guide further radiologic evaluation.

Computed Tomography of the Abdomen. The major advantages of CT are that it is not hindered by obesity or by bowel gas patterns, it is not operator dependent, and it is generally more sensitive and specific than ultrasonography in diagnosing extrahepatic biliary obstruction.[185] The disadvantages include expense, nonportability, and the requirement of intravenous contrast. Computed tomography is not as accurate as ultrasonography for diagnosing cholelithiasis because only calcified stones are imaged.

Endoscopic Retrograde Cholangiopancreatography and Percutaneous Transhepatic Cholangiography. Endoscopic retrograde cholangiopancreatography (ERCP) and percutaneous transhepatic cholangiography (PTC) permit direct visualization of the biliary and pancreatic ducts and are highly sensitive and specific (99%) for detecting obstructive disease. Both modalities also can identify the site and character of obstruction in 90% of patients.[186] A normal cholangiogram essentially rules out extrahepatic obstruction.[187] The estimated complication rate is less than 10% with ERCP and 15 to 30% with PTC. The technical success of ERCP is greater than 90%, but the technique fails when the ampulla of Vater cannot be cannulated. Under conditions in which the level of biliary obstruction is proximal to the common hepatic duct, PTC is potentially advantageous. However, PTC may be technically limited in the absence of dilatation of the intrahepatic biliary ducts and may be unsuccessful in up to 25% of patients.[188] Both ERCP and PTC are more expensive than the noninvasive studies discussed above.

Liver Biopsy. Liver biopsy is the gold standard for detecting hepatocellular disease, but it is not always required. It is best used for patients with undiagnosed persistent jaundice. In suspected obstructive jaundice, if the ERCP is negative, one should proceed with a liver biopsy. Liver biopsy has low complication rate (mainly perforation and bleeding), a morbidity rate of < 0.5%, and a mortality rate of 0.1%.

Other Diagnostic Imaging Modalities. Biliary scintigraphy (hepatobiliary iminodiacetic acid [HIDA] scan) is an excellent modality for assessing the patency of the cystic duct but is not generally helpful in distinguishing intra- from extrahepatic jaundice. Magnetic resonance cholangiopancreatography (MRCP) is another promising noninvasive tool for assessing the biliary tree. Although promising as an imaging modality, it is expensive, and it is therefore unclear whether it will supplant abdominal ultrasonography or CT as the initial test of choice. While this procedure is safer than ERCP or PTC, it lacks therapeutic capabilities. At this time, the precise role of MRCP is being defined and is a subject of debate.

Treatment

Biliary Obstruction. Biliary obstruction can be managed by endoscopic (ERCP), radiologic (PTC), or surgical approaches. The choice of procedure or approach depends upon the likely etiology and site of obstruction. Common bile duct strictures and stones or even hilar strictures and extrinsic compression are best managed by means of therapeutic endoscopic interventions such as sphincterotomy, balloon dilatation of strictures, and stent placement. Interventional radiology is more suitable for focal intrahepatic strictures. Surgery is best

reserved for mass lesions that are resectable. In patients who have signs and symptoms of ascending cholangitis, intravenous antibiotics should be given initially, and intervention should be arranged urgently to decompress the biliary tree. Two different kinds of stents—plastic biliary stents and self-expandable metal stents (SEMS)—are available for endoscopic biliary decompression. Plastic stents have a median patency of only 3 to 4 months because they get blocked as a result of bacterial colonization and sludge formation[189] whereas SEMS are used mainly for palliation of malignant biliary obstruction in unresectable cases and have a median patency of 6 to 10 months.[190] To reduce the risk of septic complications after both surgical and nonsurgical intervention, antibiotics are given prophylactically. The duration of antibiotic therapy after the said treatment depends on whether there are signs of sepsis and the adequacy of drainage.

Pruritis. Pruritis usually disappears or is much improved within 24 to 48 hours after biliary drainage. Cholestyramine is particularly valuable for itching that is associated with primary biliary cirrhosis, primary sclerosing cholangitis, and biliary stricture. One sachet (4 gm) is usually given immediately before meals so as to coincide with the delivery of the food to the duodenum. The usual maintenance dose is 12 g per day. The most common side effects are nausea and constipation.

Other drugs that have variable effects on itching are antihistamines, ursodeoxycholic acid, and phenobarbital.

Summary

A careful history and physical examination can distinguish intra- from extrahepatic liver disease in most cases. Further judicious use of laboratory and radiologic tests can help in the differential diagnosis and in deciding the appropriate type of intervention. The algorithm presented in Figure 9–1 can be used for clinical decision making.

ASCITES

Malignant ascites is relatively uncommon but can occur in patients with colon, pancreatic, breast, and lung primaries with the development of peritoneal carcinomatosis.[191] The life expectancy of such patients is generally limited to weeks to months after the onset of ascites. Of the three major complications of liver cirrhosis (hepatic encephalopathy, ascites, and variceal hemorrhage), ascites is the most common.[192] The development of ascites in the natural history of chronic liver disease is an important landmark as approximately 50% of patients with ascites succumb in 2 years.[193]

Clinical Manifestations

The earliest evidence of ascites is an increase in abdominal girth accompanied by weight gain. Ascites is usually evi-

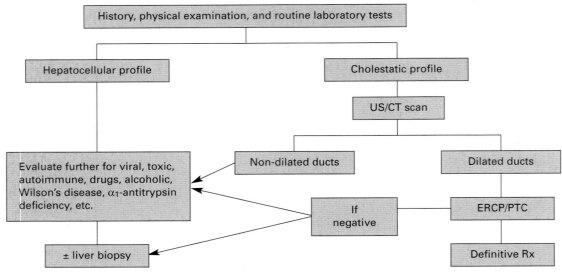

Figure 9–1. Algorithm for diagnosis in patients with jaundice. CT = computed tomography; ERCP = endoscopic retrograde cholangiopancreatography; PTC = percutaneous transhepatic cholangiography; Rx = treatment; US = ultrasonography.

dent on clinical evaluation, based on abdominal distension and flank dullness, and is frequently associated with leg edema. The presence of a full and bulging abdomen should lead to percussion of the flanks. If the flank dullness is found, then "shifting" should be checked for. Approximately 1,500 mL of fluid must be present to detect dullness.[194] In supine patients, sacral edema is an important clue. Pain accompanied by ascites suggests a malignant cause for fluid accumulation. Abdominal ultrasonography may be required to determine with certainty if fluid is present in the abdominal cavity. Ultrasonography can detect as little as 100 mL of fluid in the abdomen. About 4 to 10% of patients with ascites also develop pleural effusions, with two-thirds of the effusions being right-sided. Pleural fluid may be present with minimal or no ascites. Inguinal or umbilical hernias may accompany ascites.

Pathophysiologic Mechanisms

The pathogenesis of sodium retention and ascites formation remains controversial. One proposed theory is that a decrease in splanchnic and systemic vascular resistance leads to a reduction in the effective arterial blood volume. The patient with ascites has overall sodium and water retention and volume expansion. Peritoneal carcinomatoses cause ascites by the exudation of proteinaceous fluid from tumor cells lining the peritoneum.[191] Massive liver metastasis can cause ascites by portal hypertension. Tumor-induced portal vein thrombosis and underlying cirrhosis-related portal hypertension are also responsible for ascites in the patients with portal hypertension. Chylous ascites due to malignant lymphoma is caused by lymphatic obstruction.

Etiology

Malignancy should be suspected as a cause of ascites in patients with a history of cancer. Breast, lung, colon, and pancreatic primary malignancies are most commonly complicated by ascites.[191] Underlying liver disease is the cause of ascites formation in about 80% of cases. Approximately 5% of patients have "mixed" (ie, having two or more causes) ascites. For other causes of ascites, see Tables 9–9 and 9–10.

Diagnosis

A diagnosis of ascites is suspected on the basis of history and physical examination, but the final confirmation is based on successful abdominal paracentesis. The diagnosis of the cause of ascites is arrived at with a careful analysis of history, physical examination, and ascitic-fluid analysis. Radiologic and endoscopic procedures usually add little information in the initial evaluation of patients with ascites.

Sampling ascitic fluid in all patients with new-onset ascites is necessary. The practice of ordering every conceivable test on ascitic fluid is strongly discouraged as it can be very expensive and as it may be more confusing than helpful. A cell count with differential, albumin assessment (in addition to serum albumin), and culture in blood culture bottles should be the routine. Cytology of ascitic fluid is an important test in cancer patients. Total protein, glucose, lactate dehydrogenase (LDH), amylase, and Gram's stain tests are optional. A few other tests (eg, tuberculosis smear and culture; tests for triglyceride and bilirubin) should be ordered in the proper clinical setting.

TABLE 9–9. Subtypes of Malignancy-Related Ascites

Subtype	Prevalence (%)
Peritoneal carcinomatosis alone	53.3
Massive liver metastasis alone	13.3
Peritoneal carcinomatosis and massive liver metastasis	13.3
Hepatocellular carcinoma with portal hypertension	13.3
Malignant chylous ascites	6.7

Reproduced with permission from Runyon BA, Hoefs JC, Morgan TR. Ascitic fluid analysis in malignancy related ascites. Hepatology 1988;8:1104.

Non-neutrophilic ascitic fluid is transparent and slightly yellow to amber. The opacity of most cloudy fluid specimens is caused by neutrophils. Bloody ascites may result from traumatic tap or from ascites secondary to hepatocellular carcinoma or peritoneal carcinomatosis. Black ascites may indicate malignant melanoma. Dark brown ascitic fluid may indicate biliary perforation or leak. The upper limit of an absolute polymorphonuclear leukocyte (PMN) count in uncomplicated cirrhotic ascitic fluid is usually 250/mm^3. Any inflammatory process can result in an elevated ascitic-fluid white blood cell (WBC) count. Spontaneous bacterial peritonitis (SBP) is the most frequent cause of an increased WBC count with PMN predominance. Tuberculous peritonitis and peritoneal carcinomatosis give rise to an increased WBC count but with lymphocyte predominance. The serum-ascites albumin gradient (SAAG) has been proved in multiple studies to categorize ascites better than the total protein concentration (transudate/exudate) and other parameters. The difference between the serum and ascitic-fluid albumin concentrations correlates directly with portal pressure.[195] The calculation of the SAAG involves measuring the albumin concentration of serum and ascitic-fluid specimens and subtracting (it is not a ratio) the ascitic-fluid value from the serum value. The serum albumin is nearly always the largest value, barring laboratory error. A SAAG of > 1.1 g/dL is diagnostic of portal hypertension, with 97% accuracy.[196] Conversely, if the SAAG is < 1.1 g/dL, the patient does not have portal hypertension (with 97% accuracy). If the first value is borderline, a repeat paracentesis and analysis is usually definitive. Different causes of ascites can be classified according to whether the associated SAAG is high or low (see Table 9–10).

Ascitic-fluid culture should be done in blood culture bottles, with bedside inoculation of the bottles. Routine cultures have been found to detect bacterial growth in approximately 50% of neutrophilic samples whereas bedside inoculation of blood culture bottles with ascitic fluid detects growth in approximately 80% of cases.[197] A Gram's stain of ascitic fluid is almost never helpful except in the diagnosis of free perforation of the gut with ascites formation, when sheets of many different bacteria can be seen. Ascitic-fluid culture for mycobacteria has a 50% sensitivity; in contrast, laparoscopy with histology and culture of peritoneal biopsy specimens is approximately 100% sensitive in detecting tuberculous peritonitis. Hepatoma, massive liver metastases, and malignant lymphoma causing ascites by lymphatic obstruction, are generally not associated with positive cytology. Positive cytology of ascitic fluid for malignant cells should only be expected in cases with peritoneal carcinomatoses. Chylous ascites has a high triglyceride concentration, usually higher than the serum. A triglyceride level should be obtained routinely in the presence of milky ascitic fluid. An ascitic-fluid bilirubin level greater than the serum level of bilirubin suggests a bile leak into the ascitic fluid.

Treatment

The serum-ascites albumin gradient can be very helpful diagnostically, as well as in therapeutic decision making. Patients with low-SAAG ascites (malignant ascites falls into this category) usually do not have portal hypertension and do not respond to salt restriction or to diuretics[198] except in cases of nephrotic syndrome. The mainstay of the treatment of non-ovarian (lung, breast, colon, and pancreatic) peritoneal carcinomatosis is outpatient therapeutic paracentesis as these patients usually live for only a few weeks to months. Patients with an ovarian malignancy may respond well to surgical debulking and chemotherapy. Antituberculous therapy is the mainstay of treatment for tuberculous ascites. High-SAAG ascites usually responds well to diuretics and measures for maintaining sodium balance. Fluid loss and weight change are directly related to sodium balance. It is sodium restriction, not fluid restriction, that results in weight loss; fluid follows sodium passively. A realistic dietary sodium restriction of 2 g per day (= 2,000 mg/d

TABLE 9–10. Classification of Ascites by Serum-Ascites Albumin Gradient

High Gradient (≥ 1.1 g/dL)
    Cirrhosis
    Alcoholic hepatitis
    Cardiac ascites
    Massive liver metastases
    Budd-Chiari syndrome
    Veno-occlusive disease
    Mixed ascites
Low Gradient (< 1.1 g/dL)
    Peritoneal carcinomatosis
    Tuberculous peritonitis
    Pancreatic ascites
    Nephrotic syndrome

Adapted from Gastroenterology and hepatology: MKSAP. 2nd ed. American College of Physicians; 1997.

= 88 mmol/d) should be the goal. Fluid restriction is not necessary when treating most patients who have cirrhotic ascites. The chronic hyponatremia that is usually seen in patients with cirrhotic ascites is seldom morbid. Severe hyponatremia (eg, serum sodium < 120 mmol/L) does warrant fluid restriction in these patients.

Spironolactone is the mainstay of the treatment of cirrhotic ascites. It is slow to increase natriuresis, usually requiring about 2 weeks to take effect.[199] Single-agent spironolactone is recommended for patients with minimal fluid overload. Single-agent furosemide has been shown in a randomized controlled trial to be less efficacious than spironolactone.[200] Single daily doses are most appropriate and enhance compliance. The usual diuretic regimen consists of single morning doses of oral spironolactone (100 mg) and furosemide (40 mg). If this combination is ineffective in increasing urinary sodium or in decreasing body weight, the doses of both drugs should be simultaneously increased as needed (eg, 200 and 80 mg, 300 and 120 mg, 400 and 160 mg maximum, respectively). The 100:40 ratio of spironolactone to furosemide in the daily doses usually maintains normokalemia. The use of diuretic therapy is not without complications. Electrolyte abnormalities and intravascular volume contraction leading to prerenal azotemia can precipitate hepatic encephalopathy in the susceptible patient. The monitoring of electrolytes, renal function, blood pressure, weight, and mental status is necessary. This approach is effective in controlling ascites in 90% of patients.

About 10% of patients with cirrhotic ascites are refractory to standard medical treatment with diuretics and salt and fluid restrictions. Patients who cannot tolerate diuretics because of complications are also regarded as having refractory ascites. Large-volume paracentesis is safe and effective for the treatment of refractory ascites. The incidences of hyponatremia, hypotension, hepatic encephalopathy, and renal impairment are lower for patients treated with paracentesis than for those treated with diuretics. The use of volume expanders during paracentesis has been a controversial issue. The current recommendations are that a volume expander may be unnecessary for a paracentesis of < 5 L but should be considered when large-volume paracentesis is repeatedly performed. Peritoneovenous shunting has fallen out of favor due to excessive complications and poor patency rates. Transjugular intrahepatic portal systemic shunts (TIPS) can also be considered in patients with refractory ascites. Finally, liver transplantation is the only lifesaving therapy for all patients who present with refractory ascites and severe liver dysfunction in the absence of underlying malignancy. Patients with ascitic-fluid PMN counts of ≥ 250 cells/mm^3 or with PMN counts of < 250 cells/mm^3 with signs and symptoms suggestive of infection (temperature > 100°F; abdominal pain or tenderness) should receive empiric antibiotic therapy.

Summary

The development of ascites in the natural history of liver disease is an important landmark as 50% of patients succumb to their disease at the end of 2 years after the onset of ascites. The characteristics of ascitic fluid and the treatment of ascites depend on the pathophysiology of ascites formation. The concept of low SAAG and high SAAG enables clinicians to diagnose causes of ascites with greater accuracy and to direct the appropriate treatment. In the setting of portal hypertension, dietary sodium restriction and diuretics are the mainstay of treatment in the majority of patients, although a few patients require frequent large-volume paracentesis and TIPS. Orthotopic liver transplantation should be considered early rather than late in the course of nonmalignant liver disease once ascites develops. For malignant ascites, large-volume paracentesis is recommended; timing and frequency are dictated by the patient's symptoms.

The authors wish to thank Nagla Karim, MD, for her contributions to the section on nausea and vomiting.

REFERENCES

1. Twycross R, Back I. Nausea and vomiting in advanced cancer. Eur J Palliat Care 1998;5:39–45.
2. Davis MP, Walsh D. Treatment of nausea and vomiting in advanced cancer. Support Care Cancer 2000;8:444–52.
3. Griffin AM, Butow PN, Coastes AS, et al. On the receiving end. V: Patient perceptions of the side effects of cancer chemotherapy in 1993. Ann Oncol 1996;7:189–95.
4. Lembersky BC, Ramesh K, Ramanathan RK. Gastrointestinal toxicities. In: Current cancer therapeutics. 3rd ed. 1998. p. 362–74.
5. Morrow GR. Prevalence and correlates of anticipatory nausea and vomiting in chemotherapy patients. J Natl Cancer Inst 1982;68:585–8.
6. Loprinzi CL, Alberts SR, Christensen BJ, et al. History of the development of antiemetic guidelines at Mayo Clinic Rochester. Mayo Clin Proc 2000; 75:303–9.
7. Gralla RJ, Itri LM, Pisko SE, et al. Antiemetic efficacy of high dose metoclopramide: randomized trials with placebo and prochlorperazine in patients with chemotherapy-induced nausea and vomiting. N Engl J Med 1981;305:905–9.
8. Allen JC, Gralla R, Reily L, et al. Metoclopramide: dose-related toxicity and preliminary antiemetic studies in children receiving cancer chemotherapy. J Clin Oncol 1985; 3:1136–41.
9. Balfour JA, Goa KL. Dolasetron: a review of its pharmacology and therapeutic potential in the management of nausea and vomiting induced by chemotherapy, radiotherapy or surgery. Drugs 1997;54:273–98.

10. Abbott B, Ippoliti C, Bruton J, et al. Antiemetic efficacy of granisetron plus dexamethasone in bone marrow transplant patients receiving chemotherapy and total body irradiation. Bone Marrow Transplant 1999;23:265–9.

11. Lacerda JF, Martins C, Carmo JA, et al. Randomized trial of ondansetron, granisetron, and tropisetron in the prevention of acute nausea and vomiting. Transplant Proc 2000;32:2680–1.

12. Scarantino CW, Ornitz RD, Hoffman LG, Anderson RF Jr. Radiation induced emesis: effects of ondansetron. Semin Oncol 1992;19(6 Suppl 15):38–43.

13. Borison HL, Borison R, McCarthey LE. Role of the area postrema in vomiting and related functions. Fed Proc 1984;43:2955–8.

14. Borison HL. Area postrema: chemoreceptor circumentricular organ of the medulla oblongata. Prog Neurobiol 1989;32:351–90.

15. Gonzales-Rosales F, Walsh D. Intractable nausea and vomiting due to gastrointestinal mucosal metastases relieved tetra hydrocannabinol (Dronabinol). J Pain Symptom Manage 1997;14:311–4.

16. Navari R, Hesketh P, Grote T, et al. A double blind, randomized, comparative IV study of single dose dolasetron vs. ondansetron in preventing cisplatin-related emesis. Proc Am Soc Clin Oncol 1995;14:522.

17. Grunberg SM, Gala KV, Lampenfeld M, et al. Comparison of the antiemetic effect of high-dose intravenous metoclopramide and high-dose intravenous haloperidol in a randomized double-blind cross over study. J Clin Oncol 1984;2:782–7.

18. Twycross R, Wilcock A, Thorp S, editors. Palliative care formulary 1998. Oxford: Radcliffe Medical Press; 1998.

19. Axelrod R. Antiemetic therapy. Comp Ther 1997;23:539–45.

20. Bateman D, Croft A, Nicholson E, Pearson A. Dystonic reactions and the pharmacokinetics of metoclopramide in chlidren. Br J Clin Pharmacol 1983;15:557–9.

21. Bruera E, Roca E, Cedaro L. Improved control of chemotherapy-induced emesis by the addition of dexamethazone to metoclopramide. Cancer Treat Rep 83:1214–23.

22. DiLoreenzo C, Lucanto C, Flores AF, et al. Effect of sequential erythromycin and octreotide on antroduodenal manometry. J Pediatr Gastroenterol Nutr 1999;23:293–6.

23. Gardner C, Armour D, Beattie D, et al. GR205171: a novel antagonist with high affinity for the tachkinin NK1 receptor, and potent broad-spectrum antiemetic activity. Regul Pept 1996;65:45–53.

24. Diemunsch P, Schoeffler P, Bryssine B, et al. Antiemetic activity of NK1 receptor antagonist Gr205171 in the treatment of established postoperative nausea and vomiting after major gynecological surgery. Br J Anaesth 1999;82:274–6.

25. Kris MG, Gralla RJ, Tyson LB, et al. Controlling delayed vomiting: double blind randomised trial comparing placebo dexamethazone alone and metoclopramide plus dexamethazone in patients receiving cisplatin. J Clin Oncol 1992;7:1012–6.

26. Boley SJ, Agarwal GP, Warren AR, et al. Pathophysiologic effects of bowel distension on intestinal blood flow. Am J Surg 1969;117:228–34.

27. Heneghan JB, Robinson JW, Menge H, Winistorfer B. Intestinal obstruction in germ-free dogs. Eur J Clin Invest 1981;11:285–90.

28. Shields R. The absorption and secretion of fluid and electrolytes by the obstructed bowel. Br J Surg 1965;52:774–9.

29. Mucha P. Small intestinal obstruction. Surg Clin North Am 1987;67:597–620.

30. Dunn JT, Halls JM, Berne TV. Roentgenographic contrast studies in acute small bowel obstruction. Arch Surg 1984;119:1305–8.

31. Lo AM, Evans WE, Carey LC. Review of SBO at Milwaukee County General Hospital. Am J Surg 1966;111:884–7.

32. Balthazar EJ. CT of SBO. AJR Am J Roentgenol 1994;162:255–61.

33. Mainar A, Ariza MA, Tejero E, et al. Acute colorectal obstruction: treatment with self-expandable metal stents before scheduled surgery—results of a multicenter study. Radiology 1999;210:65–9.

34. Saunders MD, Kimmey MB. Acute colonic pseudoobstruction. Clin Perspective Gastroenterol 2000;3:156–62.

35. Ponec R, Saunders MD, Kimmey MB. Neostigmine for the treatment of acute colonic pseudo-obstruction. N Engl J Med 1999;341:137–41.

36. Winters WL, Egan S. The incidence of hemorrhage occurring with perforation in peptic ulcer. JAMA 1938;113:2199–204.

37. Albo R, Delorimier AA, Silen W. Spontaneous rupture of the stomach in the adult. Surgery 1963;53:797.

38. Parker GJ. The radiology of perforated esophagus. Clin Radiol 1973;24:324–32.

39. Miller RE, Nelson SW. The roentgenographic demonstration of tiny amounts of free intraperitoneal gas: experimental and clinical studies. AJR Am J Roentgenol 1971;112:574–85.

40. Boey J, Choi SK, Poon A, Alagaratnam TT. Risk stratification in perforated duodenal ulcers. A prospective validation of predictive factors. Ann Surg 1987;205:22–6.

41. Baehr PH, McDonald GB. Esophageal disorders caused by infection, systemic illness, medications, radiation, and trauma. In: Feldman M, Scharschmidt BF, Sleisenger MH, editors. Sleisenger and Fordtran gastrointestinal disease. 6th ed. Philadelphia: W.B. Saunders Company; 1997. p. 519–39.

42. Otero Lopez-Dubero S, Sale GE, McDonald GB. Acute graft-versus-host disease of the esophagus. Endoscopy 1997;29:535–6.

43. Goodman JL, Winston DJ, Greenfield RA, et al. A controlled trial of fluconazole to prevent fungal infections in patients undergoing bone marrow transplantation. N Engl J Med 1992;326:845–51.

44. Goodrich JM, Mori M, Gleaves CA, et al. Early treatment with ganciclovir to prevent cytomegalovirus disease after allogenic bone marrow transplantation. N Engl J Med 1991;325:1601–7.

45. Silverstein FE, Tytgat GNJ. Gastrointestinal endoscopy. 3rd ed. London: Mosby-Wolfe; 1997.

46. Wilcox CM, Alexander LN, Clark WS, Thompson SE 3rd. Fluconazole compared with endoscopy for human

immunodeficiency virus-infected patients with esophageal symptoms. Gastroenterology 1996;110: 1803–9.

47. Spencer GD, Hackman RC, McDonald GB, et al. A prospective study of unexplained nausea and vomiting after marrow transplantation. Transplantation 1986; 42:602–7.

48. McDonald GB, Sharma P, Hackman RC, et al. Esophageal infections in immunosuppressed patients after marrow transplantation. Gastroenterology 1985;88:1111–7.

49. McBane RD, Gross JB Jr. Herpes esophagitis: clinical syndrome, endoscopic appearance, and diagnosis in 23 patients. Gastrointest Endosc 1991;37:600–3.

50. McDonald GB, Shulman HM, Sullivan KM, Spencer GD. Intestinal and hepatic complications of human bone marrow transplantation. Transplantation 1986;42:602–7.

51. Hackman RC, Wolford JL, Gleaves CA, et al. Recognition and rapid diagnosis of upper gastrointestinal *Cytomegalovirus* infection in marrow transplantation recipients. A comparison of seven virologic methods. Transplantation 1994;57:231–7.

52. Reed EC, Wolford JL, Dopecky KJ, et al. Ganciclovir for the treatment of *Cytomegalovirus* gastroenteritis in bone marrow transplantation patients. A randomized, placebo-controlled trial. Ann Intern Med 1990;112: 505–10.

53. Nelson MR, Connolly GM, Hawkins DA, Gazzard BG. Foscarnet in the treatment of *Cytomegalovirus* infection of the esophagus and colon in patients with the acquired immune deficiency syndrome. Am J Gastroenterol 1991;86:876–81.

54. Walsh TJ, Belitsos NJ, Hamilton SR. Bacterial esophagitis in immunocompromised patients. Arch Intern Med 1986;146:1345–9.

55. Maguire PD, Sibley GS, Zhou SM, et al. Clinical and dosimetric predictors of radiation-induced esophageal toxicity. Int J Radiat Oncol Biol Phys 1999;45:97–103.

56. Byhardt RW, Scott C, Sause WT, et al. Response, toxicity, failure patterns, and survival in five Radiation Therapy Oncology Group (RTOG) trials of sequential and/or concurrent chemotherapy and radiotherapy for locally advanced non-small-cell carcinoma of the lung. Int J Radiat Oncol Biol Phys 1998;42:469–78.

57. Choy H, LaPorte K, Knoll-Selby E, et al. Esophagitis in combined modality therapy for locally advanced non-small cell lung cancer. Semin Radiat Oncol 1999;9 (2 Suppl 1):90–6.

58. Ng TM, Spencer GM, Sargeant IR, et al. Management of strictures after radiotherapy for esophageal cancer. Gastrointest Endosc 1996;43:584–90.

59. Sullivan KM, Agura E, Anasetti C, et al. Chronic graft-versus-host disease and other late complications of bone marrow transplantation. Semin Hematol 1991;28: 249–58.

60. McDonald GB, Sullivan KM, Schuffler MD, et al. Esophageal abnormalities in chronic graft-versus-host disease in humans. Gastroenterology 1981;80:914–21.

61. Viner CV, Selby PJ, Zulian GB, et al. Ondansetron—a new safe and effective antiemetic in patients receiving high-dose melphelan. Cancer Chemother Pharmacol 1990; 25:449–53.

62. Spencer GD, Hackman RC, McDonald GB, et al. A prospective study of unexplained nausea and vomiting after marrow transplantation. Transplantation 1986; 42:602–7.

63. Shivshanker K, Chu DZ, Stroehlein JR, Nelson RS. Gastrointestinal hemorrhage in the cancer patient. Gastrointest Endosc 1983;29:873–8.

64. Zuckerman GR, Cort D, Shuman RB. Stress ulcer syndrome. J Intern Care Med 1988;3:21–14.

65. Wilcox CM, Spenney JG. Stress ulcer prophylaxis in medical patients: who, what and how much? Am J Gastroenterol 1988;83:1199–211.

66. Cook DJ, Reeve BK, Guyatt GH, et al. Stress ulcer prophylaxis in critically ill patients. Resolving discordant meta-analyses. JAMA 1996;275:308-14.

67. Kaur S, Cooper G, Gakult S, et al. Incidence and outcome of overt gastrointestinal bleeding in patients undergoing bone marrow transplantation. Dig Dis Sci 1996;41:598–603.

68. Laine L, Peterson W. Medical progress: bleeding peptic ulcer. New Engl J Med 1994;331:717–27.

69. Saperas E, Pique JM, Perez-Ayuso R, et al. Somatostatin compared with cimetidine in the treatment of bleeding peptic ulcer without visible vessel. Aliment Pharmacol Ther 1988;2:153–9.

70. Cleary RK. *Clostridium difficile*-associated diarrhea and colitis: clinical manifestations, diagnosis, and treatment. Dis Colon Rectum 1998;41:1435–49.

71. Fainstein V, Bodey GP, Fekety R. Relapsing pseudomembranous colitis associated with cancer chemotherapy. J Infect Dis 1981;143:865.

72. Cudmore MA, Silva J Jr, Fekety R, et al. *Clostridium difficile* colitis associated with cancer chemotherapy. Arch Intern Med 1982;142:333–5.

73. Anand A, Glatt AE. *Clostridium difficile* infection associated with antineoplastic chemotherapy: a review. Clin Infect Dis 1993;17:109–13.

74. Tedesco FJ. Pseudomembranous colitis: pathogenesis and therapy. Med Clin North Am 1982;66:655–64.

75. Tedesco FJ, Gordon D, Fortson WC. Approach to patients with multiple relapses of antibiotic-associated pseudomembranous colitis. Am J Gastroenterol 1985; 80:867–8.

76. Silva J, Fekety R. Clostridia and antimicrobial enterocolitis. Ann Rev Med 1981;32:327–33.

77. Taylor NS, Thorne G, Bartlett JG. Comparison of two toxins produced by *Clostridium difficile*. Infect Immun 1981;34:1036–43.

78. Bartlett JG. *Clostridium difficile*: history of its role as an enteric pathogen and the current state of knowledge about the organism. Clin Infect Dis 1994;18:S265.

79. Rybolt AH, Bennett RG, Laughon BE, et al. Protein-losing enteropathy associated with *Clostridium difficile* infection. Lancet 1989;1;1353–5.

80. George WL. Antimicrobial agent-associated colitis and diarrhea: historical background and clinical aspects. Rev Infect Dis 1984;6:S208–13.

81. George WL, Rolfe RD, Finegold SM. *Clostridium difficile*

and its cytotoxin in feces of patients with antimicrobial agent-associated diarrhea and miscellaneous conditions. J Clin Microbiol 1982;15:1049–53.

82. Mulligan ME. Epidemiology of *Clostridium difficile*-induced intestinal disease. Rev Infect Dis 1984;6:S222–8.

83. Miles BL, Siders JA, Allen SD. Evaluation of a commercial latex test for *Clostridium difficile* for reactivity with *C. difficile* and cross-reactions with other bacteria. J Clin Microbiol 1988;26:2452–5.

84. Teasley DG, Gerding DN, Olson MM, et al. Prospective, randomized trial of metronidazole versus vancomycin for *Clostridium difficile*-associated diarrhea and colitis. Lancet 1983;2:1043–6.

85. Fekety R, Silva J, Kauffman C, et al. Treatment of antibiotic-associated *Clostridium difficile* colitis with oral vancomycin: comparison of two dosage regimens. Am J Med 1989;86:15–9.

86. Bradley SJ, Weaver DW, Maxwell NP, Bouwman DL. Surgical management of pseudomembranous colitis. Am Surg 1988;54:329–32.

87. Alt B, Glass NR, Sollinger H. Neutropenic enterocolitis in adults. Am J Surg 1985;149:405–8.

88. Williams N, Scott ADN. Neutropenic colitis: a continuing surgical challenge. Br J Surg 1997;84:1200–5.

89. Dosik GM, Luna M, Valdivieso M, et al. Necrotizing colitis in patients with cancer. Am J Med 1979;67:646–56.

90. Sherman NJ, Woolley MM. The ileocecal syndrome in acute childhood leukemia. Arch Surg 1973;107:39–42.

91. Varki AP, Armitage JO, Feagler JR. Typhlitis in acute leukemia. Cancer 1979;43:695–7.

92. McNamara MJ, Chalmers AG, Morgan M, Smith SEW. Typhlitis in acute childhood leukaemia: radiological features. Clin Radiol 1986;37:83–6.

93. Meyerovitz MF, Fellows KE. Typhlitis: a cause of gastrointestinal hemorrhage in children. AJR Am J Roentgenol 1984;143:833–5.

94. Shamberger RC, Weinstein HJ, Delorey MJ, Levey RH. The medical and surgical management of typhlitis in children with acute nonlymphocytic (myelogenous) leukemia. Cancer 1986;57:603–9.

95. Wagner ML, Rosenberg HS, Fernbach DJ, Singleton EB. Typhlitis: a complication of leukemia in childhood. Am J Roentgenol Rad Ther Nucl Med 1970;109:341–50.

96. Keidan RD, Fanning J, Gatenby RA, Weese JL. Recurrent typhlitis. A disease resulting from aggressive chemotherapy. Dis Colon Rectum 1989;32:206–9.

97. Matolo NM, Garfinkle SE, Wolfman EF Jr. Intestinal necrosis and perforation in patients receiving immunosuppressive drugs. Am J Surg 1976;132:753–4.

98. Ryan ME, Morrissey JF. Typhlitis complicating methimazole-induced agranulocytosis. Gastrointest Endosc 1983;29:299–302.

99. Katz JA, Wagner ML, Gresik MV, et al. Typhlitis. An 18-year experience and postmortem review. Cancer 1990;65:1041–7.

100. King A, Rampling A, Wight DG, Warren RE. Neutropenic enterocolitis due to *Clostridium septicum* infection. J Clin Pathol 1984;37:335–43.

101. Frick MP, Maile CW, Crass JR, et al. Computed tomogra-phy of neutropenic colitis. AJR Am J Roentgenol 1984;143:763–5.

102. Slavin RE, Dias MA, Saral R. Cytosine arabinoside induced gastrointestinal toxic alterations in sequential chemotherapeutic protocols. A clinico-pathologic study of 33 patients. Cancer 1978;42:1747–59.

103. Dworkin B, Winawer SJ, Lightdale CJ. Typhlitis. Report of a case with long-term survival and a review of the recent literature. Dig Dis Sci 1981;26:1032–7.

104. Gootenberg JE, Abbondanzo SL. Rapid diagnosis of neutropenic enterocolitis (typhlitis) by ultrasonography. Am J Pediatr Hematol Oncol 1987;9:222–7.

105. McNamara MJ, Chalmers AG, Morgan M, Smith SE. Typhlitis in acute childhood leukaemia: radiological features. Clin Radiol 1986;37:83–6.

106. Musher DR, Amorosi EL, Gouge T, et al. Neutropenic typhlitis simulating carcinoma of the cecum. Gastrointest Endosc 1989;35:449–51.

107. Del Fava RL, Cronin TG Jr. Typhlitis complicating leukemia in an adult: barium enema findings. AJR Am J Roentgenol 1977;129:347–8.

108. Kingry RL, Hobson RW, Muir RW. Cecal necrosis and perforation with systemic chemotherapy. Am Surg 1973;39:129–33.

109. Garewal HS, Dalton WS. Metoclopramide in vincristine-induced ileus. Cancer Treat Rep 1985;69:1309–11.

110. Ogilvie H. Large intestine colic due to sympathetic deprivation: a new clinical syndrome. BMJ 1948;2:671–3.

111. Laine L. Management of acute colonic pseudo-obstruction. New Engl J Med 1999;341:192–3.

112. Johnson CD, Rice CP, Kelvin FM, et al. The radiologic evaluation of gross cecel distension: emphasis on cecal ileus. AJR Am J Roentgenol 1985;145:1211–4.

113. Vanek VW, Al-Salti M. Acute pseudo-obstruction of the colon (Ogilvieís syndrome): an analysis of 400 cases. Dis Colon Rectum 1986;29:203–10.

114. Fausel CS, Goff JS. Nonoperative management of acute idiopathic colonic pseudoobstruction (Ogilvieís syndrome). West J Med 1985;43:50–6.

115. Bachulis BL, Smith PE. Pseudoobstruction of the colon. Am J Surg 1985;149:405–9.

116. Nanni G, Carbini A, Luchetti P, et al. Ogilvieís syndrome (acute colonic pseudoobstruction of the colon). Am J Surg 1985;149:405–9.

117. Sloyer AF, Panella VS, Demas BE, Shike M, et al. Ogilvieís syndrome: successful management without colonoscopy. Dig Dis 1988;33:1391–6.

118. Rex DK. Colonoscopy and acute colonic pseudoobstruction. Gastrointest Endosc Clin N Am 1997;7:499–508.

119. Dorudi S, Berry AR, Kettlewell MG. Acute colonic pseudo-obstruction. Br J Surg 1992;89:88–103.

120. Anuras S, Shirazi SS. Colonic pseudoobstruction. Am J Gastroenterol 1984;79:525–30.

121. Smit JM, Mulder NH, Sleijfer DT, et al. Evaluation of gastrointestinal toxicity following cytostatic chemotherapy. J Cancer Res Clin Oncol 1996;111:59–61.

122. Ikuno N, Soda H, Watanabe M, et al. Irinotecan (CPT-11) and characteristic mucosal changes in the mouse ileum and cecum. J Natl Cancer Inst 1995;87:1876–83.

123. The Meta-Analysis Group in Cancer. Toxicity of fluo-

rouracil in patients with advanced colorectal cancer:effect of administration schedule and prognostic factors. J Clin Oncol 1998;16:3537–41.

124. Grem JL, Shoemaker DD, Petrelli NJ, Douglass HO Jr. Severe and fatal toxic effects observed in treatment with high-and low-dose leucovorin plus 5-fluorouracil for colorectal carcinoma. Cancer Treat Rep 1987;71:1122.

125. Stein BN, Petrelli NJ, Douglass HO, et al. Age and sex are independent predictors of 5-fluorouracil toxicity. Cancer 1995;75:11–7.

126. Kris MG, Gralla RJ, Clark RA, et al. Control of chemotherapy-induced diarrhea with the synthetic enkephalin BW942C: a randomized trial with placebo in patients receiving cisplatin. J Clin Oncol 1998;6:663–8.

127. Bleiberg H, Cvitkovic E. Characterization and clinical management of CPT-11 (irinotecan)-induced adverse events: the European perspective. Eur J Cancer 1996; 32A:S18–23.

128. Shimada Y, Yoshino M, Wakui A, et al. Phase II study of CPT-11, a new camptothecin derivative, in metastatic colorectal cancer. J Clin Oncol 1993;11:909–13.

129. Cunningham D, Pyrhbnen S, James R, et al. Randomized trial of irinotecan plus supportive care versus supportive care alone after fluorouracil failure for patients with metastatic colorectal cancer. Lancet 1998;352:1413–8.

130. Petrelli NJ, Douglass HO Jr, Herrera L, et al. The modulation of fluorouracil with leucovorin in metastatic carcinoma: a prospective randomized phase III trial. J Clin Oncol 1989;7:1419–26.

131. Abigerges D, Chabot GG, Armand J-P, et al. Phase I and pharmacologic studies of the camptothecin analog irinotecan administered every 3 weeks in cancer patients. J Clin Oncol 1995;13:210–21.

132. Kudoh S, Fukuoka M, Masuda N, et al. Relationship between the pharmacokinetics of irinotecan and diarrhea during combination chemotherapy with cisplatin. Jpn J Cancer Res 1995;86:406–13.

133. Rothenberg ML, Meropol NJ, Poplin EA, et al. Mortality associated with irinotecan plus bolus fluorouracil/leucovorin: summary findings of an independent panel. J Clin Oncol 2001;19:3801–7.

134. Sargent DJ, Niedzwiecki D, O'Connell MJ, Schilsky RL. Recommendation for caution with irinotecan, fluorouracil, and leucovorin for colorectal cancers. N Eng J Med 2001;345:144–5.

135. Palmer KR, Corbett CL, Holdsworth CD. Double-blind cross-over study comparing loperamide, codeine, and diphenoxylate in the treatment of chronic diarrhea. Gastroenterology 1980;79:1272–5.

136. O'Connell MJ, Martenson JA, Wieand HS, et al. Improving adjuvant therapy for rectal cancer by combining protracted-infusion fluorouracil with radiation therapy after curative surgery. N Engl J Med 1994;331:502–7.

137. Slavin RE, Dias MA, Saral R. Cytosine arabinoside induced gastrointestinal toxic alterations in sequential chemotherapeutic protocols: a clinical-pathologic study of 33 patients. Cancer 1978;42:1747–59.

138. Schiffman KS, Bensinger WI, Appelbaum FR, et al. Phase II study of high-dose busulfan, melphalan and thiotepa with autologous peripheral blood stem cell support in patients with malignant disease. Bone Marrow Transplant 1996;17:943–50.

139. McDonald GB, Shulman HM, Sullivan KM, Spencer GD. Intestinal and hepatic complications of human bone marrow transplantation. Gastroenterology 1986;90: 460–77, 770–84.

140. Slattery JT, Kalhorn TF, McDonald GB, et al. Conditioning regimen-dependent disposition of cyclophosphamide and hydroxycyclophosphamide in human marrow transplantation patients. J Clin Oncol 1996;14:1484–94.

141. Gouyette A, Hartmann O, Pico JL. Phamacokinetics of high-dose melphalan in children and adults. Cancer Chemother Pharmacol 1986;16:184–9.

142. Epstein RJ, McDonald GB, Sale GE, et al. The diagnostic accuracy of the rectal biopsy in graft-versus-host disease: a prospective study of thirteen patients. Gastroenterology 1980;78:764–91.

143. Ponec RL, Hackman RC, McDonald GB. Endoscopic and histologic diagnosis of intestinal graft-versus-host disease after marrow transplantation. Gastrointest Endosc 1999;49:612–21.

144. Cox GJ, Matsui SM, Lo RS, et al. Etiology and outcome of diarrhea after marrow transplantation: a prospective study. Gastroenterology 1994;107:1398–407.

145. Martin PJ, Schoch G, Fisher L, et al. A retrospective analysis of therapy for acute graft-versus-host disease: initial treatment. Blood 1990;76:1464–72.

146. Weisdorf SA, Salati LM, Longsdorf JA, et al. Graft-vs-host disease of the intestine: a protein-losing enteropathy characterized by fecal alpha1-antitrypsin. Gastroenterology 1983;85:1076–81.

147. Einsele H, Ehninger G, Hebart H, et al. Incidence of local CMV infection and acute intestinal GVHD in marrow transplantation recipients with severe diarrhoea. Bone Marrow Transplant 1994;14:955–63.

148. Roy J, Snover DC, Weisdorf S, et al. Simultaneous upper and lower endoscopic biopsy in the diagnosis of intestinal graft-vs-host disease. Transplantation 1991;51:642–6.

149. Spencer GI, Shulman HM, Myerson D, et al. Diffuse intestinal ulceration after marrow transplantation: a clinical-pathological study of 13 patients. Hum Pathol 1986;17:621–33.

150. McDonald GB, Sale GE. The human gastrointestinal tract after allogenic marrow transplantation. In: Sale GE, Shulman HM, editors. The pathology of bone marrow transplantation. New York: Masson; 1984. p. 77–103.

151. Saito H, Oshimi K, Nagasako K, et al. Endoscopic appearance of the colon and small intestine of a patient with hemorrhagic enteric graft versus host disease. Dis Colon Rectum 1990;33:695–7.

152. Maile CW, Frick MP, Crass JR, et al. The plain radiograph in acute intestinal graft-versus-host disease. AJR Am J Roentgenol 1985;145:289–92.

153. Jones B, Fishman EK, Kramer SS, et al. Computed tomography of gastrointestinal inflammation after marrow transplantation. AJR Am J Roentgenol 1986;146:691–6.

154. Fisk JID, Shulman HM, Greening RR, et al. Gastrointestinal radiographic features of human graft versus-host disease. AJR Am J Roentgenol 1981;136:277–81.

155. Mowat A. Intestinal graft-versus-host disease. In: Ferrara JLM, Deeg HJ, Burakoff SJ, editors. Graft-vs-host disease. 2nd ed. New York: Marcel Dekker; 1997. p. 337–84.

156. Suzuki M, Suzuki Y, Ikeda H, et al. Apoptosis of murine large intestine in acute graft-versus-host disease after allogenic bone marrow transplantation across minor histocompatibility barriers. Transplantation 1994;57:1284–7.

157. Snover DC, Weisdorf SA, Vercellotti GM, et al. A histopathologic study of gastric and small intestine graft-versus-host disease following allogeneic bone marrow transplantation. Hum Pathol 1985;16:387–92.

158. Washington K, Bentley RC, Green A, et al. Gastric graft-versus-host disease: a blinded histological study. Am J Surg Pathol 1997;21:1037–46.

159. Ely P, Dunitz J, Rogosheske J, et al. Use of a somatostatin analogue, octreotide acetate, in the management of acute gastrointestinal graft-versus-host disease. Am J Med 1991;90:707–10.

160. Bianco JA, Higano C, Singe J, et al. The somatostatin analog octreotide in the management of the secretory diarrhea of acute intestinal gaft-versus-host disease in patients after bone marrow transplantation. Transplantation 1990;49:1194–5.

161. Singh C, Gooley T, McDonald GB. Octreotide treatment for secretary diarrhea caused by graft-vs.-host disease: a dose escalation study [abstract]. Gastroenterology 1996;110:A1016.

162. West JC, Armitage JO, Mitros FA, et al. *Cytomegalovirus* cecal erosion causing massive hemorrhage in a bone marrow transplantation recipient. World J Surg 1982;6:252–5.

163. Apperley JF, Goldman JM. *Cytomegalovirus*: biology, clinical features and methods for diagnosis. Bone Marrow Transplant 1988;3:253–64.

164. Lepinski SM, Hamilton JW. Isolated *Cytomegalovirus* ileitis detected by colonoscopy. Gastroenterology 1990;98:1704–6.

165. Hackman RC, Wolford JL, Gleaves CA, et al. Recognition and rapid diagnosis of upper gastrointestinal *Cytomegalovirus* infection in marrow transplantation recipients. A comparison of seven virologic methods. Transplantation 1994;57:231–7.

166. Naik HR, Chandrasekar PH. Herpes simplex virus (HSV) colitis in a bone marrow transplantation recipient. Bone Marrow Transplant 1996;17:285–6.

167. Kanfer EJ, Abrahamson C, Taylor J, et al. Severe rotavirus-associated diarrhoea following bone marrow transplantation: treatment with oral immunoglobulin. Bone Marrow Transplant 1994;14:651–2.

168. Yolken RH, Bishop CA, Townsend TR, et al. Infectious gastroenteritis in bone marrow transplantation recipients. N Engl J Med 1982;306:1010–2.

169. Townsend TR, Bolyard EA, Yolken RH, et al. Outbreak of Coxsackie A1 gastroenteritis: a complication of bone marrow transplantation. Lancet 1982;1:820–3.

170. Bromiker R, Korman SH, Or R, et al. Severe giardiasis in two patients undergoing bone marrow transplantation. Bone Marrow Transplant 1989;4:701–3.

171. Bavaro P, Di Girolamo G, Di Bartolomeo P, et al. Amebiasis after bone marrow transplantation. Bone Marrow Transplant 1994;12:213–4.

172. Collier AC, Miller RA, Meyers JD. Cryptosporidiosis after marrow transplantation: person-to-person transmission and treatment with spiramycin. Ann Intern Med 1984;101:205–6.

173. Kane JG, Chretien JH, Garagus VE. Diarrhea caused by *Candida*. Lancet 1976;1:335–6.

174. Gupta Tll, Ehrinpreis MN. *Candida*-associated diarrhea in hospitalized patients. Gastroenterology 1990;98:780–5.

175. Gauvreau JM, Lenssen P, Cheney CL, et al. Nutritional management of patients with intestinal graft-versus-host disease. J Am Diet Assoc 1981;79:673–7.

176. Geller RB, Gilmore CE, Dix SP, et al. Randomized trial of loperamide versus dose escalation of octreotide acetate for chemotherapy-induced diarrhea in bone marrow transplantation and leukemia patients. Am J Hematol 1995;50:167–72.

177. Morton AJ, Durrant ST. Efficacy of octreotide in controlling refractory diarrhea following bone marrow transplantation. Clin Transplant 1995;9:205–8.

178. Crouch MA, Restino MS, Cruz JM, et al. Octreotide acetate in refractory bone marrow transplant-associated diarrhea. Ann Pharmacother 1996;30:331–6.

179. Baillie-Johnson HP. Octreotide in the management of treatment-related diarrhoea. Anticancer Drugs 1996;7 (Suppl 1):11–5.

180. Harris AG, O'Dorisio TM, Woltering EA, et al. Consensus statement: octreotide dose titration in secretory diarrhea: Diarrhea Management Consensus Development Panel. Dig Dis Sci 1995;40:1464–73.

181. Fiori E, Atella F, Gazzanelli S, et al. The usefulness of biliary drainage for restoring liver function in obstructive jaundice. Panminerva Med 1994;36:171-8.

182. Scharschmidt BF, Goldberg HI, Schmid R. Approach to the patient with cholestatic jaundice. N Engl J Med 1983;308:1515–9.

183. Schenker SM, Balint J, Schiff L. Differential diagnosis of jaundice: report of prospective study of 61 proved cases. Am J Dig Dis 1962;7:449–63.

184. Anciaux ML, Pelletier G, Attali P, et al. Prospective study of clinical and biochemical features of symptomatic choledocholithiasis. Dig Dis Sci 1986;31:449–53.

185. Blackbourne LH, Earnhardt RC, Sistrom CL. The sensitivity and role of ultrasound in biliary obstruction. Am Surg 1994;60:683–90.

186. Matzen P, Malchow-Moller A, Brun B, et al. Ultrasonography, computed tomography and cholescintigraphy in suspected obstructive jaundice—a prospective comparative study. Gastroenterology 1983;84:1492–7.

187. Burcharth F. Approach to the jaundiced patient: diagnosis and treatment. Ann Radiol 1985;28:170–4.

188. Cotton PB. ERCP. Progress report. Gut 1977;18:316.

189. Teplick SK, Flick P, Brandon JC. Transhepatic cholangiography in patients with suspected biliary disease and non-dilated intrahepatic bile ducts. Gastrointest Radiol 1991;16:193–7.

190. Morb Mortal Wkly Rep 1994;43:916–7.

191. Runyon BA, Hoefs JC, Morgan TR. Ascitic fluid analysis in malignancy related ascites. Hepatology 1988;8:1104.

192. Gines P, Quintero E, Arroyo V, et al. Compensated cirrhosis: natural history and prognostic factors. Hepatology 1987;7:12–8.

193. D'Amico G, Morabito A, Pagliaro L, Marubini E. Survival and prognostic indicators in compensated and decompensated cirrhosis. Dig Dis Sci 1986;31:468–75.

194. Cattau EI, Benjamin SB, Knuff TE, et al. The accuracy of physical exam in the diagnosis of suspected ascites. JAMA 1982;247:1164–6.

195. Hoefs JC. Serum protein concentration and portal pressure determine the ascitic fluid protein concentration in patients with chronic liver disease. J Lab Clin Med 1986;102:260.

196. Runyon BA, Montano AA, Akriviadis EA, et al. The serum-ascites albumin gradient is superior to exudate-transudate concept in the differential diagnosis of ascites. Ann Intern Med 1992;117:215–20.

197. Guarner C, Runyon BA. Spontaneous bacterial peritonitis: pathogenesis, diagnosis and treatment. Gastroenterologist 1995;3:311–28.

198. Pockros PJ, Esrason KT, Nguyen C, et al. Mobilization of malignant ascites with diuretics is dependent on ascitic fluid characteristics. Gastroenterology 1992;103:1302–6.

199. Fogel MR, Sawhney VK, Neal EA, et al. Diuresis in the ascitic patient: a randomised controlled trial of three regimens. J Clin Gastroenterol 1981;3(Suppl 1):73–80.

200. Perez-Ayuso RM, Arroyo V, Planas R, et al. Randomized comparative study of efficacy of furosemide vs. spironolactone in nonazotemic cirrhosis with ascites. Gastroenterology 1983;84:961–8.

CHAPTER 10

NONINFECTIOUS PULMONARY EMERGENCIES

VICKIE R. SHANNON, MD
AMELIA NG, BS, MD

Pulmonary medicine is inextricably intertwined with oncologic emergencies and oncologic urgencies because of the propensity for cancer therapy or the disease itself to affect the lungs. For instance, the unique capacity of cancer to invade and obstruct contiguous structures may result in acute airway obstruction, superior vena caval syndrome, atelectasis, massive hemoptysis, and chylous and nonchylous pleural effusions. Necrosis of tumor in the periphery of the lung may produce pneumothorax, hemothorax, empyema, or pneumomediastinum. Pneumothorax and empyema may also occur as a consequence of the occlusion of a bronchus by tumor, resulting in distal emphysema or abscess formation that may rupture into the pleural space. Prolonged bed rest, major surgery, and hypercoagulability associated with malignancy are predisposing factors to pulmonary embolism. Analgesia and excessive sedation are major factors that render the debilitated cancer patient at risk for aspiration. The spectrum of toxic lung diseases associated with radiation and chemotherapeutic agents is broad and includes pulmonary edema, alveolar hemorrhage, bronchospasm, interstitial pneumonitis, bronchiolitis, and pneumonia. Finally, cancer as well as the treatment modalities of radiation, chemotherapy, and hematopoietic stem cell transplantation (HSCT) may cause severe depression of host defense mechanisms and inexorable pulmonary infections triggered by opportunistic and nosocomial pathogens. Thus, lung disease is a significant source of both acute and chronic morbidity in the cancer patient, and a considerable number of these patients succumb to respiratory failure as an end point of complex underlying disorders. This chapter reviews the current state of the art in regard to acute and subacute pulmonary emergencies in clinical oncology. The information provided is designed to highlight practical algorithms for the diagnosis and treatment of respiratory emergencies in clinical oncology while underscoring areas of uncertainty that warrant further study and investigation.

PULMONARY EMBOLIC EVENTS

Thromboembolism

Pulmonary embolism (PE) results from the migration of a thrombus from the deep venous circulation into the central pulmonary arteries. Venous thromboembolism represents a spectrum of disorders that range from localized deep venous thrombosis to massive pulmonary embolism. Massive pulmonary embolism (MPE) is usually a castastrophic entity, resulting in acute elevations in pulmonary vascular resistance, altered right ventricular performance, severe hypoxemia, and sudden death. Submassive PE may have an equally catastrophic outcome, depending on the underlying cardiopulmonary status of the patient. Early diagnosis and treatment has a significant impact on patient outcome. The overall in-hospital mortality rate for untreated clinically apparent cases of PE is 30%, but falls to less than 3% when PE is recognized early and appropriately treated.[1] Case fatality rates range from 8 to 23% for recurrent thromboembolism.[2,3] Thus, diligent efforts to confirm the diagnosis and initiate proper therapy are critical. In the cancer patient, in whom comorbid illnesses may mask, mimic, or simply coexist with thromboembolic disease, the diagnosis of PE presents even more of a clinical challenge. Missed diagnoses in this group of patients carry a significantly greater risk of potentially fatal consequences.

Predisposing Factors for Pulmonary Embolism in the Cancer Patient. Risk factors for thromboembolism are listed in Table 10–1. Acute arterial thrombosis may be the sentinel presentation in patients who subsequently develop malignancy.[4–7] Patients with concurrent cancer

TABLE 10–1. Stratification of Risk for Thromboembolic Disease

Variable	Low Risk	Intermediate Risk	High Risk	Comments
Incidence of PE(%)				
Nonfatal	0.02	1–2	5–10	Case fatality rate for treated stable PE is 5%.
Fatal	0.002	0.1–0.8	1–5	Rates increase to ≥ 20% with persistent hypotension despite therapy.
Condition				
Age (yr)	< 40	41–60	> 60	Risk nearly doubles with each decade after age 40 yr.
Type of surgery or trauma	Other than hip or pelvic	Lower-extremity fracture requiring cast (other than hip)	Hip/knee or pelvic surgery Hip fracture Spinal cord injury with associated paralysis	Risk of PE following hip surgery with PE prophylaxis is 20%; approximately 50% will be fatal. Risk of PE persists for 4 weeks following major surgery.
Length of anesthesia (min)	< 30	31–60	> 60	Increased risk associated with length but not type of general anesthetic.
Prior history of thromboembolism?	No	Yes	Yes	Hospitalized patients with history of PE/DVT have eightfold risk of recurrence.
Active cancer?*	No	Yes	Yes	Higher risk with advanced cancer
Other medical conditions	Pregnancy; obesity; cigarette smoking; hypertension	Stroke; congestive heart failure; indwelling central lines; right heart catheters; thrombocytopenia; thrombocytosis; postsplenectomy; BCPs with high estrogen content	Prolonged immobility; deficiencies of AT-III, Proteins C and S, antiphospholid antibody; HIT; thrombophilia	Risk of PE with third-generation BCPs is 1.5–2 times that of second-generation preparations.

AT-III = antithrombin III; BCPs = birth control pills; DVT = deep venous thrombosis; HIT = heparin-induced thrombocytopenia; PE = pulmonary embolism.
*Therapy within 6 months.

and thromboembolic disease have increased rates of recurrent thrombosis and a threefold increased rate of fatal PE when compared to patients without underlying malignancy.[8,9] Primary carcinoma of the brain, lymphoma, and adenocarcinomas of the lung, pancreas, stomach, colon, prostate, and kidneys are the most frequently reported types of malignancy associated with recurrent thromboembolic disease[6,9] (Table 10–2). Early reports noted a preponderance of thrombotic complications in patients with mucin-secreting adenocarcinomas.[10,11] This observation led to the suggestion that mucin-secreting tumors may express procoagulant substances that directly induce thrombin generation. However, many non-mucin-producing tumors are also associated with hypercoagulable states.[10,11] Furthermore, a unique procoagulant moiety in mucin has not been identified.

The triad of intimal injury, venous stasis, and alterations in coagulability enunciated by Virchow over 150 years ago remains central to the pathogenesis of thromboembolic disease. The association of malignancy with hypercoagulability is well established but poorly understood (Table 10–3). Trousseau's syndrome, a disorder in which the diagnosis of gastrointestinal malignancy is heralded by migratory thrombophlebitis, is a classic example of hypercoagulability. Early investigations into the pathogenesis of hypercoagulable states in cancer patients implicated the overexpression of fibrinogen and

clotting factors V, VIII, IX, and XI by tumor cells, as well as reduced levels of protein C, protein S, and antithrombin III. More recent work has focused on the capacity of tumor cells to produce thrombin, tissue factor, and other procoagulants that initiate blood coagulation by the activation of factor X.[12]

It is likely that the pathogenesis of the hypercoagulable state in malignancy involves the interplay of multiple variables. Clinical manifestations of an otherwise asymptomatic hypercoagulable state may be conditioned by comorbid factors, such as prolonged bed rest or major surgery, that lead to venous stasis. Central venous catheters, commonly used in cancer patients, may predispose to thrombosis by providing a nidus for clot formation.[13,14] Although more than 90% of thrombi originate in the large-capacitance vessels of the pelvis and lower extremities,[4,15] recent studies have clearly demonstrated other contributing sites for clot formation. These observations have included upper-extremity thrombi in patients with central venous catheters and right ventricular thrombi in patients with cor pulmonale or indwelling right atrial catheters.[14]

Notably, risk factors for the development of thromboembolism exert their effects cumulatively, not independently. For instance, a cancer patient with no other underlying comorbid illnesses has a modest 15 to 20% risk of thromboembolic disease. If that patient is 70 years

TABLE 10–2. Types of Cancer with the Highest Rates of Thromboembolic Disease

Cancer Type	Incidence (%)
Adenocarcinoma of	
Lung	25.0
Pancreas	17.0
Stomach	16.0
Colon	15.0
Prostate	7.0
Ovary	6.0
Gallbladder	3.0
Breast	2.0
Kidney	0.4
Primary CNS tumors	—
Non-Hodgkin's lymphoma	—

Adapted from Levitan N, et al;[9] Sorenson H, et al.[6]
CNS = central nervous system.

of age, develops congestive heart failure after receiving cardiotoxic alkylating agents for treatment of her breast cancer, or is receiving tamoxifen chemotherapy, her risk is substantially higher. A pathologic fracture of the hip from metastatic disease raises her risk for a thromboembolic event to 60 to 70%.[16] These are, unfortunately, scenarios that are all too real for the cancer patient. They create a reasonable risk profile, which should heighten the clinician's suspicion for thromboembolic events and also condition the intensity of prophylactic initiatives.

Pathophysiology. Much of the tremendous redundant vasculature of the lung is nonperfused. The pulmonary vasculature is selectively recruited in response to rising cardiac outputs. This permits optimization of the ventilation-perfusion (V/Q) balance during all phases of exercise. These compensatory mechanisms underlie the lung's tremendous capacity to tolerate clots that truncate significant portions of the normal pulmonary circulation. Up to 50% of the normal pulmonary vasculature may be obliterated with little change in pulmonary hemodynamics, right-heart performance, or V/Q match. Massive PEs may overwhelm these compensatory mechanisms, causing a progressive rise in pulmonary vascular resistance and right ventricular afterload. The right ventricle (RV) has a very limited capacity to increase its stroke volume against acute escalations in RV afterload. As RV afterload increases, parallel increases in RV wall tension above 40 to 50 mm Hg cause the RV to progressively dilate and ultimately fail. A series of hemodynamic events including ischemia, dysfunction of the RV, tricuspid regurgitation, and failure of forward flow may ensue, leading to cardiovascular collapse. Right atrial pressures in the setting of MPE may become sufficiently elevated to cause the opening of a patent foramen ovale. Intractable hypoxemia refractory to supplemental oxygen therapy may ensue as a consequence of the right-to-left intracardiac shunt. In addition, para-

doxical embolization through a patent foramen ovale or atrial septal defect may occur in the setting of severe pressure elevations. Platelet–associated serotonin and bradykinin released by the thrombus may cause further elevations of pulmonary vascular resistance as well as pulmonary vascular redistribution and local bronchial constriction. These physiologic changes create large areas of dead space that further aggravate the V/Q imbalance and contribute to poor gas exchange and worsened hypoxemia.

Clinical Presentation and Diagnostic Evaluation. Clinical evidence of PE is notoriously imprecise and cannot be solely relied on to establish or exclude the diagnosis. Patients may present with marked clinical symptoms but no objective signs of thrombosis. In only 25% of patients who present with a high clinical suspicion of PE is the diagnosis proven. Likewise, clinical signs of deep venous thrombosis (DVT) are nonspecific and cannot be relied on in the work-up and evaluation of PE. Although evidence of an association between DVT and subsequent PE is substantial, clinical findings of simultaneous PE and DVT are unusual. More than 50% of patients with documented DVT have clinically silent PE detected by V/Q scintigraphy. Conversely, 40 to 50% of patients with symptomatic PE have an asymptomatic thrombus involving the proximal vessels of the lower extremities.[17] Rarely, patients may present with symptoms of unexplained hypoxemia, acute pleuritic chest pain, arrhythmias, and hemodynamic instability, making the diagnosis intuitively obvious. In most cases, however, the presentation is sufficiently vague to warrant further test-

TABLE 10–3. Pathogenesis of Thromboembolism in Cancer Patients

Condition	Pathogenesis
Venous stasis	Venous obstruction by tumor Decreased mobility Increased blood viscosity Increased venous pressure
Vessel wall injury	Direct tumor injury to endothelium Chemotherapy-induced (BCNU, bleomycin, vincristine, doxorubicin, taxanes?)
Hypercoagulability	Direct and indirect tumor-cell activation of clotting factors Overexpression of other procoagulants? Chemotherapy-induced reductions in protein C and protein S (cyclophosphamide, methotrexate, 5-fluorouracil) Antithrombin III reductions caused by surgery, chemotherapeutic agents (taxanes, L-asparaginase) and heparin
Platelet abnormalities	Reactive thrombocytosis (carcinomas of breast, lung, stomach, ovary, and colon) Spontaneous platelet aggregation Increased thrombopoietin

BCNU = carmustine.

ing. Cancer patients may have hemostatic defects that predispose them to hemorrhagic complications associated with anticoagulation. For this reason, the risk of empiric anticoagulant therapy for thromboembolic disease should be carefully weighed against the risk of an extensive diagnostic work-up. An algorithm for the diagnostic evaluation of PE is shown in Figure 10–1. The optimal approach is one that integrates a thorough history with the physical examination, supplemented by selective diagnostic tests.

Dyspnea occurs in 70 to 90% of patients with angiographically proven PE and is the most common presenting symptom. Patients with a small clot and normal underlying cardiopulmonary function may have transient dyspnea and no significant alterations in gas exchange or cardiovascular hemodynamics. At the opposite end of the clinical spectrum is syncope and hemodynamic collapse from MPE. Patients with MPE may present with angina from right ventricular ischemia. In the Prospective Investigation of Pulmonary Embolism Diag-

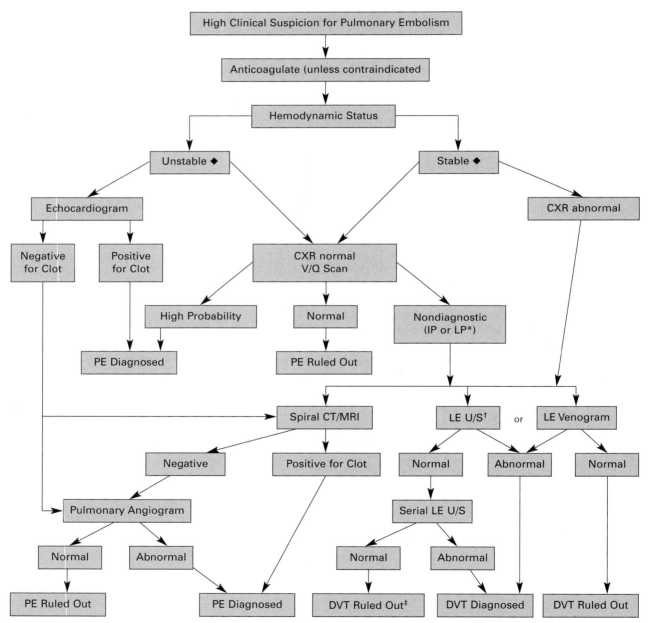

Figure 10-1. A suggested algorithm for the evaluation of pulmonary embolism. *IP = Intermediate Probability; LP = Low Probability; †LE U/S = Lower extremity ultrasound; ‡May proceed to Spiral CT/MRI or pulmonary angiogram if clinical suspicion remains high. ◆ Spiral CT may replace V/Q scan or echocardiogram as initial study in some patients.

nosis (PIOPED) study,[18,19] the symptom complex of dyspnea, pleuritic chest pain, and/or tachypnea (respiratory rate > 20 breaths per minute) was noted in 97% of patients with PE documented by angiography. Hemoptysis associated with PE indicates infarction. This rare event tends to occur in patients with prior cardiac and/or pulmonary disease, at 12 to 36 hours following the embolic event. The lungs receive their oxygen supply from the airway and from the pulmonary and bronchial circulation. Pulmonary infarction requires significant compromise of two out of three of these potential sources of oxygen. In the general population, therefore, pulmonary infarction is a rare complication of PE, but it may occur in up to 20% of patients with significant prior pulmonary or cardiac disease. Episodic dyspnea and symptoms that mimic unresolving or indolent pneumonia or refractory heart failure are atypical symptoms of PE that more often occur in elderly persons.

The physical examination may elicit nonspecific but suggestive symptoms and signs of acute PE. Unexplained tachypnea and tachycardia occur most often. Other physical findings include modest elevations in temperature (up to 38.5°F), sinus tachycardia, and pleural rub. Inspection of the lower extremities may reveal clinical evidence of DVT in less than 50% of patients. Sinus tachycardia is the most common finding by electrocardiography. Acute (usually atrial) arrhythmias are unusual presentations of PE and are typically associated with a large clot burden. Patients with massive PE may have signs of increased pulmonic second heart sound (P_2), jugular venous distension, and parasternal lift on physical examination. Findings of right axis shift (pulmonale) and T-wave inversion on the precordial leads are typical of massive PE. T-wave inversion was the most common electrocardiographic abnormality in one study[20] and was the sign that most closely paralleled PE severity. In the PIOPED[18] study, blood gas analyses, including arterial oxygen partial pressure (PaO_2) and alveolar arterial PO_2 difference ($P[A-a]O_2$) gradients, were normal in 38% of patients without prior cardiopulmonary disease and 14% of patients with pre-existing disease. Acute respiratory acidosis is typical; however, respiratory alkalosis may be seen in patients with MPE and in patients with antecedent severe cardiopulmonary disease.

Chest radiography is critical for excluding competing pathology. In the PIOPED study, 12% of patients with PE had a normal chest radiograph. Abnormal radiographic findings include focal infiltrates and atelectasis, elevation of the ipsilateral hemidiaphragm, and hypoperfusion of the involved lung, associated with enlargement of the pulmonary artery (Westermark's sign). The wedge-shaped infiltrate, felt to be characteristic of PE with infarction, has been given much attention; however, infarction-related infiltrates may be of any configuration. Cardiac echocardiography with Doppler studies via the transthoracic or transesophageal routes provides indirect evidence of hemodynamically significant PE and permits rapid bedside evaluation of the unstable patient. Echodense material representing retained right-sided mobile thrombi are occasionally visualized by echocardiography. More than 40% of patients with documented PE may have echocardiographic evidence of right ventricular strain. This finding is associated with a poor outcome. Kasper and colleagues[21] reported that mortality rates among patients with echocardiographic evidence of increased afterload was 13-fold higher than those of patients with normal right ventricular findings. Echocardiographic changes include dilated right ventricle, cor pulmonale, and dilated right pulmonary artery.

The usefulness of the above findings is in helping to exclude alternative diagnoses. However, these findings alone cannot establish the diagnosis of PE specifically. Specific diagnostic tools for the work-up of PE include V/Q scintigraphy, spiral computed tomography (CT), magnetic resonance imaging (MRI), and pulmonary angiography. Despite newer imaging modalities, V/Q scintigraphy remains the standard screening test in the initial work-up for PE. A V/Q scan demonstrating two or more moderate to large perfusion defects (occupying > 25% of a lung segment) with intact ventilation in radiographically normal areas of the lung is regarded as a "high-probability" lung scan and is evidence to treat in most cases. A normal perfusion study effectively excludes PE with a degree of certainty similar to that of pulmonary angiography.[22] Unfortunately, most V/Q studies yield intermediate probability reports. In the PIOPED study, nearly 60% of all of the patients with PE documented by pulmonary angiography had intermediate probability studies.[18] The combination of probability assessment by clinical evaluation and identification of risk factors and lung scan assessment are complementary for the diagnosis of PE and can predict PE in 60% of patients. The presence of PE can also be inferred in symptomatic patients who have abnormal lower-extremity Doppler venous ultrasonography, impedence plethysmography (IPG), contrast venography, or radioisotopic studies. The detection of DVT by one of these studies not only supports the diagnosis of PE in patients with clinical symptoms but also provides prognostic information regarding the risk of recurrent PE. Thus, investigative work-up for venous thromboembolism is an important component of the diagnostic armamentarium for patients for whom there is high clinical suspicion and who have equivocal imaging studies.[23] Stable patients with suspected PE but whose V/Q scans are nondiagnostic should undergo 4 to 6 sequential noninvasive studies of the lower extremities over 7 to 14 days. Repeated negative studies (usually IPG or lower-extremity Doppler examination) may reduce the requirement for angiography and abrogate the need for long-term anticoagulation. This combined approach of lung scanning and noninvasive studies of the lower extremities has been recently advocated for patients with adequate cardiopulmonary reserve.[24,25] In patients with suspected PE and poor cardiopulmonary reserve, the safety of withholding anticoagulation on the basis of serial negative lower-extremity findings is unproven. Those patients should undergo pulmonary angiography for diagnosis unless contraindicated.

Spiral CT and MRI are promising newer imaging modalities in the work-up of PE (Figure 10–2). These studies reliably depict clotting in the central (second- to fourth-order) pulmonary arteries, with sensitivities and specificities of more than 80% and 90%, respectively.[26–28] In addition, lung windows obtained during both MRI and spiral CT offer additional information regarding competing diagnoses. The risk of subsequent PE in patients with abnormal spiral CT studies during 3 months of follow-up (< 2%) compares favorably with with the risk of PE determined by pulmonary angiography, although the sample size of most studies has been small.[29] Two major shortcomings of both of the newer imaging techniques are recognized. Accurate detection of emboli is heavily operator dependent. In addition, clots located in the distal (subsegmental) pulmonary vasculature cannot be reliably identified by either of these methods.[30,31] The prevalence of subsegmental pulmonary emboli has been reported to vary by between 5 and 36%.[32,33] The clinical significance of small subsegmental pulmonary emboli has been a matter of much debate in the literature.[32,33] It is generally agreed that these clots may presage more serious events and that treatment may result in improved clinical outcome, especially in patients with underlying respiratory disease. Spiral CT may be

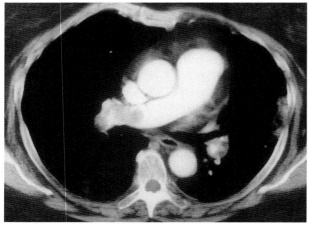

Figure 10–2. A 36-year-old woman with breast cancer and acute dyspnea. Computed tomographic angiography showed hyperlucent intraluminal filling defects in the right segmental pulmonary arteries consistent with pulmonary embolism.

slightly more accurate than MRI in identifying pulmonary emboli.[30,34] However, MRI offers cinematic images of the lung and lower-extremity vessels without exposing the patient to ionizing radiation. Patients with high clinical suspicion and abnormal spiral CT or MRI studies should undergo pulmonary angiography for definitive diagnosis.

Despite major advances in the development of less invasive tests for the study of PE, pulmonary angiography remains the "gold standard". Angiographic findings of intravascular filling defects on two or more projections are diagnostic of PE. Nonspecific and less reliable observations on angiography include vascular cutoffs, hypovascularity, and vascular pruning.[18] Pulmonary angiography is often touted as a high-risk procedure. In the PIOPED investigation, however, mortality rates were less than 0.5%, with a procedure-related morbidity of 5%.[18] Complications are primarily related to renal function or associated with catheter insertion or contrast reactions. Four injections of intravenous contrast with four views (right and left apical-posterior views and right and left oblique views) are necessary for a complete study. Partial studies with vessel injection based on V/Q findings are acceptable and help to limit the patient's exposure to contrast.

Among the various assays available for the detection of PE, the D-dimer assay has received the most scrutiny. In a recent meta-analysis pooling 29 studies, D-dimer levels of < 500 ng/mL were associated with a negative predictive value of 94%, regardless of pretest probabilities for emboli.[35] D-dimer, the crossed-linked degradation product of fibrin, has been studied extensively as a potential marker with predictive value for the diagnosis of thromboembolic disorders. D-dimer levels are virtually always elevated to > 500 ng/mL in the setting of acute thrombosis. An increased level of D-dimer is nonspecific, however, and the level may be increased in a variety of nonthrombotic disorders, particularly malignancy, recent surgery, pneumonia, myocardial infarction, hemorrhage, trauma, and sepsis.[36] The specificity of the D-dimer assay may also deteriorate with increasing patient age. Thus, D-dimer assays may be of only incremental utility in the diagnostic work-up of the hospitalized elderly patient with malignancy or other concomitant illness. Sensitivities and specificities may vary from 19 to 100% and from 10 to 68%, respectively, depending on the type of assay for detecting D-dimer and the patient population studied.[37–40]

Management. Treatment of the hypoxemic hypotensive patient with acute PE centers on several therapeutic principles: stabilization of cardiovascular hemodynamics, treatment of the clot, prevention of further clot formation, and prevention of clot migration. A therapeutic strategy for the treatment of MPE is outlined in Figure 10–3. Clot burden and the patient's underlying cardiovascular status condition the initial approach to the patient with PE. Hemodynamic stabilization is critical, independent of clot dynamics and thrombolysis. Fluid resuscitation may serve several functions; volume repletion may augment right ventricular preload and improve systemic hypotension. Caution in the use of intravenous fluids is imperative in this setting, however, as excessive increases in preload may further distend the RV, precipitating right ventricular ischemia and further deterioration in RV function. Hemodynamically unstable patients should be closely monitored in the intensive-care unit. Right atrial pressures of 15 to 20 mm Hg by central venous monitoring are usually sufficient to maintain adequate RV preload. Inotropic agents may be used to augment RV contractility. There are no randomized controlled studies that have specifically evaluated the optimal vasoactive agents in patients with MPE complicated by shock. Recent investigations have shown a favorable effect of dobutamine on RV contractility and cardiac output (CO). Dobutamine is a potent vasodilator of both the systemic and pulmonary vascular beds. In addition, it possesses inotropic properties and may decrease right-sided filling pressures. With dobutamine administration, PaO_2 may occasionally worsen because of increased blood flow through a fixed shunt. Norepinephrine, an α- and β-adrenoreceptor agonist, may enhance coronary blood flow by increasing cardiac contractility and RV perfusion pressure; as a result, systemic blood pressure (BP), CO, peripheral vascular resistance (PVR), and RV pressures may be improved. This agent, in combination with dobutamine, may also hold promise in the treatment of shock-related MPE. The vasoconstrictor effects

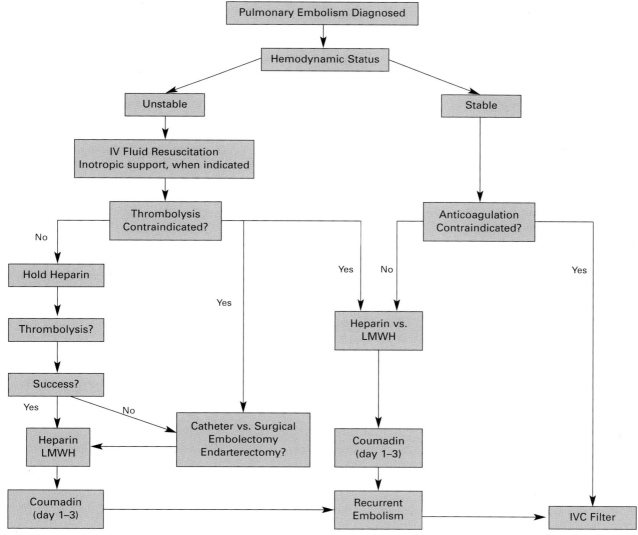

Figure 10–3. An algorithm for the treatment of pulmonary embolism. LMWH = Low molecular weight heparin.

of epinephrine and dopamine are also mediated through α-adrenergic receptors and may improve CO. Epinephrine possesses potent β1-mediated inotropic effects, which may reduce PVR. The efficacy of dopamine is limited by the adverse effect of tachycardia. Although isoproterenol is a potent pulmonary artery vasodilator, its potential to markedly reduce RV preload may have disastrous consequences. Isoproterenol administration is therefore not considered safe for the treatment of shock secondary to MPE. Two other vasoactive agents, milrinone and amrinone, have been studied in the canine model and do not appear to be indicated in the setting of MPE with severe hemodynamic irritability.

Heparin and (now) the low-molecular-weight heparin (LMWH) derivatives, are the mainstays of treatment of the stable patient with PE. Unless contraindicated, these agents should be administered immediately to patients with high clinical suspicion for PE, even before the results of diagnostic studies are obtained. Initial treatment with oral anticoagulation alone may paradoxically increase the hypercoagulable state and increase the rate of recurrent events. Unfractionated heparin is usually given as a bolus of 5,000 to 10,000 U followed by continuous infusion at 18 U/kg/h. Rapid achievement of therapeutic levels of partial thromboplastin time (PTT) is seen in most patients on this regimen. Adequate anticoagulation is usually indicated by a PTT of 60 to 80 seconds or when the patient's PTT is 1.5 to 2 times control. Heparin resistance, arbitrarily defined as the requirement of > 50,000 units of heparin per 24 hours, is rare. In patients with heparin resistance, the monitoring of plasma heparin levels rather than PTT may avoid unnecessary dose escalations. Recent studies have shown LMWH to be as effective and safe as unfractionated heparin in the treatment of the stable patient with PE.[8,41–43] The advantages of LMWH include simple administration and less frequent dosing without the need for vigilance in the monitoring of blood coagulation profiles. Warfarin sodium (Coumadin) may be administered 2 to 3 days after therapeutic levels of PTT have been achieved. A 5-mg loading dose followed by 5-mg daily is usually sufficient to attain adequate oral anticoagulation.[44] Full anticoagulation requires the depletion of both factor VII, which has a half-life of 6 hours, and thrombin, which has a half-life of 5 days. Therefore, heparin administration should continued at least through the initial 5 days of warfarin sodium therapy. Heparin reduces the international normalized ratio (INR) by approximately 0.5. Thus, an optimal targeted initial INR of 3.0 on combined warfarin sodium and heparin therapy yields an effective INR of 2.5 with warfarin sodium alone. The intent of anticoagulation in the treatment of PE is to prevent recurrence. Approximately 8% of pulmonary emboli treated with conventional anti-

coagulation therapy will recur, usually within the first 6 weeks after the initiation of therapy.[1]

The optimal duration of anticoagulation therapy remains sharply debated. Anticoagulation is usually continued for a minimum of 3 months after a single event, at which time the risk of bleeding and the risk of recurrence generally offset each other.[2,45] Prolonged therapy (6 to 12 months) is recommended for patients with active cancer or until the cancer has resolved. In patients with recurrent embolism, lifelong therapy should be considered. Patients with deficiencies of antithrombin III, protein C, or protein S may require several years of anticoagulation. The need for an indefinite treatment course in patients with factor V deficiency remains in question.

Thrombolytic agents have proven efficacy in the acceleration of clot lysis, which results in substantial improvements in RV hemodynamic parameters.[3,46,47] Accelerated thrombolysis clearly results in early improvements in radiographic and hemodynamic derangements. In a small study of 40 patients treated with thrombolysis versus heparin for MPE, however, no significant difference in RV hemodynamics or long-term survival was demonstrated at 7 days after the initiation of therapy.[48] No clinical trial to date has been large enough to conclusively demonstrate a survival advantage for patients with MPE who receive thrombolytics versus conventional heparin therapy. The indications for thrombolysis in the treatment of MPE are a source of debate (Table 10–4). It is generally agreed that thrombolysis should be considered for the hemodynamically unstable patient with MPE. A National Institutes of Health (NIH) consensus conference on MPE recommended thrombolysis in all patients in whom greater than 40% of the pulmonary vasculature is occluded by clot.[49] Other authorities include echocardiographic evidence of RV dysfunction or severe hypoxemia as indications for thrombolysis.[50]

Among the thrombolytic agents, urokinase, streptokinase, and tissue plasminogen activator (t-PA) are currently approved for use in the treatment of MPE in the United States (Table 10–5). The thrombolytic efficacies of the available agents are roughly the same although t-PA is infused over a shorter period and may cause more rapid thrombolysis.[51] The local administration of thrombolytical agents directly into selected pulmonary arteries has the theoretical advantage of inducing more rapid and complete clot lysis with lower concentrations of the drug.[52,53] The risk of systemic bleeding, therefore, appears intuitively to be less with this treatment approach. However, limited available data suggest that locally infused thrombolytic agents do not confer any advantage over systemic administration with regard to rates of clot lysis, bleeding, or induction of systemic fibrinolysis.[54] Therefore, this mode of administration is not generally recommended. Direct intraembolic infusion of

TABLE 10–4. Indications and Contraindications to Thrombolytic Therapy

Indications
- PE with shock physiology
- Failure of conventional anticoagulation
- Clot obstructing more than 50% of vessel lumen?

Contraindications
- Absolute
  - Major intracranial surgery or trauma within prior 2 months
  - Cerebrovascular hemorrhage within prior 3–6 months
  - Active intracranial neoplasm
  - Major internal hemorrhage within prior 6 months
  - Severe bleeding diatheses, including those associated with severe liver or renal disease
- Relative
  - Prolonged cardiopulmonary resuscitation
  - Pregnancy or postpartum period within prior 10 days
  - Nonhemorrhagic stroke within prior 2 months
  - Major trauma or surgery (excluding CNS) within prior 10 days
  - Thrombocytopenia (platelet count < 100,000/mm^3)
  - Hemorrhagic retinopathy
  - Allergies to thrombolytic agents
  - Minor surgery to noncompressible vessels within prior 10 days
  - Tissue biopsy within prior 10 days
  - Peptic ulceration within prior 3 months
  - Infective endocarditis/pericarditis
  - Uncontrolled hypertension (systolic BP ≥ 200 or diastolic BP ≥ 110 mm Hg)
  - Aortic aneurysm

BP = blood pressure; CNS = central nervous system; PE = pulmonary embolism.

low-dose thrombolytics (t-PA or urokinase) has recently emerged as an alternative to systemic thrombolysis. This approach may prove to be superior to the intravenous route of administration; however, larger randomized studies are needed.[52]

The contraindications to thrombolysis are primarily centered around the risk of bleeding (see Table 10–4). The extensive list of absolute and relative contraindications to thrombolysis is derived from the experience of thrombolytic therapy for the treatment of myocardial infarction. In this setting, the risk of intracranial hemorrhage (ICH), the most devastating complication, is 0.6 to 1.5%.[55,56] In a series of smaller studies, the cumulative incidence of ICH in patients treated with thrombolytic

agents for PE was slightly higher, at 1.9 to 2.1%.[3,18,57] The occurrence of ICH following thrombolytic therapy for PE is significantly greater than the reported 0.2% incidence of ICH in patients treated with heparin alone.[3] Local bleeding from arterial or venous puncture sites is a common problem. This problem can be avoided by minimizing invasive procedures around the time of thrombolysis. Patients frequently undergo pulmonary arteriography for diagnosis before starting thrombolytic therapy. Bleeding from the venous puncture site may be managed by removing the introducer sheath after thrombolytic therapy has been completed. Overt gastrointestinal bleeding can also be significant. Serious bleeding from a venous puncture site is usually controlled by local compression. If local compression fails to control the bleeding or if major bleeding occurs in a noncompressible site, the lytic agent should be discontinued. In most instances, the removal of the lytic agent suffices to control the bleeding as the half-life of these agents is short. In rare cases, reversal of the lytic state with fresh frozen plasma, platelet transfusion, and/or antifibrinolytic agents may be necessary.

Novel methods for clot removal are used when traditional approaches fail or are contraindicated. Both surgical and catheter embolectomy in this setting have had anecdotal success. However, large controlled studies evaluating the safety and efficacy of these treatment modalities are not available. The accepted indications for surgical embolectomy include refractory systemic hypotension, echocardiographic evidence of right atrial thrombi, pulmonary artery pressures > 35 mm Hg, and contraindicated or failed thrombolytic therapy.[58] Surgical or catheter embolectomy should be reserved for the removal of large centrally located clots. In the absence of MPE-associated cardiac arrest, survival rates after emergency embolectomy may exceed 80%. Mortality rates after emergency embolectomy in the setting of cardiac arrest, however, remain dismal.[59,60] Indications for surgical versus catheter embolectomy depend on available resources and the experience of the clinician. The overall experience with pulmonary embolectomy using transvenous catheters has been favorable. Greenfield reported a 76% success rate and a 70% survival rate among 46 patients with MPE who

TABLE 10–5. Thrombolytic Agents Used in the Treatment of Massive Pulmonary Embolism

Drug	Mechanism of Action	Comments
Tissue plasminogen activator (t-PA)	Cleaves plasminogen within clot	Rapid clot lysis Systemic fibrinolysis may cause excessive bleeding
Streptokinase	Cleaves circulating plasminogen	Systemic fibrinolysis may cause excessive bleeding Dissolves clots more slowly than the other two agents Degree of clot resolution after 24 hours similar to that of other agents Antigenic (may be used only once?) Least expensive agent
Urokinase	Cleaves circulating plasminogen	Rapid clot lysis Systemic fibrinolysis may cause excessive bleeding

underwent catheter embolectomy using a suction catheter. The rheolytic embolectomy catheter technology continues to evolve. Recent developments include the development of catheters with rotating heads, self-expanding stents, and rheolytic saline jets.[61] A common complication of catheter embolectomy includes hematoma formation at the catheter insertion site. Pulmonary and myocardial infarction have also been reported.

Nonthrombotic Embolism in the Cancer Patient

The normal pulmonary vasculature acts as an efficient sieve to trap and filter foreign substances of > 10 mm in diameter that gain access to the venous circulation. The classic examples of the filtering capacity of the pulmonary circulation are venous thromboembolism and pulmonary artery thrombosis. Other nonthrombotic sources of emboli, including air, tumor, fat, and bone marrow, may also become trapped within the pulmonary circulation. In addition to the elevated risk of thrombotic abnormalities also noted with cancer, the cancer patient is at risk for nonthromboembolic episodes. These unusual forms of embolism, some of which may be life threatening, are briefly discussed below.

Fat Embolism Syndrome. The triad of global neurologic impairment, acute respiratory insufficiency, and petechial rash is generally held as a vigorous criterion for the diagnosis of fat embolism syndrome (FES). The clinical presentation of FES may be quite varied, making estimations of true incidence difficult. Fat embolism syndrome typically occurs in the setting of trauma to long bones; however, clinically significant FES has been reported in the cancer patient after bone marrow transplantation,[62] in bone tumor lysis,[63] and in nontraumatic orthopedic procedures. The diagnosis of FES is based on the clinical findings of respiratory insufficiency, neurologic impairment, and petechiae. The finding of stainable fat in serum or urine or by BAL is neither sensitive nor specific for the diagnosis.[64] Ventilation-perfusion studies typically demonstrate mottled perfusion defects with normal ventilation. The clinical features of FES typically occur within 24 to 72 hours after the initiating event. Similarly to MPE, massive fat embolism may result in dramatic increases in pulmonary pressures, acute cor pulmonale, and sudden death. Acute obstruction caused by submassive fat embolization may be well tolerated because of pulmonary vascular autoregulation. Tissue injury, presumably caused by the release of fatty acids into the lung parenchyma, occurs later, usually 24 to 72 hours after the initiating event, and accounts for the delay in clinical presentation. Increased pulmonary pressures and intrapulmonary shunt formation may occur with as little as 20 cm^3 of bone marrow fat embolization.[65] These intra-arterial

shunts account for the neurologic and dermatologic manifestations of the disease. Fat globlules shunted through the pulmonary circulation may lodge in microvessels of the cerebral circulation and cause neurologic impairments. Typically, patients present with acute confusion and may progress to seizures and coma. Focal neurologic deficits, including scotomata, anisocoria, hemiplegia, aphasia, dysconjugate eye movements, and apraxia, have been reported. Permanent deficits are unusual, and neurologic recovery is expected, even in severe cases. Petechial rash distributed over the axilla, anterior chest, and head and neck are nearly pathognomonic of FES. Dermatologic manifestations may be late findings; they are seen in only 20 to 50% of cases and thus may not help in establishing the diagnosis. Overall, clinical outcome is quite good, and full recovery can be expected.[66] The indication for (and the efficacy of) steroids as either prophylaxis or definitive treatment of established FES has been sharply debated. Currently, steroid treatment is not recommended for the prophylaxis or definitive treatment of FES because no study has clearly demonstrated that this intervention improves outcome.

Tumor Embolism. Microvascular tumor embolization is usually secondary to hematogenous seeding of tumor cell clusters that are eventually trapped within the pulmonary circulation. The cancer patients with the highest risk for tumor embolization mirror those at highest risk for thromboembolic events. In particular, patients with mucin-producing adenocarcinomas of the breast, colon, and stomach are at greatest risk for tumor embolization. Autopsy evidence of tumor embolism is also frequently observed in patients with mucin-secreting adenocarcinomas of the liver, kidneys, and prostate. The incidence of microembolization of solid tumors at autopsy is 0.9 to 6%.[67] The clinical presentation mimics that of pulmonary thromboembolic disease. Thus, correct antemortem diagnosis is difficult and is observed in only 6% of patients.[68] For most patients, the diagnosis of cancer is well established. A few patients, however, may present subacutely with dyspnea, cough, and echocardiographic evidence of pulmonary hypertension, without an antecedent diagnosis of cancer. Mean pulmonary artery pressures > 50 mm Hg are typical and suggest chronic disease. Echocardiography is therefore useful in sorting acute from chronic processes and helps in establishing the severity of pulmonary hypertension as well as the degree of right ventricular dysfunction. The typical clinical presentation is the patient with a known solid tumor, insidious dyspnea, and hypoxemia that ultimately leads to cor pulmonale and death. Chest radiographs (CXRs) are usually normal but may demonstrate diffuse interstitial opacities suggestive of lymphangitic spread. Ventilation-perfusion scanning typically shows normal ventilation with mottled subsegmental perfusion defects similar to those seen in FES. Pulmonary angiograms are usually normal or near normal. Cytologic analysis of blood aspirated from pulmonary artery catheters may identify malignant cells and help with the diagnosis. Because the majority of diagnoses of microvascular tumor embolism are made post mortem, appropriate therapy has not been established. Chemotherapy, embolectomy, and surgical resection of the primary tumor source have met with limited success.

Venous Air Embolism. Venous air embolism (VAE) results from inadvertent communication between the atmosphere and the venous system, which permits the rapid ingress of atmospheric air into the venous circulation. Intravenous pressure may fall below atmospheric pressure during deep inspiration, hypovolemia, or upright positioning. This permits the ingress of air along a negative pressure gradient. Clinical situations that favor the development of VAE include central venous catheter insertions, positive pressure ventilation, surgical procedures, or any procedure in which air is insufflated into a body cavity.[69,70] Cancer patients routinely undergo central venous catheterization and surgical and gynecologic procedures that place them at risk for VAE. The incidence of catheter-related VAE in the general patient population ranges from 1 in 47 to 1 in 3,000 catheter insertions. Air in the venous circulatory system causes an acute obstruction to blood flow, with a concomitant rise in pulmonary artery pressure and right ventricular pressure; hypoxemia invariably ensues along with hypotension. Pulmonary edema may occur as a consequence of increased capillary permeability. The body position at the time of air embolization, the volume of air, and the rate with which the air is infused are three factors that determine the severity of VAE. As little as 300 to 500 mL of air infused at a rate of 100 mL/s may cause fatal embolization in humans.[71] Upright positioning at the time of air insufflation facilitates the development of catastrophic air embolization. Clinically important VAE may present as acute cardiopulmonary collapse. Vague symptoms of light-headedness, chest pain, and dyspnea are frequent. The auscultatory finding of a rhythmic "mill wheel" murmur on cardiac examination is a relatively specific but infrequent sign of VAE. Livedo reticularis, cerebral infarction, and findings of myocardial ischemia may also occur in patients with massive VAE. A definitive diagnosis of VAE requires a high index of suspicion. An accurate history in the appropriate clinical setting may yield critical clues to the diagnosis. A rise in pulmonary artery pressure and a fall in end-tidal carbon dioxide ($ETCO_2$) during a surgical procedure may suggest the diagnosis. Precardial Doppler monitoring or $ETCO_2$ monitoring with continuous measurements of pulmonary artery pressures during surgical procedures is advocated. An air-fluid level in the pulmonary artery on chest radiography is a rare but pathognomic finding for VAE. Contrast echocardiography may detect intracardiac air. Rare findings of intracerebral air by head contrast tomography has also been reported.[72] Because intravascular air is quickly reabsorbed, however, documentation by radiographic studies is unusual and may inappropriately delay urgent therapy. The goals of therapy are to restore blood flow and facilitate the resorption of intravascular air. At the first sign of VAE, patients should be placed in the left lateral decubitus position. This positioning facilitates the migration of intravascular air into the RV and improves blood flow. Aspiration of intravascular air and closed-chest cardiac massage are additional measures used in the treatment of massive VAE. Hyperbaric oxygen (HBO) therapy has been proposed for the treatment of patients with persistent hemodynamic or cerebrovascular compromise despite initial therapeutic measures. The initiation of HBO therapy may require the transfer of the patient to a hyperbaric facility. Although early aggressive therapy is recommended, the efficacy of HBO therapy, even when treatment is delayed by 30 to 40 hours, has been documented in numerous case reports.[73] Mortality rates may exceed 90% for patients with massive untreated VAE. Conventional supportive care may reduce mortality rates to 30%. Therapy with HBO has been shown to further reduce mortality rates to less than 10%.[74]

MASSIVE HEMOPTYSIS

The dual blood supply to the lungs carries out independent and specialized functions. The pulmonary circulation travels alongside the bronchial tree but interacts with the airway only at the level of the terminal bronchiole, where it participates in critical functions of gas exchange. The bronchial circulation most often branches from the aorta but may arise from the intercostal arteries in a minority of individuals. These vessels arborize extensively along the airway and provide nutrient support to the bronchi and mediastinal structures. The dominant drainage system for the bronchial arteries is the vena cava and azygos veins, with a small amount of bronchial arterial supply draining into the pulmonary veins. The bronchial circuit is under high systemic pressure and may bleed profusely in disease states. Indirect evidence implicating the bronchial circuit as the usual source of massive hemoptysis comes from studies demonstrating feeding vessels from enlarged bronchial arteries to chronically inflamed airways. Pulmonary arterial vessels in the same area tend only to develop early thrombosis.[75,76] More direct evidence has come from studies that demonstrate the successful control of bleeding by embolization of the bronchial artery.[77,78]

Bleeding into the lungs of the cancer patient may have many causes; sepsis, chemotherapy, massive blood transfusions, drug effects, and organ damage from infiltration by tumor cells are known risk factors for hemorrhage in this setting. Circulatory tumor procoagulants cause activation of the clotting cascade and chronic consumption with disseminated intravascular coagulation (DIC). Derangements in both the fibrinolytic and coagulation pathways are common in the cancer patient, resulting in an increased risk of both hemorrhage and thrombosis.

The volume of expectorated blood that distinguishes massive from submassive hemoptysis has not been firmly established. Massive hemoptysis is variably defined in the literature as the expectoration of 100 mL of blood in a single episode to more than 600 mL of blood within a 24-hour period.[75,79,80] The hemodynamic and pulmonary responses to hemoptysis also help to define massive hemoptysis. Thus, any volume of bleeding in the airways that causes life-threatening airway obstruction, hypotension, aspiration, or anemia may be regarded as massive hemoptysis. Whether massive or submassive, this sentinel event is important not only because of its potential life-threatening consequences but also because it is a sign of underlying disease.

Bleeding into the lungs warrants a thorough initial evaluation, even when the amount of blood expectorated is small. Although the volume of expectorated blood may not necessarily parallel the seriousness of the underlying disease, the risk of death from massive hemoptysis does correlate strongly with the amount of blood expectorated. The rate of hemoptysis, the underlying pulmonary reserve, and the amount of blood retained in the lungs are also associated with the risk of death from massive hemoptysis, regardless of the cause of bleeding. Approximately 5% of patients with hemoptysis experience massive hemoptysis. Nearly one-third of patients with massive hemoptysis may have a fatal hemorrhage.[75] Death from endobronchial bleeding and alveolar hemorrhage usually results from asphyxiation rather than exsanguination.

Cancer-Related Etiologies

The major causes of massive hemoptysis are listed in Table 10–6. Several factors predispose the cancer patient to hemoptysis. Hematologic derangements, including severe neutropenia and thrombocytopenia, may occur as a consequence of chemotherapy or radiation therapy or may result from cancer infiltration of the bone marrow and the liver. Both neutropenia and granulocyte recovery may potentiate alveolar hemorrhage. Prolonged neutropenia after chemotherapy is common, especially after hematopoietic stem cell transplant (HSCT) and in patients with hematologic malignancies. Neutropenic patients are at risk for the development of necrotizing fungal infections such as aspergillosis and mucormycosis.

These angioinvasive organisms may cause vascular necrosis, leading to pulmonary infarction and hemorrhage. Increased local airway inflammation during the period of granulocyte recovery further propagates vascular damage by these fungal organisms. Viral and bacterial infections, irradiation injury, sepsis, and lung injury secondary to certain cytotoxic agents are common in patients undergoing chemotherapy for leukemia or in those who have received HSCT. Postmortem pathology suggests that any of these events may provoke the development of diffuse alveolar damage (DAD). In the setting of thrombocytopenia in these patients, DAD may be the cause of intractable hemoptysis and death.

Both primary bronchogenic carcinoma and metastatic disease to the lungs are potential sources of hemoptysis

TABLE 10–6. Conditions Associated with Massive Hemoptysis and Alveolar Hemorrhage in Patients with Cancer

Infectious
    Necrotizing pneumonia (*Staphylococcus, Legionella, Klebsiella*)
    Fungal pneumonia (*Aspergillus, Mucor, Coccidioides, Histoplasma*)
    Mycetoma
    Parasitic infection (strongyloidiasis, amebiasis, ascariasis)
    Viral infection (varicella, influenza)
    Mycobacterial pneumonia (tuberculosis; atypical mycobacteria)
    Lung abscess

Malignant
    Primary bronchogenic carcinoma
    Metastatic disease

Pulmonary
    Bronchiectasis
    Bronchopleural fistula
    Bullous emphysema
    Chronic bronchitis

Hematologic
    Neutrophil recovery following severe neutropenia
    Severe thrombocytopenia
    Platelet dysfunction
    Coagulopathy

Pharmacologic/toxic
    Anticoagulants
    Thrombolytic agents
    Radiation

Vascular
    Pulmonary embolism with infarction
    Pulmonary hypertension
    Fat embolism
    Vascular prosthesis

Iatrogenic
    Bronchoscopy
    Endobronchial laser (APC, cryotherapy, brachytherapy)
    Lung biopsy
    Transtracheal needle aspiration
    Swan-Ganz catheter placement

APC = argon plasma coagulation.

(Table 10–7). Although hemoptysis occurs in 10 to 20% of patients with primary bronchogenic carcinoma, fatal massive hemoptysis is rare. Approximately 3% of study patients with primary bronchogenic carcinoma developed fatal hemoptysis.[80,81] Eighty-three percent of patients with cancer-related hemoptysis have large centrally located tumors. Small-cell and squamous cell bronchogenic carcinomas are the most frequent histologic types of lung carcinoma associated with bleeding, followed by adenocarcinoma of the lung.[80,81] By virtue of their central endobronchial location and marked vascularity, bronchial carcinoid tumors are frequently associated with hemoptysis. Hemoptysis occurs in 83% of patients with central bronchial carcinoid tumors, and the volume of blood expectorated may vary from trace amounts of blood-streaked sputum to massive fatal hemoptysis. Hemoptysis from lung metastases occurs most often in those tumors with the highest propensity to endobronchial spread of disease. These include melanoma and primary tumors of the breast, kidneys, larynx, and colon. The direct extension of tumor into the tracheobronchial tree from contiguous sites within the mediastinum may also cause massive hemoptysis; esophageal carcinoma is one such tumor, and bleeding from this source may be fatal.

Management

The debilitated cancer patient is particularly at risk for respiratory failure and death caused by alveolar hemorrhage or endobronchial bleeding because of an inability to produce an effective cough to maintain a patent airway. In patients with rapid ongoing bleeding, hemodynamic instability, ventilation impairment, severe dyspnea, or hypoxemia, early intubation to protect the airway is recommended. Lateral decubitus positioning with the bleeding lung in dependent position may minimize the aspiration of blood into the contralateral lung. Volume resuscitation, supplemental oxygen, correction of pre-existing coagulopathy, and cough suppression are also important in the initial management of the unstable patient. Protection of the nonbleeding lung requires localization of the bleeding site, which may not always be readily obvious on clinical examination. Unstable patients should undergo selective occlusion of the right or left mainstem bronchus to prevent the aspiration of blood into the contralateral lung and to preserve gas exchange. Unilateral intubation may be accomplished by using a fiberoptic bronchoscope to guide the proper positioning of the endotracheal tube. For massive bleeding from a right-sided source, the left mainstem bronchus is electively intubated over the bronchoscope. This is accomplished by passing the bronchoscope through the endotracheal tube and advancing both scope and tube into the left mainstem bronchus. The bronchoscope is then withdrawn, and the tube cuff is inflated,

effectively isolating the normal (nonbleeding) lung. Because of the risk of occluding the right upper lobe, unilateral intubation of the right lung in the case of massive left-sided bleeds is not recommended. In this case, the trachea is intubated over the bronchoscope. Under bronchoscopic guidance, a 14 French (F) 100-cm Fogarty catheter is advanced into the left mainstem bronchus and inflated. The bronchoscope is then withdrawn, leaving the catheter in the left mainstem bronchus to occlude the bleeding left lung and leaving the endotracheal tube in the trachea to ventilate the right lung. Alternatively, intubation using a double-lumen endotracheal tube may be used to selectively isolate the nonbleeding lung. Double lumen endotracheal tubes are often cumbersome to place in proper position and may easily become displaced with movement. In addition, the smaller caliber of the double-lumen tube may predispose to airway obstruction by blood clots and may preclude the passage of a bronchoscope. For these reasons, the use of double-lumen tubes should be reserved for the critically unstable patient with severe bleeding or refractory hypoxemia.

Both rigid and fiberoptic bronchoscopy are important tools in the acute evaluation and management of massive hemoptysis. Balloon catheters may be passed through either the rigid or the fiberoptic bronchoscope for attempted endobronchial tamponade to control bleeding. The rigid bronchoscope provides better airway control, permits greater access for suctioning, and is far more effective than fiberoptic bronchoscopes in removing large clots from the airway. Because of the larger diameter of the rigid bronchoscope, visualization is limited to the mainstem bronchi. On the other hand, the fiberoptic bronchoscope allows greater access and better visualization of the distal airway.[75] The choice of bronchoscopic technique is primarily dictated by the clinician's training and comfort in using these instruments. Concurrent use of the flexible scope with the rigid bronchoscope has also been reported. Once the rigid scope is

TABLE 10–7. Types of Malignancies Associated with Massive Hemoptysis

Primary bronchogenic carcinoma
    Squamous cell carcinoma
    Bronchial carcinoid
Metastatic carcinoma
    Endobronchial spread of disease
    Hodgkin's lymphoma
    Breast carcinoma
    Colon carcinoma
    Melanoma
    Sarcoma
    Renal carcinoma
Mediastinal tumors with contiguous spread into the airways
    Esophageal carcinoma
    Lymphoma

positioned in the airway, the fiberoptic scope may be advanced through its lumen, allowing maximal suctioning capacity and visualization of the distal airway.

Bronchoscopic treatment modalities for the management of massive hemoptysis include the instillation of topical agents through a bronchoscope to reduce bleeding, iced saline lavage, and endobronchial tamponade.[82–84] Iced saline lavage acts as a vasoconstrictor to promote hemostasis in the bleeding airway. Several older reports supported the efficacy of this treatment modality, however recent controlled studies are lacking.[85] Topical epinephrine (1:20,000 dilution), thrombin, and fibrinogen-thrombin combinations have been used as hemostatic agents to control bleeding. These agents are instilled directly into the bleeding bronchus through a fiberoptic bronchoscope. Obtaining the maximal effectiveness of these drugs requires the identification of the bleeding site and endobronchial instillation with the bronchoscope in a wedged position against the bleeding bronchus. The usefulness of these agents in the treatment of massive hemoptysis has not been proved in controlled trials. Nonetheless, the topical application of hemostatic agents may be helpful in the acute management of the patient with massive endobronchial bleeds. The pharmacologic treatment of massive hemoptysis is based primarily on small uncontrolled studies and individual case reports. Systemic vasopressin,[75] corticosteroids,[86,87] and oral tranexamic acid [88] have been used in the treatment of massive hemoptysis, with anecdotal success. Because of its potent vasoconstrictor properties, intravenous vasopressin should be used with caution in patients with coronary artery disease or hypertension. In a recent review by Rumbak, patients with cavitary aspergilloma were treated with direct intracavitary instillation of the antifungal drug sodium or potassium iodide, with excellent control of hemoptysis.[83] Similar results have been reported with the local instillation of amphotericin B although systemic amphotericin therapy in the treatment of acute mycetoma-related hemoptysis has been disappointing. These antifungal agents are administered by local intracavitary instillation. The catheters may be placed either percutaneously or transbronchially. Local intracavitary treatment of mycetomas may represent a viable option for patients with massive hemoptysis when surgical intervention is not feasible.

Massive hemoptysis may also be controlled by using endobronchial tamponade. Fiberoptic bronchoscopy is used to identify the bleeding site. A Fogarty 200-cm balloon catheter (ranging in size from 4 to 7 French) is advanced through the working chamber of the scope into the bleeding bronchus and is inflated under direct visualization. The inflated balloon may remain in position for 24 to 48 hours. Double-lumen balloon catheters for the treatment of massive endobronchial bleeds have recently been developed.[84] At their proximal end, these catheters have a detachable valve that facilitates the withdrawal of the bronchoscope. The catheter also has an additional inner channel that can be used to administer vasoactive and hemostatic topical agents. Prolonged tamponade using endobronchial balloon catheters raises theoretic concerns regarding ischemia of the bronchial mucosa and postobstructive pneumonia. These complications, however, have not been reported in the literature.

Laser photocoagulation and electrocautery have had mixed results in the treatment of patients with massive hemoptysis. Laser photocoagulation using neodymium: yttrium-aluminum-garnet (Nd:YAG) laser phototherapy has been used with both palliative and curative intent in the treatment of hemoptysis from endobronchial tumors.[89,90] These lasers possess photocoagulative, photoresective, and vaporization properties, which permit the laser resection of central exophytic intraluminal tumors while controlling bleeding. Rigid bronchoscopy with general anesthesia is preferred although the procedure may be performed successfully through a fiberoptic bronchoscope, using topical anesthesia and conscious sedation only. The complications of Nd:YAG laser therapy may be catastrophic. These include tissue perforation, rupture, hemorrhage, airway combustion, and death.[90] The patient as well as the clinician and other team members should use protective eyewear to avoid injury from accidental laser scatter. Operators of Nd:YAG lasers should be very familiar with the technique and potential complications of this procedure. Argon plasma coagulation (APC) is a form of noncontact electrocoagulation that is also used in the definitive and palliative treatment of proximal endobronchial lesions. Unlike Nd:YAG laser therapy, APC is routinely performed through a flexible bronchoscope. The procedure may be safely performed without the need for endotracheal intubation or general anesthesia.[91] The depth of tissue penetration is smaller for APC (3 mm) than for Nd:YAG laser therapy (5 mm), thus minimizing the risk of airway perforation. The safe use of both instruments requires that supplemental oxygen be kept at a minimal level (preferably below 40%) to avoid collateral thermal tissue damage.[91,92]

As previously mentioned, the bronchial circulation is the source of massive hemoptysis in most patients. Cannulation of the bronchial artery with selective angiography is diagnostic in identifying the bleeding source in a majority of patients with massive hemoptysis. Embolization of the identified source vessels may be accomplished by using polyvinyl alcohol foam, Gianturco steel coils, isobutyl-2-cyanoacrylate, or absorbable gelatin pledgets. Short-term success in controlling bleeding is achieved in 85 to 98% of patients.[77,93] Treatment failures are primarily due to an inability to cannulate the bronchial artery or due to bleeding from a nonbronchial artery source. Collateral arteries arising from the intercostal, subclavian, phrenic, and mammary arteries are the source of bleeding in 45% of patients.[94] In addition, the pulmonary artery may be the source of massive hemoptysis on rare occasions.[75] This rare event may occur following placement or manipulation of a Swan-Ganz catheter and is signaled by a herald bleed. Pulmonary artery puncture or rupture is usually the cause of hemoptysis in this setting and may be fatal. Recurrent bleeding after successful embolotherapy may occur in 23 to 46% of patients within the year following initial therapy.[78,95,96] Fortunately, serious complications of vessel cannulation and embolization occur infrequently. These include vessel perforation, intimal tears, and inadvertent embolization of the spinal artery. Spinal artery embolization is seen in less than 1% of patients undergoing embolotherapy and occurs when the anterior spinal artery arises from the bronchial circulation. The unfortunate sequelae of this complication include spinal cord infarction and paraparesis. Radiation therapy may have a role in the acute treatment of massive hemoptysis after failed embolization. This treatment modality induces vascular thrombosis and necrosis of feeding vessels, leading to the reduction of bleeding. Successful control of bleeding with radiation therapy has been described in patients with persistent bleeding secondary to vascular tumors and in patients with bleeding caused by rupture of a mycetoma.[97]

Finally, surgical treatment is primarily reserved for those patients with refractory hemoptysis unresponsive to other therapeutic measures and for patients with life-threatening cardiovascular compromise related to persistent bleeding. Profuse bleeding (as from the rupture of a mycetoma) and pulmonary artery rupture or perforation are also indications for surgical therapy.[98,99] Reported mortality rates in medically and surgically treated patients with massive hemoptysis are highly variable: mortality rates range from 0.9 to 50% among surgically treated patients and from 1.6 to 80% among patients treated medically.[99–101] Randomized controlled trials comparing mortality rates from medical versus surgical management of massive hemoptysis, however, are lacking. Clinicians considering patients for surgical candidacy must carefully weigh the additional operative risks in the setting of severely compromised cardiopulmonary reserve against the potential surgical benefits. The assessment of eligibility for lung resection is often based on historical data and clinical examination as these patients are usually too unstable for physiologic testing. The approach to the cancer patient with massive hemoptysis is summarized in Table 10–8.

TOXIC LUNG INJURY

As the list and complexity of therapeutic regimens for the treatment of cancer has grown, so has the incidence and spectrum of associated lung diseases. The susceptibility of tissue to cytotoxic and radiation-induced injury varies from one organ system to the next. The lungs, however, appear to be particularly vulnerable. Interstitial pneumonitis and pulmonary fibrosis are potentially fatal adverse reactions to radiation and to cytotoxic chemotherapy. In addition, bronchiolitis obliterans, alveolar hemorrhage, noncardiogenic pulmonary edema, pulmonary veno-occlusive disease, alveolar lipoproteinosis, hypersensitivity pneumonitis, and pleural diseases are well-recognized potentially life-threatening syndromes of cancer treatment.

Anecdotal reports of lung injury caused by chemotherapeutic agents date back to Oliner's description of "busulfan lung" in 1961.[102] The literature has been replete with reports of chemotherapy-induced lung toxicity since then. In addition, recent developments in the emerging understanding of the biochemical and molecu-

---

TABLE 10–8. General Principles in the Management of Patients with Massive Hemoptysis

General measures
    Lateral decubitus positioning
    Supplemental oxygen
    Volume resuscitation
    Cough suppression
    Control of pre-existing coagulopathy
    Quantitation of volume/rate of hemoptysis

Localization of Bleeding
    History and physical examination
    Rigid/flexible bronchoscopy

Systemic Control of Bleeding
    Vasopressin
    Corticosteroids
    Tranexamic acid

Endobronchial therapy
    Topical hemostatic agents
        Epinephrine
        Thrombin
        Thrombin-fibrin solution
        Iced saline lavage?
    Endobronchial tamponade
        Fogarty catheter
        Intubation using double-lumen tube
    Nd:YAG laser
    Argon plasma coagulation/electrocautery
    Photocoagulation
    Cryotherapy*

Other measures
    Radiation
    Embolotherapy with angiography
    Positive-end-expiratory pressure (PEEP)
    Direct instillation of antifungal agents (sodium or potassium iodide)
    Surgical repair/resection

Nd:YAG = neodymium:yttrium-aluminum-garnet.
*Not for acute treatment of bleeding.

lar determinants of cancer have paved the way for new classes of antineoplastic agents, including the biologic response modifiers. Some of these newer agents are also implicated in treatment-related lung damage. Because the lung is a targeted organ in the development of treatment-related disease, the amount of literature on this subject is staggering. The following discussion is not an encyclopedic treatise on all of the cytotoxic chemotherapeutic agents that are suspected of causing adverse lung effects but rather an attempt to concisely review those chemotherapeutic agents that are known to induce clinically relevant syndromes of lung disease and to summarize recent progress in this field. Table 10–9 lists these agents and their associated major patterns of lung injury. Lung toxicity is also the principal dose-limiting factor in radiotherapy. The adverse consequences of radiation therapy on the lung and the spectrum of radiation-induced lung diseases are also discussed in this section.

Cytotoxin-Related Lung Injury

Incidence. Precise estimates of the incidence of adverse pulmonary reactions caused by individual cytotoxic agents vary widely. In general, lung toxicity occurs in 3 to 30% of patients treated with chemotherapy.[103] These rates may exceed 75% in the setting of combined-modality and multidrug therapy. Identifying the responsible individual chemotherapeutic agent is even more of a diagnostic challenge. Individual drugs are usually given as part of a multidrug regimen or in conjunction with other therapeutic modalities. In addition, the clinical and radiographic manifestations of drug-induced lung disease in cancer patients may mimic a variety of other diagnoses, including pulmonary infection. Thus, in the absence of specific biologic markers for early lung injury, definitive identification of lung damage due to an individual agent is based on histologic confirmation and the exclusion of alternative diagnoses.

Pathogenesis. Two major mechanisms in the pathogenesis of cytotoxin-related lung damage have been advanced. Direct toxicity of type II pneumocytes and endothelial cells may impair cellular reparative processes and lead to lung injury. Free oxygen radicals (metabolites of molecular oxygen that damage cellular deoxyribonucleic acid [DNA]), may mediate direct toxic reactions to the lungs. Type II pneumocytes and endothelial cells are particularly susceptible to this type of insult. Chemotherapeutic agents, including bleomycin, cyclophosphamide, and busulfan, induce breaks in cellular DNA, resulting in the formation of free oxygen radicals that ultimately lead to cellular metaplasia and dysplastic changes in type II pneumocytes.[104,105] Radiation therapy and high-inspired oxygen may induce direct toxic lung reactions.[104,105] Thus, synergistic interactions that occur in multimodal-

ity therapy using certain cytotoxic drugs and radiation or high-inspired oxygen may be explained on the basis of similar mechanisms of injury.

A hypersensitivity or idiosyncratic reaction is the second major mechanism that underlies chemotherapy-induced lung injury. This mechanism of injury has been implicated in lung disease induced by bleomycin, methotrexate, procarbazine, and microtubule stabilizing agents (taxanes).[105–109] Hypersensitivity reactions tend to be dose independent. Interference with collagen metabolism may underlie other toxic lung reactions. Bleomycin has been shown to alter the collagenesis-collagenolysis balance by stimulating fibroblast proliferation. Finally, immunologic mechanisms of lung injury have been implicated. Immunomodulating agents such as cyclophosphamide, bleomycin, and methotrexate may cause lung tissue damage by altering the normal effector/suppressor immune balance within the lung. Hypersensitivity pneumonitis may occur as a result of this mechanism.

Clinical Presentation and Effects of Specific Agents. The recognition of cytotoxin-induced lung injury requires a high index of suspicion coupled with a full awareness of early signs, symptoms, and risk factors associated with the disease. The clinical manifestations of lung toxicity commonly occur during drug administration but may develop months to years later. Three major patterns of lung injury predominate: (1) chronic pneumonitis with or without fibrosis, (2) noncardiogenic pulmonary edema, and (3) acute hypersensitivity pneumonitis. Lung injuries from cytotoxic agents share common characteristic signs and symptoms, regardless of the category of the individual agent. The clinical presentation is frequently characterized by the insidious onset of dyspnea, dry cough, fever, anorexia, and malaise. Bibasilar rales on lung examination are common but nonspecific findings. Symptoms of fever, dyspnea on exertion, and dry cough usually occur 2 weeks after the initiation of therapy. A bibasilar reticular pattern, similar to that noted after the administration of other cytotoxic agents, is the usual radiographic finding. Histopathologic findings are those that are common to other types of cytotoxic lung injury; fibroblast proliferation, dysplastic type II pneumocytes, and endothelial swelling are noted routinely. A lymphocytic and histiocytic inflammatory response in the airway is also commonly found. Pulmonary function abnormalities are unreliable early predictors of lung injury. A restrictive lung defect and a decreased diffusion capacity of the lung for carbon monoxide (DL_{CO}) may be seen. This finding may not necessarily correlate with radiographic findings or the development of pulmonary symptoms.

Cytotoxic Antibiotics. *Bleomycin.* Bleomycin, a polypeptide antitumor antibiotic, exerts broad activity against

TABLE 10–9. Cancer Therapy and Major Associated Lung Toxicities

Agent	NCPE	IP	Bronchospasm	Pleural Effusion	Lung Fibrosis	ARDS	PTX	PE	Hilar LN	Other
Alkylating Agents										
Busulfan	—	Yes	—	Rare	Yes	—	—	—	—	PAP, BAC (rare)
Cyclophosphamide	Yes	Yes	—	—	Yes	—	—	—	—	—
Antimetabolites										
Cytosine arabinoside	Yes	—	—	Yes	Yes	Yes	—	—	—	—
Fludarabine monophosphate	Yes	Yes	—	Yes	—	—	—	—	—	*Pneumocystis carinii* pneumonia, other infections
Methothrexate	Yes	Yes	—	Yes	Yes	Yes	—	—	Yes	NC granulomas, nodules
Azathioprine	—	Rare	—	—	—	—	—	—	—	Airway edema
6-Mercaptopurine	—	Rare	—	Yes	—	—	—	—	—	—
Gemcitabine	Yes	—	Yes	Yes	—	—	—	—	—	—
Biologic response modifiers										
Interleukin-2	Yes	—	—	Yes	—	—	—	—	—	Pulmonary hypertension
Tumor necrosis factor	Yes	—	—	Yes	—	—	—	—	—	Pulmonary hypertension
G-CSF/GM-CSF	Yes	—	—	Yes	—	—	—	Yes	—	Peripheral eosinophilia
Trastuzumab	—	—	—	—	—	—	—	—	—	Cardiogenic pulmonary edema
Rituximab	Rare	—	Yes	—	—	—	—	—	—	Angioedema
Cytotoxic antibiotics										
Bleomycin	—	Yes	—	Yes	Yes	Yes	Yes	—	—	BOOP, lung nodules, VOD, acute chest pain
Mitomycin	Yes	Yes	Yes*	Yes	Yes	Yes	—	—	Yes	HUS/TTP
Nitrosoureas										
Carmustine	—	Yes	—	—	Yes	—	Yes	—	—	VOD (rare), granulomas mimicking WGM
Lomustine	—	Yes	—	—	Yes	—	Yes	—	—	VOD (rare), granulomas mimicking WGM
Taxanes										
Paclitaxel	—	Yes	Yes	—	—	—	—	—	—	Hypersensitivity reaction, anaphylaxis
Docetaxel	—	Yes	Yes	—	—	—	—	—	—	Hypersensitivity reaction, anaphylaxis
Other chemotherapeutic agents										
Procarbazine	—	Yes	—	Yes	Yes	—	—	—	—	NC granulomas, hypersensitivity reaction
Tamoxifen citrate	—	—	—	—	—	—	—	Yes	—	—
L-Asparaginase	—	—	—	—	—	—	—	Yes	—	—
Retinoic Acid	Yes	—	—	—	—	Yes	—	—	—	Diffuse alveolar hemorrhage
Vinblastine	Yes	—	Yes†	—	—	—	—	—	—	—
Radiation	—	Yes	—	Yes	Yes	—	Yes	—	—	Bronchiectasis, volume loss, VOD

ARDS = adult respiratory distress syndrome; BAC = bronchoalveolar cell carcinoma; BOOP = bronchiolitis obliterans and organizing pneumonia; G-CSF = granulocyte colony-stimulating factor; GM-CSF = granulocyte-macrophage colony-stimulating factor; Hilar LN = hilar lymphadenopathy; HUS = hemolytic uremic syndrome; IP = interstitial pneumonitis; NC = noncaseating; NCPE = noncardiogenic pulmonary edema; PAP = pulmonary alveolar proteinosis; PE = pulmonary embolism; PTX = pneumothorax; TTP = thrombocytopenic thrombotic purpura; VOD = veno-occlusive disease; WGM = Wegener's granulomatosis.

*In association with vinca alkaloids.

†In association with mitomycin.

germ cell tumors, malignant lymphoma, and a variety of squamous cell carcinomas. Bleomycin exerts its toxic effects where it concentrates: in the skin, mucous membranes, and lungs. The lungs and skin are particularly susceptible to bleomycin toxicity, perhaps because of the paucity of the inactivating enzyme, bleomycin hydrolase, at these sites. The principal dose-limiting factor in bleomycin administration is lung toxicity. Several distinct clinical syndromes of bleomycin-related lung toxicity exist. These include (1) a predictable dose-dependent interstitial pneumonitis that may progress to chronic fibrosis, (2) an acute chest pain syndrome, (3) bronchiolitis obliterans with organizing pneumonia, (4) acute hypersensitivity pneumonitis with peripheral eosinophilia resembling eosinophilic pneumonia syndrome, and (5) pulmonary veno-occlusive disease.[108,110] Bleomycin remains the prototypical chemotherapeutic agent for studying the pathogenesis of interstitial pneumonitis and subsequent fibrosis. Pneumonitis-fibrosis is the most common reaction in the lungs and occurs in 3 to 40% of recipients of the drug.[111,112]

The rates of bleomycin-related lung disease vary with the total cumulative dose of the drug, the route of administration, supplemental oxygen therapy, concurrent or prior irradiation, multidrug therapy, granulocyte colony-stimulating factor administration, age (higher risk with age greater than 70 years), and the presence of uremia. Although fatal pulmonary fibrosis has been reported with as little as 50 U (total) of bleomycin, the risk of lung injury increases precipitously with total cumulative levels > 450 U. The toxic effects of bleomycin on the lung are potentiated by the radiosensitizing and radio-recall properties of this drug. Lung disease following combined radiation and bleomycin chemotherapy occurs more frequently and is of greater severity than lung disease resulting from bleomycin treatment alone. Rates of lung toxicity among patients who are receiving combined bleomycin and radiation may be as high as 43% in some studies.[113] Samuels and colleagues reported increased rates of clinically significant lung disease in up to 50% of patients who received high-dose bleomycin within 12 months of prior radiation.[114] The time interval between sequential multimodality therapy with bleomycin and radiotherapy that would mitigate the risk of lung damage has not been clearly established. The coadministration of bleomycin with other chemotherapeutic agents also facilitates lung injury. Bleomycin-based regimens such as ABVD (doxorubicin [Adriamycin], bleomycin, vincristine, and dacarbazine) and M-BACOD (methotrexate, bleomycin, Adriamycin, cyclophosphamide, vincristine [Oncovin], and dexamethasone) may enhance the frequency of lung toxicity and amplify the severity of the disease.[115,116] Synergistic interactions between bleomycin and high-inspired oxygen augment

lung injury.[117,118] In landmark studies by Goldinger, patients with prior bleomycin exposure who were treated with hyperoxia (inspired fraction of oxygen [FIO2] ≥ 30%) during surgery developed excess rates of adult respiratory distress syndrome (ARDS), respiratory failure, and death.[118] Postoperative morbidity and mortality were greatly reduced when supplemental oxygen was restricted to an FIO2 ≤ 25%. In bleomycin-treated patients, ARDS may occur as early as 12 to 18 hours after hyperoxia exposure. Although the interval between bleomycin and oxygen administration that minimizes the risk of lung injury has not been clearly defined, patients with prior exposure to bleomycin within a 1- to 3-month period appear to be at greatest risk.[117] These unresolved issues pose interesting challenges for the clinician treating bleomycin-exposed patients who require mechanical ventilation or those patients who are anticipating surgical procedures with general anesthesia. Patients with recent bleomycin exposure, prior evidence of lung disease, or other identified risk factors are at greatest risk for hyperoxic-lung toxicity. In these patients, continuous invasive monitoring of mixed venous oxygen saturations is recommended to optimize oxygen saturation while minimizing oxygen requirements.

Radiographic findings of bibasilar reticular infiltrates mimic the changes seen in other types of cytotoxin-induced lung injury. In addition, pleural disease (including pleural thickening) is common. Subpleural blebs are occasionally seen and may give rise to spontaneous pneumothorax and pneumomediastinum. The presence of pleural effusions is extremely uncommon and suggests an alternative diagnosis. Bleomycin-induced lung disease may occasionally appear as discrete nodules simulating metastatic disease or infection.[119] A restrictive lung defect and a fall in DL_{CO} are the most common changes in physiologic parameters with bleomycin therapy. The DL_{CO} appears to be the most sensitive parameter and may be used to guide therapy. Reductions in the DL_{CO} are dose dependent and may precede the development of clinical symptoms and radiographic findings by 2 to 3 weeks. The early recognition of bleomycin toxicity is crucial as prompt withdrawal and treatment are associated with improvement in lung function.[120] A decline in DL_{CO} from pretreatment values of 10 to 15% or greater should prompt the withdrawal of the drug and the initiation of a work-up for possible bleomycin-induced lung injury. Linear reductions in DL_{CO} of more than 60% from baseline herald fatal pulmonary toxicity.[121] Initial therapy for patients with bleomycin toxicity is cessation of the drug; spontaneous improvement in lung function may occur with simple drug withdrawal.

Corticosteroids appear to be of variable benefit in the treatment of bleomycin-induced lung disease.[119] The recommended dosages of prednisone have ranged from

60 to 100 mg/d. Guidelines regarding the administration and withdrawal of steroid therapy have not been clearly delineated. Bleomycin-associated hypersensitivity pneumonitis with eosinophilia usually responds promptly to steroids. The value of steroids in the treatment of pneumonitis-fibrosis and other forms of bleomycin toxicity is less clear. In steroid-responsive patients, improvements in lung function and/or radiographic findings usually occur within the first 3 months of therapy. The efficacy of prophylactic steroid therapy in the treatment of bleomycin-exposed patients who subsequently require mechanical ventilation or general anesthesia has not been proved. Mortality rates for bleomycin-related lung disease vary widely, depending on the patient population studied and the criteria used in making the diagnosis. Case fatality rates range from 13 to 83% in the literature.[122]

Peplomycin. Peplomycin is a newer bleomycin analogue with extended antitumor activity. Early reports suggested lower rates of pulmonary toxicity.[122,123] Studies are needed to determine whether synergistic toxicities exist between peplomycin and hyperoxia.

Mitomycin. Mitomycin is an antitumor antibiotic that exerts its effect through cell-cycle-specific alkylation and inhibition of DNA synthesis. This agent has broad application in the treatment of carcinomas of gastrointestinal, gynecologic, breast, prostatic, and (more recently) primary bronchogenic origin. Mitomycin-induced pulmonary toxicity occurs in 3 to 12% of patients. As with bleomycin, the incidence and spectrum of lung toxicity sharply rises with multimodality or multiagent therapy. Rates of lung injury with concomitant or sequential use of the vinca alkaloids or 5-fluorouracil may approach 35%.[124] Several potentially life-threatening patterns of pulmonary toxicity have been observed. The most common pattern, interstitial pneumonitis-fibrosis, characteristically occurs 2 to 4 months after chemotherapy. Acute bronchospasm with or without pulmonary infiltrates has also been described in patients who are receiving concurrent or sequential vinca alkaloid therapy. These symptoms may develop in approximately 5% of patients receiving this combination of drugs and may be severe. Symptoms may persist for 24 hours and resolve with steroid therapy. Derangements evident on pulmonary function testing may persist despite the resolution of clinical symptoms. The recommended interval of delay in sequential mitomycin/vinca alkaloid therapy that would limit the risk of lung damage is unknown. Mitomycin also causes an acute noncardiogenic pulmonary edema when used in combination with vinca alkaloids.[125,126] Hemolytic uremic-like syndrome (HUS) has also been observed in patients with combined mitomycin/vinca alkaloid therapy and is the most life-threatening pattern of lung injury. Patients may present with microangiopathic hemolytic anemia, thrombocytopenia, and renal insufficiency in varying degrees of severity. Mortality rates may approach 90% in patients with full-blown mitomycin-induced HUS. Early discontinuation of the drug and steroid therapy may alter the outcome.[126]

Alkylating Agents. *Busulfan and Cyclophosphamide.* The alkylating agents busulfan and cyclophosphamide are antineoplastic and anti-inflammatory drugs that exert their therapeutic effects through the alkylation of cellular DNA. The earliest descriptions of cytotoxin-related lung injury implicated busulfan in the development of pulmonary fibrosis.[102] Lung toxicity due to other alkylating agents, including cyclophosphamide, melphalan, and chlorambucil, has also been documented.[127,128] Alkylating agents primarily cause excess lung injury when given in high doses or as part of a multidrug or multimodality regimen. With the exception of busulfan, these agents rarely cause lung damage as single-drug therapy. Considering the widespread use of these agents in the treatment of myeloproliferative disorders and as part of the conditioning regimen for HSCT, the incidence of pulmonary toxicity is rare. The estimated incidence of busulfan-induced lung toxicity in accumulated reports is 4 to 10%.[129,130] Subclinical toxicity does occur and is noted to be as high as 46% in autopsy studies.[130]

Busulfan lung is characterized by the insidious onset of unexplained fever, dry cough, dyspnea, weight loss, and fatigue. Symptoms tend to occur late, on average, approximately 36 months after the initiation of treatment. Radiographic findings of ill-defined bibasilar infiltrates are characteristic, and the absence of changes on chest radiography should suggest an alternative diagnosis. Pleural effusions rarely occur. The diagnosis is based on the findings of histopathologic changes present in sputum or bronchoalveolar lavage (BAL) fluid. Bizarre-shaped dysplastic pneumocytes are consistently noted in the sputum and BAL fluid and suggest the diagnosis. Histologic changes common to other cytotoxic agents are also observed and include fibroblast proliferation, mononuclear cell infiltration, and desquamation of type II pneumocytes. Pulmonary function testing usually reveals a restrictive lung defect with a reduction in DL_{CO}. Synergistic interactions between busulfan with other alkylating agents or with radiotherapy have been reported in the literature.[131] Both prior and concomitant therapy with radiotherapy or other alkylating agents may result in acute diffuse lung damage and respiratory decompensation. Although busulfan-associated lung toxicity appears to be an idiosyncratic reaction, there seems to be a threshold dose of 500 mg, above which the risk of lung damage is greatly increased. Fully developed lung injury due to busulfan carries a poor prognosis, with mortality rates as high as 90%. The average life span after the diagnosis of severe busulfan-related lung injury is only 5 months. Definitive therapy has not been established. Supportive measures, including drug withdrawal, remain the mainstays of treatment. Anecdotal reports of symptom improvement with corticosteroid therapy have been described, but no associated improvement in mortality has been systematically documented in the literature.

Cyclophosphamide, a nitrogen mustard, has efficacy in the treatment of a variety of malignant and nonmalignant diseases. This agent is cleaved to the active metabolites acrolein and phosphoramide mustard. Both of these metabolites may cause oxidant lung injury through their participation in redox reactions. In addition, cyclophosphamide's immunomodulatory effects on T cells and alveolar macrophages may indirectly contribute to lung toxicity. Accurate estimates of the incidence of cyclophosphamide-induced lung injury are difficult to assess as this agent is usually administered in conjunction with other potentially cytotoxic drugs. Nonetheless, accumulated reports suggest that 2% of patients that receive cyclophosphamide-based chemotherapy may develop lung damage. The rate may be much higher (31 to 44%) in the setting of multiagent chemotherapy regimens that contain cyclophosphamide in combination with bleomycin, vincristine, etoposide, carmustine, or mitoxanthone.[132,133] The appearance of lung injury is not directly related to dose, although more frequent toxicity has been demonstrated with high-dose therapy (50 to 150 mg/kg/d for 4 days). The clinical, radiographic, and pathologic findings of lung injury after cyclophosphamide use are similar to those seen in association with other cytotoxin-induced lung diseases. Bibasilar reticular infiltrates are common radiographic findings; noncardiogenic pulmonary edema has also been described. Symptom onset may vary widely. Patients may present with symptoms of progressive dyspnea, dry cough, and low-grade fever 2 weeks to 13 years after the initial administration of the drug. Pulmonary function testing may reveal a restrictive lung defect and decreased DL_{CO}. The degree of pulmonary function derangement may not correlate with clinical or radiographic observations. The prognosis for patients with cyclophosphamide-induced lung injury is highly variable. Mortality rates may exceed 40% and are dictated by the presence of other confounding risk factors. As with lung injury caused by other cytotoxic agents, the value of steroid therapy in altering patient outcome has not been firmly established.

Antimetabolites. *Methotrexate.* The folate antagonist methotrexate demonstrates activity in a wide range of malignant and inflammatory disorders, including acute leukemias, sarcomas, breast carcinoma, psoriasis, asthma, primary biliary cirrhosis, and rheumatoid arthritis. Sostman and colleagues reported the incidence of lung toxicity among cancer patients receiving high-dose methotrexate at 7%, with a case fatality rate of 11%.[133a] Increased rates of methotrexate toxicity are demonstrated with multidrug regimens containing etoposide or cyclophosphamide. Frequent dosing schedules also confer an increased risk. Monthly or bimonthly dosing is associated with fewer toxic lung effects than daily or weekly administration of the drug.[110] Other factors, including patient age, total cumulative dose, supplemental oxygen therapy, multimodality therapy, and preexisting underlying lung disease, do not appear to be precipitating factors in the development of lung injury. Severe toxicity has been reported after adrenalectomy and with rapid steroid withdrawal.[108] Methotrexate-induced injury is postulated to occur as a result of a hypersensitivity reaction within the lungs. Evidence in support of this theory is derived from the presence of an exuberant peripheral eosinophilia and a T-helper lymphocyte alveolitis and granuloma formation on BAL fluid analysis. Blood eosinophilia is noted in approximately 40% of patients with lung injury. Rechallenge with methotrexate, however, does not reliably reproduce lung disease, suggesting that additional mechanisms may contribute to the development of disease. Lung injury has been described with all forms of methotrexate administration (oral, intravenous, intrathecal, and intramuscular). Thus, a direct toxic effect that targets the lungs is suggested.

Several clinical patterns exist. Noncardiogenic pulmonary edema is the hallmark of the acute form of the disease, which may progress to respiratory failure and death. More commonly, patients present with a constellation of subacute symptoms including low-grade fever, nonproductive cough, dyspnea, fatigue, headache, malaise, and an erythematous skin rash. Clinical symptoms of chronic methotrexate toxicity tend to occur within 3 to 4 weeks after the initiation of the drug and may wax and wane without adjustments in therapy. Acute pleuritis occurs rarely, usually in association with pleural effusions. Diffuse bibasilar reticular infiltrates typical of other cytotoxin-related lung diseases are common. Bilateral and unilateral effusions may occur as isolated findings or in conjunction with parenchymal lung disease. Hilar adenopathy, ascinar shadows, and nodular opacities have been reported and may mimic the underlying disease.[108] Histologic findings of a mononuclear cell infiltrate, interstitial eosinophilia, and noncaseating granulomas may help to distinguish methotrexate-induced lung toxicity from other etiologies. Methotrexate-induced lung toxicity usually portends a favorable prognosis. Spontaneous remission does occur, usually in the setting of pneumonitis. Clinical remissions may occur even with continuation of therapy. The indication for steroid administration in this subgroup of patients has therefore been questioned. Corticosteroid therapy is indicated in the treatment of acute fulminant lung toxicity although no prospective studies have examined the impact of supplemental steroid therapy on outcomes. Mortality rates of 10% have been reported among patients with acute fulminant disease.

Fludarabine Monophosphate. Fludarabine, an analogue of arabinoside A, is currently the most active agent used in the treatment of chronic lymphocytic leukemias. It also has proven efficacy for the treatment of other lymphoid malignancies, including promyelocytic leukemia, cutaneous T-cell lymphoma, indolent non-Hodgkin's lymphoma, and Waldenström's macroglobulinemia. Lung toxicity and increased rates of pneumonia, pleural effusions, and interstitial pneumonitis have been observed in 14 to 69% of patients. Among the associated lung infections, *Pneumocystis carinii* pneumonia is of particular concern and occurs in 10 to 20% of patients.[134] Spontaneous remissions commonly occur with simple drug withdrawal. The overall prognosis and the response to corticosteroids are generally favorable.

Cytosine Arabinoside. Cytosine arabinoside (ara-C) is a pyrimidine nucleoside analogue that inhibits DNA. This agent is used in conventional adjuvant chemotherapy regimens primarily for the treatment of acute leukemias. High-dose ara-C may result in severe pulmonary toxicity. Noncardiogenic pulmonary edema and ARDS has been described with 14-day dosage schedules of 3 mg/m^2 per 12 hours. Estimates of lung toxicity range from 5 to 32% and vary with the dosage of the drug.[135,136] The potential pathogenic mechanism underlying lung toxicity related to ara-C has not been completely elucidated. It is thought, however, that ara-C induces a capillary leak syndrome that involves the lung parenchymal, pleural, pericardial, and peritoneal surfaces. Patients usually present with abrupt symptoms of respiratory distress at 2 to 21 days into therapy. Despite severe toxicity, the overall prognosis is good. Mortality rates of 10% are reported in the literature. Recovery is usually complete within 10 days of the onset of symptoms. Anecdotal evidence supports the use of steroid therapy in these patients.

Gemcitabine. Gemcitabine (2′,2′-difluoro-2′-deoxycytidine) is a relatively new nucleoside analogue that exerts its effect through the inhibition of DNA synthesis. This agent has proven clinical benefit in the treatment of pancreatic cancer and a variety of common epithelial solid tumors. Gemcitabine has been used extensively in the palliative treatment of advanced non-small-cell lung cancers. Lung cytotoxicity is schedule-dependent (ie, it correlates with the duration of exposure) but not distinctly dose-dependent. Two major patterns of lung toxicity have been described in patients taking this drug. Acute dyspnea with bronchospasm may occur within the first few hours of

drug infusion. This adverse reaction tends to be mild and usually remits without the discontinuation of therapy. Severe life-threatening noncardiogenic pulmonary edema reminiscent of capillary leak syndrome has also been described. The latter condition requires drug withdrawal and is (fortunately) rare. Rechallenge with this agent in patients with a prior history of gemcitabine-related pulmonary edema is not recommended.[137]

Azathioprine and 6-Mercaptopurine. 6-Mercaptopurine is the major metabolic product of azathioprine. Both drugs have been used in the treatment of hematologic malignancies as well as non-neoplastic inflammatory processes. Rare cases of acute pneumonitis associated with restrictive lung disease have been reported after treatment with each of these agents. Lung toxicity improves with the substitution of alternate therapy and the institution of corticosteroid therapy.

Nitrosoureas. The nitrosoureas are a group of agents that are used in the treatment of a variety of malignant diseases, including hematologic malignancies (multiple myeloma and lymphoma), melanoma, and carcinomas of the gastrointestinal tract, central nervous system, and lungs. These agents exert antineoplastic activity through the alkylation and carbamylation of cellular macromolecules and the inhibition of glutathione disulfide reductase. The inhibition of glutathione disulfide reductase may theoretically play a critical role in the development of lung toxicity by sensitizing normal tissues to oxidant damage. Among the six different nitrosoureas that are currently available on the market, only carmustine (BCNU), lomustine (CCNU), and semustine (methyl CCNU) have been associated with pulmonary toxicity. Most of the reports of nitrosourea-related lung injury have been due to BCNU therapy. The following discussion summarizes the current knowledge regarding BCNU-related lung disease.

Carmustine (1,3-bis[2-chloroethyl]-1-nitrosourea) is commonly used as single-agent therapy in the treatment of malignant brain tumors. The treatment of patients with BCNU as single-agent therapy permits the direct assessment of the cytotoxic effects of this drug on the lungs as most patients with glioma have no underlying lung disease at initial presentation. Rates of pulmonary toxicity with single-agent therapy vary with dosage and with the duration of treatment but generally range from 20 to 30%. Risk factors underlying BCNU-related lung disease have been clearly defined. For patients with pre-existing lung disease, including bronchiectasis, chronic obstructive pulmonary disease (COPD), asthma, or recurrent pneumonia, the risk of lung toxicity is amplified. Excessively high rates of fatal lung injury have been observed among female patients.[138] The cytotoxicity of BCNU increases linearly with increasing doses of the drug.

Cumulative doses of BCNU that exceed 1,500 mg/m^2 are associated with a 10-fold increase in the incidence of BCNU-induced lung injury. Patients younger than 7 years of age appear to be at greater risk for BCNU toxicity. This may reflect the larger numbers of cycles of the drug received in younger patients and thus greater total cumulative doses of the drug. Combined therapy with other cytotoxic agents (including cyclophosphamide and mitomycin) may aggravate BCNU cytotoxicity.[139] A synergistic relationship between BCNU and hyperoxia or radiation therapy has not been firmly established.

The signs and symptoms of BCNU lung toxicity usually occur during treatment. Occasional reports, however, have noted the insidious onset of dyspnea and dry cough years after the completion of therapy. Acute presentations that may progress to ARDS and death have also been reported and usually correlate with higher cumulative doses of the drug. The radiographic and histologic findings of BCNU toxicity are similar to those reported with other cytotoxic agents. In addition to reticular infiltrates and fibrosis, bilateral as well as unilateral pneumothorax may be seen on chest radiographs. Chest radiography cannot be relied on to assist with the diagnosis because radiographic changes tend to occur late, well after changes in pulmonary function and clinical symptoms have appeared. Occasionally, CXRs may be normal despite pathologic evidence of lung damage. The pathologic features of BCNU toxicity are similar to those already discussed. In addition, morphologic features suggesting pulmonary veno-occlusive disease and angiocentric necrotizing granulomas that mimic Wegener's granulomatosis have been reported. Histopathologic features suggesting interstitial fibrosis without accompanying inflammatory changes are typical of advanced BCNU-related lung injury. A reduction in DL$_{CO}$ represents the earliest physiologic change and may precede clinical symptoms or alterations detected by chest radiography or histopathology by several weeks. Fatal BCNU-related lung disease occurs in 30 to 40% of affected patients with full-blown disease. The disease may run a recalcitrant course despite the cessation of the drug and the institution of steroid therapy. The efficacy of prophylactic steroid administration in curtailing lung toxicity has not been proved.

Taxanes. Taxanes are microtubule-stabilizing agents that are relatively new drugs in the growing armamentarium against cancer. The two major taxane agents, paclitaxel (Taxol) and docetaxel (Taxotere) are used primarily in the treatment of solid tumors, including carcinomas of the breasts and ovaries and non-small-cell carcinoma of the lung. Myelosuppression is the major dose-dependent toxicity of taxanes. As this adverse reaction has been ameliorated with the concomitant use of growth factors, new toxicities resulting from more aggressive dose escalation

strategies have emerged. Early clinical trials described idiosyncratic hypersensitivity reactions, including anaphylaxis, in 15 to 20% of patients who take these drugs.[140] Patients developed acute flushing, bronchospasm, urticaria, angioedema, pruritis, and hemodynamic instability, usually within the first hour of drug administration. The incidence of these life-threatening symptoms has waned significantly with the routine use of prophylactic corticosteroids, epinephrine, H$_2$ antagonists and H$_1$ antagonists. Severe reactions now occur in only 2 to 3% of patients.[140] Mild hypersensitivity reactions still occur, however, despite premedication in as many as 40% of patients. Taxol and Taxotere are formulated in polyoxyethylated castor oil (cremophor EL) and polysorbate solvents that trigger the release of histamines. Mast cell activation with histamine release is thought to underlie the hypersensitivity reactions of the taxanes. Mild reactions may only warrant the administration of appropriate supportive therapy. More severe reactions, however, require drug cessation and the initiation of additional aggressive intervention with steroids, bronchodilators, epinephrine, and antihistamines. Recrudescence of symptoms may occur with redosing. Therefore, extreme caution is warranted in treating patients with an antecedent history of taxane-related hypersensitivity reactions.

Miscellaneous Cytotoxics. Procarbazine is a methylhydrazine derivative typically used in combination with other chemotherapeutic agents in the treatment of lymphoma. A hypersensitivity pneumonitis has been described in patients who are receiving procarbazine-based chemotherapy. The recurrence of symptoms after the re-institution of this drug lends support to procarbazine-induced hypersensitivity reactions. Clinical manifestations of acute fever, dyspnea, dry cough, and skin rash usually occur during drug administration. Histopathologic changes include blood and tissue eosinophilia, noncaseating granulomas, and mononuclear cell infiltration. Withdrawal of the drug may suffice to ameliorate symptoms.

L-asparaginase is an antineoplastic agent derived from *Escherichia coli* and has activity against acute lymphocytic leukemia. Reductions in antithrombin III, leading to increased rates of thromboembolic disease, have been reported with the use of this agent.[141]

Tamoxifen citrate is an antiestrogen agent with activity against breast carcinoma. This chemotherapeutic agent is associated with a slightly increased risk of venous thrombosis disease, possibly owing to its ability to decrease levels of antithrombin III.[142]

All-*trans*-retinoic acid is of proven efficacy in the treatment of acute promyelocytic leukemia. Lung toxicity (most notably noncardiogenic pulmonary edema, diffuse alveolar hemorrhage, and ARDS) has been reported in up to 25% of patients who were taking this drug.[143] Reversal of the parenchymal infiltrative processes and dramatic reductions (66%) in the incidence of lung injury have been reported with corticosteroid administration. Pretreatment strategies now include steroid administration as standard practice at most institutions.[140]

Biologic Response Modifiers. Biologic response modifiers (BRMs) make up a relatively new class of agents that target specific cellular sites that are critical to the growth, survival, and metastasis of malignant cells. This class of drugs includes a growing list of cytokines, growth factors, and synthetic compounds, including interleukin-2, trastuzumab (Herceptin), tumor necrosis factor (TNF), granulocyte macrophage colony-stimulating factor (GM-CSF), granulocyte-colony-stimulating factor (G-CSF), and the monoclonal antibody rituximab. Pulmonary toxicity has been documented with some of these agents; however, understanding of the full efficacy and toxic potential of each of these agents is still evolving.

Adoptive immunotherapy with interleukin-2 (IL-2) may cause severe cardiovascular collapse accompanied by acute severe respiratory distress and noncardiogenic pulmonary edema secondary to capillary leak syndrome. Hemodynamic derangements may mimic septic shock with reduced peripheral vascular resistance, increased cardiac output (CO), and hypotension. Approximately 11% of patients need mechanical ventilation and hemodynamic support.[144] The up-regulation of TNF-dependent cellular cytokines may underlie the expression of IL-2–related pulmonary disease. Lung toxicity and disease severity vary with the total dose of IL-2 and with the route of administration. Reduced rates of toxicity are seen with continuous IL-2 infusion. Rapid recovery is expected with the cessation of therapy and aggressive hemodynamic support. Fatal IL-2 pulmonary toxicity occurs in approximately 2% of patients. Severe bronchospasm with IL-2 therapy has also been described.[145]

The clinical manifestations of TNF toxicity mimic those of IL-2 toxicity. This cytokine may damage capillary endothelial cells through the overproduction of superoxides and hydrogen peroxide by neutrophils. Fulminant cardiovascular collapse with noncardiogenic pulmonary edema, hypotension, respiratory failure, and weight gain may occur with the same frequency and severity as with IL-2 therapy and may resolve with the withdrawal of therapy.

Granulocyte colony-stimulating factor is a growth factor that is primarily used to facilitate neutrophil recovery after myelosuppressive chemotherapy and stem cell transplantation. The spectrum of lung toxicity associated with G-CSF therapy includes venous thrombosis and noncardiogenic pulmonary edema, which may be associated with peripheral eosinophilia. Damage to the pulmonary endothelium and pooling of aggregated neutrophils are felt to underlie the development of toxicity related to G-CSF. Drug withdrawal is usually sufficient to ameliorate clinical symptoms.

Monoclonal antibodies make up a relatively new class of anticancer agents that includes rituximab and trastuzumab. Rituximab is an anti-CD20 monoclonal antibody with efficacy against non-Hodgkin's lymphoma. Rare adverse pulmonary events (including bronchospasm and angioedema) have been associated with the infusion of this agent. Rates of rituximab-related pulmonary toxicities tend to occur with initial infusions and to wane with subsequent administration of the drug.[146] Trastuzumab is a recombinant monoclonal antibody that targets the HER-2 receptor. This drug is used either as single-agent therapy or in combination with paclitaxel for the treatment of patients with stage IV breast cancer. Cardiogenic pulmonary edema has been reported following the infusion of trastuzumab. Pulmonary events are rare and tend to occur in patients who have underlying significant cardiac disease or who have had prior anthracycline therapy.[147]

Thoracic Radiation

Clinically significant lung injury occurs as a sequela to thoracic radiation in 5 to 15% of patients that undergo thorac radiation. Like cytotoxic lung injury, radiation toxicity is an elusive entity, and its precise incidence and clinical diagnosis are difficult to define. Dose-dependent pneumonitis and pulmonary fibrosis are recognized complications and limit therapy. Despite animal models of radiation-induced lung injury, the complex pathogenic events that lead to lung damage remain incompletely described. Locally released growth factors and cytokines, including transforming growth factor beta (TGF-β), interleukin-1β (IL-1β), tumor necrosis factor alpha (TNF-α), and intercellular adhesion molecule 1 (ICAM-1), trigger an exuberant inflammatory reaction in the lungs in response to thoracic irradiation. In addition, oxidative lung injury caused by the release of reactive free radicals also likely contributes to the development of radiation toxicity.

The toxic manifestations of radiation in the lungs may be divided into two clinical phases, both of which typically occur well after the completion of therapy. The early phase is heralded by the development of clinical pneumonitis, which usually appears 1 to 3 months after the completion of radiotherapy. Symptoms of pneumonitis (including fever, exertional dyspnea, and nonproductive cough), peak at 3 to 4 months after radiotherapy. The late phase is characterized by the insidious development of pulmonary fibrosis 6 months to 1 year after thoracic irradiation. The radiographic appearance of fibrosis typically stabilizes over the ensuing 1 to 2 years and persists unchanged thereafter. Both the onset and the severity of radiation toxicity are influenced by risk factors that include the dose of radiation, the volume of lung irradiated, dose fractionation, underlying pulmonary reserve, prior radiotherapy, and concomitant chemotherapy. Synergistic effects have been reported with sequential or concurrent use of doxorubicin, vincristine, bleomycin, cyclophosphamide, mitomycin C, and actinomycin D. These drugs may also shorten the period of latency after radiation exposure. Radiographic manifestations of radiation toxicity appear at doses of $\geq$ 4,000 cGy. Radiographic and histologic evidence of radiation-induced pulmonary fibrosis occurs regardless of prior clinical manifestations of pneumonitis. Radiographic changes are predominantly confined to areas of previously irradiated lung.[148] Changes on conventional chest radiography that suggest pneumonitis range from indistinct vascular margins to frank consolidation with or without air bronchograms. Ipsilateral pleural thickening, volume loss, bronchiectasis, retraction of the lung parenchyma, tenting and elevation of the hemidiaphragm, and linear densities are characteristic of radiation fibrosis (Figure 10–4). Pneumothorax, hyperlucency of the ipsilateral lung, and pulmonary veno-occlusive disease have also been

reported. Effusions may also occur. The absence of malignant cells on pleural fluid cytology, spontaneous remission, clinical and radiographic evidence of pneumonitis, and the appearance of fluid within 6 months of the completion of radiotherapy help to distinguish malignant from radiation-induced effusions. Histopathologic changes suggesting pneumonitis tend to occur early, usually within the first 2 months after radiation exposure. These changes are marked by damage to the capillary endothelium, resulting in increased vascular permeability and congestion. Hyperplasia of type II pneumocytes and marked cellular infiltration into the alveolar interstitium by neutrophils, lymphocytes, fibroblasts, and macrophages are also common. Morphologic changes consistent with pulmonary fibrosis usually occur after the first 6 months of chest radiotherapy. These changes may evolve over a 6-month period and are usually complete 1 year after radiation exposure (Figure 10–5).

The overall prognosis for radiation-induced lung disease is good. Case fatality rates of 2 to 3% are reported in the literature. Steroids are indicated for moderate to severe disease. Therapy is generally initiated with 0.5 to 1.0 mg/kg/d of prednisone or with an equivalent dose of another steroid at the time of diagnosis and is tapered once a complete response is noted.

PLEURAL EFFUSIONS

Pleural effusions are an important complication of cancer and its treatment. The spectrum of cancer-related etiologies and the management of pleural effusions continue to evolve as new classes of anticancer drugs and therapeutic regimens are developed. Although pleural effusions are rarely life threatening, rapid accumulations of pleural fluid may adversely affect the quality of life. The majority of patients with cancer-related effusions present with moderate to large effusions (500 to 2,000 mL of fluid). Massive effusions, or those causing complete opacification of the hemithorax, are noted in 10% of pleural effusion cases. Nearly two-thirds of these patients have underlying malignancy.[149] Both unilateral and bilateral effusions may lead to significant cardiopulmonary decompensation. Hemodynamic collapse occurs as a result of the transfer of intrapleural pressure to the pericardial space. Increased pressure within the pericardial space, especially when acute, may lead to mediastinal shift and ventricular collapse. As a result, life-threatening arterial hypotension and cardiorespiratory failure may ensue, requiring endotracheal intubation and mechanical ventilation.

Direct Cancer-Related Processes

The diagnosis of a malignant pleural effusion is established when exfoliated malignant cells are found in pleural fluid or tissue. Annually, approximately 200,000

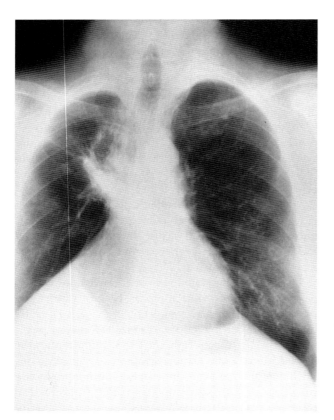

Figure 10–4. Chest radiograph showing ipsilateral tracheal deviation and tenting of the hemidiaphragm secondary to traction due to fibrotic scarring from prior radiation.

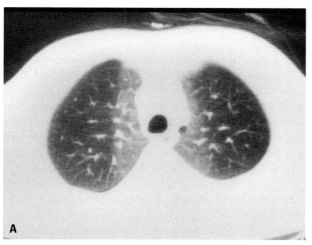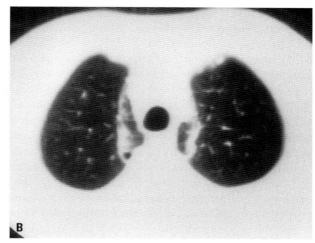

Figure 10–5. A: Early (2 months) postradiation alveolitis showing ground-glass opacities within the radiation port. B: Late (6 months) postradiation scarring and fibrosis within the radiation port.

malignant pleural effusions occur in the United States, accounting for nearly 20% of all effusions.[150] Malignancy is second only to pneumonia as a cause of exudative effusions. Transudative effusions due to an underlying neoplasm also occur and account for approximately 8 to 20% of all cytologically proven malignant effusions.[151–154] Thus, cytopathic examination of pleural fluid may be warranted in all newly diagnosed effusions. Transudative malignant effusions are felt to represent underlying comorbidities (atelectasis, congestive heart failure, and hypoalbuminemia) or early stages of lymphatic obstruction. The accumulation of protein in the pleural space usually requires several weeks to reach levels that are 50% (or more) greater than serum levels. During this period, total pleural-fluid protein concentrations will be low, consistent with transudative effusion.

Although any carcinoma can metastasize to the pleura and cause effusion, the majority (80%) of malignant effusions are caused by one of six major histologic types of cancer (Table 10–10). These include lymphoma (10%) and carcinomas of the lung (36%), breast (25%), and ovary (5%).[155] Pleural effusions associated with cancer may be serous, serosanguinous, or frankly bloody. Serous and serosanguinous malignant effusions may occur as a result of impaired lymphatic drainage from the pleural space. In most types of malignant effusions, the accumulation of pleural fluid strongly correlates with the degree of carcinomatous involvement of mediastinal lymph nodes rather than the extent of pleural metastasis.[149] Hence, those malignancies with a greater propensity for lymphatic metastasis are more likely to be associated with significant pleural effusions. The absence of pleural effusions in patients with sarcoma, which rarely metastasizes to lymph nodes but may cause extensive pleural disease, lends support to this concept.[156] This is

not the case in non-Hodgkin's lymphoma, in which pleural effusions may occur as a primary finding due to primary pleural infiltration, even in the setting of minimal mediastinal disease.[157] Capillary engorgement and lymphocytic infiltration of the pleural membrane may directly contribute to bloody pleural effusions. Several mechanisms are thought to underlie the development of malignant hemorrhagic effusions: (1) direct invasion of tumor into blood vessels, (2) tumor-induced angiogenesis, (3) the use of vasoactive substances causing increased capillary permeability, and (4) occlusion of small venules.

Indirect Cancer-Related Processes

The term "paramalignant" is applied to those pleural effusions that are cancer-related but cytopathologic analyses of pleural fluid fail to find malignant cells. Predominant carcinomatous invasion of the subserosal layer of the pleura causes minimal shedding of malignant cells into the pleural space. Thus, pleural-fluid cytology in this setting may be negative despite extensive pleural seeding. Other causes of paramalignant effusions are listed in Table 10–10. Common comorbid conditions that arise as a consequence of cancer may cause paramalignant effusions and include local and systemic tumor effects, hypoalbuminemia, complications of cancer treatment, pneumonia, and congestive heart failure.

As previously mentioned, the infiltration of hilar and mediastinal lymph nodes by tumor may lead to impaired lymphatic drainage from the pleural space. Lymphatic obstruction is the predominant mechanism responsible for pleural-fluid accumulation in malignancy and is usually associated with large-volume pleural effusions..[149,156,158] Tumors and enlarged lymph nodes may also cause bronchial obstruction, leading to atelectasis, postobstructive pneumonia, and pleural effusion. In the general population, parapneumonic effusions may occur in up to 40% of cases of pneumonia.

The term "complicated parapneumonic effusion" is used to describe those culture-negative effusions with the following pleural-fluid characteristics: (1) glucose < 40 mg/dL, (2) pH < 7.0, and (3) lactate dehydrogenase (LDH) greater than two-thirds of the upper limits of normal.[159] Empyema, defined as pus in the pleural space, typically has similar pleural-fluid characteristics, along with pleural-fluid positivity on Gram's stain or cultures. In the general population, 5 to 10% of pleural effusions are complicated by empyema. Although the exact frequency of parapneumonic effusion and empyema in cancer patients is unknown, morbidity and mortality rates among this patient population are expected to be considerably higher due to associated immunosuppression and underlying illnesses. Radiographic findings of complicated parapneumonic effusions and empyema include large multiloculated effusions with or without air-fluid levels. Pneumococci and beta-hemolytic streptococci were the most common causes of empyema in the preantibiotic era. Currently, staphylococci, anaerobes, and enteric Gram-negative bacilli have emerged as the most important pleural pathogens.

The obstruction or disruption of the thoracic duct may cause chylothorax. More than 50% of these triglyceride-rich effusions are due to neoplasms, the most common of which is lymphoma.[150] Trapped lung occurs when the atelectatic lung is prevented from re-expansion by a fibrous peel over the visceral pleura. This pleural peel is a late sequela of inflammatory reactions associated with empyema, hemothorax, pneumothorax, or thoracic operation. The presence of a pleural peel creates negative pressure in the pleural space, leading to the development of a chronic pleural effusion. Pleural effusions may also be seen in patients with superior vena caval obstruction and pericardial tamponade due to the elevated venous pressures.

Pleural effusions occurs in 30 to 50% of patients with thromboembolic disease. The majority (75%) of PE-related effusions are exudates.[160,161] Effusions usually occur early and stabilize over the first 3 days after PE. Bloody effusions and effusions that increase in size more than 4 days after the thromboembolic event suggest pulmonary infarction.

Details regarding the adverse effects of chemoradiation on the lungs have been discussed elsewhere. Both radiation and chemotherapy are capable of inducing clinically significant pleural effusions. In particular, methotrexate, procarbazine, cyclophosphamide, mitomycin, bleomycin, and interleukin-1 have been reported to cause debilitating effusions.[162] Drug-induced pleural effusions are rarely large but may be a source of significant morbidity when associated with concomitant parenchymal lung disease. The development of pleural effusions as sequelae of radiotherapy is well recognized.[163]

Clinical Presentation and Diagnostic Evaluation

At presentation, patients often appear chronically debilitated and have substantial weight loss, findings that are consistent with very advanced disease. Malignant pleural effusions may be asymptomatic in 25% of patients. In nearly half of these patients, the finding of a malignant effusion may be the earliest sign of cancer.[149] Symptoms attributable to moderate and large pleural effusions include dyspnea, orthopnea, and cough. Both the volume of pleural fluid and the rapidity with which the fluid accumulates dictate the occurrence of symptoms. Physiologic mechanisms leading to dyspnea in patients with moderate to large pleural effusions include displacement of the ipsilateral diaphragm, reduced ipsilateral lung volume and chest wall compliance, contralateral shift of the mediastinum, and altered neurogenic reflexes. The local effects of tumor on bronchi and lung parenchyma may also contribute to dyspnea and cough. Cough and dyspnea induced by these mechanisms may be unresponsive to therapeutic thoracentesis. Accompanying fever typically results from atelectasis and infection. Pleuritic chest pain and pleural friction rubs are rare findings and are usually due to pleural inflammation brought on by extensive car-

TABLE 10–10. Causes of Cancer-Related Pleural Effusions

Common cancers causing pleural effusions
    Carcinomas of lung, breast, ovary, and stomach
    Lymphoma
    Unknown primary
Indirect causes (paramalignant)
    Local effects of tumor
        Bronchial obstruction with associated pneumonia/atelectasis
        Lymphatic obstruction
        Trapped lung
        Superior vena cava syndrome
        Chylothorax
    Systemic effects of tumor
        Pulmonary embolism
        Hypoalbuminemia
    Adverse effects of treatment
        Radiation therapy
        Chemotherapy
            TNF
            IL-2
            Methotrexate
            Mitomycin
            Bleomycin
            Procarbazine
            Cyclophosphamide
            Fludarabine
            Gemcitabine
            Cytosine arabinoside

IL-2 = interleukin-2; TNF = tumor necrosis factor.

cinomatous involvement of the pleura, ribs, and chest wall.

Physical examination reveals ipsilateral dullness to percussion, decreased breath sounds, decreased diaphragmatic excursion, and decreased tactile and vocal fremitus. Crackles located immediately superior to the area of dullness may be noted in some cases. Inspiratory lag, contralateral tracheal deviation, and intercostal fullness may be seen with massive effusions (> 1,500 mL). In patients with pleural effusions due to congestive heart failure, other thoracic and extrathoracic signs (including distended neck veins, S_3 gallop, and pedal edema) may suggest the diagnosis.

Clinically significant pleural effusions warrant a rigorous diagnostic assessment. The initial step in the diagnostic evaluation is thoracentesis to obtain a sample of the pleural fluid. Thoracentesis also has great potential as a therapeutic tool. Chemical analyses of the pleural fluid permit discrimination between exudative and transudative effusions. This distinction is of fundamental value in helping to identify the underlying cause of the effusion and in guiding further therapy. In a landmark study by Light and co-workers,[164] exudative pleural effusions were defined as those with one or more of the following characterics: (1) a pleural fluid-to-serum protein ratio > 0.5, (2) a pleural fluid-to-serum LDH ratio > 0.6, or (3) a pleural-fluid LDH level greater than two-thirds of the upper limits of the normal serum value. Over the subsequent three decades, the diagnostic accuracy of "Light's criteria" has been questioned, and other discriminating biochemical markers of exudative and transudative effusions have been put forth. These have included pleural fluid-to-serum albumin gradients, bilirubin ratio, cholesterol ratio, and LDH isoenzyme analyses. However, Light's criteria remain the standard prerequisite tool for distinguishing exudative from transudative effusions.

Thoracentesis is relatively safe, is easy to perform, and is frequently the most productive initial procedure. Malignant pleural effusions are typically replete with lymphocytes, macrophages, and mesothelial cells. Pleural-fluid eosinophilia (ie, eosinophils greater than 10% of total WBCs in pleural fluid) occurs in only 8 to 10% of cases of malignant effusion.[165] The presence of pleural-fluid lymphocytosis, accompanied by a low pleural-fluid pH (< 7.3) and low glucose (< 60 mg/dL), is a helpful marker for establishing the diagnosis of malignant effusion. A low pleural-fluid pH occurs in approximately one-third of patients with malignant effusions and is predictive of both decreased survival and poor response to chemical pleurodesis.[158,166–168] High pleural salivary amylase levels in the absence of esophageal rupture is virtually diagnostic of malignancy. Disparate results of pleural-fluid protein and LDH analyses also suggest malignancy. Chylothorax is suggested when pleural-fluid triglycerides exceed 110 mg/dL. The role of tumor markers and cyto-genetic analysis of pleural fluid is still unclear. Invasive procedures, including pleural biopsy, bronchoscopy, pleuroscopy, video-assisted thoracoscopic surgery (VATS), and open biopsy of the pleura, may be used when pleural-fluid analyses fail to yield a diagnosis.

Ipsilateral effusions adjacent to the primary lung lesion are typical radiographic findings in patients with primary bronchogenic carcinoma. Cancers metastatic to the lung, however, show no ipsilateral predilection and are commonly bilateral. The finding of a normal cardiac silhouette with bilateral pleural effusions suggests malignancy as causative although other etiologies (including hypoalbuminemia, asbestos-related pleural effusions, lupus pleuritis, and cirrhosis) should be excluded. The earliest radiologic sign of pleural effusion is blunting of the posterior costophrenic angle on lateral chest radiography. Pleural-fluid accumulations of 300 to 500 mL are associated with blunting of the lateral costophrenic angle on the posteroanterior (PA) chest radiograph. Contralateral mediastinal shift is indicative of massive effusion. The absence of mediastinal shift in the setting of massive effusion suggests (1) mainstem bronchial tumor obstruction with atelectasis, (2) mediastinal fixation due to tumor or lymph nodes, or (3) extensive tumor infiltration of the ipsilateral lung by malignant mesothelioma or other tumor that radiographically mimics a large effusion. Lateral decubitus chest radiography is extremely useful for identifying small or subpulmonic effusions. This technique permits the assessment of loculated versus free-flowing fluid and may detect as little as 100 mL of pleural fluid. In severely debilitated patients, supine or semierect chest radiographs may be the only films available for review. The major finding of a pleural effusion on supine radiography is the absence of air bronchograms and increased homogeneous density over the lower lung field that does not obliterate normal bronchovascular markings. Underlying diffuse parenchymal lung disease may obscure the diagnosis. Ultrasonography or CT of the chest may be used to differentiate fluid loculations from pleural thickening or parenchymal disease and to selectively guide thoracentesis or biopsy needles to appropriate areas.

In early disease, pleural metastases tend to be focal. Thus, a blind sampling of the pleura with percutaneous needle biopsy is of lower diagnostic yield than is cytologic examination of the pleural fluid. As pleural disease progresses, however, the diagnostic sensitivity of closed needle biopsy may approach 65%.[169,170] The decision to proceed with more invasive tests in patients with suspected malignancy and negative pleural cytology should be based on available expertise and on the clinical status of the patient. Observation and repeat thoracentesis with considerations for pleural biopsy, VATS, or open pleural biopsy are viable options with some patients. Alternatively, thoracoscopic exploration via pleuroscopy or VATS is a reasonable initial diagnostic approach to patients with large undiagnosed pleural effusions. Thoracoscopic exploration with parietal pleural biopsies should be considered in patients with nondiagnostic pleural-fluid cytology and closed pleural-tissue examinations. These procedures permit direct visualization of the pleural surfaces and directed biopsy sampling of pleural tissues. The diagnostic yield of thoracoscopic biopsies (> 90%) are considerably higher than that of thoracentesis or closed pleural needle biopsy.[171] Thoracotomy with open biopsy of the pleura and lung tissue may be indicated if other invasive tests fail to yield a diagnosis. Unfortunately, even after thoracotomy, a number of patients escape diagnosis. The decision to pursue this aggressive work-up should be carefully weighed against the operative risks in these often critically ill patients. Fiberoptic bronchoscopy is of relatively little diagnostic use in the evaluation of pleural effusions in the absence of associated hemoptysis, ipsilateral mediastinal shift, or parenchymal lung disease. In the absence of any of these signs or symptoms, a pleural-fluid diagnosis is established by bronchoscopic examination in less than 10% of patients.[172]

Management

The approach to therapy is predicated upon the documentation of an etiologic diagnosis. The diagnosis of malignant effusion should not be made without definitive evidence of cytologically positive cells in the pleural fluid or tissue. Documentation of a malignant effusion helps to formulate management plans. Evidence of malignant pleural effusion in patients with carcinoma of the lung, for example, is an ominous sign and signifies inoperability. Once a definitive or presumptive diagnosis is established, appropriate therapy may be instituted. The decision to treat is dictated by several factors, including the degree of symptomatology, the rate of fluid accumulation, overall prognosis and performance status of the patient, and the relative responsiveness of the primary tumor to chemotherapy or radiation therapy (Table 10–11). These factors influence the decisions for palliation alone or for more aggressive treatment options. The risk-benefit ratio of invasive treatment modalities must be weighed very carefully. Efforts must be made to provide care with minimal discomfort, cost, and morbidity.

The overall prognosis of patients with a malignant pleural effusion is poor. Two-thirds of patients succumb to their underlying disease within 3 months, and 75% of patients are dead within 6 months of diagnosis.[149] Pleural effusions secondary to lymphoma or carcinomas of the breast and ovaries are associated with longer patient survival. In chemosensitive tumors (such as certain lymphomas, breast cancer, small-cell lung cancer, and testicular cancers), successful treatment of the underlying disease is usually associated with the regres-

sion of pleural fluid. Pleural effusions that occur as a consequence of mediastinal lymphatic obstruction may be effectively treated with mediastinal radiation; this is particularly true of lymphoma. Endobronchial tumors causing lung collapse and subsequent pleural effusion may be treated with stent placement, brachytherapy, or laser therapy. Thoracentesis is usually not indicated in the setting of congestive heart failure unless the heart failure is unresponsive to treatment or another etiology of pleural effusion is suspected. Patients usually improve with diuresis, inotropic support, and afterload reduction. Early antibiotic therapy is imperative in the treatment of pneumonia with parapneumonic effusion. Empiric antibiotic therapy is appropriate initially but should be modified according to the culture results and the *in vitro* sensitivity patterns of the infecting microorganisms. Pleural effusions that occur as a consequence of PE may resolve spontaneously or with the effective treatment of the clot. The presence of bloody pleural fluid due to PE is not a contraindication to anticoagulation or thrombolytic therapy.[160,173] Evidence of active hemorrhage into the pleural space during therapy, however, necessitates (1) discontinuation of anticoagulation, (2) tube thoracostomy, and (3) placement of a vena caval filter.

Thoracentesis and Tube Thoracostomy. Patients with significant dyspnea, hypoxemia, mediastinal shift, and hemodynamic instability should undergo emergent thoracentesis. This therapeutic maneuver can provide immediate and dramatic relief of symptoms. The decision to proceed with tube thoracostomy after the identification of a parapneumonic effusion is based on clinical features, radiographic findings, and the biochemical characteristics of the pleural fluid.[174] Evidence of purulent pleural fluid clearly establishes the need for chest tube drainage. Most experts also recommend tube thoracostomy for pleural fluid that is positive for Gram's stain or culture. Patients with complicated parapneumonic effusions may also benefit from prompt tube thoracostomy.[159] Immediate chest tube placement is recommended once a complicated parapneumonic effusion or empyema is identified because free-flowing pleural fluid may progress to loculated effusions in as little as 2 to 3 days. The presence of pleural-fluid loculations may prevent the adequate drainage of complicated pleural effusions and are associated with increased morbidity. These loculations are formed by fibrin and create limiting membranes within the pleural space. Intrapleural instillation of fibrinolytic agents such as streptokinase (250,000 U) or urokinase (100,000 U) may facilitate pleural-fluid drainage.[175–177] Thoracoscopy with adhesiolysis is indicated if tube thoracostomy and attempted thrombolysis are unsuccessful. Patients with chronic complicated parapneumonic effusions or those in whom

TABLE 10–11. Treatment Options in the Management of the Symptomatic Cancer Patient with Pleural Effusion

Treatment Option	Ideal Conditions	Comment
Thoracentesis	Large symptomatic effusions	Dramatic relief of symptoms if successful; diagnostic and therapeutic use
Tube thoracostomy	Large symptomatic effusions Empyema Complicated parapneumonic effusions	Fibrinolytic agents may be necessary for adhesiolysis; CT drainage alone usually not effective for large effusions
Thoracoscopy	Complicated parapneumonic effusions	Diagnostic and therapeutic use; may be used for talc poudrage, pleurectomy, clot removal
Pleurodesis	Recurrent malignant effusion	Offers control of effusion in > 90% of patients unless pleural fluid is acidotic (pH < 7.2) or lung is trapped
Denver catheter	Pleural fluid pH < 7.2 Failure of lung re-expansion after throracentesis Other treatment options unsuccessful	May be done on outpatient basis; may produce spontaneous pleural symphysis
Thoracotomy with decortication or pleurectomy	Trapped lung Other treatment options unsuccessful	Partial or full decortication options available; reasonable life expectancy May produce spontaneous pleural symphysis
Pleuroperitoneal shunt	Large recurrent chylous effusions Failure of other treatment options	May improve nutritional and immunologic status in patients with large recurrent chylothoraces
Radiation treatment	Pleural effusions caused by lymphoma (including chylothorax)	Regression of effusion associated with effective treatment of tumor
Chemotherapy	Malignant effusions associated with carcinomas of breast, ovaries, lung (small-cell), testicles, and lymphoma	Regression of effusion associated with effective treatment of tumor

CT = chest tube.

thoracoscopic intervention has failed should be considered for open thoracotomy with decortication.

Thoracoscopy. The role of VATS[178] in the diagnosis and treatment of certain pleuroparenchymal diseases is rapidly evolving. In addition to its use as a diagnostic instrument, thoracoscopy also has increasing therapeutic indications. The effective thoracoscopic débridement of fibrinous adhesions caused by complicated parapneumonic effusions has been well described.[178,179] The timing of thoracoscopic intervention is critical and should be considered after 3 to 5 days of inadequate chest tube drainage. Success rates for thoracoscopic débridement of complicated parapneumonic effusions approached 82% in one recent study.[180] Thoracoscopy has also been used to facilitate talc poudrage, pleurectomy, and the removal of blood clots in hemothorax (see below).

Pleurodesis. Pleurodesis has proven efficacy in controlling recurrent malignant pleural effusions. In this procedure, a sclerosing agent is instilled into the pleural cavity via a chest tube or thoracoscope in an effort to induce pleural symphysis. A variety of sclerosants (including talc, bleomycin, nitrogen mustard, minocycline, and 5-fluorouracil) are available for this procedure and have been used with variable rates of success. Doxycycline, minocycline, talc, and bleomycin are the most effective sclerosants. Success rates with these agents range from 72 to 90%.[181,182] Talc has been associated with ARDS in up to 6% of patients, which may be fatal.[183,184] Candidates for pleurodesis include those patients with symptom

relief after thoracentesis. Life expectancy should also influence the decision to proceed with pleurodesis. If the expected survival is greater than 3 months, attempted pleurodesis is reasonable. The failure of lung re-expansion after initial thoracentesis and a pleural-fluid pH of < 7.2 are associated with poor response rates to pleurodesis. In these patients, repeat thoracentesis or placement of a Denver catheter for control of recurrent pleural effusions is reasonable. The latter has been extensively used for outpatient management of malignant pleural effusions.[185–187] This technique involves the placement of a chronic indwelling catheter into the pleural space, which then drains externally. Successful Denver catheter placement results in reduced length of hospital stay, less morbidity, and lower cost in comparison to the traditional inpatient management of malignant effusions.[186,187] Denver catheter drainage may also effectively produce spontaneous pleural symphysis in 50% of patients. Increased friction between the visceral and parietal pleura occurs as the pleural effusion is diminished in volume, thus facilitating fusion of the two pleura and obliteration of the pleural space. Spontaneous pleurodesis occurs (on average) 25 days or more after the insertion of the indwelling catheter.[188]

Thoracotomy with Decortication. Therapeutic thoracotomy with pleurectomy and thoracotomy with decortication are reasonable therapeutic alternatives for a select group of patients with pleural effusions that are unresponsive to conventional management. Patients with persistent effusions secondary to trapped lung may also be suitable candidates for these surgical procedures. Several studies have documented the efficacy of these procedures in controlling recalcitrant pleural effusions.[189,190] During thoracotomy with pleurectomy, the parietal pleura may be stripped from the rib cage and mediastinum, either partially or in its entirety. Pleurectomy is effective in controlling pleural effusions in more than 90% of cases; however, a substantial morbidity and mortality must be carefully weighed against any potential benefit.[190] This procedure, therefore, should be reserved for those patients who are in otherwise good health and who have a reasonably long life expectancy. Unfortunately, few cancer patients meet these criteria. The prerequisites for thoracoscopy with decortication are similar. During decortication, purulent material and fibrinous debris are evacuated from the pleural space, permitting re-expansion of the underlying lung. Decortication is a major thoracic operation with significant morbidity and mortality. Partial decortication, which involves segmental rib resection with open drainage, may be a viable surgical option in some patients. Spontaneous resolution of the pleural peel has been reported and typically occurs within the first 6 months after treatment of the empyema.[189,190] If the pleural peel persists beyond 6 months and limits the patient's exercise capacity, full decortication should be considered.

Treatment of Chylous Effusions. The management of chylothorax is complicated by the chronic metabolic, nutritional, and immunologic consequences of prolonged chyle loss. Patients may suffer losses of large amounts of protein, fat, electrolytes, and lymphocytes by repeated thoracentesis and chest tube drainage. These nutritional and cellular deficits may lead to severe inanition and failure to thrive. Lymphocytes (particularly T lymphocytes) are the major cellular components of chyle. Although chylous effusions are bacteriostatic and therefore not likely to become infected, the loss of large amounts of lymphocytes in chylous fluid may render the patient severely immunocompromised and at risk for the development of opportunistic infections. Conservative management with chest tube drainage is appropriate for the initial management of chylous effusions. Oral dietary fats should be replaced with medium-chain triglycerides (MCTs), which are absorbed through the portal system rather than via the intestinal and thoracic route, thus minimizing the thoracic lymphatic flow. Hyperalimentation is preferred over oral nutrition, in an effort to further reduce the flow of chyle. In the absence of chylous ascites, patients with persistent chylous effusions despite conservative management should be treated by placement of a pleuroperitoneal shunt.[191] This device consists of two catheters communicating through a pumping chamber that contains two one-way valves. Fluid flows from the pleural space into the peritoneal cavity, where it is reabsorbed. Successful shunt placement abrogates any associated nutritional, immunologic, and electrolyte losses and facilitates the closure of the thoracic duct defect. The instillation of talc or other sclerosant materials should be considered with shunt failures. Exploratory thoracotomy or VATS with surgical ligation of the thoracic duct represents the definitive approach to traumatic and iatrogenic chylothorax when more conservative measures fail. Surgical intervention should be considered for average daily chyle losses of > 1,500 cc per day or if drainage persists for more than 10 days. In patients with metastatic disease or lymphoma-associated chylous effusions, the effusions may be effectively treated with mediastinal radiation. Pleuroperitoneal shunt placement or chest tube thoracostomy should be considered for these patients only if radiation fails to control the effusions.

HEMOTHORAX

Cancer-Related Etiologies

Hemothorax should be suspected whenever blood is aspirated from the pleural cavity. It is confirmed by the finding of a pleural-fluid hematocrit that is more than 50% of that of peripheral blood. The documentation of an elevated pleural-fluid hematocrit is important in the diagnosis of hemothorax since bloody-appearing effusions frequently will not meet the criterion for diagnosis. In contrast to blood that is aspirated during a traumatic tap, chronic bloody effusions are typically defibrinated, presumably secondary to the constant motion of the heart and lungs against the pleura, and therefore clot very poorly. In addition, the bloody fluid obtained during a traumatic tap rapidly clears after centrifugation whereas bloody fluid due to hemothorax may retain a reddish tint if it has been present long enough for hemolysis to occur. Several conditions may lead to hemothorax in the cancer setting (Table 10–12). Metastatic disease to the pleura is by far the most common nontraumatic cause of hemothorax in cancer patients, followed by complications of anticoagulant therapy. The latter are rare etiologies that typically occur within the first week of the initiation of anticoagulation although anecdotal reports have documented anticoagulant-induced hemothorax several months after the initiation of therapy.[192] Spontaneous hemothorax as a consequence of severe thrombocytopenia has been reported although this complication is rare.[193] Hemothorax following pulmonary embolism may occur in association with pulmonary infarction or as an iatrogenic complication of aggressive anticoagulation.[192] Bleeding from virtually any structure within the thorax may cause hemothorax. Aberrant placement of percutaneously inserted catheters into a central vein or artery may lead to iatrogenic hemothorax. Other procedures that are commonly performed in cancer patients, including thoracentesis, transbronchial biopsy, percutaneous needle aspiration or biopsy, and pleural biopsy, may cause hemothorax.

Management

In the past, hemothorax has been perfunctorily treated with chest tube thoracostomy and drainage. Blood in the pleural space is spontaneously resorbed; thus, evacuation of bloody pleural effusions may not be necessary in all cases of hemothorax.[194,195] Chest tube drainage is indicated for a large hemothorax and for an acute hemothorax from iatrogenic, traumatic, and spontaneous causes. Thoracostomy tube drainage is also mandatory if a concomitant pneumothorax (hemopneumothorax) is present. Tube thoracostomy permits quantification of the rate of bleeding. Furthermore, evacuation of the hemothorax allows the visceral and parietal pleural surfaces to approximate each other, which may help to tamponade the bleeding site. Patients with persistent bleeding (> 100 mL per hour) should be referred for emergency thoracotomy.[196] Fibrothorax is a rare complication of hemothorax, occurring in approximately 1% of patients.

PNEUMOTHORAX

Pneumothorax, or air in the pleural space, is a common disorder in the cancer patient and may result from pleural metastases, infection, underlying lung disease, cancer treatment, or an expanding variety of iatrogenic causes. Pneumothorax most commonly results from the rupture of weakened alveolar tissues, permitting the egress of extra-alveolar gas. This extra-alveolar air may track along the lower-resistance perivascular sheaths to the hilum and mediastinum before rupturing into the pleural space. Air in the mediastinum (pneumomediastinum) may freely dissect cervically along facial planes into the soft tissues of the neck, causing subcutaneous emphysema, or caudally into the retroperitoneum, causing pneumoperitoneum. Although air in these extrapleural sites is usually of no hemodynamic or physiologic significance, it is an important marker that may presage the development of pneu-

mothorax. These signs are therefore important, especially in the mechanically ventilated patient.

Two major classes of pneumothorax and attributable etiologies are listed in Table 10–13. The first, spontaneous pneumothorax, occurs without antecedent trauma. Two subcategories of spontaneous pneumothorax are recognized. Pneumothorax occurring in the absence of any apparent underlying lung disease is designated as *primary spontaneous pneumothorax*. When preexisting pulmonary or chest wall disease is known, the pneumothorax is called a *secondary spontaneous pneumothorax*. The other major class of pneumothorax is traumatic pneumothorax, which may occur (1) as a result of penetrating or blunt trauma to the airways, pulmonary parenchyma, or chest wall or (2) as a complication of invasive diagnostic and therapeutic procedures (ie, iatrogenically). Although the overall incidence of pneumothorax in cancer patients has not been reported, this group of patients is represented in the majority of invasive procedures that are associated with pneumothorax. It is generally accepted that most cancer-related pneumothoraces have iatrogenic or secondary spontaneous etiologies. This section focuses on both.

Quantifying the size of a pneumothorax is helpful in formulating management decisions. Unfortunately, methods for quantifying the degree of lung collapse have not been standardized, and the current approaches lack uniformity and precision.[150,197–199] A favored approach is the one offered by Light,[150] in which the degree of collapse (percentage pneumothorax) is estimated, based on the ratio of the cube of the diameter of the lung and hemithorax. For example, if the diameter of the collapsed lung is 8 cm and the diameter of the hemithorax is 10 cm, the collapsed lung is estimated by the following equation:

$$100\% - \left(\frac{8^3}{10^3} \times 100\% \right) = 48.8\%$$

Thus, the estimated size of the pneumothorax is 48.8%. An alternative quantification scheme was recently

TABLE 10–12. Cancer-Related Causes of Hemothorax

Nontraumatic etiologies
  Metastatic disease
  Anticoagulant therapy
  Severe thrombocytopenia
  Pulmonary embolism / infarction
Traumatic/iatrogenic etiologies
  Central venous catheter
  Thoracentesis
  Transbronchial biopsy
  Percutaneous needle aspiration
  Pleural biopsy

TABLE 10–13. Major Categories of Pneumothorax and Associated Etiologies

Spontaneous
  Primary
  Secondary
    Neoplasms (etiologies: primary bronchogenic carcinoma, metastatic pleural diseases)
    Infections (etiologies: PCP, necrotizing pneumonia, fungal pneumonia, aspiration pneumonia)
    Interstitial lung diseases (etiologies: radiation, sarcoidosis, drugs)
Traumatic
  Open
  Closed
  Iatrogenic (mechanical ventilation, thoracic procedures)

PCP = *Pneumocystis carinii* pneumonia.

put forth by the American College of Chest Physicians Pneumothorax Consensus Group.[200] In this classification scheme, small and large pneumothoraces are stratified on the basis of the distance between the apex and the cupola. Pneumothoraces with apex-to-cupola distances of < 3 cm are classified as small; those > 3 cm are considered to be large.

Iatrogenic Pneumothorax

As the frequency of invasive diagnostic and therapeutic intrathoracic procedures has increased over the past 20 years, so have the rates of iatrogenic pneumothorax. An iatrogenic etiology underlies the majority of pneumothoraces treated in most hospitals.[201,202] Procedures such as percutaneous lung biopsy, transbronchial biopsy, and the insertion of central venous lines and pulmonary artery catheters are associated with increased rates of pneumothorax. Central venous catheterization is one of the most common invasive procedures that cancer patients undergo. This procedure carries a 2 to 6% incidence of pneumothorax.[203,204] Subclavian catheterization carries a significantly higher risk than internal jugular catheterization. The risk of catheter-related pneumothorax increases with patient age and is inversely related to the patient's body mass index. Overall rates of pneumothorax following thoracentesis (12%), pleural biopsy (10%), and transbronchial biopsy (6%) are published in the literature but may vary broadly from one institution to the next, depending on the procedural acumen of the clinician.[205,206] Mechanical ventilation is a potentially lethal cause of iatrogenic pneumothorax. The overall incidence of ventilator-associated pneumothorax is 5%. This rate is much higher with the use of positive-end expiratory pressure (23%) and in patients with concomitant lung diseases such as COPD (8%).[207]

Transthoracic needle aspiration (TTNA) biopsy is the leading cause of iatrogenic pneumothorax, with rates ranging from 19 to 44%.[201,202] Rates for TTNA biopsy–associated pneumothorax are even higher among patients with underlying lung diseases such as COPD. In more than one-third of these patients, the pneumothorax is large enough to warrant chest tube placement.[208–210] The size and the location of the tumor also influence the risk of TTNA biopsy–related pneumothorax. Tumors that are < 2 cm in size and those that are deeply seated within the lung parenchyma are associated with higher rates of pneumothorax following TTNA biopsy.[211] The probability of TTNA biopsy–associated pneumothorax, based on tumor depth, is 13% at 1 cm, 49% at 4 cm, and 86% at 7 cm of depth.[206]

Secondary Spontaneous Pneumothorax

Chronic obstructive pulmonary disease is the most common cause of secondary spontaneous pneumothorax although spontaneous pneumothorax may develop in virtually any lung disease. In the Veterans Administration Cooperative Study on Pneumothorax, a direct correlation between pneumothorax rates and the severity of COPD was observed; patients in whom forced expiratory volume in 1 second (FEV_1) was < 1 L and whose mean FEV_1-to-forced vital capacity (FVC) ratios were ≤ 57% were at highest risk for spontaneous pneumothorax.[212]

Chronic obstructive pulmonary disease significantly increases the risk of spontaneous pneumothorax in cancer patients. Both metastatic and primary pulmonary neoplasms are attributable causes of pneumothorax; indeed, any tumor that metastasizes to the pleura may cause pneumothorax. Tumor-related pneumothorax occurs as a consequence of necrosis or cavitation of pleural-based tumors with secondary rupture into the pleural space. Scattered case reports document pneumothorax as the initial presentation of primary bronchogenic carcinoma, osteosarcoma, germ cell tumors, breast cancer, pancreatic cancer, and metastatic rectal cancer. Pneumothorax may complicate the treatment of highly chemo- and radiosensitive tumors such as small-cell lung cancer, germ cell tumors, lymphomas, and soft-tissue sarcomas. Chemotherapeutic agents that are associated with pneumothorax include bleomycin, BCNU, and CCNU.[105,108,115] The postulated mechanisms of treatment-associated pneumothorax include rapid tumor lysis and/or rapid rupture of chemosensitive peripheral and subpleural metastatic lesions into the pleural cavity. Multiple pleural bullae leading to spontaneous pneumothorax may occur following the development of bronchiolitis obliterans, a frequent complication of allogeneic stem cell transplantation. The hyperexpansion of distal air-spaces, secondary to obstructive or inflammatory processes, probably underlie the development of pneumothorax in this setting. Finally, a burgeoning list of pathogens that may cause necrotizing pulmonary infections are commonly associated with pneumothorax. These particular infections are seen with increased frequency in the immunocompromised host and include infections with *Staphylococcus*, *Klebsiella*, *Pseudomonas*, *Pneumocystis carinii*, and *Mycobacterium*. Pyopneumothorax (the presence of both air and pus in the pleural space) may occur as a complication of necrotizing pneumonia due to infection by *Staphylococcus*, *Klebsiella*, *Pseudomonas*, or other necrotizing organisms. Pneumothorax caused by the rupture of a mycetoma into the pleural space rarely complicates intensive cytotoxic treatment of hematologic malignancies.[213] Etiologic conditions include coccidioidomycosis, cryptococcosis, mucormycosis, and infection with *Aspergillus fumigatus*.

Tension Pneumothorax

Occasionally a ball-valve effect occurs at the site of communication between the pleural space and the alveoli, permitting only egress of air during respiratory excursions. As air accumulates in the pleural space, intrapleural pressures increase and eventually exceed atmospheric pressure, creating a tension pneumothorax. Common scenarios associated with the development of tension pneumothorax include mechanical ventilation, cardiopulmonary resuscitation, and (rarely) progression of a spontaneous pneumothorax. In mechanically ventilated patients, differential pressure gradients created by positive pressure ventilation favors the egress of intrapleural air, creating tension. The progressive increase in pleural pressures result in collapse of the ipsilateral lung, contralateral shift of the mediastinum, decreased venous return, and reduced cardiac output. Tension pneumothorax is a life-threatening event, which may result in severe hypoxemia followed by rapid cardiovascular collapse and death unless immediate medical intervention is instituted. This diagnosis should be considered (1) whenever there is a sudden unexplained deterioration of respiratory and hemodynamic status in any patient with a known pneumothorax, (2) following a procedure known to cause pneumothorax, or (3) when an abrupt increase in peak inspiratory and static pressures occurs in a patient who is on mechanical ventilation. Tension pneumothorax should also be suspected during cardiopulmonary resuscitation if ventilation suddenly becomes difficult or if the patient develops electromechanical dissociation.

Clinical Presentation and Radiologic Examination

The major physiologic alterations in pneumothorax are diminished vital capacity and reduced PaO_2. The ability of the patient to tolerate reductions in vital capacity is primarily dictated by the presence and severity of pre-existing lung disease. Thus, patients with secondary spontaneous pneumothorax are at greater risk for developing respiratory failure than those with pre-existing normal lung function. Patients typically present acutely with severe respiratory distress, tachypnea, tachycardia, cyanosis, diaphoresis, and agitation. Dyspnea in these patients is frequently out of proportion to the size of the pneumothorax. Patients with a large pneumothorax or significant concomitant lung disease may develop V/Q mismatch and shunting, leading to intractable hypoxemia, an increased alveolar-arterial oxygen gradient, and acute respiratory compromise. Arterial blood gases reflecting alveolar hypoventilation and respiratory acidosis are common in this setting.

Chest pain and dyspnea occur in nearly all patients with significant degrees of pneumothorax. The pain is characteristically acute, ipsilateral, and pleuritic. Cough, hemoptysis, and orthopnea may rarely occur. Mediastinal shift may occasionally cause Horner's syndrome due to traction of the sympathetic ganglion. The physical examination often reveals moderate tachycardia. Absent tactile fremitus, hyper-resonance on chest percussion, and absent or diminished breath sounds ipsilateral to the pneumothorax may also be noted. Contralateral deviation of the trachea, asymmetric hyperexpansion, and diminished movement of the involved hemithorax may be appreciated if the pneumothorax is sufficiently large or is under tension. Dissection of extra-alveolar air may be manifested as subcutaneous emphysema, which frequently is found upon palpation of the suprasternal notch or pericervical tissues (Figure 10–6). Hamman's sign, described as a precordial crunch or click synchronous with the heartbeat, may be detected in patients with pneumothorax as well as pneumomediastinum. Elevated central venous, pulmonary arterial, and right atrial pressures reflect tension physiology. Progressive elevations in central venous and intrapleural pressures impede venous return, causing hemodynamic collapse and refractory hypotension. Arterial blood gas derangements include severe hypoxemia and respiratory acidosis.

The patient's electrocardiogram (ECG) is typically normal. With left-sided pneumothorax, however, electrocardiographic changes mirroring acute myocardial infarction may be seen. These changes include right-axis deviation, loss of precordial R-wave progression, T-wave inversion, and a decrease in QRS amplitude. The electrocardiographic changes seen with pneumothorax, however, lack ST-segment elevation and significant Q waves. Electrocardiographic changes typically resolve with lung re-expansion.

Typical markers of pneumothorax may be found on a chest radiograph made with the patient in upright position. In a retrospective study by Tocino and colleagues, nearly one-third of pneumothoraces were not detected by radiography with the patient in the semierect and supine positions.[214] Radiographic evidence of a visceral pleural line with an absence of lung markings beyond the line confirms the diagnosis of pneumothorax in most patients. Caution must be taken, however, to exclude artifacts such as skin folds or other extrathoracic artifacts that may mimic pneumothorax. Expiratory films may facilitate the diagnosis if the evaluation remains inconclusive. Lungs that are regionally trapped by pleural adhesions may show only partial collapse, even under tension (Figure 10–7). Pleural adhesions may also cause loculated pockets of air in atypical areas, such as a sub-pulmonic location. The presence of a unilaterally depressed costophrenic sulcus ("deep-sulcus sign") may be the only roentgenographic evidence of pneumothorax in patients with extensive parenchymal infiltrates. This finding, along with radiolucency of the ipsilateral upper-abdominal quadrant, may also be seen on supine films and is a useful marker of occult pneumothorax in debilitated patients who may not be able to sit for an upright

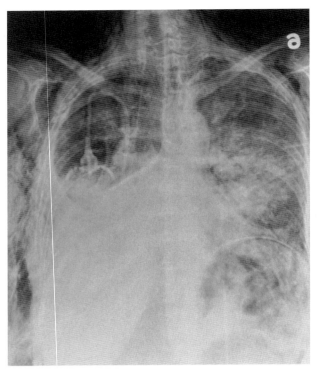

Figure 10–6. A 56-year-old woman with metastatic pancreatic cancer and severe dyspnea who developed extensive subcutaneous emphysema, pneumomediastinum, and pneumoperitoneum secondary to barotrauma following positive pressure ventilation.

film. Other roentgenographic findings that are suggestive of pneumothorax include flattening or inversion of the ipsilateral hemidiaphragm, complete diaphragm, and air-fluid levels. Small pneumothoraces (< 20%) are usually undetectable on physical examination. Large bullae in patients with COPD may mimic pneumothorax, rendering accurate diagnosis difficult in these patients. Occasionally, CT examination of the chest is necessary to differentiate pleural from parenchymal hyperlucent areas or to distinguish large thin-walled bullae in patients with COPD from pneumothorax.

The presence of mediastinal shift, rib cage expansion, and flattening or inversion of the ipsilateral diaphragm suggests tension pneumothorax. With complete lung collapse, the lung appears as a small hilar opacity. As previously mentioned, lungs that are heavily infiltrated, obstructed, or trapped may fail to collapse completely. Moreover, patients on mechanical ventilators or patients with ARDS may demonstrate little or no contralateral mediastinal shift. Intrapleural pressures may increase with smaller amounts of accumulated intrapleural air in patients with significant lung disease such as ARDS. Pneumothorax may not be readily obvious radiographically in these patients, and ipsilateral diaphragmatic depression may be the only sign of increased intrapleural pressure.

Several facts warrant emphasis. Iatrogenic pneumothorax may not be clinically or radiographically apparent for 24 or more hours following the offending procedure. Pneumothorax under tension requires immediate therapeutic intervention. Strong clinical suspicion coupled with physical findings is usually sufficient for the diagnosis of tension pneumothorax, and treatment should not be postponed in lieu of radiographic documentation of this disorder. Lung entrapment causing airway obstruction, lung parenchyma densely infiltrated by infection, or tumor and an unyielding mediastinum that is frozen by tumor, fibrosis, prior surgery, or infection may obscure the radiographic findings of tension pneumothorax. Tension may develop under these circumstances in the absence of lung collapse or significant volume loss.

Management

Conservative measures, including vigilant observation and supplemental oxygen, are appropriate therapeutic options for patients with a small pneumothorax and minimal symptoms. According to recent guidelines offered in the American College of Chest Physicians Consensus Statement on the management of spontaneous pneumothorax, such patients should be observed in the emergency department for 3 to 6 hours. Serial

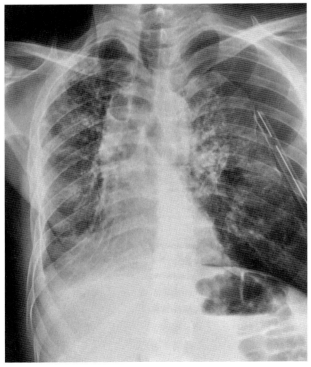

Figure 10–7. A 32-year-old man with non-Hodgkin's lymphoma, hypotension, and dyspnea. Chest radiography revealed partial left pneumothorax with mediastinal shift. Scattered heterogenous pulmonary opacities and scarring in both lungs are from old tuberculosis.

chest radiography should be performed at 3 to 6 hours. If the resulting radiograph does not demonstrate evidence of radiographic expansion of the pneumothorax, the patient may be discharged from the emergency room, with instructions for follow-up and repeat chest radiography as an outpatient 12 to 48 hours later.[200]

Hospitalized patients should be treated with supplemental oxygen to facilitate the resorption of pleural air. Spontaneous resorption of pleural air is a slow process, occurring at a rate of 1.25% per day. Thus, a 20% pneumothorax would require approximately 16 days for complete spontaneous resolution. The gas trapped in the pleural space is predominantly nitrogen. The administration of supplemental oxygen facilitates the rate of pleural resorption of air by driving down the partial pressure of arterial nitrogen (PaN_2). The increased nitrogen arterial-pleural pressure gradient promotes the resorption of the nitrogen-rich gas trapped in the pleural space. Catheter aspiration is the procedure of choice for spontaneous pneumothorax that is symptomatic, rapidly expanding, or moderate-sized (> 15% in size). Failure of lung re-expansion or recurrence after successful catheter aspiration indicates the need for chest tube thoracostomy. The placement of a Heimlich valve may be appropriate in this setting. This one-way valve is connected to a small-diameter thoracostomy tube. Heimlich-valve thoracostomy tubes are relatively easy to place and are more comfortable for the patient than chest tubes of larger diameter. Removing the thoracostomy tube is usually a two-step process. Once resolution of the pneumothorax and absence of air leak is documented, the tube is clamped for 24 hours. If subsequent chest radiography shows no evidence of re-expansion, the tube may be removed. Patients who develop iatrogenic pneumothorax with no prior underlying lung disturbance receive treatment similar to that received by patients with primary spontaneous pneumothorax. Traumatic pneumothorax, including hemothorax, usually requires the placement of a large-bore thoracostomy tube. Simple aspiration is usually ineffective for the treatment of secondary and traumatic pneumothorax. Early tube thoracostomy is indicated in patients with pneumothorax of 15 to 20% and retained secretions, ipsilateral lung infections, or other underlying parenchymal or airway disease. Early intervention with tube thoracostomy is also recommended for mechanically ventilated patients with pneumothorax because of the high potential for progression to tension. Chest tubes should remain in place in these patients until successful weaning from the ventilator is achieved. Prophylactic chest tube placement in mechanically ventilated patients with evidence of pneumomediastinum or other sites of extra-alveolar air is a source of controversy. Most experts recommend careful vigilance, with a chest tube tray at the bedside of these patients. In the case of tension pneumothorax, the immediate percutaneous placement of a large-bore needle or angiocatheter into the pleural space can be lifesaving. The needle is usually placed into the second intercostal space along the midclavicular line and is left in place until definitive tube thoracostomy is accomplished. Large-bore (36F to 40F) tube thoracostomy is usually adequate for drainage of a pyopneumothorax. Prolonged tube drainage and multiple tubes may be required to achieve adequate drainage. Pleural loculations may be managed early on with intrapleural streptokinase. A dose of 250,000 U is administered into the chest tube, and the tube is clamped for 1 to 2 hours to permit thrombolytic action.

Failed tube aspiration is usually declared if there is a persistent air leak from a bronchopleural fistula or incomplete expansion of the lung 5 to 7 days after tube thoracostomy. These patients may be considered for thoracotomy and surgical repair of the lung lesion. Both surgical approaches permit rapid re-expansion of the lung. During thoracotomy, the area causing the persistent air leak may be identified and treated directly, thereby diminishing the likelihood of recurrence. Thoracotomy may be performed via VATS or by an open procedure. A number of definitive surgical procedures may be performed through a thoracoscope as well as by open thoracotomy, including pleurodesis, surgical resection or laser ablation of blebs and bullae, parietal pleurectomy, and electrocoagulation.[215–219] The surgical management of pneumothorax by VATS has the added advantages of the avoidance of a painful postoperative thoracostomy wound, a shorter hospital stay, and lower cost. However, recurrence rates for pneumothorax are slightly lower after open thoracotomy (5 to 7%) than after VATS (10%), probably owing to the open procedure's greater exposure of the chest cavity and higher rates of detecting the offending lesion.[220–222] Thoracotomy is the preferred approach when further interventions such as wedge resection, segmentectomy, lobectomy, decortication, or pleurectomy are contemplated. The higher morbidity and mortality of thoracotomy must be weighed against these potential benefits.

The instillation of a sclerosing agent in an attempt to obliterate the pleural space with pleurodesis may represent a viable therapeutic option for some patients with a nonhealing bronchopleural fistula or recurrent spontaneous or secondary pneumothorax. Early management with pleurodesis is an attractive option, particularly for the debilitated cancer patient with poor operative risks. The types of sclerosants currently used for pleurodesis were discussed earlier (see Pleural Effusions, above). Currently, tetracycline derivatives, talc, and bleomycin are the most commonly used sclerosants in the United States.

The overall recurrence rate for spontaneous and secondary pneumothorax following chest tube thoracotomy is 36% at 5 years.[223] The rate of pneumothorax recurrence at 5 years after chest tube pleurodesis is 8 to 13%.[150,223] Rates are slightly better for pleurodesis following VATS or open thoracotomy.[181,220,222]

AIRWAY OBSTRUCTION

Upper-Airway Obstruction

Pathophysiology. Upper-airway obstruction is typically categorized on the basis of characteristic deviations from the normal flow-volume loop. The following three major patterns of airflow obstruction are recognized, based on limitations of inspiratory flow, expiratory flow, or both: (1) dynamic (variable) extrathoracic obstruction, (2) dynamic (variable) intrathoracic obstruction, and (3) fixed obstruction.

In dynamic (variable) extrathoracic airflow obstruction, intratracheal pressure exceeds the pressure around the airway (atmospheric pressure) during exhalation, lessening the obstruction. During inspiration, intratracheal pressure becomes subatmospheric, favoring a narrowing of the extrathoracic airway. Conditions that cause dynamic extrathoracic airway obstruction, therefore, result in a flattening of the inspiratory limb of the flow-volume loop (Figure 10–8). Tracheomalacia, bilateral vocal-cord paralysis, and obstructing tracheal tumors are conditions that typically cause dynamic extrathoracic obstruction.

In the presence of dynamic (variable) intrathoracic obstruction, pleural pressures exceed intratracheal pressures during exhalation and worsen the obstruction. Conversely, during inspiration, intratracheal pressures become positive relative to pleural pressures, which mitigate the obstruction. Thus, during dynamic intrathoracic obstruction, the expiratory limb of the flow-volume loop is limited. Tracheomalacia and obstructing tumors of the intrathoracic airway may cause this pattern of obstruction. Unlike the obstructing tumors of variable extrathoracic obstruction, tumors associated with variable intrathoracic airway obstruction are more often malignant.

In fixed airway obstruction, the modulating effects of transmural pressure on airway diameter are limited during both inspiration and expiration. Fixed airway obstructive lesions therefore produce a flattening of both the inspiratory and expiratory limbs of the flow-volume loop. Conditions causing this type of airflow derangement include goiter and tracheal stenosis.

Etiology. *Malignant Causes.* Upper-airway obstruction, the archetypal oncologic emergency, may result from both benign and malignant conditions (Table 10–14). Primary tumors of the base of the tongue, larynx, hypopharynx, trachea, thyroid, and lungs may cause upper-airway obstruction by direct extension into the airway. In addition, metastatic spread of tumors of the breast, esophagus, kidneys, and colon, as well as melanoma, sarcomas, and mediastinal lymphomas, are infrequent causes of upper-airway compromise. Primary lung tumors and tumors of the base of the tongue, larynx, and trachea are overwhelmingly of squamous cell histology. Both primary tumors and metastatic disease may cause airway obstruction by encroachment or invasion of the airway. Although nearly 50% of patients with lymphoma may have variable evidence of endobronchial disease, lymphomatous masses of sufficient size to cause proximal airway obstruction are rare. Slow-growing obstructive lesions of the upper airway may become acutely life threatening secondary to encroachment on the airway, associated airway edema, or hemorrhage. Most patients have a known prior history of cancer although airway obstruction may (rarely) occur as the initial clinical presentation.

Noninfectious Benign Causes. Benign conditions such as aspiration of food or other foreign body, airway edema, severe tracheomalacia, tracheal stenosis, and stricture may have a malignant impact on the airway. Tracheal

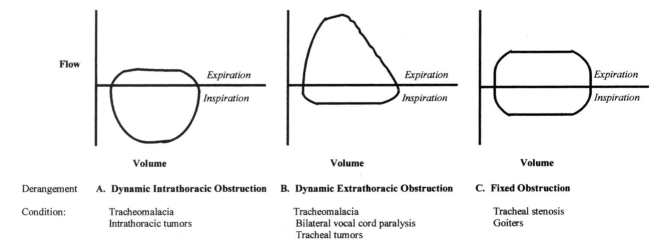

Figure 10-8. Patterns of upper airway obstruction and associated conditions.

stenosis may occur as a delayed complication of prolonged intubation. Bilateral vocal-cord paralysis may also occur, usually as a result of damage to the recurrent laryngeal nerve during thyroidectomy, carcinomatous involvement of cranial nerves, or radiation damage from treatment of head and neck cancers.[224] Unilateral vocal-cord paralysis typically does not cause airway obstruction but instead predisposes the patient to aspiration and laryngospasm.

Infectious Causes. Fungal, viral, and bacterial infections are rare causes of upper-airway obstruction in adults. In particular, invasive aspergillosis causing laryngotracheobronchitis is an uncommon but potentially fatal complication in immunocompromised patients. Candidal epiglottitis has been reported as a complication of neutropenia in leukemic patients.[225] Necrotizing laryngitis caused by herpes simplex virus (HSV) and *Cytomegalovirus* has also been documented in immunocompromised patients.[226,227] Systemic dissemination or direct extension of infection from oropharyngeal or esophageal sites accounts for most laryngeal infections caused by *Candida albicans* or HSV, although primary laryngeal infection may rarely occur. Bacteria have also been implicated in the development of an exudative laryngotracheitis and fibropurulent epiglottitis in adult patients with malignancy.[228] The predominant offending bacterial pathogens (*Haemophilus influenzae*, *Haemophilus parainfluenzae*, and various species of streptococcal and staphylococcal organisms) are isolated in culture in less than 30% of adult patients.

Cellulitis of the floor of the mouth and submandibular space (Ludwig's angina) occurs with increased frequency in malnourished patient,s and in patients with hematologic disorders such as leukemia, multiple myeloma, neutropenia, and aplastic anemia.[229] Cancer patients with dental infection or a recent tooth extraction are at increased risk of developing this infection. Approximately 25% of patients experience some degree of respiratory compromise. Complete obstruction of the posterior oropharynx may occur secondary to the posterior displacement of the tongue against the edematous and inflamed soft palate, hypopharynx, and submaxillary areas. Laryngospasm may also contribute to airway obstruction. The diagnosis is based on Grodinsky's criteria of (1) gangrenous infiltration with multifocal bilateral cellulitis of the submandibular space; (2) involvement of contiguous structures, including the fascia, muscles, and connective tissue; and (3) absence of lymphatic involvement.[230] Polymicrobial infections with streptococci, staphylococci, and anaerobes are isolated in more than 50% of patients. Gram-negative pathogens and *H. influenzae* should be considered in immunosuppressed patients and in patients with no prior history of odonto-

TABLE 10–14. Causes of Upper-Airway Obstruction in the Cancer Patient

Malignant	Benign
Primary carcinomas	Noninfectious
Trachea	Aspiration
Larynx	Airway edema
Hypopharynx	Tracheomalacia
Thyroid	Tracheal stenosis/stricture
Lung	Bilateral vocal-cord paralysis
Base of tongue	Drugs (docetaxel, paclitaxel, azathioprine)
Metastatic disease	Other (angioedema, deficiency of C1 esterase)
Breast cancer	Infectious
Sarcomas	*Candida* epiglottitis
Melanoma	*Aspergillus* laryngotracheobronchitis
Esophageal cancer	Necrotizing laryngitis (HSV, CMV)
Kidney cancer	Fibropurulent epiglottitis (*Haemophilus*
Colon cancer	*influenzae, Streptococcus, Staphylococcus*)

CMV = *Cytomegalovirus*; HSV = herpes simplex virus.

genic infections. Patients usually present with the insidious onset of neck pain and swelling, trismus, sore throat, dysphagia, drooling, and shortness of breath. The suprahyoid and submental soft tissues are brawny, painful, and indurated on physical examination. Posterior and superior displacement of the base of the tongue and floor of the mouth is readily apparent in advanced cases.

The management of Ludwig's angina involves the protection of the airway and early antibiotic therapy. Empiric therapy with penicillin and clindamycin in nonallergic patients is appropriate until cultures are available and sensitivities are determined. Aggressive antibiotic therapy and airway observation may be appropriate in some patients. The need for tracheotomy should be decided on an individual basis. Judicious surgical intervention may be warranted for selected patients with disease refractory to antibiotic therapy and for patients who develop localized abscess. Early aggressive medical management may circumvent the need for surgical intervention and has resulted in reduced mortality rates (from 50% in the preantibiotic era to 8.5% currently).[231]

Other Benign Causes. Acquired deficiency of C_1 esterase inhibitor is associated with some hematologic malignancies. This disorder is associated with the development of angioedema, which is characterized by nonpitting painless swelling of the face, eyelids, lips, tongue, and mucous membranes. Severe acute upper-airway obstruction occurs in approximately 20% of patients and can be life threatening.[232] Airway management, epinephrine, antihistamines, and corticosteroid administration are the mainstays of therapy. Fresh frozen plasma is replete with C_1 esterase inhibitor. The administration of fresh frozen plasma is advocated in cases of life-threatening angioedema. However, the theoretical risk of generating mediators with the administration of fresh frozen plasma needs to be considered. Angioedema may also (rarely) complicate paclitaxel therapy. The routine judicious use of steroids and antihistamines has reduced the incidence of taxane-induced angioedema to 2 to 3%. Finally, massive airway edema causing respiratory collapse has been documented with azathioprine administration.[233] Patients with this idiosyncratic reaction usually respond to steroids and to the withdrawal of the drug. Rechallenge with azathioprine may result in the recurrence and exaggeration of respiratory symptoms.

Clinical Presentation. The clinical examination of the patient with upper-airway obstruction may reveal only exertional dyspnea early on. Late findings include wheezing, orthopnea, tachycardia, diaphoresis, stridor, and retraction of intercostal muscles. The appearance of stridor is an ominous sign that occurs with an 80% or greater reduction in the cross-sectional area of the upper airway. This finding is best appreciated by listening near the patient's open mouth during forced exhalation. The inspiratory phase of the respiratory cycle is typically prolonged and labored. As asphyxiation progresses, stridor becomes less prominent and represents a poor prognostic sign. Bradycardia, cyanosis, obtundation, and death may ensue within minutes of initial presentation. Rapid evaluation is mandatory in this setting, and emergency intervention is often based solely on the clinical examination. In patients with bilateral vocal-cord paralysis, phonation is usually preserved. These patients usually present with gradual symptoms of increasing dyspnea on exertion and stridor. Conversely, patients with unilateral vocal-cord paralysis may present with stridor and hoarseness without dyspnea.

Management. A rapid bedside evaluation should exclude foreign-body aspiration. Particularly in the case of patients with head and neck cancers and patients with neuromuscular disease and altered mental status, foreign-body aspiration should be strongly considered. Manual removal of any evidence of foreign material in the oral cavity is recommended. Substances that are lodged more distally in the upper airway may require the Heimlich maneuver to facilitate removal. Emergent direct visualization of the larynx with laryngoscopy may facilitate the passage of an endotracheal tube. Alternatively, bronchoscopic visualization of the airway with the passage of an endotracheal tube over the bronchoscope may be accomplished by a skilled clinician. In patients with lesions involving the upper one-third of the trachea and higher, surgical management with a low tracheotomy and the placement of a long tracheostomy tube may be effective in restoring respiration. Adjunctive therapy including the use of helium-oxygen mixtures (heliox), corticosteroids, and bronchodilators may provide a temporary bridge to more definitive therapy. Air flow patterns within the prox-

imal airway are characterized by turbulent flow and dictated by the density rather than the viscosity of the inhaled gas. Gas mixtures (such as heliox) that are less dense than oxygen may theoretically offer palliation by reducing airway resistance and respiratory work.[234] Surgical management may be appropriate for some low-lying primary endotracheal tumors but is often contraindicated because of the advanced stage of the tumor or underlying disease. With the exception of slow-growing thyroid tumors, surgical resection of metastatic tracheal tumors is rarely appropriate.

Lower-Airway Obstruction

By far the most common cause of intrinsic bronchial obstruction in the cancer patient is primary bronchogenic carcinoma (Table 10–15). Squamous cell carcinoma is the most frequent histologic type of primary bronchogenic tumor causing bronchial obstruction. Other primary bronchogenic carcinomas causing endobronchial obstruction include carcinoid tumors and (occasionally) adenocarcinoma. Primary carcinoid tumors of the gastrointestinal tract with liver metastases may produce severe airway obstruction. Airway compromise in these patients is mediated by the release of secretory products that produce nonanatomic obstructions of the airway. Focal endobronchial metastases from carcinomas of the colon, breasts, thyroid, and kidneys, as well as melanoma, lymphomas, and sarcomas, are less frequent causes of lower airway obstruction. Diffuse airway narrowing secondary to extensive infiltration of the bronchial submucosa by metastatic disease has also been described. Lesions of sufficient size to obstruct the mainstem bronchi may cause complete collapse of the airway and acute symptoms of dyspnea, especially in patients with significant underlying lung disease. However, patients usually present with the gradual onset of dyspnea, cough, and focal wheezing. Postobstructive pneumonitis, fever, and hemoptysis may also occur. Unlike acute proximal airway obstruction, distal airway obstruction in the absence of significant comorbid disease is rarely fatal but may be a major cause of excess morbidity.

Chest radiography identifies abnormalities corresponding to the obstructing lesion in more than 75% of cases. Segmental consolidation, atelectasis, segmental or lobar emphysema, and narrowing of the bronchus are suggestive findings on chest radiography or CT. Bronchoscopy or fine-needle aspiration is often necessary to establish the diagnosis if sputum cytology is negative.

Interventional Pulmonology in the Treatment of Central-Airway Obstruction

The relatively new field of interventional pulmonology offers advanced bronchoscopic technology for the treatment of a variety of obstructing lesions in the airway, ranging from endotracheal and endobronchial tumors to tracheobronchial stenosis. Interventional procedures using both the rigid and the flexible bronchoscope may be used to recannalize the central airway and prevent overt respiratory failure. General anesthesia is usually required for rigid bronchoscopic examinations whereas conscious sedation is usually sufficient for fiberoptic bronchoscopy. Rigid bronchoscopy remains the instrument of choice for debulking large centrally located tracheobronchial lesions. Balloon bronchoplasty of centrally obstructing masses and stenotic lesions may be accomplished through either a rigid or flexible bronchoscope. Successful airway recannalization using balloon dilatation usually requires combined management with stent placement or endobronchial laser therapy.[235] Patients may experience chest pain and bronchospasm during balloon dilatation. More ominous complications include pneumothorax, pneumomediastinum, and perforation of the airway.[235,236]

Tracheobronchial Stent Placement. Tracheobronchial stents are indicated in the acute treatment of central-airway obstruction due to localized inoperable endobronchial disease as well as extraluminal obstruction. These devices may provide lifesaving palliation in the treatment of acute airway obstruction. Although isolated reports of attempts to maintain airway patency with the use of stents appeared in the literature as early as 1915, the use of airway stents only became standard medical practice a little over a decade ago.[237,238] The Montgomery T-tube stent of the 1960s paved the way for the Dumon silicone stent developed in 1990. Two major categories of stents currently exist (Table 10–16). The silicone stents (including the Dumon stent) are usually placed through a rigid

bronchoscope while the patient is under general anesthesia. Single-lumen and Y-shaped bifurcated silicone stents are currently approved for the treatment of proximal airway tumors, main carinal lesions, tracheobronchomalacia, and tracheoesophageal fistulae. These radiopaque prostheses may be studded to facilitate anchorage to the airway mucosa. Silicone stents may be easily repositioned or removed. In addition, their solid surfaces preclude the ingrowth of tumor along the stented lumen although tumor regrowth and the formation of granulation tissue at the ends of the stent may occur. These thick-walled stents decrease the intraluminal caliber of the airway and interfere with local mucociliary clearance. Thus, inspissation of secretions is a common problem. Stent migration and inadequate expansion of the stent (especially in the setting of extrinsic airway compression) are additional potential complications.[237,238]

Metal stents are radiopaque and consist of a flexible wire meshwork. The wire meshwork of these stents is inherently inert and may be uncovered or covered with a thin layer of nylon, polyurethane, or silicone. These prostheses may be introduced into the airway through a flexible bronchoscope. The Gianturco stent, developed at M.D. Anderson Cancer Center approximately 20 years ago, is currently the most widely used stent worldwide. These stainless steel prostheses may be passed through a rigid or fiberoptic bronchoscope. Strut fracture, migration, persistent cough, perforation, and erosion into the pulmonary artery with this type of stent have been reported in the literature. Entanglement with suction catheters, causing the dislodgment and unraveling of these stents, has also been reported.[239,240]

Newer generations of stents include the Wallstent and Ultraflex prostheses. Wallstents are cobalt based and are available in covered and uncovered varieties. The Ultraflex stent is made of a nickel-titanium meshwork and is purported to be more physiologic in that it is capable of deforming in response to changing body temperatures. Early reports suggested less tumor ingrowth along the stent lumen of the Ultraflex prosthesis than with the Gianturco stent; however, extensive experience with the Ultraflex stent is lacking.[241] All three of the above stents are self-expanding and are available in uncovered and covered varieties. The uncovered stents permit ventilation through the wall of the prosthesis and may therefore be safely placed over a patent bronchial orifice without compromising ventilation to the nonstenotic bronchus. For example, this type of stent may be used in the treatment of obstructive lesions involving the right mainstem bronchus, without occluding the right-upper-lobe bronchus. The regrowth of tumor and the formation of granulation tissue though the wire meshwork of the uncovered stent remain a problem. Covered metal stents are advocated for the management of tracheobronchial

TABLE 10–15. Causes of Lower-Airway Obstruction in the Cancer Patient

Malignancy
    Primary bronchogenic carcinoma
        Squamous cell carcinoma
        Carcinoid tumors
        Adenocarcinoma
    Metastatic disease
        Colon cancer
        Breast cancer
        Thyroid cancer
        Kidney cancer
        Melanoma
        Lymphoma
        Sarcoma
Other causes
    Asthma
    Gastrointestinal carcinoid (nonanatomic obstruction)
    Bronchiolitis obliterans

TABLE 10–16. Types of Commonly Used Airway Stents

Type of Stent	Type of Material	Ideal Condition	Advantages	Disadvantages
Tube				
Dumon	Silicone	Proximal airway tumors Main carinal lesions Tracheobronchomalacia Tracheoesophageal fistulae	Inexpensive Easily removable Protects against tumor ingrowth Minimal airway irritation	Placement usually requires rigid bronchoscopy and general anesthesia May migrate Granulation tissue formation Interferes with local mucociliary clearance Inspissation of secretions Incomplete expansion after deployment
Metal				

Gianturco	Stainless steel	Proximal airway and
		  tracheal tumors
			May be deployed through rigid or
			  flexible scope
			Self-expandable
			Covered variety now available
			Dynamic expansibility
			Radiopaque
			Ventilation maintained across lobar
			  orifices (uncovered stents)
				Most deployment has been with rigid scope
				Migration
				Dislodgment/unraveling with suctioning
				Airway irritation causing cough
				Strut fracture
				Erosion into pulmonary artery
				Tracheopharyngeal fistulae

Wallstent	Cobalt-based alloy	Proximal airway and tracheal tumors	Self-expandable May be deployed through flexible scope Covered and uncovered varieties	Limited experience
Ultraflex	Nitinol (nickel-titanium alloy)	Proximal airway and tracheal tumors	Self-expandable May be deployed through flexible scope Covered and uncovered varieties Less tumor ingrowth than Gianturco? "Shape memory" More physiologic than other stents?	Limited experience

stenosis secondary to malignancy and for the management of tracheoesophageal or esophagobronchial fistulae. The ease of placement of metal stents offers a significant advantage over silicone stents although metal stents are more difficult to remove or reposition, once placed. Metal stents are also more irritating to the airway; thus, the increased incidence of airway compromise secondary to the exuberant formation of granulation tissue is a common problem.[237,238] Multimodality therapy combining stent placement with endoscopic laser surgery, argon plasma coagulation, balloon bronchoplasty, or endobronchial brachytherapy is increasingly used in the treatment of locally advanced tracheobronchial masses and fibrotic strictures.[91,237,242] Successful placement of airway stents may provide immediate symptomatic relief in 78 to 98% of patients[238,239] (Figure 10–9). In addition, stent placement in patients with respiratory failure secondary to large centrally obstructing tumors may facilitate successful extubation.[243] The mean survival rate of patients with malignant airway obstruction is only 3 to 4 months. Thus, large studies demonstrating the long-term benefits of stent placement in patients with malignant disease are not available.

Laser Bronchoscopy. Endobronchial laser surgery may provide invaluable palliative treatment to patients with symptomatic endobronchial disease. It is indicated in the acute treatment of severe airway obstruction secondary to endobronchial disease. The benefits of this tool in the treatment of benign tracheobronchial conditions (including inflammatory strictures, overgrowth of obstructive granulation tissue, and some benign tumors) are also well established.[244,245] Several types of lasers exist; they vary in depth of penetration, photocoagulation, tissue vaporization, and hemostatic properties. The type of laser primarily used in bronchoscopic laser resection is the Nd:YAG laser. This laser is ideal for the ablation of proximal endobronchial lesions because of its superior depth of penetration and tissue vaporization and its reliability for photocoagulation and hemostasis. Although Nd:YAG laser therapy may be performed though a flexible bronchoscope, rigid bronchoscopy is preferred. Potential complications of Nd:YAG laser therapy include hemorrhage, hypoxemia, and pneumothorax. In addition, cardiac arrhythmias, fatal pulmonary edema, and air embolism have been reported.[246] Fistula formation may occur after attempted laser ablation of structures that are in close proximity to blood vessels or to the esophagus. Endobronchial fires have been reported with the use of Nd:YAG laser therapy, especially in the setting of high inspired oxygen. Oxygen flow rates should be kept to a minimum (preferably below 40%) during laser firing.[247] Laser bronchoscopy is contraindicated in the treatment of airway obstruction caused by extrinsic compression because of the increased risk of tissue perforation and airway rupture. In general, laser bronchoscopy appears to be relatively safe. Overall complication rates are less than 0.1%, and the rate of fatal complications directly attributable to laser bronchoscopy is less than 0.5%.[246]

The value of Nd:YAG laser therapy in ablating central endobronchial lesions is quite good. In one large study, intraluminal recanalization rates of 90% were noted with tumors obstructing the proximal airway, mainstem bronchi, and right bronchus intermedius.[246] Rates of recanalization were substantial. Less impressive recanalization rates were noted with more distal lesions and with lesions causing combined endobronchial and extrinsic compression (50 to 70%). The usefulness of emergent laser bronchoscopy is also reflected in improved overall survival and increased rates of successful weaning from mechanical ventilation in those patients with respiratory failure secondary to malignant airway obstruction.[92,248] It is felt that multimodality therapy that uses laser bronchoscopy with brachytherapy, stent placement, or phototherapy may improve overall outcome although no large prospective studies are available.

Endobronchial Argon Plasma Coagulation. Argon plasma coagulation (APC), a form of electrocoagulation, is an excellent and cost-effective alternative to laser bronchoscopy in the acute management of central endobronchial disease causing significant airway obstruction. This treatment modality may be applied with a flexible bronchoscope, thereby avoiding the added risks and expense of general anesthesia. This type of electrocoagulation uses argon, which forms plasma when ionized. Argon plasma is an electrically conductive medium that permits the flow of an electrical current from the tip of a probe to target tissues. Argon plasma coagulation has been used extensively in the treatment of lesions in the gastrointestinal tract and by otolaryngologists for the treatment of head and neck lesions. The efficacy of this treatment modality in hemostasis and tissue ablation in these areas is well documented.[91,249] It has only recently evolved, however, as a tool in the treatment of tracheobronchial disease. A recent small study demonstrated effective tumor ablation and control of bleeding with APC.[91] Depth of penetration is less in comparison with Nd:YAG laser therapy; therefore, the risk of tissue perforation and rupture is less with APC. Because thermal

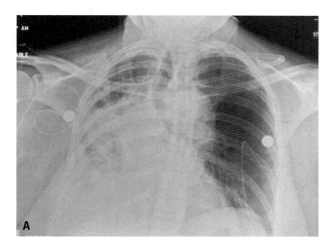

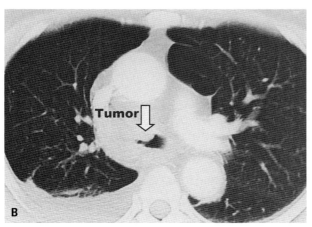

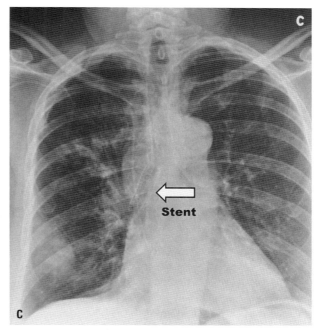

Figure 10–9. A 60-year-old woman with non-small-cell lung cancer and acute shortness of breath. A: Chest radiography revealed near-complete collapse of the right lung and postobstructive consolidation with pleural effusion. B: Chest computed tomography showed a right hilar mass contiguous with right paratracheal and subcarinal adenopathy causing narrowing of the right mainstem bronchus, with postobstructive pneumonitis. C: Stents were placed in the distal trachea and right mainstem bronchus, with successful re-inflation of the right lung seen by follow-up chest radiography.

reactions with airway devices that do not conduct electricity are minimal, the risk of endobronchial fires is much less with APC than with Nd:YAG laser bronchoscopy. Supplemental oxygen should be kept at a minimum ($FiO_2 < 40\%$) during firing of the probe, however. Large prospective studies comparing APC to laser therapy are currently not available.

Cryosurgery. Cryosurgery offers an excellent alternative in the subacute management of endobronchial lesions when surgical, laser, or radiation therapy is not an option. This technique may be successfully employed for the treatment of both benign and malignant intraluminal obstructive lesions that are cryosensitive and therefore susceptible to hypothermia-induced tissue necrosis.[250] Cryosensitive tissues include skin, mucous membranes, endothelium, nerves, and granulation tissue. Cryoablation may be accomplished through a flexible bronchoscope using a closed-tip liquid-nitrogen cryoprobe. Involved tissues must be cooled to temperatures of $-15°C$ to $-40°C$ to effect cell death. Tissue necrosis is achieved through selective cellular crystallization and microthrombosis.[250] Because the effects of cryotherapy are delayed, this treatment modality should not be used in the treatment of acute airway obstruction. Subjective improvement in respiratory function has been reported following cryoablation of endobronchial lesions; however, studies have been small, and unequivocal results are not available.[250] Although the hemostatic properties of hypothermia are well established, hemostatic control with cryotherapy is inferior to that achieved with laser bronchoscopy. The risk of severe airway hemorrhage, however, is less than 3%. The advantages of cryotherapy include a superior safety margin over laser therapy and a lower risk of airway perforation in the treatment of more distal lesions. Cryotherapy may act synergistically when used in combination with other therapeutic measures such as radiation or certain forms of chemotherapy,[251] with improved outcome. Large studies documenting these benefits, however, are not available.

Brachytherapy. Endobronchial brachytherapy is a particularly attractive therapeutic option for selected patients with endobronchial disease causing airway obstruction. The procedure involves the bronchoscopic placement of catheters adjacent to the obstructing lesion and the implantation of radioactive pellets (usually iridium-192) into the catheters. Fluoroscopy and radiography are employed to verify the proper positioning of the catheter. Low-dose-rate brachytherapy was favored up until the 1980s. This approach involved the delivery of up to 1,500 to 5,000 Gy of radioactive material in fractions of only 2 Gy/h. The more recent development of high-dose-rate (HDR) brachytherapy permits larger single doses of radiation (10 to 12 Gy/hr). The total dose and fraction of radiation given varies from one institution to the next. High-dose-rate brachytherapy has resulted in significant decrements in cost and treatment time, as well as the transfer of a previously inpatient procedure to the outpatient setting. Treatment schedules of one treatment per week to one treatment every 2 weeks are designed primarily for patient comfort.

The tumors that are best suited for brachytherapy include any centrally obstructing endobronchial mass for which surgical resection is not feasible. These include both primary or recurrent non-small-cell bronchogenic carcinomas and metastatic disease. The palliation of obstructive symptoms is the usual goal of brachytherapy although a curative potential of brachytherapy as single-modality therapy has been reported.[252] Although patient populations and techniques vary widely, most large studies report a 50% or greater increase in intraluminal caliber after brachytherapy in 50 to 80% of patients.[252,253] The effects of successful brachytherapy may be maintained for 6 months or longer after therapy. In several small studies, the control of hemoptysis and obstructive symptoms with HDR brachytherapy appeared similar to that seen with external-beam radiation.[254] Controlled studies comparing the efficacy of external-beam radiation to HDR brachytherapy in the palliation of obstructive symptoms are not available. The efficacy of brachytherapy is augmented when brachytherapy is used as adjunctive therapy with other therapeutic measures. Brachytherapy may be coupled with external-beam radiation for the treatment of some non-small-cell bronchogenic carcinomas with curative intent. In a large study by Miller and Phillips, a greater survival advantage was demonstrated with HDR brachytherapy and Nd:YAG laser resection than with brachytherapy alone.[255] The complication rate of brachytherapy ranges from 0 to 42%. Adverse effects may be categorized as early (cough, bronchospasm, pneumothorax, infection, bleeding, catheter displacement) and late (fistula formation, radiation-induced bronchitis, and stenosis) events. Hemoptysis may be massive, especially when associated with tumors of the upper lobes and mainstem bronchi in close proximity to the pulmonary arteries. Imaging with CT or MRI is indicated in these patients before initiating brachytherapy, to rule out invasion of tumor though the bronchial walls and into the major pulmonary vessels. Post-radiation edema associated with endobronchial radiation may transiently make airway obstruction worse. Patients with high-grade obstructing endotracheal masses, therefore, should first undergo treatment with laser bronchoscopy and possible stent placement before brachytherapy is attempted.

Asthma in the Cancer Patient

The reversible airflow obstruction that defines asthma is characterized by an excessive production of mucus and by airway hyperirritability. Patients typically present with episodic shortness of breath, coupled with cough and wheezing. Wheezing in the cancer patient should be distinguished from upper-airway stridor caused by proximal airway obstruction and focal wheezing caused by endobronchial disease (Figure 10–10). Wheezing and obstructive physiology on pulmonary function testing may also occur in association with bronchiolitis obliterans.

Asthma deserves separate recognition in the cancer patient for two reasons. Uncontrolled asthma may preclude the use of aggressive chemotherapy. In addition, the incidence of bronchospasm complicating cancer chemotherapy has steadily increased as newer agents and multi-drug combinations are introduced for cancer treatment. A prior history of well-controlled asthma does not contraindicate the administration of chemotherapy for most patients. In fact, studies have indicated that symptoms of asthma may remit during treatment with chemotherapy, perhaps due to diminished airway inflammation secondary to chemotherapy-related immunosuppression.[256] Patients with poorly controlled asthma and who are on optimal therapy, however, are particularly challenging, especially when certain chemotherapeutic agents known to cause bronchospasm are anticipated as part of the treatment regimen. Chemotherapeutic agents that are known to induce bronchospasm include paclitaxel, interferon, IL-2, gemcitabine, and aerosolized pentamidine.[105,145] In addition, severe bronchospasm associated with combined chemotherapy with mitomycin and vinca alkaloids is well described.[125] Airflow limitation may be monitored with pulmonary function testing and with outpatient peak flow measurements. Stepwise pharmacologic therapy should be instituted in accordance with symptom severity and NIH guidelines.[257] Drug withdrawal and premedication with a β-agonist and corticosteroids may alleviate the symptoms of bronchospasm induced by some drugs.

PULMONARY EDEMA IN THE CANCER PATIENT

Pathophysiology

Pulmonary edema, the pathologic flow of liquid from the intravascular to the interstitial spaces, may occur as a consequence of a variety of cardiogenic and noncardiogenic disorders. In both cases, the transudation of fluid from the pulmonary vessels exceeds the resorptive capacity of the pulmonary lymphatics and vasculature, resulting in the abnormal accumulation of extravascular fluid and solute in the lung. Advances in the understanding of the pathophysiology of pulmonary edema over the past 25 years have identified two fundamentally different types of this disorder. These two types of pulmonary edema are identified according to the permeability characteristics of the microvascular endothelium.

Normal microvascular-permeability pulmonary edema is usually associated with high-pressure edema and occurs primarily as a result of an imbalance of Starling forces within the lung microvasculature. This type of pulmonary edema may result from three overlapping mechanisms. Increased hydrostatic pressure favors extravascular lung water filtration. Conditions causing left ventricular dysfunction or mechanical obstruction to the left atrial outflow tract, volume overload, and increased lymphatic outflow pressures may elevate hydrostatic pressures and cause pulmonary edema secondary to this mechanism. Pulmonary venous hypertension is also a rare cause of increased microvascular hydrostatic pressure and high-pressure pulmonary edema. Pulmonary veno-occlusive disease occasionally occurs as a consequence of bleomycin-induced lung disease. This condition results in the obliteration of upstream vasculature and the subsequent elevation of pulmonary venous pressures with normal permeability pulmonary edema. In addition, decreased perimicrovascular hydrostatic pressures limit fluid and protein resorption at the level of the microvascular barrier in the lungs. Re-expansion pulmonary edema is partly due to pressure fluctuations at the perimicrovascular level. Finally, increased alveolar surface tension (as seen in patients with re-expansion pulmonary edema) and inspiratory airway obstruction are also causes of normal-pressure pulmonary edema.

Increased-permeability pulmonary edema is commonly referred to as primary or noncardiogenic pulmonary edema and is often considered with acute lung injury or ARDS. The

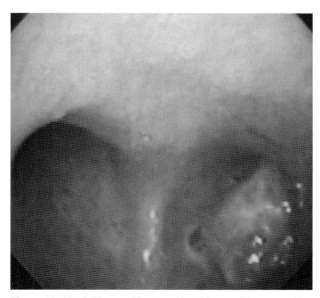

Figure 10–10. A 58-year-old man with a history of heavy smoking who presented with wheezing and right lung collapse. Bronchoscopy revealed an endobronchial mass obstructing the right mainstem bronchus.

hallmark of this type of pulmonary edema is the accumulation of a proteinaceous fluid in the interstitium as a result of a breach in the integrity of the alveolar and microvascular barriers within the lungs. The distinction between hydrostatic and increased-permeability pulmonary edema is often blurred by clinical syndromes causing pulmonary edema due to an overlap of both pathophysiologies. Neurogenic and re-expansion pulmonary edema are examples of pulmonary edema resulting from normal or increased permeability. Increased-permeability pulmonary edema/ARDS is covered in the acute lung injury and ARDS section of this chapter.

Normal-Permeability Pulmonary Edema

Etiologies. *Cardiogenic Pulmonary Edema.* The cancer patient is particularly susceptible to normal-permeability pulmonary edema resulting from a variety of cardiogenic and noncardiogenic sources (Table 10–17). The hallmark of cardiogenic normal-permeability pulmonary edema is increased pulmonary hydrostatic pressures. Potentially cardiotoxic chemotherapeutic agents such as the anthracyclines may cause cardiogenic normal-permeability pulmonary edema. The new recombinant monoclonal antibody, trastuzumab (Herceptin), has also been associated with cardiogenic pulmonary edema, especially in the setting of prior anthracycline therapy.[147] The mechanisms involved in the development of cardiogenic normal-permeability pulmonary edema with these classes of drugs are myocardial dysfunction leading to decreased left ventricular function and increased left ventricular end-diastolic pressure (LVEDP). Similarly, radiation therapy may precipitate accelerated coronary artery disease, resulting in increased LVEDP and cardiogenic normal-permeability pulmonary edema. Left atrial myxomas may cause normal-permeability pulmonary edema owing to elevated left atrial pressures. Elevated LVEDP is also seen in diastolic dysfunction; in this disorder, the normal diastolic pressure-volume relationship is shifted, resulting in a decreased end-diastolic volume for a given diastolic filling pressure. Elevated intrathoracic pressures, left ventricular ischemia, mechanical ventilation, and pericardial effusions may underlie the development of diastolic dysfunction. Each of these conditions is noted with increased frequency in patients with cancer.

Cardiogenic pulmonary edema has a diverse presentation. The acuity of the symptoms is dictated by the underlying cause. Symptoms range from cough, dyspnea, chest pain, and wheezing to syncopal episodes and sud-

TABLE 10–17. Cancer-Related Causes of Pulmonary Edema

I. Normal permeability	II. Increased permeability
Increased intravascular hydrostatic pressure	ALI/ARDS
Increased left ventricular end-diastolic pressure	Infection/inflammation
Systolic dysfunction	Sepsis syndrome
Arrhythmias	Pneumonia
Coronary artery disease	Aspiration of gastric contents
Cardiomyopathy (congestive, restrictive, hypertrophic)	Pancreatitis
High-output states (severe anemia)	Shock
Constrictive pericarditis	Disseminated intravascular coagulation
Diastolic eysfunction	Transfusion-related
Left ventricular hypertrophy	Massive blood transfusion
Ischemia	Leukoagglutination reaction
Pericardial effusion	Drugs
Volume overload or renal failure	Chemotherapy (IL-2, bleomycin, mitomycin, ara-C)
Constrictive pericarditis	Narcotics (oral and intravenous)
Mechanical ventilation (elevated intrathoracic pressure)	Radiologic contrast media
Increased left atrial pressure	Aspirin
Left atrial myxoma	Tricyclic antidepressants
Mitral/aortic valve disease	Embolic phenomenon
Increased pulmonary venous pressure	Thromboembolism
Pulmonary veno-occlusive disease	Fat embolism
Fibrosing mediastinitis	Air embolism
Neurogenic edema	Other
Seizures	Diffuse alveolar hemorrhage
Head trauma/spinal-cord injury	Trauma
Hemorrhagic/embolic strokes	Post relief of upper-airway obstruction
Decreased interstitial hydrostatic pressure	Trauma
Mechanical ventilation/PEEP	Neurogenic
Re-expansion edema	Re-expansion edema
Surfactant depletion	

ALI = acute lung injury; ara-C = cytosine arabinoside; ARDS = adult respiratory distress syndrome; PEEP = positive end-expiratory pressure.

den death, depending on the underlying cause. Tachypnea and wheezing may represent early clinical signs that may progress to diaphoresis, peripheral cyanosis, and frothy sputum production as edema progresses. A new or changing murmur may signal valvular disease as the etiology of cardiogenic pulmonary edema. The definitive diagnosis relies on the physical examination, chest radiography and echocardiographic data. Left heart or pulmonary artery catheterization may be necessary for diagnosis in some cases.

Neurogenic Pulmonary Edema. Neurogenic pulmonary edema may arise as a direct result of complications related to primary central nervous system (CNS) malignancy or metastatic CNS disease. Acute CNS events, including seizures and cerebrovascular accidents, are known causes of neurogenic pulmonary edema. The pathogenesis of neurogenic pulmonary edema has not been firmly established although hydrostatic mechanisms and changes in vascular permeability have been implicated.[258,259] Mortality rates associated with neurogenic pulmonary edema are high, primarily due to underlying CNS disease.

Re-expansion Pulmonary Edema. Re-expansion pulmonary edema is a rare and potentially fatal complication following the sudden re-inflation of a collapsed lung. The associated lung collapse is usually present for several days prior to treatment and typically involves more than 50% of the lung. Edema formation is commonly limited to the involved lung but may (rarely) progress to the contralateral side.[260] Pulmonary edema may arise after the drainage of a large pleural effusion or pneumothorax or after the removal of an obstructing tumor.[261] Pernicious coughing and chest tightness may occur during or immediately after thoracentesis or chest tube thoracostomy and may progress to severe hypoxemia, respiratory failure, cardiovascular collapse, and death. The clinical presentation may develop abruptly during or immediately following lung re-inflation and evolves over a 24- to 48-hour period. This type of pulmonary edema theoretically occurs as a result of a significant drop in perimicrovascular hydrostatic pressure that may occur with lung re-expansion. Increased microvascular permeability and lung ischemia-reperfusion injury have also been implicated in the development of this type of pulmonary edema. Supportive care with supplemental oxygen, hemodynamic support, and intubation with mechanical ventilation when necessary are the mainstays of treatment. Judicious use of diuretics is recommended. Aggressive diuresis may result in further decreases in intravascular volume and tissue perfusion. Suggested measures to prevent re-expansion pulmonary edema include the use of underwater-seal drainage during the first 24 to 48 hours after chest tube thoracostomy. The application of negative pressure to the chest tube is appropriate if lung re-expansion has not occurred after 24 hours of drainage with underwater seal. Light and colleagues advocate pleural-pressure monitoring during the evacuation of chronic, large-volume pleural effusions. Thoracentesis may safely continue as long as pleural pressures do not fall below −20 cm H_2O. In the absence of pleural-pressure monitoring, pleural-fluid evacuation should be limited to 1,000 mL of fluid.[262] The incidence of re-expansion pulmonary edema in the general population is unknown. Mahfood and colleagues reported overall mortality rates of 21%.[263] Mortality rates among cancer patients with re-expansion pulmonary edema may be even higher because of underlying comorbid conditions.

Postobstructive Pulmonary Edema. Large negative pressure swings may also underlie the development of pulmonary edema following the evacuation of pericardial effusions and in patients with severe laryngospasm, bronchospasm, or neoplastic obstruction of the upper airway. Although the exact mechanisms involved in the development of postobstructive pulmonary edema are unclear, the generation of marked negative pressures during inspiration in patients with upper-airway obstruction and the loss of intrinsic positive end-expiratory pressure (PEEP) following relief of the obstruction appear to play a role. Patients may present with upper-airway stridor or severe bronchospasm and radiographic patterns consistent with pulmonary edema as seen by chest radiography. Early recognition and treatment is imperative and usually leads to prompt resolution of the edema. Treatment is primarily supportive. Early intubation and mechanical ventilation is recommended. The application of PEEP may help to treat the edema and ameliorate symptoms. Fatal outcomes are associated with delayed treatment.

Pulmonary Edema Secondary to Lymphatic Obstruction. A variety of neoplastic and non-neoplastic conditions are associated with pulmonary edema due to decreased lymphatic clearance. Among the neoplastic etiologies, lymphatic obstruction by tumor and lymphangitic spread of disease are the most common. Pulmonary edema owing to lymphangitic spread of tumor may be difficult to distinguish from the underlying disease. Although lymphangitic spread may complicate any cancer, the most frequently associated tumors include adenocarcinomas of the breast, stomach, pancreas, and prostate. Patients typically present with dyspnea. Symptoms of shortness of breath may be insidious initially but rapidly progress to disabling dyspnea over a few weeks as fluid accumulation and neoplastic infiltration of interlobular septa and lymphatics continue. Superimposed tumor microemboli further aggravate the symptoms of dyspnea. The prognosis for patients with interstitial edema secondary to lymphangitic carcinomatosis is poor, with a mean survival of only 3 months after diagnosis.

Other Causes. Decreased interstitial hydrostatic pressures may result in normal-permeability pulmonary edema, and number of conditions are associated with this (see Table 10–17). Many of these conditions complicate cancer therapy. Pulmonary edema may occur in mechanically ventilated patients with high inspiratory pressures. The mechanisms of pulmonary edema formation in these patients involve increases in PEEP and perivascular transmural pressures and concomitant decreases in interstitial hydrostatic pressures. These fluctuations in microvascular and interstitial pressure gradients favor fluid filtration into the interstitium. Loss of alveolar surfactant may also play a role in fluid accumulation in this setting. In patients who require mechanical ventilation for treatment of respiratory failure, adequate gas exchange may be achieved at the expense of increasing amounts of inspired oxygen and PEEP. The salutary effects of increased PEEP for improving oxygenation are often offset by the attendant detrimental effects of high alveolar pressures and volumes. The role of high airway pressures and volumes in the development of barotrauma and reduced cardiac output is well established.[264] Earlier studies suggesting that increasing PEEP forces edema fluid into the pulmonary vasculature have been refuted. It is now understood that excess PEEP and high airway pressures may actually promote pulmonary edema. This adverse effect may be mitigated by the use of newer mechanical-ventilation strategies that promote derecruitment of alveoli at end expiration.[264,265]

Clinical Presentation. The classic changes on chest radiographs of patients with cardiogenic normal-permeability pulmonary edema include increased cardiac silhouette, cephalization of pulmonary vessels, prominent interstitial markings, perivascular cuffing, and the appearance of Kerley's B lines (Figure 10–11). Pleural effusions may occur as edema progresses. Central distribution of pulmonary edema fluid, cephalization of pulmonary vessels, increased cardiac size, and the presence of peribronchial cuffing, septal lines, and pleural effusions are often used to suggest cardiogenic pulmonary edema. Aberle and colleagues have shown that these radiographic findings are nonspecific and cannot be solely relied on to determine the cause of edema formation.[266] Sampling of the alveolar edema fluid by BAL may differentiate cardiogenic from increased-permeability pulmonary edema. This can usually be safely performed in the intubated patient once the patient is stabilized. Studies by Fein and colleagues suggested that pulmonary edema fluid with an alveolar protein-to-plasma protein ratio of 0.6 is diagnostic of cardiogenic pulmonary edema.[267] Hemodynamic data obtained from pulmonary artery catheterization have been traditionally used as a definitive diagnostic tool for distinguishing the cardiogenic causes of pulmonary edema from its noncardiogenic causes. Differentiating cardiogenic from noncardiogenic pulmonary edema by using this technique, however, may be difficult because of the overlap of underlying causes. Cardiogenic pulmonary edema typically shows high pulmonary capillary wedge (PCW) pressures on invasive monitoring. These pressures may be low, however, in the setting of very low osmotic pressures. Conversely, increased-permeability pulmonary edema typically demonstrates normal to low PCW pressures on Swan-Ganz monitoring. In the setting of acute lung injury with volume overload, however, these pressures may be high. The difficulty in interpreting hemodynamic data was underscored in a recent study that demonstrated

Figure 10–11. An 80-year-old man with coronary artery disease who developed acute shortness of breath following total gastrectomy for gastric cancer. Chest radiography revealed bilateral pleural effusions with consolidation consistent with pulmonary edema.

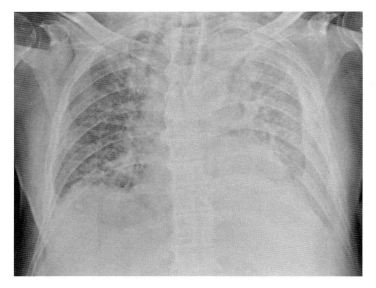

that physicians' skill in interpreting hemodynamic wave-forms was no better than random guessing.[268] Thus, hemodynamic monitoring should be used only as an adjunctive tool in the evaluation of selected patients with pulmonary edema. The interpretation and appropriate handling of hemodynamic data requires input from trained knowledgeable individuals. Although no definitive study has demonstrated a survival benefit in pulmonary artery–guided management of critically ill patients, these catheters may be of clinical benefit in the management of selected patients with pulmonary edema.

Management. Initial therapeutic options in patients with life-threatening edema are directed toward the stabilization of the patient. Immediate supportive measures may include diuresis, inotropic support, afterload reduction, supplemental oxygenation, vasodilators, morphine administration, and intubation with mechanical ventilation if indicated. Afterload reduction may be achieved with one of the ACEIs or an ACE receptor blocker. Sublingual or intravenous nitroglycerin has efficacy in decreasing preload and increasing venous capacitance in this setting and may be used if hypotension is not a problem. Low-dose dopamine has been advocated, especially for the treatment of pulmonary edema complicated by hypotension. The benefits of dopamine at low doses include increased cardiac contractility, reduced systemic vascular resistance, increased renal blood flow, and improved cardiac output without attendant increases in myocardial oxygen consumption or heart rate. Sodium nitroprusside is a potent vasodilator and may be ideal in treating the hypertensive patient who has severe pulmonary edema. These measures may help to minimize edema formation and hydrostatic pressures and thereby reduce cardiac work and improve cardiac efficiency. Judicious use of diuretics is imperative to avoid untoward effects of treatment. The sedating agents to be used during intubation must be chosen wisely as many of the standard sedating medications may decrease venous return and aggravate hypotension.

ACUTE LUNG INJURY AND ACUTE RESPIRATORY DISTRESS SYNDROME

A diverse list of insults to the pulmonary endothelial and epithelial surfaces may result in increased-permeability pulmonary edema. Primary and noncardiogenic pulmonary edema are descriptions ascribed to this type of pulmonary edema, and the associated clinical syndromes are known as acute respiratory distress syndrome (ARDS) or severe acute lung injury (ALI).[269] The two terms are often used interchangeably. More accurately, ALI and ARDS should be viewed as entities at opposite ends of a spectrum, with ARDS representing the more severe disorder. The standard definition of ARDS includes four strict criteria: (1) diffuse parenchymal infiltrates, (2) hypoxemia ($PaO_2/FiO_2 \leq 200$ torr for ARDS and ≤ 300 torr for ALI), (3) the absence of congestive heart failure (pulmonary artery occlusion pressure < 18 torr), and (4) acute onset. An expanded definition of ARDS (proposed by Murray) classifies patients according to the severity of lung injury, associated clinical disorder(s), and the presence of nonpulmonary organ dysfunction. Severity of lung injury is established by the lung injury score, which quantifies lung injury on the basis of the extent of the abnormalities seen on chest radiographs, the degree of hypoxemia, respiratory system compliance, and the amount of PEEP used.[270]

The wide variety of pathologic conditions that result in ALI/ARDS render the cancer patient distinctly susceptible to this type of lung injury (see Table 10–17). The major categories of risk factors that account for most of the reported cases of ALI/ARDS include infection, sepsis, chemotherapeutic agents, trauma, and aspiration of gastric contents. In addition, multiple conditions may act synergistically to increase the risk of ALI/ARDS. In a study by Pepe and Marini,[271] the risk of ALI/ARDS was 25% in patients with a single risk factor but increased to 85% when three or more underlying risk factors were present. Each of the categories for ALI/ARDS in Table 10–17 is over-represented in the cancer patient; thus, the incidence of ALI/ARDS in these patients is high. Death is the usual outcome for the cancer patient with severe ARDS, especially in the patient with hematologic malignancy who develops respiratory failure and ARDS following marrow transplantation.

The true incidence of sepsis causing ALI/ARDS in the cancer patient is unknown. In the general patient population, ARDS is thought to complicate 10 to 38% of all cases of sepsis.[271,272] Various degrees of ALI may be seen in an additional 35% of patients with sepsis. Thus, the incidence of some degree of lung injury in patients with sepsis syndrome is not trivial and may occur in approximately 60% of patients at some point during the course of their illness. Mortality rates exceeding 90% in these patients have not changed significantly over the past decade despite advances in therapy.[273,274] Death rates from sepsis and ALI/ARDS are higher than that from either syndrome alone. Infectious causes of ALI/ARDS are extensive. In the cancer patient, sepsis syndrome, infections caused by Gram-negative sepsis, and other bacterial, fungal, and viral pneumonias predominate.

Pathophysiology and Clinical Presentation

Acute lung injury is characterized by the sequential development of exudative, proliferative, and fibrotic changes within the lung parenchyma. Manifestations of these three stages of ALI may occur regardless of the underlying cause. Damage to the pulmonary epithelial and endothelial surfaces is the initial phenomenon that triggers a cascade of events in the evolution of ALI/ARDS. Loss of integrity of the epithelial and endothelial barriers results in the extravasation of large amounts of protein-rich fluid into the alveolar space. The edema fluid also contains large amounts of inflammatory cells (primarily neutrophils), platelets, red blood cells, fibrin, and debris that obliterate alveoli, creating large areas of V/Q inequality or shunt formation. Histologic changes consistent with diffuse alveolar damage are observed. These changes herald the earliest stage of ALI, referred to as the exudative stage. The type I epithelial cell is exquisitely sensitive to this type of lung injury, and widespread but patchy areas of destruction to alveolar type I epithelial cells is a common histologic finding. Injury to the type II cell results in reduced surfactant turnover and the disruption of normal epithelial ion transport activity. The loss of epithelial cell ion transport further impairs the removal of edema fluid from the airway. Hyaline membrane formation, composed of precipitated plasma proteins, fibrin, and necrotic debris, occurs early. Loss of normal surfactant activity by activated polymorphonuclear neutrophils and plasma proteins contributes to microatelectasis and shunt formation.

Neutrophils, complement, and humoral inflammatory mediators have been implicated in the pathogenesis of ALI/ARDS. However, ARDS is known to occur in patients with profound neutropenia, which suggests that additional mechanisms of ALI are also important. Furthermore, stimulation of neutrophil production with G-CSF does not appear to aggravate the symptoms of ALI/ARDS, again, indicating that other mediators must also play a role in the pathogenesis of this disorder.[275] The direct toxic action of oxygen metabolites, ionizing radiation, and certain chemotherapeutic agents may putatively induce lung injury by mechanisms independent of inflammation. The role of cytokines in promoting lung injury is poorly understood. A number of different pro-inflammatory cytokines, including macrophage inhibitory factor, tumor necrosis factor alpha (TNF-α), and interleukin-8, have been identified in the airways of patients with lung injury. These agents may either initiate or amplify the inflammatory response. The anti-inflammatory activities of TNF receptor (TNFr), interleukin-1 receptor antagonist, interleukin-10, and interleukin-11 may also have a modulating effect on the development of ALI/ARDS.[276,277] Alterations in the balance between pro- and anti-inflammatory cytokines in the airway may play a critical role in the development of this disorder.

Acute respiratory failure with refractory hypoxemia is typical of the exudative stage of ALI/ARDS. Patients commonly develop clinical manifestations of lung injury early, usually within 24 hours of exposure to the injurious agent.

Ninety percent of patients who ultimately develop ARDS are intubated within 72 hours of onset.[278] Chest radiography typically demonstrates patchy peripheral areas of airspace consolidation, with normal cardiac silhouette and the absence of Kerley's B lines. The radiographic findings, however, may be indistinguishable from those seen in cases of cardiogenic pulmonary edema. Patchy areas of atelectasis, alveolar filling, and consolidation seen by CT typically occur within dependent areas of the lungs. Lung injury may resolve after the exudative stage, or it may progress to fibrosing alveolitis. Disease progression is primarily dictated by the severity of the lung insult and the efficacy of the therapeutic intervention rather than by the type of the initial insult to the lungs. The proliferative phase of ALI may be as much of a response to therapeutic measures (such as oxygen toxicity) as it is to the initial underlying injury. This phase typically follows the exudative phase within 7 to 10 days. The hallmark of the proliferative phase is exuberant infiltration of fibroblasts and inflammatory cells into the alveoli and interstitium. Edema fluid is now minimal, and the pulmonary vascular bed may be extensively disrupted. Abnormalities of coagulation give rise to platelet-fibrin microthrombi, which may be extensive. Disruption of the pulmonary capillary bed, coupled with the formation of extensive microvascular thrombosis, may precipitate pulmonary hypertension. Elevations in pulmonary vascular resistance may be significant enough to induce cor pulmonale in some patients. Evidence of substantial inflammation on BAL is seen even in areas that are radiographically normal.[276] Replacement of the normal type I epithelial alveolar cells by cuboidal or bizarrely shaped type II cells is seen. A neutrophilic exudate is typically seen on BAL fluid. Fever, leukocytosis, diminished systemic vascular resistance, and diffuse areas of alveolar and interstitial consolidation on chest radiographs are common during this phase and suggest clinical infection although documentation of infection is rarely found. During the final fibrotic phase, extensive intra-alveolar and interstitial fibrosis obliterates the air space and further promotes dead-space ventilation and hypoxemia (Figure 10–12). Recovery or death may occur at any stage of ARDS. Prognosis is dependent on severity, chronicity, and treatment rather than on the etiology of the lung injury.

Management and Outcome

Although dramatic reductions in ARDS-related mortality in the general population have been reported over the past decade, mortality rates among cancer patients remain high, especially among those with hematologic malignancy and respiratory failure following stem cell transplantation.[274,279] Death rates among this cohort of patients may exceed 90%. Sepsis, age greater than 65 years, multisystem organ failure, renal insufficiency, and poor static compliance (< 25 L/cm H_2O) are poor prognostic factors. Persistent PaO$_2$-to-FiO$_2$ ratios of > 150 torr adversely influence patient outcome. Sepsis, intractable respiratory failure, and cardiac dysfunction are the leading causes of ARDS-related deaths. Early mortality (within the first 3 days) is directly attributable to the underlying illness or injury. Beyond this period, ARDS-related deaths are more often associated with the development of sepsis and/or multisystem organ failure.[280,281]

Improved survival among patients with ARDS has been attributed primarily to improvements in supportive care as no therapeutic interventions have convincingly altered the underlying pathophysiology. Prevention and early treatment of infections favorably impact survival.[280] Patients with persistent sepsis syndrome without identification or control of the underlying cause carry the highest rates of multisystem organ failure and death. Thus, an aggressive search for underlying infections and other causes of ARDS is imperative.

Fluid management in the critically ill patient with ARDS has been a source of much controversy. One strategy supports the maintenance of a low intravascular blood volume with vasopressor support as needed to maintain adequate cardiac output and blood pressure. Advocates of this strategy claim higher survival rates and fewer days on mechanical ventilation for patients treated in this manner versus those treated with conventional fluid management strategies.[282,283] Opponents of this approach have pointed out theoretical concerns regarding the potential adverse affects of vasopressors in promoting myocardial ischemia, aggravating shunt fraction, and decreasing perfusion to vital organs such as the kidneys. The latter effect could conceivably precipitate organ failure and accelerate the downhill clinical course. Additionally, fluid loading may improve oxygen consumption and tissue oxygen delivery. Although the data supporting the use of fluid restriction and vasopressors in the treatment of ARDS appear compelling, most of the data are derived from retrospective studies. The benefits of restricted versus liberal fluid management are currently under investigation by the NIH. Until data from this prospective trial are available, current recommendations support the restriction of intravenous fluids to maintain the lowest intravascular volume that permits adequate systemic tissue perfusion.

Vasopressors should be added as needed to facilitate end-organ tissue perfusion and normalize oxygen delivery. The use of vasopressors to achieve supraphysiologic levels of oxygen delivery may be detrimental and is therefore not recommended. The initial enthusiasm for the use of nitric oxide for treatment of ARDS was derived from the known effects of this agent as a selective vasodilator of the pulmonary vasculature. The results of several large randomized double-blind controlled trials, however, have been disappointing.[284,285] Inhaled nitric oxide was shown to have little effect on mortality and a

transient effect on overall length of time on the ventilator or no effect on these parameters at all. Initial attempts to control the inflammatory response in ARDS with steroids were similarly discouraging. More recent reports, however, have demonstrated potential beneficial effects of high-dose steroids administered during the fibroproliferative phase of ARDS.[286] Larger studies are needed to convincingly document a survival benefit for the use of steroid therapy. Surfactant replacement therapy has also been proposed for the treatment of patients with ARDS, based on its beneficial effects on the survival of infants with neonatal respiratory distress syndrome. So far, the results of this treatment modality have also

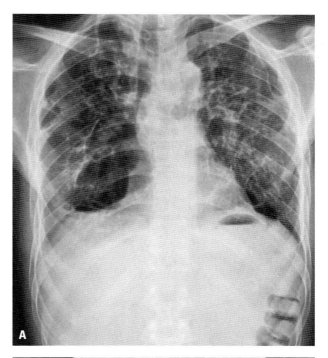

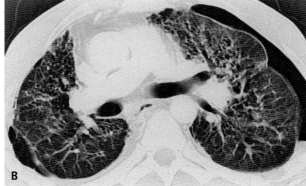

Figure 10–12. A 32-year-old man whose treatment for non-Hodgkin's lymphoma was complicated by pneumonia and adult respiratory distress syndrome (ARDS). A, B: Chest radiography (A) and computed tomography (B) showed bilateral cystic air-space disease and extensive parenchymal fibrosis.

been disappointing. Newer preparations of surfactant and methods of delivery are currently being evaluated.[287]

Noninvasive positive pressure ventilation (NPPV) may be appropriate for patients with milder levels of respiratory distress.[288] Patients with hypercapneic respiratory failure and limited acute hypoxemic failure show the highest success rates with this mode of ventilation. In patients with hemodynamic instability, a high risk of aspiration, difficulty in clearing secretions, significant gastrointestinal bleeding, uncontrolled arrhythmias, or poor compliance, NPPV should be avoided. Large controlled studies comparing NPPV with conventional mechanical ventilation in patients with ALI are unavailable.

Mechanical ventilation may be a lifesaving therapeutic intervention in patients with respiratory failure secondary to ARDS. Several patterns of ventilator-associated lung injury have been documented, including barotrauma and a pattern of lung damage that is histologically similar to ARDS. These patterns of lung injury are typically seen with conventional modes of ventilation. A variety of ventilation strategies in ARDS have been proposed, which profess reductions in these untoward effects. The optimal method of mechanical ventilation in patients with ARDS, nonetheless, is a matter of intense and ongoing controversy. The goals of all forms of artificial ventilation are to achieve normal or near-normal oxygenation while minimizing the adverse effects of mechanical ventilation on the lungs. As ARDS progresses and the lungs become less compliant, adequate oxygenation and ventilation may become exceedingly difficult to achieve. Attempts to optimize these goals by using conventional ventilation may sometimes be achieved with various combinations of tidal volumes, PEEP, and FiO2. Lung injury related to further upward adjustments of the ventilator may result in volutrauma or toxic effects of high FiO2 on the lungs. Several protective ventilatory strategies have been proposed and are currently being studied. At present, the most popular strategies include inverse ratio ventilation (IRV) and bilevel ventilation. Both of these ventilator modalities are designed to limit tidal volumes and plateau pressures in an effort to minimize the adverse effects of the ventilator on the lungs.[289] A recent NIH multicenter trial confirmed the efficacy of this approach. In bilevel or "open-lung" ventilation, recruitment of atelectatic lung is augmented by raising the level of PEEP above the level at which alveoli collapse, defined as the lower inflection point on a pressure-volume curve.[290] Amato and co-workers documented a reduction in overall mortality in a small group of patients treated with this mode of ventilation.[290] These results appear promising although larger studies are needed.

Inverse ratio ventilation exploits the effect of sustained elevations in airway pressure in the recruitment of collapsed alveoli. This may be achieved by extending the inspiratory time (I:E ratio) to greater than 50% of the res-

piratory cycle. The prolongation of inspiratory time may augment mean airway pressures while simultaneously reducing PEEP requirements and peak airway pressures. The recommended upper pressure limit for plateau pressures in mechanically ventilated patients is 35 to 40 cm H_2O, based on animal models of increased rates of lung injury with plateau pressures exceeding this range. Volume-cycled or pressure-controlled ventilation may be used for IRV. Airway pressures in IRV are limited at the expense of the tidal volume. Reductions in the delivered tidal volume result in progressive elevations in the partial pressure of carbon dioxide (PCO_2) (ie, permissive hypercapnia). Contraindications to permissive hypercapnia include increased intracranial pressure, severe pulmonary hypertension or cardiac decompensation, and profound metabolic acidosis. Permissive hypercapnia is otherwise fairly well tolerated in most patients as long as an adequate pH is maintained. Acceptable pH levels are another source of debate. In general, however, pH should be maintained above 7.2.[291] Inverse ratio ventilation promotes the development of auto-PEEP. Significant levels of auto-PEEP may be associated with hemodynamic compromise and the development of barotrauma. Patients usually require full sedation and chemical paralysis to optimize patient-ventilator synchrony. Reductions in mortality rates have been described in several small studies that have examined the efficacy of IRV in patients with ARDS. Prospective randomized trials designed to compare the influences of IRV, bilevel ventilation, and conventional ventilator strategies on patient outcomes have not been undertaken.

Lung rest using extracorporeal membrane oxygenation (ECMO) has been proposed for the treatment of patients with severe ARDS. Survival benefits of ECMO have not been borne out in any recent studies. Several studies have documented variable degrees of increased arterial oxygenation with prone positioning. This approach is based on the knowledge that fluid tends to accumulate in the gravity-dependent areas of the lung. No prospective randomized trial, however, has shown a beneficial effect of prone positioning on patient outcome. Dislodgment of catheters and endotracheal tubes and worsening oxygenation may occur during the process of repositioning the patient. Thus, nursing management plays a critical role in the success of this therapeutic intervention.

SUMMARY

The lungs are particularly vulnerable to a variety of local and systemic insults that arise as a consequence of cancer or its treatment. These insults underlie a diverse group of acute and subacute pulmonary oncologic emergencies. Damage to the lungs may not only dictate the limits of cancer therapy but also may trump otherwise successful cancer treatment strategies. Increases in the types and complexity of lung injury are expected as more aggressive therapies challenge the limits of tolerance. Aggressive immunosuppressive and multimodality cytoreductive therapies and newer agents such as immunomodulators and hematopoietic cytokines have contributed to considerable progress in antineoplastic therapy. In addition, the expanded use of stem cell transplants in the treatment of neoplastic disease offers the prospect of long-term disease-free survival for patients previously considered ineligible for this type of therapy. Advances in the local treatment of intrathoracic tumors with interventional bronchoscopic techniques may offer more complete palliation as well as definitive treatment to some patients with advanced cancers. Unfortunately, these achievements have been met with pulmonary complications that contribute significantly to the overall morbidity and mortality of the cancer patient.

The monumental challenge to the oncologist and other clinicians caring for patients with cancer is to integrate new aggressive treatment modalities with pre-emptive strategies that minimize lung injury. The timely use of empiric antimicrobials after myeloablative therapy is one such example that has led to significant improvements in the rates of infectious complications in this group of patients. Advances in cytokine and cellular therapies have added to the armamentarium of treatment strategies available for stem cell support and have reduced the morbidity of cytotoxic therapy. Standard prophylaxis against thromboembolism in cancer patients, especially those undergoing general or orthopedic surgery, has markedly reduced the incidence of thromboembolic disease in these patients.

Many questions remain unanswered. Increased insight into the pathogenic mechanisms that underlie the different patterns of cancer-related lung damage such as ARDS, diffuse alveolar hemorrhage (DAH), and cytotoxin-induced lung injury may lead to novel treatment strategies and improved outcomes.

REFERENCES

1. Carson J, Kelley M, Duff A, et al. The clinical course of pulmonary embolism. N Engl J Med 1992;326:1240–5.
2. Douketis J, Kearon C, Bates S, et al. Risk of fatal pulmonary embolism in patients with treated venous thromboembolism. JAMA 1998;279:458–62.
3. Dalen J, Joseph A, Hirsh J. Thrombolytic therapy for pulmonary embolism: is it effective? Is it safe? When is it indicated? Arch Intern Med 1997;157:2550–6.
4. Prudoni P, Lensing A, Buller H. Deep vein thrombosis and the incidence of subsequent symptomatic cancer. N Engl J Med 1992;327:1128–33.
5. Levine M. Treatment of thrombotic disorders in cancer patients. Haemostasis 1997;27(Suppl 1):38–43.
6. Sorensen H, Mellenkjaer L, Steffensen F, et al. The risk of a diagnosis of cancer after primary deep venous thrombosis or pulmonary embolism. N Engl J Med 1998;338:1167–73.
7. Solymoss S. Risk factors for thromboembolism: pathophysiology and detection. Can Med Assoc J 2000;163:991–4.
8. Columbus. The Columbus investigators: low-molecular-weight heparin in the treatment of patients with venous thromboembolism. N Engl J Med 1997;337:657–62.
9. Levitan N, Doulato A, Rencick S, et al. Rates of initial and recurrent thromboembolic disease among patients with malignancy versus those without malignancy. Medicine 1999;78:285.
10. Amico L, Caplan L, Thomas C. Cerebrovascular complications of mucinous cancers. Neurology 1989;39:522–6.
11. Pinzon R, Drewinko B, Trujilio J, et al. Pancreatic carcinoma and Trousseau's syndrome: experience at a large cancer center. J Clin Oncol 1986;4:509–14.
12. Callander N, Varki N, Rao L. Immunohistochemical identification of tissue factor in solid tumors. Cancer Chemother Pharmacol 1992;70:1194–201.
13. Monreal M, Fernandez-Llamanzares J, Pereandreau J. Occult cancer in patients with venous thromboembolism: which patients, which cancers? Thromb Haemost 1997;78:1316.
14. Wanscher B, Frifelt J, Smith-Silverstein C. Thrombosis caused by polyurethane double-lumen subclavian superior vena cava catheter and hemodialysis. Crit Care Med 1988;16:624–8.
15. Moser K. Venous thromboembolism: state of the art. Am Rev Respir Dis 1990;141:235–49.
16. Salzman E, Harris W. Prevention of venous thromboembolism in orthopaedic patients. J Bone Joint Surg 1976; 58:903–13.
17. Davidson B, Elliott C, Lensing A. Low accuracy of color Doppler ultrasound in the detection of proximal leg vein thrombosis in asymtomatic high-risk patients. Ann Intern Med 1992;117:735–8.
18. PIOPED. The PIOPED investigators: tissue plasminogen activator for the treatment of acute pulmonary embolism. Chest 1990;97:528.
19. Stein P, Saltzman H, Weg J. Clinical characteristics of patients with acute pulmonary embolism. Am J Cardiol 1991;68:1723–4.
20. Ferrari E, Imbert A, Chevalier T, Mihoubi A. The ECG in pulmonary embolism. Predictive value of negative T waves in precordial leads—80 case reports. Chest 1997;111:537–43.
21. Kasper W, Konstantinides S, Geibel A. Prognostic significance of right ventricular afterload stress detected by echocardiography in patients with clinically suspected pulmonary embolism. Heart 1997;77:346–9.
22. Hull R, Raskob G, Rosenbloom D. Heparin for 5 days as compared with 10 days in the initial treatment of proximal venous thrombosis. N Engl J Med 1990;322:1260–4.
23. Stein P, Hull R, Saltzman H, Pineo G. Strategy for diagnosis of patients with suspected acute pulmonary embolism. Chest 1993;103:1553–9.
24. Ginsberg JS. Management of venous thromboembolism. N Engl J Med 1996;335:1816–28.
25. Hyers T. Diagnosis of pulmonary embolism. Thorax 1995;50:930–2.

26. Ferretti G, Byanian D, Pison J, et al. Acute pulmonary embolism: role of helical CT in 164 patients with intermediate probability on ventilation-perfusion scintigraphy for the diagnosis of pulmonary embolism. Radiology 1998;205:453–8.

27. Garg K, Kemp J, Wojcik D. Thromboembolic disease: comparison of combined CT pulmonary angiography and venography with bilateral leg sonography in 70 patients. AJR Am J Roentgenol 2000;175:997–1001.

28. Van Rossum A, Treurnet F, Rieft G, et al. Role of spiral volumetric computed tomography in the assessment of patients with clinical suspicion of pulmonary embolism and abnormal ventilation-perfusion scan. Thorax 1996;51:23–8.

29. Goodman L, Lipchik R, Kuzo R. Subsequent pulmonary embolism: risk after a negative helical CT pulmonary angiogram. Prospective comparison with scintigraphy. Radiology 2000;132:227.

30. Sostman H, Layish D, Tapson V. Prospective comparison of helical CT and MR imaging in clinically suspected acute pulmonary embolism. J Magn Reson Imaging 1996;6:275–81.

31. Cross J, Kemp P, Walsh C. A randomized trial of spiral CT and ventilation perfusion scintigraphy for the diagnosis of embolism. Clin Radiol 1998;53:177–82.

32. Hull R, Raskob G, Ginsberg J. A noninvasive strategy for the treatment of patients with suspected pulmonary embolism. Arch Intern Med 1994;154:289–97.

33. Remy-Jardin M, Remy J, Deschildre F, et al. Diagnosis of pulmonary embolism with spiral CT. Comparison with pulmonary angiography and scintigraphy. Radiology 1996;200:699–706.

34. Meaney J, Weg J, Chenevert T. Diagnosis of pulmonary embolism with magnetic resonance angiography. N Engl J Med 1997;336:1422–7.

35. Bounameaux H, De Moerloose P, Perrier A, Miron M. D-dimer testing in suspected venous thromboembolism: an update. QJM 1997;90:437–42.

36. Goldhaber SZ, Simons G, Elliot C. Quantitative plasma D-dimer levels among patients undergoing pulmonary angiography for suspected pulmonary embolism. JAMA 1993;270:2819–22.

37. Oger E, Leroyer C, Bressollette L. Evaluation of a new, rapid, and quantitative D-dimer test in patients with suspected pulmonary embolism. Am J Respir Crit Care Med 1998;158:65–70.

38. Ginsberg J, Wells P, Kearon C. Sensitivity and specificity of a rapid whole-blood assay for D-dimer in the diagnosis of pulmonary embolism. Ann Intern Med 1998;129:1006–11.

39. Becker D, Philbrick J, Bachhuber T. D-dimer testing and acute venous thromboembolism. A shortcut to accurate diagnosis? Arch Intern Med 1996;156:939–46.

40. Kollef M, Zahid M, Eisenberg P. Predictive value of a rapid semiquantitative D-dimer assay in critically ill patients with suspected venous thromboembolic disease. Crit Care Med 2000;28:414–20.

41. Prandoni P, Lensing A, Buller HR, et al. Comparison of subcutaneous low-molecular-weight heparin with intraveneous standard heparin in proximal deep-vein thrombosis. Lancet 1992;339:441–5.

42. Hull R, Raskob G, Pineo GF, et al. Subcutaneous low-molecular-weight heparin compared with continuous intravenous heparin in the treatment of proximal vein thrombosis. N Engl J Med 1992;26:975–82.

43. Simmoneau G, Sors H, Charbonnier B. A comparison of low-molecular-weight heparin with unfractionated heparin for acute pulmonary embolism. N Engl J Med 1997;337:663–9.

44. Harrison L, Johnston M, Massicotte M. Comparison of 5-mg and 10-mg loading doses in initiation of warfarin therapy. Ann Intern Med 1997;126:133–6.

45. Schulman S, Granqvist S, Holmstrom M. The duration of oral anticoagulant therapy after a second episode of venous thromboembolism. N Engl J Med 1997;336:393–8.

46. UPET. UPET investigators: urokinase pulmonary embolism trial. Phase I results: a cooperative study. JAMA 1970;214:2163–72.

47. Thomas M, Chauhan A, More R. Pulmonary embolism-an update on thrombolytic therapy. QJM 2000;93:261–7.

48. Konstantinides S, Tiede N, Giebel A. Comparison of alteplase versus heparin for resolution of major pulmonary embolism. Am J Cardiol 1998;82:966.

49. NIH. NIH Concensus Development Conference: thrombolytic therapy in thrombosis. Ann Intern Med 1980;93:141.

50. Goldhaber S, Haire W, Feldstein M. Alteplase versus heparin in acute pulmonary embolism: randomized trial assessing right-ventricular function and pulmonary perfusion. Lancet 1993;341:507–11.

51. Goldhaber S, Heit J, Sharma G. Randomized controlled trial of recombinant tissue plasminogen activator versus urokinase in the treatment of acute pulmonary embolism. Lancet 1988;2:293–8.

52. Tapson V, Davidson C, Bauman R. Rapid thrombolysis of massive pulmonary emboli without systemic fibrinogenolysis: intra-embolic infusion of thrombolytic therapy. Am Rev Respir Dis 1992;146:A719.

53. Leeper K, Popvich J, Lesser B. Treatment of massive acute pulmonary embolism. The use of low doses of intra-pulmonary arterial streptokinase combined with full doses of systemic heparin. Chest 1988;98:234.

54. Verstraete M, Miller G, Bounameaux H, et al. Intravenous and intrapulmonary recombinant-tissue-type plasminogen activator in the treatment of acute massive pulmonary embolism. Circulation 1988;77:353–60.

55. Aylward P, Wilcox R, Horgan J. Relation of increased arterial blood pressure to mortality and stroke in the context of contemporary thrombolytic therapy for acute myocardial infarction. Ann Intern Med 1996;125:891–900.

56. Gore J, Sloan M, Price T. Intracerebral hemorrhage, cerebral infarction and subdural hematoma after acute myocardial infarction and thrombolytic therapy in the Thrombolysis in Myocardial Infarction Study: Thrombolysis in Myocardial Infarction, Phase II, pilot and clinical trial. Circulation 1991;83:448–59.

57. Kanter D, Mikkola K, Patel S, et al. Thrombolytic therapy

for pulmonary embolism: frequency of intracranial hemorrhage and associated risk factors. Chest 1997; 111:1241–5.

58. Saveyev V. Massive pulmonary embolism: embolectomy or thrombolysis. Int Angiol 1985;4:137–40.

59. Clark D, Abrams L. Pulmonary embolectomy: a 25-year experience. J Thorac Cardiovasc Surg 1986;92(3 Pt 1): 442–5.

60. Meyer G, Sors H, Charbonnier B. The European Cooperative Study Group for Pulmonary Embolism. J Am Coll Cardiol 1992;19:239–45.

61. Koning R, Cribier A, Gerber L. A new treatment for severe pulmonary embolism: percutaneous rheolytic thrombectomy. Circulation 1997;96:2498–500.

62. Lipton J, Russell J, Burgess K, et al. Fat embolization and pulmonary infiltrates after bone marrow transplantation. Med Pediatr Oncol 1987;15:24–7.

63. Menendez L, Bacon W, Kempf R, et al. Fat embolism syndrome complicating intraarterial chemotherapy with cisplatinum. Clin Orthop 1990;254:294–7.

64. Vedrinne J, Guillaume C, Gagnieu M, et al. Bronchoalveolar lavage in trauma patients for diagnosis of fat embolism syndrome. Chest 1992;102:1323–7.

65. Nijsten M, Mamer J, Ten Duis H, et al. Fat embolism and patent foramen ovale. Lancet 1989;1:1271.

66. Guenter C, Braun T. Fat embolism syndrome: changing prognosis. Chest 1981;79:143–5.

67. Veinot J, Ford S, Price R. Subacute cor pulmonale due to tumor embolization. Chest 1992;102:323–7.

68. Goldhaber S, Dricker E, Buring J, et al. Clinical suspicion of autopsy-proven thrombotic and tumor pulmonary embolism in cancer patients. Am Heart J 1987;114: 1432–5.

69. Orebaugh S. Venous air embolism: clinical and experimental considerations. Crit Care Med 1992;20:1169–77.

70. Ulyatt D, Judson J, Trubuhovich R, et al. Cerebral arterial air embolism associated with coughing on a continuous positive airway pressure circuit. Crit Care Med 1991;19:985–7.

71. Black M, Calvin J, Chan K, et al. Paradoxic air embolism in the absence of an intracardiac defect. Chest 1991;99: 754–5.

72. Golish J, Pena C, Mehta A. Massive air embolism complicating Nd-YAG laser endobronchial photoresection. Lasers Surg Med 1992;12:338–42.

73. Marini J, Culver B. Systemic gas embolism complicating mechanical ventilation in the adult respiratory distress syndrome. Ann Intern Med 1989;110:699–703.

74. Layon A. Hyperbaric oxygen treatment of cerebral air embolism: where are the data? Mayo Clin Proc 1991; 66:641–6.

75. Stoller J. Diagnosis and management of massive hemoptysis: a review. Respir Care 1992;37:564–81.

76. Deffenbach M, Charan N, Lakshiminarayan S, et al. The bronchial circulation: small but a vital attribute of the lung. Am Rev Respir Dis 1987;135:463–81.

77. Uflaker R, Laemmerer A, Neves C, et al. Bronchial artery embolization in the management of hemoptysis: the clinical aspects and long-term results. Radiology 1985; 157:637–44.

78. Rabkin J, Astafjev V, Gothman L. Transcatheter embolization in the management of pulmonary hemorrhage. Radiology 1987;163:361–5.

79. Cahill BC, Ingbar DH. Massive hemoptysis. Clin Chest Med 1994;15:147–68.

80. Hirshberg B, Biran I, Glazer M, Kramer M. Hemoptysis: etiology, evaluation, and outcome in a tertiary referral hospital. Chest 1997;112:440–4.

81. Miller R, McGregor D. Hemorrhage from carcinoma of the lung. Cancer 1980;46:200–5.

82. Tsukamoto T, Sasaki H, Nakamura H. Treatment of hemoptysis patients by thrombin and fibrinogen-thrombin infusion therapy using a fiberoptic bronchoscope. Chest 1989;96:473–6.

83. Rumbak M, Kohler G, Eastrige C. Topical treatment of life threatening haemoptysis from aspergillomas. Thorax 1996;51:253–5.

84. Freitag L. Development of a new balloon catheter for management of hemoptysis with bronchofiberscopes. Chest 1993;103:593.

85. Conlan A, Hurwitz S. Management of massive hemoptysis with the rigid bronchoscope and cold saline lavage. Thorax 1980;35:901–4.

86. Metcalf J, Rennard S, Reed E, et al. Corticosteroids as adjunctive therapy for diffuse alveolar hemorrhage associated with bone marrow transplantation. Am J Med 1994;94:327–34.

87. Haselton D, Klekamp J, Christman B. Use of high-dose corticosteroids and high-frequency oscillatory ventilation for treatment of a child with diffuse alveolar hemorrhage after bone marrow transplantation: case report and review of the literature. Crit Care Med 2000;28(1):245–8.

88. Wong L, Lillquist Y, Culham G, et al. Treatment of recurrent hemoptysis in a child with cystic fibrosis by repeated bronchial artery embolization and long-term tranexamic acid. Pediatr Pulmonol 1996;22:275–9.

89. Dweik R, Mehta A. Bronchoscopic management of malignant airway disease. Clin Pulm Med 1996;3:43–51.

90. Colt H. Laser bronchoscopy. Chest Surg Clin North Am 1996;6:277–91.

91. Morice R, Ece T, Ece F, Keus L. Endobronchial argon plasma coagulation for treatment of hemoptysis and neoplastic airway obstruction. Chest 2001;119:781–7.

92. Colt HG, Harrell JH. Therapeutic rigid bronchoscopy allows level of care changes in patients with acute respiratory failure from central airways obstruction. Chest 1997;112(1):202–6.

93. Osaki S, Nakanishi Y, Wataya H, et al. Prognosis of bronchial artery embolization in the management of hemoptysis. Respiration 2000;67:412–6.

94. Keller F, Rosch J, Loflin TG, et al. Nonbronchial systemic collateral arteries: significance of percutaneous embolotherapy for hemoptysis. Radiology 1987;164: 687–92.

95. Brinson G, Noone P, Mauro M, et al. Bronchial artery embolization for the treatment of hemoptysis in patients with cystic fibrosis. Am J Respir Crit Care Med 1998;157:1951–8.

96. Tanaka N, Yamakado K, Murashima S, et al. Superselective bronchial artery embolization for hemoptysis with

a coaxial microcatheter system. J Vasc Interv Radiol 1997;8:65–70.

97. Shneerson J, Emerson P, Phillips R. Radiotherapy for massive hemoptysis from an aspergilloma. Thorax 1980;35:953-4.

98. Kay PH. Surgical treatment of pulmonary aspergilloma. Thorax 1997;52:753–4.

99. Chen J-C, Yih-Leong L, Luh S-P, et al. Surgical treatment for pulmonary aspergilloma: a 28 year experience. Thorax 1997;52:810–3.

100. Knott-Craig C, Oostuizen G, Rossouw G, et al. Management and prognosis of massive hemoptyis: recent experience with 120 patients. J Thorac Cardiovasc Surg 1993;105:394–7.

101. Corey R, Hla KM. Major and massive hemoptysis: reassessment of conservative management. Am J Med Sci 1987;294:301–9.

102. Oliner H, Schwartz R, Rubio F. Interstitial pulmonary fibrosis following busulfan therapy. Am J Med 1961;31:134–9.

103. Tanoue L. Pulmonary toxicity associated with chemotherapeutic agents. I. Fishman's pulmonary diseases and disorders. St. Louis: McGraw-Hill Inc; 1998. p. 1003–16.

104. Deneke S, Fanburg B. Normobaric oxygen toxicity of the lung. N Engl J Med 1980;303:76–86.

105. Rosenow E. Drug-induced pulmonary disease. Dis Mon 1994;40:253–310.

106. Jones S, Moore M, Blank N. Hypersensitivity to procarbazine (matulane) manifested by fever and pleuropulmonary reaction. Cancer 1972;29:498–500.

107. Cooper J, White D, Matthay R. State of the art: drug-induced pulmonary disease. Am Rev Respir Dis 1986;133:321–40.

108. Aronchick J, Gefter W. Drug-induced pulmonary disorders. Semin Roentgenol 1995;15:18–34.

109. Sackett DL, Fojo T. Taxanes and other microtubule stabilizing agents. Cancer Chemother Biol Response Modif 1999;18:59–80.

110. Shannon V, Price K. Pulmonary complications of cancer therapy. Anesthesiol Clin North Am 1998;16:563–85.

111. Jules-Elysee K, Stover D, Yahalom J, et al. Pulmonary complications in lymphoma patients treated with high-dose therapy and autologous bone marrow transplantation. Am Rev Respir Dis 1992;146:485–91.

112. Steijfer S. Bleomycin-induced pneumonitis. Chest 2001;120:617–24.

113. Kreisman H, Wolkove N. Pulmonary toxicity of antineoplastic therapy. Semin Oncol 1992;19:508–20.

114. Samuels M, Johnson D, Holoye P. Large-dose bleomycin therapy and pulmonary toxicity: a possible role of prior radiotherapy. JAMA 1976;235:1117–20.

115. Bauer K, Skarin A, Balikian J. Pulmonary complications associated with combination chemotherapy programs containing bleomycin. Am J Med 1983;74:557–63.

116. Hirsch A, Els NV, Straus DJ. Effect of abvd chemotherapy with and without mantle or mediastinal irradiation on pulmonary function and symtoms in early-stage Hodgkin's disease. J Clin Oncol 1996;14:1297–305.

117. Mathes DD. Bleomycin and hyperoxia exposure in the operating room. Anesth Analg 1995;8:624–9.

118. Goldiner P, Rooney S. In defense of restricting oxygen in bleomycin-treated surgical patients. Anesthesiology 1984;61:225–7.

119. White D, Rankin J, Stover D. Severe bleomycin–induced pneumonitis: clinical features and response to corticosteroids. Chest 1984;86:723–8.

120. van Barneveld P, Veenstra G, Sleijfer D, et al. Changes in pulmonary function during and after bleomycin treatment in patients with testicular carcinoma. Cancer Chemother Pharmacol 1985;14:168–71.

121. Luursema P, Kroesen-Star M. Bleomycin-induced changes in the carbon monoxide transfer factor of the lungs and its components. Am Rev Respir Dis 1983;128:880–3.

122. Comis R. Bleomycin pulmonary toxicity: current status and future directions. Semin Oncol 1992;19 (2 Suppl 5): 64–70.

123. Takita T, Ogino T. Peplomycin and liblomycin, a new analogues of bleomycin. Biomed Pharmacother 1987;41: 219–26.

124. Chambers S, Flynn S, Prete SD. Bleomycin, vincristine, mitomycin C, and cisplatinum in gynecologic squamous cell carcinomas: a high incidence of pulmonary toxicity. Gynecol Oncol 1989;32:303–9.

125. Rivera NP, Kris MG, Gralla RJ. Syndrome of acute dyspnea related to combined mitomycin plus vinca alkaloid chemotherapy. Am J Clin Oncol 1995;18:245–50.

126. Jolivet J, Giroux L, Lauring S. Microangiopathic hemolytic anemia, renal failure, and noncardiogenic pulmonary edema. Cancer Treat Rep 1983;67:429–34.

127. Goucher G, Rowland V, Hawkins J. Melphalan-induced pulmonary interstitial fibrosis. Chest 1980;77:805–6.

128. Carr M. Chlorambucil induced pulmonary fibrosis: report of a case and review. Va Med Q 1986;113:667–80.

129. Zitnick R. Drug-induced lung disease: cancer chemotherapy agents. Respir Dis 1995;16:855–65.

130. Massin F. Busulfan-induced pneumopathy. Rev Mal Respir 1987;3:3–10.

131. Schallier D, Ipens N, Warson F. Additive pulmonary toxicity with melphalan and busulfan therapy. Chest 1983;84:492–3.

132. Quigley M, Brada M, Heron C, Horwich A. Severe lung toxicity with a weekly low dose chemotherapy regimen in patients with non-Hodgkins lymphoma. Hematol Oncol 1988;6:319–24.

133. Ahmed T, Ciavarella D, Feldman E. High-dose potentially myeloablative chemotherapy and autologous bone marrow transplantation for patients with advanced Hodgkin's disease. Leukemia 1989;3:223–9.

133a. Sostman HD, Matthay RA, Putman CE. Methotrexate-induced pneumonitis. Medicine 1976;55:371–88.

134. Hurst P, Habib M, Garewell H. Pulmonary toxicity associated with fludarabine monophosphate. Invest New Drugs 1987;5:207–10.

135. Andersson B, Cogan B, Keating M. Subacute pulmonary failure complicating therapy with high-dose ara-C in acute leukemia. Cancer 1985;56:2181–4.

136. Jehn U, Goldel N, Rienmuller R. Non-cardiogenic pulmonary edema complicating intermediate and high-dose ara C treatment for relapsed acute leukemia. Med Oncol Tumor Pharmacother 1988;5:41–7.

137. Pavlakis N, Bell D, Millward M. Fatal pulmonary toxicity resulting from treatment with gemcitabine. Cancer 1997;80:286–91.

138. Rubio C, Hill M, O'Brien M, Cunningham D. Idiopathic pneumonia syndrome after high-dose chemotherapy for relapsed Hodgkin's disease. Br J Cancer 1997;75:1044–8.

139. Durant J, Norgard M, Murad TM, et al. Pulmonary toxicity associated with bis-choloroethylnitrosourea (BCNU). Ann Intern Med 1979;90:191–4.

140. White D. New chemotherapy-induced pulmonary syndromes. Pulm Perspect 1995;12:4–5.

141. Pitney W, Phadke K, Dean S. Antithrombin III deficiency during asparaginase therapy. Lancet 1980;1:493–4.

142. Lipton A, Harvey H, Hamilton R. Venous thrombosis as a side effect of tamoxifen treatment. Cancer Treat Rep 1984;68:887–9.

143. Wiley J, Firkin F. Reduction of pulmonary toxicity by prednisone prophylaxis during all-trans-retinoic acid treatment of acute promyelocytic leukemia. Leukemia 1995;9:774–8.

144. Lee R, Lotze M, Skibber J. Cardiorespiratory effects of immunotherapy with interleukin-2. J Clin Oncol 1989; 7:7–20.

145. Margolin KA. Interleukin - 2 in the treatment of renal cancer. Semin Oncol 2000;27:194–203.

146. Albanell J, Baselga J. Systemic therapy emergencies. Semin Oncol 2000;27:347–61.

147. Baselga J. Multinational studies of Herceptin (humanized anti-HER2 antibody) in HER2+ metastiatic breast cancer: phase III of Herceptin plus chemotherapy (CRx) vs. CRx alone in first-time and large phase II of Herceptin alone in advanced disease. Ann Oncol 1998;9:47.

148. Putnam JB, Dignani C, Mehra RC, et al. Acute airway obstruction and necrotizing tracheobronchitis from invasive mycosis. Chest 1994;106:1265–7.

149. Chernow B, Sahn S. Carcinomatous involvement of the pleura: an analysis of 96 patients. Am J Med 1977;63: 695–702.

150. Light R. Pleural diseases. 3rd ed. Philadelphia: Lea & Febiger; 1990. p. 237–62.

151. Assi Z, Caruso J, Herdon J, Patz E. Cytologically proved malignant pleural effusions: distribution of transudates and exudates. Chest 1998;113:1302–4.

152. Aschi M, Golish J, Eng P, O'Donovan P. Transudative malignant pleural effusions: prevalence and mechanisms. South Med J 1998;91:23–6.

153. Vives M, Porcel M, Vera MVD, et al. A study of Light's criteria and possible modifications for distinguishing exudative from transudative effusion. Chest 1996;109:1503–7.

154. Romero S, Candela A, Martin C, et al. Evaluation of different criteria for the separation of pleural transudates and exudates. Chest 1993;104:339–404.

155. Sahn S. Fishman's pulmonary diseases and disorders. In: Fishman JA, editor. St. Louis: McGraw-Hill Inc; 1998. p. 1430.

156. Meyer P. Metastic carcinoma of the pleura. Thorax 1966;21:437–43.

157. Good J, Moore J, Fowler A, Sahn S. Superior vena cava syndrome as a cause of pleural effusion. Am Rev Respir Dis 1982;125:246–7.

158. Sahn S. Pleural diseases related to metastatic malignancies. Eur Respir J 1997;10:1907–13.

159. Light R. Pleural disease. Baltimore: Williams and Wilkins; 1995.

160. Bynum L, Wilson JE 3rd. Characteristics of pleural effusions associated with pulmonary embolism. Arch Intern Med 1976;136:159–62.

161. Bynum L, Wilson J. Radiographic features of pleural effusions in pulmonary embolism. Am Rev Respir Dis 1978;117:829–34.

162. Morelock S, Sahn S. Drugs and the pleura. Chest 1999; 116:212–21.

163. Libshitz H. Radiation changes in the lung. Semin Roentgenol 1993;28:303–20.

164. Light R, Erozan Y, Ball WC Jr. Cells in pleural fluid. Their value in differential diagnosis. Arch Intern Med 1973; 132:854–60.

165. Rubins J, Rubins H. Etiology and prognostic significance of eosinophilic pleural effusions. A prospective study. Chest 1996;110:1271–4.

166. Sahn S. Malignancy metastatic to the pleura. Clin Chest Med 1998;19:351–61.

167. Rodriguez-Panadero F, Lopez-Mejias J. Survival time of patients with pleural metastatic carcinoma predicted by glucose and pH studies. Chest 1989;95:320–4.

168. Sanchez-Armengol A, Rodriguez-Panadero F. Survival and talc pleurodesis in metastatic pleural carcinoma, revisited. Chest 1993;104:1482–5.

169. Prakash U, Reiman H. Comparison of needle biopsy with cytologic analysis for the evaluation of pleural effusion: analysis of 414 cases. Mayo Clin Proc 1985;60: 158–64.

170. Poe R, Israel R, Utell M. Sensitivty, specificity, and predictive value of closed pleural biopsy. Arch Intern Med 1984;144:325–8.

171. Harris R, Kavuru M, Mehta A, et al. The impact of thoracoscopy on the management of pleural disease. Chest 1995;107:845–52.

172. Feinsilver S, Barrows A, Braman S. Fiberoptic bronchoscopy and pleural effusion of unknown origin. Chest 1986;90:516–9.

173. Brown S, Light R. Pleural effusion associated with pulmonary embolization. Clin Chest Med 1985;6:77–81.

174. Heffner J. Indications for draining a parapneumonic effusion: an evidence based approach. Semin Respir Infect 1999;14:48–58.

175. Davies R, Traill Z, Gleeson F. Randomized controlled trial of intrapleural streptokinase in community acquired pleural infection. Thorax 1997;52:416–21.

176. Jerjes-Sanchez C, Ramirez-Rivera A, Elizalde J, et al. Intrapleural fibrinolysis with streptokinase as an adjunctive treatment in hemothorax and empyema: a multicenter trial. Chest 1996;109:1514–9.

177. Bouros D, Schiza S, Tzanakis N, et al. Intrapleural urokinase vs normal saline in the treatment of complicated parapneumonic effusions and empyema: a randomized, double-blind study. Am J Respir Crit Care Med 1999;159:37–42.

178. Colt H. Thoracoscopy: window to the pleural space. Chest 1999;116:1409–15.

179. Landreneau R, Keenan R, Hazelrigg S, et al. Thorascopy for empyema and hemothorax. Chest 1996;109:18–24.

180. Cassina P, Hauser M, Hillejan L, et al. Video-assisted thoracoscopy in the treatment of pleural empyema: stage-based management and outcome. J Thorac Cardiovasc Surg 1999;117:234–8.

181. De Campos J, Vargas F, DeCampos E, et al. Thoracoscopy talc poudrage: a 15-year experience. Chest 2001;119:801–6.

182. Viallat J, Rey F, Astoul P, Boutin C. Thoracoscopic talc poudrage pleurodesis for malignant effusions. A review of 360 cases. Chest 1996;110:1387–93.

183. Light R. Diseases of the pleura: the use of talc for pleurodesis. Curr Opin Pulm Med 2000;6:255–8.

184. Rehse D, Aye R, Florence M. Respiratory failure following talc pleurodesis. Am J Surg 1999;177:437–40.

185. Pien G, Gant M, Washam C, Sterman D. Use of an implantatble pleural catheter for trapped lung syndrome in patients with malignant pleural effusion. Chest 2001;119:1641–6.

186. Putnam J, Walsh G, Swisher S, et al. Outpatient management of malignant pleural effusion by a chronic indwelling pleural catheter. Ann Thorac Surg 2000;69:369–75.

187. Putnam JB, Light R, Rodriguez R, et al. A randomized comparison of indwelling pleural catheter and doxycycline pleurodesis in the management of malignant pleural effusions. Cancer 1999;86:1992–9.

188. Light R, Rodriguez R. Factors predicting spontaneous pleurodesis in patients with indwelling pleural catheters. Eur Respir J 1998;12:238S.

189. Martini N, Bains M, Beattie EJ Jr. Indications for pleurectomy in malignant effusion. Cancer 1975;35:734–8.

190. Fry W, Khadekar J. Parietal pleurectomy for malignant pleural effusion. Ann Surg Oncol 1995;2:160–4.

191. Murphy M, Newman B, Rodgers B. Pleuroperitoneal shunts in the management of persistent chylothorax. Am Thorac Surg 1989;48:195–200.

192. Rostand R, Feldman R, Block E. Massive hemothorax complicating heparin anticoagulation for pulmonary embolus. South Med J 1977;70:1128–30.

193. Fromke V, Schmidt W. Hemothorax in idiopathic thrombocytopenic purpura (ITP). J Thorac Cardiovasc Surg 1972;63:962–7.

194. Weil P, Margolis B. Systematic approach to traumatic hemothorax. Am J Surg 1981;142:692–4.

195. Wilson J, Boren C, Peterson S, et al. Traumatic hemothorax: is decortication necessary? J Thorac Cardiovasc Surg 1979;77:489–95.

196. Carillo E, Richardson J. Thoracoscopy in the management of hemothorax and retained blood after trauma. Curr Opin Pulm Med 1998;4:243–6.

197. Collins C, Lopez A, Wood V, et al. Quanitification of pneumothorax size on chest radiographs using interpleural distances: regression analysis based on measurements from helical CT. AJR Am J Roentgenol 1995;165:1127–30.

198. Rhea J, DeLuca S, Greene R. Determing the size of pneumothorax in the upright patient. Radiology 1982;144:733–6.

199. Axel L. A simple way to estimate the size of a pneumothorax. Invest Radiol 1981;16:165–6.

200. Baumann M, Strange C, Heffner J, et al. AACP Pneumothorax Consensus Group. Management of spontaneous pneumothorax: an American College of Chest Physicians Delphi consensus statement. Chest 2001;119:590–602.

201. Despars J, Sassoon C, Light R. Significance of iatrogenic pneumothorax. Chest 1994;105:1147–50.

202. Sassoon C, Light R, O'Hara V, Moritz T. Iatrogenic pneumothorax: etiology and morbidity. Results of a Department of Veterans Affairs Cooperative Study. Respiration 1992;59:215–20.

203. Conces D, Holden R. Aberrant locations and complications in initial placement of subclavian vein catheters. Arch Surg 1984;119:293–5.

204. Broadwater J, Henderson M, Bell J, et al. Outpatient percutaneous central venous access in cancer patients. Am J Surg 1990;160:676–80.

205. Collins T, Sahn S. Clinical value, complications, technical problems and patient experience. Chest 1987;91:817–22.

206. Poe R, Kallay M, Wicks CM, et al. Predicting risk of pneumothorax in needle biopsy of the lung. Chest 1984;85:232–5.

207. Zwillich C, Pierson D, Creagh C, et al. Complications of assisted ventilation: a prospective study of 354 consecutive episodes. Am J Med 1974;57:161–70.

208. Larscheid R, Thorpe P, Scott W. Percutaneous transthoracic needle aspiration biopsy: a comprehensive review of its current role in the diagnosis and treatment of lung tumors. Chest 1998;114:704–9.

209. Westcott J, Rao N, Colley D. Transthoracic needle biopsy small pulmonary nodules. Radiology 1997;202:97–103.

210. Shepherd J. Complications of percutaneous needle aspiration biopsy of the chest: prevention and management. Semin Interv Radiol 1994;11:181–5.

211. Bergquist T, Bailey P, Cortese D, et al. Transthoracic needle biopsy: accuracy and complications in relation to location and type of lesion. Mayo Clin Proc 1980;55:475–81.

212. Light R, O'Hara V, Moritz T, et al. Department of Veterans Affairs Cooperative Study Group on spontaneous pneumothorax: intrapleural tetracyline for the prevention of recurrent spontaneous pneumothorax: results of a Department of Veterans Affairs cooperative study. JAMA 1990;264:2224–30.

213. Martino P, Girmenia C, Venditti M, et al. Spontaneous pneumothorax complicating pulmonary mycetoma in patients with acute leukemia. Rev Infect Dis 1990;12:611–7.

214. Tocino I, Miller M, Fairfax W. Distribution of pneumothorax in the supine and semirecumbent critically ill adult. AJR Am J Roentgenol 1985;144:901–5.

215. Chan P, Clarke P, Daniel F, et al. Efficacy study of video-assisted thoracoscopic surgery pleurodesis for spontaneous pneumothorax. Ann Thorac Surg 2001;71:452–4.

216. Liu H, Lin P, Hsieh M, et al. Thoracoscopic surgery as a routine procedure for spontaneous pneumothorax. Results from 82 patients. Chest 1995;107:559–62.

217. Waller D. Video-assisted thoracoscopic surgery for spontaneous pneumothorax—a 7-year learning experience. Ann R Coll Surg Engl 1999;81:387–92.

218. Torre M, Grassi M, Nerli F, et al. Nd-YAG laser pleurodesis via thoracoscopy. Endoscopic therapy in spontaneous pneumothorax Nd-YAG laser pleurodesis. Chest 1994;106:338–41.

219. Maier A, Anegg U, Renner H, et al. Four-year experience with pleural abrasion using a rotating brush during video-assisted thoracoscopy. Surg Endosc 2000;14:75–8.

220. Bertrand P, Regnard J, Spaggiari L, et al. Immediate and long-term results after surgical treatment of primary spontaneous pneumothorax by VATS. Ann Thorac Surg 1996;61:1641–5.

221. Hurtgen M, Linder A, Friedel G, Toomes H. Video-assisted thoracoscopic pleurodesis. A survey conducted by the German Society of Thoracic Surgery. Thorac Cardiovasc Surg 1996;44:199–203.

222. Mouroux J, Elkaim D, Padovani B, et al. Video-assisted thoracoscopic treatment of spontaneous pneumothorax: technique and results of one hundred cases. J Thorac Cardiovasc Surg 1996;112:385–91.

223. Almind M, Lange P, Viskum K. Spontaneous pneumothorax: comparison of simple drainage, talc pleurodesis, and tetracycline pleurodesis. Thorax 1989;44:627–30.

224. Stern Y, Marshak G, Shiptzer T, et al. Vocal cord palsy: possible late complication of radiotherapy for head and neck cancer. Ann Otol Rhinol Laryngol 1995;104:294–6.

225. Cole S, Zawin M, Lundberg B, et al. *Candida* epiglottitis in an adult with acute nonlymphocytic leukemia. Am J Med 1987;82:662–4.

226. D'Angelo A, Zwillenberg S, Olekszyk J, et al. Adult supraglottitis due to herpes simplex virus. J Otolaryngol 1990;19:179–81.

227. Lopez-Amado M, Yebra-Pimentel M, Garcia-Sarandeses A. *Cytomegalovirus* causing necrotizing laryngitis in a renal and cardiac transplant recipient. Head Neck 1996;18:455–7.

228. Lederman M, Lowder J, Lerner P. Bacteremic pneumococcal epiglottitis in adults with malignancy. Am Rev Respir Dis 1982;125:117–8.

229. Marple B. Ludwig angina: a review of current airway management. Arch Otolaryngol Head Neck Surg 1999;125:596–9.

230. Fritsch D, Klein D. Ludwig's angina. Heart Lung 1992;21:39–46.

231. Moreland L, Corey J, McKenzie R. Ludwig's angina. Report of a case and review of the literature. Arch Intern Med 1988;148:461–6.

232. Megerian C, Arnold J, Berger M. Angioedema: 4 year's experience, with a review of the disorder's presentation and treatment. Laryngoscope 1992;102:256–60.

233. Jungling A, Shangraw R. Massive airway edema after azathioprine. Anesthesiology 2000;92:888–90.

234. Rodrigo G, Rodrigo C. Heliox effect of rapid-onset acute severe asthma. Chest 2000;117:1212–3.

235. Sheski F, Mathur P. Long-term results of fiberoptic bronchoscopic balloon dilation in the management of benign tracheobronchial stenosis. Chest 1998;114:796–800.

236. Noppen M, Schlesser M, Meysman M, et al. Bronchoscopic balloon dilation in the combined management of postintubation stenosis of the trachea in adults. Chest 1997;112:1187–8.

237. Colt H. Thorascopic management of malignant pleural effusions. Clin Chest Med 1995;16:505–18.

238. Mehta A, Dasgupta A. Airway stents. Clin Chest Med 1999;20:139–51.

239. Carrasco C, Nesbitt J, Charnsangavej C, et al. Management of tracheal and bronchial stenosis with the Gianturco stent. Ann Thorac Surg 1994;58:1012–7.

240. Freitag L, Tekolf E, Stamatis G, Greschuchna D. Clinical evaluation of a new bifurcated dynamic ariway stent: a 5-year experience with 135 patients. Thorac Cardiovasc Surg 1997;45:6–12.

241. Yanagihara K, Mizuno H, Wada H, Hitomi S. Tracheal stenosis treated with self-expanding nitinol stent. Ann Thorac Surg 1997;63:1789–90.

242. Shapshay S. Endoscopic treatment of tracheobronchial malignancy. Experience with Nd-YAG and CO2 lasers in 506 operations. Otolaryngol Head Neck Surg 1987;93:205–10.

243. Shaffer J, Allen J. The use of expandable metal stents to facilitate extubation in patients with large airway obstruction. Chest 1998;114:1378–82.

244. Shah H, Garbe T, Nussbaum E, et al. Benign tumors of the tracheobronchial tree. Endoscopic characteristics and role of laser resection. Chest 1995;107:1744–5.

245. Turner J, Wang K. Endobronchial laser therapy. Clin Chest Med 1999;20:107–22.

246. Cavaliere S, Venuta F, Foccoli P, et al. Endoscopic treatment of malignant airway obstructions in 2,008 patients. Chest 1996;110:1536–42.

247. Scherer T. Nd-YAG laser ignition of silicone endobronchial stents. Chest 2000;117:1449–54.

248. Stanopoulos I, Beamis JJ, Martinez F, Shapshay S. Laser bronchoscopy in respiratory failure from malignant airway obstruction. Crit Care Med 1993;21:386–91.

249. Bergler W, Riedel F, Baker-Schreyer A, et al. Argon plasma coagulation for the treatment of hereditary hemorrhagic telangiectasia. Laryngoscope 1999;109:15–20.

250. Mathur P, Wolf K, Busk M, et al. Fiberoptic bronchoscopic cryotherapy in the management of tracheobronchial disorder. Chest 1996;110:718–23.

251. Vergnon J, Schmitt T, Alamartine E, et al. Initial combined cryotherapy and irradiation for unresectable non small cell lung cancer. Chest 1992;102:1436–40.

252. Nori D, Allison R, Kaplan B, et al. High dose–rate intraluminal irradiation in bronchogenic carcinoma. Chest 1993;104:1006–11.

253. Schray M, McDougall J, Martinez A, et al. Management of malignant airway obstruction: clinical and dosimetric consideration using an iridium–192 afterloading technique in conjunction with the neodymium-YAG laser. Int J Radiat Oncol Biol Phys 1985;11:403–9.

254. Burt P, O'Driscoll B, Notely H, et al. Intraluminal irradiation for the palliation of lung cancer with the high dose rate microselection. Thorax 1990;45:765–8.

255. Miller J, Phillips T. Neodymium:YAG laser and brachytherapy in the management of inoperable bronchogenic carcinoma. Ann Thorac Surg 1990;50:190–5.

256. Jones P, Henry R, Francis L, Gibson P. Chemotherapy reduces the prevalence of asthma symptoms in children with cancer: implications for the role of airway

257. Anonymous. New NHLBI guidelines for the diagnosis and management of asthma. National Heart, Lung and Blood Institute. Lippincott Health Promot Lett 1997;2:8–9.

258. Smith S, Matthay M. Evidence for a hydrostatic mechanism in human neurogenic pulmonary edema. Chest 1997;111:1326–33.

259. Maron M. Analysis of airway fluid protein concentration in neurogenic pulmonary edema. J Appl Physiol 1987;62:470–6.

260. Ozlu O, Kilie A, Cengizlier R. Bilateral re-expansion pulmonary edema in a child: a reminder. Acta Anaesthesiol Scand 2000;44:884–5.

261. Tremey B, Guglielminotti J, Belkacem A, et al. Acute respiratory failure after re-expansion pulmonary edema localized to a lobe. Intensive Care Med 2001;27:325–6.

262. Light R, Girard W, Jenkinson S, George R. Parapneumonic diseases. Am J Med 1980;69:507–12.

263. Mahfood S, Hix W, Aaron B, et al. Reexpansion pulmonary edema. Ann Thorac Surg 1988;45:340–5.

264. Parker J, Hernandez L, Peevy K. Mechanisms of ventilator–induced lung injury. Crit Care Med 1993;21:131–43.

265. Marcy T, Marini J. Inverse ratio ventilation in ARDS: rationale and implementation. Chest 1991;100:494–504.

266. Aberle D, Wiener-Kronish J, Webb W, Matthay M. Hydrostatic versus increased permeability pulmonary edema: diagnosis based on radiographic criteria in critically ill patients. Radiology 1988;168:73–9.

267. Fein A, Grossman R, Jones J, et al. The value of edema fluid protein measurement in patients with pulmonary edema. Am J Med 1979;67:32–8.

268. Komadina K, Schenk D, LaVeau P, et al. Interobserver variability in the interpretation of pulmonary artery catheter pressure tracings. Chest 1991;100:1647–54.

269. Bernard G, Artigas A, Brigham K, et al. The American-European Consensus Conference on ARDS: definitions, mechanisms, relevant outcomes, and clinical trial coordination. Am J Respir Crit Care Med 1994;149:818–24.

270. Murray J, Mathay M, Luce J, et al. An expanded definition of the adult respiratory distress syndrome. Am Rev Respir Dis 1988;138:720–3.

271. Pepe P, Marini J. Occult positive end-expiratory pressure in mechanically ventilated patients with airflow obstruction: the auto-PEEP effect. Am Rev Respir Dis 1982;126:166–70.

272. Bone R, Fisher C, Clemmer T, et al. Early methylprednisolone treatment for septic syndrome and the adult respiratory distress syndrome. Chest 1987;92:1032–6.

273. Seidenfeld J, Pohl D, Bell R, et al. Incidence, site, and outcome of infections in patients with the adult respiratory distress syndrome. Am Rev Respir Dis 1986;134:12–6.

274. Price K, Thall P, Kish S, Shannon V. Prognostic indicators for blood and marrow transplant patients admitted to an intensive care unit. Am J Respir Crit Care Med 1998;158:876–84.

275. Nelson S, Belknap S, Carlson R, et al. A randomized controlled trial of filgrastim as an adjunct to antibiotics for treatment of hospitalized patients with community-acquired pneumonia. J Infect Dis 1998;1998:1075–80.

276. Pittet J, MacKersie R, Martin T, Matthay M. Biological markers of acute lung injury: prognostic and pathogenetic significance. Am J Respir Crit Care Med 1997;155:1187–205.

277. Matthay M, Geiser T, Matalon S, Ischiropoulos H. Oxidant-mediated lung injury in the acute respiratory distress syndrome. Crit Care Med 1999;27:2028–30.

278. Fowler A, Hamman R, Good J, et al. Adult respiratory distress syndrome: risk with common predispositions. Ann Intern Med 1983;98:593–7.

279. Millberg J, Davis D, Steinberg K, Hudson L. Improved survival of patients with acute respiratory distress syndrome (ARDS). JAMA 1995;273:306–9.

280. Montgomery A, Stager M, Coalson J, Hudson L. Causes of mortality in patients with the adult respiratory distress syndrome. Am Rev Respir Dis 1985;132:485–9.

281. Suchya M, Clemmer T, Elliott C, et al. The adult respiratory distress syndrome: a report on survival and modifying factors. Chest 1992;101:1074–9.

282. Humphrey H, Hall J, Sznajder I, et al. Improved survival in ARDS patients associated with a reduction in pulmonary capillary wedge pressure. Chest 1990;97:1176–80.

283. Schuller D, Mitchell J, Calandrino F, Schuster D. Fluid balance during pulmonary edema. Is fluid gain a marker or a cause of poor outcome? Chest 1991;100:1068–75.

284. Dellinger R, Zimmerman J, Taylor R, et al. Effects of inhaled nitric oxide in patients with acute respiratory distress syndrome: results of a randomized phase II trial. Inhaled Nitric Oxide in ARDS Study Group. Crit Care Med 1998;26:15–23.

285. Troncy E, Collet J, Shapiro S, et al. Inhaled nitric oxide versus conventional therapy: effect on oxygenation in ARDS. Am J Respir Crit Care Med 1998;157:1372–80.

286. Meduri G, Headley A, Golden E, et al. Effect of prolonged methylprednisolone therapy in unresolving acute respiratory distress syndrome: a randomized controlled trial. JAMA 1998;280:159–65.

287. Long W, Thompson T, Sundell H, et al. Effects of two rescue doses of a synthetic surfactant on mortality rate and survival without bronchopulmonary dysplasia in 700- to 1350-gram infants with respiratory distress syndrome. J Pediatr 1991;118:595–605.

288. Ambrosino N. Noninvasive mechanical ventilation in patients with acute respiratory failure. Crit Care Med 1996;24:705–15.

289. Anonymous. Ventilation with lower tidal volumes as compared with traditional tidal volumes for acute lung injury and the acute respiratory distress syndrome. The Acute Respiratory Distress Syndrome Network. N Engl J Med 2000;134:1301–8.

290. Amato M, Barbas C, Medeiros D, et al. Effect of a protective-ventilation strategy on mortality in the acute respiratory distress syndrome. N Engl J Med 1998;338:347–54.

291. Stoller J, Kacmarek R. Ventilatory strategies in the management of the respiratory distress syndrome. Clin Chest Med 1990;11:755–72.

inflammation in asthma. J Paediatr Child Health 1999;35:269–71.

Chapter 11

Emergent Pulmonary Infections

Vickie R. Shannon, MD
Amelia Ng, BS, MD

PNEUMONIA IN THE CANCER PATIENT

The recognition, diagnosis, and successful treatment of cancer patients with pneumonia remain pervasive and complex clinical challenges. Despite major advances in the diagnosis and treatment of pneumonia in general, mortality rates for cancer-related pulmonary infection remain high. Pneumonia in the cancer patient may develop as a consequence of the cancer itself or as a result of its treatment. Absolute neutropenia is defined as an absolute neutrophil count (ANC) of < 500/mm^3 or an ANC of 1,000 that falls to < 500/mm^3 within 48 hours. Both absolute and functional neutropenia are well-established risk factors for the development of pneumonia. The risk of developing pneumonia is further heightened by the impact of radiation and cytotoxic drugs on normal tissues, local lung defense mechanisms, and the immune system. This chapter focuses on some of the diagnostic dilemmas and advancements in the treatment of lung infections in the cancer patient.

Pneumonia in the cancer patient may have an explosive onset with an inexorable and rapid downhill course. Unless promptly recognized and aggressively treated, this complication may be fatal. The difficulties in diagnosing pneumonia in the general population are magnified in the cancer patient. The conventional clinical symptoms of cough, fever, and sputum production may be absent. Furthermore, chest radiography may be normal despite overwhelming pneumonia in severely neutropenic patients and abnormal despite the absence of any detectable infection during the period of marrow recovery. In the latter scenario, the radiographic appearance of pulmonary infiltrates after a period of severe neutropenia may represent an inflammatory response to cytokine release during marrow recovery. Radiation therapy and a growing number of chemotherapeutic agents may induce clinical and radiographic signs and symptoms

that closely mimic opportunistic pulmonary infections. Comorbid illnesses such as adult respiratory distress syndrome (ARDS), pulmonary edema, alveolar hemorrhage, atelectasis, leukoagglutinin transfusion reaction, or pulmonary infarction, all of which occur at increased rates in the cancer patient, further amplify the difficulty in making the diagnosis and confound therapy. The approach to the cancer patient with suspected pneumonia, therefore, requires knowledge of the atypical presentation of pneumonia in these patients and an understanding of the common cancer comorbidities that may mimic and/or obscure the diagnosis.

Incidence of Pneumonia in Patients with Cancer

Pneumonia is the overall leading infectious cause of death in cancer patients.[1–3] The reported incidence of pneumonia in patients with cancer varies widely with the diagnostic criteria, study population, and nature of the underlying neoplasm. In the bone marrow transplantation population, estimates of pulmonary infection range from 40 to 60% although rates may be lower in recipients of stem cell transplants with growth factor administration.[4–7] Nearly 66% of leukemic patients will develop pneumonia during the course of their illness. Postobstructive pneumonia in patients with centrally obstructing bronchogenic carcinoma or metastatic disease decisively contributes to the overall morbidity and mortality in this group of patients. Aspiration pneumonia, putatively due to the effects of sedatives and narcotics, mucositis, or the mechanical effects of tumor in the proximal airway, are also common and may be life threatening. Pneumonia is the attributable cause of all deaths in nearly 60% of patients with leukemia, 40% of patients who have undergone hematopoietic stem cell transplantation (HSCT), and 40% of patients with solid tumors.[8]

Host Defenses and Pneumonia

Local Defenses. The incidence of pneumonia and other types of infection has steadily ballooned as increasingly aggressive radiation and chemotherapeutic protocols for the treatment of cancer have been implemented. These protocols result in the further suppression of an already impaired host defense system. Local defenses as well as all three components of the immune system (granulocytes and humoral and cellular immunity) may be profoundly affected by cancer and its treatment. The skin and mucous membranes represent the first line of defense against bacterial and fungal organisms. These mechanical barriers are often breached in patients with cancer. Mucositis, resulting from chemotherapy or from the disruption of anatomic barriers by local invasion of tumor into the airway, may predispose the cancer patient to the development of pneumonia. Iatrogenic alterations in mechanical barriers (eg, by hyperalimentation or by the placement of central venous lines, endotracheal tubes, or Foley catheters) also facilitate the development of local bacterial infections and bacteremia.

Granulocyte Deficiency. The critical phagocytic function of neutrophils is frequently compromised in cancer patients. Polymorphonuclear neutrophils are the primary cellular defense against infections caused by bacterial and fungal organisms.[3] The development of serious infection is not only conditioned by the degree of neutropenia but also by its duration and phagocytic function. Neutrophils are avidly phagocytic. Neutrophil numbers and activity may be profoundly affected by cancer, chemotherapy, radiation treatment, or infectious infiltration of the bone marrow. As a result, severe infections that are often refractory to standard antibiotic therapy may occur. Profound neutropenia in patients with acute myeloid leukemia is extremely common. The incidence of lung infection in these patients may exceed 80%.[8] Resident neutrophils exist in both intravascular and extravascular sites, including subepithelial areas of the skin and the submucosa of the gastrointestinal (GI) tract. Loss of the mechanical barriers of the skin and gut mucosa is frequent in patients who receive certain types of chemotherapy. These patients are particularly susceptible to the development of blood stream and pulmonary infections caused by Gram-negative and fungal pathogens. Specific pathogens that cause pneumonia and that are commonly encountered in neutropenic patients are listed in Table 11–1. Bacterial infections in neutropenic patients typically originate from skin and gut flora. This observation is consistent with the loss of subepithelial and submucosal polymorphonuclear leukocytes from these sites. Among the species of Enterobacteriaceae that cause pneumonia (*Klebsiella*, *Escherichia coli*, *Pseudomonas aeruginosa*, *Proteus*, *Serratia*, *Enterobac-*

ter), *Pseudomonas aeruginosa* is the most life-threatening pathogen. Thus, empiric antibiotic therapy in the febrile neutropenic patient should include coverage for *Pseudomonas*. Although Gram-negative pneumonias remain common in neutropenic patients, the incidence of Gram-positive pathogens has been increasingly recognized. Lung infections due to *Staphylococcus aureus*, *Streptococcus viridans*, and *Streptococcus pneumoniae* have increased by nearly 40% in neutropenic patients over the past few years.[9] This change is a reflection of the increased use of intravascular catheters and the expanded use of antimicrobial prophylaxis directed at aerobic Gram-negative organisms. Neutropenia that persists for more than 7 days is associated with increased rates of severe fungal pneumonias that are often fatal. Specific fungal infections may be secondary to opportunistic nosocomial pathogens (*Aspergillus*, *Candida*, Mucoraceae, and *Cryptococcus*) and/or the re-activation of indolent endemic organisms (*Histoplasma capsulatum*, *Coccidioides immitis*, *Paracoccidioides brasiliensis*, *Blastomyces dermatidides*).

Deficiencies of Humoral Immunity. Cancer patients, particularly those with lymphoreticular malignancies and those who have had cytoreductive chemotherapy and HSCT, commonly develop deficiencies in B-cell function. As a result, a profound impairment of humoral immunity occurs, leading to impaired neutralization of toxins, disorders of immunoglobulin production, and hypocomplementemia. In addition, patients with lymphoreticular malignancies are often either functionally or anatomically asplenic. Both conditions are associated with defects in opsonization by the alternative complement pathway, which is housed in the spleen. The major pathogens causing pneumonia in patients with defective humoral immunity are listed in Table 11–1. Bacterial infections that cause pneumonia in patients with impaired humoral immunity are characteristically those caused by encapsulated organisms. Among these, *Streptococcus pneumoniae* is the most life-threatening. *Neisseria meningitidis*, *Pseudomonas aeruginosa*, *Haemophilus influenzae*, and encapsulated strains of Gram-negative bacilli are also important pulmonary pathogens in this group of patients. In addition, viral pneumonias caused by influenza viruses and enteroviruses are noted with increased frequency.

Defects in Cell-Mediated Immunity. The integrity of the cell-mediated immune system is dependent on intact macrophage and T-lymphocyte interactions. These cells function in concert to facilitate macrophage killing of organisms by phagocytosis. Consequently, disorders that affect either T-lymphocyte and macrophage function or total cell counts profoundly affect this host defense mechanism. Prolonged administration of corticosteroids or other immunosuppressive therapies, lymphoreticular malignancies of T-cell origin, and viral illnesses may depress the cellular arm of the immune system. Infections by unusual pathogens are common among this group of patients. Most notably, patients with defects in cell-mediated immunity are susceptible to bacterial infections by intracellular bacteria, including *Mycobacterium* species, *Legionella*, and *Listeria monocytogenes*. Other unusual pathogens that can cause infection among patients is the defective cell-mediated immunity of increased rates include *Nocardia*, *Salmonella*, *Brucella*, and *Rhodococcus*. Opportunistic and endemic filamentous fungi, viruses, parasites, and protozoa make up the remaining list of offending organisms. Viral pneumonias, including those caused by *Cytomegalovirus*, herpesviruses, respiratory syncytial virus (RSV), influenza virus and adenovirus, may be particularly virulent in the setting of depressed cell-mediated immunity. The serious nature of lung infections caused by these pathogens is underscored by mortality rates of 50 to 90%.[10–12] Viral infections causing pneumonia in patients with defects in humoral immunity may occur as a result of the re-activation of latent infection or as primary disease.

Common Pulmonary Pathogens in Cancer Patients

The diverse group of opportunistic pathogens causing pulmonary infection in the immunocompromised patient is extensive. Common infections in this group of patients often reflect the individual ecology of the hospital. Overall rates of fatal pneumonias in immunocompromised patients are significantly higher than in the general population. This section focuses only on those common pathogens that frequently cause life-threatening pulmonary infections.

Common Bacterial Pneumonias. Bacterial pneumonia remains the most common source of infection during the early stages of immune compromise. The early empiric use of broad-spectrum antibiotics during episodes of neutropenic fever renders precise estimates of the incidence of bacterial pneumonia in this setting difficult.

TABLE 11–1. Important Pathogens Causing Infection in the Immunocompromised Patient

Defect	Condition	Bacteria	Fungi	Viruses	Protozoa/Parasites
Local defenses	Mucositis Indwelling catheter Intubation Venipuncture	*Streptoccoccus* *Staphylococcus* Enterobacteriaceae *Pseudomonas* *Corynebacterium*	*Aspergillus* *Candida* Mucoraceae Fusaria	Herpes simplex virus Varicella-zoster virus	
Neutropenia	Mucositis Acute leukemia Chemotherapy	*Staphylococcus aureus* Coagulase-negative staphylococci Enterococci *Streptococcus viridans* *Corynebacterium jeikeium* Enterobacteria *Pseudomonas aeruginosa* *Bacteroides fragilis* *Treponema pallidum* *Rickettsia* *Chlamydia*	*Candida* *Aspergillus* Mucoraceae Fusaria *Pseudallescheria boydii*		
Humoral	CLL Corticosteroids Chemotherapy Multiple myeloma	*Streptococcus pneumoniae* *Haemophilus influenzae* Encapsulated strains of GNRs *Neisseria* species *Salmonella* *Escherichia coli* *Pseudomonas* *Plasmodium* species	*Pneumocystis carinii*	Influenza virus Arbovirus Echovirus	
CMI	Hodgkin's disease Non Hodgkin's disease Hairy cell leukemia Corticosteroids Chemotherapy	*Mycobacteria* *Listeria* *Nocardia* *Rhodococcus* *Legionella* *Brucella* *Bartonella* *Salmonella*	*Cryptococcus* *Histoplasma* *Coccidioides* *Blastomyces* *Candida* *Aspergillus* *Pneumocystis*	Herpes simplex virus Varicella-zoster virus *Cytomegalovirus* Epstein-Barr virus *Polyomavirus* Adenovirus Measles virus	*Toxoplasma* *Amoeba* *Strongyloides* *Giardia* *Cryptosporidium* *Isospora* *Microsporidium*

CCL = chronic lymphocytic leukemia; CMI = cell-mediated immunity; GNRs = Gram-negative rods.

Nonetheless, pneumonia due to bacterial organisms accounts for 12 to 50% of lung infections during the first 100 days post transplantation in published reports.[4,7,13,14] Rates of bacterial infection are higher in allogeneic transplant recipients than in autologous transplant recipients.

Gram-negative pneumonias caused by *Pseudomonas* and organisms of the family Enterobacteriaceae are the most common and the most virulent. *Streptococcus pneumoniae*, *Staphylococcus*, and a growing number of other Gram-positive organisms have emerged as significant pathogens in the immunocompromised patient. This shift in the microbial spectrum of immunocompromised patients is primarily due to the widespread use of indwelling central venous catheters and the use of antibiotic prophylaxis against Gram-negative organisms. Both *Staphylococcus* and *Streptococcus pneumoniae* may also re-emerge as the dominant causes of late infection in HSCT patients with chronic graft-versus-host disease (GVHD). Mixed bacterial infections have also been increasingly isolated in the compromised host. Aspiration of Gram-positive and anaerobic organisms is of particular concern in neutropenic patients who require narcotic analgesics or in those with oral mucositis. Increased rates of antibiotic resistance to *Staphylococcus* and *Streptococcus pneumoniae* have been reported in recent literature. Pneumonia caused by *Streptococcus viridans* has also become more prevalent in recent years. This organism is responsible for viridans streptococcal toxic shock syndrome, characterized by the development of palmar desquamation, hypotension, rash, and an aggressive pneumonia leading to ARDS and death. This syndrome has been described in leukemia patients with severe oropharyngeal mucositis following the administration of high-dose arabinoside C.[15] Neutropenic patients who receive prophylactic antibiotic coverage with trimethoprim/sulfamethoxazole (TMP/SMX) or fluoroquinolones are at higher risk for the development of streptococcal toxic shock syndrome because of the less predictable coverage of these antibiotics against Gram-positive organisms. Mortality rates for pneumonia caused by *S. viridans* are higher than those for pneumonia caused by any of the other Gram-positive organisms.

Bacterial pneumonia in neutropenic patients may have an atypical presentation and a fulminant course. Fever and cough may be absent, and sputum production may be negligible. The classic pattern of lobar consolidation that is typical of many bacterial pneumonias is less common in this setting. Instead, chest radiography more often reveals diffuse interstitial infiltrates or patchy areas of dense alveolar consolidations in the setting of neutropenia (Figure 11–1). Nodular lesions suggestive of *Staphylococcus*, *Nocardia*, *Pseudomonas*, or fungal infections may occur. Normal chest radiographs in severely neutropenic patients with fulminant disease have also been described.

Nocardia Pneumonia. *Nocardia asteroides* is a filamentous slow-growing Gram-positive bacillus found in soil. This opportunistic organism is weakly acid-fast. Patients with lymphoreticular malignancies or other causes of defective cell-mediated immunity are susceptible to infection by these organisms. Neutropenia is not a common precursor, but a history of prolonged steroid administration is commonly reported. Fever and a nonproductive cough are typical presenting symptoms. The classic radiographic pattern of nocardial pneumonia is a slowly progressive nodular infiltrate that may cavitate. Diffuse disease is associated with spread of infection to the central nervous system (CNS) and carries a poor prognosis. Pleural effusions occur in nearly 50% of patients. Nocardial empyema and abscess formation have also been described. The diagnosis is suggested by the triad of pustular skin lesions, neurologic disease (encephalitis, brain abscess), and nodular lesions on chest radiography. In clinical and radiographic evaluation, *Nocardia* may mimic *Mycobacterium tuberculosis*; however, fibrocavitary disease is less prominent in *Nocardia* pneumonia. The organism may be isolated in cultures of sputum although colonies may not be apparent for 6 to 8 weeks. Lung aspiration and biopsy are often diagnostic when sputum cultures are negative. Local infection from transcutaneous inoculation after transtracheal aspiration has been described; therefore, transtracheal aspiration in suspected cases of nocardiosis should be avoided.

Sulfonamides remain the first-line therapy. Antibiotic therapies with amikacin, imipenem, cefuroxime, cefotaxime, or minocycline are viable alternatives for persons intolerant of sulfa drugs. Prolonged antibiotic

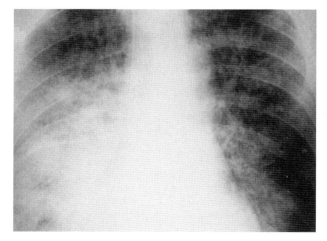

Figure 11–1. 65-year-old woman with renal cell carcinoma presented with fever and bilateral pulmonary infiltrates. Sputum culture grew *Pseudomonas aeruginosa*.

therapy (8 to 12 months) is required in all patients to prevent disease relapse. Immunosuppressed patients with nocardiosis require at least a year of therapy. The treatment course may be extended beyond a year in settings of severe immunosuppression and CNS disease. Surgical drainage is indicated for empyemas. Antibiotic therapy alone may be sufficient for the treatment of abscesses. Early diagnosis and treatment carries a 95% cure rate.

Legionella pneumophila **Pneumonia.** These fastidious Gram-negative bacilli are found in contaminated potable water. *Legionella* is a particularly virulent pathogen. The virulence of this pathogen is underscored by its high rate of hastening respiratory failure. *Legionella pneumophila* pneumonia represents the second most common cause of community-acquired pneumonia in patients admitted to intensive-care units. The primary sources of infection in humans include water distribution systems and water-containing respiratory devices. Contaminated cooling towers have also been implicated as a source of *Legionella* although this has been hotly debated in the literature. Lower water temperatures (< 60°C or < 140°F), sediment accumulation, and the presence of commensal organisms facilitate the colonization of water distribution systems by *Legionella*. Aspiration is the major mode of transmission from water to humans. Patients with defects in specific cellular and humoral immunity have an increased predilection for legionnaires' disease. The role of neutropenia in the development of this disease is not clearly understood. Major risk factors for the development of *Legionella* infection include cigarette smoking, chronic pulmonary disease, organ transplantation, and immunosuppressive therapy. Cancer patients, especially those on long-term steroid therapy, patients with hairy cell leukemia, and those with head and neck cancer are particularly susceptible to infections caused by this organism. Patients with head and neck cancer have higher rates of cigarette smoking and an almost universal propensity for aspiration.

Of the forty different species of *Legionella* that have been identified, *L. pneumophila* is the species implicated in the overwhelming majority of infections. Named after the outbreak of severe pneumonia at an American Legion convention in 1976, *Legionella pneumophila,* literally translated, means "lung loving." Two diverse forms of *Legionella* infection exist. Pontiac fever, characterized by fatigue, malaise, myalgias, and fever, is usually a self-limited disease. Pneumonia is not a prominent feature of this disease although a dry cough may occur. In legionnaires' disease, however, pneumonia predominates. Immuno-compromised patients with this syndrome may present with various manifestations of multisystem disease. After a 2- to 10-day incubation period, patients typically pre-

sent with nonspecific symptoms of fever, malaise, lethargy, and weakness. A dissociation between high fever and pulse has been reported in the literature but is probably overstated. Cough is dry early on but gradually becomes productive of mucopurulent and blood-streaked sputum. Extrapulmonary symptoms, including nausea, vomiting, diarrhea, abdominal pain, headache, change in mental status, and pleuritic chest pain, are frequent complaints. Extrathoracic complications, including pericarditis, endocarditis, sinusitis, pancreatitis, and cellulitis, are believed to be secondary to bacteremic spread of the organism. Hyponatremia (serum sodium < 130 mEq/L) occurs more freqently in legionnaires' disease than in other types of pneumonia and is a bad prognostic sign. Other reported findings (rash, rhabdomyolysis, disseminated intravascular coagulation, and neuropathy) are nonspecific features of pneumonia that may be found in severe disease. Virtually all patients have abnormalities on chest radiographs at the time of presentation. Progression of infiltrates (as seen by chest radiography) despite antibiotic therapy is suggestive of legionnaires' disease in the appropriate clinical setting.

A variety of radiographic presentations exist. These include unilateral segmental or lobar alveolar opacities that may progress to mutilobar bilateral disease. Pleural effusions, empyemas, and pleural-based densities resembling pulmonary infarction are also common presentations. Pleural effusions may precede the development of parenchymal infiltrates. Circumscribed nodular densities are common in the immunosuppressed patient; these nodular densities may progress rapidly. Abscess formation and cavitation are not uncommon. Cavitation may occur despite appropriate antibiotic therapy. The identification of *Legionella* by Gram's stain in sputum or otherwise sterile sites such as pleural fluid or lung tissue suggests the diagnosis. Examination of bronchoalveolar lavage (BAL) fluid may yield the organism when sputum is not available. Culture of *Legionella* from specialized culture media is definitive. However, the 3 to 5 days that are required for growth in culture may cause an unacceptable delay in the diagnosis and treatment of these critically ill patients. Several specialized tests have been developed that are capable of providing accurate and rapid identification of *Legionella*. These include direct fluorescent antibody (DFA) staining of clinical specimens, indirect staining using enzyme-linked immunosorbent assay (ELISA) of serologic specimens, radioimmunoassay (RIA) of urine samples for soluble *Legionella pneumophila* antigen, and radiolabeled deoxyribonucleic acid (DNA) probes. Of these, DFA and RIA detection of urinary antigen are most widely used. The sensitivities and specificities of urinary antigen testing for *L. pneumophila* rival those of culture. This diagnostic tool has recently emerged as a very useful study with very high sensitivity and specificity for *L. pneumophilia* serogroup 1, the pathogenic subtype that is responsible for more than 80% of *Legionella* infections.

The newer macrolides (clarithromycin and azithromycin) and the quinolones (gemifloxacin, ofloxacin, levofloxacin, gatifloxacin, moxifloxacin, and ciprofloxacin) are highly active against *Legionella*. These antibiotics have superior *in vitro* activity and pharmacokinetics when compared with erythromycin and are currently the drugs of choice for the treatment of this disease. Other drugs with suggested efficacy against *Legionella* include tetracycline, TMP/SMX, clindamycin, and imipenem. Monotherapy using one of the newer macrolides or quinolones is approved for the treatment of legionnaires' disease. The addition of rifampin to erythromycin has been demonstrated to improve erythromycin's efficacy. Intravenous therapy is initially preferred because of the potential for incomplete GI absorption. Immunosuppressed patients should be treated with 21 days of antimicrobial therapy. In immunocompetent patients, early and appropriate antibiotic therapy is usually associated with full recovery. Mortality rates may approach 50% in immunosuppressed patients, however, especially in the setting of treatment delay.

Mycobacterial Pneumonia. Rates of infections by tuberculous (TB) and nontuberculous (NTB) mycobacteria are increased in the cancer patient. Both TB and NTB typically present as lung disease although disseminated disease does occur. Cancer patients who are at highest risk for mycobacterial infection include those with chronic T-cell suppression secondary to corticosteroids or other treatment modalities. Disseminated TB with spread to the brain, pleura, pericardium, peritoneum, kidneys, bones, or skin may be rapidly fatal. Prolonged fever, unexplained weight loss, and demonstration of upper-lobe-predominant disease by chest radiography suggest the diagnosis. Although many studies have questioned the usefulness of purified protein derivative (PPD) evaluation in patients with cancer because of associated anergy, at least one study supports this practice, citing positive PPDs in up to 65% of cancer patients, despite immunosuppression.[16] Bronchoscopy or open lung biopsy is commonly required for diagnosis. Polymerase chain reaction (PCR) may expedite the diagnosis and facilitate early therapeutic strategies. Delayed diagnosis may result in fatal outcomes and permit the spread of tuberculous infection within the hospital. Triple or quadruple antibiotic therapy may be indicated, depending on the characteristic sensitivities of the region in which the patient lives.

Among NTB pneumonias, those caused by *Mycobacterium avium-intracellulare* (MAI) complex, *Mycobacterium chelonai*, and *Mycobacterium kansasii* are the most

common. The clinical manifestations of NTB infection may mimic those of TB infection. Risk factors for the development of MAI pneumonia include Hodgkin's and non-Hodgkin's lymphomas, hairy cell leukemia, and long-term steroid therapy. Abnormalities on chest radiographs may mimic TB pneumonia and may range from minimal changes to diffuse pulmonary involvement with cavitation (Figure 11–2). Bronchoscopy or open lung biopsy is required for diagnosis. Sputum cultures are often negative. Pneumonias caused by MAI are typically treated with multidrug therapy that includes a macrolide (clarithromycin or azithromycin), a fluroquinolone (ciprofloxacin or ofloxacin), a rifamycin (rifampin or rifabutin), and clofazamine or ethambutol. The approach to *Mycobacterium kansasii* is similar to the approach to *Mycobacterium tuberculosis*. Prolonged treatment is usually indicated for both.

Fungal Pneumonias. A resurgence of pathogenic fungal organisms causing recalcitrant infections has been seen over the past decade. Both the incidence of fungal infections and resistant fungal organisms are on the rise, partly due to the widespread use of aggressive antibiotic therapy for established infections and prophylaxis. Treatment protocols that prolong the duration of neutropenia have also contributed to the increased incidence of fungal infections among cancer patients. In addition, patient age, history of prior lung infection, presence of GVHD, and corticosteroid administration following marrow engraftment contribute to the appearance of fungal infections. Pneumonia is the most common and the most

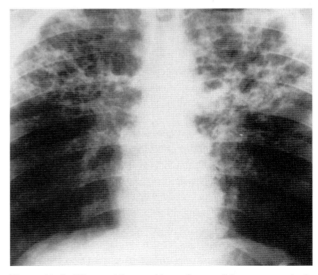

Figure 11–2. 54-year-old man with carcinoma of the tongue and a 2-month history of low-grade fever, night sweats, weight loss, and dry cough. Chest radiography revealed bilateral apical thin-walled cavitary lesions. Culture from bronchoalveolar lavage (BAL) grew *Mycobacterium avium-intracellulare.*

virulent type of infection caused by fungus in the immunocompromised patient. Prolonged neutropenia plays a critical pathogenic role in the development of opportunistic fungal pneumonias caused by *Aspergillus, Candida,* fungi of the family Mucoraceae (*Mucor, Rhizopus,* and *Absidia),* *Fusaria* and *Cryptococcus.* In patients who are compromised predominantly by cellular immunity, re-activations of infections with *Histoplasma capsulatum, Coccidioides immitis, Paracoccidioides brasiliensis,* and *Blastomyces dermatitidis* may be seen. Both *Candida* and *Aspergillus* may colonize the proximal airway. The presence of filamentous fungi in sputum or BAL fluid from febrile neutropenic patients with lung infiltrates is highly suggestive of the diagnosis of fungal pneumonia and represents sufficient evidence to initiate treatment in most patients. The diagnosis of *Candida* pneumonia based on the recovery of yeast from upper-respiratory secretions is difficult because of the frequent colonization of the oropharynx and proximal airway by this organism. Amphotericin B and its liposomal derivatives target *Aspergillus* as well as candidal pneumonias and are the current drugs of choice for the empiric treatment of neutropenic fever that persists beyond 7 days despite antibiotic therapy.[17]

Aspergillus Pneumonia. Aspergillus pneumonia is the most common fungal pneumonia in patients with neutropenia and in those who have undergone stem cell transplantation. Susceptibility to *Aspergillus* infection correlates with the degree of immunosuppression. Thus, recipients of allogeneic stem cell transplants are at highest risk for the development of invasive aspergillosis. Other risk factors include the administration of high-dose steroids, prolonged neutropenia, the development of GVHD, and T-cell depletion of harvested marrow. Neutropenia lasting more than 7 days is associated with an increased risk. Increased susceptibility to invasive aspergillosis occurs in recipients of T-cell-depleted marrow, presumably on the basis of an associated delay in engraftment.

Pathologic changes include a necrotizing bronchopneumonia, tracheobronchitis, and sinopulmonary disease. Pulmonary infarction as a result of vascular invasion may occur. Bronchoscopic examination may reveal pseudomembranes lining the bronchial mucosa and necrotic endobronchial disease (Figure 11–3, A–B). Although the isolation of *Aspergillus* from sputum or BAL fluid is usually treated as a contaminant in the normal host, the detection of this organism in oral or airway

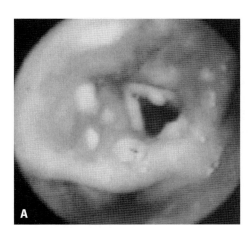

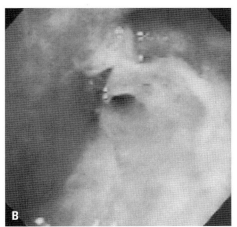

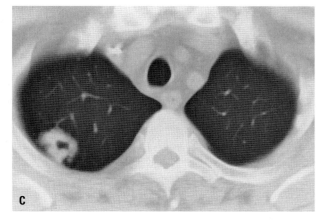

Figure 11–3. 29-year-old male with prolonged neutropenia and hemoptysis 3 weeks after receiving an allogeneic stem cell transplant for acute myelogenous leukemia. A, B: Bronchoscopic images showing mucosal erythema, ulcerations (A), and pseudomembranes (B) in the supraglottic, tracheal, and bronchial airways. C: Chest computed tomography (CT) reveals a cavitary lesion in the right apex. Silver stain from BAL showed *Aspergillus* hyphae with branching at 45°.

secretions in patients who have undergone HSCT should signal invasive disease.

Bronchoscopy with BAL is an effective diagnostic procedure in HSCT patients with diffuse disease, with sensitivities approaching 100%.[18] Transbronchial biopsies typically are not feasible because of prohibitive thrombocytopenia. Primary infection may occasionally begin in sinuses, skin, frontal cortex, or periorbital areas and spread to the lungs. Skin lesions are characterized by concentrically enlarging nodules with central necrosis. Biopsy of the skin lesions may yield the diagnosis. Almost all patients present with nonspecific symptoms of fever, dry cough, and dyspnea. Focal wheezing, hemoptysis, pleuritic chest pain, and a pleural friction rub are highly suggestive although this constellation of symptoms is seen in only 30% of patients.[1,19] Death from a rapidly progressive hemorrhagic pneumonia with infarction and fungemia may ensue. Chest radiographs of patients with severe neutropenia may be normal; more often, however, focal or diffuse infiltrates and nodules with or without cavitation are described (see Figure 11–3, C). Wedge-shaped pleural-based infiltrates may occur occasionally, suggesting pulmonary infarction. The radiographic finding of an air-crescent sign is also highly suggestive of *Aspergillus* pneumonia (Figure 11–4). Aggressive therapy at the first sign of invasive aspergillosis is recommended. Amphotericin B and its liposomal derivatives remain the cornerstone of therapy. The efficacy of azole compounds (such as itraconazole) in the treatment of invasive aspergillosis is currently being studied. Recently, a cell

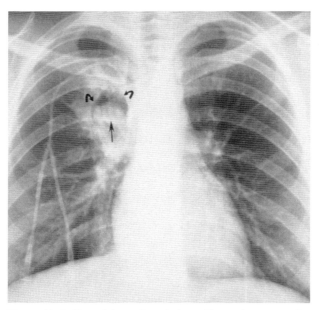

Figure 11–4. Upper-lobe cavitary lesion with an air-crescent sign consistent with *Aspergillus* pneumonia. *Curved arrows* = air crescent sign; ↑ = fungus ball.

wall active agent, caspofungin acetate (Cancidas), was approved for the treatment of severe *Aspergillus* infections and holds promise in the treatment of other types of fungal diseases as well. Despite aggressive therapy, mortality rates among patients with invasive aspergillosis following HSCT remain high. The most effective intervention is prevention. *Aspergillus* infections are primarily nosocomially acquired. Nosocomial dissemination via airborne contamination in buildings undergoing renovation or construction and in contaminated air conditioning units is common. Laminar airflow and high efficiency particulate air (HEPA) filtration of patients' rooms have been shown to be highly protective, lowering the incidence of invasive *Aspergillus* infections in the HSCT population.

Candida *Pneumonia.* Together, *Candida* and *Aspergillus* species are the predominant fungal pathogens in patients with malignant disease and account for more than 90% of fungal infections in cancer patients. Candidal pneumonias occur via one of two major routes: (1) aspiration of upper-airway contents or (2) hematogenous dissemination. Hematogenous dissemination from concomitant sources such as the GI or genitourinary tract is the more typical route. Pure pneumonias caused by *Candida* are so rare and the clinical and radiographic pictures are so varied that no typical presentation can be offered. Establishing the diagnosis is rendered more problematic by the fact that isolates from sputum or even BAL that reflect true disease are difficult to distinguish from upper-airway contamination. Unlike aspergillosis, primary infection involving the skin or sinuses is unusual. The diagnosis is suggested by local invasion of GI or genitourinary mucosal surfaces in a patient with pulmonary infiltrates that are unresponsive to antibiotic therapy. Histopathologic studies demonstrating tissue invasion may be necessary for definitive diagnosis. Evidence of spread to the skin or retina also helps with the diagnosis. *Candida albicans* is the most common pathogenic candidal species causing lung infection although resistant *Candida glabrata*, *Candida tropicalis*, and *Candida krusei* have been noted recently with increasing frequency. Amphotericin B, lipid-complexed amphotericin B, and triazole compounds have been tried in the treatment of *Candida* pneumonia with fungemia, with varying success.

Pneumocytis carinii *Pneumonia.* The incidence of *Pneumocystis carinii* pneumonia (PCP) among cancer and HSCT patients has dropped dramatically with the routine use of aggressive prophylactic therapy. The current rate of PCP among patients post HSCT is less than 10%.[17,19] The pneumonia characteristically occurs approximately 2 months after bone marrow transplantation in those patients who are either noncompliant with prophylactic therapy or allergic to sulfa drugs. Patients typically present with fever, nonproductive cough, dyspnea and cyanosis. The clinical picture may progress rapidly to respiratory failure and death, especially in the post-transplantation patient. Laboratory evidence of elevated lactate dehydrogenase, erythrocyte sedimentation rate, angiotensin-converting enzyme levels, and fibrinogen levels are nonspecific but helpful findings. The classic radiographic appearance includes perihilar infiltrates, which may progress to diffuse alveolar consolidation. Air bronchograms may be seen in more than half of the patients. Predominantly upper-lobe infiltrates mimicking tuberculosis are common in patients who are receiving aerosolized pentamidine prophylaxis. Nodular densities, cavitation, lobar distribution, abscess formation, unilateral predominance, and even normal chest radiographs have been described.[19,20] Diffuse ground-glass attenuations on CT is characteristic (Figure 11–5).

The diagnosis of PCP is clinched with the identification of intracytoplasmic cysts and trophozoites attached to cells on silver staining, DFA staining, or histopathologic analysis of respiratory secretions or biopsy specimen tissue. The mainstay of therapy is high-dose TMP/SMX (dosed at 20 mg/kg/d of the trimethoprim [TMP] component). Alternatively, intravenous pentamidine is offered to patients with prior history of allergy to sulfa-containing medications. Adjuvant corticosteroid therapy has proven efficacy in reducing inflammation and in improving hypoxemia, azotemia, hypoglycemia,

abnormalities of liver function, and rash. Severe bronchospasm has been reported with aerosolized pentamidine therapy. Other treatment options for mild to moderate disease include atovaquone, trimetrexate, or combined therapy with dapsone/TMP or clindamycin/primaquine. Early institution of therapy is critical. Untreated disease and delayed therapy in immunocompromised patients are almost uniformly fatal.

Other Invasive Mycoses. Pneumonias caused by other invasive fungi (including *Fusaria, Pseudallescheria boydii, Penicillium, Cladosporium,* and *Trichosporon* organisms) have been reported, especially in patients with leukemia, lymphoma, and severe neutropenia and in those taking corticosteroids. *Fusarium* is a filamentous fungus with a predilection for vascular infarction and disseminated invasion similar to that of *Aspergillus.* Concomitant involvement of the sinuses and skin is common. Radiographic changes are nonspecific. The identification of filamentous fungi in blood cultures or the observation of subcutaneous nodules on physical examination suggests the diagnosis. Mortality rates are high despite aggressive antifungal therapy. The organisms that cause mucormycosis belong to the class Zygomycetes and are broadbased fungi found in soil. These ubiquitous fungi are responsible for several clinically important infections. Three distinct clinical syndromes of mucormycosis exist:

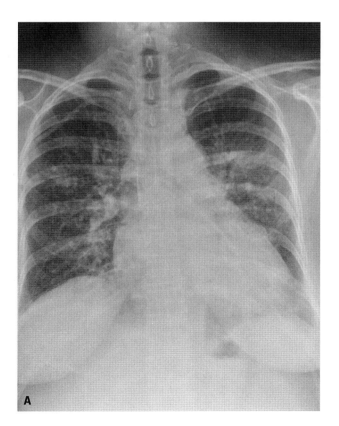

A

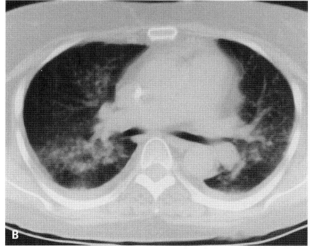

B

Figure 11–5. 40-year-old woman with chronic myelogenous leukemia with progressive cough and dyspnea 6 months after bone marrow transplantation from a human leukocyte antigen (HLA)–matched unrelated donor. A: Chest radiography reveals diffuse bilateral patchy air-space opacities consistent with multifocal pneumonia. B: Computed tomography (CT) reveals ground-glass opacities with patchy areas of consolidation and small bilateral pleural effusions. Clusters of trophozoites and cysts on methenamine silver stain confirmed the diagnosis of *Pneumocystis carinii* pneumonia.

(1) rhinocerebral mucormycosis, which primarily involves the sinuses, the vestibule, or both and which tends to occur particularly in poorly controlled diabetic patients; (2) pulmonary mucormycosis, a devastating infection with a predilection for cancer patients, particularly post-transplantation patients and those with leukemia or lymphoma; and (3) gastrointestinal mucormycosis, which is a rare complication of diabetes, solid-organ transplantation, and corticosteroid treatment and presents as hemorrhagic ulceration and infarction. Pulmonary mucormycosis is the only clinical syndrome that primarily involves the lungs. Transmission of infection presumably occurs by the inhalation of spores by a susceptible host. Prior deferoxamine therapy increases the risk and severity of invasive mucormycosis.[21] Pulmonary mucormycosis may be rapidly fatal. Patients commonly present with a diffuse pneumonia with infarction and necrosis. The clinical presentation may be indistinguishable from that of invasive aspergillosis. Fever and hemoptysis are usual presenting symptoms. Fatal hemoptysis has been described. Local spread of infection to contiguous structures (such as the heart and mediastinum) and hematogenous spread to the brain have been reported. Surgical resection of early pulmonary infection may be curative; however, most patients present with advanced multilobar disease. Overall, prognosis is poor despite therapy with amphotericin B. Mortality rates of 80% have been reported.[22]

Viral Pneumonias. Viral infections occur in 35 to 50% of patients, usually within the first year following HSCT. Disseminated disease to the GI tract, lungs, brain, and liver occurs in approximately 10% of affected patients. The major viral pneumonias among hospitalized cancer patients include those caused by members of the Herpesviridae family (herpes simplex virus [HSV], *Cytomegalovirus* [CMV], Epstein-Barr virus [EBV], varicella-zoster virus [VZV], and human herpesvirus-6), measles virus, influenza virus, RSV, and adenovirus. Herpes viral pneumonia occurs in a well-defined group of cancer patients and particularly in patients with severe and prolonged immunosuppression and patients who have undergone HSCT. With the exception of those caused by HSV and several community-acquired viral pathogens, viral pneumonias are unusual during the initial 30 days after HSCT but become increasingly important causes of treatment failure after the first month of transplantation. Increased rates of CMV pneumonia during this period correlate with episodes of graft rejection and periods of severe immunosuppression. With the exception of CMV pneumonia, viral infections in cancer patients overwhelmingly reflect the re-activation of latent disease.

Cytomegaloviral Pneumonia. *Cytomegalovirus* is one of the most important causes of interstitial pneumonitis following transplantation[23,24] and is a major cause of morbidity and mortality. Fatal CMV pneumonitis has been reported in 80 to 90% of patients who develop interstitial pneumonitis.[24] Effective prophylaxis and pre-emptive treatment have resulted in a sharp decline in the rates of CMV pneumonia to approximately 4% for both allogeneic and autologous transplant recipients. Reactivation of latent disease accounts for the predominant source of CMV infection, with a minority of cases attributable to transfusions. A disordered immune response may underlie the development of CMV pneumonia. Abnormalities of the immune system, coupled with an apparent tropism of CMV for the lung, may explain the higher rates of CMV pneumonia in patients with GVHD and in recipients of allogeneic transplants. Increased rates of CMV pneumonitis also correlate with the intensity of the preconditioning regimen, methotrexate prophylaxis for GVHD, pretransplant conditioning with high-dose radiation, and pretransplant seropositivity for CMV.[19,24]

Only approximately 25 to 33% of patients with serologic evidence of CMV infection develop clinical syndromes of CMV disease. The manifestations of these clinical syndromes include fever, hypoxia, atypical lymphocytosis, leukopenia, pneumonitis, hepatitis, arthritis, and GI ulcerations. Radiographic changes are nonspecific and include diffuse interstitial infiltrates (Figure 11–6). Isolation of CMV from cultures of peripheral-blood buffy coat suggests the diagnosis. The definitive diagnosis of CMV pneumonitis relies on sputum and BAL cytopathology or lung biopsy specimens demonstrating intranuclear inclusion bodies in association with an inflammatory reaction and tissue destruction. Standard therapy includes intravenous ganciclovir together with unselected immune globulin or CMV-specific immune globulin. Six weeks of therapy is usually indicated for definitive treatment. The routine use of CMV prophylactic strategies has significantly reduced the incidence of disease.[24,25] Preventive measures include the use of CMV-seronegative blood products for seronegative patients, prophylactic therapy with ganciclovir, or weekly administration of intravenous immunoglobulin or acyclovir. Ganciclovir administration has been limited by the development of severe neutropenia.[24] Foscarnet has been used for definitive treatment and prophylaxis of CMV pneumonitis. Nephrotoxicity and poor GI absorption of the oral formulation have limited the widespread use of this drug.

Herpes Simplex Virus Pneumonia. Herpes simplex virus has been implicated as a rare cause of pneumonia in post-transplantation and severely immunosuppressed patients. Pneumonias due to HSV infection may be rapidly fatal. Diagnoses are rarely made ante mortem. Infection tends to occur early, within the first 3 to

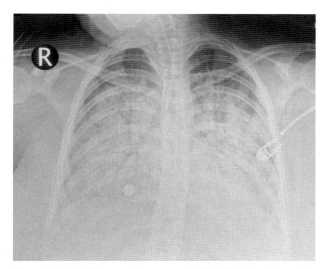

Figure 11–6. A 22-year-old woman with Hodgkin's lymphoma who developed acute respiratory deterioration 2 months after allogeneic peripheral stem cell transplantation complicated by acute graft-versus-host disease (GVHD) of the skin. Chest radiography reveals diffuse bilateral alveolar opacities consistent with adult respiratory distress syndrome (ARDS). Bronchoalveolar lavage was positive for *Cytomegalovirus* antigen by shell vial.

4 weeks after HSCT. Although HSV-related gingivostomatitis is common following HSCT, associated pneumonias are rare, and cultures of HSV from the oropharynx do not automatically imply causality. Re-activation of latent disease, usually from an oropharyngeal source, is the rule. Histopathologic evidence of intranuclear inclusion bodies on lung biopsy specimens is usually necessary for diagnosis. Chest radiography may demonstrate focal or multifocal opacities or (more commonly) diffuse interstitial infiltrates. Antiviral therapy for full-blown disease has been wholly inadequate. Intravenous acyclovir is the mainstay of therapy.

Varicella-Zoster Virus Pneumonia. Varicella-zoster virus pneumonia occurs most commonly among children with acute lymphocytic leukemia but has also been described in adult patients with lymphoma and following allogeneic transplantation. The re-activation of VZV typically occurs late, between 3 months and 2 years after transplantation, and correlates with the period of the most severe humoral deficiency. Disseminated disease to the skin, lungs, brain, and liver has been described. The appearance of GVHD augments the risk of VZV infection. Pulmonary symptoms of dry cough, dyspnea, and pleuritic chest pain usually occur 2 days after the onset of rash. Extensive nodular and interstitial infiltrates in a peribronchial distribution are characteristic findings by chest radiography. Patients may present with a high fever, a dry cough, dyspnea, and pleuritic chest pain. The physical examination may reveal rales, wheezes, or rhonchi. Pulmonary lesions tend to occur during the period of cutaneous dissemination, and the characteristic rash of VZV infection is helpful in establishing the diagnosis. Treatment consists of high-dose acyclovir (10 to 15 mg/kg every 8 hours). Mortality remains high despite aggressive therapy.

Human Herpesvirus-6 Pneumonia. Human herpesvirus-6 (HHV-6) is rarely isolated in lung biopsy specimens of HSCT patients. The pathogenic role of this virus in the development of pulmonary disease is not well understood, but HHV-6 is thought to cause an interstitial pneumonitis that is indistinguishable from that caused by CMV. Human herpesvirus-6 is inherently immunosuppressive. This property may contribute to the polymicrobial infections with EBV or CMV that are occasionally observed in patients with HHV-6 infection. Graft-versus-host disease appears to be a risk factor for the development of disease. Clinical manifestations of fever, encephalitis, and rash may suggest the diagnosis. Adequate therapy for HHV-6 pneumonitis is not available. Limited experience with ribavirin, acyclovir, and foscarnet suggest that these agents may have some therapeutic efficacy against this infection.[26]

Respiratory Syncytial Virus Pneumonia. Patients with T-cell deficiency have a higher propensity to develop RSV pneumonia. Infections tend to occur during the immediate postengraftment period following HSCT. Infection with RSV typically begins as an upper respiratory infection (with sinusitis, rhinitis, fever, and cough) and progresses to pneumonitis. Bilateral interstitial infiltrates, indistinguishable from pneumonitis secondary to other causes, are typical chest radiographic findings. Symptoms may quickly progress to respiratory failure in the HSCT patient, and mortality rates in this group of patients are high. Diagnosis relies on viral cultures, immunofluorescent staining, antigen testing, or direct tissue examination. Standard treatment with aerosolized ribavirin and immunoglobulin G (IgG) may effect an uneventful recovery if administered early, before respiratory failure.

Other Viral Pneumonias. Pneumonias caused by parainfluenza virus, influenza virus, and adenovirus are rare complications of HSCT. Among these, adenoviral infection is the most common and occurs in approximately 5% of HSCT recipients. Approximately 20% of affected patients will develop pneumonia. Although the re-activation of latent adenovirus is almost universal following HSCT, pulmonary infection occurs in only 2% of patients. Graft-versus-host disease represents a dominant risk factor for this disease. Re-activation typically occurs 3 months after HSCT. The clinical syndromes of adenovirus infection include interstitial pneumonitis, hemorrhagic cystitis, nephritis, hepatitis, and hemorrhagic colitis. Multiorgan failure is seen with disseminated disease. Pneumonias caused by influenza and parainfluenza viruses peak during the immediate postengraftment period. Influenza virus infection occurs with seasonal variations. The peak periods of infection are during the late fall through winter. Patients typically present with fever and upper-respiratory-tract symptoms. Nonspecific opacities and interstitial infiltrates may be observed on chest radiographs. Mortality rates associated with influenza and parainfluenza virus pneumonia are high. Aerosolized ribavirin may be of some clinical benefit.

Aspiration Pneumonia

Owing to a number of factors, debilitated cancer patients have an increased predilection to aspirate oropharyngeal and gastric contents. An ineffective cough reflex, impaired respiratory mucociliary clearance, altered mental status, and abnormalities of airway cellular and immune function may all contribute to an increased propensity to aspirate. The volume of the aspirate as well as the content determines the likelihood of developing clinically significant pulmonary disease. Prompt suctioning of aspirated material may prevent significant lung injury. Large-volume aspirates typically incite bronchospasm followed by hypoxemia, hypercapnia, and severe respiratory distress. Arterial blood gas values may improve after 3 to 4 hours as bronchospasm resolves. Loss of surfactant and the destruction of type II pneumocytes occur approximately 36 to 48 hours after the initial event and correspond with further respiratory deterioration. If mechanical ventilation is required, the application of positive end-expiratory pressure (PEEP) is recommended to minimize airway collapse. Continuous positive airway pressure (CPAP) may be administered to nonintubated patients with mild to moderate respiratory distress. Antibiotics chosen should include those that are bactericidal for Gram-negative and anaerobic organisms. As with other serious pneumonias, empiric therapy with two parenteral antibiotics is reasonable, pending the results of diagnostic studies.

Role of Myeloid Growth Factors and Granulocyte Transfusions

The significant improvements in survival outcomes in the treatment of cancer patients over the past decade have been partly attributable to advancements in the management and prevention of infectious complications of cancer. One area of major progress has been in the area of hematologic supportive care. In particular, the purification of myeloid growth factors, including granulocyte colony-stimulating factor (G-CSF), granulocyte-macrophage colony-stimulating factor (GM-CSF), interleukin-3, and macrophage colony-stimulating factor (M-CSF), has led to effective approaches to the supportive care of patients who

are undergoing myeloablative therapy. Granulocyte-macrophage colony-stimulating factor stimulates the proliferation and maturation of polymorphonuclear leukocytes (PMNs), monocytes, and eosinophils within the bone marrow and augments specific PMN functions, including bactericidal activity, cellular adhesion, chemotaxis, and phagocytosis.[27–29] Granulocyte colony-stimulating factor has a more narrow target of activity, stimulating only the proliferation and maturation of neutrophil colonies.[29] Both GM-CSF and G-CSF augment the fungicidal activity of PMNs against *Aspergillus* and *Candida*.[29–31] These activities suggest an important role for myeloid growth factors in the treatment of cancer patients with both neutropenic and nonneutropenic infections. Evidence demonstrating clear benefit in the prevention of neutropenic infections is mounting. Recent investigations have demonstrated unequivocal reductions in both the duration and severity of neutropenia after stem cell transplantation and in patients treated with chemotherapy for solid tumors and hematologic malignancies.[32,33] These favorable results were associated with fewer infections and reduced rates of postchemotherapy-induced mucositis. These benefits, however, have not resulted in reduced mortality rates in any subset of cancer patients.[34] The clinical benefits of other growth factors, including M-CSF, interleukin-3, interferon-α, and tumor necrosis factor alpha (TNF-α [cachectin]) and beta (TNF-β [lymphotoxin]) are still being evaluated.

Nonneutropenic cancer patients with open wounds, mucositis, and bronchial obstruction are at increased risk of developing recalcitrant infections that may be resistant to single-modality therapy with antibiotics. Because of the impact of growth factors in enhancing neutrophil activity, these patients may also benefit from the initiation of therapy with these agents. Clear data demonstrating definitive benefit in this group of patients, however, are not available. The current recommendations for myeloid growth factor administration include its use for the prevention and treatment of infection in patients with prolonged neutropenia or in patients in which prolonged neutropenia is anticipated after further courses of chemotherapy.[35,36] The risk of developing serious infection with prolonged neutropenia varies with the type of malignancy being treated. Knowledge of the associated infection risk should also influence decisions to initiate G-CSF therapy. Myeloid growth factors may also be used to treat prolonged neutropenia associated with established soft-tissue infections although the benefits of therapy in this setting are not as clearly defined.[37]

Passive immunization with intravenous immune globulin (IVIG) has been used, most notably in conjunction with ganciclovir in the treatment of CMV-related pneumonitis following stem cell transplantation. Intravenous immune globulin treatment of active CMV infection presumably exerts its effect through immunomodulation. Intravenous immune globulin has also been used with some success as prophylaxis against respiratory infections in patients with chronic lymphocytic leukemia (CLL).[38] The use of granulocyte transfusions in the prevention and treatment of serious infections associated with neutropenia is steeped in controversy. Earlier attempts to augment numbers of circulating PMNs with granulocyte transfusions were hampered by the inability to collect sufficient numbers of donor PMNs, coupled with the perceived higher risk for CMV infection, GVHD, and the development of ARDS following granulocyte transfusions. More recently, pharmacologic stimulation of donor PMNs with G-CSF and the use of sedimenting agents during centrifugation leukapheresis have been used to optimize PMN collection. In addition, the standard use of human leukocyte antigen (HLA) or leukocyte antigen–matched products has improved donor-recipient compatibility. Currently, granulocyte transfusions are considered to represent a reasonable adjunctive therapy in patients with severe neutropenia secondary to myeloid hypoplasia and bacterial sepsis unresponsive to conventional management. Isolated case reports also support the use of granulocyte transfusions in the treatment of severe fungal infections[39,40] although the benefits of granulocyte transfusions in this setting have not been proven in any large prospective studies.

PULMONARY EMERGENCIES FOLLOWING HEMATOPOIETIC STEM CELL TRANSPLANTATON

Infectious Complications

Chemotherapeutic regimens for the treatment of hematologic malignancies, as well as chemoablative regimens used in the preparation of patients for HSCT, result in a severe and predictable decline in immune function. All three arms of the immune system are profoundly affected by HSCT. The chronologic development of pneumonia in these patients is tightly linked to their dynamically changing immunologic status during the course of treatment. Susceptibility to infection is roughly predictable, based on the amount of time that has elapsed since transplantation. Periods of increased susceptibility to infection may be divided to reflect three stages of major impairment of specific arms of the host defense system. These three stages correlate with periods of highest vulnerability to specific organisms. The pre-engraftment stage usually occurs within the first 3 weeks after transplantation and correlates with the period of neutropenia. Profound neutropenia and lymphopenia occur early after cytoablative chemotherapy and usually persist for 14 to 21 days.[3,10] The risk of infection increases with both the duration and degree of neutropenia and is greatest when the neutrophil count falls to $< 1,000/mm^3$. The intermediate postengraftment stage follows and may last from 3 weeks to 3 months after transplantation. This period is marked by profound suppression of both the cellular and humoral arms of the host defense system. Reconstitution of lymphocytes and partial recovery of nonspecific cytotoxic and proliferative activity of lymphocytes may be seen within the first 3 months after transplantation. The activity of tissue and blood lymphocytes and macrophages may remain impaired, however, for approximately 12 months after transplantation. The development of infectious complications during the late postengraftment period is tightly linked to the appearance of chronic GVHD. Late-postengraftment infections are therefore typically seen only in recipients of allogeneic transplants. This period characteristically occurs 3 months or more after transplantation. Mucocutaneous damage and severe persistent dysfunction of the cellular and humoral immune arms of the host defense system mark this stage of transplantation. Evaluation of the HSCT patient requires an understanding of the specific host immune defects that occur as a consequence of therapy. Diagnostic strategies in the evaluation of the HSCT patient for pneumonia should exploit the unique susceptibility of these patients to the sequential pathogens that emerge during the evolution of immune reconstitution (Figure 11–7). The temporal sequence of pulmonary complications that regularly occur following transplantation may vary significantly, however, depending on the rate of immune recovery.

Pre-engraftment Period. During the neutropenic pre-engraftment period, the patient is susceptible to infections by a variety of predominantly endogenous, extracellular, and pyogenic organisms. Gram-negative pneumonias are the most common bacterial infections during this period although Gram-positive pathogens such as *Streptococcus pneumoniae* and *Staphylococcus aureus* have been increasingly isolated over the past decade.[41] Documented infections by Gram-negative pathogens such as *Legionella, Pseudomonas,* bacteria of the family Enterobacteriaceae, and *Stenotrophomonas maltophilia* may cause fatal pneumonias during this period. Methotrexate administration and T-cell depletion of the donor marrow may prolong the period of neutropenia. As neutropenia persists, the risk of mucormycosis or infection by opportunistic filamentous fungal pathogens such as *Aspergillus* and *Fusarium* increases. Deficiencies in the humoral immune system are also seen, and these deficiencies render the patient susceptible to infections by Gram-negative rods (such as *Haemophilus influenzae, Neisseria meningitis,* and *Pseudomonas*) and by encapsulated organisms (including *Streptococcus*). Candidal pneumonia is also seen early on although diligent prophylaxis with azole derivatives after

alternative to vancomycin for the treatment of suspected resistant Gram-positive organisms. An antipseudomonal β-lactam antibiotic may be used in combination with a quinolone or an aminoglycoside when initial therapy with vancomycin is not indicated. Alternatively, monotherapy with cefepime or a carbapenem may provide reasonable coverage in this setting. In the absence of prior quinolone prophylaxis, quinolones are excellent alternatives to aminoglycosides and may be used for patients with altered renal function. Definitive treatment should be initiated once the offending pathogen is identified. Antibiotic selections for definitive therapy should

be chosen on the basis of their maximal curative effect, cost-effectiveness, and safety. Combination drug therapy may be warranted in some cases for synergy to achieve bactericidal activity against the pathogen. Antifungal coverage may be added at day 3 to day 5 of empiric therapy in culture-negative patients with persistent fever. Parenteral antifungal choices include amphotericin B, one of its liposomal derivatives, or the newer cell-wall agent, caspofungin. Although amphotericin is the most cost-effective of the available parenteral antifungal agents, it is associated with the highest rates of renal toxicity. Other antifungal agents may be preferred in this set-

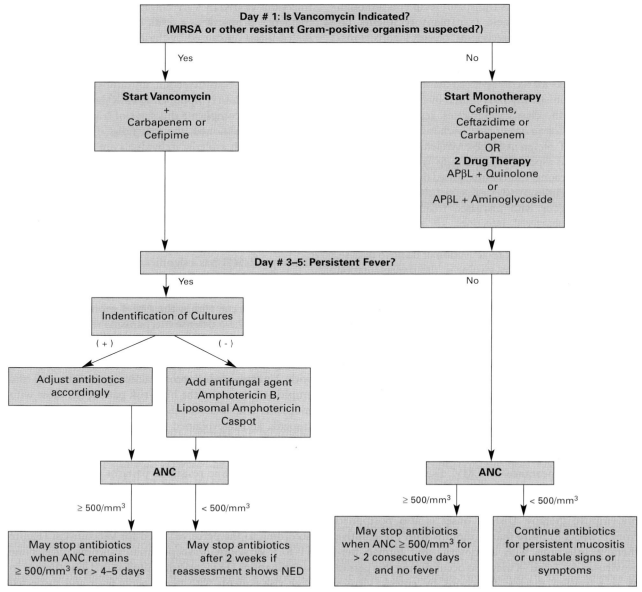

Figure 11–8. Empiric therapy for high risk patients with neutropenic fever.[45] ANC = absolute neutrophil count; APβL = Antipseudomonal β lactam; MRSA = methicillin-resistant *staphylococcus aureus*; NED = no evidence of disease.

ting. The duration of antibiotic therapy is influenced in part by the ANC. Antibiotic therapy should continue for an additional 2 days in patients who defervesce after 3 days of antibiotic therapy and whose ANC remains > 500/mm³ for 2 consecutive days. Unstable patients who are afebrile by day 3 of empiric antibiotic therapy but whose ANC remains < 500/mm³ should be reassessed after 14 days of antibiotic therapy. In patients with persistent fever after 3 days of antibiotic therapy, antibiotics may be discontinued after 4 to 5 days of documented elevations of the ANC to > 500/mm³. Finally, a full 2-week course of antibiotics is recommended for patients with persistent fever and an ANC of < 500/mm³. Adjunctive therapy with G-CSF is generally added around day 3 to day 5 in patients with established soft-tissue infections and persistent neutropenia.

Prophylactic Strategies. A variety of antimicrobial strategies for prophylaxis against infectious organisms has been proposed. In general, antibiotic coverage of Gram-positive and Gram-negative pathogens and antifungal therapy are routinely given through the time of engraftment. Antiviral therapy is typically initiated during the pretransplantation period and is continued up through the first 100 days after transplantation. Thereafter, adjustments in antimicrobial prophylaxis are made on the basis of the individual's state of immune recovery and the presence of GVHD.

Noninfectious Complications

Most of the noninfectious complications of HSCT, including diffuse alveolar hemorrhage, pulmonary edema, and ARDS, are covered in chapter 10. Other disease entities that may mimmic pulmonary infections, including idiopathic pneumonia syndrome, bronchiolitis obliterans, and GVHD, are discussed below.

Idiopathic Pneumonia Syndrome. Interstitial pneumonia that occurs without an apparent cause is often referred to as idiopathic pneumonia syndrome (IPS). This term is applied to approximately 30 to 50% of patients with interstitial pneumonia.[46] Infectious and toxic etiologies are eventually identified in only a minority of patients with interstitial pneumonia. These etiologies, including viral, fungal, and drug-induced interstitial pneumonitis, are discussed in detail elsewhere in this chapter. Both secondary and idiopathic interstitial pneumonias may be associated with a rapid decline in pulmonary function and with death. Recipients of allogeneic transplants are at greatest risk for IPS. The rates of IPS following allogeneic transplantation range from 33 to 50% but are much lower (20%) among recipients of autologous or syngeneic transplants.[47,48] High-dose radiation, a low pretransplantation Karnofsky score,

older age, and methotrexate administration are strongly correlated with the occurrence of IPS in both allogeneic and autologous transplant recipients. These observations implicate the cumulative toxic effects of radiation and chemotherapy on the lungs in the development of IPS. Severe GVHD is also an important independent risk factor in the development of secondary interstitial pneumonia among recipients of allogeneic transplants. An insidious onset of fever, dry cough, and hypoxemia, coupled with diffuse interstitial infiltrates as seen by chest radiography, suggests the diagnosis. Symptoms usually occur 40 to 75 days (median, 42 to 49 days) after grafting.[49] The diagnosis is made by histologic evidence of diffuse alveolar damage on a biopsy specimen and the absence of obvious infectious or toxic etiologies. No specific therapy for IPS exists. Although corticosteroids are often used in the treatment of this disease, the clinical benefit of this therapy has not been proved in any large prospective studies. Patients who receive cyclosporine or intravenous immunoglobulin (IVIG) prophylaxis for GVHD appear to have less severe disease. Thus, an immunopathologic mechanism for IPS has been advanced. Mortality rates for IPS may exceed 70% despite corticosteroid therapy.

Diffuse Alveolar Hemorrhage. Diffuse alveolar hemorrhage (DAH), resulting in intraparenchymal bleed, is a major challenge, especially in the severely thrombocytopenic leukemic patient. It also threatens the success of autologous as well as allogeneic stem cell transplants in 8 to 33% of patients.[19,50] Patients with DAH typically develop acute symptoms of cough, progressive dyspnea, and low-grade fever. Intraparenchymal bleeding may pool within the alveoli without ready access to the central bronchi. Therefore, hemoptysis is not a reliable index of the presence or degree of intraparenchymal bleeding. Even in the setting of severe pulmonary hemorrhage, hemoptysis occurs in fewer than 25% of patients.[51,52] Chest radiography typically shows patchy areas of central infiltrates that progress to bilateral areas of alveolar consolidation (Figure 11–9, A and B). The diagnosis is made on the basis of bronchoscopic examination, which demonstrates progressively bloody aspirates in BAL. The identification of hemosiderin-laden macrophages on BAL fluid is helpful in making the diagnosis, but they may not be present in acute bleeds. The etiology of DAH is unclear. Radiation injury to the lungs, prior treatment for solid tumors, sepsis, cytotoxic lung injury, pneumonia (especially of fungal origin), severe mucositis, and renal insufficiency have been implicated.[51,53] Although most patients are thrombocytopenic, with platelet counts of < 20,000 cells/μL, the correction of thrombocytopenia alone does not eliminate the syndrome.[49,54] Furthermore, the appearance of thrombocytopenia or coagulopathy does not correlate with the development or the severity of this disorder.[54] Interestingly, the occurrence of DAH is commonly coincident with marrow recovery, which typically occurs 12 days (range of 7 to 40 days) after HSCT.[53,54] Respiratory failure secondary to DAH heralds a poor prognosis, with in-hospital mortality rates between 50 and 82%.[54–56] Recent reports have supported the use of high-dose steroids in efforts to favorably alter the outcome of patients with DAH.[50,57] Anecdotal evidence of decreased rates of respiratory failure and improved survival were associated with dosages of 500 to 1,000 mg/d of intravenous methyprednisolone in two reports.[50,57] Lower dosages of corticosteroids did not alter outcomes in these patients.

Bronchiolitis Obliterans. Bronchiolitis obliterans (BO) occurs as a late complication in recipients of allogeneic hematopoietic stem cell transplants but may also (rarely) occur as a nonspecific response to chemotherapy or infection following autologous HSCT.[58] The reported incidence of BO among allogeneic transplant recipients ranges from 2 to 13%.[59] The development of GVHD is a strong risk factor for this disease. Viral infections and the development of autoimmune processes that specifically target the small airways are postulated etiologies for the development of BO.[48] The appearance of a new or changing obstructive lung defect, coupled with a reduction in the diffusion capacity of the lung for carbon monoxide (DL_{CO}) on pulmonary function tests, suggests the diagnosis. Occasionally, a mixed obstructive-restrictive pattern or a pure restrictive pattern suggesting bronchiolitis obliterans with organizing pneumonia (BOOP)

is observed. A nonproductive cough, dyspnea, inspiratory rales, and expiratory wheezes make up the constellation of clinical findings. Chest radiography may demonstrate hyperinflation with or without parenchymal infiltrates. Patchy areas of consolidation and decreased peripheral vascular markings may be demonstrated on high-resolution CT. Histologic confirmation of BO on transbronchial biopsy (TBB) specimens or open lung biopsy specimens may be necessary for diagnosis; however, this may not be feasible in many cases because of low platelet counts (Figure 11–10, A and B). The diagnosis is often inferred and treatment initiated based on suggestive clinical findings, the results of the pulmonary function test (PFT), and the exclusion of competing infectious etiologies. The impact of high-dose steroids on outcomes has not been defined.

Impact of Graft-versus-Host Disease

Graft-versus-host disease and its associated intensive immunosuppressive treatment further challenge the allogeneic stem cell transplant by amplifying the associated incidence and severity of both infectious and noninfectious complications. Graft-versus-host disease arises when immune donor cells are transfused into a nonidentical recipient. This initiates a series of reactions resulting in injury to targeted host tissues. The skin, GI tract, and liver are particularly vulnerable to this type of immune assault and are the most common sites of injury in both acute and chronic GVHD. In order for GVHD to occur, the following prerequisite conditions must exist: (1) the donor graft must contain immunocompetent cells, (2) the recipient (host) must possess antigenically distinct

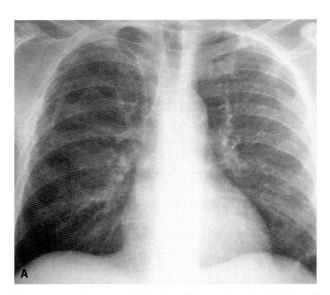
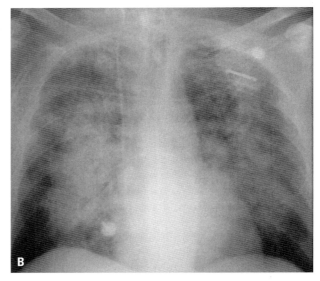

Figure 11–9. A 22-year-old female with acute lymphocytic leukemia and fever, pancytopenia, and blood-tinged sputum, 2 weeks following an allogeneic stem cell transplant. A normal chest radiograph (A) rapidly progressed to bilateral dense alveolar consolidation (B) 24 hours after presentation. Bronchoscopy results were consistent with diffuse alveolar hemorrhage.

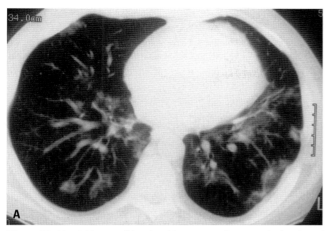
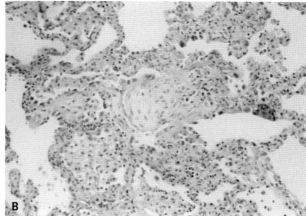

Figure 11–10. A 42-year-old male with acute myelogenous leukemia and chronic graft-versus-host disease (GVHD) following hematopoietic stem cell transplantation (HSCT). A: Chest computed tomography (CT) showed diffuse patchy alveolar opacities at both lung bases and in the periphery. The diagnosis of bronchiolitis obliterans with organizing pneumonia (BOOP) was confirmed with open lung biopsy (B) which showed bronchioles and alveoli plugged with fibrous exudates and a dense inflammatory cell infiltrate in the surrounding alveolar and interstitial spaces.

properties that allow the donor cells to recognize it as foreign, and (3) the immunologic response of the recipient cells to the graft must be weak and ineffective.

Acute GVHD typically occurs between 20 and 100 days following HSCT and complicates 25 to 75% of all stem cell transplantations.[4,60] Clinical features that include exfoliative skin rash, liver dysfunction, and diarrhea may signal the development of this syndrome, which usually occurs between day 20 and day 100 after transplantation. Chronic GVHD occurs in roughly one-third of patients who survive beyond the first 3 months of transplantation and is the most common late complication of allogeneic transplantation.[4] The incidence of chronic GVHD strongly correlates with prior acute GVHD. Approximately 65% of patients with chronic GVHD had a prior acute form of the disease. This inherently immunonodeficient syndrome is characterized by the development of immunoglobulin A (IgA) deficiency, functional asplenia, and a sicca-like syndrome. Scleroderma-like changes and clinical features that resemble those of a variety of other autoimmune multisystem diseases (including Sjögren's syndrome, autoimmune hemolytic anemia, abnormal gastrointestinal motility, malabsorption, primary biliary cirrhosis, and ophthalmic and sinopulmonary sicca) are prominent features of this disease. The lungs are commonly involved in chronic GVHD. Associated pathologic diagnoses include lymphoid interstitial pneumonia, chronic aspiration, and sinopulmonary infections due to encapsulated bacteria, *Pneumocystis carinii,* and *Aspergillus.* In addition, severe progressive obstruction due to chronic bronchitis or BO may occur, usually 6 months or more after allogeneic transplantation. The association between lymphocytic bronchitis with chronic GVHD has been questioned.

A variety of immunosuppressive strategies are used for prophylaxis against the development of GVHD. These usually entail the use of combinations of antilymphocyte preparations, cyclosporine, azathioprine, methotrexate, and high-dose steroids. The appearance of GVHD prompts the escalation of immunosuppressive therapy and further predisposes these patients to infectious complications. These patients frequently have significant disruptions of mucosal barriers of the gut and skin secondary to GVHD. Thus, infections in patients with established GVHD are almost universal and are frequently fatal. It is estimated that approximately 50% of affected patients will succumb to the disease or to infectious complications associated with therapy.[4,19]

SUMMARY

Lung injury due to infectious and noninfectious etiologies remains a critical limiting factor in the overall successful outcome of the cancer patient and the patient following HSCT. The diagnosis of pneumonia has played a persistent and substantive role as the proximal cause of death in the majority of studies on HSCT outcomes over the past $2^1/_2$ decades. The development of preemptive strategies designed limit pulmonary infectious complications following cancer treatment is therefore pivotal to the overall successful outcome of these patients. Effective prophylactic strategies have significantly diminished the incidence of certain infections following HSCT. However, these protocols must continue to evolve as more resistant strains of pathogens emerge. In addition, more effective antimicrobial therapy and the use of less toxic conditioning regimens may also help to mitigate the incidence of infections in these patients.

REFERENCES

1. Aronchick J. Pulmonary infections in cancer and bone marrow transplant patients. Semin Roentgenol 2000; 35:140–51.

2. Bergen G, Shelhamer J. Pulmonary infiltrates in the cancer patient. New approaches to an old problem. Infect Dis Clin North Am 1996;10:297–325.

3. Collin BA, Ramphal R. Lower respiratory tract infections. Infect Dis Clin North Am 1998;12:781–805.

4. Krowka MJ, Rosenow EC, Hoagland HC. Pulmonary complications of bone marrow transplantation. Chest 1985;87:237–46.

5. Kolbe K, Domkin D, Derigs H, et al. Infectious complications during neutropenia subsequent to peripheral blood cell transplantation. Bone Marrow Transplant 1997;19:143–7.

6. Mossad S, Longworth D, Goormastic M, et al. Early infectious complications in autologous bone marrow transplantation. A review of 219 patients. Bone Marrow Transplant 1996;18:265–71.

7. Raad I, Whimbey E, Rolston K, et al. A comparison of aztreonam plus vancomycin and imipenem plus vancomycin as initial therapy for febrile neutropenic cancer patients. Cancer 1996;77:1386–94.

8. Tenholder M, Hooper R. Pulmonary hemorrhage in the immunocompromised host—an elusive reality. Am Rev Respir Dis 1980;121:A198.

9. Marschmeyer G, Link H, Hiddemann W, et al. Pulmonary infiltrations in febrile patients with neutropenia. Cancer 1994;73:2296–304.

10. Meyers J, Thomas E. Infection complicating bone marrow transplantation. Clinical approach to infection in the compromised host. In: Rubin R, Young L, editors. 1988. p. 525–55.

11. Emanuel D, Cunningham L, Jules-Elysee K, et al. *Cytomegalovirus* pneumonia after bone marrow transplantation successfully treated with the combination of ganciclovir and high dose intravenous immune globulin. Ann Intern Med 1988;109:777–82.

12. Wendt C, Hertz M. Respiratory syncytial virus and parainfluenza virus infections in the immunocompromised host. Semin Respir Infect 1995;10:224–31.

13. Lossos I, Breuer R, Or R, et al. Bacterial pneumonia in recipients of bone marrow transplantation: a five year prospective study. Transplantation 1995;60:672–8.

14. Cordonnier C, Bernaudin J, Bierling P, et al. Pulmonary complications occurring after allogeneic bone marrow transplantation. Cancer 1986;58:1047–54.

15. Bochud P, Calandra T, Francioli P. Bacteremia due to viridans streptococci in neutropenic patients. A review. Am J Med 1997;3:256–64.

16. Fled R, Bodey G, Groschel D. Mycobacteriosis in patients with malignant disease. Arch Intern Med 1976;136:67.

17. Vartirarian S, Anaissie E, Bodey G. Emerging fungal pathogens in immunmocomprised patients: classification, diagnosis, and management. Clin Infect Dis 1993; 17:S487.

18. McWhinney P, Kibbler C, Hamon M, et al. Progress in the diagnosis and management of aspergillosis in bone marrow transplantation: 13 years' experience. Clin Infect Dis 1993;17:397–404.

19. Soubani O, Miller K, Hassoun P. Pulmonary complications of bone marrow transplantation. Chest 1996; 109:1066–77.

20. McCloud T, Naidich D. Thoracic disease in the immunocompromised patient. Radiol Clin North Am 1992;30: 525–54.

21. Boelaert J, Fenves AZ, Coburn JW. Deferoxamine therapy and mucormycosis in dialysis patients: report of an international registry. Am J Kidney Dis 1991;18:660–7.

22. Kontoyiannis D, Wessel V, Bodey G, Rolston K. Zygomycosis in the 1990s in a tertiary-care cancer center. Clin Infect Dis 2000;30:851–6.

23. Jules-Elysee K, Stover D, Yahalom J, et al. Pulmonary complications in lymphoma patients treated with high-dose therapy and autologous bone marrow transplantation. Am Rev Respir Dis 1992;146:485.

24. Winston D, Ho W, Champlin R. *Cytomegalovirus* infections after allogenic bone marrow transplantation. Rev Infect Dis 1990;12:S776.

25. Meyers J, Leszezynski J, Zaia J, et al. Prevention of *Cytomegalovirus* infection by *Cytomegalovirus* immune globulin after marrow transplantation. Ann Intern Med 1983;98:442.

26. Kadakia M, Rybka W, Stewart J, et al. Human herpesvirus 6: infection and disease following autologous and allogeneic bone marrow transplantation. Blood 1996;87: 5341–54.

27. Dale D, Liles W, Summer W, et al. Granulocyte colony-stimulating factor: role and relationships in infectious diseases. J Infect Dis 1995;172:1061–75.

28. Yong K, Rowles P, Patterson K, et al. Granulocyte macrophage colony-stimulating factor induces neutrophil adhesion to pulmonary vascular endothelium in vivo: role of beta 2 integrins. Blood 1992;80:1565–75.

29. Roilides E, Uhlig K, Venzon D, et al. Neutrophil oxidative burst in response to blastoconidia and pseudohyphae of *Candida albicans*: augmentation by granulocyte colony-stimulating factor and interferon-gamma. J Infect Dis 1992;166:668–73.

30. Vadhan-Raj S, Buescher S, Broxmeyer H. Stimulation of myelopoiesis in patients with aplastic anemia by recombinant human granulocyte-macrophage colony stimulating factor. N Engl J Med 1988;319:1628–34.

31. Roilides E, Walsh T, Pizzo P, Rubin M. Granulocyte colony-stimulating factor enhances the phagocytic and bactericidal activity of normal and defective human neutrophils. J Infect Dis 1991;163:579–83.

32. Roilides E, Pizzo P. Modulation of host defenses by cytokines: evolving adjuncts in prevention and treatment of serious infections in immunocompromised hosts. Clin Infect Dis 1992;15:508–24.

33. Nemunaitis J, Rabinowe S, Singer J, et al. Recombinant granulocyte-macrophage colony-stimulating factor after autologous bone marrow transplantation for lymphoid cancer. N Engl J Med 1991;324:1773–8.

34. Vellenga E, Uyl-de-Groot C, Wit RD, et al. Randomized

placebo-controlled trial of granulocyte-macrophage colony-stimulating factor in patients with chemotherapy-related febrile neutropenia. J Clin Oncol 1996;14:619–27.

35. Nelson S. Novel nonantibiotic therapies for pneumonia: cytokines and host defense. Chest 2001;119 (2 Suppl): 419S–25S.

36. Pizzo P. Management of fever in patients with cancer and treatment-induced neutropenia. N Engl J Med 1993; 328:1323–32.

37. Crawford J, Ozer H, Stoller R, et al. Reduction by granulocyte colony-stimulating factor of fever and neutropenia induced by chemotherapy in patients with small-cell lung cancer. N Engl J Med 1991;325:164–70.

38. Weeks J, Tierney M, Weinstein M. Cost effectiveness of prophylactic intravenous immune globulin in chronic lymphocytic leukemia. N Engl J Med 1991;325:81–6.

39. Spielberger R, Falleroni M, Coene A. Concomitant amphotericin B therapy, granulocyte transfusions, and GM-CSF administration of disseminated infection with *Fusarium* in a granulocytopenic patient. Clin Infect Dis 1993;16:528–30.

40. Strauss R. Therapeutic granulocyte transfusions in 1993. Blood 1993;81:1675–8.

41. Spanik S, Kukuckova E, Pichna P, et al. Analysis of 553 episodes of monomicrobial bacteraemia in cancer patients: any association between risk factors and outcome to particular pathogen? Support Care Cancer 1997;5:330–3.

42. Clark J. The challenge of bone marrow transplantation [editorial]. Mayo Clin Proc 1990;65:111–4.

43. Fetscher S, Mertelsmann R. Supportive care in hematological malignancies: hematopoietic growth factors, transfusion therapy. Curr Opin Hematol 1999;6:262–73.

44. Winston D, Territo M, Ho W, et al. Alveolar macrophage dysfunction in human bone marrow transplant recipients. Am J Med 1982;73:859–66.

45. Zinner S. Relevant aspects in the Infectious Diseases Society of America (IDSA) guidelines for the use of antimicrobial agents in neutropenic patients with unexplained fever. Int J Hematol 1998;68:1:S31–4.

46. Meyers J, McGuffin R, Bryson Y, et al. Treatment of *Cytomegalovirus* pneumonia after marrow transplant with combined vidarabine and human leukocyte interferon. J Infect Dis 1982;146:80–4.

47. Weiner R, Horowitz M, Gale R, et al. Risk factors for interstitial pneumonia following bone marrow transplantation for severe aplastic anemia. Br J Haematol 1989;71:535.

48. Holland H, Wingard J, Beschorner W, et al. Bronchiolitis obliterans in bone marrow transplantation and its relationship to chronic graft-vs-host disease and low serum IgG. Blood 1988;72:621–7.

49. Clark JG, Hansen JA, Hertz MI, et al. Idiopathic pneumonia syndrome after bone marrow transplantation. Am Rev Respir Dis 1993;147:1601–6.

50. Metcalf J, Rennard S, Reed E, et al. Corticosteroids as adjunctive therapy for diffuse alveolar hemorrhage associated with bone marrow transplantation. Am J Med 1994;94:327–34.

51. Smith L, Katzenstein A. Pathogenesis of massive pulmonary hemorrhage in acute leukemia. Arch Intern Med 1982;142:2149–52.

52. Hildebrand FL Jr, Rosenow EC 3rd, Haberman TM, Tazelaar HD. Pulmonary complications of leukemia. Chest 1990:1233–9.

53. Sisson J, Thompson A, Anderson J. Airway inflammation predicts diffuse alveolar hemorrhage during bone marrow transplantation in patients with Hodgkin disease. Am Rev Respir Dis 1992;146:439–43.

54. Robbins R, Linder J, Stahl M. Diffuse alveolar hemorrhage in autologous bone marrow transplant recipients. Am J Med 1989;87:511–8.

55. Price K, Thall P, Kish S, Shannon V. Prognostic indicators for blood and marrow transplant patients admitted to an intensive care unit. Am J Respir Crit Care Med 1998;158:876–84.

56. Srivastava A, Gottlieb D, Bradstock K. Diffuse alveolar haemorrhage associated with microangiopathy after allogeneic bone marrow transplantation. Bone Marrow Transplant 1995;15:863–7.

57. Haselton D, Klekamp J, Christman B. Use of high-dose corticosteroids and high-frequency oscillatory ventilation for treatment of a child with diffuse alveolar hemorrhage after bone marrow transplantation: case report and review of the literature. Crit Care Med 2000;28(1):245–8.

58. Paz H, Crilley P, Patchefsky A, et al. Bronchiolitis obliterans after autologous bone marrow transplantation. Chest 1992;101:775–8.

59. Theodore J, Starnes V, Lewiston N. Obliterative bronchiolitis. Clin Chest Med 1990;11:309–21.

60. Ferrara J, Deeg H. Graft-versus-host disease. N Engl J Med 1991;324:667–74.

CHAPTER 12

NEUROLOGIC EMERGENCIES

ELLEN F. MANZULLO, MD
LAURENCE D. RHINES, MD
ARTHUR D. FORMAN, MD

Neurologic emergencies are common in the cancer population. Frequently patients with cancer will present to the emergency center with a neurologic sign or symptom that will require a thoughtful evaluation. This chapter focuses on the areas of brain metastasis, cerebrovascular disease, and spinal cord compression. Leptomeningeal disease rarely constitues a true emergency and thus will not be discussed in this chapter. The evaluation of cancer patients with altered mental status is discussed in Chapter 4.

BRAIN METASTASIS

Metastases to the brain are the most common intracranial tumors in adults and occur up to 10 times more frequently than primary brain tumors.[1] Each year, approximately 17,500 patients in the United States are diagnosed with primary brain tumors,[2] and 66,000 patients are diagnosed with brain metastases that are symptomatic.[3] In addition, the most common neurologic complication of systemic cancer is metastasis to the brain. Brain metastases are second only to metabolic encephalopathies as a cause of central nervous system dysfunction in cancer patients. In one study, neurologic signs and symptoms were present in 38% of oncology-related emergency-department visits at a community teaching hospital.[4] If a patient with known systemic cancer develops new neurologic abnormalities, brain metastasis should be suspected.

Clinical Manifestations

Most brain metastases are symptomatic, and over two-thirds of patients with brain metastases develop neurologic symptoms during the course of their illness.[5,6] In approximately 35% of patients who have brain tumors, the presenting complaint is a headache, and approximately 70% of patients with brain tumors will have a headache at some time during the course of their illness.[7] Headaches from brain tumors have been classically described as occurring predominantly in the morning upon awakening and improving after the patient arises, but this type of headache occurs in only a minority of the affected patients. More commonly, patients with central nervous system lesions will experience a dull nonthrobbing headache that gradually increases in duration and severity and is associated with other symptoms such as nausea, vomiting, and impaired consciousness.[8]

The second most common complaint in patients with brain tumors is focal deficits. Patients can experience a change in mental status or have focal motor and sensory deficits. The deficits will depend on the location of the tumor and the amount of surrounding edema. In 30% of patients, cognitive disturbances will occur. For example, affected patients may display a memory deficit, a change in personality, or apathy. Seizures are the presenting symptom in 33% of patients who have gliomas and in 15 to 20% of patients who have brain metastases. In addition, seizures occur at some time in 40 to 60% of patients who have gliomas and in 30 to 40% of patients who have brain metastases.[7,9]

Pathophysiologic Mechanisms

Most cases of brain metastasis are a result of the hematogenous spread of cancer cells to the brain. The dissemination of malignant cells can also occur through the vertebral venous system (Batson's plexus). Because the cerebral hemispheres receive most of the blood flow to the brain, they are the site of approximately 80% of brain metastases. The cerebellum is the site of 15% of metastases, and the brain stem is the site of 5%.[10,11] About two-thirds to three-fourths of patients with brain metastases have multiple lesions.

The clinical features of brain tumors are a result of either direct destruction or displacement of normal brain tissue by the tumor and associated edema. In addition, the tumor and its associated edema can cause compression of vascular structures and can interfere with neuronal pathways. Headaches are a very common chief complaint because of pressure on pain-sensitive intracranial structures such as the dura mater, certain cranial nerves, and large venous sinuses.[11]

Etiology

Cancer from any organ may metastasize to the brain. The majority of brain metastases are from cancers of the lung, breast, skin (malignant melanoma), genitourinary tract, and gastrointestinal tract. [3, 9] In adults, melanoma is the tumor most likely to metastasize to the brain; however, more cases of brain metastases are caused by lung and breast cancer because of the greater frequency of these malignancies compared with other cancers. Metastases from breast, renal, and colon cancer tend to be single whereas lung cancer and melanoma tend to produce multiple cerebral lesions.

Diagnosis

The possibility of a brain lesion should be considered in any cancer patient presenting with a headache. A careful history and physical examination are required. In particular, a detailed neurologic evaluation including a mental status examination should be performed. To make the diagnosis of a brain tumor, contrast-enhanced computed tomography (CT) or magnetic resonance imaging (MRI) is usually performed. Of these two diagnostic studies, MRI may be more sensitive, especially when performed with high doses of gadolinium as a contrast agent. [12–15]

It is important to distinguish a metastatic lesion from a primary brain tumor, abscess, hemorrhage, or infarct. At times, a biopsy is required to establish the diagnosis.

Treatment

Unfortunately, brain metastases are associated with a poor prognosis. Untreated patients have a median survival of approximately 1 month. A variety of factors must be taken into consideration when determining the best treatment plan for an individual patient; these factors are the patient's neurologic status at the time of diagnosis, the extent of systemic disease, and the number and sites of metastases.

Patients with brain tumors who are symptomatic usually benefit from glucocorticoid therapy. Kofman and colleagues were the first to demonstrate the benefit of steroid therapy in patients with metastatic brain tumors. [16] Galicich and French introduced dexamethasone therapy as the standard treatment for tumor-associated edema, [17] and dexamethasone is currently routinely used for the treatment of patients with brain tumors. Approximately 70 to 80% of the patients with brain metastases will improve with dexamethasone therapy. [11] However, the optimal dose has not yet been determined. The usual starting dose is 10 mg orally, followed by 4 mg four times a day. [18] It should be noted that lower doses of steroids given less frequently have been demonstrated to be efficacious. [19] Patients should be treated with the smallest effective dose and for the shortest period of time. However, if the standard dose fails to produce a clinical response within 48 hours, then the dose should be doubled every 48 hours until a response occurs. At times, up to 100 mg of dexamethasone over 24 hours is required. [20]

Dexamethasone therapy offers several benefits. One benefit is the minimization of the mineralocorticoid effect; dexamethasone makes salt retention and peripheral edema less likely. In addition, dexamethasone is less likely to be associated with infection and cognitive impairment than other drugs are. [18] However, like other fluorinated steroids, dexamethasone is more likely to cause myopathy.

Patients who have a rapid clinical response to steroid therapy usually have symptoms that are related to tumor-associated edema rather than to the actual tumor mass. In particular, patients experiencing headache and lethargy are more likely to respond to steroid therapy than are individuals with focal neurologic deficits. Patients' symptoms begin to improve within hours of an intravenous injection of corticosteroids. Positron emission tomography in humans with brain tumors reveals an effect of steroids on the blood-brain barrier as early as 6 hours after an intravenous bolus. [21] Maximal clinical improvement usually occurs in 24 to 72 hours. The median survival of patients treated with steroids alone is usually 2 months.

As mentioned previously, patients with brain lesions can have associated seizures. In fact, seizures are the initial manifestation of cerebral metastases in 15 to 20% of patients, and 30 to 40% of patients will have at least one seizure during their illness. [22] Patients with cerebral metastases are most likely to have seizures of the simple or complex partial type, which are more likely to result in Todd's paralysis. [23, 24] Anticonvulsant therapy is indicated for patients with seizures from a brain tumor. Phenytoin is often chosen first; other agents commonly used are carbamazepine, phenobarbital, and valproate. Valproate is increasingly being used as a first-choice drug because it has fewer interactions with other therapies and because it may be less sedating than phenytoin. It is important to monitor the blood levels of anticonvulsants in patients with cerebral metastases because these patients are often also receiving other medications such as dexamethasone, which could cause variations in the anticonvulsant levels. For brain tumor patients without seizures, prophylactic anticonvulsant therapy has not been shown to reduce the incidence of subsequent seizures. Prophylactic anticonvulsant therapy is therefore not indicated for patients who have brain metastases and who are without a history of seizures. [23]

Radiotherapy plays a key role in the treatment of patients with brain metastases. There is a lack of consensus regarding the optimal radiation dose and schedule for these patients. The standard approach is treatment of the whole brain because two-thirds to three-fourths of patients have multiple metastases. [25] Symptoms improve in more than 80% of patients within 3 weeks of treatment.[26] The median survival of patients treated with whole-brain radiation is 3 to 6 months.

Stereotactic radiosurgery, which is a method of delivering intense focal radiation by using a linear accelerator or a gamma knife, has been used to treat metastatic brain tumors.[27,28] This type of procedure does not replace whole-brain radiotherapy but can be a substitute for surgical therapy, particularly for lesions in surgically inaccessible areas.

Because most patients with brain metastases have multiple lesions or extensive systemic cancer, surgery is not always feasible. However, for patients in whom brain metastases are the only site of metastasis or whose systemic disease is otherwise controlled, the treatment of the brain lesions may be the determining factor in the length of their survival. The best surgical results are seen in patients who have a single accessible lesion; however, surgery is occassionally performed for multiple metastases if doing so can improve the patient's quality of life and potentially affect survival.[29] In addition, surgery also benefits patients who have impending herniation due to increased intracranial pressure.

Some patients will require emergency treatment of cerebral edema to prevent herniation and possibly death. The most rapid method for decreasing a patient's intracerebral pressure is hyperventilation. Hyperventilation decreases the partial pressure of carbon dioxide (PCO_2), which results in cerebral vasoconstriction in undamaged portions of the brain and in a decrease in cerebral blood volume and intracranial pressure. The patient is intubated and ventilated to decrease the PCO_2 to 25 to 30 mm Hg. The intracranial pressure decreases within 30 seconds of lowering the PCO_2; it remains low for 15 to 20 minutes but usually returns to the original level in 1 hour.[30] Another modality for decreasing the intracerebral pressure is a hyperosmolar agent such as mannitol. A solution (20 to 25%) of mannitol may be given at a dose of 0.5 to 2.0 g/kg intravenously over 10 to 20 minutes. The effect usually begins within minutes and can persist for several hours.[31] The mode of action of hyperosmolar agents is not entirely known. It is thought that their effect is partly due to their creation of an osmotic gradient between the blood and the part of the brain with an intact blood-brain barrier, resulting in the movement of water from the brain to the site of higher osmolarity in the blood.[1] Currently, there is controversy regarding the use of hypertonic saline solution in the treatment of increased intracranial pressure. Further studies need to be performed to address the role of this agent. Diuretics, especially the loop diuretics such as furosemide (20 to 40 mg), are effective for the short-term treatment of increased intracranial pressure. Finally, dexamethasone can also help to decrease high intracranial pressure; an intravenous bolus of 40 to 100 mg of dexamethasone followed by 40 to 100 mg per day is used. If these measures fail, emergent surgery to remove the tumor and decompress the brain can be considered.

Summary

Brain metastases are the most common intracranial tumors in adults, and most are symptomatic. The most common complaints are headache and a change in mental status, with focal motor and sensory deficits. Most brain metastases are a result of hematogenous spread of cancer cells to the brain, and the majority are seen in patients with cancers of the lung, breast, skin, genitourinary tract, and gastrointestinal tract. This diagnosis should be considered in cancer patients who present with a headache, and a careful history and physical examination should be performed. To make the diagnosis, contrast-enhanced CT or MRI is usually performed. The mainstay of treatment is usually steroid therapy. If the patient has seizures, anticonvulsant therapy is warranted. An individualized treatment plan is formulated, based on the patient's neurologic status, the extent of systemic disease, and the number and sites of metastases.

CEREBROVASCULAR DISEASE

Cerebrovascular disease (CVD) is the second most common central nervous system abnormality found in cancer patients at autopsy. In an autopsy study by Graus and colleagues, CVD was present in 500 (14.6%) of 3,426 patients who died of systemic cancer. Of those 500 patients, 255 patients (51% of the patients with CVD, or 7.4% of the total autopsy series) experienced clinical symptoms related to CVD. It should be noted that the frequency of cerebral hemorrhage and the frequency of infarction were equal; however, the hemorrhages were more symptomatic.[32]

Cerebrovascular disease in cancer patients differs somewhat from CVD in noncancer patients. First, the risk factors for CVD in cancer patients are unique. The predisposing risk factors are based on the effects of the primary tumor, cancer therapies, coagulation disorders, and infections. In addition, hypertension is a rare cause of intracerebral hemorrhage in cancer patients; hypertension accounted for only 6% of such cases in the series by Graus and colleagues.[32] Furthermore, cancer patients with cerebrovascular events often present with encephalopathy instead of the acute focal neurologic signs that are usually present in noncancer patients.

Intracerebral Hemorrhage

Brain Metastasis. The most common cause of brain hemorrhages in patients with solid tumors is metastatic brain tumors.[32]

Clinical Manifestations. A patient with an intracerebral hemorrhage caused by a metastatic tumor usually has acute symptoms such as headache, nausea, vomiting, seizure, or obtundation. These symptoms are usually accompanied by focal neurologic findings that are revealed by physical examination.

Pathophysiology. A multitude of factors can contribute to intracerebral hemorrhages caused by metastatic tumors. These factors can be classified into (a) the effects of the tumor on the surrounding tissue and blood vessels, (b) the effects of tumor necrosis, and (c) the effects of the rupture of neoplastic vessels.[33]

Etiology. Hemorrhages from metastatic brain tumors have been reported in patients with many tumor types, but they are most commonly observed in patients with metastatic melanoma, lung cancer, and germ cell tumors (such as choriocarcinoma).[32,34]

Diagnosis. To make the diagnosis of intracerebral hemorrhage, noncontrast CT is usually the initial choice of study. These imaging studies usually show a multitude of hemorrhages, with early edema and enhancement adjacent to the hemorrhages. In addition, the hemorrhages are located in areas different from those in which hypertensive hemorrhages are seen.[35] Spin echo MRI is one modality that is used to distinguish neoplastic from non-neoplastic hematomas.[36] Neoplastic hematomas usually show a heterogeneous pattern of signal intensity, with delayed or atypical patterns of evolution, and they lack the well-defined complete hemosiderin rim that is visible on MRI and that is characteristic of non-neoplastic hematomas.

Treatment. Patients with intracerebral hemorrhages that are associated with metastatic brain tumors usually have a poor prognosis. A patient with a single hemorrhage may benefit from the evacuation of the hematoma (depending on its location). In such a case a neurosurgical consultation should be considered.[34,37]

Dural/Arachnoid Metastasis. *Clinical Manifestations.* A patient with a subdural hemorrhage due to a dural metastasis usually has acute symptoms such as confusion, lethargy, nausea, and vomiting. The patient is not likely to have acute focal neurologic signs; instead, the signs may develop insidiously.

Pathophysiology. Neoplastic involvement of the dura and arachnoid areas is usually due to hematogenous metastasis to those regions. Another possibility is the extension of a skull metastasis into those regions. The hemorrhage may be a tumoral hemorrhage, or it may be due to the dilatation and rupture of the capillaries of the inner dural layer caused by the obstruction of the vessels of the outer layer by a tumor.

Etiology. Subdural hemorrhages are seen in patients with cerebral dural metastases from lymphoma, leukemia (especially acute lymphocytic leukemia), or carcinoma (especially gastric and prostate carcinoma).[32,38,39]

Diagnosis. To make the diagnosis of a subdural hemorrhage, CT or MRI can be used to detect the presence of a hematoma or a skull metastasis. Histologic examination of the dural membrane or cytologic examination of the subdural fluid will be necessary to make the diagnosis if a dural metastasis is not apparent.

Treatment. Symptomatic patients may require craniotomy for evacuation of acute blood and for resection of metastases. If the disease is diffuse, radiation should be considered. Patients who are asymptomatic can be observed as their treatment proceeds. Acute or subacute blood will eventually liquify and can be drained via simple bur holes if symptoms develop.

Coagulopathy and Thrombocytopenia. *Clinical Manifestations.* A patient with an intracerebral hemorrhage resulting from a coagulopathy usually has symptoms that are acute and potentially quite severe. Symptoms include vomiting, headache, a decreased level of consciousness, and focal neurologic signs revealed at physical examination. Patients with acute disseminated intravascular coagulation (DIC) can have evidence of bleeding at other sites, such as the retina, the mucosa, the skin, and the gastrointestinal and genitourinary tracts.

Pathophysiology and Etiology. A patient with an intracerebral hemorrhage due to a coagulopathy will most commonly have leukemia.[32] Acute promyelocytic leukemia (APML) is frequently associated with intracerebral hemorrhage as a complication of acute DIC.[40] This usually occurs after the beginning of cancer treatment. In the other types of leukemia, an intracerebral hemorrhage may be associated with DIC, but the hemorrhage occurs at relapse or with the failure to induce a complete remission. In the series by Graus and colleagues, thrombocytopenia and sepsis were present in all leukemia patients who had subdural hematomas, with or without DIC. This was in contrast to the few carcinoma patients in the study, who had a subdural hematoma with a coagulopathy.[32]

In a small percentage of patients with leukemia, especially newly diagnosed patients with acute myelogenous leukemia, an intracerebral hemorrhage is associated with hyperleukocytosis (a white blood count above 100,000). Intracerebral hemorrhages due to hyperleukocytosis have been declining because of more effective treatment of this disease.

Diagnosis and Treatment. A diagnosis can be based on CT or MRI of the brain, which can reveal evidence of single or multiple parenchymal hemorrhages.

For patients who develop a cerebral hemorrhage from coagulopathy, treatment should be focused on controlling the tumor, the coagulopathy, and any other conditions that may be contributing factors. The incidence of intracerebral hemorrhages in APML can be reduced with prophylactic heparin, chemotherapy,[41,42] and all-trans retinoic acid.[43]

Cerebral Infarction

When a patient with cancer has a cerebral infarction, there are several possible etiologies to consider. In the autopsy series performed by Graus and colleagues,[32] atherosclerosis was found to be the most common cause of cerebral infarction in cancer patients. The most commonly associated malignancies with atherosclerotic brain infarctions are of the lung and the head and neck. However, these represented only 14.5% of the symptomatic infarctions in that study.[32]

Direct Effects of Tumor. *Clinical Manifestations.* Patients who have a tumor-related cerebral infarction can have a variety of symptoms. For example, a patient with a metastatic superior sagittal sinus occlusion can have subacute symptoms such as headache, vomiting, or papilledema. In contrast, a patient with a cerebral infarction due to tumor embolism can have an abrupt onset of focal symptoms or seizures.

Pathophysiology. A patient can have a cerebral infarction from the direct effect of a tumor as a result of any of the following three mechanisms: leptomeningeal metastasis, a tumor embolism to the brain, or a venous occlusion due to a dural or skull tumor that is compressing or infiltrating the sinus, which would result in thrombosis and stasis.

Etiology. Patients with cerebral infarctions caused by a tumor embolism usually have solid tumors with lung or cardiac metastasis. Metastatic venous occlusion can occur with a variety of tumors but occurs most commonly in patients with lung cancer, lymphoma, and neuroblastoma.[32,44]

Diagnosis and Treatment. Computed tomography or MRI of the brain is usually required to make the diagnosis of a tumor-related cerebral infarction.

The treatment of metastatic superior sagittal sinus occlusion is brain irradiation and corticosteroids. When sagittal sinus occlusion is due to coagulopathy, heparin use is controversial due to fears of extending the hemorrhages associated with venous infarction. Recent clinical evidence supports the use of endovascular thrombolytic therapies.[45–47]

Treatment-Related Cerebral Infarction. Cancer patients who are receiving therapy can experience cerebral infarction when the therapy results in a coagulopathy or in direct toxicity to the intra- or extracranial cerebral vessels.

Clinical Manifestations. Patients can have a variety of central nervous system manifestations, such as those that are classic for an infarction or a transient ischemic attack. These patients can also have seizures.

Pathophysiology. The mechanism of chemotherapy-related complications is not well understood. Possible causes of cerebral thrombosis include vasospasm, endothelial cell damage, and coagulation abnormalities. Radiation therapy has been thought to produce or to accelerate the development of atherosclerosis, as described in more detail below.

Etiology. An association between the administration of chemotherapy and the occurrence of cerebrovascular events has been observed. For example, systemic, cerebral venous, and arterial thromboembolic complications were observed in women who were receiving multiagent chemotherapy for breast cancer.[48] An association between cerebral infarction and combination chemotherapy containing cisplatin has also been noted.[49,50] In addition, leukemia patients who are receiving induction therapy with L-asparaginase may experience cerebral infarction or cerebral venous thrombosis.[51] Finally, patients who develop a cardiomyopathy from doxorubicin (Adriamycin) are predisposed to the development of ventricular mural thrombi that can embolize and cause a cerebral infarction.[44,52]

An association between radiation therapy and the development of carotid artery disease has been noted.[53,54] The time between the administration of radiation and the development of carotid artery disease can vary considerably. A recent review by Murros and Toole[55] reported a range of 6 months to 57 years between radiation therapy and the development of extracranial vascular disease.[55]

Diagnosis and Treatment. Given the appropriate clinical setting, angiography can suggest the diagnosis as radiation vasculopathy which often involves a longer segment of the vessel and a more distinct margin at the edges of the irradiated field than does atherosclerosis.

The ideal treatment for patients with radiation-induced carotid disease is not known. At this time, no prospective medical trials have been reported. The favorable performance of endarterectomy in a small number of patients has been reported, but it was technically difficult.[56]

Nonbacterial Thrombotic Endocarditis. In the study performed by Graus and colleagues, the most common cause of symptomatic cerebral infarction in cancer patients was nonbacterial thrombotic endocarditis.[32]

Clinical Manifestations. Patients with nonbacterial thrombotic endocarditis usually have neurologic symptoms that are focal and that begin abruptly. A common symptom is aphasia. The neurologic deficits are usually progressive, but recovery can occur between episodes.[57,58]

Pathophysiology. Nonbacterial thrombotic endocarditis is a result of the formation of platelet-fibrin vegetations that develop on cardiac valves and other large and medium-sized arteries. Cerebral vessels are occluded as a result of the embolization of cardiac vegetations to the brain. In addition, occlusion of the cerebral vessels can be a result of the associated coagulation disorder. With thrombotic endocarditis, small or medium-sized cerebral vessels are occluded more often than large vessels. As a result, patients have cerebral infarctions that are multiple and that can be hemorrhagic.

Etiology. Nonbacterial thrombotic endocarditis occurs most commonly in patients with adenocarcinomas (especially of the lung or gastrointestinal tract). It usually occurs in patients with widely disseminated cancer, but it can also occur at any stage, and it can be the first sign of malignancy.

Diagnosis and Treatment. It can be a challenge to make the diagnosis of nonbacterial thrombotic endocarditis. Patients can present with a variety of symptoms, such as neurologic changes, evidence of systemic bleeding, or thromboembolism. It is rare for patients to have a new or changing cardiac murmur, and echocardiography is usually not helpful. Computed tomography or MRI of the brain will reveal evidence of cerebral infarction, but cerebral angiography is the most specific test for patients with focal neurologic symptoms.

The therapy for nonbacterial thrombotic endocarditis should be focused on the cause of the coagulation disorder, such as the tumor or an infectious process. There have been no prospective studies evaluating the use of anticoagulation therapy.

Intravascular Coagulation. The second most common cause of symptomatic cerebral infarction in patients with cancer is thrombotic occlusion of cerebral vessels as a result of a coagulopathy.[32]

Clinical Manifestations. The neurologic symptoms usually begin abruptly and commonly produce a diffuse encephalopathy. In approximately one-half of patients, focal neurologic signs are also present, but these signs are often transient.[59] The clinical course is often progressive, and there may be fluctuations in the patient's neurologic status.

Pathophysiologic Mechanisms. Cerebral intravascular coagulation is thought to result most likely from a chronic form of DIC. The neuropathologic findings are cerebral arterial, arteriolar, capillary, and/or venular occlusion by fibrin, with adjacent microinfarction or petechiae. Often, multiple vessels in more than one major vessel territory are thrombosed.

Etiology. This disorder occurs most commonly in patients with leukemia, breast cancer, and lymphoma.[44,52,59] It is usually seen in the setting of advanced cancer and sepsis.

Diagnosis and Treatment. Diagnosing this disorder can be quite challenging. There is no definitive laboratory test. The only way to make a definite diagnosis is to confirm the diagnosis at autopsy.

The appropriate treatment of this disorder is unknown. Usually, patients with this disorder have a very poor prognosis, and they live only a few weeks. They usually die as a result of bleeding, sepsis, and disseminated cancer.

SPINAL-CORD COMPRESSION

Spinal-cord compression is one of the most common reasons for emergency neurologic consultation in cancer patients.[60] The vast majority of patients with spinal-cord compression present with back pain as their chief complaint, which is unfortunate because back pain is a common acute problem, and its symptoms are often nondescript. Intervention prior to the development of signs of neurologic dysfunction affords the best outcome in patients with epidural spinal-cord compression from a malignancy. Therefore, any cancer patient who has back pain deserves a thoughtful evaluation, given the consequences of a late diagnosis of epidural spinal-cord compression.

Clinical Manifestations and Etiology

As stated previously, back pain is the most common symptom of epidural spinal-cord compression, and patients often have back pain for many months prior to a proper evaluation. Patients or their caregivers often minimize the symptoms, as back pain is common and is frequently dismissed as minor trauma or arthritis. Such delay is particularly unfortunate because treatment prior to developing incontinence or the inability to walk is the most important variable in a successful outcome.[61–64] Pain that worsens on recumbence is unusual in degenerative disk disease and should raise the concern that the patient has an epidural metastasis. Patients may have difficulty localizing their pain, especially when the pain is severe, so analgesics should be prescribed generously.

Direct metastasis to the spinal cord is uncommon, and most cases of cord compression result from metastasis to vertebral bodies or adjacent structures. Palpation and percussion along the vertebral column frequently help to localize metastatic deposits. Paravertebral masses such as those occurring in lung cancer, retroperitoneal sarcoma, and lymphoma may grow along nerve roots and follow them into the spinal canal, with little if any involvement of the surrounding bones. Lung, prostate, and breast cancers are the most common primary tumors causing epidural spinal-cord compression, but any type of malignancy can be responsible.

Ending at the lower thoracic or upper lumbar vertebral region, the spinal cord is much shorter than the spinal canal. The thoracic spine is the most common site of vertebral-body metastasis,[65] and unfortunately, the thoracic cord's blood supply is precarious, being both prone to atherosclerotic disease and highly variable in its anatomy.[66] Pain from spinal-cord compression arises less from spinal-cord injury and much more from the disturbance of the adjacent nerve roots. As the spinal cord ends before reaching the lumbar nerve roots, leg and buttock pains cannot be symptoms of spinal-cord compression although they frequently prompt urgent consultation to rule out cord compression. Metastasis to a thoracic vertebral body produces less compelling symptoms than does metastasis to cervical or lumbar vertebral bodies, but thoracic metastasis is far more dangerous because, in addition to the region's vulnerable blood supply, the width of the thoracic spinal canal relative to the width of the cord is the smallest among the three areas.

Ironically, the thoracic spine (which harbors most vertebral-body metastases and which has the greatest predilection for myelopathy) has nerve roots that are small, forming the intercostal nerves whose injury causes relatively innocuous symptoms. Bandlike paresthesias (sometimes described by the patient as a feeling of being "squeezed, like a belt being pulled tight" or as a "band of numbness about my waist") are a particularly ominous sign of epidural spinal-cord compression. As vertebral-body metastases are often multiple and as patients complain only about the most painful areas of bone disease, clinicians should specifically question patients about these symptoms even when the chief complaint is pain that is referable to the legs.

Patients' sensory levels should be checked ventrally and dorsally. This is best accomplished by using the wood from a broken cotton swab, which is less threatening and more hygienic than a pin. A metal tuning fork may be more useful than a pin for testing a patient's sensitivity to cold. Vibration levels over bone prominences can be tested as well, but these thick dorsal columns may be more resistant to compressive myelopathy than other tracts are. Sensory testing requires concentration on the part of the patient and patience on the part of the examiner. Sensory testing is very unreliable when patients are in pain and should be done while the patient is relaxed and comfortable.

Leg ataxia may be present before weakness arises in patients with epidural spinal cord compression and may even occur without pain.[67] Using a standardized strength scale (Table 12–1) at the initial evaluation greatly aids in monitoring the clinical course of the patient's disease. Each muscle group should be tested separately, and the results from each side of the body should be compared.[68] Rectal sphincter tone should be checked in all patients suspected of having epidural spinal-cord compression. Patients who are immunosuppressed or at risk for bleeding can be safely tested by placing a cotton-wrapped examining finger adjacent to but not in the anal meatus and having the patient gently squeeze on it. Observing the umbilical movement while the recumbent patient flexes his or her head forward against resistance helps in detecting lower thoracic nerve root dysfunction. The umbilicus may move caudad if the root dysfunction is above T10 and cephalad if involvement is below T10 (Beevor's sign).

Babinski's sign is sensitive and specific evidence of corticospinal-tract dysfunction, but the interpretation of this valuable sign requires experience. While most clinicians observe the great toe's movement during noxious stimulation along the lateral aspect of the bottom of the foot, the movement of the four smaller toes is a more reliable indicator. As Babinski observed, "The toes, instead of flexing, develop an extension movement at the metatarsal joint."[69] Checking for the presence of Babinski's sign should be done at the end of the examination, and the patient should be warned that the maneuver will be unpleasant.

Pathophysiologic Mechanisms

"Epidural spinal-cord compression" is a pathophysiologic misnomer. Normally, venous blood from the spinal cord drains into a venous plexus within the overlaying vertebral bodies. When a tumor invades these vertebral bodies, however, it induces inflammatory mediators within the bone and soft tissues, which causes venous stasis.[70] Animal models demonstrate that obliteration of the vertebral venous plexus occurs early in epidural spinal-cord compression and is followed by diminished spinal-cord blood flow owing to venous stasis, which is worsened by mechanical compression.[71,72]

Diagnosis

Magnetic resonance imaging is the best method for evaluating epidural spinal cord compression. The study takes

TABLE 12–1. Medical Research Council Muscle Testing Scale

Grade	Criterion
0	No contraction
1	Flicker or trace of contraction
2	Active movement, with gravity eliminated
3	Active movement against gravity
4	Active movement against gravity and resistance*
5	Normal power

Adapted from Medical Research Counil of the UK.[68]
*Grades 4–, 4, and 4+ may be used to indicate movement against slight, moderate, and strong resistance, respectively.

about 45 minutes to complete and requires the patient to fit into the scanner, lie flat, and be absolutely still. Open scanners can accommodate larger patients and those who are claustrophobic, but these scanners are not widely available, and they deliver suboptimal (but usually adequate) images. Myelography, when performed by an experienced physician and coupled with CT, can be done on any patient, with relatively little discomfort. This technique yields cerebrospinal fluid and takes very little time, but in cases in which metastatic disease completely blocks the spinal cord, myelography will not define the upper margin of tumor involvement, and further imaging studies will be necessary.

Treatment

Corticosteroid therapy should be commenced upon suspicion of malignant epidural spinal-cord compression. Dexamethasone is extremely well absorbed from the gut and has a half-life of more than 36 hours, but most patients are started with a high (100 mg) intravenous bolus dose and are then placed on a maintenance dose (16 mg every 6 hours) for the first few days. This concurs with widely used treatment protocols,[63,73] but other studies suggest that much lower doses are equally effective and are less likely to cause toxic effects.[74,75] As steroid toxicity relates to the total dose given as well as to the duration of therapy,[76] administering a bolus of 10 to 40 mg of dexamethasone followed by maintenance doses of 12 to 24 mg a day in 4 divided doses is a reasonable alternative. After a few days, this can be changed to a less toxic twice-a-day schedule. Careful clinical follow-up is essential, and the steroid dose should be increased if symptoms do not improve. Gastrointestinal hemorrhage is a common side effect of steroid therapy and should be treated with antacid therapy. A less well-known but more serious complication is lower-intestinal perforation, which can be minimized by preventing the patient from becoming constipated.

Epidural spinal-cord compression has also been treated with surgical decompression,[77] resection of the vertebral body and stabilization,[78] radiation therapy,[64] and systemic cytoreductive therapy.[79] All therapeutic decisions must take into account the state of the patient's systemic disease because epidural spinal-cord compression frequently occurs at an advanced stage of the patient's illness. Anterior vertebral-body resection with stabilization may offer the best chance for a good outcome, but the procedure is a major undertaking and requires (1) a patient with a good performance status, (2) uninvolved adjacent vertebral bodies for stabilization of the spinal canal, and (3) a skilled neurosurgical team. Surgery should particularly be considered for cases in which the cause of the compression is in doubt, the tumor is insensitive to radiation (especially if there is a paraspinal mass),[80] the involved segment has already been irradiated, or there is mechanical instability of the spinal canal. Even patients with advanced disease and a limited life expectancy can benefit from prompt therapy when it is appropriate to their circumstances.[81]

Summary

Epidural spinal-cord compression is a common problem in emergency centers and requires skilled early management and the coordination of a multidisciplinary effort. Remarkably, most cases present on Fridays,[82] which only adds to the difficulty of marshaling the appropriate diagnostic and treatment forces. This is particularly frustrating because few conditions are as amenable to clinical improvement if managed expeditiously, and few conditions have consequences as serious if unrecognized or managed inappropriately.

REFERENCES

1. Posner JB. Management of brain metastases. Rev Neurol (Paris) 1992;148:477–87.
2. Lesser GJ, Grossman S. The chemotherapy of high-grade astrocytomas. Semin Oncol 1994;21:220–35.
3. Posner JB. Brain metastases: 1995. A brief review. J Neurooncol 1996;27:287–93.
4. Swenson KK, Rose MA, Ritz L, et al. Recognition and evaluation of oncology-related symptoms in the emergency department. Ann Emerg Med 1995;26:12–7.
5. Cairncross JG, Posner JB. The management of brain metastases. In: Walker MD, editor. Oncology of the nervous system. Boston: Martinus Nijhoff; 1983. p. 341–77.
6. Posner JB. Clinical manifestations of brain metastasis. In: Weiss L, Gilbert HA, Posner A, editors. Brain metastasis. Boston: GK Hall; 1980. p. 189–207.
7. Wen PY. Diagnosis and management of brain tumors. In: Black PM, Loeffer JS, editors. Cancer of the nervous system. Cambridge: Blackwell Science; 1997. p. 106.
8. Forsyth P, Posner JB. Headaches in patients with brain tumors. A study of 111 patients. Neurology 1993;43:1678–83.
9. Posner JB. Brain metastases. In: Neurologic complications of cancer. Philadelphia: F.A. Davis; 1995. p. 80.
10. Delattre JY, Krol G, Thaler HT, et al. Distribution of brain metastases. Arch Neurol 1988;45:741–4.
11. Schiff D, Batchelor T, Wen PY. Neurologic emergencies in cancer patients. Neurol Clin 1998;16:449–83.
12. Tsukada Y, Fouad A, Pickren JW, Lane WW. Central nervous system metastasis from breast carcinoma: autopsy study. Cancer 1983;52:2349–54.
13. Runge VM, Kirsch JE, Burke VJ, et al. High dose gadoteridol in MR imaging of intracranial neoplasms. J Magn Reson Imaging 1992:2:9–18.
14. Akeson P, Larsson EM, Kristofferson DT, et al. Brain metastases: comparison of gadodiamide injection-enhanced MR imaging at standard and high dose, contrast-enhanced CT, and non-contrast-enhanced MR imaging. Acta Radiol 1995;36:300–6.
15. Yuh WT, Fisher DJ, Runge VM, et al. Phase III multicenter

trial of high-dose gadoteridol in MR evaluation of brain metastasis. Am J Neuroradiol 1994;15:1037–51.

16. Kofman S, Garvin JS, Nagamani D, et al. Treatment of cerebral metastases from breast carcinoma with prednisolone. JAMA 1957;163:1473.

17. Galicich JH, French LA. Use of dexamethasone in the treatment of cerebral edema resulting from brain tumors and brain surgery. Am Pract Dig Treatment 1961;12:169–74.

18. Fishman RA. Cerebrospinal fluid in diseases of the nervous system. 2nd ed. Philadelphia: W.B. Saunders; 1992.

19. Weissman DE, Janjan NA, Erickson B, et al. Twice-daily tapering dexamethasone treatment during cranial radiation for newly diagnosed brain metastases. J Neurooncol 1991;11:235–9.

20. Lieberman A, Le Brun Y, Glass P, et al. Use of high-dose corticosteroids in patients with inoperable brain tumors. J Neurol Neurosurg Psychiatry 1977;40:678–82.

21. Jarden JO, Dhawan V, Moeller JR, et al. The time course of steroid action on blood-to-brain and blood-to-tumor transport of 82Rb: a positron emission tomographic study. Ann Neurol 1989;25:239–45.

22. Cohen N, Strauss G, Lew R, et al. Should prophylactic anticonvulsants be administered to patients with newly diagnosed cerebral metastases? A retrospective analysis. J Clin Oncol 1988;6:1621–4.

23. Posner JB. Neurologic complications of cancer. Philadelphia: F.A. Davis Co; 1995.

24. Weaver S, DeAngelis LM, Fulton D, et al. A prospective, randomized study of prophylactic anticonvulsants in patients with primary brain tumors or metastatic brain tumors and without prior seizures. Ann Neurol 1997;42:430.

25. Goodheart RS, Patchell RA. Management of brain metastases. In: Wiley RG, editor. Neurological complications of cancer. New York: Marcel Dekker Inc; 1995. p. 1–21.

26. Hoskin PJ, Crow J, Ford HT. The influence of extent and local management on the outcome of radiotherapy for brain metastases. Int J Radiat Oncol Biol Phys 1990;19:111–5.

27. Leksell L. Steriotactic radiosurgery. J Neurol Neurosurg Psychiatry 1983;46:797–803.

28. Liltz W, Winston KR, Maliki PV. A system for sterotactic radiosurgery with a linear acceleration. Int J Radiat Oncol Biol Phys 1988;14:373–81.

29. Bindal RK, Sawaya R, Leavens ME, et al. Surgical treatment of multiple brain metastasis. J Neurosurg 1993;79:210–6.

30. Ropper AH. Neurological and neurosurgical intensive care. 3rd ed. New York: Raven; 1993.

31. Ropper AH. Raised intracranial pressure in neurologic disease. Semin Neurol 1984;4;397.

32. Graus F, Rogers LR, Posner JB. Cerebrovascular complications in patients with cancer. Medicine 1985;64:16–35.

33. Kondziolka D, Bernstein M, Resch L, et al. Significance of hemorrhage into brain tumors: clinicopathological study. J Neurosurg 1987;67:852–7.

34. Mandybur TI. Intracranial hemorrhage caused by metastatic tumors. Neurology 1977;27:650–5.

35. Bitoh S, Hasegawa H, Ohtsuki H, et al. Cerebral neoplasms initially presenting with massive intracerebral hemorrhage. Surg Neurol 1984;22:57–62.

36. Atlas SW, Grossman RI, Gomori JM, et al. Hemorrhagic intracranial malignant neoplasms: spin-echo MR imaging. Radiology 1987;164:71–7.

37. Little JR, Dial B, Belanger G, et al. Brain hemorrhage from intracranial tumor. Stroke 1979;10:283–8.

38. Belmusto L, Rogelson W, Owens G, et al. Intracranial extracerebral hemorrhages in acute lymphocytic leukemia. Cancer 1964;8:1079.

39. Pitner SE, Johnson WW. Chronic subdural hematoma in childhood acute leukemia. Cancer 1973;32:185–90.

40. Freireich EJ, Thomas LB, Frei E, et al. A distinctive type of intracerebral hemorrhage associated with "blastic crisis" in patients with leukemia. Cancer 1978;41:2484.

41. Drapkin RL, Gee TS, Dowling MD, et al. Prophylactic heparin therapy in acute promyelocytic leukemia. Cancer 1978;41:2484–90.

42. Gralnick HR, Bagley J, Abrell E. Heparin treatment for hemorrhagic diathesis of acute promyelocytic leukemia. Am J Med 1972;52:167–74.

43. Castaigne S, Chomienne C, Daniel MT, et al. All-trans retinoic acid as a differentiation therapy for acute promyelocytic leukemia: I, clinical results. Blood 1990;76:1704–9.

44. Packer RJ, Rorke LB, Large BJ, et al. Cerebrovascular accidents in children with cancer. Pediatrics 1985;76:194–201.

45. Chow K, Gobin YP, Saver J, et al. Endovascular treatment of dural sinus thrombosis with rheolytic thrombectomy and intra-arterial thrombolysis. Stroke 2000;31:1420–5.

46. Hsu FP, Kuether T, Nesbit G, et al. Dural sinus thrombosis endovascular therapy. Crit Care Clin 1999;15:743–53.

47. Philips MF, Bagley LJ, Sinson GP, et al. Endovascular thrombolysis for symptomatic cerebral venous thrombosis. J Neurosurg 1999;90:65–71.

48. Wall JG, Weiss RB, Norton L, et al. Arterial thrombosis associated with adjuvant chemotherapy for breast carcinoma. A cancer and leukemia Group B study. Am J Med 1989;87:501–4.

49. Doll DC, List AF, Greco FA, et al. Acute vascular ischemic events after cisplatin-based combination chemotherapy for germ-cell tumors of the testis. Ann Intern Med 1986;105:48–51.

50. Kukla LJ, McGuire WP, Lad T, et al. Acute vascular episode associated with therapy for carcinomas of the upper aerodigestive tract with bleomycin, vincristine, and cisplatin. Cancer Treat Rep 1982;66:369–70.

51. Feinberg WM, Swenson MR. Cerebrovascular complications of L-asparaginase therapy. Neurology 1988;38:127–33.

52. Schachter S, Freeman R. Transient ischemic attack and Adriamycin cardiomyopathy. Neurology 1982;32:1380–1.

53. Carmody BJ, Arora S, Avena R, et al. Accelerated carotid artery disease after high-dose head and neck radiotherapy: is there a role for routine carotid duplex surveillance? J Vasc Surg 1999;30:1045–51.

54. Lam WW, Leung SF, So NM, et al. Incidence of carotid stenosis in nasopharyngeal carcinoma patients after radiotherapy. Cancer 2001;92:2357–63.

55. Murros KE, Toole JF. The effect of radiation on carotid arteries. Arch Neurol 1989;46:449–55.

56. Atkinson JLD, Sundt TM, Dale AJ, et al. Radiation-associated atheromatous disease of the cervical carotid artery: report of seven cases and review of the literature. Neurosurgery 1989;24:171–8.

57. Reagan TJ, Okazaki H. The thrombotic syndrome associated with carcinoma. A clinical and neuropathologic study. Arch Neurol 1974;31:390–5.

58. Rogers LR, Cho ES, Kengsin S, et al. Cerebral infarction from nonbacterial thrombotic endocarditis. Am J Med 1987;83:746–56.

59. Collins RC, Al-Mondhiry H, Chernik NL, et al. Neurologic manifestations of intravascular coagulation in patients with cancer. Neurology 1975;25:795–806.

60. Quinn JA, DeAngelis LM. Neurologic emergencies in the cancer patient. Semin Oncol 2000;27:311–21.

61. Sundaresan N, Sachdev VP, Holland JF, et al. Surgical treatment of spinal cord compression from epidural metastasis. J Clin Oncol 1995;13:2330–5.

62. Makris A, Kunkler IH. The Barthel Index in assessing the response to palliative radiotherapy in malignant spinal cord compression: a prospective audit. Clin Oncol (R Coll Radiol) 1995;7:82–6.

63. Greenberg HS, Kim JH, Posner JB. Epidural spinal cord compression from metastatic tumor: results with a new treatment protocol. Ann Neurol 1980;8:361–6.

64. Janjan NA. Radiotherapeutic management of spinal metastases. J Pain Symptom Manage 1996;11:47–56.

65. Constans JP, de Divitiis E, Donzelli R, et al. Spinal metastases with neurological manifestations: review of 600 cases. J Neurosurg 1983;59:111–8.

66. Crock HV, Yoshizawa H. The blood supply of the vertebral column and spinal cord in man. Chicago: R.R. Donnelly and Sons; 1977.

67. Hainline B, Tuszynski MH, Posner JB. Ataxia in epidural spinal cord compression. Neurology 1992;42:2193–5.

68. Medical Research Council of the UK. Aids to the investigation of peripheral nerve injuries. Memorandum No. 45. London: Pendragon House; 1976.

69. Babinski J. Sur le réflexe cutané plantaire dans certaines affection organiques du système nerveux central. C R Soc Biol 1896;48:207–8.

70. Ikeda H, Ushio Y, Hayakawa T, et al. Edema and circulatory disturbance in the spinal cord compressed by epidural neoplasms in rabbits. J Neurosurg 1980;52:203–9.

71. Kato A, Ushio Y, Hayakawa T, et al. Circulatory disturbance of the spinal cord with epidural neoplasm in rats. J Neurosurg 1985;63:260–5.

72. Siegal T. Serotonergic manipulations in experimental neoplastic spinal cord compression. J Neurosurg 1993; 78:929–37.

73. Sorensen S, Helweg-Larsen S, Mouridsen H, et al. Effect of high-dose dexamethasone in carcinomatous metastatic spinal cord compression treated with radiotherapy: a randomized trial. Eur J Cancer 1994;30A: 22–7.

74. Vecht CJ, Haaxma-Reiche H, van Putten WL, et al. Initial bolus of conventional versus high-dose dexamethasone in metastatic spinal cord compression. Neurology 1989;39:1255–7.

75. Heimdal K, Hirschberg H, Slettebo H, et al. High incidence of serious side effects of high-dose dexamethasone treatment in patients with epidural spinal cord compression. J Neurooncol 1992;12:141–4.

76. Weissman DE, Dufer D, Vogel V, et al. Corticosteroid toxicity in neuro-oncology patients. J Neurooncol 1987;5: 125–8.

77. Young RF, Post EM, King GA. Treatment of spinal epidural metastases. Randomized prospective comparison of laminectomy and radiotherapy. J Neurosurg 1980;53:741–8.

78. Sucher E, Margulies JY, Floman Y, et al. Prognostic factors in anterior decompression for metastatic cord compression. An analysis of results. Euro Spine J 1994;3:70–5.

79. Pashankar FD, Steinbok P, Blair G, et al. Successful chemotherapeutic decompression of primary endodermal sinus tumor presenting with severe spinal cord compression. J Pediatr Hematol Oncol 2001;23:170–3.

80. Kim RY, Smith JW, Spencer SA, et al. Malignant epidural spinal cord compression associated with a paravertebral mass: its radiotherapeutic outcome on radiosensitivity. Int J Radiat Oncol Biol Phys 1993;27:1079–83.

81. Ingham J, Beveridge A, Cooney NJ. The management of spinal cord compression in patients with advanced malignancy. J Pain Symptom Manage 1993;8:1–6.

82. Poortmans P, Vulto A, Raaijmakers E. Always on a Friday? Time pattern of referral for spinal cord compression. Acta Oncol 2001;40:88–91.

Chapter 13

Nephrologic and Urologic Emergencies

Erik K. Johnson, MD
Adam D. Klotz, MD
Anjali A. Vaze, MD
Venera Grasso, MD

ACUTE RENAL FAILURE

Acute renal failure (ARF) occurs when renal function deteriorates over a period of hours to days, causing the retention of nitrogenous waste products and the inability of the kidneys to maintain fluid and electrolyte balance. It is a complex syndrome for which many causes have been identified. Acute renal failure is identified in 1% of patients upon admission to the hospital, occurs in 2 to 5% of patients during hospitalization, and has a frequency as high as 4 to 15% after cardiopulmonary bypass, but the incidence among oncology patients as a subset is not well characterized.[1–3]

Acute renal failure may be classified into three categories, according to etiology: prerenal, intrinsic, and postrenal. Each differs in its pathogenesis, clinical presentation, evaluation, and management. This text focuses on ARF related to cancer and cancer treatment.

Etiology and Pathophysiology

Prerenal Renal Failure. Prerenal renal failure, the most common cause of ARF, results from a decrease in renal perfusion. Numerous conditions may impair renal blood flow, including hypovolemia, hypotension, heart disease, liver disease, and localized renal ischemia. If the underlying disorder is treated expeditiously, so that the kidneys do not sustain prolonged hypoperfusion, renal parenchymal tissue should not be damaged, and the ARF may be reversed.[1–3]

Hypovolemia, an effective drop in circulatory volume, may result from acute hemorrhage or dehydration. The latter is especially common in patients with cancer and is one of the most common reasons they present to emergency departments. Dehydration may occur for several reasons, including inadequate fluid intake, excessive fluid loss from the gastrointestinal or urinary tract, and third-spacing of fluid in body cavities. Many chemotherapeutic agents (most notably carboplatin, carmustine, cisplatin, cyclophosphamide, cytarabine, dacarbazine, doxorubicin, ifosfamide, mechlorethamine, melphalan, and thiotepa) can cause intractable nausea and vomiting. Further, apathy or loss of appetite in patients with cancer may limit their ability to replenish fluids orally. Doxorubicin, 5-fluorouracil, and methotrexate may cause severe mucositis, resulting in decreased oral intake, and irinotecan and 5-fluorouracil frequently cause severe diarrhea. Other causes of gastrointestinal fluid loss include radiation therapy (which may cause mucositis, emesis, and enteritis), bowel obstruction due to adhesions from prior surgery or from abdominal metastases, and infectious gastroenteritis. Peritoneal carcinomatosis can cause ascites, which may decrease the functional intravascular volume due to third-spacing of fluid. Urinary fluid loss may occur in patients who are taking diuretics or may result from osmotic diuresis in uncontrolled diabetes (as may be seen, for example, in patients receiving prednisone for lymphoma or patients with central nervous system metastases taking dexamethasone).

Hypotension may result from hemorrhage, severe dehydration, cardiac ischemia, sepsis, and the adverse effects of certain medications. Patients with cancer are at increased risk for sepsis due to neutropenia from myelosuppressive chemotherapy. The incidence of ARF in patients with sepsis is high: 19% for patients with sepsis, 23% for those with severe sepsis, and 51% for those in septic shock. In sepsis, cytokine activation causes systemic vasodilatation and (variably) renal arteriolar vasoconstriction, resulting in renal hypoperfusion. Inflammatory mediators and products of neutrophil activation may cause capillary leak and direct damage to renal parenchyma.[4,5] Additionally, interleukin-2, which is used as immunotherapy for advanced renal cell carcinoma and melanoma, may cause capillary leak and prerenal ARF.[6]

Congestive heart failure (CHF) may occur in the setting of pre-existing cardiac disease or as the result of cardiomyopathy related to anthracycline-based chemotherapy. Decreased cardiac output results in the activation of the sympathetic nervous system and the renin-angiotensin-aldosterone axis as the body attempts to maintain systemic blood pressure and renal perfusion through vasoconstriction and sodium retention.[2,7] In severe CHF, however, these mechanisms do not adequately maintain cardiac output, and renal blood flow decreases. The glomerular filtration rate (GFR) declines, and prerenal azotemia results. Additionally, medications used in the treatment of CHF, such as diuretics and angiotensin-converting enzyme inhibitors, may worsen renal blood flow and lead to renal failure.[2,7] Nonsteroidal anti-inflammatory drugs (NSAIDs), many of which are available without a prescription and often are not mentioned by patients during the emergency-room history, inhibit prostaglandin synthesis. In patients with CHF, this loss of prostaglandin-mediated vasodilation results in unopposed systemic vasoconstriction by angiotensin II, thereby decreasing GFR and worsening renal function.[2,8]

Liver disease related to cirrhosis (due, for example, to chronic viral or alcoholic hepatitis or as a late side effect of intrahepatic arterial chemotherapy infusion for liver metastases from gastrointestinal adenocarcinomas) or metastatic deposits often results in increased hepatic sinusoidal pressure, portal hypertension, and ascites, which may decrease intravascular volume and thereby lead to prerenal renal failure. With advanced liver disease, a progressive decline in renal function may result in hepatorenal syndrome and worsened renal function. The exact mechanism of this process is unclear but is thought to involve renal vasoconstriction.[2,9]

Intrinsic Renal Failure. The etiology of intrinsic renal failure is identified by the primary site of injury in the kidney, namely, the tubules, the interstitium, or the glomerulus.

Injury to the tubules, or acute tubular necrosis (ATN), is due to either ischemia or nephrotoxic agents. The most common causes of ischemic ATN in patients with cancer are dehydration and sepsis, both of which are seen frequently in the emergency setting. As the underlying hypovolemia increases the risk of ATN, caution must be exercised when administering certain nephrotoxic diagnostic and therapeutic agents to these patients.[1,2] Radiographic contrast, for example, may cause renal vasoconstriction, which may in turn worsen ischemia in the medullary portion of the kidney in the setting of hypovolemia.[2,10]

Aminoglycosides, the most common cause of antibiotic nephrotoxicity, cause necrosis of tubular cells.[2,11] Acute tubular necrosis occurs in up to 20% of patients receiving these agents and is directly correlated with the dosage and duration of therapy.[12] Amphotericin B results in some degree of renal dysfunction in up to 80% of patients; the mechanism includes both renal vasoconstriction and direct tubular injury.[13,14] Both acyclovir and sulfonamides (particularly sulfamethoxazole and sulfadiazine) may crystallize in renal tubules and cause ATN, especially in states of volume depletion.[2,15,16] Vancomycin produces mild renal impairment in up to 15% of patients and can potentiate the nephrotoxic effects of agents like aminoglycosides when these agents are given concurrently.[2,17] Foscarnet, used to treat resistant *Cytomegalovirus* infections, causes a rise in creatinine in up to two-thirds of patients, possibly through a direct toxic effect on renal tubules.[18]

Several chemotherapeutic agents are known to cause ATN. Cisplatin is a direct tubular toxin, damaging primarily the proximal tubule and causing magnesium wasting. Up to 35% of patients may experience mild renal dysfunction that is partially reversible after the first cycle of cisplatin. Upon repeated administration, however, renal function may decline further and become irreversible.[2,19,20] Ifosfamide is also toxic to proximal tubular cells. It generally results in only mild renal dysfunction when given alone, but coadministration with other nephrotoxins may be synergistic.[2,21] Methotrexate can form crystals in renal tubules when given in high doses; the resultant renal failure is usually reversible.[22]

Multiple myeloma causes tubulointerstitial renal impairment in several ways. The filtration of light chains and cast formation can lead to tubular destruction, known as myeloma kidney. Amyloid and light-chain deposition may also occur and lead to renal failure, and hypercalcemia (which occurs commonly in patients with myeloma) may exacerbate renal insufficiency via renal vasoconstriction and intracellular calcium deposition.[23,24]

Acute interstitial nephritis (AIN) usually results from exposure to a particular drug, but certain infections (eg, streptococcal infections), infiltrative diseases (such as sarcoidosis), and autoimmune disorders (such as systemic lupus erythematosus) are also potential causes.[1,2] Numerous drugs have been implicated. Methicillin, although rarely used now, is the classic example; AIN occurs in up to 17% of patients treated with methicillin for more than 10 days.[25] Other agents known to cause AIN include other penicillin derivatives, cephalosporins, sulfonamides (including trimethoprim/sulfamethoxazole), ciprofloxacin, rifampin, allopurinol, furosemide, bumetanide, thiazides, cimetidine, certain NSAIDs, and quinine. Histologically, AIN manifests as interstitial edema and infiltration of the interstitium with T lymphocytes and monocytes.[2,26]

Glomerular diseases encompass a variety of histologic patterns, etiologies, and clinical presentations. Secondary membranous nephropathy is associated with malignancy in 5 to 10% of adult cases. This syndrome occurs most commonly in patients with solid tumors such as lung or colon adenocarcinomas, and renal injury results from tumor antigen deposition in the glomeruli, antibody deposition, complement activation, and epithelial cell and basement membrane injury.[27] Minimal change disease may be seen with hematologic malignancies, most commonly with Hodgkin's disease but also with other lymphomas and with leukemias. It is hypothesized that the tumor cells secrete cytokines that are toxic to glomeruli.[28] Focal glomerulosclerosis may be associated with both Hodgkin's and non-Hodgkin's lymphoma.[29] Immunoglobulin A (IgA) nephropathy has been described in the setting of small-cell lung carcinoma and mycosis fungoides.[30] Membranoproliferative glomerulonephritis is occasionally seen with chronic lymphocytic leukemia, melanoma, and non-Hodgkin's lymphoma.[29,31]

Acute renal failure is a common complication of both autologous and allogeneic bone marrow transplantation (BMT). Various groups have described incidences ranging from 26 to 64%.[32,33] Early post-BMT causes include tumor lysis syndrome and marrow infusion toxicity (seen within the first 5 days) as well as hepatic venoocclusive disease (seen within 7 to 21 days); because of the long hospital stays after BMT, however, these entities are seldom encountered in the emergency room.[34] Nephropathy related to BMT is seen more than 4 weeks after transplantation in 0.6 to 13.0% of adults and in up to 45% of children.[35] Its pathogenesis is unclear but may be the result of radiation nephritis from the total-body irradiation used to precondition patients before BMT. Cyclosporine, used in BMT to prevent graft-versus-host disease, may result in ARF by causing the following three mechanisms: (1) renal afferent arteriolar vasoconstriction (a prerenal cause),[36] (2) chronic progressive renal dysfunction from interstitial fibrosis and glomerulosclerosis,[37] and (3) hemolytic uremic syndrome from cyclosporine-induced injury to renal vascular endothelium and resultant thrombotic microangiopathy.[38]

Postrenal Renal Failure. Postrenal renal failure, or obstructive uropathy, refers to ARF that results from obstruction anywhere along the urinary outflow tract, from the renal pelvis to the urethra. Common causes in the patient with cancer include bladder outlet obstruction from cancers of the prostate, bladder, uterus, or cervix and ureteral obstruction from primary or metastatic cancers in the retroperitoneum. Myeloma light-chain deposition and the precipitation of crystals or proteins in the renal calyces and pelves (as with tumor lysis syndrome and with acyclovir, sulfonamide, and methotrexate toxicity) and may cause postrenal ARF. Less common causes include bilateral renal calculi, papillary necrosis, and fungal infections. Of note, patients with ureteral stents or percutaneous nephrostomy tubes that are already in place for obstruction may present to the emergency room with postrenal ARF when these devices themselves become obstructed by debris, infection, or tumor ingrowth.[1,39–41]

Clinical Manifestations

Acute renal failure itself may be asymptomatic. Oliguria, or a urine output of < 400 mL per day, is only variably present. Patients with cancer often present to the emergency room with symptoms of the underlying processes that are responsible for the decline in renal function. Complaints may include weakness, nausea, vomiting, fever, dizziness, confusion, anorexia, mucositis, melena, hematochezia, dyspnea, abdominal pain, abdominal distention, flank pain, dysuria, hematuria, oliguria, anuria, and edema. Frankly uremic patients may complain of chest pain and palpitations, or they may be encephalopathic or obtunded.

A comprehensive history is crucial. Attention must be given to any history of pelvic or retroperitoneal neoplasms; prior renal insufficiency; underlying medical conditions that may predispose to renal failure (hypertension, vascular disease, diabetes, etc); risks for urinary obstruction (presence of stones, stents, or nephrostomy tubes) or retention (recent urethral catheterization); exposure to known nephrotoxins such as chemotherapeutic agents, antimicrobials (especially aminoglycosides and amphotericin B), and intravenous contrast dyes; ingestion of chronic medications that are potentially nephrotoxic (diuretics, angiotensin-converting enzyme [ACE] inhibitors, NSAIDs, cyclosporine, etc); and radiation therapy to the abdomen, pelvis, or retroperitoneum.

The physical examination may reveal important clues as to the process involved. Orthostatic hypotension, tachycardia, and loss of skin turgor indicate hypovolemia. Fever and hypotension often indicate sepsis. Jugular venous distention, extra heart sounds (S$_3$, S$_4$), rales, and peripheral edema are found in CHF. A pericardial friction rub may be heard in cases of uremic pericarditis. Ascites, edema, and ecchymoses may be signs of liver disease. Edema (and often anasarca) and hypertension may be seen in glomerulonephritis. Suprapubic fullness may indicate bladder distention in urethral obstruction whereas suprapubic and costovertebral angle tenderness may be present in urinary-tract infections. Patients with nephrostomy tubes, chronic indwelling urethral catheters, and urostomies from ileal conduits may have little or no urine present in their collection bags.[1,2,41]

Diagnostic Evaluation

Acute renal failure is documented by a sudden increase in serum creatinine, usually with a concomitant rise in blood urea nitrogen (BUN). The underlying mechanisms must be identified because many cases of ARF in patients with cancer are reversible with prompt intervention. Laboratory tests and imaging studies are almost always required, and the results of many of these can be obtained in the emergency room.[1,2]

Blood Tests. The ratio of BUN to creatinine may suggest the type of ARF. In prerenal ARF, urea is passively reabsorbed with water and sodium whereas creatinine is not, leading to a ratio higher than 20:1. Other conditions may influence this ratio; gastrointestinal hemorrhage, high protein intake, and corticosteroids can increase the ratio whereas low protein intake, vomiting, and liver disease may decrease the ratio.

A comprehensive metabolic panel and a complete blood count with differential should be obtained. Serum sodium is an indicator of volume status. Elevated serum uric acid, phosphorus, and potassium, with decreased calcium, may indicate tumor lysis syndrome in patients who have received chemotherapy. Hypercalcemia may be present with many cancers (eg, lymphoma, myeloma, and lung cancer) and may contribute to ARF. Hypomagnesemia can be an early sign of cisplatin toxicity. Hyperkalemia often results from ARF and must be given particular attention if present. An acute drop in hemoglobin may represent hemorrhage and may be the cause of hypotension and hypovolemia. Both elevated and depressed leukocyte counts may be seen in sepsis. Eosinophilia may be seen in AIN.[1,2]

Urinalysis. Urine should be obtained from all patients. Urethral catheterization may be required and may be therapeutic in cases of acute urinary retention due to spasm, blood clots, or incomplete obstruction from tumor masses. Urinalysis in the setting of prerenal ARF may reveal a high specific gravity, low-level proteinuria, and ketonuria. With ATN, urinalysis may show mild to moderate proteinuria. Acute interstitial nephritis may also cause mild to moderate proteinuria, but it also causes hemoglobinuria. Moderate to severe proteinuria and hemoglobinuria may be seen with glomerulonephritis. In postrenal ARF, urinalysis may reveal trace proteinuria and hemoglobinuria.

Urine microscopy should also be performed. Hyaline casts may be present in prerenal ARF. Muddy brown-pigmented granular casts are typical of ATN. Leukocytes and leukocyte casts, eosinophils, and erythrocytes may be seen in AIN. Erythrocytes and erythrocyte casts may be found in glomerulonephritis. Crystals, leukocytes, and erythrocytes may all be observed in patients with postrenal ARF.[1,2]

Urine Indices. Also helpful is the measurement of urine sodium, urine creatinine, and urine osmolality. Generally, urine sodium is low (< 20 mEq/L) in prerenal ARF whereas it is high (> 40 mEq/L) in ATN. A more specific way to differentiate prerenal ARF from ATN is to calculate the fractional excretion of sodium (FENa), as follows:

$$FENa = \frac{urine\ sodium \times plasma\ creatinine}{plasma\ sodium \times urine\ creatinine} \times 100\%$$

A value < 1% can be normal or suggests prerenal ARF whereas a value > 2% in the absence of diuretic use suggests ATN.

A urine osmolality > 500 mOsm/kg is highly suggestive of prerenal ARF. In ATN, the urine concentrating ability is lost; thus, the urine osmolality is usually < 350 mOsm/kg.[1,2]

Radiologic Studies. Radiologic studies are helpful in the evaluation of postrenal ARF. Renal ultrasonography should be undertaken to look for hydronephrosis and its causes, including obstructed ureteral stents, stones, abscesses, and tumor masses. Contrast-enhanced computed tomography (CT) (eg, to evaluate tumor masses in the retroperitoneum) should be undertaken only after the acute obstruction is relieved and renal function has improved. Usually, these studies will not be ordered for this purpose from the emergency room.[1,2,42]

Renal Biopsy. Renal biopsy is not routinely used to evaluate ARF in patients with cancer.

Treatment

The treatment of ARF depends on the underlying condition.[1,2] Prerenal ARF due to hypovolemia and hypotension may be treated with intravenous fluids, blood transfusions, and antibiotics (in cases of sepsis). Patients receiving chemotherapy and radiation should receive appropriate antiemetic agents (prochlorperazine, ondansetron, granisetron, dexamethasone, metoclopramide, and lorazepam). Mucositis may be treated topically with anesthetic agents, and antifungal and antiviral agents may be added if concomitant infection is suspected. Chemotherapy-induced diarrhea may be palliated with loperamide, diphenoxylate/atropine, or (when severe) tincture of opium. Hyperglycemia in uncontrolled diabetes must be controlled with insulin or oral agents. Congestive heart failure should be treated to optimize cardiac output and renal perfusion.

Nephrotoxins must be discontinued. Aminoglycosides, vancomycin, acyclovir, foscarnet, and amphotericin B should be stopped. If amphotericin B is crucial, lipid formulations may be administered. Cyclosporine may need to be discontinued, or its dose may need to be decreased. Nephrotoxic chemotherapy should be stopped, and aggressive hydration should be begun. Hydration should also be used in the prevention and treatment of radiocontrast-induced ARF. The administration of high-dose leucovorin to patients receiving methotrexate reduces the risk of toxicity and may result in the recovery of renal function.[43] Acute renal failure from multiple myeloma may respond acutely to plasmapheresis combined with chemotherapy.[44] Glomerulopathies may require corticosteroids but often respond and entirely remit when the underlying malignancy is treated.[1,45]

Postrenal ARF requires urgent intervention.[1,2,39] Urethral catheterization may relieve urinary obstruction from spasm, blood clots, or partially obstructing tumor masses and may result in the rapid recovery of renal function. Hydronephrosis may necessitate ureteral stenting or the placement of percutaneous nephrostomy tubes. If these devices are already present, they may need to be exchanged. Relief of obstruction may cause a post-obstructive diuresis, so careful attention to volume repletion and serum electrolytes is required.

URINARY-TRACT INFECTION

Urinary-tract infection (UTI), the most common bacterial infection in humans, occurs when microorganisms gain entrance to the urinary tract, adhere to uroepithelium, and cause inflammation and destruction of host tissue. To accomplish this, organisms must overcome host defenses, which include normal perineal flora (particularly lactobacilli), normal anatomy and micturition, and inflammatory and immunologic responses. Patients with cancer may be particularly susceptible to developing UTIs because of immunosuppression, the presence of foreign bodies in the urinary tract (ie, urethral or suprapubic catheters, ureteral stents, and/or percutaneous nephrostomy tubes), or abnormal anatomy as a result of tumors or the surgical creation of ileal conduits, reservoirs, and neobladders.[46–49] Other potentially complicating factors and situations include funguria, the use of intravesical bacille Calmette-Guérin, acute bacterial prostatitis, and Fournier's gangrene.

Etiology and Pathophysiology

The most common uropathogen is the bacterium *Escherichia coli*, which is a normal resident of the colon but which may colonize the perineum when the normal flora is altered by hospitalization and the use of broad-spectrum antibiotics. Both of these factors place patients with cancer at risk for colonization with *E. coli*, other enteric bacteria and resistant nosocomial organisms (such as Enterococcus, *Pseudomonas aeruginosa*, *Klebsiella pneumoniae*, *Proteus mirabilis*, *Enterobacter cloacae*, *Staphylococcus aureus*, and *Staphylococcus epidermidis*), and yeasts (such as *Candida albicans*, *Candida tropicalis*, and *Candida [Torulopsis] glabrata*). The most common mode of entry by far is via the urinary catheter, which results in a cumulative risk for bacteriuria of 3 to 10% per day; nearly 50% of patients are infected after 1 week of closed-system catheterization drainage. The incidence of UTI is directly related to the duration of catheterization.[46–49]

The normal urinary tract is resistant to microbiologic colonization and rapidly clears organisms through micturition. Normal urine has factors that may inhibit bacterial growth, including high osmolarity, low pH, high urea content, and antibacterial prostatic secretions, all of which may be adversely affected by chemotherapy, renal disease, and prostate dysfunction. The mucopolysaccharide lining of the bladder (uromucoid) binds and traps certain bacteria, but this defense can be compromised by chemotherapy, local urinary-tract cancers, and foreign bodies such as calculi and urinary catheters. Obstruction to urine flow at any point, whether structural (as with calculi, growing tumors, or obstructed ureteral stents or nephrostomy tubes) or functional (as with neurogenic bladder), predisposes to infection. In fact, the high pressure that results from urinary obstruction yields a higher rate of tissue invasion, bacteremia, and urosepsis.[47,49,50] Polymorphonuclear leukocytes do not prevent bacterial adherence but can limit the extent of infection. They also contribute to renal tissue damage through the elaboration of lysozymes and oxygen free radicals. Interestingly, neutropenic patients with UTI, having less pyuria, therefore have less tissue destruction than hosts with normal neutrophil counts. In patients with functional lymphocytes, humoral antibody production against bacterial antigens may facilitate phagocytosis through opsonization. The roles of antibody- and cell-mediated immunities remain unclear.[47,51]

Clinical Manifestations

Infection of the bladder (cystitis) results in typical lower-tract symptoms, including dysuria, urgency, frequency, hesitancy, and suprapubic discomfort. Cystitis is not usually associated with fever or elevated leukocyte counts.[52] Patients with untreated bacteriuria or prolonged indwelling urinary catheters are at risk for ascending infection. Infection of the kidney (pyelonephritis) is characterized by fever, flank pain, rigors, nausea, vomiting, and prostration. Elevated leukocyte counts are often seen, and bacteremia is not infrequent. Patients with pyelonephritis often do not have antecedent lower-tract symptoms. The complications of pyelonephritis include renal and perinephric abscesses, calculus formation (associated with urease-producing bacteria such as *Proteus*), emphysematous pyelonephritis, xanthogranulomatous pyelonephritis, and urosepsis.[48,51]

Diagnostic Evaluation

Urinalysis and urine culture are used to diagnose UTI. A complete blood count with differential, serum chemistries, and blood cultures should be done in patients who have fever or who are systemically ill. Abdominal radiography may be useful for detecting calculi and gas collections. Renal ultrasonography and contrast-enhanced CT are the imaging tests of choice for identifying renal abscesses and other complications.[53]

Treatment

Cystitis is treated with a 3- to 5-day course of an oral antibiotic, commonly trimethoprim/sulfamethoxazole or a fluoroquinolone (eg, ciprofloxacin or ofloxacin). The choice of empiric antibiotic therapy should be based on risk factors for resistance and the resistance pattern of the local community.[54] Pyelonephritis requires a 10- to 14-day course of antibiotics, usually administered intravenously until defervescence and clinical stability are achieved. The course may then be completed with an appropriate oral agent. Parenteral regimens commonly used include ampicillin, with or without an aminoglycoside (eg, gentamicin or amikacin); a penicillinase-resistant penicillin (eg, ticarcillin/clavulanate); a third-generation cephalosporin (eg, ceftriaxone or ceftazidime); a fluoroquinolone; or trimethoprim/sulfamethoxazole.[51,52] Antibiotic therapy, of course, should be guided by urine culture and sensitivity results when available. In patients with pyelonephritis who do not defervesce and clinically improve within 48 to 72 hours, the possibility of renal or perinephric abscess or septic obstruction should be entertained, and ultrasonography or CT should be considered. Abscesses require prompt drainage, which often can be accomplished percutaneously under ultrasonographic or CT guidance. Open surgical drainage or emergent nephrectomy may rarely be required. Percutaneous nephrostomy or ureteral stent placement may be needed to relieve obstruction and hydronephrosis.[48,52] Neutropenic patients with fever and UTI should be treated along institutional guidelines for febrile neutropenia (ie, with double coverage for aerobic Gram-negative bacilli by using, for example, ticarcillin/clavulanate and amikacin, which is the most common regimen employed at Memorial Sloan-Kettering Cancer Center).

Complicating Factors

Ureteral Stents. Ureteral stents are often used in patients with cancer, to re-establish and maintain ureteral patency when malignant obstruction develops. They are available in a number of shapes and materials (eg, the commonly used polyurethane double-pigtail stent and the less commonly used stainless-steel-mesh Wallstent) and are deployed endouroscopically.[55] Ureteral stents can increase the risk of UTI. Riedl and colleagues examined 93 double-pigtail stents from 71 patients (including 27 stents used for malignant obstruction). Patients with temporary stents (average duration of 14 days) showed a stent bacterial colonization rate of 70%, a bacteriuria rate of 24%, and an overt infection rate of 6.5%. Patients with permanent stents (average duration of 40 days) showed 100% stent colonization and bacteriuria rates and an overt infection rate of 33%. Prophylactic antibiotics were not shown to be effective in preventing this colonization.[56] Comparable rates have been demonstrated elsewhere.[57] Lugmayr and Pauer looked at 30 cases in which metallic Wallstents were used for malignant ureteral obstruction, however, and found no infections after a mean follow-up of 30 weeks.[58] Wallstents rapidly encrust, however, and are thus seldom used to palliate malignant ureteral obstruction. Patients with ureteral stents and UTI should be treated aggressively with antibiotics. Bacterial adherence to stent material often results in the formation of biofilms, which afford bacteria a degree of protection against antibiotics. Because infection may be associated with stent obstruction, hydronephrosis, and renal failure, immediate ultrasonography or CT should be considered. Endouroscopic removal and replacement are frequently required when stents become infected.

Percutaneous Nephrostomy Tubes. Percutaneous nephrostomy tubes are often used to relieve hydronephrosis in patients with malignant obstruction, usually when placing a ureteral stent is unfeasible or when internal stents have failed. Nephrostomy tubes, like ureteral stents, may increase the risk of UTI. Cronan and colleagues observed 22 nephrostomy systems placed in patients with initially sterile urine and found that bacteriuria and pyuria developed in all patients by 9 weeks. Interestingly, the predominant organisms were *Pseudomonas*, *Enterococcus*, and *Candida*, rather than *Escherichia coli*.[59] Donat and Russo retrospectively looked at 78 patients with nonurologic malignancies who underwent ureteral decompression and who were observed for a median of 7.5 months.[60] Of these patients, 68% required ureteral stents placed endouroscopically or percutaneously (or both), and 32% required percutaneous nephrostomy. Urinary tract infection was the most common complication observed, and 29% of patients experienced a serious infection.

As in patients with ureteral stents, patients with nephrostomy tubes and UTI must be aggressively treated with antibiotics. Tube removal and exchange or conversion to an internalized system may be necessary.

Ileal Conduits, Reservoirs, and Neobladders. Urinary diversion after radical cystectomy, by means of a surgically implanted segment of intestine (usually ileum), can take three forms: (1) the incontinent ileal conduit, which drains through a stoma into a bag; (2) the continent reservoir,

is sometimes accompanied by microscopic hematuria.[81] Methotrexate can crystallize in the renal tubule and thereby lead to tubule dysfunction and hematuria.[82]

Erosion of neoplastic tissue into the rich vascular supply of the upper and lower genitourinary tract is probably the most common cause of hematuria in the patient with cancer. In a similar fashion, mucosal irritation by a foreign body (such as a percutaneous nephrostomy catheter, ureteral stent, or kidney stone) may also result in bleeding. Additionally, most genitourinary malignancies are invested with a network of poorly organized vascular tissues from which spontaneous microscopic or frank bleeding is common.[83] Hematuria may not necessarily be due to a solid tumor; leukemic or lymphomatous infiltration of the renal parenchyma and bladder wall are also known to cause hematuria.[84,85]

Some patients with cancer are at increased risk of kidney stone formation and subsequent hematuria.[86] Hypercalcemia is often noted in patients with malignancies that metastasize to the skeleton, as well as in those whose tumors secrete parathyroid hormone (PTH)–like peptide.[87] Hyperphosphatemia and hyperuricemia are common sequelae of cytolytic chemotherapy for acute leukemia and lymphoma.[88] Electrolyte abnormalities in conjunction with dehydration and prolonged immobility may lead to stone formation in patients who have no prior history of nephrolithiasis.

As noted above, patients with cancer are at increased risk for genitourinary infection, another common cause of hematuria.[89] Cell-mediated immunity may be suppressed by both the underlying malignancy and the effects of chemotherapy on leukopoiesis. Bacteria may be introduced into the collecting system by bladder catheterization and surgery, and a loss of local genitourinary-tract defenses occurs with any defect in urothelial integrity related to radiation, chemotherapy, indwelling foreign bodies, or cancerous growth. Like the common bacterial and fungal urinary pathogens, viral pathogens may also cause hematuria.[90] The BK type of human *Polyomavirus* is associated with a mild respiratory illness and subsequent colonization of the kidney in immunocompetent individuals.[91] Following BMT, prolonged hemorrhagic cystitis (ie, longer than 7 days in duration) was noted four times more frequently in patients who excreted the BK virus than in patients with no viruria.[92] Although a direct causal relationship has not been established, the role of prophylactic uroprotective antiviral therapy in transplant recipients is currently under investigation.[93]

Hemorrhagic cystitis, in which the bladder mucosa is diffusely inflamed, may be acute or chronic; in patients with cancer, it is usually related to exposure to urotoxins.[94] Chemotherapy, radiation, and (less commonly) viral infection can all cause mucosal edema and ulceration resulting in hemorrhage. Numerous synthetic toxins are known to cause hemorrhagic cystitis.[95] In patients with cancer, the oxazaphosphorine alkylating agents cyclophosphamide and ifosfamide are the agents most commonly associated with this condition.[96] However, oral busulfan and intravesicular thiotepa have also been associated with the development of hemorrhagic cystitis.[97,98] The toxic metabolite of the oxazaphosphorines is acrolein (and perhaps there are others), which causes the bladder wall mucosa to become edematous, hyperemic, and friable within 4 hours of exposure.[99] Early experience with these agents was associated with an incidence of hemorrhagic cystitis varying from 17 to 50%, depending on the dose, and a mortality of 4%.[100] Prophylactic measures such as concomitant infusion of mesna (which inhibits the spontaneous breakdown of cyclophosphamide to acrolein in the urine and which also complexes with the terminal methyl group of acrolein, forming a nontoxic ether) and hyperhydration with forced diuresis (which prevents significant levels of toxic urinary metabolites from accumulating in the bladder) have reduced the incidence of clinically significant hemorrhagic cystitis to < 4%.[101] Hemorrhagic cystitis from oxazaphosphorine alkylating agents is usually transient and occurs soon after exposure. It usually resolves within several days although chronic bleeding is noted in approximately 2% of patients treated with high-dose cyclophosphamide. Busulfan-induced cystitis is seen following chronic therapy, usually after several years.

Roughly 20% of patients receiving radiation therapy to the pelvis experience bladder complications (ranging from urgency and frequency to hematuria) and urinary retention.[102] Injury to small vessels by radiation leads to interstitial bladder wall fibrosis and the formation of friable, telangiectatic vessels that can spontaneously rupture and bleed.[103] Fulminant bladder hemorrhage is rare and occurs in 1.0 to 2.3% of patients, depending on radiation dose, intensity, and field of treatment.[104] These side effects are usually noted within 3 months of initiating treatment but may occur as late as 5 years after treatment has been completed.[102,105]

Transurethral resection of the prostate (TURP), transurethral resection of bladder tumors (TURBT), and ureteral stent placement may be followed by episodes of urinating frank blood.[106] Hematuria usually occurs 1 to 2 weeks after the procedure and is related to a loss of the mucosal scab. Endourologic devices such as ureteral stents and percutaneous nephrostomy catheters sometimes cause spontaneous bleeding. These episodes are usually self-limited and are managed conservatively.[107]

Defects of clotting or coagulation (such as thrombocytopenia, therapeutic anticoagulation for thromboembolic disease, or disseminated intravascular coagulation) can result in frank bleeding in a host with a defect (known or unknown) in the urothelium. As in a patient without cancer, an episode of unexplained hematuria in a patient with cancer should prompt a systematic evaluation of the genitourinary tract for sources of bleeding. Occult genitourinary malignancies must be considered in patients who have been exposed to carcinogenic therapies such as cyclophosphamide and ifosfamide.

Pseudohematuria, or a reddish discoloration of the urine that does not reflect bleeding, should always be excluded (urine microscopy will show fewer than 3 RBCs per HPF). Common causes of pseudohematuria in the patient with cancer include doxorubicin (Adriamycin), laxatives containing phenolphthalein, rifampin, pyridium, intravascular hemolysis, beets, food dyes (eg, rhodamine B), urates, and porphyrins. Contamination of the urine specimen with vaginal or rectal blood may occur, and this must also be excluded.

Clinical Manifestations

The severity of genitourinary bleeding can be highly variable. The term "microscopic hematuria" refers to urine that is yellow or clear but that contains three or more RBCs per HPF.[108] Urine that is dipstick positive for blood must be examined microscopically to exclude myoglobinuria (in which no RBCs are seen). Increasing amounts of blood will make the urine appear darker or redder. The term "frank hematuria" describes urine that obviously contains blood. As with gastrointestinal bleeding, the spectrum of hematuria ranges from chronic low-grade bleeding (possibly resulting in anemia) to acute massive hemorrhage with hemodynamic instability.

Pain associated with hematuria may be an important diagnostic clue. Suprapubic discomfort, bladder spasm, flank pain, and testicular pain associated with hematuria suggest an inflammatory etiology. Fever and genitourinary bleeding suggest infection of the bladder, ureter, or kidney. Patients with hematuria who develop urinary retention require prompt attention because large blood clots may obstruct the ureters or bladder outlet and cause hydronephrosis and renal insufficiency or failure.[109]

Diagnostic Evaluation

The primary tasks in evaluating a patient with cancer who presents with hematuria are assessing the severity of bleeding and determining its most probable source. This is usually possible if a careful history, physical examination, and basic blood and urine studies are carried out.

History. The amount of blood in the urine and the frequency of urination can help determine the severity of a bleeding episode. It is difficult, however, to quantify the amount of blood in the urine of patients with frank hemorrhage as small amounts of blood produce dramatic changes in the color and turbidity of urine specimens. Comparing the urine color to such familiar liquids as

rosé wine, tea, or punch may be helpful. Patients should be asked if they feel that the hematuria is resolving, increasing, or staying the same.

When blood appears in the urinary stream it provides a clue to its origin. Initial hematuria is blood in the early part of urination and suggests pathology within the penile or bulbous urethra. Terminal hematuria occurs at the end of urination or even afterward and is associated with abnormalities in the prostatic urethra. Total hematuria is blood that is noted throughout urination. This suggests a pathology that is above the bladder neck and that is allowing urine and blood to mix freely.

Similarly, the presence of blood clots in the urine sometimes provides a clue to the source of bleeding. Vermiform or spaghetti-like clots originate in the renal pelvis and ureters whereas bladder clots vary in size and shape. It is important to determine how long a patient has been urinating blood clots. Clots retained in the bladder for more than a few hours may require cystoscopic removal. The adequacy of urine flow relative to normal urination should be assessed because bladder clots may result in urinary retention.

Painful hematuria implies an inflammatory process. Suprapubic pain and bladder spasms may be related to tumor invading the bladder wall; cystitis due to infection, chemotherapy, or radiation; or urinary retention. Flank pain that radiates to the groin suggests an upper-tract pathology such as nephrolithiasis or pyelonephritis. Constitutional symptoms such as fever, nausea, and vomiting correlate with the severity of the underlying process to some extent and should be noted.

Physicians examining patients with cancer and hematuria should inquire about the following aspects of the oncologic history: sites of primary tumors and known metastases, chemotherapy exposure (especially to cyclophosphamide/ifosfamide, methotrexate, carboplatin/cisplatin, busulfan, intravesicular therapy, and doxorubicin [Adriamycin] [pseudohematuria]); pelvic irradiation; bone marrow transplantation; and recent urologic procedures (catheterization, stent placement, percutaneous nephrostomy tube insertion, TURP, TURBT, and urinary diversion). Additional aspects of the history that may be relevant include prior renal disease (polycystic kidneys, vasculitis, nephritis), hematuria, nephrolithiasis, benign prostatic hypertrophy, inflammatory bowel disease, diverticulitis, thromboembolic disease, and exposure to culprit medications and toxins, including anticoagulants, NSAIDs (especially tiaprofenic acid), allopurinol, danazol, penicillamine, turpentine, ether, gentian violet, and contraceptive suppositories containing nonoxynol-9.[94]

Physical Exam. One should carefully assess the patient's general appearance and vital signs; check for the presence of abdominal, suprapubic, or costovertebral angle tenderness; inspect any externally accessible indwelling urologic devices; and note any signs or symptoms of anemia or other bleeding (purpura, epistaxis). Rectal and pelvic examinations may help to exclude bleeding from the gastrointestinal or reproductive tract as sources of urinary contamination.

Laboratory Studies. Routine laboratory studies including a complete blood count, coagulation profile (prothrombin time [PT]/INR, activated partial thromboplastin time [aPTT]), BUN, serum creatinine, and urine dipstick and spun microscopy, are sufficient for documenting hematuria and assessing its severity.

In the patient with no history of cancer in the pelvis and no obvious etiology for genitourinary bleeding, an imaging study (usually CT with intravenous contrast) is indicated. This study is useful in detecting occult malignancies, nephrolithiasis, renal parenchymal abnormalities, and inflammatory conditions of the genitourinary and gastrointestinal tracts. If CT with contrast is unrevealing, cystoscopy to evaluate the bladder and ureteral mucosa may be indicated.

Treatment

The first step in treating a patient with cancer and hematuria is to irrigate the genitourinary (GU) tract. If the hematuria is mild (ie, there is no frank blood) or resolving, one can "flush" the GU tract with oral and/or intravenous hydration. Treatment with diuretics is unnecessary and is not recommended. One liter of normal saline delivered intravenously often produces enough urine to assess whether the hematuria is resolving or persistent. Patients with mild hematuria should be observed until the urine clears. Occasionally, hematuria will abate and then recur, necessitating further hydration. Vigilance for signs of CHF should be exercised while hydrating patients who are of advanced age or who have known cardiac dysfunction or extensive prior exposure to anthracyclines (eg, doxorubicin [Adriamycin] or idarubicin).

Bladder irrigation is indicated for patients with persistent gross hematuria.[48] A standard or 3-way Foley catheter (minimum, 22 French) is inserted into the bladder, and aliquots of 60 mm of normal saline are gently instilled and aspirated. If the urine fails to clear (typically because of excessively large clots), a 24 or 26 French "hematuria" catheter may be inserted after instilling lidocaine jelly into the urethra (some authors recommend a 28 French fenestrated rectal tube for severe clot retention).[110] If bleeding or clot retrieval continues after 2 L of continuous bladder irrigation, cystoscopy may be indicated, and consultation with a urologist is advised.

Cystoscopic evaluation of the GU tract enables the urologist to identify the most likely source of bleeding

and to implement appropriate therapy.[111] Bleeding from a tumor breaching the urothelium is often self-limited and may not require treatment. Active bleeding from a discrete source may warrant cautery with an electrode or laser (usually a neodymium:yttrium-aluminum-garnet [Nd:YAG] laser). Complications from endourologic procedures are relatively uncommon, occur in 1.3 to 15.3% of patients, and include perforation, recurrent or persistent bleeding, fever, infection or sepsis, colic, reflux, and ureteral or urethral stricture.[112]

Intravesicular instillation of a hemostatic agent is indicated for patients with hematuria from a bladder source that is refractory to irrigation or too diffuse for local cystoscopic therapy.[110] Many different preparations are available. At our institution, the first agent used is a 1% solution of alum that is delivered by continuous infusion until bleeding ceases; this can take up to 7 days.[113] Renal insufficiency is a contraindication to alum therapy and is associated with elevated serum aluminum levels and encephalopathy.[114] If alum therapy is unsuccessful, prostaglandin E$_2$ (PGE$_2$) or prostaglandin F$_2$ is instilled into the bladder at the bedside. These agents are considered to be safe and effective for refractory bladder hemorrhage but are associated with painful bladder spasms that can limit their use.[115] Another intravesicular agent for persistent bladder hemorrhage is silver nitrate. A 1% solution of silver nitrate is instilled at 15-minute intervals, followed by gentle saline lavage.[116]

Bladder hemorrhage that is refractory to alum, PGE$_2$, and silver nitrate may require intravesicular formalin. This agent is reported to be 80% effective in terminating bladder hemorrhage, but its administration requires regional or general anesthesia.[117] Cystography is performed beforehand to assess for ureteral reflux and pre-existing bladder perforation. If reflux is noted, a Fogarty balloon catheter is placed to protect the upper GU tract. Under spinal or general anesthesia, 500 mL to 1 L of 1% formalin is instilled under gravity (from lower than 15 cm above the pubis) and is left in the bladder for 10 to 15 minutes. This is followed by irrigation of the bladder with 1 L of distilled water; a Foley catheter is left in place for 24 hours. Repeated treatment with increasing concentrations of formalin (up to a 10% solution) may be necessary if bleeding persists after 48 hours (often the case in patients with radiation-induced hemorrhagic cystitis). The risks of using intravesicular formalin include renal papillary necrosis, renal failure, ureteral stenosis, bladder contracture, and bladder rupture with subsequent peritonitis.[118] Consequently, evidence of bladder perforation is a contraindication to using intravesicular formalin.

Surgical options that are reserved for patients with life-threatening or refractory hemorrhage include cystotomy with bladder packing or cystectomy with urinary diversion.[119] Patients for whom surgery presents unacceptable risks may benefit from the selective embolization of bleeding tumors.[120,121] Hyperbaric oxygen[122] and conjugated estrogen therapy[123] have been used successfully for the treatment of chronic hematuria secondary to radiation cystitis.

It is also important to correct any underlying defects in hemostasis. Bleeding due to thrombocytopenia usually stops when transfusion brings the platelet count to > 20,000.[124] Bleeding related to therapeutic or supratherapeutic anticoagulation with heparin or warfarin should be reversed with fresh frozen plasma when the hemorrhage is life-threatening. For milder bleeding, the risks and benefits of discontinuing and/or reversing anticoagulation should be weighed against the risk of thromboembolic disease.

Antibiotics are usually indicated when fever accompanies hematuria. Fever and hematuria in a patient with an indwelling endourologic device are an absolute indication for antibiotic therapy. Patients with obstructed pyelonephritis may require emergent surgical or percutaneous drainage in addition to antibiotics, as detailed in the Urinary-Tract Infection section in this chapter.

OBSTRUCTIVE UROPATHY

Obstructive uropathy is defined as the blockage of urinary flow along the upper or lower urinary tract. In cancer patients, this is most commonly due to (a) tumor compression, (b) retroperitoneal lymphadenopathy or fibrosis, or (c) direct tumor invasion of the ureter, bladder neck, or urethra.[48,125] The complications of obstructive uropathy range from no complications to renal failure, urosepsis, and diabetes insipidus, depending on the nature and duration of the obstruction. Though effective treatment is available, this condition often portends a poor overall prognosis.

Pathophysiology

The primary function of the kidney is to filter the end products of metabolic pathways from the blood. The ultrafiltrate is ideally free of protein and contains appropriate amounts of free water and electrolytes to maintain homeostasis. The adequate elimination of soluble wastes and toxins through the urinary tract is essential to survival. The ultrafiltrate (urine) is then channeled via the ureters to the bladder for storage until elimination takes place with micturition. On average, 1.5 to 2.0 L of urine flows through the urinary tract daily.

The normal flow of urine depends on ureteral peristalsis and on a hydrostatic pressure gradient from the renal tubules to the renal pelvis. Obstructive uropathy is the structural impedance to the flow of urine, which eventually leads to functional damage of the renal parenchyma (obstructive

nephropathy).[125] "Hydronephrosis," strictly a descriptive term, refers to the structural dilatation of the renal pelvis and calyces. Because hydronephrosis can be present without obstruction, the term should not be used interchangeably for obstructive uropathy. However, the term is often used to refer to the dilatation of the renal calyces and pelvis proximal to the point of urinary-tract obstruction.

Following the onset of obstructive uropathy, pressures increase within the renal pelvis and tubules, and this results in the dilatation of these structures. The change in the appearance of the kidney varies with the location, degree (partial or complete), and duration of the obstruction. Intrarenal obstruction may cause little hydronephrosis as the surrounding renal parenchyma may limit the degree of dilation. In contrast, extrarenal obstruction may result in the dilation of the collecting system, with little impedance from surrounding soft tissue. Regardless of the site of obstruction, renal damage results from high intratubular pressures and leads to decreased renal blood flow and resultant ischemia, cellular atrophy, and necrosis. Superimposed infection can accelerate kidney destruction secondary to parenchymal infiltration by activated leukocytes, causing inflammation and scarring.

Metabolic complications ensue with obstructive uropathy because the impaired urine flow in the urinary tract causes a rise in intratubular pressure. This increased pressure causes a decreased hydrostatic filtration pressure gradient across the glomerular capillaries, leading to a fall in the GFR. After the onset of complete obstruction, transient renal vasodilation is followed by progressive vasoconstriction, which is mediated by angiotensin II and thromboxane A_2. These vasoconstricting mediators are offset by the vasodilatory eicosanoids prostaglandin E_2 and prostacyclin, which tend to prevent a further drop in the GFR.

With partial obstruction, the GFR may also fall. Further, a decreased ability to concentrate the urine results from the decrease in medullary solute concentration that occurs as a consequence of the increased medullary blood flow that accompanies obstruction. In patients with chronic partial obstruction, the inability to form concentrated urine may be reflected clinically as polyuria and nocturia, often without elevated levels of BUN and serum creatinine.

Etiology

In the general patient population, obstructive uropathy is a relatively common disorder. Between the ages of 20 and 60 years, urinary-tract obstruction is more common in females, primarily due to pregnancy and uterine cancer. After the age of 60 years, urinary-tract obstruction is more common in men because of prostatic disease. Urolithiasis is a common cause of obstruction, and 12% of the US population form calculi at some time in their lives.[126] Other non-cancer-related causes of obstructive uropathy are well outlined elsewhere in the literature.[127]

Obstructive uropathy as a direct complication of cancer or its treatment can be devastating to the patient's quality of life and may effect treatment options. The increased incidence of pain and infection can dramatically affect performance status, and the resultant decrease in creatinine clearance can affect the dosing and choices of chemotherapeutic and supportive agents. The resultant metabolic changes, with fluid and electrolyte abnormalities and acid-base disorders, can precipitate the failure of other organ systems, and the effects of uremia on platelet function can lead to catastrophic hemorrhage. Obstructive nephropathy can develop insidiously and may be detected incidentally or may present as florid renal failure. Whenever obstructive uropathy is diagnosed, a treatment plan should be instituted urgently (and sometimes emergently) to salvage renal function.

In the cancer patient, obstructive uropathy can occur at any location in the urinary tract (eg, at the level of the renal tubules, ureter, bladder outlet, or urethral meatus). The obstruction can be partial or complete, and it can be acute or chronic. The obstruction may be intrinsic (intraluminal or intramural) or extrinsic to the urinary tract. Intraluminal obstruction is caused by impedance of urine flow by material within the collecting system itself. Intraluminal obstruction can occur intrarenally (eg, from uric acid crystals or Bence Jones protein) or extrarenally (eg, from blood clots). Intramural obstruction may be secondary to anatomic changes within the wall of the collecting system (eg, from metastatic or primary tumors, prior ureteral instrumentation, or radiation) or may result from a functional defect in peristalsis (eg, neurogenic bladder from neurologic compromise or anticholinergic medications). Extrinsic obstruction occurs through direct compression by any space-occupying lesion or fibrotic change outside the collecting system (eg, a tumor mass, retroperitoneal or pelvic lymphadenopathy, fibrosis from prior surgery, chemotherapy, or radiation) (Table 13–1).

Intrinsic Obstruction. In patients with multiple myeloma, intrinsic tubular obstruction can occur through the deposition of monoclonal light chains.[128] This Bence Jones protein precipitates as amorphous casts within the renal tubules. The chemical composition of the pathologic light-chain deposits has not yet been determined. However, recent data point to possible increased pathogenesis of certain Bence Jones proteins that co-precipitate with accessory molecules (eg, Tamm-Horsfall protein, a glycoprotein produced by cells of the thick ascending loop of Henle). These accessory molecules may initiate or facilitate aggregation.[129] Further, interleukin-6 may play an important role in the pathogenesis of myeloma cast nephropathy.[130]

Crystal nephropathy is an important cause of intrinsic obstructive uropathy in patients with aggressive hematologic malignancies, including aggressive high-grade non-Hodgkin's lymphoma (Burkitt's lymphoma or lymphoblastic lymphoma) and leukemia with hyperleukocytosis (acute lymphoblastic leukemia or accelerated chronic myelogenous leukemia). When patients with these exquisitely chemosensitive malignancies undergo treatment, tumor lysis syndrome may develop. Occasionally, this syndrome may be observed even in untreated patients with aggressive disease when a large tumor burden and high cell proliferation rates are present. Tumor lysis syndrome is a metabolic derangement that occurs when large quantities of intracellular purines, phosphate, and potassium are released from dying cancer cells. The purines are catabolized to uric acid, and urate crystals can deposit in a high concentration within tubular cells, damaging them and leading to intrarenal obstructive uropathy. Rarely, acute urate nephrolithiasis can develop, causing extrarenal obstructive uropathy.

TABLE 13–1. Causes of Cancer-Related Obstructive Uropathy

Intrinsic processes
  Intraluminal
    Intrarenal
      Multiple myeloma
      Crystal uropathy
        Uric acid crystals (tumor lysis syndrome)
        Medications (eg, acyclovir, sulfonamides, methotrexate, indinavir)
    Extrarenal
      Nephrolithiasis
      Blood clot
      Fungus ball
      Metastatic tumor
  Intramural
    Functional (neurogenic bladder secondary to spinal-cord compression, cauda equina syndrome)
    Medication (anticholinergics)
    Anatomic (prior instrumentation)
Extrinsic processes
  Ureteral
    Lower ureter: extension of pelvic tumor (eg, cervix, prostate, bladder, colo-rectal)
    Upper ureter: primary or metastatic tumor (eg, lymphoma, sarcoma, gastrointestinal, ovary)
    Retroperitoneal fibrosis
      Idiopathic
      Drugs (methysergide)
      Radiation
      Postsurgical
    Abscess
    Hematoma
  Bladder outlet
    Cancer of bladder, prostate, urethra
    Strictures from prior surgery
    Spasm after instrumentation

The medications used in the management of cancer patients can result in obstructive nephropathy. Acyclovir given at high doses can precipitate in the renal tubule. Likewise, methotrexate and sulfadiazine can precipitate in the distal tubule, leading to nephropathy.[131] Patients with coexisting human immunodeficiency virus (HIV) disease who are taking indinavir can present with renal insufficiency and renal calculi composed almost exclusively of this drug.[132]

Other intrinsic causes of obstructive uropathy include blood clots in patients with coagulopathy or tumor bleeding, and fungus balls.

Extrinsic Obstruction. Obstruction of the ureter in the cancer patient can be caused by direct compression by a retroperitoneal tumor, by encasement of the ureter by involved lymph nodes, or (very rarely) by direct metastatic involvement of the ureter.

Metastatic disease to the retroperitoneum can cause ureteral obstruction. The majority of these tumors are genitourinary in origin. Cancers of the cervix, prostate, and bladder account for 70% of secondary retroperitoneal tumors that cause extrinsic obstruction of the ureter. Cervical cancer is the most common cause of ureteral compression (30% of patients with cervical cancer have obstruction),[133] followed by bladder cancer[127] and prostate cancer. Prostate cancer can also result in obstruction at the bladder neck, invasion of the ureteral orifice, or involvement of the ureter or pelvic lymph nodes. Prostate carcinoma can also cause urethral obstruction, as can rare cases of urethral carcinoma.

To a lesser extent, colon, ovarian, endometrial, gastric, and breast cancers can metastasize to retroperitoneal and periureteral nodes and can encase and obstruct the ureters.[134] Tumors that spread by direct extension to the retroperitoneum (typically from the cervix, endometrium, bladder, prostate, sigmoid colon, or rectum) usually involve the lower third of the ureter. Ureteral obstruction can also be caused by retroperitoneal fibrosis from radiation, chemotherapy (particularly intraperitoneal chemotherapy),[135] medications (notably methysergide), and prior surgery. Additionally, coagulopathy and procedural complications can lead to retroperitoneal hemorrhage and hematoma formation, which may cause extrinsic compression of the ureter.

Radiation. Ureteral obstruction after radiation therapy is relatively uncommon compared to radiation complications involving the bladder and rectum. Overall, the ureter is relatively resistant to radiation, and studies have shown that radiation-induced stricture is unlikely in a normal ureter that is exposed to up to 600 rad.[136] The possible relationships between radiation and ureteral obstruction include the following: (1) a local desmoplastic response from an adjacent tumor that persists after the neoplasm has been eradicated; (2) postradiation tumor necrosis, with resultant fibrosis and scarring if the tumor has involved the ureter wall; (3) direct injury to the ureteral wall, particularly if the radiation was administered in the setting of existing UTI or pelvic inflammatory disease.[137]

Ureteral obstruction may occur near the end of radiation therapy, as a result of ureteral edema. Hydroureteronephrosis has been reported in 50 to 60% of patients treated with radiation therapy for carcinoma of the cervix.[138] This condition almost always resolves within 3 to 4 months after the cessation of therapy.

Hydroureteronephrosis that occurs later after radiation therapy usually portends a more chronic ureteral obstruction. Obstruction can occur 6 to 12 months to even 10 years after radiation therapy but most often becomes evident within 1 to 3 years following the completion of therapy.[139] The obstruction in these late cases is secondary to reduced vascular supply resulting from radiation-induced endarteritis obliterans and connective-tissue proliferation.[140] Prior pelvic surgery increases the patient's risk of developing radiation-induced ureteral obstruction, most likely secondary to alterations in blood supply that may occur as a result of surgery.

Functional Obstructive Uropathy. Functional uropathy may have several causes. Medications that decrease bladder contractility (these include anticholinergics, calcium channel blockers, antihistamines, and opiates) may result in obstruction.[141] Bladder neural compromise can result from local tumor progression, prior pelvic surgery, or epidural spinal-cord compression. Functional obstruction can also occur as a result of GU instrumentation such as cystoscopy, ureteroscopy, or ureterolithotomy.

Clinical Manifestations

The chief presenting symptom of obstructive uropathy is pain, the intensity of which is directly proportional to the rapidity with which the obstruction develops.[125,127] Obstruction from a slow growing pelvic tumor, for example, may be asymptomatic and may be reflected only as an increased creatinine level in blood work or as hydroureter and hydronephrosis on imaging studies. Acute obstruction from a calculus, however, may present as excruciating pain and may be the reason the patient seeks attention in the emergency room. The location of the pain often corresponds to the level of the obstruction. Typically, patients with upper-tract obstruction complain of back or flank pain and may have costovertebral angle tenderness on examination. Patients with lower-tract obstruction often report that the pain is abdominal or suprapubic, with radiation to the ipsilateral testicle or labia.

Patients with complete bilateral obstruction may additionally present with acute or chronic renal failure, again depending on the progress of the obstruction. The

Post-obstructive Diuresis. As discussed above, unilateral ureteral obstruction is often clinically silent in patients whose contralateral kidney is functioning. However, bilateral ureteral obstruction or lower-tract obstructions will lead to the accumulation of solutes and water. Following urinary decompression, a physiologic and self-limited diuresis usually takes place. Peak urine flow rates of up to 69 mL/min have been observed although most patients average 30 mL/min (1.8 L/h).[127] Patients at an increased risk for developing postobstructive diuresis can be identified by the following signs and laboratory abnormalities: hypertension, ankle edema, CHF, confusion, azotemia, hyperkalemia, hyperphosphatemia, hypocalcemia, and low serum bicarbonate. Rarely, diabetes insipidus that is unresponsive to vasopressin ensues.

We recommend frequent weight and blood pressure measurements in the supine and upright positions after decompression of the GU tract. In a conscious and alert individual, the thirst mechanism will correct any abnormal water loss. Pathologic loss of sodium with subsequent intravascular contraction will lead to orthostatic hypotension. These patients should receive 0.45% normal saline, initially at a rate that is one-half to two-thirds of their urinary output, until orthostasis resolves. More aggressive repletion may unnecessarily prolong the solute diuresis. Nephrogenic diabetes insipidus can be recognized by urine that has an unusually low specific gravity (1.000 to 1.004); its treatment is beyond the scope of this chapter, and general nephrology texts should be consulted.

MALIGNANT PRIAPISM

Priapism is defined as prolonged penile erection not due to sexual stimulation. This rare condition requires prompt evaluation and treatment to prevent subsequent erectile dysfunction. Priapism is thought to reflect several different pathophysiologic mechanisms and has been associated with a variety of malignancies. Malignant priapism carries a worse prognosis for the restoration of normal sexual function than does priapism in a patient without cancer.

Clinical Manifestations

Priapism may be acute or chronic. Patients with new-onset priapism often seek medical attention within the first 24 hours.[171] Pain may be associated with this condition and usually reflects ischemia of the corpora cavernosa. These patients are at highest risk for the subsequent complications of impotence or recurrent priapism. Chronic or recurrent priapism is often seen in patients with cancer with penile metastases; this condition may be painful or painless. Rarely, urinary retention and renal insufficiency ensue.[172] Clitoral priapism has been noted in some women with metastatic disease to the perineum.[173]

Etiology and Pathophysiology

Normal erections occur when sexual stimulation results in the relaxation of the vascular smooth musculature of the corpora cavernosa, allowing arteriolar blood into the expanding cavernosal sinusoids and leading to further trapping of blood by compression of the subtunical venular plexuses (the normal site of venous outflow). During detumescence, arteriolar tone increases, preventing further inflow of sinusoidal blood. Venous channels reopen, and blood drains from the corpora cavernosa.[171] Priapism occurs when either of these processes (ie, decreased arteriolar inflow or increased venous outflow) is altered.

Low-flow (ischemic) priapism results from decreased venous outflow from the corpora cavernosa. This may be related to anatomic obstruction of the venous channels by metastatic disease, hyperviscous blood (as in patients with chronic myelogenous leukemia or sickle cell disease), hypercoagulable blood, or medications that interfere with normal vascular physiology (especially intracavernosal agents that are used to treat impotence, such as papaverine, phentolamine, and prostaglandin E). Blood sampled from the cavernosa of patients with low-flow priapism is acidotic and has a low oxygen tension.[174] Irreversible cellular damage and fibrosis can occur if this type of priapism is left untreated for more than 24 hours.[175]

High-flow (arterial) priapism results when increased arterial inflow exceeds venous drainage. This condition is usually related to arterial trauma (specifically to the internal pudendal artery or one of its distal branches) but may also be idiopathic. Intracavernosal blood demonstrates arterial blood pH, with arterial oxygen tensions. Cellular damage and long-term complications are less common in this kind of priapism because of the high oxygen content of the trapped blood. Some authors have suggested that a "spectrum" exists between high- and low-flow states, according to the number of subtunical venules and emissary veins that are occluded.[131]

In the largest series to date, Pohl and colleagues reviewed the etiology, management, and outcome of 230 cases of priapism.[176] Idiopathic priapism was diagnosed in approximately 35% of these cases, and medications (principally antipsychotics, anticoagulants, and antihypertensives [Table 13–2]) were believed to account for another 33%. Of note, this series was published prior to the use of intracavernosal agents for the treatment of impotence; these medications are probably the most common cause of medication-associated priapism today.[177] Other important causes found in this series were trauma (12%) and sickle cell disease (11%). Malignant priapism was observed in only 7% of these cases, primarily in pediatric patients with leukemia.

Among the solid tumors that are known to cause priapism, metastatic cancer of the prostate (accounting for

26 to 32% of all cases), bladder (27 to 35% of cases), kidney (8 to 11%), and testicle (3 to 10%) are the most common. Other malignancies that are associated with priapism include malignant melanoma and carcinoma of the colon, rectum, lung, nasopharynx, and pancreas.[178–180]

In addition to penile metastases, important causes of priapism in the cancer patient include intracavernosal medications for the treatment of impotence (especially following radical prostatectomy and/or pelvic irradiation), obstruction of venous outflow from the penis by a large pelvic tumor, and the loss of central nervous system inhibition of tumescence, secondary to spinal-cord compression by metastatic disease.[181]

Diagnostic Evaluation

It is important to establish the cause of priapism promptly as the choice of treatment depends greatly on the underlying etiology. A history of cancer should not lull the clinician into assuming that a patient's priapism is related to a penile metastasis. Patients presenting with priapism should be asked about the following historical details: (1) the duration of erection (longer episodes may result in more impotence); (2) the degree of pain (pain is often associated with low-flow states); (3) recent penile or saddle-area trauma, including that related to sexual intercourse (trauma is often antecedent in high-flow states); (4) prior erectile problems; (5) exposure to culprit medications (see Table 13–2); (6) cancer history (especially of disease in the pelvis and spinal cord); and (7) history of medical problems associated with priapism (eg, sickle cell disease, thalassemia, thrombocythemia, and paroxysmal nocturnal hemoglobinuria).

On examination, patients with low-flow priapism often have a rigid and painful penile shaft with a soft glans. In high-flow priapism, the entire penis is rigid (or partially rigid) and without pain. The examining physician must be vigilant for masses, ulcers, or areas of induration that may indicate penile metastasis. Pseudopriapism is a condition in which penile rigidity and edema are caused by superficial nodular metastases rather than tumescence of the corpora cavernosa.

Intracorporal blood gas sampling is an essential part of the work-up in patients presenting with new priapism. The following results suggest a low-flow state: pH < 7.25, partial pressure of oxygen < 30 mm Hg, and partial pressure of carbon dioxide > 69 mm Hg. Doppler studies and duplex ultrasonography may aid in evaluating the penile vasculature. In high-flow priapism, these studies show normal flow in the cavernosal and dorsal arteries. In low-flow priapism, ultrasonography of the dorsal arteries of the penis shows a smaller diameter, a finding more commonly seen in the flaccid state. Penile arteriography is useful in evaluating high-flow priapism that is refractory to medical therapy. Other diagnostic modalities that may be helpful include CT or MRI of the pelvis (to look for masses obstructing venous outflow and to look for penile metastases) and core biopsy of penile tissue (to confirm metastatic disease). Hemoglobin electrophoresis is used to establish the diagnosis of sickle cell disease.

Treatment

The first step in the management of a patient who presents with priapism is corporal aspiration of 60 mL of blood by using a 21-gauge scalp vein needle. Blood gas analysis should be performed on this specimen. If the history, examination, and blood gas analysis results suggest a low-flow etiology, an intracorporal injection of 200 μg of phenylephrine should be given (although some authors recommend a trial of cavernosal lavage with normal saline prior to administering phenylephrine).[125] Detumescence usually occurs within 45 seconds and lasts between 7 and 20 minutes. If detumescence does not occur, the intracorporal administration of phenylephrine can be repeated, up to three times. Relative contraindications to intracorporal

TABLE 13–2. Medications and Substances Known to Cause Priapism

Carbon monoxide
Chlorpromazine
Clozapine
Cocaine
Diazepam
Droperidol
Ethanol
Fluphenazine
Gonadotropin-releasing hormone
Haloperidol
Heparin*
Hydralazine
Labetalol
Marijuana
Mesoridazine
Metoclopramide
Molindone
Nifedipine
Papaverine
Perphenazine
Phenoxybenzamine
Prazosin
Promazine
Prostaglandin E$_1$
Tamoxifen
Testosterone
Thiothixene
TPN
Trazodone
Triflupromazine
Warfarin

Adapted from Stackl W, Lee SL.[181]
TPN = triphosphopyridine nucleotide.
*Unfractionated; no data for low-molecular-weight preparations.

phenylephrine include heart block and bradycardia. Other intracavernosal α-adrenergic agents that are used to treat priapism include epinephrine, norepinephrine, etilefrin, ephedrine, and metaraminol. Oral terbutaline (5 mg) has been used for the treatment of intraoperative erections as well as erections caused by intracavernosal therapy.[182] Relative contraindications to terbutaline include coronary artery disease, CHF, and hypokalemia.[183]

Failure of medical therapy to induce detumescence in patients with low-flow priapism is an indication for a "corporo-glans" shunt.[184] This is performed (with the patient under local anesthesia) by inserting a narrow-bladed knife or a Tru-Cut biopsy needle through the glans, dorsal to the meatus, through the tunica albuginea and into the corpora cavernosa. Multiple incisions in each tunica albuginea are made through the same entry site in the glans, which is subsequently closed with a 5-0 or 6-0 polydioxanone (PDS) suture.[185] Failure of the corporo-glans shunt to induce detumescence may prompt one of two more extensive shunting procedures: a proximal cavernosa-to-spongiosum shunt or a cavernosa-to-saphenous vein shunt.[186]

In patients with metastatic disease limited to the glans or shaft without extension into the pelvic diaphragm, total penectomy may be performed for the relief of severe pain or urinary obstruction.[187] In patients who are poor surgical candidates, palliation with systemic chemotherapy or radiation therapy to the pelvis is recommended.[133]

The first step in the management of high-flow priapism is the identification of the arteriocavernosal fistula by selective pelvic arteriography. Once the fistula is identified, embolization is performed with an autologous blood clot or with titanium coils. This is usually followed by rapid detumescence. Recurrent priapism is not uncommon and should prompt repeat arteriography and embolization.[188] Potency is usually preserved following this procedure. Priapism that persists despite multiple attempts at embolization is an indication for open surgical ligation of the fistula.[189]

Medical therapy for priapism secondary to sickle cell anemia differs from medical therapy for other types of priapism. Hyperhydration and hypertransfusion are the cornerstones of treatment.[190,191] Intravenous fluids should be given at three times the maintenance rate. Exchange transfusions should be given to raise the hematocrit above 30%, and the liberal use of analgesics is encouraged.

The prognosis for cancer patients with priapism depends on the underlying etiology of the priapism. Long-term sequelae (ie, impotence or recurrent priapism) arise in patients with medication-induced priapism only when this condition is left untreated for a prolonged period. Priapism caused by penile metastases carries a graver prognosis; the mean survival is estimated at 3.9 months (range, 0 to 20 months) for patients with urothelial carcinoma[192] and is slightly longer for patients with prostatic and colo-rectal primaries.[193,194] The rarity of this disorder has precluded clinical trials of particular interventions, so treatment decisions should be based on an individual patient's functional status, extent of disease, and life expectancy.

The authors wish to thank Christopher Kripas, MD, Brian Meltzer, MD, and Richard Hatchett, MD, for their valued assistance.

REFERENCES

1. Thadhani R, Pascual M, Bonventre JV. Acute renal failure. N Engl J Med 1996;334:1448–60.
2. Black RM. Rose & Black's clinical problems in nephrology. Boston: Little, Brown; 1996.
3. Nissenson AR. Acute renal failure: definition and pathogenesis. Kidney Int Suppl 1998;66:S7–10.
4. Thijs A, Thijs LG. Pathogenesis of renal failure in sepsis. Kidney Int Suppl 1998;66:S34–7.
5. Karnik AM, Bashir R, Khan FA, Carvounis CP. Renal involvement in the systemic inflammatory reaction syndrome. Ren Fail 1998;20:103–16.
6. Belldegrun A, Webb D, Austin HA, et al. Effects of interleukin-2 on renal function in patients receiving immunotherapy for advanced cancer. Ann Intern Med 1987;106:817–22.
7. Dzau VJ. Renal and circulatory mechanisms in congestive heart failure. Kidney Int 1987;31:1402–15.
8. Whelton A. Nephrotoxicity of non-steroidal anti-inflammatory drugs: physiologic foundations and clinical implications. Am J Med 1999;106:13S–24S.
9. Epstein M. Hepatorenal syndrome: emerging perspectives. Semin Nephrol 1997;17:563–75.
10. Solomon R. Radiocontrast-induced nephropathy. Semin Nephrol 1998;18:551–7.
11. Humes HD. Aminoglycoside nephrotoxicity. Kidney Int 1988;33:900–11.
12. Aronson JK, Reynolds DJ. ABC of monitoring drug therapy. Aminoglycoside antibiotics. BMJ 1992;305:1421–4.
13. Zager RA, Bredl CR, Schimpf BA. Direct amphotericin B-mediated tubular toxicity: assessment of selected cytoprotective agents. Kidney Int 1992;41:1588–94.
14. Sawaya BP, Briggs JP, Schnermann J. Amphotericin B nephrotoxicity: the adverse consequences of altered membrane properties. J Am Soc Nephrol 1995;6:154–64.
15. Sawyer MH, Webb DE, Balow JE, Straus SE. Acyclovir induced renal failure. Clinical course and histology. Am J Med 1988;84:1067–71.
16. Carbone LG, Bendixen B, Appel GB. Sulfadiazine-associated obstructive nephropathy occurring in a patient with the acquired immunodeficiency syndrome. Am J Kidney Dis 1988;12:72–5.
17. Rybak MJ, Albrecht LM, Boike SC, et al. Nephrotoxicity of vancomycin, alone and with an aminoglycoside. J Antimicrob Chemother 1990;25:679–87.
18. Deray G, Martinez F, Katlama C, et al. Foscarnet nephro-

toxicity: mechanism, incidence, and prevention. Am J Nephrol 1989;9:316–21.

19. Ries F, Klastersky J. Nephrotoxicity induced by cancer chemotherapy with special emphasis on cisplatin toxicity. Am J Kidney Dis 1986;8:368–79.

20. Lam M, Adelstein D. Hypomagnesemia and renal magnesium wasting in patients treated with cisplatin. Am J Kidney Dis 1986;8:164–9.

21. Skinner R, Pearson AD, Price L, et al. Nephrotoxicity after ifosfamide. Arch Dis Child 1990; 65:732–8.

22. Abelson H, Fosberg MT, Beardsley GP, et al. Methotrexate-induced renal impairment: clinical studies and rescue from systemic toxicity with high-dose leucovorin and thymidine. J Clin Oncol 1983;1:208–16.

23. Rota S, Mougenot B, Baudouin B, et al. Multiple myeloma and severe renal failure: a clinicopathologic study of outcome and prognosis in 34 patients. Medicine 1987;66:126–37.

24. Kyle RA. Monoclonal proteins and renal disease. Ann Rev Med 1994;45:71–7.

25. Galpin JE, Shinaberger JH, Stanley TM, et al. Acute interstitial nephritis due to methicillin. Am J Med 1978;65:756–65.

26. Neilson EG. Pathogenesis and therapy of interstitial nephritis. Kidney Int 1989;35:1257–70.

27. Burstein DM, Korbet SM, Schwartz MM. Membranous glomerulonephritis and malignancy. Am J Kidney Dis 1993;22:5–10.

28. Dabbs DJ, Striker LM, Mignon F, Striker G. Glomerular lesions in lymphomas and leukemias. Am J Med 1986;80:63–70.

29. Rault R, Holley JL, Banner BF, el-Shahawy M. Glomerulonephritis and non-Hodgkin's lymphoma: a report of two cases and a review of the literature. Am J Kidney Dis 1992;20:84–9.

30. Galla J. IgA nephropathy. Kidney Int 1995;47:377–87.

31. Moulin B, Ronco PM, Mougenot B, et al. Glomerulonephritis in chronic lymphocytic leukemia and related B-cell lymphomas. Kidney Int 1992;42:127–35.

32. Kone BC, Whelton A, Santos G, et al. Hypertension and renal dysfunction in bone marrow transplant recipients. QJM 1988;69:985–95.

33. Zager RA, O'Quigley J, Zager BK, et al. Acute renal failure following bone marrow transplantation: a retrospective study of 272 patients. Am J Kidney Dis 1989;13:210–6.

34. Zager RA. Acute renal failure in the setting of bone marrow transplantation. Kidney Int 1994;46:1443–58.

35. Cruz DN, Perazella MA, Mahnensmith RL. Bone marrow transplant nephropathy: a case report and review of the literature. J Am Soc Nephrol 1997;8:166–73.

36. Shihab FS. Cyclosporine nephropathy: pathophysiology and clinical impact. Semin Nephrol 1996;16:536–47.

37. Myers BD, Newton L. Cyclosporine-induced chronic nephropathy: an obliterative microvascular injury. J Am Soc Nephrol Suppl 1991;2:S45–52.

38. Milone J, Napal J, Bordone J, et al. Complete response in severe thrombotic microangiopathy post bone marrow transplantation (BMT-TM) after multiple plasmaphereses. Bone Marrow Transplant 1998;22:1019–21.

39. Norman RW, Mack FG, Awad SA, et al. Acute renal failure secondary to bilateral ureteric obstruction: review of 50 cases. Can Med Assoc J 1982;127:601–4.

40. Platt JF, Rubin JM, Ellis JH. Acute renal obstruction: evaluation with intrarenal duplex Doppler and conventional US. Radiology 1993;186:685–8.

41. Watson G. Problems with double-J stents and nephrostomy tubes. J Endourol 1997;11:413–7.

42. Mucelli RP, Bertolotto M. Imaging techniques in acute renal failure. Kidney Int Suppl 1998;66:S102–5.

43. Kepka L, de Lassence A, Ribrag V, et al. Successful rescue in a patient with high dose methotrexate-induced nephrotoxicity and acute renal failure. Leuk Lymphoma 1998; 29:205–9.

44. Zucchelli P, Pasquali S, Cagnoli L, Ferrari G. Controlled plasma exchange trial in acute renal failure due to multiple myeloma. Kidney Int 1988;33:1175–80.

45. Cattran DC. Evidence-based recommendations for the treatment of glomerulonephritis. Introduction. Kidney Int Suppl 1999;70:S1–2.

46. Korzeniowski OM. Urinary tract infection in the impaired host. Med Clin 1991;75:391–404.

47. Tolkoff-Rubin NE, Rubin RH. Urinary tract infection in the immunocompromised host. Infect Dis Clin 1997; 11:707–17.

48. Russo P. Urologic emergencies in the cancer patient. Semin Oncol 2000;27:284–9.

49. Warren JW. Catheter-associated urinary tract infections. Infect Dis Clin 1997;11:609–22.

50. Neal DE. Host defense mechanisms in urinary tract infections. Urol Clin 1999;26:677–86.

51. Roberts JA. Management of pyelonephritis and upper tract infections. Urol Clin 1999;26:753–63.

52. Anderson RU. Management of lower urinary tract infections and cystitis. Urol Clin 1999;26:729–35.

53. Baumgarten DA, Baumgartner BR. Imaging and radiologic management of upper urinary tract infections. Urol Clin 1997;24:545–69.

54. Gupta K, Hooton TM, Stamm WE. Increasing antimicrobial resistance and the management of uncomplicated community-aquired urinary tract infections. Ann Intern Med 2001;135:41–50.

55. Adams J. Renal stents. Emerg Med Clin 1994;12:749–58.

56. Riedl CR, Plas E, Hubner WA, et al. Bacterial colonization of ureteral stents. Eur Urol 1999;36:53–9.

57. Farsi HM, Mosli HA, Al-Zemaity MF, et al. Bacteriuria and colonization of double-pigtail ureteral stents: long-term experience with 237 patients. J Endourol 1995;9:469–72.

58. Lugmayr H, Pauer W. Self-expanding metal stents for palliative treatment of malignant ureteral obstruction. AJR Am J Roentgenol 1992;159:1091–4.

59. Cronan JJ, Marcello A, Horn DL, et al. Antibiotics and nephrostomy tube care: preliminary observations. Part I. Bacteriuria. Radiology 1989;172:1041–2.

60. Donat SM, Russo P. Ureteral decompression in advanced nonurologic malignancies. Ann Surg Oncol 1996;3: 393–9.

61. Bruce AW, Reid G, Chan RC, Costerton JW. Bacterial

adherence in the human ileal conduit: a morphological and bacteriological study. J Urol 1984;132:184–8.

62. Wishnow KI, Johnson DE, Dmochowski R, Chong C. Ileal conduit in era of systemic chemotherapy. Urology 1989;33:358–60.

63. Lieskovsky G, Boyd SD, Skinner DG. Management of late complications of the Kock pouch form of urinary diversion. J Urol 1987;137:1146–50.

64. Navon JD, Weinberg AC, Ahlering TE. Continent urinary diversion using a modified Indiana pouch in elderly patients. Am Surg 1994;60:786–8.

65. Regalado Pareja R, Huguet Perez J, Errando Smet C, et al. [Orthotopic bladder replacement. II. Functional results and complications in patients with Studer-type ileal neobladder.] Arch Esp Urol 1997;50:234–41.

66. Gutierrez Banos JL, Martin Garcia B, Hernandez Rodriguez R, et al. [Studer's type ileal neobladder. Study of complications and continence.] Actas Urol Esp 1998;22:828–34.

67. Fisher JF, Newman CL, Sobel JD. Yeast in the urine: solutions for a budding problem. Clin Infect Dis 1995; 20:183–9.

68. Gubbins PO, McConnell SA, Penzak SR. Current management of funguria. Am J Health Syst Pharm 1999;56: 1929–35.

69. Garyfallou GT. Mycobacterial sepsis following intravesical instillation of bacillus Calmette-Guérin. Acad Emerg Med 1996;3:157–60.

70. Lamm DL, van der Meijden PM, Morales A, et al. Incidence and treatment of complications of bacillus Calmette-Guérin intravesical therapy in superficial bladder cancer. J Urol 1992;147:596–600.

71. Izes JK, Bihrle W, Thomas CB. Corticosteroid-associated fatal mycobacterial sepsis occurring 3 years after instillation of intravesicular bacillus Calmette-Guérin. J Urol 1993;150:1498–500.

72. Lipsky BA. Prostatitis and urinary tract infection in men: what's new; what's true? Am J Med 1999;106:327–34.

73. Vick R, Carson CC. Fournier's disease. Urol Clin 1999; 26:841–9.

74. Smith GL, Bunker CB, Dinneen MD. Fournier's gangrene. Br J Urol 1998;81:347–55.

75. Carson CC, Segura JW, Greene LF. Clinical importance of microhematuria. JAMA 1979;241:149–50.

76. Garderet L, Bittencourt H, Sebe P, et al. Cystectomy for severe hemorrhagic cystitis in allogeneic stem cell transplant recipients. Transplantation 2000;70:1807–11.

77. Howards S. Standard diagnostic considerations. In: Gillenwater J, Grayhack J, Howards S, Duckett J, editors. Adult and pediatric urology. Chicago: Year Book Medical Publishers, Inc; 1987. p. 67–8.

78. Schaeffer AJ, Del Greco F. Other renal diseases of urologic significance. In: Walsh PC, Retik AB, Stamey TA, Vaughan ED, editors. Campbell's urology. Philadelphia: W.B. Saunders Company; 1992. p. 2065–72.

79. Wagrowska-Danilewicz M, Danilewicz M. Glomerulonephritis associated with malignant diseases of nonrenal origin. A report of three cases and a review of the literature. Pol J Pathol 1995;46:195–8.

80. Usalan C, Emri S. Membranoproliferative glomerulonephritis associated with small cell lung carcinoma. Int Urol Nephrol 1998;30:209–13.

81. Schuman GB, Weiss MA. Atlas of renal and urinary tract cytology and its histopathologic bases. Philadelphia: J.B. Lippincott Company; 1981.

82. Perazella MA. Crystal-induced acute failure. Am J Med 1999;106:459–65.

83. Campbell SC. Advances in angiogenesis research: relevance to urological oncology. J Urol 1997;158:1663–74.

84. Grooms AM, Morgan SK, Turner WR. Hematuria and leukemic bladder infiltration. JAMA 1973;223:193–4.

85. Mourad WA, Khalil S, Radwi A, et al. Primary T-cell lymphoma of the urinary bladder. Am J Surg Pathol 1998;22:373–7.

86. Trinchieri A, Rovera F, Nespoli R, Curro A. Clinical observations on 2086 patients with upper tract stone. Arch Ital Urol Androl 1996;68:251–62.

87. Body JJ. Current and future directions in medical therapy: hypercalcemia. Cancer 2000;88(12 Suppl):3054–8.

88. Schilsky RL. Renal and metabolic toxicities of cancer chemotherapy. Semin Oncol 1982;9:75–83.

89. Bryan CS, Reynolds KL. Hospital-acquired bacteremic urinary tract infection: epidemiology and outcome. J Urol 1984;132:494–8.

90. Mufson MA, Belshe RB. A review of adenoviruses in the etiology of acute hemorrhagic cystitis. J Urol 1976; 115:191–4.

91. Shah KV, Daniel RW, Warzawski RM. High prevalence of antibodies to BK virus, an SV40-related papovavirus in residents of Maryland. J Infect Dis 1973;128:784–7.

92. Bedi A, Miller CB, Hanson JL, et al. Association of BK virus with failure of prophylaxis against hemorrhagic cystitis following bone marrow transplantation. J Clin Oncol 1995;13:1103–9.

93. Vianelli N, Renga M, Azzi A, et al. Sequential vidarabine infusion in the treatment of polyoma virus-associated acute haemorrhagic cystitis late after allogeneic bone marrow transplantation. Bone Marrow Transplant 2000;25:319–20.

94. deVries CR, Freiha FS. Hemorrhagic cystitis: a review. J Urol 1990;143:1–9.

95. Bramble FJ, Morley R. Drug-induced cystitis: the need for vigilance. Br J Urol 1997;79:3–7.

96. Stilwell TJ, Benson RC. Cyclophosphamide-induced hemorrhagic cystitis. A review of 100 patients. Cancer 1988;61:451–7.

97. Millard RJ. Busulfan-induced hemorrhagic cystitis. Urology 1981;18:143–4.

98. Treible DP, Skinner D, Kasimain D, et al. Intractable bladder hemorrhage requiring cystectomy after use of intravesical thiotepa. Urology 1987;30:568–70.

99. Forni AM, Koss LG, Geller W. Cytologic study of the effect of cyclophosphamide on the epithelium of the urinary bladder in man. Cancer 1964;17:1348–55.

100. Pyeritz RE, Droller MJ, Bender WL, Saral R. An approach to the control of massive hemorrhage in cyclophosphamide-induced cystitis by intravenous vasopressin: a case report. J Urol 1978;120:253–4.

101. Levine LA, Richie JP. Urologic complications of cyclophosphamide. J Urol 1989;141:1063–9.

102. Villasanta U. Complications of radiotherapy for carcinoma of the uterine cervix. Am J Obstet Gynecol 1972; 114:717–26.

103. Schoenrock GJ, Cianci P. Treatment of radiation cystitis with hyperbaric oxygen. Urol 1986;27:271–2.

104. Lupton EW. Radiation cystitis. In: Fitzpatrick JM, Krane RJ, editors. The bladder. Edinburgh: Churchill Livingstone; 1995. p. 251–6.

105. Kottmeier HL. Complications following radiation therapy in carcinoma of the cervix and their treatment. Am J Obstet Gynecol 1964;88:854–66.

106. Olapada-Olaopa EO, Solomon LZ, Carter CJ, et al. Haematuria and clot retention after transurethral resection of the prostate: a pilot study. Br J Urol 1998;82:624–7.

107. Vallejo Herrador J, Burgos Revilla FJ, Alvarez Alba J, et al. [Double J ureteral catheter. Clinical complications.] Arch Esp Urol 1998;51:361–73.

108. Corwin HL, Silverstein MD. Microscopic hematuria. Clin Lab Med 1988;8:601–10.

109. Keiller DL. Extraordinary bladder clots. J Urol 1977;117: 43–5.

110. Plawker MW, Hashmat AI. The rectal tube: an excellent catheter for severe clot retention. J Urol 1997;157:1781–2.

111. Wedderburn AW, Ratan P, Birch BR. A prospective trial of flexible cystodiathermy for recurrent transitional cell carcinoma of the bladder. J Urol 1999;161:812–4.

112. Bagley D. Treatment of hematuria. In: Smith A, editor. Controversies in endourology. Philadelphia: W.B. Saunders; 1999. p. 220–5.

113. Kennedy C, Snell ME, Witherow RO. Use of alum to control intractable vesical haemorrhage. Br J Urol 1984;56: 673–5.

114. Phelps KR, Naylor K, Brien TP, et al. Encephalopathy after bladder irrigation with alum: case report and literature review. Am J Med Sci 1999;318:181–5.

115. Mohiuddin J, Prentice HG, Schey S, et al. Treatment of cyclophosphamide-induced cystitis with prostaglandin E2. Ann Intern Med 1984;101:142.

116. Kumar AP, Wrenn EL, Jayalakshmamma B, et al. Silver nitrate irrigation to control bladder hemorrhage in children receiving cancer therapy. J Urol 1976;116:85–6.

117. Fair WR. Formalin in the treatment of massive bladder hemorrhage: techniques, results, and complications. Urolology 1974;3:573–6.

118. Donahue LA, Frank IN. Intravesical formalin for hemorrhagic cystitis: analysis of therapy. J Urol 1989;141: 809–12.

119. Golin AL, Benson RC. Cyclophosphamide hemorrhagic cystitis requiring urinary diversion. J Urol 1977;118: 110–1.

120. Appleton DS, Sibley GNA, Doyle PT. Internal iliac artery embolisation for the control of severe bladder and prostate haemorrhage. Br J Urol 1988;61:45.

121. Ferrer Puchol MD, Borrel Palanca A, Gil Romero J, et al. [Severe hematuria caused by radiation cystitis. Selective percutaneous embolization as an alternative therapy.] Actas Urol Esp 1998;22:519–23.

122. Mathews R, Rajan N, Josefson L, et al. Hyperbaric oxygen therapy for radiation induced hemorrhagic cystitis. J Urol 1999;161:435–7.

123. Miller J, Burfield GD, Moretti KL. Oral conjugated estrogen therapy for treatment of hemorrhagic cystitis. J Urol 1994;151:1348–50.

124. Medeiros D, Buchanan GR. Major hemorrhage in children with idiopathic thrombocytopenic purpura: immediate response to therapy and long-term outcome. J Pediatr 1998;133:334–9.

125. Klahr S. New insights into the consequences and mechanisms of renal impairment in obstructive nephropathy. Am J Kidney Dis 1991;18:689–99.

126. Johnson CM, Wilson DM, O'Fallon WM, et al. Renal stone epidemiology: a 25-year study in Rochester, Minnesota. Kidney Int 1979;16:624–31.

127. Curhan GC, McDougall WS, Zeidel ML. Urinary tract obstruction. In: Brenner BM, editor. Brenner and Rector's the kidney. 6th ed. Philadelphia: W.B. Saunders; 2000. p. 1820–43.

128. Dhodapkar MV, Merlini G, Solomon A. Biology and therapy of immunoglobulin deposition diseases. Hematol Oncol Clin 1997;11:89–110.

129. Sanders PW, Herrera GA, Chen A, et al. Differential nephrotoxicity of low molecular weight proteins including Bence Jones proteins in the perfused rat nephron in vivo. J Clin Invest 1988;82:2086–96.

130. Fattori E, Della Rocca C, Costa P, et al. Development of progressive kidney damage in myeloma kidney in interleukin-6 transgenic mice. Blood 1994;83:2570–9.

131. Choudhury D, Ahmed Z. Drug-induced nephrotoxicity. Med Clin 1997;81:705–17.

132. Stenzel MS, Carpenter CC. The management of the clinical complications of antiretroviral therapy. Infect Dis Clin 2000;14:851–78.

133. Jones CR, Woodhouse CR, Hendry WF. Urologic problems following treatment of carcinoma of the cervix. Br J Urol 1984;56:609–13.

134. Holden S, McPhee M, Grabstald H. The rationale of urinary diversion in cancer patients. J Urol 1979;121:19–21.

135. Fata F, Ron IG, Maluf F, et al. Intra-abdominal fibrosis after systemic and intraperitoneal therapy containing fluoropyrimidines. Cancer 2000;88:2447–51.

136. Albers DD, Dee AL, Kalmon EH, et al. Irradiation injury to the ureter and surgical tolerance. An experimental study. Invest Urol 1976;14:229–32.

137. Resnick MI, Kursh ED. Extrinsic obstruction of the ureter. In: Walsh PC, Retik AB, Vaughan ED, Wein AJ, editors. Campbell's urology. 7th ed. Philadelphia: W.B. Saunders; 1998. p. 387–422.

138. Sklaroff DM, Gnaneswaran P, Sklaroff RB. Postirradiation ureteric stricture. Gynecol Oncol 1978;6:538–45.

139. Underwood PB, Lutz MH, Smoak DL. Ureteral injury following irradiation therapy for carcinoma of the cervix. Obstet Gynecol 1977;49:663–9.

140. Alfert HJ, Gillenwater JY. The consequence of ureteral irradiation with special reference to subsequent ureteral injury. J Urol 1972;107:369–71.

141. Norris JP, Staskin DR. History, physical examination, and classification of neurogenic voiding dysfunction. Urol Clin 1996;23:337–43.

142. Shekarriz B, Shekarriz H, Upadhyay J, et al. Outcome of palliative urinary diversion in the treatment of advanced malignancies. Cancer 1999;85:998–1003.

143. Van Laecke E, Oosterlinck W. Physiopathology of renal colic and the therapeutic consequences. Acta Urol Belg 1994;62:15–8.

144. Sjodin JG, Whalberg J, Persson AE. The effect of indomethacin on glomerular capillary pressure and pelvic pressure during ureteral obstruction. J Urol 1982;127:1017–20.

145. Caine M, Raz S, Ziegler M. Adrenergic and cholinergic receptors in the human prostate, prostatic capsule, and bladder neck. Br J Urol 1975;47:193–202.

146. Taube M, Gajraj H. Trial without catheter following acute retention of urine. Br J Urol 1989;63:180–2.

147. Lepor H, Knapp-Maloney G, Wozniak-Petrofsky J. The safety and efficacy of terazosin for the treatment of benign prostatic hyperplasia. Int J Clin Pharmacol Ther Toxicol 1989;27:392–7.

148. Stoner E. Three-year safety and efficacy data on the use of finasteride in the treatment of benign prostatic hyperplasia. Urology 1994;43:284–92.

149. Bruskewitz RC, Larsen EH, Madsen PO, Dorflinger T. 3-year followup of urinary symptoms after transurethral resection of the prostate. J Urol 1986;136:613–5.

150. Lepor H, Rigaud G. The efficacy of transurethral resection of the prostate in men with moderate symptoms of prostatism. J Urol 1990;143:533–7.

151. Neal DE, Ramsden PD, Sharples L, et al. Outcome of elective prostatectomy. BMJ 1989;299:762–7.

152. Mebust WK, Holtgrewe HL, Cockett AT, Peters PC. Transurethral prostatectomy: immediate and postoperative complications. A cooperative study of 13 participating institutions evaluating 3,885 patients. J Urol 1989;141:243–7.

153. Agarwal M, Palmer JH, Mufti GR. Transurethral resection for a large prostate—is it safe? Br J Urol 1993;72:318–21.

154. Anson KM, Watson GM, Shah TK, Barnes DG. Laser prostatectomy: our initial experience of a technique in evolution. J Endourol 1993;7:333–6.

155. Bihrle R, Foster RS, Sanghvi NT, et al. High intensity focused ultrasound for the treatment of benign prostatic hyperplasia: early United States clinical experience. J Urol 1994;151:1271–5.

156. Bdesha AS, Bunce CJ, Kelleher JP, et al. Transurethral microwave treatment for benign prostatic hypertrophy: a randomised controlled clinical trail. BMJ 1993; 30:1293–6.

157. Guazzoni G, Montorsi F, Rigatti P. The use of wallstents in patients with benign prostatic hyperplasia. Arch Esp Urol 1994;47:927–31.

158. Fainsinger RL, MacEachern T, Hanson J, Bruera E. The use of urinary catheters in terminally ill cancer patients. J Pain Symptom Manage 1992;7:333–8.

159. Maynard FM, Diokno AC. Urinary infection and complications during clean intermittent catheterization following spinal cord injury. J Urol 1984;132:943–6.

160. Russo P, Packer MG, Fair WR. Prophylactic antibiotics in urological surgery. Semin Urol 1983;1:155–63.

161. Petersen TK, Husted SE, Rybro L, et al. Urinary retention during i.m. and extradural morphine analgesia. Br J Anaesth 1982;54:1175–8.

162. Dohil R, Roberts E, Jones KV, Jenkins HR. Constipation and reversible urinary tract abnormalities. Arch Dis Child 1994;70:56–7.

163. Ouslander JG. Geriatric urinary incontinence. Dis Mon 1992;38:65–149.

164. Yamanishi T, Yasuda K, Sakakibara R, et al. Urinary retention due to herpes virus infections. Neurourol Urodyn 1998;17:613–9.

165. Gasparini M, Carrol P, Stoller M. Palliative and endoscopic urinary diversion for malignant ureteral obstruction. Urology 1991;38:408–12.

166. Eiley DM, McDougall EM, Smith AD. Techniques for stenting the normal and obstructed ureter. J Endourol 1997;11:419–29.

167. Schlick RW, Seidl E, Kuster J, et al. [Improved tumor stent for internal palliative urinary diversion.] Urologe 1999;38:138–42.

168. Farrell TA, Hicks ME. A review of radiologically guided percutaneous nephrostomies in 303 patients. J Vasc Interv Radiol 1997;8:769–74.

169. Dyer RB, Assimos DG, Regan JD. Update on interventional uroradiology. Urol Clin 1997;24:623–52.

170. Hamdy FC, Williams JL. Use of dexamethasone for ureteric obstruction in advanced prostate cancer: percutaneous nephrostomies can be avoided. Br J Urol 1995;75:782–5.

171. Macaluso JN, Sullivan JW. Priapism: review of 34 cases. Urol 1985;26:233–6.

172. Bar-Moshe O, Abdul-Sater A, Vandendris M. [Acute urinary retention secondary to cavernous metastases from a prostatic tumor.] Prog Urol 1991;1:1042–5.

173. Monllor J, Tano F, Arteaga PR, Galbis F. Priapism of the clitoris. Eur Urol 1996;30:521–2.

174. Lue TF, Hellstrom WJ, McAninch JW, Tanagho EA. Priapism: a refined approach to diagnosis and treatment. J Urol 1986;136:104–8.

175. Pryor JP, Hehir M. The management of priapism. Br J Urol 1982;54:751–4.

176. Pohl J, Pott B, Kleinhans G. Priapism: a three-phase concept of management according to aetiology and prognosis. Br J Urol 1986;58:113–8.

177. Harmon WJ, Nehra A. Priapism: diagnosis and management. Mayo Clin Proc 1997;72:350–5.

178. Chan PT, Begin LR, Arnold D, et al. Priapism secondary to penile metastasis: a report of two cases and a review of the literature. J Surg Oncol 1998;68:51–9.

179. Osther PJ, Lontoft E. Metastasis to the penis. Case reports and review of the literature. Int Urol Nephrol 1991; 23:161–7.

180. Powell BL, Craig JB, Muss HB. Secondary malignancies of the penis and epididymis: a case report and review of the literature. J Clin Oncol 1985;3:110–6.

181. Stackl W, Mee SL. Priapism. In: Krane RJ, Siroky MB, Fitzpatrick JM, editors. Clinical urology. Philadelphia: J.B. Lippincott Company; 1994, p. 1245–58.

182. Shantha TR. Intraoperative management of penile erection using terbutaline. Anesthesiology 1989;70:707–9.

183. Shantha TR, Finnerty DP, Rodriquez AP. Treatment of persistent erection and priapism using terbutaline. J Urol 1989;141:1427–9.

184. Ercole CJ, Pontes JE, Pierce JM. Changing surgical concepts in the treatment of priapism. J Urol 1981;125:210–1.

185. Winter CC. Cure of idiopathic priapism: new procedure for creating fistula between glans penis and corpora cavernosa. Urol 1976;8:389–91.

186. Greyhack JT, McCullogh W, O'Connor VJ Jr, Trippel O. Venous bypass to control priapism. Invest Urol 1964; 1:509.

187. Mukamel E, Farrer J, Smith RB, de Kernion JB. Metastatic carcinoma to penis: when is total penectomy indicated? Urol 1987;29:15–8.

188. Walker TG, Grant PW, Goldstein I, et al. "High-flow" priapism: treatment with superselective transcatheter embolization. Radiology 1990;174:1053–4.

189. Harding JR, Hollander JB, Bendick PJ. Chronic priapism secondary to a traumatic arteriovenous fistula of the corpus cavernosum. J Urol 1993;150:1504–6.

190. Tarry WF, Duckett JW, Snyder HM. Urologic complications of sickle cell disease in a pediatric population. J Urol 1987;138:592–4.

191. Emond AM, Holman R, Hayes RJ, Serjeant GR. Priapism and impotence in homozygous sickle cell disase. Arch Intern Med 1980;140:1434–7.

192. Haddad FS, Kivirand AI. Metastases to the corpora cavernosa from transitional cell carcinoma of the bladder. J Surg Oncol 1986;32:19–21.

193. Whitmore WF. The rationale and results for ablative surgery for prostate cancer. Cancer 1963;16:1119–32.

194. Rees BI. Secondary involvement of the penis by rectal cancer. Br J Surg 1975;66:77–9.

CHAPTER 14

EMERGENCY CARDIAC PROBLEMS

MICHAEL S. EWER, MD, MPH, JD
JEAN BERNARD DURAND, MD
JOSEPH SWAFFORD, MD
SYED WAMIQUE YUSUF, MD, MRCP

Cardiac problems in cancer patients are true medical dilemmas for physicians in an emergency-center setting because heart-related symptoms are common, may be life threatening, and are frequently nonspecific. A symptom or sign giving rise to cardiac concerns may (but need not) be the consequence of a major medical problem, and analyzing the characteristics of a patient's complaint is especially important. Complaints typical of a serious disorder may be the result of atypical or trivial illness whereas atypical symptoms cannot be discounted as being inconsistent with a major cardiac event.

Patients have been taught by both health care professionals and extensive media educational programs that cardiac problems are poorly managed with a "wait-and-see" approach. Expedient evaluation in an emergency facility is the first priority for managing a cardiac condition that can evolve rapidly into a medical emergency with a fatal outcome.

Emergency-center physicians have developed a heightened scrutiny with regard to their approach to complaints that may be of cardiac origin. A desire to provide optimal medical care and a well-founded fear of potential litigation when a cardiac event is misdiagnosed have resulted in broadly accepted algorithms for managing patients with suspected cardiac illness in an emergency-center setting.[1,2] These algorithms have helped to standardize acute cardiac care, and they clearly need to be the basis for triaging patients into various treatment pathways, initiating care in the emergency center, and defining optimal urgent care beyond the emergency facility.

However, standardized approaches for emergency cardiac care may not always apply when cardiac patients concomitantly have cancer. First, these approaches are based on experiences with large groups of patients whose primary medical problem is cardiac (coronary artery disease, congestive heart failure, valvular heart disease, or cardiac arrhythmia); such patients may have undergone prior invasive or pharmacologic treatments of their cardiac disease. Second, large clinical trials are the basis for many of the pathways, and cancer patients have generally been excluded from such trial populations. While pathways are developed to maximize benefit and to minimize the risk of treatment for the subject population, cancer patients often do not fit standard models and may be better served through alternative approaches. The sensitivity and specificity of treatment outcomes in cancer patients may be significantly less than in the case of larger trial populations.[3] This is especially true when cancer patients who have nonspecific cardiac symptoms are treated. Laboratory tests, electrocardiographic data, and increases in plasma concentrations of cardiac enzymes, for example, provide important information that, when interpreted according to the standard algorithms, could result in a greater suspicion of cardiac disease for patients with cancer than is actually warranted. The failure to recognize this fact may result in physicians' subjecting some cancer patients to increased testing that is often painful, dangerous, and expensive. On the other hand, cancer and its treatment do not exclude patients from having the same cardiac entities as do noncancer patients, and failure to recognize concomitant serious cardiac problems can be lethal.

Treating cardiac problems in cancer patients is complicated and challenging, and increased clinical acumen is needed to evaluate these patients. When additional studies are required to help unravel the clinical problem, they should be ordered earlier for patients with cancer, but the fact that these tests may be less sensitive and specific in cancer patients should never be overlooked.

Altered threshold values and estimates for sensitivity and specificity for subgroups of patients with various stages of malignancy in addition to heart disease would be exceedingly helpful. At present, such analyses and guidelines are simply not available.

In view of these realities, how should cardiac abnormalities in cancer patients who present at the emergency center be handled? It should now be apparent that if a patient's cancer and cancer treatment are not taken into consideration, unnecessary treatments may have an increased risk or decreased benefit in view of the patient's reduced life expectancy. However, if too great an emphasis is placed on the patient's cancer, important treatment strategies may not be offered in a timely manner. In addition, physicians must keep in mind the concern of having to justify treatment that deviates from the accepted algorithms and pathways. It is often regarded as safer for a physician to follow the established pathways than to modify them, and often the patient with cancer must pay the price.

This chapter examines some of the more common cardiac conditions in cancer patients and attempts to balance the contribution of the malignancy and the underlying cardiac condition to the presentation. Clinicians must take into account risks to which patients may be exposed during treatment of cardiac problems and must attempt to optimize treatment strategies. Clearly, no set of guidelines is universally suited to all patients. Furthermore, a balance of more than one disease process should be kept in mind when treating the cardiac patient with cancer in an emergency center. The guiding principle should be that patients who have malignant disease and an excellent long-term prognosis and who have undergone treatments with limited systemic effects should be managed similarly to those who do not have cancer. On the other hand, patients who have extensive malignant disease, prior exposure to highly toxic treatment strategies, and a severely limited life expectancy may need to have their cardiac problems treated in a less aggressive manner. Conventional approaches may be too risky, and an anticipated benefit may not be realized because of the patient's reduced life expectancy due to the cancer. End-stage cancer patients who have a cardiac event may be treated with palliative measures.

ARRHYTHMIA

Arrhythmia is common in cancer patients and often requires them to seek help in the emergency center. Arrhythmia may be related to a patient's malignancy or cancer treatment, or it may be the result of unrelated medical problems. Symptoms can be subtle and have been described by patients as benignly as "occasional palpitations" or a mild "fluttering in the chest." Patients may also present with significant symptomatology and may be seen during or subsequent to an isolated or recurrent episode of loss of consciousness, lightheadedness, or dizziness. Patients sometimes present after the onset of one or more transient neurologic deficits, peripheral embolization, or acute claudication secondary to clot migration or stroke.

Arrhythmia, whether related or not related to cancer, is often transient. The normal sinus rhythm that is revealed on a single standard 12-lead electrocardiographic study, on an electrocardiographic rhythm strip, or during a brief episode of continuous electrocardiographic monitoring does not exclude the possibility of a latent and potentially serious rhythm disturbance. Even without obvious arrhythmia detected in the emergency center, a rhythm disturbance should be sought aggressively when symptoms suggest one of the entities noted above. The initial approach to arrhythmia is similar in patients with and without cancer.

However, analyzing cardiac rhythm in cancer patients may be more complicated because these patients often have exaggerated respiratory variations of the electrical axis and changes in mean QRS voltage that can be confused with arrhythmia. Such changes may be due to pleural or pericardial effusions, pulmonary resection, or radiation to the chest, with damage to the lungs.

Characterization

A somewhat restrictive categorization of arrhythmia in cancer patients includes the following two groupings: primary cardiac arrhythmia, which encompasses rhythm disturbances that arise from abnormalities within cardiac structures; and secondary arrhythmia, which includes disturbances that are due to metabolic abnormalities.

Primary Arrhythmia. Primary arrhythmia encompasses disturbances that arise from cardiac and pericardial structures and includes mechanical etiologies and local metabolic sequelae of primary cardiac disease. Primary arrhythmia may be caused by focal or diffuse abnormalities. Focal abnormalities are those that involve one or more localized areas of the myocardium; diffuse abnormalities can be found throughout the heart. The following are all common causes of primary arrhythmia in both cancer patients and noncancer patients: ischemic disease; increased intracardiac pressure and wall stress; congestive, hypertrophic, and infiltrative cardiomyopathy; and fibrosis related to aging. A number of other abnormalities, however, are more likely to be found in patients with cancer, and these include intracardiac thrombi (Figure 14–1), primary or metastatic malignant intracardiac tumors, amyloid infiltration, myopericarditis, pericardial constriction, and cardiomyopathy related to antitumor agents.

pericardiocentesis. The pleuropericardial-window procedure is usually done in an operating room, but it can be performed under local anesthesia with the patient in a hospital room or in an intensive-care unit.

Long-term management of malignant pericardial effusion focuses on preventing the reaccumulation of fluid, which occurs in more than 50% of patients. Because the long-term survival for most patients with malignant effusion is limited, an effective therapy that limits discomfort and that is not associated with excessive risk to the patient should be used. For patients with severe hemodynamic compromise and a rapid reaccumulation of fluid, the pleuropericardial window offers the most definitive therapy. In stable patients, systemic chemotherapy or thoracic irradiation may be used for tumors that are still sensitive to these treatment modalities. Additional radiation should be avoided in patients who have already received significant amounts of radiotherapy involving the heart. The use of local chemotherapeutic agents or agents given to sclerose the pericardium will prevent fluid reaccumulation in many patients. Sclerosis may be painful and often requires analgesia. The use of a percutaneous intrapericardial balloon catheter to create a pleuropericardial window has had some success. The results from a large series of patients treated with this modality are not yet available.[15,16]

ISCHEMIC HEART DISEASE

Cancer patients frequently present with symptoms of chest pain, and ischemic heart disease is often an initial concern for both the patient and the emergency physician. The terms "unstable angina" and "acute coronary syndrome" refer to the more serious cardiac etiologies of ischemic heart disease seen in the emergency center. Unstable angina includes new-onset angina, angina at rest, acceleration of angina, and postinfarction angina. Acute coronary syndrome also encompasses unstable angina but additionally includes non-ST-segment-elevation and ST-segment-elevation myocardial infarction.[17]

Management approaches to these syndromes that do not take the patient's cancer into account may expose the patient to unnecessary invasive procedures or to a course of action that can delay crucial early interventions. Coronary occlusion due to arterial embolism[18,19] and coronary artery spasm that may or may not be related to anticancer therapy are among the entities that are considerably more common in the cancer patient than in the general population.

Several chemotherapy agents have been noted to induce ischemia. The most notable is 5-fluorouracil.[20–27] Several cases of ventricular fibrillation temporally related to the infusion time of 5-fluorouracil also have been noted. The mechanism is presumed to be an acute coronary syndrome that is probably triggered by coronary vasospasm.

Patients with significant pre-existing coronary disease appear to be more susceptible, as are patients who have received the drug by continuous infusion.

The acute coronary syndrome may also be initiated or exacerbated by anemia, fever, infection, and concomitant treatment with other drugs. Previous clinical investigations have suggested that radiation therapy may lead to the development of early advanced coronary disease or accelerated restenosis in epicardial arteries within the radiation field; it has been suggested that microvascular injury may lead to fibrosis and ischemic cardiomyopathy. An increased incidence of ostial left main lesions and right coronary artery disease has been reported following radiotherapy.[28–33]

Conventional approaches to revascularization that are considered appropriate for noncancer patients with atherosclerotic coronary disease may have much less overall benefit for the patients with advanced cancer. Patients with a poor long-term prognosis may be unable to benefit from these interventions and are often at a much higher risk for the early complications of attempted revascularization.

Widely metastatic malignant disease may cause electrocardiographic and echocardiographic abnormalities that are indistinguishable from the findings in patients with typical myocardial ischemia, despite a lack of vascular involvement (Figure 14–4). Q waves and an altered R-wave progression may be seen in such patients, albeit with evolution over a longer period than is otherwise typical.[34] Symmetrically inverted T waves are sometimes seen in patients with central nervous system abnormalities and also may be confused with coronary artery disease (Figure 14–5).

Coronary insufficiency in cancer patients should be viewed as a disruption in oxygen supply or as a manifestation of increased oxygen demand. Unstable coronary disease may develop in patients with previously stable coronary disease because of anemia, hyperadrenergic states, and hormonal imbalances. Stabilizing strategies aimed at the problem of increasing oxygen requirements rather than revascularization may by prudent.

In an emergency-center setting, a two-pronged approach should be used for treating a patient who presents with symptoms consistent with ischemic heart disease. The priorities of the first prong are to diagnose or exclude an acute ischemic event, to stratify risk, and to plan and initiate urgent care based on guidelines from the American College of Cardiology and the American Heart Association. Even in the emergency center, the physician must explore and anticipate essential modifications in the usual approach because of the patient's decreased life expectancy, the patient's wishes for intensive treatment, and increased risk of complications associated with invasive procedures. Potentially correctable coexisting conditions that exacerbate the ischemic process (anemia, hyper-

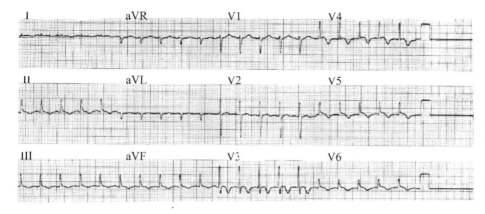

Figure 14–4. Electrocardiogram from a 26-year-old patient with metastasis to the myocardium, simulating the electrocardiographic findings of ischemia. This patient's angiogram showed no evidence of coronary artery disease.

thyroidism, or the shunting of blood through a vascular tumor) and the increased risk of thrombolysis or revascularization (owing to increased bleeding or intracranial metastatic disease) must be considered, and the treatment plan should be implemented accordingly. Thrombolytic agents are absolutely contraindicated in the presence of primary or metastatic brain lesions. These agents are associated with an increased risk of bleeding in all patients with widespread malignancy, and the use of thrombolytic agents in such patients should be approached with caution. Aspirin can be used unless specific contraindications for its use exist.[35–38] The overall benefit of aspirin is clearly established, and unpublished data from our institution suggest that even patients with platelet counts ≤ 50,000 and who experience manifestations of the coronary syndrome have a significantly lower 24-hour survival rate when they are not treated with aspirin.

Conventional or low-molecular-weight heparin, agents of the glyroprotein IIb IIIa class, and clopidogrel (Plavix) may also be used, with the caveat that many cancer patients have coagulopathies, decreased platelet counts, and primary and metastatic lesions that are prone to hemorrhage. Angiotensin-converting enzyme inhibitors, β-adrenergic blocking agents, and nitrates can be used in cancer patients with the same precautions that are appropriate for noncancer patients. The long-term effects of prior radiation for malignancy, however, may increase the risk of revascularization by complicating the

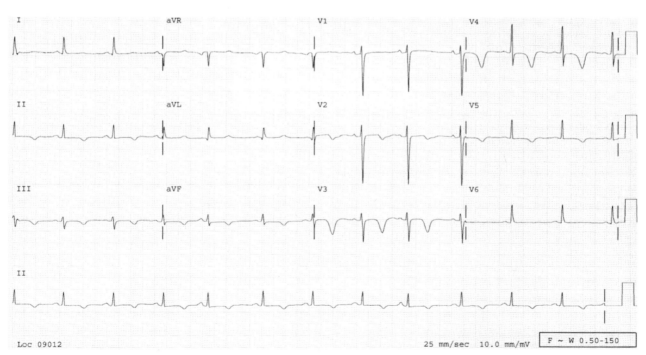

Loc 09012   25 mm/sec 10.0 mm/mV   F ~ W 0.50-150

Figure 14–5. Electrocardiogram from a breast cancer patient with central nervous system manifestations of metastatic disease and without evidence of coexisting coronary artery disease. Note deeply inverted T waves in the inferior and septal leads.

surgical approach or by making vessel dilatation, stenting, or grafting more difficult or impossible.

The second prong of emergency care for patients who are being evaluated for symptoms of ischemia is to attempt to rule in or rule out nonischemic causes of chest pain.

Musculoskeletal pain related to a tumor or to a prior surgery is common in patients with chest malignancies, as is pleural or pericardial pain, which may accompany or be independent of effusions. The discomfort associated with these entities may be clinically indistinguishable from that caused by ischemia. Pulmonary embolism, pain from acute or chronic pericarditis, and aneurysmal dissection also may be difficult to distinguish from ischemia. All of these entities are emergencies, and a delay in diagnosis may be life threatening; each entity can masquerade as ischemic heart disease, each is seen more frequently in cancer patients, and each requires a very different management strategy. A nonsequential approach should be used, and the emphasis should shift as the predominant risk emerges as being more typical of classic arteriosclerotic disease or as some other condition requiring very different urgent intervention. An initial approach to the management of chest pain in such patients is suggested in Figure 14–6.

HEART FAILURE

Heart failure is an extraordinarily common condition in the general population. An estimated 700,000 new cases of heart failure are diagnosed in the United States per year. Although increased awareness among physicians and other health care providers accounts for some of the apparent increase, the actual prevalence of heart failure continues to rise. Heart failure in the cancer patient may or may not be related to the malignancy or its treatment. Many causes of heart failure are seen more often in cancer patients than in the general population. Frequently, effects from several coexisting factors, any of which alone might not result in recognizable cardiac dysfunction, occur concurrently or sequentially and result in clinically symptomatic problems. Diagnosis and treatment options in cancer patients with multifactorial etiologies of heart failure produce dilemmas for physicians, especially in the setting of the emergency center, where therapeutic decisions must sometimes be made without the benefit of the results of extensive or invasive testing.

It is extremely important to think of cardiac dysfunction as a continuum rather than as a threshold phenomenon in which heart failure suddenly becomes relevant when the systolic function deteriorates below some trigger value. Modern therapeutic guidelines suggest that there is considerable benefit from early pharmacologic intervention. Heightened awareness of the possibility of a cardiac contribution to a nonspecific symptom may help the physician to establish the diagnosis of heart failure sooner and to suggest appropriate intervention. Traditional screening tests may not be sufficiently sensitive to suggest the presence of congestive heart failure; in some instances, the chest roentgenograph and the electrocardiogram may be normal despite significant systolic and/or diastolic cardiac dysfunction. Etiology is seldom suggested by these studies, and the definitive cause or causes of congestive heart failure often remain speculative.

Etiology

The most common cancer-specific etiology of heart failure in patients who have been treated with anthracyclines is chemotherapy-induced cardiomyopathy. Although methods for protecting the myocardium from damage are in increasingly wider use, this entity is still a problem and should be considered whenever a patient has received previous chemotherapy with an anthracycline or a related compound and subsequently presents without other obvious etiology for cardiac dysfunction. In the case of anthracyclines, the cardiac damage is related to the cumulative dose, and sequential insults and subsequent injury (even those that occur years after the initial treatment) may result in the clinical manifestations of heart failure with little warning. We and previous authors have observed that as many as 5 to 10% of patients who have received doxorubicin in cumulative doses of ≥ 450 mg/m^2 by rapid infusion have significant cardiac dysfunction. With a higher dose, the incidence rises exponentially.[39] Sporadic cases of heart failure have been observed at much lower cumulative doses, but this is rare in patients with no preexisting cardiac damage. Patients who are at highest risk include those with a history of significant coronary artery disease, those who have had prior radiation to the thorax, those at the extremes of age, and those with increased wall stress in the cardiac chambers. The relative contribution of each of many factors is not yet well defined.

The mechanism for anthracycline cardiomyopathy is complex, but it has been thought to be related to the formation of metabolically active free radicals. Doxorubicin has been studied more extensively than related agents, but daunorubicin, epirubicin, and mitoxantrone hydrochloride all demonstrate a similar cumulative dose–related toxicity. The concurrent administration of dexrazoxane may partially protect the myocardium but has raised concerns about a reduction in the efficacy of anthracycline.[40,41]

Management

Well-established guidelines for the management of heart failure in the general population exist, and these measures should form the basis for treatment for patients with cancer as well.[42] Randomized placebo-controlled trials for angiotensin-converting enzyme inhibitors,

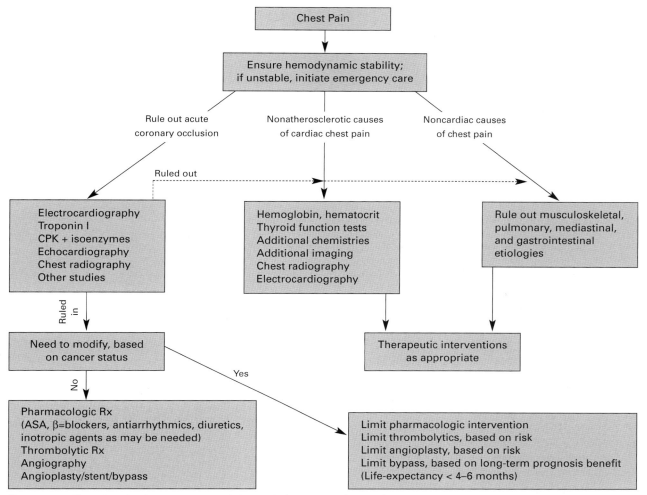

Figure 14–6. Flow chart for the management of chest pain in cancer patients. ASA = acetylsalicylic acid; CPK = creatine phosphokinase; Rx = therapy.

digoxin, or β-blockers for patients with suspected chemotherapy-induced heart failure are not available. For asymptomatic patients with clearly reduced systolic function, the early and judicious use of β-adrenergic blocking agents and angiotensin-converting enzyme inhibitors should be considered. Such therapy should be started at a very low dose and gradually increased. Our preference is to use a starting dose of 3.125 mg of carvedilol (Coreg) twice daily, gradually increasing the dose to 25 mg twice daily. β-Adrenergic blockade should not be used in an initial attempt to control symptoms in patients who have florid congestive heart failure, who have acute pulmonary edema, or who are severely hypotensive. Once stable, however, these patients may be started on β-blockers, and such patients often have a very beneficial and enduring response. Reduction of cardiac afterload is also very helpful in treating congestive heart failure. Enalapril (Vasotec), captopril (Capoten), and hydralazine (Apresoline) have all been used extensively

with significant benefit. Digitalis preparations are sometimes used and may offer symptomatic benefit. Unfortunately, unlike the β-blockers and the angiotensin-converting enzyme inhibitors, digitalis preparations do not appear to prolong life in patients with heart failure.

REFERENCES

1. Braunwald E, Antman EM, Beasley JW, et al. ACC/AHA guidelines for the management of patients with unstable angina and non-ST-segment elevation myocardial infarction: executive summary and recommendations. Circulation 2000;102:1193–209.

2. Antman EM, Brooks NH, Califf RM, et al. 1999 update: ACC/AHA guidelines for the management of patients with acute myocardial infarction. J Am Coll Cardiol 1999;34:1016–30.

3. Ewer MS, Benjamin RS. Cardiac complications. In: Holland J, Frei E, editors. Cancer medicine. 5th ed. Hamilton and London; BC Decker, Inc.; 2000. p. 2324–39.

4. Drugs causing prolongation of QT interval and torsades de pointes. Canadian Adverse Drug Reaction Newsletter. Can Med Assoc J 1998;8:103–4.

5. Hazinski MF, Cummins RO, Field JM, editors. 2000 Handbook of emergency cardiovascular care for healthcare providers. Dallas; American Heart Association; 2000.

6. Kern KB, Halperin HR, Field J. New guidelines for cardiopulmonary resuscitation and emergency cardiac care: changes in the management of cardiac arrest. JAMA 2001;284:1267–9.

7. Tieleman RG, Gosselink AT, Crijns HJ, et al. Efficacy, safety, and determinants of conversion of atrial fibrillation and flutter with oral amiodarone. Am J Cardiol 1997;79:53–7.

8. Vaughn Williams EM. A classification of antiarrhythmic action as reassessed after introduction of new drugs. J Clin Pharmacol 1984;24:129–47.

9. Gibbs HR, Swafford J, Nguyen HD, et al. Postoperative atrial fibrillation in cancer surgery: preoperative risks and clinical outcome. J Surg Oncol 1992;50:224–7.

10. Fuster V, Ryden LE, Asinger RW, et al. ACC/AHA/ESC guidelines for the management of atrial fibrillation: executive summary. J Am Coll Cardiol 2001;38:1231–65.

11. McKenna RJ Jr, Ali MK, Ewer MS, Frazier OH. Pleural and pericardial effusions in cancer patients. Curr Probl Cancer 1985;9:1–44.

12. Kralstein J, Frishman W. Malignant pericardial diseases: diagnosis and treatment. Am Heart J 1987;113:785–90.

13. Zepf RE, Johnston WW. The role of cytology in the evaluation of pericardial effusions. Chest 1972;62:593.

14. Reyes CV, Strinden C, Banerji M. The role of cytology in neoplastic tamponade. Acta Cytol 1982;26:299.

15. Ziskind A, Pearce A, Lemmon C, et al. Percutaneous balloon pericardiotomy for the treatment of cardiac tamponade and large pericardial effusions: descriptions of technique and report of the first 50 cases. J Am Coll Cardiol 1993;21:1–5.

16. Galli M, Politi A, Pedretti F, et al. Percutaneous balloon pericardiotomy for malignant pericardial tamponade. Chest 1995;108:1499–501.

17. Theroux P, Fuster V. Acute coronary syndromes: unstable angina and non-Q-wave myocardial infarction. Circulation 1998;97:1195–206.

18. Ali MK, Ewer MS, Cangir A, Fisher DJ. Coronary artery embolism following cancer chemotherapy. J Pediatr Hematol Oncol 1987;9:200–3.

19. Prizel KR, Hutchins GM, Bulkley BH. Coronary artery embolism and myocardial infarction: a clinicopathologic study of 55 patients. Ann Intern Med 1978;88:155–61.

20. De Forni M, Malet-Martino MC, Jaillas P, et al. Cardiotoxicity of high-dose continuous infusion fluorouracil: a prospective clinical study. J Clin Oncol 1992;10:1795–801.

21. Freeman NJ, Costanza ME. 5-Fluorouracil associated cardiotoxicity. Cancer 1998;61:36–45.

22. Labianca R, Beretta G, Clerici M, et al. Cardiac toxicity of 5-FU: a study of 1083 patients. Tumori 1982;68:505–10.

23. Keefe DL, Roistacher N, Pierri MK. Clinical cardiotoxicity of 5-fluorouracil. J Clin Pharmacol 1993;33:1060–70.

24. Ensley J, Kish J, Tapazoglou E, et al. 5-Fluorouracil infusions associated with an ischemic cardiotoxicity syndrome [abstract 554]. Proc Am Soc Clin Oncol 1986;5:142.

25. Jakubowski AA, Kemeny N. Hypotension as a manifestation of cardiotoxicity in 3 patients receiving cisplatin and 5-fluorouracil. Cancer 1988;62:266–9.

26. Anand AJ. Fluorouracil cardiotoxicity. Ann Pharmacother 1994;28:374–8.

27. Ewer MS, Benjamin RS, Hong WK, et al. Electrocardiographic changes in patients receiving chemotherapy with 5-fluorouracil and cis-platinum with and without diethyldithiocarbamate. Abstract 555. Proceedings of the 15th International Congress of Chemotherapy; July 19–24; Istanbul, Turkey. Federal Republic of Germany: Ecomed Verlagsgesellschaft mgh; 1987. p. 717–719.

28. McEniery PT, Dorosti K, Schiavone WA, et al. Clinical and angiographic features of coronary artery disease after chest irradiation. Am J Cardiol 1987;60:1020–4.

29. Tracy GP, Brown DE, Johnson LW, Gottlieb AJ. Radiation-induced coronary artery disease. JAMA 1974;228:1660–2.

30. Dollinger MR. Myocardial infarction due to postirradiation fibrosis of the coronary arteries. JAMA 1966;195:316–9.

31. Simon EB, Ling J, Mendizabal RC, Midawell J. Radiation-induced coronary artery disease. Am Heart J 1984;108:1032–4.

32. Silverberg GD, Britt RH, Goffinet DR. Radiation induced carotid artery disease. Cancer 1978;41:130–7.

33. Stewart JR, Fajardo LF. Radiation-induced heart disease: an update. Prog Cardiovasc Dis 1984;27:173–94.

34. Ewer MS, Ali MK. Critical cardiologic considerations in the cancer patient. Crit Care Clin 1988;13:41–60.

35. Lewis HD, Davis JW, Archibald DG, et al. Protective effects of aspirin against acute myocardial infarction and death in men with unstable angina: results of a Veterans Administration Cooperative Study. N Engl J Med 1983;309:396–403.

36. Cairns JA, Gent M, Singer J, et al. Aspirin, sulfin-pyrazone, or both in unstable angina. N Engl J Med 1985;313:1369–75.

37. Theroux P, Ouimet H, McCans J, et al. Asprin, heparin, or both to treat acute unstable angina. N Engl J Med 1988;319:1105–111.

38. The RISC Group. Risk of myocardial infarction and death during treatment with low dose aspirin and intravenous heparin in men with unstable coronary artery disease. Lancet 1990;336:827–30.

39. Ewer MS, Benjamin RS. Cardiotoxicity of chemotherapeutic drugs. In: Perry MC, editor. The chemotherapy source book. Philadelphia: Lippincott Williams & Wilkins; 2001. p. 458–68.

40. Swain SM, Whaley FS, Gerber MC, et al. Cardioprotection with dexrazoxane for doxorubicin-containing therapy in advanced breast cancer. J Clin Oncol 1997;15:1318–32.

41. Swain SM, Whaley FS, Gerber MC, et al. Delayed administration of dexrazoxane provides cardioprotection for patients with advanced breast cancer treated with doxorubicin-containing therapy. J Clin Oncol 1997;15:1333–40.

42. Pacher M, Cohn JN. Consensus recommendations for the management of chronic heart failure. Am J Cardiol 1999;83(2A):1A–38A.

CHAPTER 15

VASCULAR EMERGENCIES

SHUWEI GAO, MD
VICKI R. SHANNON, MD

ACUTE DEEP VENOUS THROMBOSIS

Venous thromboembolism (VTE) represents a spectrum of disease that includes both deep venous thrombosis (DVT) and pulmonary embolism (PE). Venous thromboembolism has long been recognized to be associated with malignancy. Symptomatic DVT occurs in up to 15% of patients with clinical overt cancer[1] whereas the prevalence of asymptomatic DVT is even higher, being reported in up to 50% of patients with advanced malignancy.[2] Deep venous thrombosis may lead to pulmonary embolism and cause significant morbidity and mortality if not diagnosed and treated promptly. However, the clinical diagnosis of DVT cannot be established with certainty without objective testing. Cancer patients tend to have more complications associated with treatment of DVT compared to non-cancer patients.

Etiology and Pathophysiology

There are a number of risk factors that can lead to venostasis, hypercoagulability, and endothelial injury (Virchow's triad) and thus lead to venous thrombosis. These risk factors can be hereditary or acquired. The most common risk factors are listed in Table 15–1. Most patients with DVT have multiple risk factors.[3,4]

Cancer has long been recognized as a major factor for VTE. Hypercoagulability is often seen in cancer patients because cancer cells can produce substances with procoagulant activity.[5,6] In addition, chemotherapy can decrease levels of the naturally occurring anticoagulant proteins.[7–9] Venous blood flow and vascular endothelium integrity are frequently disrupted by extrinsic compression due to bulky tumor masses, direct tumor invasion, or other risk factors frequently found in cancer patients, such as surgery, immobility, infection, and indwelling central venous catheters.[10,11]

Venous thrombosis usually occurs in the deep venous system of the lower extremities, but it may occur in the pelvic veins, renal veins, vena cava, or veins of the upper extremities.[12,13] Deep venous thrombosis of the lower extremities is subdivided into proximal (thigh) vein thrombosis and distal (calf) vein thrombosis. Proximal vein thrombosis is considered to be of more importance clinically because thrombi in proximal veins nearly always embolize and because more than 90% of cases of acute PE are due to emboli emanating from the proximal veins of the lower extremities.[14,15] The importance of isolated calf vein thrombosis is still a subject of debate. Most studies indicate that untreated calf vein thrombi do not lead to significant PE or to death.[16,17] However, some studies indicate that more than 20% of calf vein thrombi will propagate proximally above the knee,[18] and most deaths from PE are preceded by multiple smaller and silent embolic events.[19]

Central venous catheters are commonly used in cancer patients for chemotherapy, delivery of parenteral nutrition, blood transfusion, and the drawing of blood for laboratory tests. Thrombosis is one of the most common complications of central venous catheter use since central venous catheters may provide a nidus for clot formation. Thrombi can involve the catheter tip only or can occlude the superior vena cava or the main vessels of the

TABLE 15–1. Common Risk Factors for the Development of Venous Thromboembolism

Inherited thrombophilia
    Factor V Leiden mutation (activated protein C resistance)
    Prothrombin gene mutation
    Protein S deficiency
    Protein C deficiency
    Antithrombin III deficiency
    Increased factor VIII coagulant activity

Acquired predisposing factors
    Prolonged immobilization
    Surgery within the last 3 months
    History of venous thromboembolism
    Intravenous procedure or devices
    Malignancy
    Oral contraceptives or hormone replacement therapy
    Antiphospholipid antibody syndrome
    Myeloproliferative disorders
    Hyperhomocysteinemia
    Obesity

neck or upper extremities. The reported incidence of asymptomatic catheter-related thrombosis ranges from 13 to 56%;[20–22] the incidence of symptomatic catheter-related thrombosis is approximately 20%.[22,23] Pulmonary embolism occurs in up to 20% of patients with symptomatic catheter-related thrombosis, and fatal PE is not uncommon in these patients.[24]

Clinical Manifestations

The classic symptoms and signs of lower-extremity DVT include pain, swelling, erythema, warmth, tenderness, and palpable cord in the involved extremity. However, none of these symptoms or signs are specific to DVT; a significant percentage of patients with proved proximal DVT have no symptoms or signs,[25] and the majority of patients with these symptoms or signs do not have DVT.[26,27] Common clinical conditions that may mimic lower-extremity DVT include muscle strain, malignancy with venous or lymphatic obstruction, Baker's cyst, cellulitis, superficial phlebitis, and venous insufficiency.

Catheter-related upper-extremity thrombosis may manifest as pain or swelling of the neck or upper extremity. More often, however, patients with catheter-related upper-extremity thrombosis are totally asymptomatic or have only a catheter malfunction.[20,28]

Routine laboratory findings in patients with DVT are neither sensitive nor specific; this includes findings of leukocytosis, increased erythrocyte sedimentation rate, and elevated serum levels of lactate dehydrogenase and aspartate aminotransferase. Clotting function is normal in most patients with DVT, but thrombosis can occur in patients who are fully anticoagulated.

D dimer, a degradation product of cross-linked fibrin, has been extensively studied for its potential value in the diagnosis of DVT. When reliable assays are used, D-dimer levels are elevated in virtually all patients with clinically significant thrombosis. However, D-dimer levels may be elevated in a number of other clinical conditions, such as recent surgery, sepsis, and malignancy.[29] Therefore, a negative D-dimer test may be used to exclude significant thrombosis, but a positive D-dimer test is not sufficient to diagnose thrombosis.

Conventional enzyme-linked immunosorbent assay (ELISA) for D dimer has been the reference standard for D-dimer measurement. However, ELISA is performed in batches and is time-consuming and therefore unsuitable for use in emergency settings. The latex agglutination D-dimer assay routinely used in most hospitals has been proved to be not sufficiently sensitive to reliably exclude the presence of thrombosis. Newer rapid D-dimer assays developed in recent years have been extensively studied and are believed to be as reliable as conventional ELISA. Studies have shown that D-dimer levels of < 500 ng/mL as measured by rapid

quantitative D-dimer assay have an 81 to 99% negative predictive value for acute DVT.[30–33]

Despite promising data, the usefulness of D-dimer measurement in the diagnosis of DVT in patients with cancer has not been well studied. Limited data indicate that D-dimer measurement for the diagnosis of DVT may not be as helpful for patients with cancer as it is for patients without cancer.[34] At present, the D-dimer test cannot be recommended as a standard part of the diagnostic algorithm for cancer patients with suspected VTE.

Diagnosis

Clinical Evaluation. A detailed clinical history, including risk factors for DVT, should be obtained, and a complete physical examination should be performed. Objective imaging studies should be sought to establish or exclude the diagnosis as soon as DVT is clinically suspected because untreated acute DVT may lead to thrombus extension or PE, and administering anticoagulation to a patient without VTE may cause hemorrhagic complications since cancer patients often have hemostatic defects.

Compression Ultrasonography. In most circumstances, compression ultrasonography (US) or compression US with color Doppler (duplex US) is the noninvasive diagnostic approach of choice in patients with clinically suspected DVT. Compression US has been proved to be very accurate for diagnosing acute symptomatic proximal lower-extremity DVT; with reported sensitivities of 88 to 100% and specificities of 90 to 100%.[35,36] However, compression US has much lower sensitivity in the diagnosis of asymptomatic proximal lower-extremity DVT[37] or isolated calf vein DVT[35,38] although the specificity of compression US in these settings remains excellent. Therefore, positive findings on compression US are diagnostic of acute lower-extremity DVT in patients with or without symptoms, but negative findings on compression US cannot be relied on to exclude asymptomatic proximal lower-extremity DVT or calf vein DVT. Compression US may have to be repeated at 7 to 10 days if the initial studies are negative, because proximal propagation of undetected calf vein DVT occurs in 15 to 25% of cases, usually within 1 week.[39,40] The incidence of VTE during 3 to 6 months of follow-up being less than 1.5%, it is considered safe to withhold anticoagulation and to follow the case clinically if findings on repeat US remain negative.[39–41]

Compression US is not reliable for diagnosis of recurrent DVT unless findings on US have normalized prior to the suspected recurrence because it is not possible to accurately discriminate between acute and chronic thrombosis on the basis of clot echogenicity. The rate of normalization after abnormal findings on US after a first episode of acute DVT is only 60% after 1 year,[42,43] compared to more than 90% with impedance plethysmography (IPG).[44,45] It may be appropriate to perform follow-up compression US after 3 to 6 months of anticoagulation to serve as a baseline study in case symptoms recur.

Duplex US is the initial study of choice for the diagnosis of symptomatic upper-extremity DVT. This examination has a sensitivity of 93% and a specificity of 95% in symptomatic patients if the study is adequate.[46,47] The sensitivity of duplex US is lower in asymptomatic patients with catheter-related thrombosis.[48]

Impedance Plethysmography. Compared with other diagnostic tests for DVT, IPG is less expensive and requires less technical training. However, this technique does not distinguish between venous obstruction due to DVT and venous obstruction caused by nonthrombotic entities. False-positive results may occur with any disorder that impairs venous flow, such as venous compression by tumor or lymph node, congestive heart failure, increased intra-abdominal pressure, obesity, or decreased arterial blood flow due to arterial insufficiency. False-negative results may occur in patients with non-occlusive thrombi.[44,49]

Despite these limitations, IPG has proved to be very useful in the detection of proximal lower-extremity DVT in symptomatic patients, for which it has with a sensitivity of 91% and a specificity of 96%.[50] However, the sensitivity of IPG in the detection of isolated calf vein thrombosis and upper extremity thrombosis has been reported to be very low.[50–52] Serial IPG over 10 to 14 days has been used to improve the sensitivity of the test by detecting the extension of calf thrombi into the proximal veins. The positive conversion rate was reported to be 15%.[16]

Impedance plethysmography may be especially useful for the evaluation of suspected recurrent proximal DVT because, compared with compression US, findings on IPG normalize at a much more rapid and predictable rate after a first occurrence of DVT.[44]

Radionuclide Venography and Scintigraphy. Although the accuracy of radionuclide venography in the diagnosis of acute DVT has not been proved by large prospective studies, this technique has been routinely used at many institutions for many years for the detection of both lower- and upper-extremity DVT. Using contrast venography as the reference standard, several small studies revealed an 86% overall accuracy of radionuclide venography for the detection of acute lower-extremity DVT.[53–56] The sensitivity of radionuclide venography was higher for the detection of proximal major vein thrombosis, especially in the iliac vein or vena cava.[54–56] Radionuclide venography has also been used in the evaluation of upper-extremity thrombosis,[28] but there have been very few studies comparing it with contrast venography in this setting, and the reported accuracy of radionuclide venography is only 73%.[57]

Because radionuclide venography has not been validated satisfactorily against contrast venography, radionu-clide venography should not be included in the standard diagnostic work-up of acute lower- or upper-extremity DVT at present. Both positive and negative findings on radionuclide venography should be confirmed by other validated measures if these findings are not strongly concordant with clinical suspicion.

Other nuclear studies focus on direct "imaging" of the thrombi. In the iodine 125 fibrinogen uptake test, fibrinogen labeled with iodine 125 is injected into the peripheral vein, and the extremities are scanned 24 and 72 hours later for evidence of new deposition of fibrin. This test is no longer used in clinics because it is time-consuming and has significant false-positive and false-negative rates.[58]

Several newly developed thromboscintigraphic tests use radiolabeled antifibrin monoclonal antibody,[59] radiolabeled tissue plasminogen activator,[60] or radiolabeled apcitide (a synthetic peptide with a high affinity to glycoprotein IIb/IIIa receptors expressed on the surface of activated platelets)[61] to quickly detect newly formed thrombi. Although these new measures have not been tested extensively, limited data have shown these measures to have great potential in the diagnosis of acute DVT. Compared with contrast venography, technetium-99m (Tc-99m) apcitide thromboscintigraphy had a specificity of 84 to 88% and a sensitivity of 86 to 91% for the detection of acute DVT in phase III studies.[61,62]

Contrast Venography. Contrast venography remains the "gold standard" for the diagnosis of symptomatic DVT. This test is nearly 100% sensitive and specific, provided that it is technically adequate and that strict diagnostic criteria are adhered to.[63] Unlike compression US or IPG, contrast venography is also sensitive in the detection of asymptomatic proximal lower-extremity DVT, calf DVT, and upper-extremity DVT. However, one study found that contrast venography could not be performed in up to 20% of patients with clinically suspected DVT because of contraindications or technical difficulties.[64]

Contrast venography is currently reserved for situations in which US or IPG is not feasible or in which the results of noninvasive studies are either equivocal or discordant with a strong clinical impression.

Magnetic Resonance Venography. Magnetic resonance imaging (MRI) is increasingly used in the diagnosis of DVT. Preliminary studies suggest that magnetic resonance (MR) venography has excellent sensitivity and specificity for proximal lower-extremity DVT and upper-extremity DVT.[65–67] The accuracy of MR venography for the diagnosis of pelvic noniliac DVT is even superior to that of contrast venography.[68] MR venography may be a useful alternative approach when contrast venography is required but precluded because of contraindications or technical difficulties.

Other advantages of MR venography include the avoidance of patient exposure to ionized contrast, the opportunity to diagnose nonthrombotic conditions that may mimic DVT,[65] the potential to distinguish acute from chronic thrombosis,[69] and the ability to simultaneously scan both the lungs and the lower extremities for clots.[70]

Summary: Diagnostic Approach to Acute Deep Venous Thrombosis. Acute lower-extremity DVT should be suspected in any cancer patient with a new onset of leg pain, swelling, or discoloration, even if an alternative diagnosis seems obvious. The diagnostic work-up should begin with a complete history and physical examination, followed by compression US or by IPG if US is not feasible. A positive finding on either of these studies is considered to be diagnostic of DVT, and anticoagulation should be initiated in this case. If findings on compression US or IPG are negative, the diagnostic approach should be individualized. For most patients, repeat compression US 5 to 7 days later or serial IPG over 7 to 10 days should be performed. If findings on repeat US or serial IPG remain negative, the patient can be observed clinically without anticoagulation measures.

If neither compression US nor IPG can be performed, if the diagnosis remains in question after US or IPG, or if the findings on US or IPG conflict with strong clinical suspicion, then contrast venography or MR venography should be performed. A suggested diagnostic approach to suspected acute DVT is shown in Figure 15–1.

The diagnostic approach to suspected recurrent DVT should be individualized. No single test is ideal. Compression US and IPG are the preferred noninvasive screening tests. If the resolution of previous DVT has been documented, compression US or IPG can be used to confirm the recurrence. Compression US can also be diagnostic if the noncompressible segment is in a new location. Contrast venography should be performed if US or IPG is not diagnostic. If the differentiation of old clots from new clots remains unclear and if the technique is available, radionuclide scintigraphy to specifically probe the fresh clot may be considered.

Treatment

The goals of the treatment of DVT are to prevent the occurrence of PE, to prevent recurrent thrombosis, and to minimize long-term morbidity. The treatment of DVT in patients with cancer can be especially challenging. As a group, cancer patients have an elevated incidence of anticoagulant-related bleeding and an elevated incidence of recurrent VTE; in addition, cancer patients often undergo frequent invasive procedures and have a limited life expectancy. Therefore, the treatment of DVT in cancer patients must be individualized on the basis of the overall therapeutic and palliative goals of care.

Most patients with acute DVT can be managed on an outpatient basis if the risk of PE is believed to be low. Bed rest for the first 24 hours, with both lower extremities elevated, is desirable. However, in a recent study, prolonged bed rest after an occurrence of acute lower-extremity DVT did not reduce the incidence of PE.[71]

Anticoagulation has been the mainstay of therapy for DVT. When there is a high clinical suspicion of concurrent PE, anticoagulation should be started before investigation because the risk of recurrent PE outweighs the risk of complications secondary to anticoagulation. Other treatment modalities available are interruption of the venous pathway, thrombectomy, and thrombolysis.

Anticoagulation. Anticoagulation prevents the progression of clots and reduces the risk of further thromboembolic events. Anticoagulation is carried out by an initial treatment with unfractionated heparin (hereafter referred to simply as heparin) or fractionated low-molecular-weight (LMW) heparins to achieve immediate antithrombotic effects, followed by long-term maintenance treatment with oral coumadin derivatives (eg, Warfarin) or LMW heparins to prevent the recurrence of VTE.

Absolute contraindications to anticoagulation include active bleeding, recent intracranial surgery, a history of hemorrhagic stroke, and severe thrombocytopenia. The presence of a primary brain tumor or brain metastases is not an absolute contraindication if there is no evidence or history of intracranial hemorrhage and if the brain lesions are not highly vascular lesions (such as those from melanoma). Advanced age is not a contraindication to anticoagulation, but more intensive monitoring is required for elderly patients because of the increased risk of both bleeding and thrombotic complications.

The duration of anticoagulation should be based on thromboembolic risk factors and clinical situations. In patients with transient risk factors such as surgery or cured malignancy, 3 to 6 months of anticoagulation may be sufficient.[72,73] In patients with irreversible risk factors such as active malignancy or hereditary thrombophilia, indefinite anticoagulation may be required.[74] In patients with advanced malignancy and limited life expectancy, quality of life is a major factor to be considered, and the benefits of anticoagulation must be weighed against the ongoing risk of bleeding associated with indefinite anticoagulation.

Unfractionated Heparin. Heparin is the anticoagulant that is most often used for initial anticoagulation. It inhibits thrombin and other clotting factors by potentiating antithrombin III. Heparin is usually given as an initial intravenous loading bolus, followed by continuous infusion. The infusion is adjusted every 4 to 6 hours to maintain the activated partial thromboplastin time (aPTT) at 1.5 to 2.5 times the control value (Table 15–2). The half-life of heparin is 90 minutes, and a stable therapeutic level

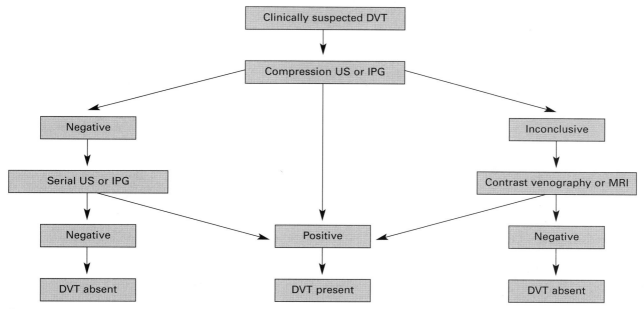

Figure 15–1. Diagnostic approach to patients with suspected acute deep venous thrombosis. DVT = deep venous thrombosis; IPG = impedance plethysmography; MRI = magnetic resonance imaging; US = ultrasonography.

can be achieved within 5 hours with an appropriate bolus and infusion. However, in many patients with acute VTE, the aPTT does not reach a therapeutic level within 24 hours due to an insufficient starting bolus dose or an insufficient initial infusion rate.[75] Oral warfarin is usually started on the 2nd day after a patient's aPTT has reached a therapeutic level, and heparin infusion is continued for 5 to 7 more days until warfarin has remained at therapeutic levels for 2 consecutive days.

Patients with an excess of plasma heparin-binding proteins require a larger dose of heparin. For these patients, monitoring the heparin concentration is preferable to monitoring aPTT, in terms of avoiding heparin overdose.[76] Clinically effective anticoagulation is achieved with serum heparin levels of 0.4 to 0.7 U/mL as measured by anti-factor-Xa assay.[77]

The advantages of heparin infusion include rapid therapeutic effects and rapid reversal of anticoagulant effects by stopping the infusion or by infusing 15 mg of protamine sulfate over 3 minutes. The disadvantages of heparin infusion include the need for intravenous administration, the need for frequent laboratory monitoring, and the uncommon but fatal complication of heparin-induced thrombocytopenia.

Subcutaneous unfractionated heparin has been used for initial anticoagulation treatment of DVT at some centers, and a weight-based algorithm has been suggested.[78] However, there is no validated guideline for this usage, and it is difficult to reach or maintain a therapeutic aPTT with the use of subcutaneous heparin.

Fractionated Low-Molecular-Weight Heparins. LMW heparins are fractionated products of standard heparin that are produced by the enzymatic or chemical depolymerization of unfractionated heparin. These heparins have many advantages over unfractionated heparin, including a longer plasma half-life, better bioavailability after subcutaneous injection, and a more predictable anticoagulant dose response.[79] These pharmacokinetic properties make it possible to give LMW heparins subcutaneously once or twice daily without the need for laboratory monitoring of the anticoagulant effect.[77]

LMW heparins have been demonstrated to be at least as effective and safe as "standard" dose-adjusted intravenous unfractionated heparin for the initial treatment of established DVT.[80–83] They have also been demonstrated to be safe, effective, and convenient for treatment of DVT on an outpatient basis.[84–86] As is the case with unfractionated heparin, oral warfarin is usually started on the 2nd day of LMW heparin use, and LMW heparin is continued for 5 to 7 more days until therapeutic warfarin levels have been reached and have been maintained for 2 consecutive days.

Large clinical trials comparing LMW heparins with warfarin in cancer patients have yet to be completed. Available data from studies involving patients both with and without cancer have proved that LMW heparins as long-term anticoagulation are at least as effective and safe as warfarin.[87]

Although warfarin is still the preferred agent for maintenance anticoagulation in most patients with VTE,

TABLE 15–2. M. D. Anderson Cancer Center Weight-Based Schedule for Intravenous Heparin Infusion

1. Initial bolus dose, 80 U/kg; initial infusion dose, 18 U/kg/h
2. Check aPTT every 6 hours until stable. Adjust heparin dosage as follows:
   - aPPT < 35:80 U/kg bolus, then increase infusion rate by 4 U/kg/h
   - aPTT 35–45: 40 U/kg bolus, then increase infusion rate by 2 U/kg/h
   - aPTT 46–70: no change in infusion rate
   - aPTT 71–90: decrease infusion rate by 2 U/kg/h
   - aPTT > 90: hold infusion for 1 hour, then decrease infusion rate by 3 U/kg/h

aPTT = activated partial thromboplastin time.

LMW heparins have several advantages over warfarin. First, LMW heparins do not require laboratory monitoring since dosing is based on body weight.[79] Second, LMW heparins also have a more reliable anticoagulant effect, one that is not influenced by diet or drugs.[79] Like heparin, LMW heparins are effective for patients who have warfarin-resistant thrombosis,[88] which seems to be more common in patients with cancer than in patients without cancer.[89]

Low-molecular-weight heparins are associated with the same complications as is unfractionated heparin, but the complications of bleeding or heparin-induced thrombocytopenia may be less common or less severe with LMW heparins.[77,81–83] The long half-life of LMW heparins may not be desirable if anticoagulation needs to be reversed in case of significant hemorrhage; 1 mg of protamine sulfate may reverse the effect of 1 mg of enoxaparin.

Warfarin. The oral anticoagulant warfarin is a vitamin K inhibitor that depletes vitamin K–dependent coagulation proteins (factors II, VII, IX, and X) and anticoagulant protein (protein C). Because protein C has a shorter half-life, the exhaustion of protein C before the exhaustion of coagulation factors may cause an early hypercoagulable state that can lead to clot extension or recurrent thromboembolism if warfarin is given without full anticoagulation.

The full anticoagulant effect of warfarin may not be apparent for 5 days, even if the prothrombin time increases more rapidly.[90] Therefore, heparin infusion or subcutaneous LMW heparins should be administered concurrently with warfarin for at least 5 days, until all procoagulant factors have been depleted. A transient hypercoagulable state after the discontinuation of warfarin can also occur, due to the differential recovery of procoagulant and anticoagulant proteins. It may be rational to administer subcutaneous LMW heparins for 5 days at the end of warfarin therapy.

The anticoagulant effect of warfarin is adjusted by varying the dose to keep the International Normalized Ratio (INR) within the range of 2.5 to 3.5. Frequent laboratory monitoring may be required, especially for cancer patients, because the warfarin level is markedly influenced by diet, drugs, gastrointestinal absorption, and hepatic function, and wide fluctuations in the INR can lead to excessive bleeding or to a recurrence of VTE.[91]

Inferior Vena Cava Filtration. Inferior vena cava (IVC) filtration has often been used for prophylaxis against PE or recurrent PE in cancer patients. The main indications for the placement of an IVC filter in patients with DVT are listed in Table 15–3. An IVC filter is not a substitute for anticoagulation. When possible, anticoagulants should be given in an effort to prevent further thrombosis. This is because an IVC filter may decrease the risk of short-term recurrence of emboli, but without additional long-term anticoagulation, it may greatly increase the long-term rate of recurrent VTE.[92,93]

Although they are relatively safe, IVC filters can cause severe complications such as filter migration, caval perforation, caval thrombosis, bowel obstruction, and ureteral injury.[94,95] Temporary retrievable IVC filters may avoid some of the long-term complications and have been successfully used in patients who require a period of protection against PE, such as patients who are undergoing thrombolysis, thrombectomy, or high-dose chemotherapy and such as patients with temporary contraindications for anticoagulation.[96,97]

Thrombolysis and Thrombectomy. Thrombolysis and thrombectomy for lower-extremity DVT are rarely indicated,[98] and the potential benefit of reducing the incidence of postphlebitic syndrome is questionable.[99,100]

Treatment of Catheter-Related Thrombosis. For thrombosis of the catheter lumen or tip, the administration of a low-dose thrombolytic agent (5,000 U of urokinase or 2 mg TPA) into the catheter will usually restore catheter patency.[101] If empiric therapy fails to restore catheter function, radiologic imaging is advisable to rule out a mechanical problem such as a kink or malposition.

If the thrombus extends beyond the catheter tip and if the patient has clinical evidence of upper-extremity thrombosis, standard anticoagulation should be initiated.

TABLE 15–3. Indications for Placement of Inferior Vena Cava Filter in Patients with Deep Venous Thrombosis

Anticoagulation contraindicated
  Active bleeding
  High risk of catastrophic bleeding: post craniotomy or large brain mass
  Planned intensive chemotherapy, with anticipated severe thrombocytopenia

Anticoagulation failure despite adequate therapy

Prophylaxis in high-risk patients
  Proximal DVT with inadequate cardiopulmonary reserve
  Extensive and progressive DVT
  In conjunction with thrombectomy, embolectomy, or thrombolysis

DVT = deep venous thrombosis.

Anticoagulation as sole therapy has been successful in restoring catheter patency, reducing symptoms, and preventing embolization to the lungs.[28,102] If no improvement is noted or if a rapid result is desired, full-dose thrombolytic therapy should be considered.[103,104] The catheter, as the cause of the thrombus, should be removed if its removal does not significantly jeopardize the patient's care. To prevent thrombus extension or embolization, anticoagulation should be continued for a short period after catheter removal.

Prophylaxis with low-fixed-dose warfarin (1 mg/d) or low-dose LMW heparins in cancer patients with long-term subclavian catheters may significantly reduce the incidence of thrombotic complications.[105,106]

Summary

Deep venous thrombosis is a common complication in patients with cancer. In most cases, DVT can be reliably diagnosed or excluded with noninvasive diagnostic tests. Angiography should be used only when noninvasive testing is not clinically feasible or if the results of noninvasive tests are equivocal. In addition to the increased risks for anticoagulant-related bleeding and for failure of anticoagulation, cancer patients often are subject to other issues that complicate the treatment of their DVT. The management of DVT in patients with cancer should be individually adjusted to meet the overall therapeutic and palliative goals of care. Treatment of DVT at home with LMW heparins is an attractive option for patients with cancer.

SUPERIOR VENA CAVA SYNDROME

Superior vena cava syndrome (SVCS) comprises an array of signs and symptoms that are caused by the partial or complete obstruction of blood flow through the superior vena cava (SVC) to the right atrium as a result of the compression, invasion, thrombosis, or fibrosis of this thin-walled vessel. The primary cause of SVCS has shifted dramatically over the past 50 years; whereas infectious diseases once constituted the primary cause, malignancies now account for up to 90% of cases.[107–110] Although SVCS was once considered a medical emergency that merited immediate radiotherapy, it is now well established that SVCS rarely causes immediate life-threatening complications.[111,112]

Anatomy and Pathophysiology

The SVC is the major drainage vessel for venous blood from the head, neck, upper extremities, and upper thorax. The SVC is located in the middle mediastinum and extends from the junction of the innominate veins to the right atrium. The azygos vein, the last main auxiliary vessel of the SVC, drains blood from the chest wall and enters the SVC just above the pericardial reflection. The

SVC is thin walled and has a low intravascular pressure. It is surrounded by rigid structures such as the sternum, trachea, aorta, pulmonary artery, right bronchus, and perihilar and paratracheal lymph nodes. Therefore, the SVC is particularly vulnerable to obstruction, especially to external compression due to tumor or enlarged lymph nodes. Superior vena cava obstruction (SVCO) can also be caused by direct tumor invasion, by a thrombus, or by a fibrotic process from inflammation due to infection, chemotherapy, or radiotherapy.[113–115]

Obstruction of the SVC causes venous pressure in the SVC to rise. This increased pressure may cause extensive venous collateral circulation. The azygos venous system is the most important alternate pathway for blood flow. Obstruction below or at the entrance of the azygos vein forces blood to traverse in a retrograde manner down the azygos vein and the other chest wall veins to reach the drainage area of the IVC, thus causing more prominent symptoms of SVCS. Elevated venous pressure in the SVC and the occurrence of collateral circulation (which is more prominent in a recumbent or forward-leaning position) lead to the characteristic clinical features of SVCS: venous distention and interstitial edema of the upper body. The sudden obstruction of the SVC, which is rare, can cause the rapid elevation of intracranial pressure, resulting in cerebral edema, intracranial thrombosis or bleeding, and death.

A contiguously extended tumor can compress or invade other adjacent structures such as the trachea, the bronchus, or the spinal cord, resulting in simultaneous airway obstruction or spinal-cord compression.[116,117]

Etiology

From the first recorded description of SVCS in 1757 by William Hunter through the first half of the twentieth century, syphilitic aneurysm and tuberculous mediastinitis were the prominent etiologic factors of SVCS. With the rapid rise in the incidence of lung cancer and with the advent of better treatment modalities for infectious disease, the primary causes of SVCS have shifted dramatically to malignancy. Currently, nearly all cases of SVCS are caused by malignancy (Table 15–4).

Lung cancer is the leading cause of SVCS and accounts for 65 to 85% of all SVCS cases.[108,110,118,119] Superior vena cava syndrome is encountered as a complication in approximately 3% of all patients with lung cancer.[109] Small-cell lung cancer is the most common histologic subtype, and SVCS complicates approximately 8 to 12% of all cases of small-cell lung cancer.[120–123] In one report, up to 80% of the tumors that induced SVCS were located in the right lung.[124]

Non-Hodgkin's lymphoma is the second most common cause of SVCS and accounts for 8% of all cases of SVCS. Diffuse large-cell lymphoma and lymphoblastic lymphoma are the most common histologic subtypes associated with SVCS.[125] Although Hodgkin's lymphoma commonly involves the mediastinum, it rarely causes SVCS.[125,126]

Other primary mediastinal malignancies that may cause SVCS include thymoma and germ cell tumors, which together make up fewer than 2% of all SVCS cases.[127] Metastatic cancers account for approximately 5 to 10% of all cases of SVCS.[119] Breast cancer is the most common metastatic disease that causes SVCS.[128] Other metastatic malignancies that can cause SVCS include gastrointestinal cancers, sarcomas, prostate cancer, and melanomas.[129]

An increasing cause of SVCS in cancer patients is central venous catheter–induced thrombosis, which is the result of the frequent use of intravenous devices for chemotherapy administration, parenteral nutrition, and blood transfusion.[130,131]

Currently, fewer than 10% of SVCS cases are due to nonmalignant causes such as retrosternal goiters, teratoma, pleural calcification, constrictive pericarditis, pyogenic infections, postradiation fibrosis or obliteration, chemotherapy-induced fibrosis, silicosis, sarcoidosis, or idiopathic mediastinal fibrosis.[108,110,118]

Clinical Presentation

The manifestation of specific symptoms and signs of SVCS depends on the site and the rapidity of the obstruction. The syndrome usually develops insidiously, over a few weeks; common symptoms are dyspnea, facial swelling, head fullness, cough, chest pain, arm swelling, and dysphagia.[108,109,119,132,133] The typical signs of SVCS include venous distention of the neck and chest wall, facial edema, facial plethora, cyanosis, and upper-extremity edema.[109,119,132,133] Other physical findings may include nonpitting edema of the neck (collar of Stokes), Horner's syndrome, glossal edema, proptosis, and dilated vessels of the retina. The symptoms and signs are usually exacerbated when the patient bends forward, stoops, or lies down.

Rarely, patients may present acutely with rapidly progressive cyanotic facial and upper-body swelling, dyspnea, and distended neck veins. Stridor is an ominous sign in these patients and indicates severe airway compromise (due to proximal airway edema or obstruction) and impending respiratory failure. This complication is more often seen in pediatric patients with lymphoma. Neurologic abnormalities such as severe headaches, blurred vision, altered sensorium, and seizures secondary to increased intracranial pressure and cerebral edema are also ominous. Airway compromise, cardiovascular collapse, and neurologic abnormalities are fortunately rare but remain life-threatening manifestations of SVCS that warrant emergent medical therapy.

Diagnosis

In most cases, the characteristic signs and symptoms of SVCS easily lead to a clinical diagnosis of SVCS. In a few cases, particularly those in which the obstruction is minimal, the clinical findings may be subtle, and the diagnosis may be more difficult to establish. Many imaging modalities can be used to confirm SVCO. However, it is more important to promptly establish a histologic diagnosis of the underlying cause of SVCO since SVCS is rarely life threatening and because optimal management of SVCS depends on the underlying disease.

Imaging Studies. Confirmatory diagnostic imaging is useful for delineating the extent of tumor and for ruling out simultaneous complications such as proximal airway obstruction, spinal-cord compression, and pericardial metastasis.

Chest radiography should be the first radiographic procedure performed when SVCS is suspected. Superior vena cava syndrome is frequently accompanied by mediastinal widening or by a mass in the superior mediastinum, right hilum, or right upper lobe.[108] Less common findings include pleural effusion, right-upper-lobe collapse, or rib notching. However, up to 16% of patients with SVCS are normal on chest radiography at the time of presentation.[108]

Computed tomography (CT), especially contrast-enhanced spiral CT, is the most useful radiographic study for diagnosing SVCS. Not only can CT reveal the site of obstruction and collateral flow, but it can also differentiate extravascular tumor compression from intravascular thrombus formation.[134,135] More important, CT provides detailed information about the tumor mass and its relation to mediastinal structures, thus helping to guide fine-needle aspiration biopsy or other diagnostic procedures if a histologic diagnosis has not been previously established. Computed tomography may also provide information on other critical structures (such as the bronchi and the spinal-cord), to exclude the presence of truly emergent complications

TABLE 15–4. Common Causes of Superior Vena Cava Syndrome in 743 Patients

Cause	Percentage
Lung Cancer	70.0
(Small-cell lung cancer)	(26.0)
(Non-small-cell lung cancer)	(44.0)
Lymphoma	9.7
Other Malignancies	8.7
Nonmalignant causes	6.7
Not diagnosed	4.8

Adapted from Parish JM, et al;[108] Armstrong BA, et al;[109] Yellin A, et al;[110] Davenport D, et al;[111] Schraufnagel DE;[118] Bell DR, et al;[119] Lochridge SK, et al;[133] Scarantino C, et al;[228] Little AG, et al.[229]

(such as proximal airway obstruction, spinal-cord compression, and pericardial metastases) that frequently accompany SVCO.[118,134,136]

Radionuclide venography is useful for identifying the site of obstruction and for delineating collateral blood flow.[137,138] It may also be useful in long-term follow-up and for making serial comparisons.[138]

Magnetic resonance imaging has been increasingly used for determining the cause of SVCS. Many investors believe that MRI is more effective than CT in demonstrating the relationships among vessels, nodes, and other mediastinal structures, as well as vessel patency.[139] Magnetic resonance imaging can be used in patients for whom contrast-enhanced CT is contraindicated.

Contrast venography (CV) for diagnosis of SVCS is controversial and rarely indicated. However, CV does provide more accurate anatomic details of the obstruction site and information on the development of collateral blood flow.[140,141] Compared with other diagnostic tools, CV may also more accurately demonstrate an intravascular thrombus.[141] Common complications of CV include phlebitis, thrombosis, and prolonged bleeding secondary to increased intraluminal pressure.

Transesophageal echocardiography and duplex US may be used to distinguish thrombus formation from external compression of the SVC.[142]

Histologic Diagnosis. More than 50% of patients with SVCS in reported studies developed symptoms of the condition before the primary diagnosis was established.[116,118,143] Although imaging studies can confirm the clinical diagnosis of SVCS, priority should be given to procedures that help to establish the histologic diagnosis. The diagnostic approach may vary, depending on the working diagnosis, the location of the tumor, the physical condition of the patient, and the available expertise. The least invasive procedures should be performed first. Emergent irradiation before biopsy may preclude proper interpretation of the specimen in 50% of cases.[136]

Sputum cytology can establish the diagnosis of underlying malignancies in 27 to 59% of patients in whom bronchogenic carcinoma is suspected.[110,118]

Serum tumor markers, such as β–human chorionic gonadotropin (β-hCG) and α-fetoprotein should be checked if germ cell cancer is suspected, especially in young men.

Bronchoscopy is the most commonly performed invasive procedure used to establish the histologic diagnosis of SVCS. It may provide the diagnosis in up to 50% of patients with SVCS and in most of cases of small-cell carcinoma of the lung.[116,143,144]

Thoracentesis can be very useful in establishing the diagnosis of malignancy in patients with SVCS and pleural effusion.[143]

Lymph node biopsy of palpable supraclavicular or cervical lymph nodes can help to establish the diagnosis, with minimal morbidity in most cases.[143–145] However, fine-needle aspiration should be avoided if lymphoma is suspected.[125]

Bone marrow biopsy should be performed if lymphoma is suspected, especially in young adults. Small-cell carcinoma of the lung also often involves the bone marrow.[144]

Mediastinoscopy is much more effective than bronchoscopy in diagnosing the primary disease.[144–146] However, mediastinoscopy is also more invasive and has a higher complication rate.

Thoracostomy can determine the cause of SVCO in virtually every case in which other diagnostic procedures have failed.[144,145] It has the advantages of direct visualization, the ability to assess the extent of the disease involved, and adequate biopsy samples. However, this procedure is the most invasive of all the techniques and has significant morbidity and mortality rates; therefore, it is rarely indicated.

Percutaneous transthoracic biopsy with CT guidance is emerging as an effective and safe alternative to open lung biopsy and mediastinoscopy. It has a high diagnostic yield and relatively low morbidity and mortality rates.[145,147]

Treatment

The focus of the management of SVCS has shifted from empiric radiotherapy to careful diagnostic evaluation. The prognosis of patients with SVCS strongly correlates with the prognosis of the underlying disease. The common malignant causes of SVCS, such as small-cell lung cancer and lymphoma, are chemosensitive and potentially curable even in the presence of SVCS.[123,148] Every effort should be made to define a histologic diagnosis before treatment is initiated, except in rare emergent situations of impending airway obstruction or increased intracranial pressure. In such cases, empiric radiotherapy or intravascular stenting should be used immediately.

Supportive Measures. Patients should be closely watched while a definitive diagnosis is pending. Supplemental oxygen, sedation, and bed rest with the upper body elevated may help to lessen the symptoms by lowering venous pressure and cardiac output. The use of diuretics may transiently decrease edema, but the efficacy of this has not been proved. Diuretics may exacerbate hemodynamic instability by further reducing venous return and may increase the risk of thrombosis by causing dehydration. The use of steroid therapy in the treatment of increased intracranial pressure and SVCS secondary to lymphoma is well established. Corticosteroids are frequently used in an attempt to alleviate symptoms associated with SVCS-related airway inflammation and edema. However, controlled trials documenting objective benefits of steroid therapy in this setting are not available.[118,132] Elevated central venous pressures may cause excessive bleeding after venipuncture or venous access procedures in the upper extremities. Therefore, alternative sites for venous access should be sought.

Anticoagulation and Thrombolysis. Although superimposed thrombosis occurs in up to 50% of cases of SVCS, anticoagulation in this setting is controversial and has not been shown to confer a significant survival benefit.[149] Anticoagulation and thrombolysis may be beneficial in certain situations, such as propagation of the thrombus into the brachiocephalic or subclavicular systems or such as thrombosis induced by an indwelling catheter. The success of thrombolytic therapy in clot lysis and recannulation of the vessel approaches 73% if done early, within the first 5 days after thrombosis, but wanes significantly thereafter.[150] However, because of the risks of intracranial bleeding and impairment of diagnostic efforts, anticoagulation should be avoided unless a clear indication for its use is identified.

Chemotherapy. Chemotherapy is the preferred initial treatment of SVCS caused by chemosensitive tumors such as small-cell lung cancer (SCLC) and lymphoma. Most SCLC patients will experience partial or complete resolution of signs and symptoms within 1 to 2 weeks of the initiation of treatment.[122] Recent studies have shown no added benefit with the addition of radiotherapy after chemotherapy, versus chemotherapy alone for the specific treatment of SVCS in SCLC patients.[121,151] Although SVCO recurs in approximately 25% of all cases, re-institution of salvage chemotherapy and/or radiotherapy has effected the prompt resolution of symptoms in most patients.[148] Chemotherapy is also the treatment of choice for SVCS secondary to non-Hodgkin's lymphoma because this treatment modality provides both local and systemic therapeutic activity. However, local consolidation with radiotherapy may be beneficial in patients with large-cell lymphoma and a large mediastinal mass.[125]

Radiotherapy. Radiotherapy remains the primary treatment for patients with malignant SVCS resulting from recurrent disease after chemotherapy or nonchemosensitive tumors such as non-small-cell lung cancer.[148] It is also justified if a histologic diagnosis cannot be established. Emergent radiotherapy prior to a diagnostic work-up may be indicated in rare life-threatening situations, such as in airway obstruction, spinal-cord compression, or increased intracranial pressure.[110,116] High-dose external-beam radiation (300 to 400 cGy per day for three fractions) is relatively safe and generally well tolerated. Most patients experience relief from symptoms within 1 to 3 weeks of the initiation of treatment.[109,111]

Superior Vena Cava Stenting. Superior vena cava stenting may provide rapid relief from symptoms within 48 hours in 75 to 100% of cases.[152,153] It may be used in patients who have severe symptoms while the histologic diagnosis is pending or in patients in whom ongoing radiation or chemotherapy has not yet taken effect. However, SVC stenting is more often used as a palliative care measure in patients who have been unsuccessfully treated with conventional radiotherapy or chemotherapy.[153] Compared to palliative radiotherapy, SVC stenting provides more sustained relief of symptoms.[154] The long-term patency rates have not been established, but in cases of SVCS secondary to malignancy, stents usually remain patent for the lifetime of the patient.[152] Because this measure can dramatically improve the quality of life, SVC stenting is fully justified in those patients with severe symptoms and limited life expectancy.[152] The complications associated with use of the intravascular stent are relatively rare and include stent migration, thrombotic occlusion, emboli, and fatal arrhythmia.[152,155] The need for long term anticoagulation to reduce the risk of stent thrombosis has been debated. Although anticoagulation may prolong stent patency, the risk of long-term anticoagulation must be weighed against potential bleeding complications.[156] Anticoagulation following stent placement is generally recommended if there is a significant risk of thromboembolism.

Surgical Bypass. Surgical bypass from the internal jugular vein or innominate vein to the right atrial appendage has been used successfully in cases of SVCS resulting from benign causes[157] and in selected cancer patients who have severe acute SVCS or who are refractory to conventional definitive therapy.[158] Surgical intervention offers the dual advantage of (1) rapid resolution of symptoms with the definitive correction of the obstructing lesion and (2) the establishment of a tissue diagnosis. The morbidity and the mortality of median sternotomy and thoracotomy in these patients are significant. Surgical options should therefore be considered only for those patients who have a reasonable anticipated survival. Surgical bypass has been virtually replaced by less invasive percutaneous techniques for palliative treatment of malignant SVCO.

Summary

Superior vena cava syndrome is usually a subacute process that is caused primarily by malignancy. Because optimal therapy depends on the diagnosis of the underlying disease, every effort should be made to obtain a histologic diagnosis before initiating therapy. The least invasive diagnostic procedure that is appropriate in the individual case should be performed first. However, most diagnostic procedures, including bronchoscopy, lymph node biopsy, percutaneous lung biopsy, and mediastinoscopy, are relatively safe. Radiotherapy remains the main treatment of malignant SVCS in most cases, but chemotherapy is the treatment of choice for patients with chemosensitive tumors. Intravascular stenting is increasingly used in patients with malignant SVCS to relieve symptoms more rapidly. An algorithm for the diagnosis and management of SVCS is shown in Figure 15–2.

INFERIOR VENA CAVA SYNDROME

"Inferior vena cava syndrome" (IVCS) refers to the series of signs and symptoms caused by the obstruction of blood flow through the IVC to the right atrium. In addition to intravascular thrombosis, a variety of abdominal malignancies can cause such an obstruction by compression or invasion of the IVC. Obstruction of the IVC is less dramatic and less life threatening than obstruction of the SVC, but the rapid-onset ascites and marked lower-extremity edema may be debilitating and hazardous. Early diagnosis and better systemic therapy of the underlying tumor may result in reduced morbidity and improved survival.

Anatomy and Pathophysiology

Anatomically, the IVC may be divided into thirds. The lower third extends from the confluence of the iliac veins that form the vena cava to the renal veins; the middle third extends from the renal veins to the hepatic veins; and the upper third extends from the hepatic veins to the right atrium. The IVC is relatively fixed retroperitoneally, ascending in front of lumbar vertebrae on the right side of, and parallel with, the abdominal aorta. It passes behind the liver in a fixed position, lying in a deep groove between the right and caudate lobes. On the right, the IVC is in contact with the right adrenal gland, the right kidney, and the right ureter. These anatomic features make the IVC vulnerable to external compression from retroperitoneal masses or an enlarged liver and also make it subject to direct invasion from a right renal or adrenal malignancy.

When the IVC is obstructed, venous pressure distal to the obstruction can be significantly elevated, leading to lower-extremity swelling and edema. Suprarenal IVC obstruction and coincident renal vein obstruction cause renal congestion leading to proteinuria, hematuria, nephrotic syndrome, or renal failure. Suprahepatic IVC obstruction with concurrent hepatic vein obstruction increases intrahepatic pressure and subsequently increases portal pressure, causing ascites and tender hepatomegaly (Budd-Chiari syndrome).

Etiology

Obstruction of the infrarenal IVC most commonly occurs by the extension of a thrombus from the pelvic and thigh veins into the IVC.[159,160] Rapid blood flow from renal veins usually stops the thrombus at this level. Iatrogenic thrombosis due to surgery in the lower extremities or to direct caval manipulation (such as IVC clipping or IVC filters) has led to the formation of a significant number of IVC obstructions.

Obstruction of the midcaval IVC is usually caused by right-sided intra-abdominal malignancies, especially right renal cell carcinoma, which typically invades the IVC rather than extrinsically compressing it.[161] Other causes of midcaval IVC obstruction include right adrenal carcinoma, pancreatic cancer, lymphoma, neuroblastoma, germ cell tumor, and retroperitoneal adenopathy.[162–164]

Obstruction of the intrahepatic IVC is most frequently caused by a greatly enlarged liver due to primary or (more often) metastatic hepatic malignant neoplasms, such as melanoma and breast, colonic, pancreatic, esophageal, gastric, or ovarian cancer.[165] Rare hepatic vein thrombosis (Budd-Chiari syndrome), which is often related to myeloproliferative disease, causes IVC obstruction not only by thrombus formation in the IVC but also by external compression of the IVC from a congested caudate lobe.[166] A tumor thrombus from renal carcinoma can extend cephalically into the hepatic region of the IVC or (frequently) into the right atrium.[167,168] Primary malignant tumors of vascular origin, such as leiomyosarcoma, can also involve the IVC and other major veins, causing obstruction.[169]

Clinical Manifestations

The clinical manifestations of IVC obstruction vary, depending upon the underlying cause, the level of obstruction, the adequacy of collateral circulation, the presence of concurrent disease, and the organ system involved. The gradual formation of an obstruction allows the development of collateral circulation channels and, perhaps, less severe symptoms, regardless of the level of obstruction. It is not uncommon for asymptomatic IVC obstructions to be discovered incidentally by radiologic imaging.

Infrarenal IVC obstruction typically causes bilateral lower-extremity swelling, but unilateral swelling is not uncommon.[170] An infrarenal obstruction is usually well tolerated because the collateral circulation develops within a few months after the IVC interruption.

Midcaval IVC obstruction may cause renal damage in addition to bilateral lower-extremity edema. Proteinuria, hematuria, or nephrotic syndrome are often seen.[171] If bilateral renal veins are blocked rapidly, renal hypertension or acute renal failure will develop.

Intrahepatic or suprahepatic IVC obstruction may show features that are characteristic of Budd-Chiari syndrome: massive ascites, subdiaphragmatic edema, tender hepatomegaly, and the development of superficial abdom-

nancy, a shift in these normal functions can cause excessive bleeding. Local tumor invasion, invasive surgical procedures, or wound infections can damage vascular integrity. Because tumor infiltration of vessels causes the vessels to lose their normal elasticity, massive bleeding that results from the local invasion of vascular structures rarely stops spontaneously. The cancers that most frequently precipitate such life-threatening hemorrhage include head and neck tumors that spread to the carotid arteries, lung cancer that erodes into the bronchial arteries, and large intra-abdominal sarcomas that invade the main abdominal vessels.[191–193] In addition, thrombocytopenia can be caused by bone marrow replacement in cases of hematologic or metastatic malignancy, by platelet consumption due to disseminated intravascular coagulation (DIC), or (more often) by myelosuppression due to chemotherapy and radiation therapy.[194] Coagulopathy can be caused by metastatic liver disease, by some chemotherapy agents, by acquired anticoagulants produced by certain tumors, and by DIC.

Clinical Manifestations. The clinical manifestations of acute bleeding in cancer patients depend on the rate and site of the bleeding. In most cases, the bleeding is obvious, as in hematemesis and melena (GI-tract bleeding), hematuria (GU-tract bleeding), or hemoptysis (respiratory-tract bleeding). However, some patients may have only nonspecific signs and symptoms related to the organ system in which the bleeding occurs whereas others may show only features of hypovolemia and hypoperfusion, such as tachycardia, hypotension, oliguria, and depressed mental status. Hypotension is a relatively late sign of hemorrhage and signifies substantial blood loss.

Diagnosis. The diagnosis of internal bleeding in cancer patients can be difficult, especially in cases of bleeding into the thoracic cavity, the abdominal cavity, or the retroperitoneal space. The diagnosis of internal bleeding in these cases often requires imaging studies or specialized investigations such as CT, US, or endoscopy.

Red blood cell counts, platelet counts, hematocrit level, coagulation activity, and renal and liver functions should be examined in the patient who is at risk for blood loss or bleeding. Because the hematocrit level can remain within normal limits during the first 12 to 24 hours of acute bleeding, normal hematocrit levels do not exclude the diagnosis of acute bleeding. Series hematocrit levels should be monitored if acute bleeding is suspected.

Management. The key to the successful management of acute bleeding is rapid identification and control of the bleeding source. In cases of acute bleeding, external compression of the bleeding site should be applied immediately whenever feasible. The airway, breathing, and circulation should be assessed urgently. Intravenous access should be established, and blood should be typed and crossmatched. Fluid resuscitation is vital to restoring intravascular volume, cardiac output, and tissue perfusion. Isotonic crystalloid fluids should be used initially because colloids have not improved the mortality rate and are more expensive.[195] Any existing coagulopathy or thrombocytopenia should be corrected immediately. The decision to administer a blood transfusion must be made on an individual basis, depending on the patient's hemodynamic stability, the persistence of hemorrhage, and the presence of comorbid diseases. In cases of transfusion, typed and crossmatched packed red blood cells are preferred, but uncrossmatched type-specific blood or type O blood can be used in cases of massive life-threatening hemorrhage. Specific measures for the control of bleeding (such as endoscopy, transcatheter embolization, or surgery) should be performed early, depending on the cause and source of the bleeding.

Carotid Artery Rupture

Etiology and Pathophysiology. Most cases of carotid artery rupture, or "blowout," occur in patients with head and neck malignancies. Carotid artery rupture may result from direct tumor invasion of the carotid artery but more frequently results from complications of cancer treatment, such as postsurgical wound infection, postradiation necrosis, orocutaneous fistula, or (rarely) erosion from an intraluminal catheter.[196–198]

Clinical Manifestations. Carotid artery rupture usually presents as a sudden and massive arterial spurring. Occasionally, small and transient bleeding episodes (so-called sentinel bleeds) herald a massive blowout.[199] Some cases of bleeding through fistulae into the esophagus or trachea manifest as massive GI or respiratory bleeding. Without prompt management, the condition of the patient rapidly deteriorates, proceeding to hypotension, loss of consciousness, and death.

Diagnosis. Sudden massive carotid artery rupture is easy to recognize, especially in patients who have had neck surgery or radiation therapy for head and neck malignancy. Carotid artery rupture rarely requires any diagnostic studies before surgical management, except in cases of bleeding into the esophagus or trachea. Angiography may be performed to establish the diagnosis, but definitive repair should not be delayed for confirmatory findings.

Management. The most important therapeutic maneuver for controlling the bleeding is the continuous application of firm manual compression over the rupture site of the vessel until the patient's arrival in the operating room for definitive treatment. Fluid resuscitation, prompt blood transfusion, and catecholamines should be given to maintain blood pressure. Spontaneous cessation of bleeding occurs very rarely, and surgical treatment is almost always required. However, definitive surgical ligation is associated with a high incidence of neurologic sequelae (25%) and death (40%).[200] An intraluminal-balloon occlusion technique has been successfully used in recent years to control carotid bleeding temporarily or permanently for selected patients who are stable enough to undergo angiography.[201,202]

Spleen Ruptures

Etiology and Pathophysiology. The spleen is the intra-abdominal organ that is most vulnerable to rupture. Most cases of spleen rupture are secondary to abdominal trauma. Spontaneous rupture of the spleen is often associated with splenomegaly due to such infiltrative disease processes as infectious mononucleosis and malaria. Although splenic involvement is common in hematologic malignancies, spontaneous spleen rupture is relatively rare in those patients.[203] Acute leukemia and non-Hodgkin's lymphoma are the malignancies most commonly associated with spontaneous spleen rupture.[203] Other hematologic malignancies that are associated with spleen rupture include chronic myelogenous leukemia, chronic lymphocytic leukemia, hairy cell leukemia, and Hodgkin's lymphoma.[204,205] Splenic rupture has also been associated with metastasis to the spleen in patients with solid tumors, such as renal cell cancer, teratomas, melanoma, esophageal cancer, prostate cancer, and lung cancer.[206–208] The exact mechanism of spontaneous spleen rupture is not clear. However, minor or non-obvious trauma to the spleen may be responsible for the rupture in some cases, and splenic enlargement, leukemic infiltrate of the splenic capsule, splenic infarction, thrombocytopenia, leukemia-associated coagulopathy, and anticoagulation are considered the main contributory factors in the development of spontaneous splenic rupture.[209–211]

Clinical Manifestations. The clinical presentation of splenic rupture varies, depending on the extent of the rupture, the underlying causes, and the patient's general condition. The extent of bleeding can range from a subcapsular hematoma to full-blown laceration of the spleen with severe intraperitoneal or retroperitoneal hemorrhage. The classic clinical features of splenic rupture are pain in the left shoulder or abdomen, tachycardia, and hypotension. However, these symptoms may be confounded by other medical problems that are associated with the underlying malignancy and related treatments. Occasionally, splenic rupture may be the initial presenting feature of hematologic malignancy.[212,213]

Diagnosis. The clinical diagnosis of spontaneous splenic rupture is difficult since there are no pathognomonic signs and symptoms and since the clinical findings may mimic those of a wide variety of conditions. Differential diag-

noses include acute cardiovascular disease or other acute abdominal emergencies, such as the rupture of any other intra-abdominal organs, perforation of the bowel, rupture of an arterial aneurysm, and intraperitoneal infection.

The accurate diagnosis of splenic rupture depends on objective studies. Plain-film abdominal radiography may reveal signs that suggest splenic rupture, but it is neither sensitive nor specific for that condition.[214] Contrast-enhanced spiral CT is the most accurate noninvasive imaging study. It may not only reveal the extent of splenic rupture and intraperitoneal or retroperitoneal hemorrhage but may also allow the simultaneous evaluation of the other abdominal organs.[214,215] The use of US to diagnose splenic rupture has gained more attention because this technique is readily available and can be performed at bedside, which is advantageous for hemodynamically unstable patients. Ultrasonography may reveal the presence of an intrasplenic hematoma, a subcapsular hematoma, a rupture of the spleen, or blood collection in the peritoneal cavity.[213] Diagnostic peritoneal lavage is rarely used except in trauma patients. Technetium-99m sulfur colloid scintigraphy has occasionally been used to diagnose isolated splenic injuries.[216]

Management. Prompt splenectomy is the only effective treatment of splenic rupture in patients with hematologic malignancies. The mortality rate for those patients who do not undergo surgery is almost 100%.[209] In selected patients with tumor involvement of the spleen or with conditions that are contraindications to surgery, selective arterial embolization or irradiation of the ruptured site may temporarily control the bleeding.[209,217] Patients for whom nonsurgical treatment has been selected should be managed with supplemental oxygen, correction of thrombocytopenia and coagulopathy, and blood transfusion. The management team caring for such patients should closely monitor the vital signs, series hematocrit levels, and series imaging (such as US or abdominal CT).

Retroperitoneal Hemorrhage

Etiology and Pathophysiology. Retroperitoneal hemorrhage can be caused by a variety of disorders. Any damage to peritoneal organs or structures, such as the kidneys, adrenal glands, pancreas, major blood vessels, muscles, or bones, may cause substantial retroperitoneal bleeding. Spontaneous retroperitoneal hemorrhage due to cancer is rare; it is usually caused by primary or metastatic renal or adrenal-gland tumors.[218–220] Thrombocytopenia, coagulopathy, and anticoagulation are precipitating factors for spontaneous retroperitoneal hemorrhage.[221,222] Retro- and intraperitoneal procedures and the insertion of an intravascular catheter through a femoral vessel can also cause severe retroperitoneal bleeding.[223]

Clinical Manifestations. The clinical manifestations of retroperitoneal bleeding are nonspecific and may vary, depending on the rate of the bleeding and on the underlying disease. Typically, patients with retroperitoneal bleeding present with abdominal pain, a tender mass in the flank, and hypotension. Some may have hematuria or hemotochezia if bleeding into the ureter or colon occurs.

Diagnosis. It is difficult to establish a clinical diagnosis of retroperitoneal hemorrhage on the basis of clinical findings. Maintaining a high clinical suspicion and performing early imaging studies are the keys to diagnosing and successfully treating patients with retroperitoneal hemorrhage. Computed tomography of the abdomen and pelvis is the most commonly used noninvasive study for the diagnosis of retroperitoneal bleeding and also helps to differentiate this condition from other clinical conditions with similar clinical manifestations. Ultrasonography can be performed at bedside and is useful in establishing a rapid diagnosis in some cases.[219] Angiography may help to identify the site of bleeding and may also be of help in the embolization, if necessary, of the bleeding vessel.[224]

Management. The management of retroperitoneal hemorrhage depends on the severity of the bleeding and on the underlying cause. Routine measures for acute hemorrhage, such as fluid resuscitation, blood transfusion, and the correction of coagulopathy and thrombocytopenia, should be initiated immediately. Most patients require emergent surgery to remove bleeding tumors or organs, especially in life-threatening situations.[225,226] Selective arterial embolization has been proposed as a means to control the bleeding of renal lesions.[225] Irradiation of the bleeding tumor is an option for patients with subacute bleeding and relatively stable hematocrit levels.[227]

REFERENCES

1. Mateo J, Oliver A, Borrell M, et al. Laboratory evaluation and clinical characteristics of 2,132 consecutive unselected patients with venous thromboembolism—results of the Spanish Multicentric Study on Thrombophilia (EMET-Study). Thromb Haemost 1997;77:444–51.

2. Johnson MJ, Sproule MW, Paul J. The prevalence and associated variables of deep venous thrombosis in patients with advanced cancer. Clin Oncol 1999;11:105–10.

3. Cogo A, Bernardi E, Prandoni P, et al. Acquired risk factors for deep-vein thrombosis in symptomatic outpatients. Arch Intern Med 1994;154:164–8.

4. Samama MM. An epidemiologic study of risk factors for deep vein thrombosis in medical outpatients: the sirius study. Arch Intern Med 2000;160:3415–20.

5. Donati MB, et al. Cancer procoagulant in human tumor cells: evidence from melanoma patients. Cancer Res 1986;46:6471–4.

6. Edwards RL, Silver J, Rickles FR. Human tumor procoagulants: registry of the Subcommittee on Haemostasis and Malignancy of the Scientific and Standardization Committee, International Society on Thrombosis and Haemostasis. Thromb Haemost 1993;69:205–13.

7. Love RR, Surawicz TS, Williams EC. Antithrombin III level, fibrinogen level, and platelet count changes with adjuvant tamoxifen therapy. Arch Intern Med 1992;152:317–20.

8. Rogers JS 2nd, Murgo AJ, Fontana JA, Raich PC. Chemotherapy for breast cancer decreases plasma protein C and protein S. J Clin Oncol 1988;6:276–81.

9. Priest JR, Ramsay NK, Steinherz PG, et al. A syndrome of thrombosis and hemorrhage complicating L-asparaginase therapy for childhood acute lymphoblastic leukemia. J Pediatr 1982;100:984–9.

10. Marras LC, Geerts WH, Perry JR. The risk of venous thromboembolism is increased throughout the course of malignant glioma: an evidence-based review. Cancer 2000;89:640–6.

11. Levitan N, Dowlati A, Remick SC, et al. Rates of initial and recurrent thromboembolic disease among patients with malignancy versus those without malignancy. Risk analysis using Medicare claims data. Medicine (Baltimore) 1999;78:285–91.

12. Prandoni P, Polistena P, Bernardi E, et al. Upper-extremity deep vein thrombosis. Risk factors, diagnosis, and complications. Arch Intern Med 1997;157:57–62.

13. Moser KM. Venous thromboembolism. Am Rev Respir Dis 1990;141:235–49.

14. Stamatakis JD, Kakkar VV, Lawrence D, Bentley PG. The origin of thrombi in the deep veins of the lower limb: a venographic study. Br J Surg 1978;65:449–51.

15. Havig O. Deep vein thrombosis and pulmonary embolism. An autopsy study with multiple regression analysis of possible risk factors. Acta Chir Scand 1977;478(Suppl 1):–120.

16. Huisman MV, Buller HR, ten Cate JW, Vreeken J. Serial impedance plethysmography for suspected deep venous thrombosis in outpatients. The Amsterdam General Practitioner Study. N Engl J Med 1986;314:823–8.

17. Barnes RW, Nix ML, Barnes CL, et al. Perioperative asymptomatic venous thrombosis: role of duplex scanning versus venography. J Vasc Surg 1989;9:251–60.

18. Philbrick JT, Becker DM. Calf deep venous thrombosis. A wolf in sheep's clothing? Arch Intern Med 1988;148:2131–8.

19. Morpurgo M. Pulmonary embolism: the dimensions of the problem. G Ital Cardiol 1984;14(Suppl 1):3–5.

20. Balestreri L, De Cicco M, Matovic M, et al. Central venous catheter-related thrombosis in clinically asymptomatic oncologic patients: a phlebographic study. Eur J Radiol 1995;20:108–11.

21. Horne MK 3rd, May DJ, Alexander HR, et al. Venographic surveillance of tunneled venous access devices in adult oncology patients. Ann Surg Oncol 1995;2:174–8.

22. Lokich JJ, Becker B. Subclavian vein thrombosis in patients treated with infusion chemotherapy for advanced malignancy. Cancer 1983;52:1586–9.

23. Anderson AJ, Krasnow SH, Boyer MW, et al. Thrombosis: the major Hickman catheter complication in patients with solid tumor. Chest 1989;95:71–5.

24. Monreal M, Lafoz E, Ruiz J, et al. Upper-extremity deep venous thrombosis and pulmonary embolism. A prospective study. Chest 1991;99:280–3.

25. Flinn WR, Sandager GP, Silva MB Jr, et al. Prospective surveillance for perioperative venous thrombosis. Experience in 2643 patients. Arch Surg 1996;131:472–80.

26. Barnes RW, Wu KK, Hoak JC. Fallibility of the clinical diagnosis of venous thrombosis. JAMA 1975;234:605–7.

27. Kahn SR, Joseph L, Abenhaim L, Lecierc JR. Clinical prediction of deep vein thrombosis in patients with leg symptoms. Thromb Haemost 1999;81:353–7.

28. Frank DA, Meuse J, Hirsch D, et al. The treatment and outcome of cancer patients with thromboses on central venous catheters. J Thromb Thrombolysis 2000;10:271–5.

29. Goldhaber SZ, Simons GR, Elliott CG, et al. Quantitative plasma D-dimer levels among patients undergoing pulmonary angiography for suspected pulmonary embolism. JAMA 1993;270:2819–22.

30. Becker DM, Philbrick JT, Bachhuber TL, Humphries JE. D-dimer testing and acute venous thromboembolism. A shortcut to accurate diagnosis? Arch Intern Med 1996;156:939–46.

31. Ginsberg JS, Kearon C, Douketis J, et al. The use of D-dimer testing and impedance plethysmographic examination in patients with clinical indications of deep vein thrombosis. Arch Intern Med 1997;157:1077–81.

32. Bates SM, Grand'Maison A, Johnston M, et al. A latex D-dimer reliably excludes venous thromboembolism. Arch Intern Med 2001;161:447–53.

33. van der Graaf F, van den Borne H, van der Kolk M, et al. Exclusion of deep venous thrombosis with D-dimer testing—comparison of 13 D-dimer methods in 99 outpatients suspected of deep venous thrombosis using venography as reference standard. Thromb Haemost 2000;83:191–8.

34. Lee AY, Julian JA, Levine MN, et al. Clinical utility of a rapid whole-blood D-dimer assay in patients with cancer who present with suspected acute deep venous thrombosis. Ann Intern Med 1999;131:417–23.

35. Habscheid W, Hohmann M, Wilhelm T, Epping J. Real-time ultrasound in the diagnosis of acute deep venous thrombosis of the lower extremity. Angiology 1990;41:599–608.

36. Lensing AW, Prandoni P, Brandjes D, et al. Detection of deep-vein thrombosis by real-time B-mode ultrasonography. N Engl J Med 1989;320:342–5.

37. Davidson BL, Elliott CG, Lensing AW. Low accuracy of color Doppler ultrasound in the detection of proximal leg vein thrombosis in asymptomatic high-risk patients. The RD Heparin Arthroplasty Group. Ann Intern Med 1992;117:735–8.

38. Rose SC, Zwiebel WJ, Nelson BD, et al. Symptomatic lower extremity deep venous thrombosis: accuracy, limitations, and role of color duplex flow imaging in diagnosis [published erratum appears in Radiology 1990 Sep;176:879]. Radiology 1990;175:639–44.

39. Birdwell BG, Raskob GE, Whitsett TL, et al. The clinical validity of normal compression ultrasonography in outpatients suspected of having deep venous thrombosis. Ann Intern Med 1998;128:1–7.

40. Cogo A, Lensing AW, Koopman MM, et al. Compression ultrasonography for diagnostic management of patients with clinically suspected deep vein thrombosis: prospective cohort study. BMJ 1998;316(7124):17–20.

41. Kearon C, Ginsberg JS, Hirsh J. The role of venous ultrasonography in the diagnosis of suspected deep venous thrombosis and pulmonary embolism. Ann Intern Med 1998;129:1044–9.

42. Prandoni P, Cogo A, Bernardi E, et al. A simple ultrasound approach for detection of recurrent proximal-vein thrombosis. Circulation 1993;88:1730–5.

43. Heijboer H, Jongbloets JM, Buller HR, et al. Clinical utility of real-time compression ultrasonography for diagnostic management of patients with recurrent venous thrombosis. Acta Radiol 1992;33:297–300.

44. Huisman MV, Buller HR, ten Cate JW. Utility of impedance plethysmography in the diagnosis of recurrent deep-vein thrombosis. Arch Intern Med 1988;148:681–3.

45. Koopman MM, van Beek EJ, ten Cate JW. Diagnosis of deep vein thrombosis. Prog Cardiovasc Dis 1994;37:1–12.

46. Knudson GJ, Wiedmeyer DA, Erickson SJ, et al. Color Doppler sonographic imaging in the assessment of upper-extremity deep venous thrombosis. AJR Am J Roentgenol 1990;154:399–403.

47. Koksoy C, Kuzu A, Kutlay J, et al. The diagnostic value of colour Doppler ultrasound in central venous catheter related thrombosis. Clin Radiol 1995;50:687–9.

48. Haire WD, Lynch TG, Lieberman RP, Edney JA. Duplex scans before subclavian vein catheterization predict unsuccessful catheter placement. Arch Surg 1992;127:229–30.

49. Keefe DL, Roistacher N, Pierri MK. Evaluation of suspected deep venous thrombosis in oncologic patients. Angiology 1994;45:771–5.

50. Hull R, van Aken WG, Hirsh J, et al. Impedance plethysmography using the occlusive cuff technique in the diagnosis of venous thrombosis. Circulation 1976;53:696–700.

51. Agnelli G, Cosmi B, Ranucci V, et al. Impedance plethysmography in the diagnosis of asymptomatic deep vein thrombosis in hip surgery. A venography-controlled study. Arch Intern Med 1991;151:2167–71.

52. Horne MK 3rd, Mayo DJ, Alexander HR, et al. Upper extremity impedance plethysmography in patients with venous access devices. Thromb Haemost 1994;72:540–2.

53. Ennis JT, Elmes RJ. Radionuclide venography in the diagnosis of deep vein thrombosis. Radiology 1977;125:441–9.

54. Bentley PG, Hill PL, de Haas HA, et al. Radionuclide venography in the management of proximal venous occlusion. A comparison with X-ray contrast venography. Br J Radiol 1979;52:289–301.

55. Kilpatrick TK, Lichtenstein M, Andrews J, et al. A comparative study of radionuclide venography and con-

trast venography in the diagnosis of deep venous thrombosis. Aust N Z J Med 1993;23:641–5.

56. Mangkharak J, Chiewvit S, Chaiyasoot W, et al. Radionuclide venography in the diagnosis of deep vein thrombosis of the lower extremities: a comparison to contrast venography. J Med Assoc Thai 1998;81:432–41.

57. Podoloff DA, Kim EE. Evaluation of sensitivity and specificity of upper extremity radionuclide venography in cancer patients with indwelling central venous catheters. Clin Nucl Med 1992;17:457–62.

58. Moser KM, Brach BB, Dolan GF. Clinically suspected deep venous thrombosis of the lower extremities. A comparison of venography, impedance plethysmography, and radiolabeled fibrinogen. JAMA 1977;237:2195–8.

59. Bautovich G, Angelides S, Lee FT, et al. Detection of deep venous thrombi and pulmonary embolus with technetium-99m-DD-3B6/22 anti-fibrin monoclonal antibody Fab' fragment. J Nucl Med 1994;35:195–202.

60. Butler SP, Rahman T, Boyd SJ, et al. Detection of postoperative deep-venous thrombosis using technetium-99m-labeled tissue plasminogen activator. J Nucl Med 1997;38:219–23.

61. Taillefer R, Therasse E, Turpin S, et al. Comparison of early and delayed scintigraphy with 99mTc-apcitide and correlation with contrast-enhanced venography in detection of acute deep vein thrombosis. J Nucl Med 1999;40:2029–35.

62. Taillefer R, Edell S, Innes G, Lister-James J. Acute thromboscintigraphy with (99m)Tc-apcitide: results of the phase 3 multicenter clinical trial comparing 99mTc-apcitide scintigraphy with contrast venography for imaging acute DVT. Multicenter Trial Investigators. J Nucl Med 2000;41:1214–23.

63. Hull R, Hirsh J, Sackett DL, et al. Clinical validity of a negative venogram in patients with clinically suspected venous thrombosis. Circulation 1981;64:622–5.

64. Heijboer H, Cogo A, Buller HR, et al. Detection of deep vein thrombosis with impedance plethysmography and real-time compression ultrasonography in hospitalized patients. Arch Intern Med 1992;152:1901–3.

65. Erdman WA, Jayson HT, Redman HC, et al. Deep venous thrombosis of extremities: role of MR imaging in the diagnosis. Radiology 1990;174:425–31.

66. Carpenter JP, Holland GA, Baum RA, et al. Magnetic resonance venography for the detection of deep venous thrombosis: comparison with contrast venography and duplex Doppler ultrasonography. J Vasc Surg 1993;18:734–41.

67. Spritzer CE, Norconk JJ Jr, Sostman HD, Coleman RE. Detection of deep venous thrombosis by magnetic resonance imaging. Chest 1993;104:54–60.

68. Montgomery KD, Potter HG, Helfet DL. Magnetic resonance venography to evaluate the deep venous system of the pelvis in patients who have an acetabular fracture. J Bone Joint Surg Am 1995;77:1639–49.

69. Moody AR, Pollock JG, O'Conner AR, Bagnall M. Lower-limb deep venous thrombosis: direct MR imaging of the thrombus. Radiology 1998;209:349–55.

70. Meaney JF, Weg JG, Chenevert TL, et al. Diagnosis of pulmonary embolism with magnetic resonance angiography. N Engl J Med 1997;336:1422–7.

71. Schellong SM, Schwarz T, Kropp J, et al. Bed rest in deep vein thrombosis and the incidence of scintigraphic pulmonary embolism. Thromb Haemost 1999;82 (Suppl 1):127–9.

72. Schulman S, Rhedin AS, Lindmarker P, et al. A comparison of six weeks with six months of oral anticoagulant therapy after a first episode of venous thromboembolism. Duration of Anticoagulation Trial Study Group. N Engl J Med 1995;332:1661–5.

73. Kearon C, Gent M, Hirsh J, et al. A comparison of three months of anticoagulation with extended anticoagulation for a first episode of idiopathic venous thromboembolism [published erratum appears in N Engl J Med 1999 Jul 22;341:298]. N Engl J Med 1999;340:901–7.

74. Schulman S, Granqvist S, Holmstrom M, et al. The duration of oral anticoagulant therapy after a second episode of venous thromboembolism. The Duration of Anticoagulation Trial Study Group. N Engl J Med 1997;336:393–8.

75. Wheeler AP, Jaquiss RD, Newman JH. Physician practices in the treatment of pulmonary embolism and deep venous thrombosis. Arch Intern Med 1988;148:1321–5.

76. Levine MN, Hirsh J, Gent M, et al. A randomized trial comparing activated thromboplastin time with heparin assay in patients with acute venous thromboembolism requiring large daily doses of heparin. Arch Intern Med 1994;154:49–56.

77. Hirsh J, Warkentin TE, Raschke R, et al. Heparin and low-molecular-weight heparin: mechanisms of action, pharmacokinetics, dosing considerations, monitoring, efficacy, and safety [published erratum appears in Chest 1999 Jun;115:1760]. Chest 1998;1145 Suppl):489S–510S.

78. Prandoni P, Bagatella P, Bernardi E, et al. Use of an algorithm for administering subcutaneous heparin in the treatment of deep venous thrombosis. Ann Intern Med 1998;129:299–302.

79. Weitz JI. Low-molecular-weight heparins. [published erratum appears in N Engl J Med 1997 Nov 20;337:1567]. N Engl J Med 1997;337:688–98.

80. Hull RD, Raskob GE, Pineo GF, et al. Subcutaneous low-molecular-weight heparin compared with continuous intravenous heparin in the treatment of proximal-vein thrombosis. N Engl J Med 1992;326:975–82.

81. Lensing AW, Prins MH, Davidson BL, Hirsh J. Treatment of deep venous thrombosis with low-molecular-weight heparins. A meta-analysis. Arch Intern Med 1995;155:601–7.

82. Dolovich LR, Ginsberg JS, Douketis JD, et al. A meta-analysis comparing low-molecular-weight heparins with unfractionated heparin in the treatment of venous thromboembolism: examining some unanswered questions regarding location of treatment, product type, and dosing frequency. Arch Intern Med 2000;160:181–8.

83. Leizorovicz A, Simonneau G, Decousus H, Boissel JP. Comparison of efficacy and safety of low molecular weight heparins and unfractionated heparin in initial

treatment of deep venous thrombosis: a meta-analysis. BMJ 1994;309:299–304.

84. Levine M, Gent M, Hirsh J, et al. A comparison of low-molecular-weight heparin administered primarily at home with unfractionated heparin administered in the hospital for proximal deep-vein thrombosis. N Engl J Med 1996;334:677–81.

85. Harrison L, McGinnis J, Crowther M, et al. Assessment of outpatient treatment of deep-vein thrombosis with low-molecular-weight heparin. Arch Intern Med 1998; 158:2001–3.

86. Koopman MM, Prandoni P, Piovella F, et al. Treatment of venous thrombosis with intravenous unfractionated heparin administered in the hospital as compared with subcutaneous low-molecular-weight heparin administered at home. The Tasman Study Group. N Engl J Med 1996;334:682–7.

87. Monreal M, Roncales FJ, Ruiz J, et al. Secondary prevention of venous thromboembolism: a role for low-molecular-weight heparin. Haemostasis 1998;28:236–43.

88. Walsh-McMonagle D, Green D. Low-molecular-weight heparin in the management of Trousseau's syndrome. Cancer 1997;80:649–55.

89. Chan A, Woodruff RK. Complications and failure of anti-coagulation therapy in the treatment of venous thromboembolism in patients with disseminated malignancy. Aust N Z J Med 1992;22:119–22.

90. Harrison L, Johnston M, Massicotte MP, et al. Comparison of 5-mg and 10-mg loading doses in initiation of warfarin therapy. Ann Intern Med 1997;126:133–6.

91. Bona RD, Sivjee KY, Hickey AD, et al. The efficacy and safety of oral anticoagulation in patients with cancer. Thromb Haemost 1995;74:1055–8.

92. Decousus H, Leizorovicz A, Parent F, et al. A clinical trial of vena caval filters in the prevention of pulmonary embolism in patients with proximal deep-vein thrombosis. Prevention du Risque d'Embolie Pulmonaire par Interruption Cave Study Group. N Engl J Med 1998; 338:409–15.

93. Yazu T, Fujioka H, Nakamura M, et al. Long-term results of inferior vena cava filters: experiences in a Japanese population. Intern Med 2000;39:707–14.

94. Schwarz RE, Marrero AM, Conlon KC, et al. Inferior vena cava filters in cancer patients: indications and outcome. J Clin Oncol 1996;14:652–7.

95. Becker DM, Philbrick JT, Selby JB. Inferior vena cava filters. Indications, safety, effectiveness. Arch Intern Med 1992;152:1985–94.

96. Linsenmaier U, Rieger J, Schenk F, et al. Indications, management, and complications of temporary inferior vena cava filters. Cardiovasc Intervent Radiol 1998;21:464–9.

97. Lorch H, Zwaan M, Siemens HJ, et al. Temporary vena cava filters and ultrahigh streptokinase thrombolysis therapy: a clinical study. Cardiovasc Intervent Radiol 2000;23:273–8.

98. Piccioli AP, Prandoni P, Goldhaber SZ. Epidemiologic characteristics, management, and outcome of deep venous thrombosis in a tertiary-care hospital: the Brigham and Women's Hospital DVT registry. Am Heart J 1996;132:1010–4.

99. Rogers LQ, Lutcher CL. Streptokinase therapy for deep vein thrombosis: a comprehensive review of the English literature. Am J Med 1990;88:389–95.

100. Hyers TM, Agnelli G, Hull RD, et al. Antithrombotic therapy for venous thromboembolic disease. Chest 1998; 114(5 Suppl):561S–78S.

101. Haire WD, Atkinson JB, Stephens LC, Kotulak GD. Urokinase versus recombinant tissue plasminogen activator in thrombosed central venous catheters: a double-blinded, randomized trial. Thromb Haemost 1994;72:543–7.

102. Gould JR, Carloss HW, Skinner WL. Groshong catheter-associated subclavian venous thrombosis. Am J Med 1993;95:419–23.

103. Fraschini G, Jadeja J, Lawson M, et al. Local infusion of urokinase for the lysis of thrombosis associated with permanent central venous catheters in cancer patients. J Clin Oncol 1987;5:672–8.

104. Schindler J, Bona RD, Chen HH, et al. Regional thrombolysis with urokinase for central venous catheter-related thrombosis in patients undergoing high-dose chemotherapy with autologous blood stem cell rescue. Clin Appl Thromb Hemost 1999;5:25–9.

105. Bern MM, Lokich JJ, Wallach SR, et al. Very low doses of warfarin can prevent thrombosis in central venous catheters. A randomized prospective trial. Ann Intern Med 1990;112:423–8.

106. Monreal M, Alastrue A, Rull M, et al. Upper extremity deep venous thrombosis in cancer patients with venous access devices—prophylaxis with a low molecular weight heparin (Fragmin). Thromb Haemost 1996;75:251–3.

107. Fincher RM. Superior vena cava syndrome: experience in a teaching hospital. South Med J 1987;80:1243–5.

108. Parish JM, Marschke RF Jr, Dines DE, Lee RE. Etiologic considerations in superior vena cava syndrome. Mayo Clin Proc 1981;56:407–13.

109. Armstrong BA, Perez CA, Simpson JR, Hederman MA. Role of irradiation in the management of superior vena cava syndrome. Int J Radiat Oncol Biol Phys 1987;13:531–9.

110. Yellin A, Rosen A, Reichert N, Lieberman Y. Superior vena cava syndrome. The myth—the facts. Am Rev Respir Dis 1990;141:1114–8.

111. Davenport D, Ferree C, Blake D, Raben M. Radiation therapy in the treatment of superior vena caval obstruction. Cancer 1978;42:2600–3.

112. Lokich J, Goodman R. Superior vena cava syndrome: clinical management. JAMA 1975;231:58–60.

113. Puel V, Caudry M, Le Metayer P, et al. Superior vena cava thrombosis related to catheter malposition in cancer chemotherapy given through implanted ports. Cancer 1993;72:2248–52.

114. Woodyard TC, Mellinger JD, Vann KG, Nisenbaum J. Acute superior vena cava syndrome after central venous catheter placement. Cancer 1993;71:2621–3.

115. Lee Y, Doering R, Jihayel A. Radiation-induced superior vena cava syndrome. Tex Heart Inst J 1995;22:103–4.

116. Ahmann FR. A reassessment of the clinical implications of the superior vena caval syndrome. J Clin Oncol 1984;2:961–9.

117. Rubin P, Hicks GL. Biassociation of superior vena caval obstruction and spinal-cord compression. N Y State J Med 1973;73:2176–82.

118. Schraufnagel DE, Hill R, Leech JA, Pare JA. Superior vena caval obstruction. Is it a medical emergency? Am J Med 1981;70:1169–74.

119. Bell DR, Woods RL, Levi JA. Superior vena caval obstruction: a 10-year experience. Med J Aust 1986;145:566–8.

120. Salsali M, Cliffton EE. Superior vena caval obstruction with lung cancer. Ann Thorac Surg 1968;6:437–42.

121. Sculier J, Evans W, Feld R. Superior vena caval obstruction syndrome in small cell lung cancer. Cancer 1986; 15:847–51.

122. Urban T, Lebeau B, Chastang C, et al. Superior vena cava syndrome in small-cell lung cancer. Arch Intern Med 1993;153:384–7.

123. Wurschmidt F, Bunemann H, Heilmann HP. Small cell lung cancer with and without superior vena cava syndrome: a multivariate analysis of prognostic factors in 408 cases. Int J Radiat Oncol Biol Phys 1995;33:77–82.

124. Salsali M, Cliffton EE. Superior vena caval obstruction in carcinoma of lung. N Y State J Med 1969;69:2875–80.

125. Perez-Soler R, McLaughlin P, Velasquez WS, et al. Clinical features and results of management of superior vena cava syndrome secondary to lymphoma. J Clin Oncol 1984;2:260–6.

126. Lazzarino M, Orlandi E, Paulli M, et al. Primary mediastinal B-cell lymphoma with sclerosis: an aggressive tumor with distinctive clinical and pathologic features. J Clin Oncol 1993;11:2306–13.

127. Sumiyoshi Y, Kikuchi M. Leiomyosarcoma of the superior vena cava producing superior vena cava syndrome and heart tamponade. Pathol Int 1995;45:691–4.

128. Chen JC, Bongard F, Klein SR. A contemporary perspective on superior vena cava syndrome. Am J Surg 1990; 160:207–11.

129. Montalban, C, Moreno MA, Molina JP, et al. Metastatic carcinoma of the prostate presenting as a superior vena cava syndrome. Chest 1993;104:1278–80.

130. Schwarz RE, Groeger JS, Coit DG. Subcutaneously implanted central venous access devices in cancer patients: a prospective analysis. Cancer 1997;79:1635–40.

131. Bertrand M, Presant CA, Klein L, Scott E. Iatrogenic superior vena cava syndrome. A new entity. Cancer 1984;54:376–8.

132. Maddox AM, Valdivieso M, Lukeman J, et al. Superior vena cava obstruction in small cell bronchogenic carcinoma. Clinical parameters and survival. Cancer 1983; 52:2165–72.

133. Lochridge SK, Knibbe WP, Doty DB. Obstruction of the superior vena cava. Surgery 1979;85:14–24.

134. Yedlicka JW Jr, Cormier MG, Gray R, Moncada R. Computed tomography of superior vena cava obstruction. J Thorac Imaging 1987;2:72–8.

135. Schwartz EE, Goodman LR, Haskin ME. Role of CT scanning in the superior vena cava syndrome. Am J Clin Oncol 1986;9:71–8.

136. Loeffler JS, Leopold KA, Recht A, et al. Emergency prebiopsy radiation for mediastinal masses: impact on subsequent pathologic diagnosis and outcome. J Clin Oncol 1986;4:716–21.

137. Van Houtte P, Fruhling J. Radionuclide venography in the evaluation of superior vena cava syndrome. Clin Nucl Med 1981;6:177–83.

138. Mahmud AM, Isawa T, Teshima T, et al. Radionuclide venography and its functional analysis in superior vena cava syndrome. J Nucl Med 1996;37:1460–4.

139. Weinreb JC, Mootz A, Cohen JM. MRI evaluation of mediastinal and thoracic inlet venous obstruction. AJR Am J Roentgenol 1986;146:679–84.

140. Dyet JF, Moghissi K. Role of venography in assessing patients with superior caval obstruction caused by bronchial carcinoma for bypass operations. Thorax 1980;35:628–30.

141. Stanford W, Jolles H, Ell S, Chiu LC. Superior vena cava obstruction: a venographic classification. AJR Am J Roentgenol 1987;148:259–62.

142. Ayala K, Chandrasekaran K, Karakis DG, et al. Diagnosis of superior vena caval obstruction by transesophageal echocardiography. Chest 1992;101:874–6.

143. Shimm DS, Logue GL, Rigsby LC. Evaluating the superior vena cava syndrome. JAMA 1981;245:951–3.

144. Painter TD, Karpf M. Superior vena cava syndrome: diagnostic procedures. Am J Med Sci 1983;285:2–6.

145. Porte H, Metois D, Finzi L, et al. Superior vena cava syndrome of malignant origin. Which surgical procedure for which diagnosis? Eur J Cardiothorac Surg 2000;17:384–8.

146. Jahangiri M, Goldstraw P. The role of mediastinoscopy in superior vena caval obstruction. Ann Thorac Surg 1995;59:453–5.

147. Cosmo L, Haponik EF, Dariak JJ, Summer WR. Neoplastic superior vena caval obstruction: diagnosis with percutaneous needle aspiration. Am J Med Sci 1987;293:99–102.

148. Chan RH, Dar AR, Yu E, et al. Superior vena cava obstruction in small-cell lung cancer. Int J Radiat Oncol Biol Phys 1997;38:513–20.

149. Adelstein DJ, Hines JD, Carter SG, Sacco D. Thromboembolic events in patients with malignant superior vena cava syndrome and the role of anticoagulation. Cancer 1988;62:2258–62.

150. Greenberg S, Kosinski R, Daniels J. Treatment of superior vena cava thrombosis with recombinant tissue type plasminogen activator. Chest 1991;99:1298–301.

151. Shah R, Sabanathan S, Lowe RA, Mearns AJ. Stenting in malignant obstruction of superior vena cava. J Thorac Cardiovasc Surg 1996;112:335–40.

152. Oudkerk M, Heystraten FM, Stoter G. Stenting in malignant vena caval obstruction. Cancer 1993;71:142–6.

153. Hennequin LM, Fade O, Fays JG, et al. Superior vena cava stent placement: results with the Wallstent endoprosthesis. Radiology 1995;196:353–61.

154. Nicholson AA, Ettles DF, Arnold A, et al. Treatment of malignant superior vena cava obstruction: metal stents or radiation therapy. J Vasc Interv Radiol 1997;8:781–8.

155. Zhang C, et al. Ultrasonically guided inferior vena cava stent placement: experience in 83 cases. J Vasc Interv Radiol 1999;10:85–91.

156. Kee S, Fu L, Zhang G, et al. Superior vena cava syndrome:

treatment with catheter-directed thrombolysis and endovascular stent placement. Radiology 1998;206:187–93.

157. Magnan PE, Thomas P, Giudicelli R, et al. Surgical reconstruction of the superior vena cava. Cardiovasc Surg 1994;2:598–604.

158. Avasthi RB, Moghissi K. Malignant obstruction of the superior vena cava and its palliation: report of four cases. J Thorac Cardiovasc Surg 1977;74:244–8.

159. Pleasants J. Obstruction of the inferior vena cava with a report of 18 cases. Johns Hopkins Hosp Rep 1911;16:363–548.

160. Farber SP, O'Donnell TF Jr, Deterling RA, et al. The clinical implications of acute thrombosis of the inferior vena cava. Surg Gynecol Obstet 1984;158:141–4.

161. Madayag MA, Ambos MA, Lefleur RS, Bosniak MA. Involvement of the inferior vena cava in patients with renal cell carcinoma. Radiology 1979;133:321–6.

162. Cahill PJ, Sukov RJ. Inferior vena caval involvement by adrenal cortical carcinoma. Urology 1977;10:604–7.

163. Benderev TV, Grayhack JT, Bockrath JM, Uke ET. Inferior vena cava obstruction secondary to adenocarcinoma of the prostate. Role of orchiectomy in treatment. Arch Intern Med 1986;146:598–9.

164. Hassan B, Tung K, Weeks R, Mead GM. The management of inferior vena cava obstruction complicating metastatic germ cell tumors. Cancer 1999;85:912–8.

165. Hartley JW, Awrich AE, Wong J, et al. Diagnosis and treatment of the inferior vena cava syndrome in advanced malignant disease. Am J Surg 1986;152:70–4.

166. Valla D, Benhamou JP. Obstruction of the hepatic veins or suprahepatic inferior vena cava. Dig Dis 1996;14:99–118.

167. Yamana D, Yanagi T, Nanbu I, et al. Intracaval invasion of left adrenal cortical carcinoma extending into the right atrium. Radiat Med 1997;15:327–30.

168. Babu SC, Mianoni T, Shah PM, et al. Malignant renal tumor with extension to the inferior vena cava. Am J Surg 1998;176:137–9.

169. Pollanen M, Butany J, Chiasson D. Leiomyosarcoma of the inferior vena cava. Arch Pathol Lab Med 1987;111:1085–7.

170. Ranniger K. Obstruction of the inferior vena cava with edema or thrombophlebitis of the lower extremities. Am J Roentgenol Radium Ther Nucl Med 1970;109:563–7.

171. Piessens WF, Zeicher M. Hodgkin's disease causing a reversible nephrotic syndrome by compression of the inferior vena cava. Cancer 1970;25:880–4.

172. Singh V, Sinha SK, Nain CK, et al. Budd-Chiari syndrome: our experience of 71 patients. J Gastroenterol Hepatol 2000;15:550–4.

173. Sonin AH, Mazer MJ, Powers TA. Obstruction of the inferior vena cava: a multiple-modality demonstration of causes, manifestations, and collateral pathways. Radiographics 1992;12:309–22.

174. Pittman C, Reddy M, Reddy ER. Radiological evaluation of inferior vena cava obstruction: pictorial essay. Can Assoc Radiol J 1999;50:376–83.

175. Rahmouni A, Mathieu D, Berger JF, et al. Fast magnetic resonance imaging in the evaluation of tumoral

obstructions of the inferior vena cava. J Urol 1992;148:14–7.

176. Ng CS, Husband JE, Padhani AR, et al. Evaluation by magnetic resonance imaging of the inferior vena cava in patients with non-seminomatous germ cell tumours of the testis metastatic to the retroperitoneum. Br J Urol 1997;79:942–51.

177. Gehl HB, Bohndorf K, Klose KC. Inferior vena cava tumor thrombus: demonstration by Gd-DTPA enhanced MR. J Comput Assist Tomogr 1990;14:479–81.

178. Park JH, Lee JB, Han MC, et al. Sonographic evaluation of inferior vena caval obstruction: correlative study with vena cavography. AJR Am J Roentgenol 1985;145:757–62.

179. Didier D, Racle A, Etievent JP, Weill F. Tumor thrombus of the inferior vena cava secondary to malignant abdominal neoplasms: US and CT evaluation. Radiology 1987;162(1 Pt 1):83–9.

180. Habboub HK, Abu-Yousef MM, Williams RD, et al. Accuracy of color Doppler sonography in assessing venous thrombus extension in renal cell carcinoma. AJR Am J Roentgenol 1997;168:267–71.

181. Dhekne RD, Moore WH, Long SE. Radionuclide venography in iliac and inferior vena caval obstruction. Radiology 1982;144:597–602.

182. Powell-Jackson PR, Karani J, Ede RJ, et al. Ultrasound scanning and 99mTc sulphur colloid scintigraphy in diagnosis of Budd-Chiari syndrome. Gut 1986;27:1502–6.

183. Raju GS, Felver M, Olin JW, Satti SD. Thrombolysis for acute Budd-Chiari syndrome: case report and literature review. Am J Gastroenterol 1996;91:1262–3.

184. Neglen P, Nazzal MM, Al-Hassan HK, et al. Surgical removal of an inferior vena cava thrombus. Eur J Vasc Surg 1992;6:78–82.

185. Angle JF, Matsumoto AH, Al Shammari M, et al. Transcatheter regional urokinase therapy in the management of inferior vena cava thrombosis. J Vasc Interv Radiol 1998;9:917–25.

186. Fletcher WS, Lakin PC, Pommier RF, Wilmarth T. Results of treatment of inferior vena cava syndrome with expandable metallic stents. Arch Surg 1998;133:935–8.

187. Spitz A, Wilson TG, Kawachi MH, et al. Vena caval resection for bulky metastatic germ cell tumors: an 18-year experience. J Urol 1997;158:1813–8.

188. Sarkar R, Eilber FR, Gelabert HA, et al. Prosthetic replacement of the inferior vena cava for malignancy. J Vasc Surg 1998;28:75–83.

189. Klastersky J, Daneau D, Verhest A. Causes of death in patients with cancer. Eur J Cancer 1972;8:149–54.

190. Chang HY, Rodriguez V, Narboni G, et al. Causes of death in adults with acute leukemia. Medicine (Baltimore) 1976;55:259–68.

191. Suarez Nieto C, Estevan Solano JM, Buron Martinez G, et al. Invasion of the carotid artery in tumours of the head and neck. Clin Otolaryngol 1981;6:29–37.

192. Miller RR, McGregor DH. Hemorrhage from carcinoma of the lung. Cancer 1980;46:200–5.

193. Reina AJ, Fuentes O, Garcia A, et al. Intestinal leiomyosarcoma as the cause of severe hemoperitoneum. Dig Surg 1998;15:69–71.

194. Mac Manus M, Lamborn K, Khan W, et al. Radiotherapy-associated neutropenia and thrombocytopenia: analysis of risk factors and development of a predictive model. Blood 1997;89:2303–10.

195. Bisonni RS, Holtgrave DR, Lawler F, Marley DS. Colloids versus crystalloids in fluid resuscitation: an analysis of randomized controlled trials. J Fam Pract 1991;32:387–90.

196. Fajardo LF, Lee A. Rupture of major vessels after radiation. Cancer 1975;36:904–13.

197. Maran AG, Amin M, Wilson JA. Radical neck dissection: a 19-year experience. J Laryngol Otol 1989;103:760–4.

198. Chaloupka JC, Roth TC, Putman CM, et al. Recurrent carotid blowout syndrome: diagnostic and therapeutic challenges in a newly recognized subgroup of patients. AJNR Am J Neuroradiol 1999;20:1069–77.

199. Walker AT, Chaloupka JC, Putman CM, et al. Sentinel transoral hemorrhage from a pseudoaneurysm of the internal maxillary artery: a complication of CT-guided biopsy of the masticator space. AJNR Am J Neuroradiol 1996;17:377–81.

200. Heller KS, Strong EW. Carotid arterial hemorrhage after radical head and neck surgery. Am J Surg 1979;138:607–10.

201. Chaloupka JC, Putman CM, Citardi MJ, et al. Endovascular therapy for the carotid blowout syndrome in head and neck surgical patients: diagnostic and managerial considerations. AJNR Am J Neuroradiol 1996;17:843–52.

202. Morrissey DD, Andersen PE, Nesbit GM, et al. Endovascular management of hemorrhage in patients with head and neck cancer. Arch Otolaryngol Head Neck Surg 1997;123:15–9.

203. Giagounidis AA, Burk M, Meckenstock G, et al. Pathologic rupture of the spleen in hematologic malignancies: two additional cases. Ann Hematol 1996;73:297–302.

204. Brissette M, Dhru RD. Hodgkin's disease presenting as spontaneous splenic rupture. Arch Pathol Lab Med 1992;116:1077–9.

205. Von der Walde J, Mashiah A, Berrebi A. Spontaneous rupture of the spleen in hairy cell leukemia. Clin Oncol 1981;7:241–4.

206. Cook AM, Graham JD. Spontaneous rupture of the spleen secondary to metastatic teratoma. J R Soc Med 1996;89:710.

207. Lam KY, Tang V. Metastatic tumors to the spleen: a 25-year clinicopathologic study. Arch Pathol Lab Med 2000;124:526–30.

208. Van Poppel H, Aswarie H, Vandenhove J, Baert L. Spontaneous rupture of splenomegaly due to disseminated bone metastases from prostatic carcinoma. Br J Urol 1991;67:653–4.

209. Bauer TW, Haskins GE, Armitage JO. Splenic rupture in patients with hematologic malignancies. Cancer 1981;48:2729–33.

210. Jabbour M, Tohme C, Ingea H, Farah P. [Spontaneous splenic rupture due to heparin. Report of a case and review of the literature]. J Med Liban 1995;43:107–9.

211. Weiss SJ, Smith T, Laurin E, Wisner DH. Spontaneous splenic rupture due to subcutaneous heparin therapy. J Emerg Med 2000;18:421–6.

212. Haj M, Zaina A, Wiess M, et al. Pathologic-spontaneous-rupture of the spleen as a presenting sign of splenic T-cell lymphoma—case report with review. Hepatogastroenterology 1999;46:193–5.

213. Bernat S, Garcia Boyero R, Guinot M, et al. Pathologic rupture of the spleen as the initial manifestation in acute lymphoblastic leukemia [letter]. Haematologica 1998;83:760–1.

214. Paivansalo M, Myllyla V, Siniluoto T, et al. Imaging of splenic rupture. Acta Chir Scand 1986;152:733–7.

215. Mall JC, Kaiser JA. CT diagnosis of splenic laceration. AJR Am J Roentgenol 1980;134:265–9.

216. Kienzle GD, Stern J, Cooperberg A, Osborne CA. Spontaneous rupture of the spleen in primary plasma cell leukemia. Scintigraphic-pathologic correlation. Clin Nucl Med 1985;10:639–41.

217. Athale UH, Kaste SC, Bodner SM, Ribeiro RC. Splenic rupture in children with hematologic malignancies. Cancer 2000;88:480–90.

218. Heyman J, Leiter E. Spontaneous retroperitoneal hemorrhage: unusual presentation of renal cancer. Urology 1987;30:259–61.

219. Machuca Santa Cruz J, Julve Villalta E, Galacho Bech A, et al. [Spontaneous retroperitoneal hematoma: our experience]. Actas Urol Esp 1999;23:43–50.

220. Yamada AH, Sherrod AE, Boswell W, Skinner DG. Massive retroperitoneal hemorrhage from adrenal gland metastasis. Urology 1992;40:59–62.

221. Casella R, Staedele H, von Weymarn A, et al. Life-threatening spontaneous retroperitoneal bleeding: a rare complication of oral anticoagulation. Urol Int 1999;63:247–8.

222. Di Rosa C, Venora S, Monterosso N, et al. [Retroperitoneal hematoma during heparin therapy. Comments on 3 cases]. Minerva Chir 1997;52:493–7.

223. Lodge JP, Hall R. Retroperitoneal haemorrhage: a dangerous complication of common femoral arterial puncture. Eur J Vasc Surg 1993;7:355–7.

224. Morettin LB, Kumar R. Small renal carcinoma with large retroperitoneal hemorrhage: diagnostic considerations. Urol Radiol 1981;3:143–8.

225. Pummer K, Lammer J, Wandschneider G, Primus G. Renal cell carcinoma presenting as spontaneous retroperitoneal haemorrhage. Int Urol Nephrol 1990;22:307–11.

226. Chang SY, Ma CP, Lee SK. Spontaneous retroperitoneal hemorrhage from kidney causes. Eur Urol 1988;15:281–4.

227. Berney CR, Roth AD, Allal A, Rohner A. Spontaneous retroperitoneal hemorrhage due to adrenal metastasis for non-small cell lung cancer treated by radiation therapy. Acta Oncol 1997;36:91–3.

228. Scarantino C, Salazar OM, Rubin P, et al. The optimum radiation schedule in treatment of superior vena caval obstruction: importance of 99mTc scintiangiograms. Int J Radiat Oncol Biol Phys 1979;5:1987–95.

229. Little AG, Golomb HM, Ferguson MK, et al. Malignant superior vena cava obstruction reconsidered: the role of diagnostic surgical intervention. Ann Thorac Surg 1985;40:285–8.

Chapter 16

Hematologic Emergencies

Mary Ann Weiser, MD, PhD
Susan O'Brien, MD
Aida B. Narvios, MD

TRANSFUSION REACTIONS

Transfusion reactions are less frequent in cancer patients than in noncancer patients (< 1% compared withapproximately 3%, of all blood product infusions).[1] However, blood component therapy is often used in the supportive care of cancer patients, so transfusion reactions are not uncommon in this patient population and frequently require urgent or emergent evaluation and treatment. It is important that both clinical staff and laboratory staff understand the different types of transfusion reactions so that a proper diagnosis can be made, effective treatment can be given, and possible preventive measures can be taken.

In the past, the vast majority of transfusion reactions were thought to be antibody mediated, resulting from the response of recipient antibodies to donor products or vice versa. However, recent observations have led to an alternative hypothesis for the most frequently seen type of reaction, the febrile nonhemolytic transfusion reaction (FNHTR). This type of reaction originally was thought to be caused by recipient antibodies directed against donor leukocytes. While this is probably true for red blood cell transfusions, recent studies have shown that in platelet transfusions, biologic response modifiers accumulated during platelet storage most often cause FNHTRs.[2] Acute and delayed hemolytic transfusion reactions, anaphylaxis, and urticaria are caused by recipient antibodies to donor products. Transfusion-related acute lung injury is the result of donor antibodies to recipient leukocytes. Although not a true transfusion reaction, bacterial contamination of donor products must also be considered when assessing and treating a patient with a suspected transfusion reaction and is therefore included in the classification scheme presented here (Table 16–1).

Acute Hemolytic Transfusion Reactions

Most acute hemolytic transfusion reactions (AHTRs) involve ABO blood group incompatibility, in which case they can be severe and life threatening. However, the severity of alloimmune-mediated hemolytic reactions depends on many factors, such as the class, subclass, and plasma concentration of the immunoglobulin causing the event; the red blood cell antigen density; the amount of incompatible red blood cells transfused; and whether hemolysis is predominantly intravascular or extravascular. Extravascular reactions are usually less severe because the rate of hemolysis is slower. Hemoglobinemia and hemoglobinuria are also relatively rare with extravascular hemolysis, as are renal failure and death. Antibodies directed against antigens of the Kell, Duffy, and Rh systems usually cause extravascular rather than intravascular hemolysis.

The incidence of immune-mediated AHTRs is approximately 1 per 25,000 units transfused, and the mortality rate is estimated at 5 to 10%.[3] The incidence of fatal hemolytic reactions is estimated at 1 per 100,000 units transfused. The most common causes of AHTRs are misidentification of the recipient and clerical error at the time of type and crossmatch.

Because of suppressed isoagglutinin in titers, AHTRs may be less severe and may therefore be under-reported in oncology patients. A retrospective study of 100,177 transfused units of red blood cells given to 25,477 cancer patients over 4 years included only 4 acute hemolytic reactions (1 per 25,044 transfused units, or 0.004%) and 13 delayed hemolytic reactions (1 per 7,705 transfused units, or 0.013%).[1] All acute reactions resulted from human error. All delayed reactions occurred in patients who had a history of blood transfusion. There were no deaths.

The most common presenting signs and symptoms of AHTRs are fever and chills. Nausea, vomiting, flushing, dyspnea, chest pain, back or flank pain, vague uneasiness, discomfort at the site of infusion, and hypotension occur less frequently. Patients who are unconscious or under general anesthesia and undergoing surgery might present only with uncontrolled bleeding secondary to disseminated intravascular coagulation (DIC). The risk of renal failure and death increases with increasing amounts of

TABLE 16–1. Classification of Transfusion Reactions

Type of Reaction	Mechanism	Incidence	Intravascular or Extravascular	Timing	Potential Complications
Acute hemolytic	Recipient antibodies to antigens (usually ABO) on donor RBCs	1/1,417 to 1/21,000	Either	Usually within minutes or hours of transfusion	Hemoglobinuria, DIC, renal failure, hypotension; 5–10% mortality
Delayed hemolytic	Previously undetected or newly formed recipient antibodies to donor RBCs (usually non-ABO)	1/2,500	Usually extravascular	Within 7–14 days after transfusion; range, 3–21 days	Usually minor, as in drop in hemoglobin level; hemoglobinuria is rare
Febrile nonhemolytic	Recipient antibodies to passenger donor leukocytes/platelets or pyrogenic cytokines accumulated during storage	1/100 RBC transfusions; 1/5 platelet transfusions	Intravascular	Within 1 hour of transfusion	Usually none
Anaphylaxis	Recipient antibodies interact with donor plasma proteins to form immune complexes that activate complement	1/150,000	Intravascular	Within minutes of starting transfusion	Hypertension followed by hypotension, laryngeal edema, bronchospasm, gastrointestinal distress
Urticaria	Incomplete manifestations of anaphylaxis	1/1,000	Intravascular	Within minutes of starting transfusion	Urticaria, pruritis
Acute lung injury	Donor antibodies, usually HLA, react against recipient leukocytes	1/5,000	Intravascular	Within 6 hours of transfusion	Noncardiogenic pulmonary edema
Bacterial contamination	N/A	1/2,500,000 RBCs; 1/350 platelets	Intravascular	Within hours of transfusion	Hypotension, severe sepsis, shock

DIC = disseminated intravascular coagulation; HLA = human leukocyte antigen; N/A = not applicable; RBC = red blood cells.

mismatched blood transfused and higher plasma concentrations of immunoglobulin. Fortunately, the most feared complications (hemoglobinuria, intravascular coagulation, and renal failure) are uncommon in cancer patients.[1]

The laboratory evaluation of patients with AHTRs should include a search for possible clerical errors, a serologic check for incompatibility, done by performing a direct antiglobulin (Coombs') test; a complete blood count to determine the presence or absence of schistocytes; and a comparison of pre- and postreaction specimens for hemoglobinemia and hemoglobinuria. Other causes of hemoglobinemia and hemoglobinuria include sepsis, DIC, and the infusion of hypotonic saline. Hemoglobinemia may also be caused ex vivo as a result of venipuncture.

The goal of treatment of an AHTR should be to minimize exposure as well as potential complications. The transfusion should be stopped immediately, and venous access should be maintained. Intravenous fluids, mannitol, and furosemide should be used as necessary, to maintain blood pressure and urine output and to minimize renal injury.

Delayed Hemolytic Transfusion Reactions

Delayed hemolytic transfusion reactions typically occur within 7 to 14 days after a transfusion (range, 3 to 21 days). In delayed reactions, previously undetected or newly formed recipient antibodies directed against donor red blood cells cause hemolysis. The antibodies are typically noncomplement-binding immunoglobulin G (IgG) and are directed against any of the non-ABO red blood cell antigens. The antigens most commonly involved are Rh (c and E), Kidd, Duffy, and Kell. Identifying new alloantibodies in a newly transfused patient is not uncommon. In contrast to acute reactions, the hemolytic process in delayed reactions is usually slower, less severe, and extravascular. Delayed reactions often go undetected because of their mildness. The estimated overall incidence is 1 per 2,500 units of transfused red blood cells (0.04%), and the incidence in oncology patients is slightly lower (around 0.01%). This, again, is likely due to the tumor or to treatment-related suppression of alloimmunization.[1]

Patients with a delayed hemolytic reaction typically present with fever, a drop in hemoglobin with or without jaundice, and a positive direct antiglobulin test. Hemoglobinuria is rare. Treatment is supportive and is rarely required. Preventing delayed hemolytic reactions involves asking prospective recipients about their transfusion history and about any symptoms that are suggestive of a delayed reaction. Antigens associated with any previously detected antibodies should be avoided, even if the antibody is no longer detectable.

Febrile Nonhemolytic Transfusion Reactions

A febrile nonhemolytic transfusion reaction is defined as an increase of 1°C in body temperature within 2 hours after infusion, unattributable to causes other than infusion. This type of reaction is a fairly common complication of transfusion therapy and occurs in up to 1% of all blood component transfusions and in as much as 30% of all platelet transfusions.[4]

Such reaction are caused by the actions of recipient antibodies (stimulated by previous transfusions or pregnancy) directed against passenger leukocytes in donor blood and by pyrogenic cytokines, which have been shown to increase in concentration during platelet blood storage.

Most red blood cell FNHTRs are thought to be antibody mediated. With cancer patients, this type of reaction occurs in approximately 0.16% of red blood cell transfusions. Leukocyte reduction has been shown to reduce the rate of this type of red blood cell transfusion reaction from 0.3 to 0.1% in all transfusion patients. However, because of the logistic problems and cost considerations involved in preparing leukocyte-poor RBCs (LPRBCs) and the relatively low morbidity associated with this type of reaction, the use of LPRBCs should be limited to selected patients with a history of severe or repeated FNHTRs.[1,3]

Most FNHTRs that are associated with platelet transfusions do not involve an immune-mediated event but are caused by the accumulation of biologic response modifiers during platelet storage. At least two studies have shown an association between this type of reaction and high levels of interleukin-1β, interleukin 6, and tumor necrosis factor-α.[5,6]

The transfusion of single-donor platelets rather than pooled platelets may reduce the risk of antibody-mediated febrile reactions.[7] Several approaches have been suggested for preventing FNHTRs caused by cytokine accumulation, including reduction of the platelet storage time to 3 days, prestorage leukoreduction, and plasma removal before transfusion. A recent randomized controlled study of 380 platelet transfusions to 30 patients demonstrated that plasma removal prior to transfusion was more effective than poststorage white blood cell reduction for preventing reactions (17% vs 25.8%, $p < .008$), most (88%) of which were FNHTRs. A prospective study comparing plasma depletion to prestorage white blood cell reduction is under way.[8] Transfusing fresh platelet concentrates when available is also considered by some investigators to be an effective way to minimize the risk for this type of reaction.

As for most transfusion reactions, treatment is supportive. Antipyretics, meperidol, and histamine blockers are useful for symptomatic treatment.

Antibody-mediated FNHTRs are unlikely to recur if a different donor is used, so a change in transfusion practice after a first FNHTR is not required. For patients who have repeated FNHTRs despite risk-reduction measures, the decision to discontinue a transfusion should be made on a case-by-case basis. The transfusion of fresh platelet concentrates (when available) is considered an effective alternative.

Anaphylaxis and Urticarial Reactions

Anaphylactic transfusion reactions are similar to hypersensitivity reactions to insect stings or foods but do not involve immunoglobulin E (IgE). These reactions are rare, occurring in less than 0.001% of all transfusions.[9] These reactions are caused by the interaction between recipient antibodies and donor plasma proteins, which combine to form immune complexes that activate complement. Activated complement components directly trigger the release of mediators from mast cells and basophils. Hence, this type of reaction is sometimes referred to as anaphylactoid rather than as anaphylactic. This type of reaction is also commonly seen in patients with congenital immunoglobulin A (IgA) deficiency, who can become sensitized to IgA in donor blood products.

The clinical symptoms of transfusion-related anaphylaxis occur shortly after the transfusion is started and include transient hypertension followed by hypotension, flushing, chills, laryngeal edema, bronchospasm, and gastrointestinal distress. Treatment consists of immediately stopping the transfusion and administering H$_1$ and H$_2$ histamine blockers. Bronchodilators, nebulized racemic epinephrine, and parenteral epinephrine should be used as indicated. Corticosteroids may also be of benefit to patients with severe reactions. Patients with a history of anaphylactic transfusion reaction should be given only washed blood products. Because it is impossible to verify the absence of responsible antigens, such patients should not be given fresh-frozen plasma unless absolutely necessary.

Urticarial reactions are incomplete manifestations of anaphylactic reactions and are much more common. They are estimated to occur once for every 1,000 units of transfused blood products.[9] The incidence of progression to hypotension, laryngeal edema, and bronchospasm is unknown. In most cases of isolated urticaria, the transfusion can be continued after treatment with antihistamines. Patients with a history of transfusion-related urticaria should be premedicated with antihistamines before transfusion.

Transfusion-Related Acute Lung Injury

Transfusion-related acute lung injury differs from other immune-mediated transfusion reactions in that most cases (nearly 90%) are thought to be caused by antibodies in the donor unit reacting against recipient leukocytes. These reactions are estimated to occur in less than 0.01% of red blood cell transfusions.[9] The causative antibodies are typically antibodies to class I human leukocyte antigens (HLAs). Antibodies to neutrophil-specific antigens are less commonly involved. Donated blood products from multiparous women (who are most likely to be alloimmunized)[10] are most likely to lead to acute lung reactions. This type of reaction is likely to be less severe, and therefore under-reported, in oncology patients who are neutropenic as a result of chemotherapy.

The clinical presentation of transfusion-related acute lung injury is adult respiratory distress syndrome that develops within 6 hours after a transfusion of plasma-containing blood components. A diagnosis can be made by ruling out other causes of acute respiratory distress, such as cardiogenic pulmonary edema. Unlike patients with cardiogenic pulmonary edema, patients with transfusion-related acute lung injury have low or normal pulmonary wedge pressure and normal central venous pressure. The diagnosis can be confirmed retrospectively by testing the donor blood for antileukocyte antibodies. Donors with clinically significant antileukocyte antibody titers should not participate in routine blood donation.

Treatment is supportive. Oxygen, intubation, and ventilation are frequently required. However, the prognosis is good, and most patients recover fully within 48 to 96 hours. The mortality rate is approximately 5%.[10]

Bacterial Contamination

The bacterial contamination of donated blood is considered rare and is estimated to occur once in every 2,500,000 units of red blood cell transfusion and once in every 350 units of platelet transfusion. However, there has been recent concern over a reported rise in the number of bacterially contaminated units in blood bank inventories.[11,12]

Because they must be stored at 22°C to maintain function, platelets are more commonly associated with bacterial contamination than are other blood products. Potential sources of blood product contamination include incompletely sterilized venipuncture sites, asymptomatic donor bacteremia at the time of collection, leaky collection or storage equipment, and equipment contaminated at the time of manufacture. The risk of contamination also increases with platelet storage time. *Yersinia enterocolitica*, a cold-loving bacterium with the ability to proliferate at refrigerated temperatures (1° to 6°C) and a predilection for an iron-rich environment, is a leading cause of concern in many blood product contamination studies.[13,14]

A rise in the bacterial contamination of blood products would have a particularly detrimental effect on cancer patients, especially those who are transfusion dependent and immunosuppressed. Fortunately, a recent retrospective study of bacterial cultures performed on over 1,200 units of "at-risk" blood products at the University of Texas M.D. Anderson Cancer Center demonstrated that bacterial contamination remains a rare complication of transfusion therapy.[15] In 25 culture-positive units (2%), the most common organism identified was coagulase-negative *Staphylococcus* (present in 18 units, 3 of which were polymicrobial). The other organisms identified were *Enterobacter agglomerans* (1 unit), *Enterococcus* (1 unit), *Pseudomonas paucimobilis* (1unit), and Gram-variable or Gram-negative bacilli (4 units). Single-donor platelets that had been stored for more than 24 hours had the highest percentage of positive cultures (4.7%). In this series, none of the patients who experienced transfusion reactions after receiving culture-positive units showed evidence of sepsis, and all blood cultures obtained post-transfusion were negative for bacterial contamination.

The clinical presentation of bacterial contamination is the same as for sepsis: fever, tachycardia, tachypnea, and leukocytosis or leukopenia with or without hypotension and end-organ damage. Fever is usually higher than fever in acute hemolytic reactions or FNHTRs (2°C vs 0.9°C above normal) and peaks later, up to 4 hours after transfusion. Gram's stain and culture of the remaining donor blood are helpful only when the suspicion of bacterial contamination is high or when platelets that were stored for more than 4 or 5 days have been transfused. Treatment includes broad-spectrum antibiotics and intravenous fluids. Vasopressors such as dopamine and epinephrine are required when hypotension does not respond to intravenous-fluid challenge.

ANEMIA

Anemia is common in cancer patients. It occurs at some point in nearly all patients with leukemia; in 50% of patients with lymphoma, after chemotherapy; and in up to 50% of patients with solid tumors.[16] When anemia occurs, it is usually chronic, but it is not unusual for patients to become symptomatic with anemia, a development that may require urgent evaluation and treatment.

The symptoms of anemia include fatigue, generalized weakness, headache, tinnitus, dyspnea, palpitations, and light-headedness or dizziness. Patients with underlying coronary artery disease may also present with worsening angina; those with peripheral vascular disease may present with worsening claudication; and those with dementia may present with worsening confusion, agitation, and memory loss. Occasionally, patients may develop symptoms of high-output congestive heart failure.

To some degree, the physical findings are a function of the cause of the anemia. Patients with chronic anemia typically present with pallor, tachycardia, increased pulse pressure, systolic ejection murmurs, and mild peripheral edema. Anemia secondary to acute blood loss may also cause hypotension and in severe cases, shock or death.

The evaluation of patients with anemia should include a careful history and physical examination, with close attention paid to signs and symptoms of acute blood loss. Red blood cell indices, reticulocyte count, ferritin or serum iron level, and total iron-binding capacity should be included in the initial evaluation. The reticulocyte count is considered a key test because it distinguishes anemia secondary to bone marrow failure from anemia secondary to acute blood loss or hemolysis. Further evaluation depends on the suspected cause of anemia; however, the cause might be multifactorial.

Anemia Due to Bone Marrow Failure

Bone marrow failure always leads to a decrease in the absolute reticulocyte count; however, red blood cells may be microcytic, normocytic, or macrocytic (Table 16–2). The diagnostic evaluation of microcytic and normocytic anemia due to bone marrow failure differs significantly from that of macrocytic anemia. However, it should be kept in mind that determining mean corpuscular volume by using electronic counters is subject to error and that the readings can be falsely elevated by the presence of cold agglutinins, marked hyperglycemia, or extreme leukocytosis.

Normocytic and Microcytic Anemia: Anemia of Chronic Disease. Anemia of chronic disease is the most common type of anemia seen in patients with solid tumors. It is usually mild and primarily caused by the failure of red blood cell production. However, the life span of red blood cells is also decreased, probably because of extravascular hemolysis. The exact cause of bone marrow failure is unknown although several causes have been postulated, including the relative lack of erythropoietin, the sequestration of iron in macrophages, and the inhibitory effects of cytokines on the responsiveness of erythroid progenitor cells to erythropoietin.[17]

Red blood cell morphology is usually normochromic and normocytic in anemia of chronic disease but may be microcytic in 30 to 40% of cases. The absolute reticulo-cyte count, serum iron (Fe) concentration level, total iron-binding capacity (TIBC), and Fe-to-TIBC ratio are decreased while iron stores (ferritin) remain normal. The severity of anemia typically correlates with the extent of the underlying disease; however, the development of this type of anemia does not imply bone marrow invasion by tumor.

Anemia of chronic disease in patients with cancer should respond to treatment of the underlying malignancy. Blood transfusions are of limited value but may be used as a temporary measure. Erythropoietin, 100 U/kg subcutaneously three times weekly, has been shown to be of benefit, resulting in an increase in hematocrit, a decrease in transfusion requirements, and improved quality of life. However, these treatment effects are not seen for at least several weeks. Administration of iron, vitamin B_{12} and folate are of no value for these patients.[18]

Macrocytic Anemia. Macrocytic anemia due to bone marrow failure is a common disorder. Among cancer patients, the most common causes are drugs and primary marrow disturbances. Other common causes of macrocytic anemia include alcoholism, liver disease, and hypothyroidism.

Marrow Invasion and Primary Marrow Disorders. The malignancies most commonly associated with marrow invasion include small-cell carcinoma of the lung, adenocarcinoma of the breast and prostate, and lymphoma. Immature white blood cells and nucleated red blood cells are frequently present, and severe cases may result in pancytopenia.[19]

Aplastic anemia and pure red cell dysplasias are rare disorders in which developing red cells are absent or markedly diminished in the bone marrow. Myelodysplastic syndrome, refractory anemia, refractive anemia with ringed sideroblasts, refractory anemia with excess blasts, refractory anemia with excess blasts in transition,

TABLE 16–2. Anemias Associated with Decreased Red Blood Cell Production*

Type of Anemia	MCV	Diagnostic Studies	Treatment
Chronic disease	Normal or low	Low Fe, low TIBC, increased ferritin	Underlying disease if possible; transfusions of limited value; erythropoietin
Iron deficiency	Normal or low	Low Fe, normal or high TIBC, low or normal ferritin	Iron supplement
Marrow invasion/ primary marrow failure	Normal or high; other cell lines frequently depressed	Normal or high Fe, above-normal Fe/TIBC ratio	Primary disorder; transfusion support; erythropoietin
Treatment-related	High	Same as chronic disease	Transfusion support; erythropoietin
Megaloblastic	High	High Fe, decreased or normal cobalamin or folate, decreased RBC folate, increased homocysteine, increased or normal methylmalonic acid	Replacement with cobalamin and/or folate; appropriate drug antidote or removal of offending drug

Fe = serum iron concentration; MCV = mean corpuscular volume; RBC = red blood cell; TIBC = total iron-binding capacity.
*Low or normal reticulocyte count.

TABLE 16–3. Characteristics of Autoimmune Hemolytic Anemias

AIHA Subtype	Antibody Type	Clinical Presentation	Coombs' Test, DAT Results	Treatment Options
WAIHA	Usually IgG	Idiopathic Lymphoproliferative disorders (CLL, lymphoma) Autoimmune diseases drugs: fludarabine, 2-CdA, 6-mercaptopurine, carboplatin, a-methyldopa, quinidine, penicillin Postviral infection Solid tumors (rare) of breast, lung, colon, ovary, testis, thymus, kidney	Positive for IgG and C	Steroids; splenectomy; immunosuppressive therapy (cyclophosphamide, azathioprine [Imuran]), IV γ-globulin; bood transfusion (with caution)
CAIHA				
Acute/transient	IgM, IgG	Usually younger patients, in association with *Mycoplasma* or EBV infection; polyclonal	IgG negative (usually)	Supportive
Chronic	IgM, IgG	Idiopathic or associated with lymphoproliferative disorders (including lymphoma, CLL, myeloma, and Waldenströms macroglobulinemia); monoclonal	C3d=positive	Treat underlying malignancy
Paroxysmal cold hemoglobinuria	IgG	Postinfection pediatric patients	C-positive; IgG-negative	Usually self-limiting
AIHA with BMT	Early onset: IgM; late onset: IgG	Status post BMT; usually T-cell-depleted graft	—	Steroids, alone or combined with Ig; staphylococcal protein A column; azathioprine, lymphoid radiation

Adapted from Hashimoto C.[29]

2-CdA = 2-chlorodeoxyadenosine; AIHA = autoimmune hemolytic anemia; BMT = bone marrow transplantation; C = complement; CAIHA = cold autoimmune hemolytic anemia; CLL = chronic lymphocytic leukemia; DAT = direct antiglobulin test; Ig = immunoglobulin; EBV = Epstein-Barr virus; IV = intravenous; WAIHA = warm autoimmune hemolytic anemia.

(2-CdA), and 6-mercaptopurine, have been reported to cause WAIHA.[24,25] Carboplatin, among other agents used in the treatment of solid tumors, has also been reported to cause WAIHA.[26] The mechanism is unknown.

In patients with tumor-related WAIHA, successful treatment of the primary tumor often leads to the resolution of WAIHA. Corticosteroid treatment is usually less effective with WAIHA than with idiopathic autoimmune hemolysis.[27] In cases of recurrent or unresponsive tumors, splenectomy is a reasonable treatment option. Intravenous immunoglobulins (400 mg/kg/d for 5 days) may be indicated for patients with CLL and severe hypogammaglobulinemia; however, most studies have failed to show that this treatment has a benefit for patients with classic AIHA associated with CLL.[28] Blood transfusions increase the risk for alloantibody-induced hemolytic transfusion reactions and require complicated pretransfusion testing; they should therefore be avoided.[29]

In cases of chemotherapy-related AIHA, the drug should be discontinued. In severe cases, intravenous high-dose steroids (prednisone, 1 to 2 mg/kg/d or equivalent)[28] and/or cyclophosphamide may be required, along with red blood cell transfusion.

Cold Autoimmune Hemolytic Anemia. Cold autoimmune hemolytic anemia is the second most common form of AIHA and accounts for approximately 20 to 25% of all cases. It has two types of clinical presentations: a transient form and a chronic form. The autoantibody is IgM, which optimally binds to red blood cells at 4°C. Because of the low affinity of IgM to red blood cells at 37°C, Coombs' test is usually negative.

Transient CAIHA occurs in younger patients as a rare complication of infections such as *Mycoplasma* or Epstein-Barr virus infections. Although the anemia may be abrupt in onset (2 to 3 weeks following infection) and occasionally severe, it usually resolves spontaneously. In addition to hemolysis, patients with CAIHA may develop acrocyanosis or marked purpling of the extremities, ears, and nose, which occurs when the blood becomes cold enough to agglutinate in the veins.

Treatment of the acute form of CAIHA is supportive and includes hydration, avoidance of cold (or maintenance of a warm environment), and blood transfusion. Splenectomy is usually not of value in the treatment of this disorder.

The chronic form of CAIHA usually presents as mild to moderate stable anemia. It is considered a rare complication of malignancy and is typically seen in older patients with lymphoproliferative diseases such as lymphoma, CLL, myeloma, and Waldenström's macroglobulinemia. Hemolysis may be intravascular, extravascular, or both. Patients without an established cancer diagnosis should be evaluated for underlying B-cell lymphoma.

The chronic form of CAIHA usually responds to the appropriate treatment of the malignant neoplasm responsible for the production of the cold agglutinin.

Autoimmune Hemolytic Anemia Associated with Bone Marrow Transplantation. In bone marrow transplantation patients, immune-mediated hemolytic anemia may be alloimmune in origin, owing to red blood cell incompatibility between donor and host, or autoimmune, which is thought to result from a transient immune system imbalance that occurs during recovery of normal immune and hematopoietic systems.

Autoimmune hemolytic anemia is typically seen in patients who are receiving T-cell-depleted grafts and has been reported in up to 3% of bone marrow transplantation cases. The onset can occur anytime from 2 to 25 months after transplantation. In one study, early-onset hemolysis (2 to 8 months post transplantation) was found to be caused by autoantibodies of the cold-reactive type, and late-onset hemolysis (6 to 18 months post transplantation) was caused by autoantibodies of the warm-reactive type.[29]

Treatments for AIHA associated with bone marrow transplantation include steroids (alone or in combination with immunoglobulin), staphylococcal protein A, azathioprine, and lymphoid radiation therapy. The response to treatments has been variable, but the overall prognosis for patients is poor, with a mortality rate of nearly 60%.[29]

Microangiopathic Hemolytic Anemia

Microangiopathic hemolytic anemia (MAHA) associated with renal failure (thrombotic thrombocytopenic purpura [TTP] or hemolytic uremic syndrome [HUS]) complicates almost 6% of cases of metastatic malignancy (Table 16–4).[30] It occurs most commonly in gastric adenocarcinoma, followed by breast cancer, colon cancer, unknown primary cancer, and lung cancer.[31]

Chemotherapeutic agents have also been implicated in the development of MAHA. This is especially so of mitomycin C, which has been reported to cause MAHA in up to 10% of treated patients; its toxic effect is related to the cumulative dose and can develop even months after mitomycin C has been discontinued. There have also been reports of MAHA related to cisplatin-based chemotherapy given with bleomycin[32] and as a complication of treatment with gemcitabine.[33,34]

Target-organ dysfunction in MAHA is caused by marked platelet aggregation in the microcirculation, most commonly involving the kidneys, brain, heart, and adrenal glands; central nervous system involvement is more predominant in TTP whereas renal involvement predominates in HUS. The pathophysiology of MAHA is complicated and has not been fully explained. Possible pathophysiologic mechanisms include abnormalities in fibrinolysis and prostacyclin release, as well as the absence or presence of unknown mediators of platelet aggregation.

In addition to the typical abnormalities seen with hemolytic anemia, marked thrombocytopenia and renal insufficiency characterize this syndrome. Symptoms are abrupt in onset, with hemolytic anemia preceding renal dysfunction by 1 to 2 weeks. Anemia and thrombocytopenia are usually severe, with hemoglobin values typically < 8 g/dL and the platelet count < 25,000/L. Although immune complexes are present in plasma, Coombs' test is negative. Unlike DIC, there is no coagulopathy; coagulation times, fibrinogen, fibrin-split products, and D-dimer levels are normal. Rash, fever, arterial hypertension, central neurologic dysfunction, pericarditis, interstitial pneumonitis, hematuria, and proteinuria may occur. In chemotherapy-related MAHA, fever is uncommon, and respiratory dysfunction may be more prominent than in the classic form.[32]

TABLE 16–4. Microangiopathic Hemolytic Anemia in Cancer Patients

Most common malignancies associated with MAHA
  Gastric
  Breast
  Colon
  Unknown primary
  Lung

Most common chemotherapeutic agents implicated in MAHA
  Mitomycin C
  Cisplatin with bleomycin
  Cisplatin with gemcitabine

Clinical features
  Purpura, fever, hypertension
  Pericardial friction rub/pericardial effusion, atrial arrhythmias
  Neurologic symptoms (headache, aphasia, stupor [more common in TTP])
  Respiratory symptoms/pneumonitis (may be more prominent in chemotherapy-related MAHA)
  Acute renal failure (more common in HUS)
  Thrombocytopenia (platelet count usually < 25,000/L)
  Anemia (hemoglobin concentration usually < 8 g/L)
  Schistocytes
  Elevated reticulocyte count, total bilirubin, lactic dehydrogenase
  Decreased haptoglobin
  Hematuria, proteinuria
  Negative Coombs' test
  Coagulation times, fibrinogen, fibrin split products, and D dimer usually normal

Treatment
  Prednisone, 200 mg/d
  Plasmapheresis

HUS = hemolytic uremic syndrome; MAHA = microangiopathic hemolytic anemia; TTP = thrombocytopenic purpura.

MAHA carries a poor prognosis; without treatment, the mortality rate is close to 100%. However, appropriate therapy can improve the mortality rate, perhaps to as low as 10%.[35] Treatment with high-dose steroids (prednisone at 200 mg/d) has been effective in patients with mild disease (ie, minimal symptoms and no neurologic abnormalities other than a mild headache). Prednisone plus plasmapheresis and replacement with fresh frozen plasma is indicated for patients presenting with central nervous system symptoms and rapidly declining hematocrit values and platelet counts. Plasmapheresis plus plasma replacement is also indicated for patients with mild disease that does not respond within 48 hours to initial high-dose steroids. Infusion with fresh frozen plasma alone is not efficacious for most patients. The use of antiplatelet agents in the treatment of this disease is controversial, and there is little evidence to support it. Relapse can occur in up to 64% of cases.[35,36]

Anemia from Blood Loss

Blood loss is another common cause of anemia in patients with malignancy. With chronic blood loss and normally functioning bone marrow, the absolute reticulocyte count will be increased; however, this may not be the case in patients with cancer-related or treatment-related bone marrow suppression. Red blood cell morphology is either hypochromic or normochromic.

Blood loss related to solid tumors may be chronic or acute; common causes include locally advanced and superficial tumors, such as breast carcinoma or advanced cervical carcinoma, and gastrointestinal tumors or metastases. Nongastrointestinal tumors that tend to involve the gastrointestinal tract and that cause bleeding include melanoma and lymphoma. Renal cell carcinoma and transitional cell carcinoma of the bladder may also cause significant blood loss as a result of hematuria.

Massive life-threatening hemorrhages usually result from local invasion of the blood vessels by tumor; the most frequent sites are the neck and chest. The local invasion of head and neck tumors into a carotid artery or jugular vein typically presents as massive epistaxis or carotid artery "blowout." The local invasion of lung tumors near the hilum or bronchial arteries can also cause massive hemoptysis. In such cases, the surgical occlusion of major vessels may temporarily stop a massive hemorrhage; however, this type of bleeding is often fatal.

THROMBOCYTOPENIA

Thrombocytopenia may result from decreased bone marrow production, increased splenic sequestration, accelerated destruction, or a combination of these. In cancer patients, thrombocytopenia is usually disease related or treatment related.

Disease-related causes of thrombocytopenia include marrow replacement by primary or metastatic tumors and physiologic derangements which may involve peripheral destruction, splenic sequestration, or abnormal production of platelets. Potential causes of abnormal platelet production include nutritional deficiencies, abnormal feedback, or bone marrow reaction as in fibrosis. Splenic sequestration may occur in the setting of primary splenic involvement of lymphoproliferative disorders such as chronic myelogenous leukemia (CML), CLL, lymphoma, or hairy cell leukemia. It is also seen as a result of metastases from solid tumors (especially carcinomas of the breast, lung, prostate, colon, and stomach) or congestive splenomegaly resulting from splenic vein obstruction in pancreatic cancer or extensive hepatic metastases.[37,38]

Treatment-related thrombocytopenia can be caused by chemotherapy or radiation therapy. In addition to chemotherapeutic agents, a variety of common drugs, including heparin and phenytoin, have also been implicated in thrombocytopenia (Table 16–5).

Thrombocytopenia resulting from chemotherapy usually occurs on day 9 or 10 of treatment, with nadirs on days 14 to 18 although the nadir is more delayed with some agents (eg, carmustine [BCNU] and busulfan) and can occur as late as week 4 or 5 of treatment. The onset and severity of radiation-induced thrombocytopenia depends on the dose and timing of therapy.

Thrombocytopenia may result in spontaneous retroperitoneal hemorrhaging or bleeding from the mucous membranes, gastrointestinal tract, or urinary tract. The most feared complication is a fatal intracerebral hemorrhage, which is often preceded by a spontaneous retinal hemorrhage. Several factors can increase the risk of spontaneous bleeding, including fever and the presence of microangiopathic coagulopathy.

The trigger level for prophylactic platelet transfusion remains highly controversial and currently ranges from 5,000 to 20,000/L.[39] The decision to transfuse platelets prophylactically ultimately rests on the consideration of various factors, including the presence of fever, the likelihood of endogenous bone marrow recovery, platelet level stability, history of bleeding, the presence of concurrent neutropenia and risk of infection, platelet availability, and access to health care. In the absence of risk factors or extenuating circumstances, the threshold for prophylactic transfusion can usually safely be set at 10,000/L, and there is evidence that it may be as low as 5,000/L.[40,41] Patients with thrombocytopenia and active bleeding should be transfused until the bleeding stops or until the bleeding time is less than two times the upper limit of normal.

Platelet transfusion carries several risks, including transfusion reactions (see previous section), infection,

TABLE 16–5. Drugs and Substances Implicated in Thrombocytopenia

Suppression of platelet production
  Myelosuppressive drugs
    Severe: cytosine arabinoside, daunorubicin
    Moderate: cyclophosphamide, busulphan, methotrexate,
      6-mercaptopurine
    Mild: vinca alkaloids
  Thiazide diuretics
  Ethanol
  Estrogens

Immunologic platelet destruction
  Clinical suspicion plus convincing experimental evidence
    Antibiotics: sulfathiazole, novobiocin, p-aminosalicylate
    Cinchona alkaloids: quinidine, quinine
    Foods: beans
    Sedatives, hypnotics, anticonvulsants (apronalide,
      carbamazepine)
    Arsenical drugs used to treat syphilis
    Digitoxin
    Methyldopa
    Stibophen
  Clinical suspicion (major drugs and substances implicated)
    Aspirin
    Chlorpropamide
    Chlorothiazide, hydrochlorothiazide
    Gold salts
    Insecticides
    Sulfadiazine, sulfisoxazole, sulfamerazine, sulfamethazine,
      sulfamethoxypyrazinamide, sulfamethoxazole, sulfatolamide

and transfusion-associated graft-versus-host disease, which usually occurs in immunocompromised hosts who receive a blood component transfusion from donors sharing HLA antigens. Therefore, the effectiveness of platelet transfusion should always be assessed with a 1-hour post-transfusion platelet count. Patients with an abnormally low increment (10,000/L per unit of platelets) after transfusion of pooled platelets should be considered for transfusion of single-donor platelets. Those whose condition remains refractory should be evaluated for the cause. Prolonged or improper storage of platelets is an uncommon cause of poor platelet survival. Clinical conditions that can lead to poor platelet survival include fever, prior bone marrow transplantation, disseminated intravascular coagulation, concurrent infusion of amphotericin B, drug-induced platelet antibodies, autoantibodies, and HLA antibodies.[41]

HYPERLEUKOCYTOSIS

Hyperleukocytosis (extreme elevation in the white blood cell count) is usually defined by a peripheral white blood cell count > 100,000/L. Diseases that are associated with this disorder include CML (in the chronic, accelerated, and

blast crisis phases) acute myelogenous leukemia (AML), acute lymphocytic leukemia, and CLL (Table 16–6).

Hyperleukocytosis poses the greatest danger in patients with AML when the circulating white blood cells consist primarily of blast cells. In such cases, the risk of early death (within 7 days) is much higher (20% for patients with a white blood count > 100,000/L, as opposed to 5% for those with a white blood count < 100,000/L).[42] Typically, hyperleukocytosis is best tolerated by patients with CLL because the lymphocytes are usually small and deformable and do not stick or become lodged in the microvasculature (as do leukocytes in other leukemias).

Symptoms related to hyperleukocytosis include headache, dizziness, confusion, dyspnea, and hemoptysis. They are usually a result of increased blood viscosity, and the most pronounced changes are seen when there are large numbers of circulating myeloblasts and promyelocytes. For this reason, symptoms are more common in patients with AML or with CML in blast crisis than in patients with CML in chronic phase or with ALL, and symptoms are usually absent in patients with leukocytosis due to infection or a leukemoid reaction.[43]

Complications

Pulmonary Complications. Pulmonary congestion is a common complication of hyperleukocytosis and occurs in up to 35% of patients with AML who have an initial white blood cell count > 100,000/L.[44] Respiratory com-

TABLE 16–6. Associated Malignancies, Clinical Features, and Treatment of Hyperleukocytosis

Associated malignancies
  Acute myelogenous leukemia (poses the most danger)
  Chronic myelogenous leukemia: chronic, accelerated, and blast crisis
    phases
  Acute lymphocytic leukemia
  Chronic lymphocytic leukemia (best tolerated)

Clinical features
  Peripheral white blood cell count > 100,000/L
  Headache, dizziness, confusion, blurred vision, ataxia, stupor
  Dyspnea, hemoptysis
  Hypoxemia, hypotension
  Hyperkalemia, hypocalcemia, hyperuricemia, lactic acidosis
  Pulmonary congestion, capillary leak (ARDS), ventilation-perfusion
    mismatch
  CNS hemorrhage
  Acute renal failure

Treatment
  Supportive measures
  Chemotherapy
  Leukapheresis

ARDS = acute respiratory distress syndrome; CNS = central nervous system.

promise results from blockage of the pulmonary vasculature by leukostasis within the capillaries; diffuse capillary leakage and adult respiratory distress may follow.[45]

In some cases, hyperleukocytosis may mimic acute pulmonary embolism, with sludging in small vessels that causes ventilation-perfusion mismatches and significant hypoxemia while chest radiographs are normal.[46] Hyperleukocytosis may also result in the direct lowering of oxygen partial pressure (PO_2) by consumption of oxygen in blood samples obtained for analysis.[47]

Immediate management involves reducing the white blood cell count and increasing the inspired oxygen tension. Aggressive diuresis is not recommended because it can raise the white blood cell concentration and increase sludging in the pulmonary vasculature.

Central Nervous System Complications. The pathophysiology of leukostasis in the central nervous system is similar to that seen in the lungs (ie, leukostatic plugging of the capillaries, followed by endothelial damage and leakage involving small or large vessels). Signs and symptoms include blurred vision, dizziness, ataxia, stupor, coma, and hemorrhage.[45,48] Because a similar presentation can occur with meningeal leukemia, the evaluation of patients with neurologic signs and symptoms should include an imaging study of the brain, preferably magnetic resonance imaging with gadolinium contrast. Patients with evidence of leptomeningeal leukemia on magnetic resonance imaging of the brain should also have a lumbar puncture for cytologic examination of the cerebrospinal fluid, the results of which are usually negative in patients with central nervous system leukostasis. Intrathecal chemotherapy should be administered at the time of a diagnostic lumbar puncture.

Tumor Lysis Syndrome. Tumor lysis syndrome results from the rapid turnover of myeloid or lymphoid blast cells and is characterized by hyperkalemia, hypocalcemia, hyperuricemia, lactic acidosis, hypotension, and hypoxemia. Tumor lysis syndrome can exacerbate acute respiratory diseases and lead to the onset of urate nephropathy and acute renal failure. It can occur even before treatment of leukocytosis is initiated and can be exacerbated by the use of cytotoxic drugs.

Treatment

The treatment of hyperleukocytosis remains controversial, and two recent studies reported conflicting results regarding the efficacy of leukapheresis. One study of 48 patients with hyperleukocytosis and newly diagnosed AML or CML in blast crisis who were treated with leukapheresis demonstrated no correlation between the degree of leukoreduction and the early mortality rate.[49] However, a more recent study, of 53 patients with hyperleuko-

cytosis and newly diagnosed AML, showed that patients treated with therapeutic leukapheresis resulting in a 50% reduction in the initial white blood cell count had an early mortality rate that was much lower than the previously published rate (4% versus 30 to 50%).[50]

Based on these results, therapeutic leukapheresis is recommended in those patients who are most likely to benefit, including those with signs or symptoms of organ dysfunction (particularly neurologic or pulmonary), a white blood count $> 100 \times 10^9$/L, and a high percentage of blasts and promyelocytes (50 to 100×10^9/L). Under appropriate conditions, leukapheresis will rapidly reduce the white blood count to 30 to 60% below pretreatment levels, with a dramatic improvement in symptoms. However, the beneficial effect is usually brief, and repeated daily treatments are often necessary, so prompt treatment of the underlying leukemia with chemotherapy is also required.

The treatment of hyperleukocytosis must also include minimizing the adverse effects of the metabolic imbalances that accompany extreme leukocytosis and tumor lysis. Basic therapeutic measures include adequate hydration and the avoidance of unnecessary red blood cell transfusions that might further increase blood viscosity. Alkalinization of the urine and control of uric acid production with allopurinol may be required to minimize the effects of urate nephropathy. Severe cases may require hemodialysis.[43]

HYPERVISCOSITY SYNDROME

The malignant clones of the plasma cell disorders multiple myeloma and Waldenström's macroglobulinemia secrete monoclonal immunoglobulins (M proteins). High serum concentrations of these immunoglobulins can lead to hyperviscosity syndrome (HVS), as can an increase in the concentration of red blood cells, as in polycythemia vera. Hyperviscosity also occurs in patients with acute leukemia; however, it is less common in these patients because they often have severe anemia, which counteracts the effect of the hyperleukocytosis on whole-blood viscosity (Table 16–7).[51]

Hyperviscosity occurs in 8 to 40% of patients with Waldenström's macroglobulinemia.[52,53] It is much less common in patients with multiple myeloma and occurs in less than 5% of cases of that disorder. The syndrome is caused by the increased concentration of plasma immunoglobulins, which impedes capillary blood flow, leading to ischemia and organ dysfunction. Plasma volume is also expanded, which may result in congestive symptoms.

The dominant clinical features of HVS are bleeding, retinopathy, and neurologic signs and symptoms. Cardiac complications associated with hypervolemia and increased vascular resistance also occur but are less common. Bleed-

TABLE 16–7. Associated Malignancies, Clinical Features, and Treatment of Hyperviscosity Syndrome

Associated malignancies
   Waldenström's macroglobulinemia (8 to 40% of WM cases)
   Multiple myeloma (< 5% of MM cases)
   Acute leukemia (uncommon)
Clinical features
   Bleeding
      Oral and nasal mucous membranes
   Ocular symptoms
      Blurred vision, double vision, vision loss
      Retinal venous dilatation
      Retinal hemorrhage
      Central retinal vein occlusion
      Papilledema
   Neurologic symptoms
      Headache, pressure, light-headedness, unsteadiness, hearing loss
      Ataxia
      Seizures, chorea, dementia
Treatment
   Intravenous hydration and diuresis
   Plasma-exchange apheresis
   Phlebotomy (100–200 mL of whole blood)
   Chemotherapy

MM = multiple myeloma; WM = Waldenström's macroglobulinemia.

ing usually originates from the oral and nasal mucous membranes. Ocular manifestations of HVS include retinal venous dilatation, sometimes followed by retinal hemorrhage, central retinal vein occlusion, and papilledema. Early on, patients may be asymptomatic for ocular involvement but may subsequently develop blurred vision, diplopia, and loss of vision. Common neurologic symptoms include headache, pressure in the head, light-headedness, unsteadiness, and hearing loss. Neurologic signs are ataxia, seizures, chorea, and (rarely) dementia. Common cardiac manifestations of HVS include congestive heart failure, arrhythmias, and angina.[51,54]

The goal of the treatment of HVS is to lower plasma viscosity and thereby to improve capillary blood flow and organ function. Initial treatment consists of rehydration with intravenous fluids and diuresis.[54] Plasma-exchange apheresis rapidly reduces plasma viscosity by removing plasma containing M protein and replacing it with 5% albumin and normal saline. The symptoms of hyperviscosity are usually relieved after the first plasma-exchange treatment. The need for further treatment and the frequency of maintenance therapy depend on the response to treatment and the type of M protein causing the disease. In HVS caused by multiple myeloma (IgM protein), only one or two exchange procedures are required to return the plasma viscosity to near normal, but more procedures are necessary for HVS caused by IgG or IgA M proteins.[51,55] When plasmapheresis is not available, phlebotomy of 100 to 200 mL of blood may be performed to relieve symptoms in cases of acute severe

HVS.[55] Chemotherapy should also be initiated as soon as possible to reduce the production of M protein and to reduce the tumor burden.

REACTIVE AND PRIMARY THROMBOCYTOSIS

Reactive thrombocytosis can occur as a result of stress, iron deficiency anemia, acute blood loss, splenectomy, or any acute or chronic inflammatory process. It is rarely an emergency and does not always require treatment, even when the platelet count is > 1,000,000/L.

Primary thrombocytosis is usually associated with a myeloproliferative disorder. Patients frequently have severe symptoms and require emergent and aggressive treatment. Primary, or clonal, thrombocytosis can occur with any of the myeloproliferative disorders. It is commonly seen in cases of polycythemia vera, myelofibrosis, chronic myelogenous leukemia, and essential thrombocythemia. However, the symptoms and complications are usually seen only in patients with polycythemia vera and essential thrombocythemia (Table 16–8).[41]

The major causes of morbidity and mortality in patients with primary thrombocytosis are hemorrhage

TABLE 16–8. Associated Disorders, Clinical Features, and Treatment of Thrombocytosis

Associated malignancies/disorders
   Symptomatic
      Polycythemia vera
      Essential thrombocythemia
   Usually asymptomatic
      Myelofibrosis
      Chronic myelogenous leukemia
Clinical features
   Microvascular thrombosis
      Transient cerebral ischemia
      Migraine headache
      Visual disturbance
      Digital ischemia
      Erythromelalgia
   Macrovascular thrombosis
      Coronary artery occlusion syndrome
      Pulmonary embolism
   Bleeding
      Bruising
      Epistaxis
      Superficial gastrointestinal hemorrhage
Treatment
   Thrombosis with bleeding
      Plateletpheresis
   Thrombosis
      Plateletpheresis and aspirin,[*] 75–100 mg/d
      Anagrelide
      Hydroxyurea, busulfan, pipobroman, interferon–α

*Used with caution in patients with essential thrombocythemia.

and thrombosis. Thrombosis can involve large or small vessels and may occur in up to 15% of patients with essential thrombocythemia. Older patients (> 60 years of age) and those with a history of a prior thrombotic event are at increased risk for thrombosis. Involvement of the microvasculature is common and typically presents as transient cerebral ischemia, migraine and visual dysfunction, digital ischemia, or erythromelalgia (localized burning pain, redness, and warm congestion of the extremities). Larger peripheral and coronary artery occlusion syndromes, as well as deep venous thrombosis and pulmonary embolism, are not uncommon.[56,57]

Bleeding in association with thrombocytosis may occur spontaneously as a result of platelet-mediated occlusion (usually of the microvasculature, followed by ischemia and vascular leakage) or as a result of trauma. It typically presents as bruising, epistaxis, or superficial gastrointestinal hemorrhage. Major bleeding complications are less common than thrombosis and usually occur in patients with profound platelet function defects such as those seen with the chronic use of aspirin.[41,56]

The treatment of patients who have isolated and asymptomatic thrombocytosis can usually be safely postponed until the underlying etiology can be determined. Furthermore, asymptomatic patients with essential thrombocythemia who are at low risk for developing thrombosis (ie, those who are less than 60 years of age and who have no prior history of thrombosis) can be observed without treatment until they become symptomatic.[56]

Patients with primary thrombocytosis and acute serious bleeding should be treated by reducing the platelet count with plateletpheresis; those with thrombosis should be treated with plateletpheresis and aspirin (75 to 100 mg/d). In patients with essential thrombocythemia, aspirin should be used with caution since platelet function defects are not uncommon in this disorder.

Although effective, plateletpheresis provides only temporary control of the platelet count; therefore, symptomatic patients usually will also require treatment with anagrelide.[58,59] Hydroxyurea, busulfan, pipobroman, and interferon-α have also been shown to be efficacious in treating clonal thrombocytosis.[41,56]

DISSEMINATED INTRAVASCULAR COAGULATION

Disseminated intravascular coagulation (DIC) is a systemic thrombohemorrhagic disorder that is seen in association with several well-defined clinical disorders (Table 16–9). It is characterized by the widespread activation of coagulation which through the formation of fibrin results in thrombotic occlusion of small and mic-size vessels. Compromise in blood supply may lead to end-organ damage. Simultaneous consumption of platelets and coagulation factors may induce severe bleeding and further complicate decisions about treatment (Figure 16–1).[60]

DIC maybe acute or chronic among cancer patients, DIC is most often seen in association with widely disseminated metastatic solid tumors, acute leukemia, infection, and transfusion reactions.[61]

The chronic form of DIC often presents as a coagulation abnormality that can be detected only by laboratory tests. The malignancies most commonly associated with chronic or compensated DIC are adenocarcinomas of the gastrointestinal tract, lung, and breast. Although bleeding does occur, the chronic form of DIC is more often manifested clinically by thrombosis, which may be

TABLE 16–9. Oncologic and Related Conditions Associated with Disseminated Intravascular Coagulation

Obstetric accidents
    Amniotic-fluid embolism
    Abruptio placentae
    Retained-fetus syndrome
    Eclampsia
    Abortion
Intravascular hemolysis
    Hemolytic transfusion reactions
    Minor hemolysis
    Massive transfusion
Septicemia
    Gram-negative (endotoxin)
    Gram-positive (mucopolysaccharides)
Viremias
    HIV infection
    Hepatitis
    Varicella
    Cytomegalovirus infection
Metastatic malignancy
    Prostate
    Melanoma
    Lung
    Gallbladder
    Stomach
    Colon
    Breast
    Ovary
Leukemia
    Acute myelogenous leukemia
    Acute promyelocytic leukemia
Initiation of chemotherapy
Burns, crush injuries, trauma
Acute liver disease
    Obstructive jaundice
    Acute hepatic failure
Prosthetic devices
    LeVeen or Denver shunts
    Aortic balloon assist devices
Vascular disorders, autoimmune disease

Adapted from Bick RL.[68]

migratory (as in Trousseau's phenomenon) or which may involve unusual sites such as the upper extremities or such as the portal or hepatic veins.[38,60]

In acute DIC, the derangement of coagulation and fibrinolysis is mediated by proinflammatory cytokines. Interleukine-6 is considered the principal mediator of activation of coagulation. Tumor necrosis factor-α indirectly influences the activation of coagulation and mediates dysregulation of the anticoagulation pathway and fibrinolysis.[60]

Acute or uncompensated DIC is seen less often in patients with solid tumors but can complicate the course of acute leukemia in approximately 50% of patients. It is observed frequently during therapy for acute promyelocytic leukemia and in patients with severe sepsis. Among patients with solid tumors, acute DIC occurs most commonly in those with carcinoma of the prostate but also occurs in those with malignant melanoma and with carcinomas of the lung, gallbladder, stomach, colon, breast, and ovary. The initiation of chemotherapy has also been associated with the precipitation or acceleration of DIC.[37]

Diagnosis

The systemic signs and symptoms of DIC include fever, hypotension, proteinuria, and hypoxia. Petechiae, purpura, hemorrhagic bullae, acral cyanosis, wound bleeding, and oozing from venipuncture sites or intra-arterial lines are also common findings. The most common sites of bleeding are the skin, the lungs, and the gastrointestinal and genitourinary tracts.[37] The clinical manifestations of microvascular or even large-vessel thrombosis may be subtle and could be missed if not specifically sought. The most common vessels involved are those of the cardiac, pulmonary, renal, hepatic, and central nervous systems.

Many tests of varying degrees of usefullness have been developed for diagnosing DIC. Highly specific and sensitive tests that are considered useful but are not generally available include the measurement of soluble fibrin and assays that measure the generation of thrombin such as prothrombin activation fragment F(1 + 2) or thrombin/antithrombin complexes. In clinical practice, DIC can be diagnosed on the basis of the following findings: (a) an underlying disease known to be associated with DIC; (b) an initial platelet count of less than 100,000/L (or a rapid decline in platelet count); (c) prolongation of clotting times, such as the partial thromboplastin time; (d) the presence of fibrin degration products in plasma; (e) and low plasma levels of coagulation inhibitors, such as antithrombin III.[61]

Treatment

The appropriate therapy for DIC depends on the underlying clinical disorder, the site and severity of hemorrhage and thrombosis, and whether the condition is acute or chronic.

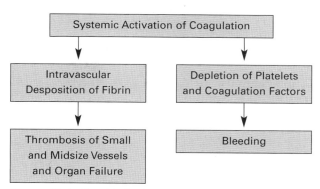

Figure 16–1. The Mechanism of Disseminated Intravascular Coagulation. Systemic activation of coagulation leads to widespread intravascular deposition of fibrin and depletion of platelets and coagulation factors. As a result, thrombosis of small and midsize vessels may occur, contributing to organ failure, and there may be severe bleeding.

Chronic Form. In general, the coagulopathy of chronic DIC is well compensated, and many patients remain asymptomatic. However, any stress, such as infection or surgery, may perturb the compensated state and cause bleeding. Therefore, treatment should be approached with caution. Patients with symptomatic thrombosis will probably require chronic heparin therapy since anticoagulation with warfarin is often inadequate.[38] Patients who are asymptomatic may be observed, and their treatment may be deferred until signs or symptoms of thrombosis or bleeding occur.[19]

Acute Form. The first step in the treatment of decompensated DIC is to determine and treat the probable precipitating cause. This includes administering antibiotics, correcting shock and acidosis in the setting of sepsis, and (when possible) treating the underlying malignancy. Heparin use remains controversial. In patients with acute promyelocytic leukemia, heparin has been shown to improve coagulation abnormalities (see below). There is no consensus on the use of heparin in patients with solid tumors. In patients with bleeding, many clinicians advocate starting low-dose heparin (5 to 10 U/kg/h) by continuous infusion. Platelets and plasma (up to 6 units per 24 hours) should also be administered in patients with severe bleeding or who require an invasive procedure. There is no evidence to support the prophylactic administration of platelets or plasma in patients who are not bleeding.

The goal of treatment of acute DIC is to achieve a platelet count of 50×10^9/L and a fibrinogen level of 125 to 150 mg/dL. These parameters should be measured every 4 to 6 hours, and if therapeutic levels cannot be achieved or if rapid decline occurs, the dose of heparin should be increased cautiously, in small increments.[38]

In recent trials, the administration of supraphysiologic concentrations of antithrombin III has been shown to be of benefit and therefore may also be considered a supportive therapeutic option.[61]

ACUTE PROMYELOCYTIC LEUKEMIA

Acute promyelocytic leukemia (APL) (French-American-British classifications M3) occurs in approximately 10% of adults with newly diagnosed leukemia. A bleeding diathesis, usually attributed to DIC, occurs in most patients and is often exacerbated by cytotoxic chemotherapy.

Early fatal hemorrhage occurs in 8 to 47% of patients.[62] Central nervous system bleeding, in particular, is more common in patients with APL than in those with other diseases associated with DIC.[63] The risk factors for early fatal hemorrhage include thrombocytopenia (platelet count < 30,000/L), elevated absolute blast and promyelocyte counts (≥ 1,000/L), age (≥ 50 years), anemia (Hgb < 11.0 gm/dL), and hypofibrinogenemia (< 150 mg/dL).[64,65]

Several processes (including accelerated intravascular coagulation, hyperfibrinolysis, and thrombocytopenia) are involved in the hemorrhagic diathesis that occurs in patients with APL. The intravascular clotting in these patients is caused by procoagulants associated with the malignant promyelocytes. In the subset of patients with systemic fibrinolysis, the malignant cells are also probably the source of fibrinolytic enzymes, including plasminogen activators and elastase. The depletion of homeostatic fibrinolytic inhibitors such as α-antiplasmin, plasminogen activator inhibitor, and C1 esterase inhibitor also probably contributes to the fibrinolytic process.[62]

The severity of DIC in patients with APL varies, depending partly on the hemostatic activity of the malignant cells and on the timing of cytoreductive therapy. Severity does not correlate with the peripheral blood promyelocyte cell counts. The prothrombin time is elevated in up to 90% of cases; although occasionally prolonged, the partial thromboplastin time is often normal and may even be shortened because of circulating clotting factors. The fibrinogen level is typically low, but since fibrinogen levels are frequently elevated in patients with untreated acute leukemia, a normal fibrinogen level in a patient with APL is compatible with the accelerated fibrinogen consumption due to DIC. The platelet count is also moderately or markedly reduced. Fibrin degradation products, as measured by assay of plasma D dimer, are usually moderately or markedly elevated and are an excellent marker for the activity of DIC. A stable or rising concentration of fibrin degradation products suggests persistent DIC; falling levels reflect a slowing of intravascular clotting. Other tests (outlined above) for detecting low levels of DIC include fibrinopeptide (FPA) assays and tests for thrombin/antithrombin complexes and prothrombin fragment F(1+2).[63]

Systemic fibrinolytic activity is seen in approximately 20% of patients with untreated APL. Plasma levels of α2 plasmin inhibitor are reduced in many patients with fibrinolysis, and this assay has been used to guide antifibrinolytic therapy.[63]

In the past, treatment of APL with an anthracycline and cytosine arabinoside was effective but often worsened the coagulopathy. Now, almost all patients are treated with all-trans retinoic acid, which has been shown to be highly effective and to induce remission in up to 94% of patients. Furthermore, the coagulopathy tends to improve rather than get worse when all-trans retinoic acid is administered. Unfortunately, improvement in DIC may take several days, and hemorrhagic deaths can still occur. In addition, reports of thrombotic complications are increasing.[66] Therefore, patients treated with all-trans retinoic acid require close observation.

Another complication of all-trans retinoic acid use is the retinoic acid syndrome seen in up to 25% of cases and characterized by fever, dyspnea, pleural and pericardial effusion, pulmonary infiltrates, peripheral edema, and transient myocardial infarction. This syndrome is usually seen in the first 2 weeks of treatment and may respond to dexamethasone.[63] Other adverse reactions, including headache, skin reactions, nausea and vomiting, and bone pain, are not uncommon.[67]

The treatment of DIC in the setting of APL is the same as for DIC in other conditions. As outlined above, it includes intravenous heparin and the replacement of clotting factors with cryoprecipitate, fresh frozen plasma, and platelets. Low-molecular-weight heparin (specifically enoxaparin, 40 mg subcutaneously every 12 hours) has also been shown to be a feasible alternative to heparin in patients with APL. Antifibrinolytic agents such as α-aminocaproic acid or tranexamic acid should only be used for patients who exhibit clear evidence of systemic fibrinolysis (eg, shortened whole-blood or euglobulin clot lysis time or α2-plasmin inhibitor levels < 40% of normal) and in conjunction with heparin if DIC is present.[63]

REFERENCES

1. Huh YO, Lichtiger B. Transfusion reactions in patients with cancer. Am J Clin Pathol 1987;87:253–7.
2. Heddle NM. Febrile nonhemolytic transfusion reactions to platelets. Curr Opin Hematol 1995;2:478–83.
3. Dodd RY. Adverse consequences of blood transfusion: quantitative risk estimates. In: Nance ST, editor. Blood supply: risks, perceptions and prospects for the future. Bethesda: American Association of Blood Banks; 1994.
4. Heddle NM, Klama LN, Griffith L, et al. A prospective study to identify the risk factors associated with acute reactions to platelet and red cell transfusions. Transfusion 1993;33:794–7.
5. Muylle L, Joos M, Wouters E, et al. Increased tumor

necrosis factor alpha (TNF alpha), interleukin 1, and interleukin 6 (IL-6) levels in the plasma of stored platelet concentrates: relationship between TNF alpha and IL-6 levels and febrile transfusion reactions. Transfusion 1993;33:195–9.

6. Heddle NM, Klama L, Singer J, et al. The role of the plasma from platelet concentrates in transfusion reactions. N Engl J Med 1994;331:625–8.

7. Chambers LA, Kruskall MS, Pacini DG, Donovan LM. Febrile reactions after platelet transfusion: the effect of single versus multiple donors. Transfusion 1990;30:219–21.

8. Heddle NM, Klama L, Meyer R, et al. A randomized controlled trial comparing plasma removal with white cell reduction to prevent reactions to platelets. Transfusion 1999;39:231–8.

9. Walker RH. Special report: transfusion risks. Am J Clin Pathol 1987;88:374–8.

10. Popovsky MA, Chaplin HC Jr, Moore SB. Transfusion-related acute lung injury: a neglected, serious complication of hemotherapy. Transfusion 1992;32:589–92.

11. Braine HG, Kickler TS, Charache P, et al. Bacterial sepsis secondary to platelet transfusion: an adverse effect of extended storage at room temperature. Transfusion 1986;26:391–3.

12. Goldman M, Blajchman MA. Blood product-associated bacterial sepsis. Transfusion Med Rev 1991;5:73–83.

13. Aber RC. Transfusion-associated *Yersinia enterocolitica*. Transfusion 1990;30:193–5.

14. Tipple MA, Bland LA, Murphy JJ, et al. Sepsis associated with transfusion of red cells contaminated with *Yersinia enterocolitica*. Transfusion 1990;30:207–13.

15. Alvarez FE, Rogge KJ, Tarrand J, Lichtiger B. Bacterial contamination of cellular blood components. A retrospective review at a large cancer center. Ann Clin Lab Sci 1995;25:283–90.

16. Coiffier B. The impact and management of anaemia in hematological malignancies. Med Oncol 2000;17:S2–10.

17. Spivak JL. The blood in systemic disorders. Lancet 2000;355:1707–12.

18. Henry DH. Recombinant human erythropoietin treatment of anemic cancer patients. Cancer Pract 1996;4:180–4.

19. Dutcher JP. Hematologic abnormalities in patients with nonhematologic malignancies. Hematol Oncol Clin North Am 1987;1:281–99.

20. Hofmann WK, Ottmann OG, Ganser A, Hoelzer D. Myelodysplastic syndromes: clinical features. Semin Hematol 1996;33:177–85.

21. Estey EH, Keating MJ, Dixon DO, et al. Karyotype is prognostically more important than the FAB system's distinction between myelodysplastic syndrome and acute myelogenous leukemia. Hematol Pathol 1987;1:203–8.

22. Henry DH. The management of cancer anemia. Support Care Cancer 1994;2:403–4.

23. Rytting M, Worth L, Jaffe N. Hemolytic disorders associated with cancer. Hematol Oncol Clin North Am 1996;10:365–76.

24. Robak T, Blasinska-Morawiec M, Krykowski E, et al. Autoimmune haemolytic anaemia in patients with chronic lymphocytic leukaemia treated with 2-chlorodeoxyadenosine (cladribine). Eur J Haematol 1997;58:109–13.

25. Pujol M, Fernandez F, Sancho JM, et al. Immune hemolytic anemia induced by 6-mercaptopurine. Transfusion 2000;40:75–6.

26. Marani TM, Trich MB, Armstrong KS, et al. Carboplatin-induced immune hemolytic anemia. Transfusion 1996;36:1016–8.

27. Spira MA, Lynch EC. Autoimmune hemolytic anemia and carcinoma: an unusual association. Am J Med 1979;67:753–8.

28. Gonzalez H, Leblond V, Azar N, et al. Severe autoimmune hemolytic anemia in eight patients treated with fludarabine. Hematol Cell Ther 1998;40:113–8.

29. Hashimoto C. Autoimmune hemolytic anemia. Clin Rev Allergy Immunol 1998;16:285–95.

30. Lohrmann HP, Adam W, Heymer B, Kubanek B. Micro-angiopathic hemolytic anemia in metastatic carcinoma. Report of eight cases. Ann Intern Med 1973;79:368–75.

31. Lesesne JB, Rothschild N, Erickson B, et al. Cancer-associated hemolytic-uremic syndrome: analysis of 85 cases from a national registry. J Clin Oncol 1989;7:781–9.

32. van der Heijden M, Ackland SP, Deveridge S. Haemolytic uraemic syndrome associated with bleomycin, epirubicin and cisplatin chemotherapy—a case report and review of the literature. Acta Oncol 1998;37:107–9.

33. Brodowicz T, Breiteneder S, Wiltschke C, Zielinski CC. Gemcitabine-induced hemolytic uremic syndrome: a case report. J Nat Cancer Inst 1997;89:1895–6.

34. Nackaerts K, Daenen M, Vansteenkiste J, et al. Hemolytic-uremic syndrome caused by gemcitabine. Ann Oncol 1998;9:1355.

35. Bell WR, Braine HG, Ness PM, Kickler TS. Improved survival in thrombotic thrombocytopenic purpura-hemolytic uremic syndrome. Clinical experience in 108 patients. New Engl J Med 1991;325:398–403.

36. Rock GA, Shumak KH, Buskard NA, et al. Comparison of plasma exchange with plasma infusion in the treatment of thrombotic thrombocytopenic purpura. Canadian Apheresis Study Group. New Engl J Med 1991;325:393–7.

37. Bick RL, Strauss JF, Frenkel EP. Thrombosis and hemorrhage in oncology patients. Hematol Oncol Clin North Am 1996;10:875–907.

38. Rosen PJ. Bleeding problems in the cancer patient. Hematol Oncol Clin North Am 1992;6:1315–28.

39. Beutler E. Platelet transfusions: the 20,000/microL trigger. Blood 1993;81:1411–3.

40. Bick RL. Coagulation abnormalities in malignancy: a review. Semin Thromb Hemost 1992;18:353–72.

41. Gerson SL, Lazarus HM. Hematopoietic emergencies. Semin Oncol 1989;16:532–42.

42. Dutcher JP, Schiffer CA, Wiernik PH. Hyperleukocytosis in adult acute nonlymphocytic leukemia: impact on remission rate and duration, and survival. J Clin Oncol 1987;5:1364–72.

43. Grima KM. Therapeutic apheresis in hematological and oncological diseases. J Clin Apheresis 2000;15:28–52.

44. Lester TJ, Johnson JW, Cuttner J. Pulmonary leukostasis as the single worst prognostic factor in patients with acute myelocytic leukemia and hyperleukocytosis. Am J Med 1985;79:43–8.

45. Vernant JP, Brun B, Mannoni P, Dreyfus B. Respiratory distress of hyperleukocytic granulocytic leukemias. Cancer 1979;44:264–8.

46. Kaminsky DA, Hurwitz CG, Olmstead JI. Pulmonary leukostasis mimicking pulmonary embolism. Leukemia Res 2000;24:175–8.

47. Fox MJ, Brody JS, Weintraub LR. Leukocyte larceny: a cause of spurious hypoxemia. Am J Med 1979;67:742–6.

48. McKee LC, Collins RD. Intravascular leukocyte thrombi and aggregates as a cause of morbidity and mortality in leukemia. Medicine 1974;53:463–78.

49. Porcu P, Danielson CF, Orazi A, et al. Therapeutic leuka-pheresis in hyperleucocytic leukaemias: lack of correlation between degree of cytoreduction and early mortality rate. Br J Haematol 1997;98:433–6.

50. Thiebaut A, Thomas X, Belhabri A, et al. Impact of pre-induction therapy leukapheresis on treatment outcome in adult acute myelogenous leukemia presenting with hyperleukocytosis. Ann Hematol 2000;79:501–6.

51. Gertz MA, Kyle RA. Hyperviscosity syndrome. J Intensive Care Med 1995;10:128–41.

52. Facon T, Brouillard M, Duhamel A, et al. Prognostic factors in Waldenstrom's macroglobulinemia: a report of 167 cases. J Clin Oncol 1993;11:1553–8.

53. Case DC, Ervin TJ, Boyd MA, Redfield DL. Waldenstrom's macroglobulinemia: long-term results with the M-2 protocol. Cancer Invest 1991;9:1–7.

54. Pimentel L. Medical complications of oncologic disease. Emerg Med Clin North Am 1993;11:407–19.

55. Geraci JM, Hansen RM, Kueck BD. Plasma cell leukemia and hyperviscosity syndrome. South Med J 1990;83:800–5.

56. Barbui T, Finazzi G. Management of essential thrombo-cythemia. Crit Rev Oncol Hematol 1999;29:257–66.

57. Chistolini A, Mazzucconi MG, Ferrari A, et al. Essential thrombocythemia: a retrospective study on the clinical course of 100 patients. Haematologica 1990;75:537–40.

58. Pescatore SL, Lindley C. Anagrelide: a novel agent for the treatment of myeloproliferative disorders. Expert Opin Pharmacother 2000;3:537–46.

59. Gilbert HS. Diagnosis and treatment of thrombocythemia in myeloproliferative disorders. Oncology (Huntingt) 2001;8:989–1008.

60. Gregory SA, McKenna R, Sassetti RJ, Knospe WH. Hematologic emergencies. Med Clin North Am 1986;70:1129–49.

61. Bick RL. Disseminated intravascular coagulation. Objective criteria for diagnosis and management. Med Clin North Am 1994;78:511–43.

62. Warrell RP, de The H, Wang ZY, Degos L. Acute promyelocytic leukemia. New Engl J Med 1993;329:177–89.

63. DeLoughery TG, Goodnight SH. Acute promyelocytic leukaemia in the all trans retinoic acid era. Med Oncol 1996;13:233–40.

64. Kantarjian HM, Keating MJ, Walters RS, et al. Acute promyelocytic leukemia. M.D. Anderson Hospital experience. Am J Med 1986;80:789–97.

65. Cunningham I, Gee TS, Reich LM, et al. Acute promyelo-cytic leukemia: treatment results during a decade at Memorial Hospital. Blood 1989;73:1116–22.

66. Escudier SM, Kantarjian HM, Estey EH. Thrombosis in patients with acute promyelocytic leukemia treated with and without all-trans retinoic acid. Leuk Lymphoma 1996;20:435–9.

67. Frankel SR, Eardley A, Heller G, et al. All-trans retinoic acid for acute promyelocytic leukemia. Results of the New York Study. Ann Intern Med 1994;120:278–86.

68. Levi M, Ten Cate H. Current concepts: disseminated intravascular coagulation. NEJM 1999;341:586–92.

CHAPTER 17

CANCER PAIN EMERGENCIES

NICOLE D. SWITZER, MD
ARUN RAJAGOPAL, MD

Unlike other emergencies that are described in relation to specific organ systems (eg, neurologic emergencies, cardiac emergencies, hematologic emergencies, etc), the term "pain emergency" refers only to an acute exacerbation of a symptom that may pose significant distress or problems for the patient if left untreated. The exacerbation of pain that necessitates a trip to the emergency department poses special problems for the clinician. The reasons for the sudden increase in pain are diverse and need to be ascertained before the problem can be properly addressed. Often, the pain is a pre-existing symptom that has simply worsened due to chronic undertreatment. However, the development of a sudden and unexplained pain can be a warning of an impending medical catastrophe needing immediate attention. In this chapter, the emphasis is on the approach to the patient with a pain emergency in the emergency department. Certain specific pain syndromes are also discussed, as well as related topics such as pseudoaddiction syndrome, depression and anxiety, intractable pain, and opioid withdrawal.

INITIAL ENCOUNTER

Assessment

The experience of pain includes nociception (pain from actual tissue damage), perception, and expression. Since nociception and perception cannot be measured directly, expression of pain is the main target of assessment and treatment. Pain is a multidimensional experience affected by physical, psychological, spiritual, and cultural factors, and the expression of pain varies tremendously from patient to patient. The assessment of the patient with a pain emergency begins with a series of questions to elucidate the nature of the pain (Table 17–1).[1] It is important to qualify the pain as well as possible since the treatment for one type of pain may not be appropriate for another. Obviously, if the patient is in too much distress to answer questions, one or two breakthrough doses of opioid may be needed to control the pain quickly. The need for a proper assessment must be balanced with the

need to render the patient comfortable enough to tolerate the history and physical examination.

Hill has described a "morphine test," a simple method for attaining rapid pain relief in the cancer patient.[2] Before the assessment, the patient presenting with uncontrolled pain is administered intravenous boluses of morphine sulfate, initially in 5- to 15-mg boluses, followed every 15 minutes by repeat doses until either satisfactory analgesia is achieved or unacceptable side effects

TABLE 17–1. Multidimensional Pain Assessment

General[*]
- Where does it hurt? (location and radiation, more than one location?)
- Onset and time course of pain?
- How much does it hurt? (Use a visual analog scale of 1 to 10.)
- Factors that exacerbate or relieve pain?
- Current and past pain medication regimen?
- Other treatments in the past for pain relief?
- Are the treatments/medications effective?

Psychological[†]
- Is the patient cognitively impaired or delirious? (Use the Mini–Mental State Questionnaire.)
- Is the patient experiencing major psychological distress? (Look for somatization, the expression of suffering as physical pain.)
- How has the patient coped with stress in the past?
- Is there a history of alcohol or drug addiction? (Use the CAGE questionnaire as a screening tool.)[††]

Social [†]
- How does the pain influence the patient's daily living?
- How effective is the patient's social support network?
- Are there financial stressors?

Cultural[†]
- What are the cultural traditions, customs, beliefs, and values that influence the patient's expression of pain?

Spiritual[†]
- What is the meaning of pain to this patient?
- Are there any other spiritual issues affecting the patient?

CAGE = **C**utdown on drinking, being **A**nnoyed at criticisms about drinking, feeling **G**uilty about drinking, using alcohol as an **E**ye-opener.
*These questions are required.
†These questions may be optional, depending on the situation.
††Bruera E, Moyano J, Seifert L, et al. The frequency of alcholism among patients with pain due to terminal cancer. J Pain Symptom Manage 1995;10:599–603.

develop. The relatively recent introduction of oral transmucosal fentanyl may provide an acceptable noninvasive alternative to intravenous morphine.

Physical Examination

A thorough physical examination including a complete neurologic examination complements the history. Certain pain emergencies present with definite physical findings, and the examination can facilitate making the correct diagnosis and deciding what diagnostic tests need to be ordered. The importance of a complete neurologic examination cannot be overstated. Several potentially catastrophic medical conditions present only with nonspecific pain and subtle neurologic findings. Specific correlations between physical examination findings and diagnoses are outlined later in the chapter.

Psychological Evaluation, Psychosocial Assessment, and Diagnostic Studies

Although a psychological evaluation and a psychosocial assessment are extremely important in managing pain, the diagnoses of somatization, anxiety, depression, or other forms of psychological distress are diagnoses of exclusion in the emergency department. Occasionally, patients may develop a sudden anxiety attack, worsening depression, an episode of fear about their illness, or other psychological stressors that can manifest as an acute increase in pain. The clinician should still follow the same general strategy of trying to identify the more common causes of increased pain (recurrence, opioid tolerance, delirium, infection, etc) before considering psychological distress. If no identifiable cause can be found and if the clinician suspects that the increased pain is a manifestation of psychological distress, the clinician should carefully ask the patient if there are suicidal plans or ideation. A consultation with the psychiatry service in the emergency department may also be helpful, especially if the patient has ideas of harming him- or herself.

Diagnostic studies should be ordered based on the information obtained in the history and physical examination. (Relevant diagnostic studies are detailed later in this chapter under each diagnosis heading.)

Treatment Plan

Once the assessment is complete, a pain management plan should be outlined with the patient. The patient may need outpatient follow-up with a specialty service, or a referral to hospice may be indicated. If the patient is to follow up with the pain service, a consultation in the emergency department may be needed to outline interventional options (if any). If the patient needs a multidisciplinary assessment for palliative care issues, consultation with the palliative service may be needed. Consultation with the psychiatry service may alleviate symptoms of anxiety and depression. Overall, the goal of outlining the treatment plan with the patient is to set reasonable expectations for the treatment to be initiated.

PHARMACOLOGIC EVALUATION

When a patient presents to the emergency department complaining of increasing pain, the clinician must keep in mind the distinction between a true increase in nociception and the development of tolerance. The development of tolerance is a natural consequence of being on opioids for a prolonged period of time, and the patient may now simply be undertreated. The pharmacologic evaluation allows the clinician to assess the patient's opioid and adjuvant medications.

Morphine Equivalent Daily Dose

The pharmacologic evaluation begins with the calculation of the morphine equivalent daily dose (MEDD). If a patient has been on several different opioids over time, it may be difficult to ascertain a trend in the patient's consumption of opioids from which to determine whether the overall dosage is increasing or decreasing. Standardizing the patient's opioid dose to the MEDD allows the clinician to compare one opioid to another, allows the clinician to follow a trend in the patient's consumption of opioid during opioid rotations and changes in the route of administration, and facilitates rotation to a different opioid if needed. Using the conversion table shown in Table 17–2, the patient's current opioid dose is converted to the equivalent daily dose of oral morphine. Dose adjustments or rotations are made to the MEDD, and the MEDD is then converted back to the desired opioid.

An example of how to calculate and use the MEDD is as follows: A 35-year-old man complaining of pain presents to the emergency department. When he increases his opioid intake, he experiences severe side effects, but he cannot decrease his dosage because of significant breakthrough pain. His current regimen is sustained-release morphine, 200 mg orally twice daily, with immediate-release morphine, 2 to 3 15-mg tablets every 3 hours. The patient states that he takes 20 tablets of immediate-release morphine per day.

Since the patient cannot decrease his dosage because of pain and cannot increase his dosage because of intolerable side effects, you decide that an opioid rotation is the best recourse (see next section). You decide to rotate the patient's opioid medication to oxycodone.

To calculate the optimal dosage, start by calculating the patient's MEDD:

$$(200 \text{ mg} \times 2 \text{ tablets}) + (15 \text{ mg} \times 20 \text{ tablets}) = 700$$

TABLE 17–2. Opioid Conversion Table

Opioid	Parenteral Opioid to Parenteral Morphine	Parenteral Opioid to Same Oral Opioid	Oral Opioid to Oral Morphine	Oral Morphine to Oral Opioid
Morphine	1	2.5	1	1
Hydromorphone (Dilaudid)	5	2	5	0.2
Meperidine (Demerol)	0.13	4	0.1	10
Levorphanol	5	2	5	0.2
Codeine	N/A	N/A	0.15	7
Oxycodone	N/A	N/A	1.5	0.7
Hydrocodone	N/A	N/A	0.15	7

N/A = not applicable.

Convert the oral morphine dose into oxycodone (refer to the opioid conversion table):

$$700 \times 0.7 = 490$$

To avoid partial cross-tolerance to the new opioid, give 30% less initially:

$$490 \times 0.7 = 343$$

Thus, approximately 340 mg of oxycodone represents the daily dose of opioid that is equivalent to this patient's oral morphine dose. Deciding the rationale for dividing this dosage into sustained-release and immediate-release tablets depends largely on patient compliance and convenience. A reasonable division between sustained-release and immediate-release tablets is about 70:30, so this patient should receive approximately 240 mg of sustained-release oxycodone (eg, 80 mg orally three times daily) and 100 mg of immediate-release oxycodone (eg, 3 to 4 5-mg tablets every 4 to 6 hours) daily.

Rationale for Opioid Rotation

Some patients who are on chronic opioid therapy develop intolerable side effects such as myoclonus, delirium, nausea, emesis, or sedation, before satisfactory analgesia is achieved. Some of these side effects may be managed by the concurrent administration of other medications (antiemetics, psychostimulants, etc). However, when these attempts to control side effects fail, an opioid rotation may be warranted.

Opioid rotation is based on the premise that different opioids have different side effects for a variety of reasons[3] such as differences in receptor activity, differences in cross-tolerances between opioids, different intrinsic efficacies, and different metabolites. With rotation to a different opioid, better analgesia may be achieved with relatively fewer side effects. The choice of which opioid to rotate to is empirical and depends on the clinical situation. In general, a patient on a strong opioid should be rotated to another strong opioid.

Breakthrough Pain

Breakthrough pain is defined as a "transitory exacerbation of pain that occurs on a background of otherwise stable persistent pain."[4] Breakthrough pain may be caused by somatic, visceral, or neuropathic nociceptive input and is most often in the same area as the baseline pain. The episodes are severe and paroxysmal and may last from a few minutes to a few hours. Breakthrough pain may be related to movement (incident pain), occur without provocation (spontaneous pain), or occur toward the end of a dosing interval (end-of-dose failure). Treatment is largely by supplemental opioid medication although if breakthrough pain is caused by neoplastic progression, antineoplastic therapy should also be considered.[5]

SPECIFIC EMERGENCIES AND PAIN SYNDROMES

Spinal-Cord Compression

Metastatic disease to the bony skeleton involves the vertebral column more than any other part of the body. Metastases to the pedicles or laminae can enlarge and lead to cord injury by direct compression of the dura. The most common cancers that metastasize to the vertebrae are lung, breast, prostate, and renal cancers. Additionally, tumor extension through the intervertebral foramina can also lead to cord compression; multiple myeloma and certain lymphomas are usually the culprits in these cases.

Presentation and Assessment. The initial presenting symptom in greater than 90% of patients with spinal-cord compression is pain. Usually, the pain begins as an area of tenderness over the affected vertebra. This is most common in the thoracic spine (70% of cases), followed by the lumbar spine (20%) and cervical spine (10%).[6] The pain may have a gradual course with slight progression and may be worse when the patient is lying supine. The pain may follow either a unilateral or bilateral radicular distribution. The development of other neurologic signs and symptoms such as numbness, tingling, weakness, loss of anal sphincter tone, and/or urinary retention usually occurs later in the course of cord compression although any of these may present by themselves.

TABLE 17–3. Physical Examination Findings Suggestive of Spinal-Cord Compression

Tenderness to vertebral palpation or percussion
Numbness or paresthesias in a radicular distribution
Muscle weakness or spasticity
Diminished or absent anal "wink" reflex
Postvoid bladder residual volume > 150 mL

The clinician may find that the physical examination is completely normal, even in a patient with risk factors for cord compression such as known cancer with new-onset back pain. Despite the normal examination, a high index of suspicion should be maintained in regard to such patients. Physical findings that are suggestive of cord compression are outlined in Table 17–3.

Treatment. Obviously, the goal of treatment in the emergency department is to prevent further neurologic compromise. In general, patients can be quickly stratified on the basis of the history and the neurologic examination (Figure 17–1).[7] If the examination is normal, plain-film radiography of the spine should be ordered in the emergency department, with symptomatic management if the films are normal. However, even if the plain radiographs are normal, an outpatient magnetic resonance imaging (MRI) scan should be done on a semiemergent basis.

If the films or neurologic examination are abnormal, steroid therapy should be initiated immediately and MRI of the spine should be ordered. Although there is no specific upper limit to steroid therapy, dexamethasone, 10 to 100 mg via the intravenous or oral route, may generally be needed initially. Depending on the results of the MRI, further consultation may be needed. If MRI shows epidural metastases, immediate radiation therapy and high-dose intravenous steroids are usually the initial treatments of choice. Neurosurgical consultation may also be considered, especially if the neurologic picture is rapidly evolving, if a pathologic fracture is evident, if the etiology of the metastasis is unknown, or if the type of tumor is known to be radioresistant.

Headache

Presentation and Causes. Since headaches are one of the most common complaints patients bring to physicians, the emergency-department clinician must be able to quickly differentiate among literally hundreds of causes for head and facial pain and decide whether the presenting complaint is indeed an emergency. In general, headaches can be classified into two groups: chronic headaches (migraines, cluster headaches, tension-type headaches, and cranial neuralgias) and acute headaches (those caused by exacerbation of chronic headache, raised intracranial pressure, intracranial hemorrhage, infection, trauma, or withdrawal). Of all causes of headaches, the two that require the most immediate attention, especially in the cancer pain setting, are raised intracranial pressure (whether from a mass, hemorrhage, or thrombosis[8]) and infection. (A complete discussion of infectious causes of headaches is beyond the scope of this chapter, but those causes that relate to cancer are discussed in the next section.)

About 25% of cancer patients have intracranial metastases, and the three most common cancers that metastasize to the brain are lung cancer, breast cancer, and melanoma. The gradual increase in the size and number of metastases can cause progressive symptoms of headache, nausea, vomiting, altered cognition, seizures, and focal neurologic symptoms. The sudden development of a severe headache is usually due to a hemorrhagic event in a metastasis. Severely thrombocytopenic patients are also at risk for developing intracranial hemorrhage, either spontaneously or with minimal trauma. Findings consistent with this picture include neck stiffness, visual changes, altered mentation, and papilledema; however, a patient may present with a severe headache in the absence of any of these.

A patient may present to the emergency department with a history of a headache that has been gradually worsening over weeks to months. In addition to intracranial malignancies, many extracranial head and neck malignancies can also present with headaches (eg, sinus tumors;[9] carcinomas of the head and/or neck, with cranial nerve involvement;[10] bone metastases).

Treatment. Once the cause (or suspected cause) of the headache has been determined, treatment depends on the severity of the diagnosis.

In the case of acute intracranial hemorrhage, although a computed tomography (CT) scan is desirable in order to establish the diagnosis, stabilization of the patient's "ABCs" (airway, breathing, and circulation) is vital before the patient is transported to the radiology department. If signs and symptoms of raised intracranial pressure and impending brain herniation are evident (eg, drowsiness, papilledema, severe headache, or pupillary dilation) the patient's airway should be protected by intubation if necessary, and infusions of mannitol (1 to 1.5 g/kg) should be started. (Although it has been generally accepted that hyperventilation of intubated patients improves neurologic outcome, it should be noted that there have been recent reports suggesting *adverse* outcomes when hyperventilation is instituted.)[11,12] An initial intravenous dose of dexamethasone (10 to 100 mg) should also be given. Neurosurgical consultation should be sought immediately to explore surgical options to relieve intracranial pressure.

For the patient presenting with a gradually worsening headache over several weeks to months, if the clinician is satisfied that there are no signs or symptoms of raised intracranial pressure and no new neurologic deficits, MRI or CT of the head may be ordered as an outpatient procedure as soon as possible, with follow-up. Pharmacologic therapy may be deferred until the imaging study is completed. If the clinician is satisfied that there are no cancer-related causes of the headache (eg, intracranial tumor, hemorrhage, leptomeningeal disease), chronic headaches of "benign" origin may be managed conservatively. Discussion of these headaches (ie, tension headaches, migraines, cluster headaches, etc) is beyond the scope of this chapter.

Epidural Abscess

Features and Causes. The epidural space is the potential space located just outside or above the dura. It may be bordered superficially by the ligamentum flavum in the spinal column or by the calvarium in the skull. An infection in this space presents with a triad of increasing pain, fever, and neurologic signs. The history of pain may be of gradual onset (over several months), or it may be acute (over just a few days). Fever is common although the absence of fever does not rule out an epidural abscess. The white blood cell count and sedimentation rate may also be elevated. Initially, pain (headache or back pain) and fever may be the only signs, but as the abscess enlarges, venous congestion along the spinal cord can lead to injury and the development of focal neurologic signs. The most common organism found in epidural abscesses is *Staphylococcus aureus* although *Streptococcus*, anaerobes, fungi, and Gram-negative bacilli have also been implicated.[13]

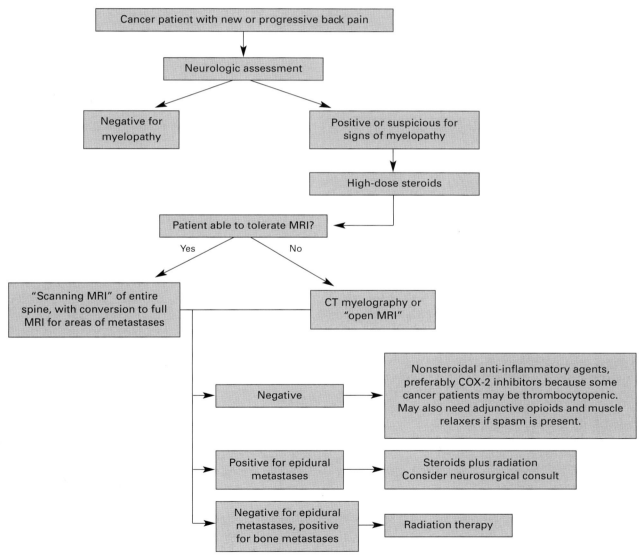

Figure 17–1. Algorithm for treatment of a cancer patient with new or progressive back pain. COX-2 = cyclooxygenase-2; CT = computed tomography; MRI = magnetic resonance imaging.

Risk factors for the development of an epidural abscess include immunocompromised status, intravenous drug abuse, and concurrent infections. In the cancer setting, the presence of a malignancy and/or treatment with chemotherapy can render patients immunocompromised. Although the majority of epidural abscesses occur via hematogenous spread, iatrogenic causes must also be considered, especially in the cancer setting, where the blood-brain barrier is often violated during treatment (eg, by intrathecal chemotherapy, lumbar puncture, epidural catheterization for pain control,[14,15] spinal anesthesia, spinal surgery, or placement of ventriculoperitoneal shunts).

Treatment. Treatment of an epidural abscess is a true surgical emergency; thus, the following should be kept in mind when treating this condition:

1. The presence of fever, pain and neurologic signs necessitates CT or preferably MRI, along with neurosurgical consultation.
2. Blood cultures should be obtained, and appropriate antibiotics should be started empirically in the emergency department.
3. In the presence of fixed neurologic deficits, surgery is unlikely to improve neurologic outcome although it may still be necessary to drain and débride the abscess to effectively treat the infection, in addition to starting antibiotic therapy.
4. In the presence of evolving neurologic deficits, an emergency decompressive laminotomy may improve or completely reverse paralysis.

Bone Pain and Pathologic Fracture

Mechanism and Presentation. Some types of cancer commonly metastasize to the bony skeleton (eg, melanoma and lung, breast, and prostate cancers.) Nociception in bone pain is thought to be due to the tumor invasion resulting in invasion or stretching of the periosteum and the sensitization of nerves in bony tissue by the production of autocoids during osteoclastic activity.[16]

Not only does the presence of disease in the bone cause pain, the integrity of the bones can be compromised by the presence of metastatic disease or prior radiation. In these weakened areas, the sudden development of severe localized pain should alert the clinician to the possibility of a pathologic fracture. The patient usually presents to the emergency department with a complaint of sudden-onset pain that may or may not have been preceded by a fall or some trauma. Plain radiography can usually confirm the diagnosis.

Treatment. Treatment in the emergency department involves the following:

1. For bone pain, opioid therapy should be initiated, and the radiation oncology service should be consulted for consideration of palliative radiotherapy. Steroids may also be indicated for relief of bone pain.[17]
2. Pathologic fractures should be immobilized with a noncircumferential splint. Analgesic medication should be administered, after which an orthopedic consultation may be requested.
3. If movement-related pain (incident pain) is very severe, consultation with the pain management service may be indicated for epidural analgesia or other interventional procedures (eg, intercostal nerve blocks for rib fractures).
4. The patient may benefit from (1) nonsteroidal anti-inflammatory drugs (NSAIDs) (intravenous [15 to 30 mg] or intramuscular [30 to 60 mg] ketorolac; celecoxib [100 to 200 mg]) given in the emergency department and (2) initiation of bisphosphonate therapy. Although most of the current literature supports the use of bisphosphonates, mainly for breast cancer with bone metastases,[18,19] it is also used in patients with myeloma and prostate cancer. There are reports suggesting a therapeutic benefit for other malignancies as well.[20]
5. Consultation with the neurosurgical service may be indicated for pathologic vertebral compression fractures that result in severe incident pain.

Abdominal Pain

Underlying Causes in the Cancer Patient. The cancer patient who presents with abdominal pain to the emergency department poses a unique challenge to the clinician because of the wide spectrum of cancer-related diagnoses that can cause pain in the abdomen (Table 17–4). (A complete discussion on managing abdominal emergencies is found in Chapter 9). It is, however, incumbent on the emergency room physician, when first evaluating a cancer patient with abdominal pain, to rule out an acute emergent problem first. The clinician should maintain a low threshold for considering acute processes such as intra-abdominal infections, bowel obstruction or perforation, or hemorrhage. A complete blood count with differential; liver function tests; assays of bilirubin, electrolytes, creatinine, and blood urea nitrogen; urinalysis; and cultures are indicated, as are imaging studies (an acute abdominal series, with upright chest radiography to rule out free air). More-detailed imaging such as CT or ultrasonography may also be necessary to clarify the diagnosis. Until the clinician is fairly sure that the patient does not have an acute problem that requires surgical intervention, opioids should be used judiciously prior to establishing a diagnosis.

Other common causes of abdominal pain that frequently bring the patient to the emergency department are the following:

TABLE 17–4. Cancer-Related Causes of Abdominal Pain

Pancreatic cancer
Gastric cancer
Lymphoma/retroperitoneal mass
Constipation
Hepatic cancer, primary or metastatic (distension of hepatic capsule)
Acute urinary retention
Bowel ischemia
Abdominal distension (ascites, abdominal carcinomatosis)
Retroperitoneal metastases
Perforated viscus
Bowel obstruction

- Constipation. Many cancer patients develop profound constipation from opioid use, chemotherapeutic interventions, dehydration, and autonomic dysfunction from advanced cancer. They may present with a history of no (or inadequate) bowel movements for lengthy periods. Abdominal pain is usually crampy and may radiate to the back or shoulders.
- Abdominal distension from carcinomatosis or ascites. Abdominal distension causes visceral pain from irritation of the gut and somatic pain from stretching of the abdominal wall.
- Acute urinary retention, which may develop secondary to (a) pharmacologic therapy, (b) obstruction secondary to tumor, or (c) neurogenic bladder secondary to the central spread of malignancy.
- Pancreatic cancer. Patients with pancreatic cancer may complain of achy intense pain in the upper abdomen or lower back. Low back pain is secondary to malignancy that has spread to the retroperitoneum and may involve the celiac plexus.
- Hepatic capsular distension. Hepatic tumors can cause the liver to enlarge and distend the hepatic capsule. Patient complains of visceral pain (achy, intense, and poorly localized) in the right upper quadrant and lower chest area and may also complain of pain in the shoulders.

Treatment of Abdominal Pain from Specific Causes. In the emergency department, treatment of the above conditions is largely conservative.[21] The clinician is assumed to have ruled out an acute abdomen.

Constipation. Constipation may be treated by administering an enema, by increasing the dosage of oral laxatives, by optimizing electrolyte status, and by increasing hydration. Note that in the cancer setting, many patients are thrombocytopenic or leukocytopenic. Both of these conditions are contraindications for administering an enema due to the increased risks of bleeding and of translocating bacteria into the peritoneal cavity. If relief of constipation improves pain, the patient may be discharged with appropiate follow-up.

Ascites. The clinician should consider a paracentesis in the emergency department for diagnostic purposes if an infection is suspected. If the patient is dyspneic and the clinician feels that the dyspnea is secondary to increased abdominal pressure from ascites, a paracentesis should be done in the emergency department; otherwise, (in non-emergent situations), therapeutic paracentesis may be scheduled on an outpatient basis.

Pancreatic Cancer. In the emergency department, pancreatic cancer pain may be managed conservatively with intravenous opioids. Consider consultation with the pain management service for evaluation for a splanchnic nerve block or celiac plexus block, especially if the patient is intolerant to the side effects of opioids.

Hepatic Distension. Management of pain from hepatic distention is similar to management of pain from pancreatic cancer. This pain is also primarily visceral pain and responds favorably to a splanchnic nerve block.

Urinary Retention. Pain from urinary retention may be managed by placement of a Foley catheter. Bladder irrigation may have to be implemented as well in the case of urinary retention secondary to bleeding and/or clots. If obstruction is suspected as the cause of urinary retention, consider a urologic consultation. If a neurogenic bladder is suspected as the cause of the urinary retention, a complete neurologic examination is indicated, and the treatment scheme is the same as that previously outlined in the section about treatment of spinal-cord compression.

Phantom Limb Pain and Stump Pain

"Phantom limb pain" refers to the experience of pain in a limb that has been amputated. It should be noted that "phantom" refers to the limb and not the pain; some patients have reported problems dealing with other clinicians, families, or friends who may not have taken the pain seriously because they thought it was "phantom pain." The majority of patients who have undergone an amputation will develop phantom limb pain, and studies have reported an incidence of nearly 80%.[22,23] In most patients, phantom limb pain begins to resolve with a "telescoping" sensation of the amputated limb shortening, with a decrease in pain. Although many trials have been conducted with various nerve blocks, antidepressants, antiepileptics, transcutaneous electrical nerve stimulation (TENS), and physical therapy, most patients report marginal to no benefit from any of these interventions. "Stump pain" refers to neuropathic pain at the site of amputation. Stump pain can be easily reproduced by palpation or percussion of the stump.

For the emergency department clinician, the two most common reasons for these patients to present at the emergency department are an increase in pain from a recurrence and the development of a tolerance to pain medications. Less common but treatable causes include angina presenting as pain in the amputated left arm,[24,25] acute herpes zoster presenting as radicular pain in the amputated limb,[26] and disc herniation presenting as radicular lower-extremity pain. For phantom limb pain, treatment is usually conservative; opioids, antiepileptics, and tricyclic antidepressants are the most common agents used. Whether or not phantom limb pain responds to opioid therapy on a chronic basis remains controversial. For stump pain, consultation with the pain management service may be considered for injection of the painful area, or consultation with the physical medicine and rehabilitation service may be considered if there are issues of functional limitation with pain.

The treatment of angina is described in Chapter 14. The treatment of acute herpes zoster or shingles is described below. If disc herniation is suspected, outpatient imaging studies and follow-up with the orthopedic service or pain management service is usually adequate.

Postmastectomy Pain Syndrome

Postmastectomy pain syndrome affects about 5 to 10% of women after breast surgery and axillary lymph node dissection.[27] It is thought to be due to damage to the intercostobrachial nerve during surgery. The intercostobrachial nerve has a superficial course in the axilla and can be easily damaged during axillary node dissections. Damage to this nerve may result in chronic burning pain in the medial aspect of the arm to the elbow, the lateral and anterior chest wall, and axilla. Lancinating pain is not uncommon in the area of distribution, and there may be components of severe allodynia to light touch. Since any movement can worsen the pain, the patient often keeps the affected extremity voluntarily immobile.

Patients with postmastectomy pain do not usually seek treatment in the emergency department unless there has been some acute change in the quality of the pain. The emergency-department clinician should be aware that brachial plexopathies from tumor infiltration can also present with similar pain and should consider the possibility of a recurrent tumor at the site. A careful history and physical examination should be performed, with attention paid to whether the pain has changed in intensity or duration and to whether there are any progressive neurologic symptoms. Changes in the type of pain and the development of neurologic deficits necessitate the use of imaging studies to rule out a recurrence. In the absence of a recurrence, the clinician should consider the possibility of tolerance, opioid withdrawal, or psychosocial stressors as possible causes of increased pain. Symptomatic management with follow-up appointments is usually sufficient if there is no recurrence.

Post-thoracotomy Pain Syndrome

Following thoracotomy, some patients complain of persistent pain in a distribution that parallels the intercostal nerves at the level of the incision. In most patients, post-thoracotomy pain resolves within 2 weeks to 2 months. In about 20% of patients, pain persists well beyond the usual convalescent period. Kanner and colleagues[28] have shown that the majority of these patients have persistent pain because of cancer recurrence. However, there are a small number of patients who have persistent neuropathic pain at the surgical site without recurrent disease.

There are two types of post-thoracotomy patients who present to the emergency department: patients in whom a recurrence has suddenly caused an increase in pain and patients who are discharged from the hospital with inadequate opioid coverage for the convalescent period.

The emergency-department clinician should review the patient's medical record to determine how many days have elapsed in the postoperative period and which opioid medications the patient was receiving while in the hospital. A quick comparison of the MEDD while the patient was in the hospital with the patient's current MEDD usually identifies the patient who is relatively underdosed. If the patient is receiving adequate medication and is still complaining of increased pain, consideration should be given to a recurrence versus an abscess at the site. It may be possible to rule out an infectious etiology of the increase in pain by checking the patient's white blood cell count and temperature and by obtaining the result of imaging studies (eg, a chest radiograph or a CT scan).

For the patient who is underdosed, symptomatic management and a follow-up appointment are usually sufficient. If the pain is very severe, the Hill "morphine test" (described earlier) may be used to assess the patient's opioid requirements. For the patient who may have a recurrence or an infection, consultation with the surgical team is needed.

Postradiation Pain Syndrome

Radiation therapy is used for a variety of cancers, for both curative and palliative reasons. In general, the overall dose of radiation is higher when radiation therapy is used for curative intent although individual fractions may be higher when used for palliation. Of all patients treated by radiotherapy, approximately 40% are treated for pain control. Paradoxically, radiation therapy can acutely decrease pain while potentially increasing pain in the long-term period by causing radiation-induced nerve damage. The mechanism for nerve damage is either a direct effect of demyelination and focal necrosis of neural matter or an indirect effect of fibrosis and scarring in surrounding connective tissue, leading to pain.[29]

Presentation. Patients with acute postradiation pain syndrome present to the emergency department with primarily nociceptive pain from acute tissue injury and breakdown (eg, esophagitis, oral mucositis, skin burns, and gastrointestinal (GI) and/or vaginal mucosal injury). Patients with severe esophagitis may have a normal-appearing oral and pharyngeal mucosa with severe dysphagia/odynophagia and may complain of an inability to swallow. Patients with skin burns may present with anything from mild erythema to frank blistering and sloughing of skin with severe hyperalgesia. Patients who have had radiation to the pelvic area may present with severe vaginitis or proctitis with associated bleeding.

Since the onset of pain is usually gradual, patients with chronic postradiation pain syndrome present to the emergency department less commonly. In the weeks to months (and sometimes, even years) after radiation therapy is administered, the patient may develop a burning or lancinating neuropathic pain in the affected area. Deep, achy, myofascial pain may also develop because of direct muscle damage by the radiation or because of secondary muscle spasm from injury to the nerves.

Treatment. The treatment of acute postradiation injury is significantly different from that of chronic postradiation injury. In acute radiation-induced esophagitis or mucositis, treatment should include coating agents (eg, sucralfate, 1 g orally three to four times a day), acid blockers (eg, famotidine, 20 to 40 mg orally; ranitidine, 150 to 300 mg orally; or omeprazole, 20 mg orally), topical anesthetics, and opioids (see section on mucositis, below). At the M. D. Anderson Cancer Center (Houston, Texas), the pharmacy extemporaneously prepares a topical anesthetic solution for mucositis and/or pharyngitis; each 15 mL contains 10 mg of diphenhydramine syrup (12.5 mg/5 mL), 15 mg of viscous lidocaine (20 mg/mL), and an aluminum hydroxide and magnesium hydroxide suspension (9.5 mL).

For chronic postradiation pain, the clinician should consider the possibility of recurrence. If there is no recurrence of cancer, the clinician may manage myofascial pain by the judicious use of opioids and other adjuvant analgesics. Neuropathic pain may respond to antiepileptics (see below) or tricyclic antidepressants (eg, amitryptyline, 10 to 25 mg orally at bedtime).[30,31] As an antiepileptic, gabapentin has a favorable side effect profile and may be started at 100 to 300 mg orally at bedtime, with a gradual escalation (300 to 600 mg per week) in dose until satisfactory analgesia is achieved. There is no maximum dose of gabapentin per se, but in general, if analgesia is not achieved by 3,600 mg, switching to another antiepileptic may be considered. Examples of other antiepileptics used are lamotrigine and oxcarbazepine. If the affected area includes a joint that has begun to show a limited range of motion because of fibrosis or pain, a consultation may be arranged with a rehabilitation service.

Chemotherapy-Induced Neuropathic Pain

Mechanism and Presentation. Certain types of antineoplastic agents are known to cause pain. The mechanism of this pain is thought to be neuropathic pain from interruption of the axonal microtubular transport system. This creates a deafferentation-like pain syndrome manifested by burning, tingling, numbness, and dysesthesias most commonly seen in the feet and hands.[32] The most common agents that cause chemotherapy-induced neuropathic pain are listed in Table 17–5.

Patients with neuropathic pain from chemotherapy most commonly present to the emergency department with complaints of burning and tingling pain in the extremities. Less commonly, patients may present with other neurologic deficits such as nerve palsies, altered mental status, ototoxicity, cerebellar dysfunction, or weakness.

Treatment. Unless there is a recurrence of cancer, the management of chemotherapy-induced neuropathic pain is conservative, with the following features:

1. Opioids and adjuvants (antiepileptics, tricyclic antidepressants) are usually the mainstay of therapy.
2. The patient's primary oncologist should be notified because early detection of neurotoxicity and a subsequent decrease in dosage or the cessation of the drug may reverse symptoms in many cases.
3. A starting dose of gabapentin (100 mg orally three times daily) may be given, with gradual escalation every 3 to 4 days as tolerated. If the total daily dose reaches 3,600 mg without a significant reduction in pain, switching to a different antiepileptic may be considered.
4. A consultation with the physical medicine and rehabilitation service may be indicated to assist the patient in managing his or her functional limitations.
5. If the pain is severe, consultation with a pain management service may be indicated for opioid and adjuvant adjustment and for consideration of interventional blocks. Certain mononeuropathies may respond favorably to peripheral neurolytic blocks.[33]

TABLE 17–5. Chemotherapeutic Agents Known to Cause Neurotoxicity

High-dose cytarabine	Cisplatin
High-dose methotrexate	Carboplatin
Vincristine	Paclitaxel
Vinblastine	Procarbazine
Vinolrebine	Interleukin-2
Ifosfamide	Interferons

Pain from Hematopoietic Growth Factors

Up to 20% of patients receiving granulocyte colony-stimulating factor (G-CSF) can develop transient bone pain that can be severe enough to necessitate a trip to the emergency room. Similarly, granulocyte-macrophage colony-stimulating factor (GM-CSF) causes a flulike syndrome with myalgias and arthralgias that can be severe enough for the patient to go to the emergency room. Both of these conditions are transient and respond favorably to opioids.

Herpes Zoster (Shingles) and Postherpetic Neuralgia

Course and Presentation. After a childhood bout of chickenpox, the varicella-zoster virus lies dormant in the dorsal root ganglia for decades. A decline in immunity usually triggers a flare of acute herpes zoster (also known as shingles) along one or more dermatomes. Common risk factors for the decline in immunity are malignancy, immunosuppressant therapy, and increasing age.

Patients with shingles present with pain along one or more dermatomes. Vesicular eruptions along the dermatome develop 2 to 5 days after the onset of pain and can persist for weeks. Usually, the more immunocompromised a person is, the longer the rash persists. The pain is described (in terms that confirm its neuropathic nature) as burning, shooting, itching, sharp, and worsening with light touch.

Postherpetic neuralgia is a sequela of acute herpes zoster. After the lesions have healed, many patients experience excruciating neuropathic pain in the affected dermatome. This pain is described as a burning pain with exquisite allodynia to light touch in the affected area. Postherpetic neuralgia seems to be an age-related phenomenon, and older patients are more prone to developing chronic pain after an outbreak of shingles.[34]

Treatment. Patients presenting to the emergency department with complaints of burning pain along one or more dermatomes with the development of a rash should be presumed to have an acute outbreak of herpes zoster, and antiviral therapy should be started immediately. Acyclovir (800 mg by mouth five times daily for 5 to 7 days), famciclovir (500 mg by mouth three times daily for 5 to 7 days), or valacyclovir (1 g by mouth three times daily) can accelerate the time for healing and may reduce the zoster-associated pain of the lesions. Data are mixed with regard to the efficacy of one antiviral agent over the other, but in general, famciclovir and valacyclovir may be more effective than acyclovir for pain and are easier to take.[31,35,36] Note that shingles can present with severe pain in the absence of a rash. If this is the case, acyclovir and famciclovir may be started empirically although the presence of pain in a dermatomal distribution should alert the clinician to consider a recurrence.

In addition to starting antiviral therapy, the clinician should provide the patient with adequate opioid analgesics. Topical application of a eutectic mixture of local anesthetics (EMLA) or capsaicin (0.025% cream) may be helpful in alleviating symptoms. Tricyclic antidepressants or a TENS unit may also be of some benefit in treating zoster-associated pain. Consideration should be given to consulting a pain management service since studies have shown that sympathetic blockade, somatic nerve blocks, or intralesional injections early in the course of the flare-up can provide symptomatic relief.[37,38] The role of sympathetic ganglion blocks in treating acute outbreaks of shingles to prevent the development of postherpetic neuralgia is controversial.[39,40] The role of opioids in treating postherpetic neuralgia also has been controversial, but newer antiepileptic drugs have shown some promise in treating this condition.[30,41]

Mucositis

Mucositis is a commonly occurring side effect of certain types of chemotherapy and can be a dose-limiting complication of treatment (Table 17–6). In addition, mucositis is commonly seen in patients who are receiving high doses of chemotherapy in preparation for bone marrow transplantation. Radiation to the oral cavity can also cause mucositis, xerostomia, and tissue necrosis (see Postradiation Pain Syndrome, above).

The patient presenting to the emergency department will complain of severe pain in the oral cavity and an inability to eat or swallow. Treatment should include coating agents, acid blockers, topical anesthetics, and opioids (see section on treatment under Postradiation Pain Syndrome for specific doses). Opioids should be administered as elixirs or as immediate-release potent opioids (these are smaller tablets and are thus easier to swallow). Initial treatment of pain may also be via the subcutaneous or intravenous route.

Mucosal damage predisposes the patient to yeast overgrowth, which can worsen the tissue damage; the clinician should thus maintain a low threshold for treating for yeast infections in these patients (eg, nystatin solution or fluconazole). Often, patients with acute esophagitis or mucositis arrive severely dehydrated and

TABLE 17–6. Chemotherapeutic Agents Known to Cause Mucositis

Antimetabolites (methotrexate, fluorouracil, cytarabine, irinotecan)
Antitumor antibiotics (doxorubicin, dactinomycin, mitomycin, bleomycin)
Plant alkaloids (vincristine, vinblastine, etoposide)
Others (alkylating agents at high doses)
Biologic agents (interleukins, lymphokine-activated killer cells)

may need to be admitted for intravenous hydration, pain control, and consideration of placement of a feeding tube. Interruption of the mucosal barrier, along with myelosuppression from chemotherapy, may predispose the patient to sepsis.

Analgesia in the patient who is admitted for pain control is best achieved by using patient-controlled analgesia (PCA). Initially, the patient's previous dose of opioids should be calculated (as the MEDD), and this should be instituted as a basal rate. Additional doses of opioids may be self-administered by the patient as needed. In the opioid-naive patient, the use of a basal infusion is not recommended due to the risk of accidental overdosage. Studies have shown that in general, patients with mucositis use less overall opioid and report the same pain scores with a better side effect profile if opioids are administered only as needed, with no continuous infusion.[42]

Steroid-Induced Pain Syndromes

Steroid therapy or the cessation of steroid therapy can cause a variety of pain syndromes, most of which are self-limiting. The acute administration of 100 mg of intravenous dexamethasone has been associated with burning perineal pain that is transient. Rapid or slow withdrawal of steroids may cause steroid pseudorheumatism, a pain syndrome manifested by diffuse myalgias and arthralgias. The mechanism of steroid pseudorheumatism may be the sensitization of joint mechanoreceptors and nociceptors after steroid withdrawal. Chronic administration of steroids may be associated with aseptic necrosis of the femoral or humeral head. Pain usually begins before radiologic changes are evident.

In the case of the patient presenting to the emergency department, a careful history may elicit the diagnosis of one of the above steroid-associated pain syndromes. As usual, the presence of recurrent disease must be ruled out. The treatment of perineal pain from acute steroid administration is conservative since the condition is self-limiting. Steroid pseudorheumatism responds to restarting steroids at higher doses and then a more gradual tapering down of the dose. The treatment of aseptic necrosis of the humeral or femoral head involves radiographic determination of the problem with supportive care, using appropriate analgesics and anti-inflammatory agents. Orthopedic consultation may be necessary if joint destruction is severe enough to warrant replacement.

CANCER PAIN–RELATED ISSUES

Delirium

Delirium is an acute confusional state that results from global brain dysfunction and often presents with an exaggerated expression of pain. There are many causes of delirium, and it is estimated that some 80% of cancer patients will develop delirium in the last week of life. Delirium can manifest earlier in the trajectory of the illness; its causes are listed in Table 17–7. In the absence of identifiable organic causes for the increase in pain, consideration should be given to delirium as a possible etiology of the pain complaint. A diagnosis of delirium is especially challenging for the clinician and family since confusion and agitation are expressions of brain malfunction and not necessarily increased pain or suffering. In this setting, increasing the dose of opioids may paradoxically increase the expression of "pain" as displayed by increased grimacing or moaning.[43]

The presence of disinhibition with delirium is usually the most distressing aspect of delirium for the family. The patient may express what seems to be pain and suffering in a manner that is grossly exaggerated in comparison with earlier expression. The patient may also make unreasonable requests, such as "I want to go home," and may become hostile if his or her wishes are not acceded to immediately. To minimize distress to the family, patient, and staff, delirium (especially hyperactive delirium) should be managed as quickly as possible while reassuring the family that most patients do not remember their behavior once the delirium has resolved.[44]

The key to identifying and treating delirium is to follow a systematic approach to assessing and correcting the underlying problem, as follows:

1. The assessment begins with the Mini–Mental State Examination (MMSE);[45] a score of < 24 indicates significant cognitive impairment, even in a patient who may appear to be lucid.
2. Ask the patient about hallucinations (especially tactile hallucinations).
3. Specific tests (such as the complete blood count; electrolyte screen; tests for ammonia level [if liver dysfunction is suspected], calcium, and oxygen saturation; and chest radiography) may need to be ordered. After appropriate tests are completed, the underlying problems should be corrected if possible.
4. If an underlying problem is not discovered or is not treatable or if the patient is very agitated, the symp-

TABLE 17–7. Common Causes of Delirium

Opioid toxicity
Hypoxia
Brain tumor, metastasis, or leptomeningeal disease
Cancer treatment
Drug reaction
Thyroid or adrenal dysfunction
Metabolic derangements
Nutritional deficits
Paraneoplastic syndromes
Infection, sepsis
Dehydration

toms of delirium can be managed with haloperidol (1 to 2 mg orally, subcutaneously, or intravenously, every 15 minutes to 4 hours as needed to bring agitation under control).

5. Rarely, more aggressive sedation may be needed, using midazolam at continuous doses of approximately 1 to 2 mg/h via the subcutaneous or intravenous route.

Depression and Anxiety

A significant number of patients with cancer have major depression, and this number increases with the severity of disease, degree of functional impairment, and presence of pain. Unfortunately, pain and depression occur simultaneously in many patients, and determining a cause-and-effect relationship is not always straightforward. Some patients become severely depressed because of inability to control pain, and some patients express pain as the only symptom of depression. The somatic symptoms typically associated with depression in the nonmalignant population (ie, anorexia, anhedonia, fatigue, insomnia, and weight loss) may not reliably indicate depression in the cancer population because these symptoms can develop secondary to the disease or treatment. As a result, the diagnosis and management of depression and/or pain can be particularly challenging.[46]

Anxiety in the cancer patient can be a normal reaction to being confronted with the diagnosis; it can also occur secondary to cancer treatment. With some patients, generalized anxiety or phobias could have predated the cancer. Anxiety can lead to increased nociception by several mechanisms, and stress can accentuate the central nervous system's ability to provoke muscle tension and spasm. Anxiety can also increase the individual's perception of noxious stimuli.[47]

In the emergency department, the clinician should keep anxiety and depression in mind as possible reasons for an exacerbation in the patient's pain presentation. However, depression and anxiety should be considered as diagnoses of exclusion and should be considered only if organic causes have been satisfactorily ruled out. Consultation with the psychiatry service can be particularly helpful if the patient is severely anxious or depressed and expressing hopelessness or suicidal ideation. Although there are a variety of medications that have shown efficacy in treating anxiety, the drugs of choice in the emergency-department setting are benzodiazepines (alprazolam, 0.25 to 0.5 mg two to three times daily; oxazepam, 10 to 30 mg three to four times daily; or lorazepam, 1 to 2 mg two to three times daily).

Pain from Opioid Withdrawal or Underdosage

Pain from opioid withdrawal is a relatively rare presentation in the emergency department. A history of running out of opioids in the 2 to 3 days prior to the emergency department visit with a corresponding increase in pain, rebound diarrhea, sweating, piloerection "goosebumps," and mild increases in blood pressure, heart rate, and respiratory rate confirm the diagnosis. A more common presentation in the emergency department is the patient who gradually builds up a tolerance to opioids (whether or not nociception from the underlying cancer is increasing) and suddenly realizes that the pain is intolerable. Some patients may be receiving chronic opioid therapy by alternate routes of administration (eg, epidural catheters, implanted intrathecal pumps, or subcutaneous infusions), and a problem may have developed in the dispensing equipment.

If the clinician suspects underdosage or equipment malfunction as the cause of the increased pain, a systematic evaluation of the patient's medications and an assessment of the equipment may diagnose the problem. Consultation with the pain service or neurosurgery service may be needed to assess the patency of an indwelling catheter or intrathecal pump. Until the problem is resolved, the patient may be at risk for developing symptoms of withdrawal, and opioids should be given by alternative routes (oral, transmucosal, rectal, intravenous, or subcutaneous).

Intractable Pain

Patients with cancer pain sometimes present to the emergency department with a complaint of severe pain that seemingly has no identifiable cause. The usual scheme for assessing and treating pain is unsuccessful in treating this pain, and the patient continues to complain of severe refractory pain. This type of pain is termed "intractable pain" and is often used as a criterion for admitting the patient. Intractable pain can occur for the usual reasons for a sudden increase in pain (ie, increase in not readily identifiable nociception, worsening depression, acute anxiety attack or panic attack, side effects of medications, brain metastasis, metabolic derangement, or tolerance to medications).

If no etiology for the pain can be identified, the patient should be admitted, and consultation with the pain management service or psychiatry service, or both, should be considered.

Tolerance, Physical Dependence, and Psychological Dependence (Addiction)

Assuming that the level of nociception remains constant, most patients will need to gradually increase their opioid regimen to maintain the same degree of pain relief. This phenomenon is referred to as tolerance and is thought to be due to changes at the opioid receptor level or to changes in opioid metabolism. Once the body is exposed to opioids for a long period of time, sudden cessation can precipitate withdrawal symptoms. This is called physical dependence, and it is seen with a variety of non-opioid medications as well (eg, antihypertensives). Psychological dependence (or addiction) is the compulsion to use a substance resulting in physical, psychological or social harm. There is a large body of evidence that in the absence of a history of substance abuse, cancer patients exposed to opioid therapy for prolonged periods are at virtually no risk for developing addiction;[48–50] they will, however, develop tolerance and physical dependence. The development of withdrawal symptoms with drug cessation is not an indication of addiction.

Pseudoaddiction Syndrome

Pseudoaddiction is a condition characterized by drug-seeking behavior that is caused by unrelieved pain. The condition may be iatrogenic because of chronic under-dosage. The clinician should assess the degree of true drug-seeking behavior as opposed to pseudoaddiction syndrome by reviewing the patient's records to identify sources of nociception, a history of chemical coping, a history of depression or anxiety, or an escalation of drug dosage. Consultation with the pain management or psychiatry service may be beneficial in differentiating drug-seeking behavior from pseudoaddiction syndrome.

CONCLUSION

In summary, the following cancer pain management "pearls" are offered:

- In a cancer patient, a new or progressive complaint of pain is always a recurrence until proved otherwise.
- Ask the patient about his or her pain, and always believe what they report. However, not all expression of pain is nociception. The assessment should consider nociception, psychosocial stressors, delirium, and somatization.
- *Always* conduct a thorough neurologic examination.
- Know the patient's MEDD, and always treat pain promptly and aggressively. Use potent short-acting opioids to titrate effective pain control. The fentanyl patch should not be used in the emergency-department setting to treat an acute pain exacerbation because of the amount of time (24 to 72 hours) it takes to achieve stable blood levels.
- Always provide adequate follow-up appointments.
- Do not overlook constipation as a major cause of abdominal pain.
- Because opioid conversion tables are inexact, patients should be observed closely after an opioid conversion.

REFERENCES

1. Bruera E, Watanabe S. New developments in the assessment of pain in cancer patients. Support Care Cancer 1994;2:312–8.

2. Hill CS, Thorpe DM, McCrory L. A method for attaining rapid and sustained pain relief and discriminating nociceptive from neuropathic pain in cancer patients. Pain 1990;(Suppl 5):S498.

3. Mercadante S. Opioid rotation for cancer pain: rationale and clinical aspects. Cancer 1999;86:1856–66.

4. Portenoy RK, Hagen NA. Breakthrough pain: definition, prevalence, and characteristics. Pain 1990;41:273–81.

5. Simmonds MA. Management of breakthrough pain due to cancer. Oncology 1999;13(8):1103–8.

6. Boogerd W, van der Sande JJ. Diagnosis and treatment of spinal cord compression in malignant disease. Review. Cancer Treat Rev 1993 April;19(2):129–50.

7. Ruckdeschel JC. Spinal cord compression. In: Abeloff MD, Armitage JO, Lichter AS, Niederhuber JE, editors. Clinical oncology. New York: Churchill Livingstone, 2000. p. 814–5.

8. Raizer JJ, De Angelis LM. Cerebral sinus thrombosis diagnosed by MRI and MR venography in cancer patients. Neurology 2000;54(6):1222–6.

9. Abrahao M, Goncalves AP, Yamashita R, et al. Frontal sinus adenocarcinoma. Sao Paulo Med J 2000;118(4):118–20.

10. Agut Fuster M, Riera Sala C, Aldasoro Martin J, et al. Meningeal carcinomatosis in cancer of the larynx [Spanish]. Acta Otorrinolaringol Esp 2000;51(3):267–70.

11. Manley GT, Hemphill JC, Morabito D, et al. Cerebral oxygenation during hemorrhagic shock: perils of hyperventilation and the therapeutic potential of hypoventilation. J Trauma Injury Infect Crit Care 2000;48(6):1025–32.

12. Schierhout G, Roberts I. Hyperventilation therapy for acute traumatic brain injury [computer file]. Cochrane Database of Systematic Reviews 2000;(2):CD000566.

13. Hauser SL. Diseases of the spinal cord. In: Fauci AS, Braunwald E, Isselbacher KJ, et al. editors. Harrison's principles of internal medicine. New York: McGraw-Hill, 1998. p. 2385–6.

14. Sillevis Smitt P, Tsafka A, van den Bent M, et al. Spinal epidural abscess complicating chronic epidural analgesia in 11 cancer patients: clinical findings and magnetic resonance imaging. J Neurol 1999;246(9):815–20.

15. Okano K, Kondo H, Tsuchiya R, et al. Spinal epidural abscess associated with epidural catheterization: report of a case review of the literature [review]. Jpn J Clin Oncol 1999;29(1):49–52.

16. Portenoy RK. Cancer pain: pathophysiology and syndromes. Lancet 1992;339:1026.

17. Johnson BW, Parris WCV. Mechanisms of cancer pain. In: Parris WCV, editor. Cancer pain management: principles and practice. Boston: Butterworth-Heinemann; 1997. p. 31.

18. Hilner BE, Ingle JN, Berenson JR, et al. American Society of Clinical Oncology guideline on the role of bisphosphonates in breast cancer. J Clin Oncol 2000;18(6):1378–91.

19. Hortobagyi GN, Theriault RL, Lipton A, et al. Long-term prevention of skeletal complications of metastatic breast cancer with pamidronate. Protocol 19 Aredia Breast Cancer Study Group. J Clin Oncol 1998;16(6):2038–44.

20. Grauer A, Ziegler R. Bisphosphonate therapy in the man-

agement of skeletal metastases [review]. Orthopade 1998;27(4):231–9.

21. Tabbarah HJ, Lowitz BB. Abdominal complications. In: Casciato DA, Lowitz BB, editors. Manual of clinical oncology. Boston: Little, Brown & Company; 1995. p. 498–506.

22. Jensen TS, Krebs B, Nielsen J, et al. Phantom limb, phantom pain and stump pain in amputees during the first 6 months following limb amputation. Pain 1983;17:243.

23. Sherman RA, Sherman CJ. Prevalence and characteristics of chronic phantom limb pain among American veterans. Results of a trial survey. Am J Phys Med 1983;62:227.

24. Cohen H. Anginal pain in a phantom limb [letter]. BMJ 1976;2:475.

25. Meter SW, Clintron GB, Long C. Phantom angina. Am Heart J 1988;116:1627.

26. Wilson PR, Person JR, Su DW, et al. Herpes zoster reactivation of phantom limb pain. Mayo Clin Proc 1978;53:336.

27. Hord AH. The sympathetic nervous system. In: Parris WCV, editor. Cancer pain management: principles and practice. Boston: Butterworth-Heinemann;1997. p. 110.

28. Kanner R, Martini N, Foley KM. Nature and incidence of postthoracotomy pain. Proc Am Soc Clin Oncol 1982;1:152.

29. Johnson BW, Parris WCV. Mechanisms of cancer pain. In: Parris WCV, editor. Cancer pain management: principles and practice. Boston: Butterworth-Heinemann; 1997. p. 37.

30. Backonja MM. Antiepileptics (antineuropathics) for neuropathic pain syndromes. Clin J Pain 2000;16(2 Suppl):S67–72.

31. Omrod D, Goa K. Valaciclovir: a review of its use in the management of herpes zoster. Drugs 2000;59(6):1317–40.

32. Elliott K, Foley KM. Neurologic pain syndromes in patients with cancer. Neurol Clin 1989;7(2):349.

33. Abram SE. Neural blockade for neuropathic pain [review]. Clin J Pain 2000;162(2 Suppl):S56–61.

34. Raj PP. Management of pain due to herpes zoster and postherpetic neuralgia. In: Parris WCV, editor. Cancer pain management: principles and practice. Boston: Butterworth-Heinemann;1997. p. 346–7.

35. Alper BS, Lewis PR. Does treatment of acute herpes zoster prevent or shorten postherpetic neuralgia? J Fam Pract 2000;49(3):255–64.

36. Whitley RJ. Varicella-zoster virus infections. In: Fauci AS, Braunwald E, Isselbacher KJ, et al, editors. Harrison's principles of internal medicine. New York: McGraw-Hill; 1998. p. 1088.

37. Raj PP. Pain due to herpes zoster. In: Raj PP, editor. Practical management of pain. 2nd ed. St. Louis: Mosby-Year Book; 1992. p. 517–45.

38. Epstein E. Triamcinolone-procaine in the treatment of zoster and postzoster neuralgia. Calif Med 1971;115:6–10.

39. Ali NM. Does sympathetic ganglion block prevent postherpetic neuralgia? Reg Anesth 1995;20(3):227–33.

40. Wu CL, Marsh A, Dworkin RH. The role of sympathetic nerve blocks in herpes zoster and postherpetic neuralgia. Pain 2000;87(2):121–9.

41. Ross EL. The evolving role of antiepileptic drugs in treating neuropathic pain. Neurology 2000;55(5 Suppl 1):S41–8.

42. Hill HF, Chapman CR, Kornell JA, et al. Self-administration of morphine in bone marrow transplant patients reduces drug requirement. Pain 1990;40:121–9.

43. Bruera E, Lawlor P. Cancer pain management. Acta Anaesthesiol Scand 1997;41(1 Pt 2):146–53.

44. Driver LC, Bruera E. The M. D. Anderson palliative care handbook. Houston: MDACC Printing Services, 2000. p. 95–8.

45. Tombaugh TN, McIntyre NJ. The mini-mental state examination: a comprehensive review. J Am Geriatr Soc 1992;40:922–35.

46. Massie MJ, Holland JC. Depression and the cancer patient. J Clin Psychiatry 1990;51:12.

47. Holland JC. Anxiety and cancer: the patient and the family. J Clin Psychiatry 1989;50:20.

48. Portenoy RK, Lesage P. Management of cancer pain. Lancet 1999;353(9165):1695–700.

49. Paice JA, Toy C, Shott S. Barriers to cancer pain relief: fear of tolerance and addiction. J Pain Symptom Manage 1998;16(1):1–9.

50. Passik SD, Portenoy RK, Ricketts PL. Substance abuse issues in cancer patients. Part 1: Prevalence and diagnosis. Oncology (Huntingt) 1998;12(4):517–21.

CHAPTER 18

PSYCHIATRIC EMERGENCIES

MICHAEL A. WEITZNER, MD
JENNIFER STRICKLAND, PHARMD, BCPS
TERESITA SANJURJO-HARTMAN, MD

As patients with cancer become progressively ill and enter the advanced stages of illness, the burden of both physical and psychological symptoms becomes enormous.[1,2] In fact, physical symptoms such as pain, dyspnea, and constipation are not the most prevalent symptoms of patients with advanced cancer. Rather, psychological symptoms such as worrying, nervousness, lack of energy, insomnia, and sadness are among the most prevalent and distressing symptoms encountered in this population.[2] Neuropsychiatric symptoms and syndromes, such as mood disorders (ie, depression), cognitive impairment disorders (ie, delirium), anxiety, insomnia, and suicidal ideation, play a crucial role in the management in patients with advanced disease. They frequently coexist with other physical and psychological symptoms, interacting with each other and negatively impacting quality of life.

Since the patient and the family are the unit of concern, psychological symptoms and psychiatric disorders must be understood in that context. Therefore, the prompt recognition and effective treatment of both psychiatric and physical symptoms become critically important to the well-being of the patient with advanced disease, as well as to his or her family.[3] Pain and suffering are among the most feared consequences of a cancer illness. Although aggressive medical management of cancer pain often leads to profound relief of pain, many patients continue to suffer pain because of unaddressed psychiatric complications of cancer. Psychiatric symptoms and disorders in the cancer patient with pain require the same degree of aggressive attention and focus of care, particularly when they threaten compliance with treatments and the safety of the patient and staff or interfere dramatically with quality of life.[4]

A psychiatric emergency in its broadest sense can be defined as "a disruption of an individual's mental functioning to a degree that prevents the interrelated adaptation of the patient himself, his family, and representatives of his community. Intervention is required to avoid permanent harm to these people or to avoid situational deterioration to a degree that would require more conventional intervention at a later time."[5] Unfortunately, the psychiatric complications of cancer are too often ignored and are addressed only when a crisis has developed unexpectedly. Psychiatric symptoms must become as important a focus of care as pain and other physical symptoms in the advanced cancer patient. This chapter reviews the most common psychiatric emergencies encountered in the cancer setting: delirium, severe anxiety, depression, and suicidal ideation.

DELIRIUM AND COGNITIVE IMPAIRMENT DISORDERS

Delirium is extremely common in cancer patients with advanced disease, particularly in the last weeks of life. Given that delirium is associated with increased morbidity in the terminally ill, much distress is caused for patients, family members, and staff.[6–8] Delirium can interfere significantly with the identification and control of other physical and psychological symptoms, such as pain.[9–12] It is not uncommon for delirium to occur as a preterminal event and to be associated with significant physiologic disturbance. Most deliria involve multiple medical etiologies, including infection, organ failure, and medication side effects, as well as extremely rare paraneoplastic syndromes.[13–15]

The prevalence of delirium in general hospital practice is quite high, making it one of the most prevalent mental disorders in the medical setting. At greater risk for delirium are elderly, postoperative, and cancer patients.[16–19] As many as 33% of hospitalized medically ill patients have serious cognitive impairments.[20] Approximately 30 to 40% of medically hospitalized patients develop delirium,[21] and as many as 65 to 80% develop some form of organic mental disorder.[22] In cancer inpatients, the prevalence of cognitive impairment is 44%;[17] the prevalence rises to 62.1% just prior to death.

The incidence of delirium in the terminally ill cancer patient has been found to be up to 85%.[16] Delirium also occurs in up to 51% of postoperative patients.[18,23] The incidence of delirium is increasing, which reflects the growing numbers of elderly patients, a particularly susceptible group.[19]

Clinical Features and Diagnosis

The clinical features of delirium are quite numerous and include a variety of neuropsychiatric symptoms that are also common to other psychiatric disorders, such as depression, dementia, and psychosis (Table 18–1). Disordered attention and cognition, accompanied by disturbances of psychomotor behavior and the sleep-wake cycle, are symptoms that have been emphasized as pathognomonic of delirium.[23] Table 18–2 lists the criteria for delirium, from the *Diagnostic and Statistical Manual of Mental Disorders*, 4th edition (DSM-IV).[24] Two delirium subtypes clinically based on psychomotor behavior and arousal levels have been described.[23] The subtypes are the hyperactive (or agitated, or hyperalert) subtype and the hypoactive (or lethargic, or hypoalert) subtype (Table 18–3). Other researchers have proposed a "mixed" subtype[25] with features of each. Whereas the hyperactive form is most often characterized by hallucinations, delusions, agitation, and disorientation, typical of withdrawal syndromes and anticholinergic-induced delirium, the hypoactive form is characterized by confusion and sedation but is rarely accompanied by hallucinations, delusions, or illusions. The hypoactive form is

TABLE 18–1. Clinical Features of Delirium

Prodromal symptoms
    Restlessness
    Anxiety
    Sleep disturbance
    Irritability
Rapidly fluctuating course
Reduced attention (distractibility)
Altered arousal
Increased or decreased psychomotor activity
Disturbance of sleep-wake cycle
Affective symptoms
    Emotional lability
    Sadness
    Anger
    Euphoria
Altered perceptions
    Misperceptions (illusions)
    Hallucinations
Disorganized thinking (poorly formed delusions); incoherent speech
Disorientation to time, place, and/or person
Memory impairment (inability to register new information)

Adapted from Trzepacz PT, Wise MG. Neuropsychiatric aspects of delirium. In: Yudofsky SC, Hales RE, editors, Textbook of neuropsychiatry 3rd ed. Washington: American Psychiatric Press; 1997. p. 447–470.

TABLE 18–2. Criteria* for Delirium Due to General Medical Condition

A. Disturbance of consciousness (that is, reduced clarity of awareness of the environment), with reduced ability to focus, sustain, or shift attention.

B. Change in cognition (such as memory deficit, disorientation, language disturbance, or perceptual disturbance) that is not better accounted for by a pre-existing, established, or evolving dementia.

C. The disturbance develops over a short period of time (usually hours to days) and tends to fluctuate during the course of the day.

D. There is evidence from the history, physical examination, or laboratory findings of a general medical condition judged to be etiologically related to the disturbance.

Adapted from American Psychiatric Association.[24]
*From *Diagnostic and Statistical Manual of Mental Disorders*, 4th ed. (DSM-IV).

typical of hepatic or metabolic encephalopathies, acute intoxications from sedatives, or hypoxia.[26]

Instruments for the evaluation of delirium have been grouped into four categories: (1) tests that measure cognitive impairment, which are usually used to screen for delirium (ie, the Mini–Mental State Exam [MMSE]); (2) delirium diagnostic instruments based on DSM or International Classification of Diseases (ICD) criteria, which are used to make a "yes/no" judgment on the presence or absence of delirium (ie, the Confusion Assessment Method); (3) delirium-specific numerical rating scales, whose scores can be used to evaluate the likelihood of diagnosis or to estimate the severity of the delirium (ie, the Delirium Rating Scale [DRS]); and (4) delirium severity rating scales (ie, the Memorial Delirium Assessment Scale [MDAS]) (Table 18–4).[24,27–38] The MMSE, while not a screening tool specifically for delirium, has become one of the most frequently used neuropsychological tests in the clinical evaluation of delirium and has thus become the de facto reference against which other instruments are judged.[39] The DRS is a 10-item clinician-rated symptom measure that specifically integrates criteria from DSM-III (the previous edition to DSM-IV). The scale is designed to be used by the clinician to identify delirium and to reliably distinguish delirium from dementia or other neuropsychiatric disorders. The MDAS was designed to quantify the severity of the delirium and to be administered repeatedly within the same day, in order to allow for the objective measurement of changes in delirium severity in response to medical changes or clinical interventions.[33]

When diagnosing delirium in the advanced cancer patient, the clinician must formulate a differential diagnosis as to the likely etiologies. Most often, the etiology of the delirium is multifactorial or cannot be determined. A thorough diagnostic assessment should be entertained unless the patient is imminently terminal, since available diagnostic information can lead to specific therapies that may be able to reverse the delirium. One study found that 68% of delirious cancer patients could be improved

TABLE 18–3. Contrasting Features of Delirium Subtypes

| Feature | Delirium Subtype | |
	Hyperactive, Hyperalert, Agitated	Hypoactive, Hypoalert, Lethargic
Symptoms	Hallucinations, delusions, hyperarousal (eg, withdrawal syndromes from alcohol, benzodiazepines)	Sleepiness, withdrawal, slowness (eg, hepatic and metabolic encephalopathies; benzodiazepine intoxication)
Pathophysiology	Elevated or normal cerebral metabolism; fast or normal EEG; reduced GABA activity	Decreased global cerebral metabolism; diffuse slowing EEG; increased GABA activity

Adapted form Breitbart W, Cohen K.[41]
EEG = electroencephalogram; GABA = γ-aminobutyric acid.

despite a 30-day mortality rate of 31%.[40] The diagnostic work-up should include an assessment of potentially reversible causes of delirium. A full physical examination should assess for evidence of sepsis, dehydration, or major organic failure. Chemotherapeutic agents that could contribute to the delirium should be reviewed (Table 18–5). A screen of laboratory parameters will allow the assessment of the possible role of metabolic abnormalities, such as hypercalcemia, and other problems, such as hypoxia or disseminated intravascular coagulation. Imaging of the brain and assessment of the cerebrospinal fluid may be appropriate in some instances.[41]

The causes of delirium in cancer patients are listed in Table 18–6. Although delirium may occasionally be due to the direct effect of cancer on the central nervous system, it is more common for delirium to be related to the indirect effects of cancer. Electrolyte imbalance (especially of sodium, potassium, calcium, and magnesium) may constitute a metabolic cause of altered mental status.[42] Inten-

tional and oftentimes-needed polypharmacy, combined with a fragile physiologic state in the patient, can cause even routinely ordered hypnotics to precipitate an episode of delirium. Opiates may play a role in the development of a case of delirium, particularly in those patients who are elderly or have significant hepatic or renal dysfunction. The toxic accumulation of meperidine's metabolite, normeperidine, is associated with florid delirium accompanied by myoclonus and possible seizures.[10] It is extremely rare for stable regimens of oral or intravenous opioid analgesics for the control of cancer pain to induce an overt delirium or confusional state,[43] although this has been reported.[44] However, significant cognitive impairment, as well as delirium, is now commonly identified as a dose-limiting adverse effect during opioid dose titration and is observed most commonly in older patients receiving intravenous opioid infusions.[10,45–47]

Management

The approach to the management of delirium in the medically ill cancer patient includes identifying and correcting

TABLE 18–4. Methods of Assessing Delirium in Cancer Patients

Diagnostic classification system
  DSM-IV (APA, 1994)
  ICD-9, ICD-10
Diagnostic interviews/instruments
  Delirium Symptom Interview (DSI) (Albert et al, 1991)[27]
  Confusion Assessment Method (CAM) (Inouye et al, 1990)[28]
Delirium rating scales
  Delirium Rating Scale (DRS) (Trzepacz et al, 1988)[29]
  Delirium Rating Scale—Revised—98 (DRS-R-98) (Trzepacz et al, 1999)[30]
  Confusion Rating Scale (CRS) (Williams, 1991)[31]
  Saskatoon Delirium Checklist (SDC) (Miller et al, 1988)[32]
  Memorial Delirium Assessment Scale (MDAS) (Breitbart et al, 1997)[33]
  Abbreviated Cognitive Test for Delirium (CTD) (Hart et al, 1997)[34]
Cognitive impairment screening instruments
  Mini–Mental State Examination (MMSE) (Folstein et al, 1975)[35]
  Short Portable Mental Status Questionnaire (SPMSQ) (Wolber et al, 1984)[36]
  Cognitive Capacity Screening Examination (CCSE) (Jacobs et al, 1977)[37]
  Blessed Orientation Memory Concentration Test (BOMC) (Katzman et al, 1983)[38]

Adapted from Breitbart W.[12]
APA = American Psychiatric Association; DSM-IV = *Diagnostic and Statistical Manual of Mental Disorders*, 4th edition; ICD = International Classification of Diseases.

TABLE 18–5. Neuropsychiatric Side Effects of Chemotherapeutic Drugs

Drug	Neuropsychiatric Symptoms
Methotrexate (intrathecal)	Delirium, dementia, lethargy, personality changes
Vincristine, vinblastine	Delirium, hallucinations, lethargy, depression
Asparaginase	Delirium, hallucinations, depression, cognitive dysfunction
BCNU (carmustine)	Delirium, dementia
Bleomycin	Delirium
Fluorouracil	Delirium
Cisplatin	Delirium
Hydroxyurea	Hallucinations
Procarbazine	Depression, mania, delirium, dementia
Cytosine arabinoside	Delirium, lethargy, cognitive dysfunction
Hexylmethylamine	Hallucinations
Ifosfamide	Delirium, lethargy, hallucinations
Prednisone	Depression, mania, delirium, psychoses
Interferon	Flulike syndrome, delirium, hallucinations, depression
Interleukin	Cognitive dysfunction, hallucinations

Adapted from Roth AJ, Breitbart W.[72]

TABLE 18–6. Causes of Delirium

Direct
    Primary brain tumor
    Metastatic spread
        Cerebral
        Leptomeningeal
Indirect
    Metabolic encephalopathy due to organ failure
    Electrolyte imbalance
    Treatment side effects from:
        Chemotherapeutic agents
        Steroids
        Radiation
        Opiates
        Anticholinergics
        Antiemetics
    Infection
    Hematologic abnormalities
    Nutrition
    Paraneoplastic syndromes

Adapted from Breitbart W, Cohen K.[41]

the underlying cause, which is usually multifactorial (Figure 18–1). Although this process may take some time, it is important to provide relief from the behavioral symptoms the patient may be experiencing as a result of the confusion. Simple measures that can be taken include environmental manipulations (eg, keeping a dim light on in the patient's room so as to allow the patient to have the opportunity to reorient him- or herself when awakened). Frequent reorientation of the patient by the nursing staff is also helpful. In the event that a patient is agitated and may be considered a danger to him- or herself due to disinhibition, one-on-one observation by a companion may be indicated.

Physical restraint, either by a Posey vest or by hand/ankle restraints, should be avoided as these tend to add to the patient's agitation. Instead, chemical restraint with a neuroleptic will be more efficacious. Haloperidol, a high-potency neuroleptic, is the drug of choice in this situation.[48–50] It can be given orally, subcutaneously, or intravenously; the dose and route of administration will depend on the type of delirium being experienced by the patient. For the hypoalert delirious patient, low dosages of haloperidol are most often successful in relieving the confusion and may help to increase the patient's ability to focus and sustain his or her attention. If the patient can swallow and if there is no concern regarding a potentially compromised airway, then oral haloperidol, 1 mg every 8 hours, may be used, with additional doses available every 2 to 4 hours as needed. If there is concern about a potentially compromised airway or chemotherapy-related stomatitis, then the intravenous route is preferred. Haloperidol's bioavailability by the intravenous route is twice its bioavailability by the oral route.[51] For the hypoalert patient, therefore, a starting dose of 0.5 mg every 8 hours would be indicated. For the hyperalert delirious patient, in which agitation and the potential for self-harm are high, the intravenous route is indicated. The usual starting dose in this situation is 1 mg every 4 hours around the clock, with additional doses available as needed every 30 to 60 minutes, depending on the level of agitation. It is not uncommon for continuous intravenous infusions of haloperidol to be prescribed for the severely agitated delirious patient; this would be indicated for the patient who is taking multiple additional doses in addition to the scheduled doses. If intravenous access is unavailable, a subcutaneous infusion may be started and then converted to (a) an intravenous infusion when an intravenous line has been established or (b) oral administration if the patient's condition improves and the agitation lessens. In a double-blind randomized comparison trial of haloperidol versus chlorpromazine versus lorazepam, lorazepam alone (in doses up to 8 mg in a 12-hour period) was ineffective in the treatment of delirium and in fact contributed to worsening delirium and cognitive impairment.[52] However, in low doses (approximately 2 mg of haloperidol equivalent per 24 hours), both neuroleptic drugs were highly effective in controlling the symptoms of delirium and in improving cognitive function. Along with haloperidol, lorazepam at 0.5 to 1.0 mg every 1 to 2 hours (orally or intravenously) may be more effective in rapidly sedating the agitated delirious patient.[53,54]

A common approach to managing the confusion caused by opioid therapy is to lower the dose if the patient's pain is controlled or to change to another opioid if there is still pain coincident with the confusion.[55,56] An option that is becoming more widely used is the addition of a psychostimulant to offset the sedation and confusion that are related to higher doses of opiates.[57] The most commonly used psychostimulant is methylphenidate, begun in oral doses of 5 mg twice per day (at 8:00 am and 12:00 noon) and increased to 20 mg twice per day. A newer psychostimulant, modafinil, works by a totally different mechanism (ie, the hypothalamus rather than the reticular activating system), which allows the patient to have increased alertness but without increased energy and motivation.[58] This is helpful in the situation of the patient who is sedated and very confused, when it is less desirable to stimulate the patient while increasing his or her alertness. Modafinil is started at 100 mg orally once per day, usually in the morning, and can be increased to 400 mg once daily. Doses of up to 1,200 mg once daily have been given without adverse effects.[58]

States of withdrawal from alcohol, benzodiazepines, and barbiturates can be life threatening. The treatment of these withdrawal states depends on the particular

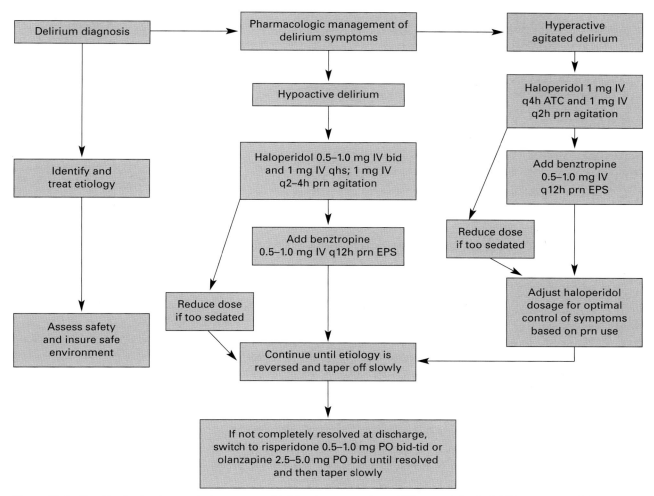

Figure 18–1. Algorithm for the pharmacologic treatment of delirium in cancer patients. ATC = around the clock; EPS = extrapyramidal symptoms; prn = as circumstances require.

agent involved. The goal sometimes may be to stabilize the patient on the agent (eg, a benzodiazepine), and sometimes the goal may be to provide a suitable substitute (eg, benzodiazepine) for the offending agent (eg, ethanol or a barbiturate). The concern with all three of these agents is that withdrawal can manifest with seizure activity. Thus, patients need to be placed on benzodiazepines quickly and titrated based on physiologic parameters. For withdrawal states caused by any of these substances, the patient needs to be administered lorazepam intravenously, starting with 1 mg every 4 hours around the clock, with additional doses available every 30 to 60 minutes on the basis of vital-sign parameters (ie, pulse > 90 bpm, diastolic blood pressure > 90 mm Hg, tremulousness, and diaphoresis).[59,60] Vital signs need to be checked hourly, and the patient needs to be vigorously hydrated unless the patient has congestive heart failure, hepatic dysfunction (as evidenced by decreased albumin or significant peripheral edema), or

renal impairment, in which case hydration is administered judiciously. The additional as-needed lorazepam doses that are administered over a 24-hour period are thus added to the scheduled doses for the next 24-hour period. The as-needed lorazepam doses are administered and added to the scheduled doses until the physiologic parameters normalize, at which point a steady state has been reached. After 24 hours, the total lorazepam dose can be decreased by 10 to 20%; this is done daily until the lorazepam is discontinued. If the withdrawal is severe, it may be necessary to administer the lorazepam in a continuous intravenous infusion ranging from 0.5 mg/h to as much as 6 mg/h, based on physiologic parameters. The addition of scheduled haloperidol (1 mg IV q4h) may help to keep down the lorazepam dose requirements.[61] The use of β-blockers for treating alcohol withdrawal is not indicated since they address only the peripheral manifestations of the withdrawal and not its central nervous system effects.[60]

ANXIETY DISORDERS

Throughout its span, cancer disrupts patients' social roles, patients' interpersonal relationships, and the ways in which these patients view their future.[62] Although anxiety, in the general population, is associated with female gender, young age, and low socioeconomic status,[63] these patterns do not appear in cancer patients since demographic factors may become less important as cancer progresses. The evaluation of anxiety symptoms is a common reason for requesting psychiatric consultations in the cancer setting and accounts for up to 16% of such requests.[64] In one study, 25% of patients referred for anxiety were diagnosed as having either an anxiety disorder (4%) or an adjustment disorder with anxious mood (21%), and 57% were diagnosed as having major depression (9%) or an adjustment disorder with depressed mood (48%). This is consistent with other studies of cancer patients that have reported a higher prevalence of mixed anxiety and depressive symptoms than of anxiety alone.[65] In two controlled studies, cancer patients have been found to have higher levels of anxiety than healthy individuals (up to 28%, compared to 15% of controls).[66,67] According to the National Comorbidity Survey, the one year point prevalence of anxiety disorders in the general population is 17%.[63]

In general, only a small number of cancer patients have anxiety disorders that predate the cancer diagnosis and that are worsened by the stress associated with cancer diagnosis and treatment.[68] Many patients with anxiety usually report subjective feelings of foreboding, apprehension, or dread. Anxiety symptoms can be either cognitive or somatic (Table 18–7). In patients who experience panic attacks, symptoms related to increased autonomic discharge increase dramatically.[69] As patients with severe anxiety experience increased fears, they may see their environment as threatening, and they are often motivated to flee, a reaction that commonly precipitates treatment refusals or demands for premature hospital discharge.[70]

When diagnosing anxiety states, it is important that the physician inquire about anxiety symptoms when distress is suspected, because patients may be embarrassed by their present concerns or by a history of phobias or panic; Table 18–8 lists some useful questions. In general, adjustment disorder, or reactive anxiety, is an exaggerated form of the "normal" anxiety related to illness. It differs from normal fears of cancer by the greater duration and intensity of symptoms, the impairment of normal function, and (if severe enough) the impairment of the patient's ability to comply with treatment.[71] It is "normal" for patients to experience fear with restlessness and insomnia before undergoing painful or stressful presurgery procedures (such as bone marrow aspiration, chemotherapy, and radiation therapy) and while awaiting test results. In these situations, most patients with

TABLE 18–7. Somatic and Cognitive Symptoms of Anxiety

Somatic
  Tachycardia
  Shortness of breath
  Diaphoresis
  Gastrointestinal distress
  Nausea
  Loss of appetite
  Diminished libido
  Insomnia
  Hyperarousal
  Irritability
Cognitive
  Recurrent unpleasant thoughts about cancer
    Fears of death
    Dependency on others
  Aberrant thinking style
    Overgeneralization
    Catastrophization
    Negative outcomes seem inevitable
    "Helpless in a hopeless situation"

mild to moderate anxiety will respond positively to being given adequate information, reassurance, and support. A significant minority of patients will require medication to control their distress. On the other hand, patients with severe anxiety and who are extremely fearful are typically unable to absorb information or to cooperate with procedures. To reduce symptoms to a manageable level, these patients require pre-emptive psychological support, medication, and/or behavioral interventions.[72]

TABLE 18–8. Questions for Querying Patients with Cancer about Anxiety Symptoms

Have you experienced any of the following symptoms since your cancer diagnosis or treatment? If yes, when do they do occur, and how long do they last?

  Do you feel nervous, shaky, or jittery?
  Have you felt fearful, apprehensive, tense?
  Have you had to avoid certain places or activities because of fear?
  Have you experienced your heart racing or pounding?
  Have you had trouble catching your breath when nervous?
  Have you had any unjustified sweating or trembling?
  Have you felt a knot in the pit of your stomach?
  Have you felt a lump in your throat when getting upset?
  Do you find yourself pacing back and forth?
  Are you afraid to close your eyes at night for fear that you will die in your sleep?
  Do you find yourself worrying about the next diagnostic test, or the results of it weeks in advance?
  Have you had the sudden onset of a fear of losing control or going crazy?
  Have you had the sudden onset of a fear of dying?
  Do you often worry about when your pain will return and how bad it will get?
  Do you worry about whether you'll be able to get your next dose of pain medication on schedule?
  Do you spend more time in bed than you should because you fear intensification of pain if you stand up or move about?

Adapted from Roth et al.[71]

Types of Disorders

Anxiety resulting from uncontrolled pain, abnormal metabolic states, pulmonary emboli, and hormone-producing tumors, for example, is referred to as an anxiety disorder due to a general medical condition. Anxiety induced by medications (eg, steroids, psychostimulants, sedatives, hypnotics, and anxiolytics) is called substance-induced anxiety disorder[24] (Table 18–9). Undermanaged pain remains a common cause of anxiety and decreased quality of life in the cancer patient. It is important to understand the specific nature of the patient's pain (ie, whether somatic, visceral, neuropathic, or neuralgic) in order to determine the most appropriate treatment for the pain and consequent anxiety. Patients who experience more "breakthrough pain" (episodes of severe or excruciating pain superimposed on relatively stable and well-controlled baseline pain) tend to report significantly more anxiety and depression than patients who do not have as many of these episodes.[73] The undermanagement of patients' pain may result from a variety of reasons,

TABLE 18–9. Criteria* for Anxiety Disorder Due to a General Medical Condition and for Substance-Induced Anxiety Disorder

Anxiety disorder due to a general medical condition
A. Prominent anxiety, panic attacks, or obsessions or compulsions predominate in the clinical picture.
B. There is evidence from the history, physical examination, or laboratory findings that the disturbance is the direct physiologic consequence of a general medical condition.
C. The disturbance is not better accounted for by another mental disorder (eg, adjustment disorder with anxiety, in which the stressor is a serious general medical condition).
D. The disturbance does not occur exclusively during the course of a delirium.
E. The disturbance causes clinically significant distress or impairment in social, occupational, or other important areas of functioning.

Substance-induced anxiety disorder
A. Same as A above.
B. There is evidence from the history, physical examination, or laboratory findings that either
  1. the symptoms in criterion A developed during or within 1 month of substance intoxication or withdrawal, or
  2. medication use is etiologically related to the disturbance.
C. The disturbance is not better accounted for by an anxiety disorder that is not substance induced. Evidence that the symptoms are better accounted for by an anxiety disorder that is not substance induced might include the following: the symptoms precede the onset of the substance use (or medication use); the symptoms (a) persist for a substantial period of time (eg, about a month) after the cessation of acute withdrawal or severe intoxication or (b) are substantially in excess of what would be expected, given the type or amount of the substance used or the duration of use; or there is evidence suggesting the existence of an independent non-substance-induced anxiety disorder (eg, a history of recurrent non-substance-related episodes).
D. Same as D above.
E. Same as E above.

Adapted from American Psychiatric Association.[24]
*From *Diagnostic and Statistical Manual of Mental Disorders*, 4th ed. (DSM-IV).

only one of which may be the lack of understanding of the most appropriate pharmacologic interventions. It is not uncommon for physicians to prescribe short-acting opioids (to be taken as needed) such as oxycodone to treat constant pain, which may result in alternating periods of oversedation and periods of pain as well as increase distress and anxiety. Instead, physicians may prescribe longer-acting opioids (to be given around the clock) for constant pain, along with shorter-acting opioids for breakthrough pain; this may provide more consistent pain relief. In such a situation, the consequence may be that not only does the patient receive more consistent pain relief, but also the patient's sense of control over the pain may alleviate his or her anxiety.[69] It is important to remember that the patient with unrelieved pain may appear tense, restless, and diaphoretic and may become agitated if adequate relief is not provided. Suicidal ideation is common with the experience of uncontrolled pain; no psychiatric diagnosis, however, can be made until the pain has been controlled.[74] If the patient remains anxious after the pain has been adequately treated, other medical or psychological factors should be considered. Many other medical conditions must be considered in the differential diagnosis of anxiety;[75] these are listed in Table 18–10.

The majority of cancer patients with phobias, panic disorder, post-traumatic stress disorder, and generalized anxiety disorder may have been treated for these disorders for years prior to the their cancer diagnosis. A small number of patients are first diagnosed with these disorders while undergoing cancer treatment. It is important to accurately diagnose and treat these disorders since they have the potential not only to cause extreme distress but also to interfere with the adequate medical management of the patient.[76] The stress of the diagnosis of cancer may activate a pre-existing phobia that was not bothersome to the person previously. Agoraphobia and phobias of blood, doctors, and hospitals are common sources of anxiety in the hospital[72] (Table 18–10).

In contrast to phobias, in which there is a clearly defined situation or object of dread, panic disorder often presents as a sudden unpredictable episode of intense discomfort and fear accompanied by shortness of breath, diaphoresis, tachycardia, feelings of choking or being smothered, and thoughts of impending doom. These symptoms may be re-activated by a cancer diagnosis or by difficult treatment. Generalized anxiety disorder is characterized by excessive worry, difficulty in controlling the worry or apprehension, and the presence of symptoms of autonomic hyperactivity and hypervigilance. Post-traumatic stress disorder (PTSD) may be activated by isolation or conditions that recall some prior highly frightening event. Holocaust survivors and Vietnam War veterans may be vulnerable to PTSD. An

TABLE 18–10. Underlying Medical Causes of Anxiety

Cardiovascular conditions	Peptic ulcer disease
Angina pectoris	Respiratory conditions
Arrhythmia	Asthma
Congestive heart failure	Chronic obstructive pulmonary disease
Hypovolemia	Pneumothorax
Myocardial infarction	Pulmonary edema
Valvular disease	Pulmonary embolism
Endocrine conditions	Immunologic conditions
Carcinoid	Anaphylaxis
Hyperadrenalism	Systemic lupus erythematosus
Hypercalcemia	Medications
Hyperthyroidism	Bronchodilators
Hypocalcemia	Corticosteroids
Hypothyroidism	Psychostimulants
Pheochromocytoma	Caffeine
Metabolic conditions	Withdrawal states
Hyperkalemia	Alcohol
Hyperthermia	Benzodiazepines
Hypoglycemia	Barbiturates
Hyponatremia	Opioids
Hypoxia	
Porphyria	
Neurologic conditions	
Akathisia	
Encephalopathy	
Mass lesion	
Postconcussion syndrome	
Seizure disorder	
Vertigo	

Adapted from Goldberg RJ, Posner DA.[75]

aspect of PTSD is the fact that both adults and children may experience PTSD following traumatic events related to cancer treatment. Such persons display an exaggerated startle response, have insomnia and nightmares, re-experience the feelings and invasive thoughts experienced at the time of the trauma, and avoid anything associated with the trauma (eg, the hospital). These conditions can lead to emergent situations. The anticipatory anxiety seen at follow-up visits after cancer treatments have ended is likely PTSD-related, the patient responding to cues that are painful reminders. Anticipatory nausea and vomiting with anxiety are conditioned responses to chemotherapy. Post-traumatic stress disorder is likely a learned response to prior trauma, which explains the symptoms that occur in cancer survivors who experience reminders of the treatment.[72] It has been reported that almost half (48%) of a group of cancer survivors reported symptoms related to PTSD; of these, 4% met the criteria for current PTSD and 22% met the criteria for a lifetime diagnosis of PTSD.[77] Among blood and marrow transplantation patients, it has been shown that lower social support and a higher degree of coping by avoidance 1 month prior to transplantation predicted a greater severity of PTSD symptoms an average of 7 months post transplantation.[78]

Management of Anxiety

At the foundation of treatment of anxiety is the provision of psychological support. Cognitive therapeutic techniques identify maladaptive automatic thoughts and underlying negative assumptions patients have about themselves that interfere with coping. Brief supportive therapy, crisis intervention, and insight-oriented psychotherapy are also used. Behavioral approaches of progressive relaxation, guided imagery, meditation, biofeedback, and hypnosis treat anxiety symptoms that are associated with painful procedures, pain syndromes, and anticipatory fears of chemotherapy and radiation therapy.[79]

Unfortunately, there are occasions when it is not possible to implement psychological interventions until the level of anxiety has been decreased. Such occasions require pharmacologic intervention. One example is the classic conditioned anxiety before chemotherapy, usually manifest as anticipatory nausea and/or vomiting. Whereas behavioral therapy (ie, relaxation therapy and guided imagery) is very helpful, anxiolytics are often used first to decrease the level of anxiety so that behavioral therapy may be more helpful. Although there are several possible pharmacologic choices for the treatment of anxiety, the most frequently used group is the benzodiazepines. The choice of medication depends on the severity of the anxiety, the desired duration of drug action, the rapidity of onset needed, the route of administration available, the presence or absence of active metabolites, and the metabolic problems that must be considered.[80] Dosing schedules depend on patients' tolerance and require individual titration (Figure 18–2).

The first factor to consider is the type of anxiety pattern that needs to be treated. In very general terms, reactive anxiety is either (1) an affective state that occurs intermittently with a "crescendo-decrescendo" pattern in which the patient experiences his or her "normal" baseline state in-between episodes or (2) an increased anxious baseline state with intermittent crescendo-decrescendo episodes (seen more commonly in cancer patients). The first pattern is best treated with short-acting (eg, alprazolam) or intermediate-acting (eg, lorazepam) benzodiazepines on an as-needed basis. The second pattern is best treated with an intermediate-acting benzodiazepine (eg, lorazepam, clonazepam) in scheduled doses given every 4 hours.[81] For those patients who need a rapid onset of anxiolytic effect or who need to experience the "on" effect of the anxiolytics, alprazolam or lorazepam are the agents of choice.[81]

Given the two patterns of reactive anxiety described above, additional considerations include the presence of active or inactive metabolites and the impact of hepatic metabolism and excretion. Three benzodiazepines (lorazepam, oxazepam, and temazepam) have no active metabolites and are not metabolized by the cytochrome P-450 system of the liver. They are considered intermedi-

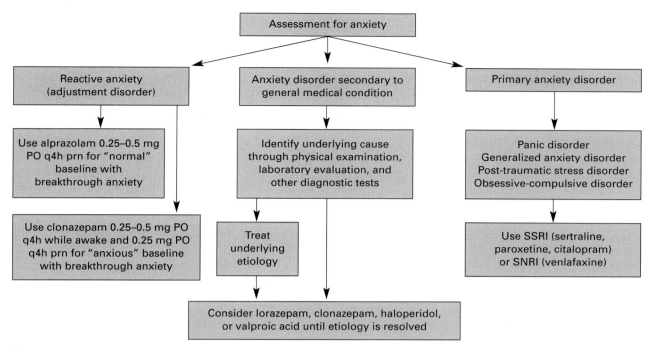

Figure 18–2. Algorithm for the assessment and management of anxiety disorders in cancer patients. prn = as circumstances require; SNRI = serotonin/norepinephrine reuptake inhibitor; SSRI = selective serotonin reuptake inhibitor.

ate-acting benzodiazepines and have an average effective half-life of 4 to 6 hours, making them useful on either a scheduled or as-needed basis.[81] These three anxiolytics are the drugs of choice for those patients with hepatic impairment related to metastatic disease or other metabolic problems. Since they have no active metabolites, these three benzodiazepines are also the drugs of choice for patients with renal impairment. It is important to remember that all benzodiazepines are renally excreted and are not dialyzable. Lorazepam has an additional benefit in that it is available for intravenous administration. Although the longer-acting benzodiazepines (ie, diazepam, chlordiazepoxide, and clorazepate) are available, their use in the treatment of reactive anxiety in the cancer patient is limited because of their very long elimination half-life (96 hours), their increased number of active metabolites, and their poor safety profile for patients with liver impairment.[81] Patients who experience end-of-dose failure and recurrence of anxiety on shorter-acting drugs find clonazepam helpful. It is not uncommon for us to switch patients from alprazolam to clonazepam when attempting to taper off alprazolam.

The most common side effects of benzodiazepines are dose dependent and are controlled by titrating the dose to avoid drowsiness, confusion, motor incoordination, and sedation. Although benzodiazepines rarely cause respiratory depression when given alone in the healthy patient, caution should be exercised in their use in patients with hepatic impairment and pre-existing cardiopulmonary disease (ie, chronic obstructive pulmonary disease, congestive heart failure, and pneumonia), since there may be a potential for increased respiratory depression in the presence of these pre-existing medical conditions. In addition, the respiratory depressant effects are additive or even synergistic in the presence of antidepressants, antiemetics, and analgesics.[82] Although rarely needed, alternatives to benzodiazepines exist. Low doses of the antihistamine hydroxyzine (12.5 to 25.0 mg every 6 hours as needed) or of the neuroleptics chlorpromazine (25 mg every 4 to 6 hours as needed) and thioridazine (10 to 25 mg every 4 to 6 hours as needed) can be used safely and relatively effectively in situations in which there is concern about depression of central respiratory mechanisms.[83] Discontinuation of a benzodiazepine in a patient who has been on a standing dose for more than 2 to 4 weeks should be done with a tapering schedule to avoid withdrawal.

Because a stigma exists about taking anxiolytic medications (both for patients and for physicians), cancer patients usually need to be encouraged to maintain compliance. Medications are readily discontinued when symptoms subside. As with all medications, tolerance and physical dependence may occur; however, addiction, which is a psychological dependence, is rare and almost never occurs in individuals who do not have a history of drug abuse prior to the cancer illness.[84]

In addition to reactive anxiety (ie, adjustment disorder), anxiety can occur as a symptom related pathophysiologically to an underlying medical condition or as an adverse effect of a drug or substance. For example, patients with respiratory distress often will experience anxiety as part of their distress related to air hunger, and patients with pain often experience anxiety as part of their pain. In both situations, the anxiety experienced by these patients adds to their perception of air hunger or pain. In other words, the anxiety that they experience effectively lowers their thresholds for symptom tolerance (ie, pain and air hunger). For both of these situations, the most effective treatments might include oxygen, diuretics, antibiotics, systemic or nebulized steroids, nebulized β-agonists, nebulized morphine (in the case of respiratory distress) and opiates, or other adjuvant pain medications for the pain.[85–87] Although opioid drugs such as the narcotic analgesics are indicated primarily for the control of pain, these drugs are also effective in the relief of dyspnea due to cardiopulmonary processes and the anxiety associated with them.[88] Opioid drugs are particularly useful in the treatment of dying patients who are in respiratory distress. Continuous intravenous infusions of morphine or other narcotic analgesics allow for careful titration and control of respiratory distress, anxiety, pain, and agitation.[45] Although the evidence remains mostly anecdotal, there is a suggestion that nebulized morphine may also be helpful for the treatment of respiratory distress in the advanced cancer patient.[85,89] Occasionally, to maximize the patient's comfort, one must maintain the patient in a state of unresponsiveness.[90] When respiratory distress is not a major problem, it is preferable to use the opioid drugs solely for analgesic purposes and to add more specific anxiolytics (such as the benzodiazepines) to control concomitant anxiety.

Akathisia is described as an inner sense of restlessness. Patients usually cannot sit still and pace or (if confined to bed) continuously move and change position. This is quickly controlled by stopping the causative drug (usually a neuroleptic antiemetic such as promethazine, perchloperazine, or metoclopramide) and by adding a benzodiazepine (ie, lorazepam, 1 mg orally four times per day), a β-blocker such as propranolol (40 to 80 mg orally once or twice per day), or an antiparkinsonian agent such as amantadine (100 to 200 mg two to three times per day).[91–93]

Last, the anxiety that can occur in the immediately terminal patient may be very difficult to manage. Midazolam, a very short-acting water-soluble benzodiazepine, is useful in controlling anxiety and agitation in patients in terminal phases of illness.[94,95] It has a short duration of action, and doses ranging from 2 to 10 mg per day have been found to be safe and effective for most patients. However, doses as high as 30 to 60 mg per day have been reported.[94]

Another type of anxiety is related to an underlying psychological disorder such as panic disorder, generalized anxiety disorder, or obsessive-compulsive disorder.

These disorders are best treated with antidepressants, particularly the selective serotonin reuptake inhibitors (SSRIs). In the emergent setting, patients with this type of anxiety respond well to anxiolytics, but their optimal treatment is with the SSRIs. Doses tend to be higher for these disorders than for major depressive disorder.

DEPRESSION

The disease trajectory for a patient with cancer progresses through well-identified stages: investigation, diagnosis, treatment, remission, relapse, and, eventually, terminal disease. Each of these phases have psychological consequences.[96] Throughout these periods, the threat of loss of physical integrity, the possibility of the deterioration of mental and functional capacities, changes in family and social roles, increasing dependence on the medical system, and the ultimate prospect of death can all serve as sources of chronic mental strain. In general, patients may turn to a variety of strategies to cope with the distress associated with these events. Although patients' ways of coping may range from frank denial to stoic acceptance, some investigators have found that those who adopt more active strategies (eg, seeking support, attempting constructive problem solving, focusing on the positive) may show a better long-term adjustment than those who rely more often on passive-avoidant strategies (eg, social withdrawal, rumination).[97–100] Nevertheless, the emotional consequences of coping with a life-threatening illness may include periods of anxiety, sadness, fatalism, and grief, all of which can be considered part of the normal adjustment process.[100] However, when the experience of depression becomes especially severe, pervasive, and prolonged to the point of interference with functional abilities, then the likelihood of a clinically significant depressive disorder is high.[101]

Diagnosis and Assessment

The incidence of depression in cancer patients ranges from 20 to 25% and increases with higher levels of disability, advanced illness, and pain.[83,102,103] The 12-month prevalence of major depression in the general population in the United States is 5%, and the lifetime prevalence is 17%.[63] The diagnosis of major depression is based on specific diagnostic criteria (the DSM-IV[24] criteria are listed in Table 18–11). For major depression to be present, the patient must admit to at least a 2-week history of depressed mood and/or loss of interest in usual activities (ie, anhedonia); without at least one of these two symptoms, the diagnosis of major depression cannot be made. The somatic symptoms of depression, such as anorexia, insomnia, fatigue, and weight loss, are unreliable and lack specificity in the cancer patient, who may have no appetite because of chemotherapy, who sleeps poorly because of pain or hospitalization, and who is fatigued because of the cancer, radiation therapy, and chemotherapy.[52] Thus, the psychological symptoms of depression can be substituted for greater diagnostic value. These include the following: dysphoric mood; feelings of hopelessness, worthlessness, and guilt; and suicidal ideation.[82,102–104] Table 18–12 highlights these somatic and cognitive symptoms. A family history of depression and a history of previous depressive episodes further suggest the reliability of the diagnosis. The evaluation should consider organic factors that can precipitate or exacerbate depression (Table 18–13).

Table 18–14 lists questions that a physician can ask when making a rapid assessment of mood. Physicians often underestimate the incidence of depression, believing

people to be more likely depressed if they have increased pain or a decreased performance status.[105] The patient's mood, physical symptoms of depression, and the severity of depression (including the risk of suicide), must be assessed. Physical symptoms must be carefully evaluated to determine whether fatigue, insomnia, and decreased libido are caused by depression, by cancer, or as a complication of treatment. When it is difficult to determine the etiology and if symptoms are impairing the patient's functioning, a trial of antidepressants is warranted.

The physician should ask about uncontrolled pain, which is a common cause of depression in cancer patients. Uncontrolled pain leads to hopeless and desperate feelings and a sense that life is intolerable unless pain is relieved. Patients interpret a new or increasingly severe pain as a sign that the cancer has progressed, and this results in greater depression and hopelessness. Suicide is a real risk with these patients, especially if they do not believe that efforts are being made to control the pain or that relief is possible. Suicidal ideation and major depressive symptoms often abate when pain is controlled.

Management

Depression in cancer patients is optimally managed by using a combination of supportive psychotherapy, cognitive-behavioral techniques, and antidepressant medications.[83] Psychotherapy and cognitive-behavioral techniques are useful in the management of psychological distress in cancer patients, and they have been applied to the treatment of depressive and anxious symptoms related to cancer and cancer pain. Psychotherapeutic interventions, in the form of either individual or group counseling, have been shown to effectively reduce psychological distress and depressive symptoms in cancer patients.[106–108] Cognitive-behavioral interventions such as relaxation and distraction with pleasant imagery have also been shown to decrease depressive symptoms in patients with mild to moderate levels of depression.[109]

TABLE 18–11. Criteria* for Major Depressive Episode

A. Five (or more) of the following symptoms have been present during the same 2-week period and represent a change from previous functioning; at least one of the symptoms is either depressed mood (1) or loss of interest or pleasure (2).
Note: Do not include symptoms that are clearly due to a general medical condition or that are mood-incongruent delusions or hallucinations.
   1. Depressed mood most of the day nearly every day, as indicated by either subjective report (eg, feels sad or empty) or observation made by others (eg, appears tearful).
   2. Markedly diminished interest or pleasure in all or almost all activities most of the day nearly every day, as indicated by either subjective report or observations made by others.
   3. Significant weight loss when not dieting or weight gain (eg, a change in more than 5% of body weight in 1 month), or a decrease or increase in appetite nearly every day.
   4. Insomnia or hypersomnia nearly every day.
   5. Psychomotor agitation or retardation nearly every day (observable by others, not merely subjective feelings of restlessness or being slowed down).
   6. Fatigue or loss of energy nearly every day.
   7. Feelings of worthlessness or excessive or inappropriate guilt (which may be delusional) nearly every day (not merely self-reproach or guilt about being sick).
   8. Diminished ability to think or concentrate or indecisiveness, nearly every day (either by subjective account or as observed by others).
   9. Recurrent thoughts of death (not just fear of dying), recurrent suicidal ideation without a specific plan, or a suicide attempt or a specific plan for committing suicide.
B. The symptoms do not meet criteria for a mixed episode.
C. The symptoms cause clinically significant distress or impairment in social, occupational, or other important areas of functioning.
D. The symptoms are not due to the direct physiologic effects of a substance (eg, a drug of abuse or a medication) or a general medical condition (eg, hypothyroidism).
E. The symptoms are not better accounted for by bereavement (ie, after the loss of a loved one, the symptoms persist for longer than 2 months or are characterized by marked functional impairment, morbid preoccupation with worthlessness, suicidal ideation, psychotic symptoms, or psychomotor retardation).

Adapted from American Psychiatric Association.[24]
*From *Diagnostic and Statistical Manual of Mental Disorders*, 4th ed.(DSM-IV).

TABLE 18–12. Somatic and Cognitive Symptoms of Major Depression

Cognitive symptoms
   Depressed mood
   Loss of interest or pleasure
   Worthlessness; guilt
   Indecisiveness
   Recurrent thoughts of death; suicidal ideation
Somatic symptoms
   Increased or decreased weight/eating
   Increased or decreased sleep
   Psychomotor agitation/retardation
   Fatigue, poor energy
   Decreased concentration

TABLE 18–13. Causes of Depression in Patients with Cancer

Uncontrolled pain
Metabolic abnormalities
    Hypercalcemia
    Sodium, potassium imbalance
    Anemia
    Deficient vitamin B_{12} or folate
Endocrinologic abnormalities
    Hyper- or hypothyroidism
    Adrenal insufficiency
Medications
    Steroids
    Interferon and interleukin-2
    Methyldopa, reserpine
    Barbiturates
    β-Blockers
    Some antibiotics (eg, amphotericin B)
    Some chemotherapeutic agents
        Vincristine
        Vinblastine
        Procarbazine
        L-Asparaginase

Adapted from Roth AJ, Holland JH.[126]

Psychopharmacologic interventions are the mainstay of management in the treatment of cancer patients with severe depressive symptoms who meet the criteria for major depressive episodes.[83] The efficacy of antidepressants in the treatment of depression in cancer patients has been well established.[110–114] The medications used for depression in patients with cancer are SSRIs, tricyclic antidepressants (TCAs), and psychostimulants (Figure 18–3).

Although TCAs have been around for a very long time, their use for the treatment of major depressive disorder, whether in healthy individuals or in patients with severe medical illness, has dramatically diminished. It may be stated that there is almost no situation in which a TCA would be the drug of choice for the treatment of major depressive disorder in a patient with cancer. Today, SSRIs are used most commonly to treat major depressive disorder.[115] The choice of antidepressant is usually dictated by the symptoms that the patient is expressing and the opportunity that the clinician has to use the side effect profile of a particular medication to enhance overall symptom control of the major depression. For example, if a patient is having a significant sleep disturbance as part of his or her presentation of depression, the use of a sedating SSRI, such as paroxetine or citalopram, may be indicated. If the patient is having somatizing symptoms associated with the depression, such as nausea or diarrhea, paroxetine (20 to 40 mg nightly) and citalopram (20 to 40 mg nightly) may be the drugs of choice, given their anticholinergic side effect profile. On the other hand, if the patient has no sleep disturbance but is acknowledging significant fatigue, then a more activating SSRI such as sertraline (50 to 200 mg in the morning) may be in order.[116] Fluoxetine (10 to 20 mg in the morning), although a good antidepressant, has rather limited usefulness in the cancer patient unless the patient is in remission, is not receiving any antineoplastic therapies, and has no other significant medical comorbidities. Simply put, fluoxetine is the most potent inhibitor of the cytochrome P-450 IID6 microenzyme, potentially causing significant

TABLE 18–14. Questions to Ask to Assess Depressive Symptoms in Patients with Cancer

Question	Symptom
Mood Evaluation	
How well are you coping with your cancer? Well? Poorly?	Well-being
How are your spirits since diagnosis? Down? Blue?	Mood
Do you cry sometimes? How often? Only alone?	—
Are there things you still enjoy doing, or have you lost pleasure in things you used to do before you had cancer?	Anhedonia
How does the future look to you? Bright? Bleak?	Hopelessness
Do you feel you can influence your care, or is your care totally under others' control?	—
Do you worry about being a burden to family and friends during treatment for cancer?	Worthlessness
Do you feel others might be better off without you?	Guilt
Physical Evaluation*	
Do you have pain that is not controlled?	Pain
How much time do you spend in bed?	Fatigue
Weak? Fatigue easily? Rested after sleep? Any relationship to change in treatment or how you feel otherwise physically?	—
How is your sleeping? Trouble going to sleep? Awake early? Often?	Insomnia
How is your appetite? Food tastes good? Weight loss or gain?	Appetite
How is your interest in sex? Extent of sexual activity?	Libido
Do you think or move more slowly?	Psychomotor slowing

Adapted from Roth AJ, Holland JH.[126]
*Evaluate in the context of cancer-related symptoms.

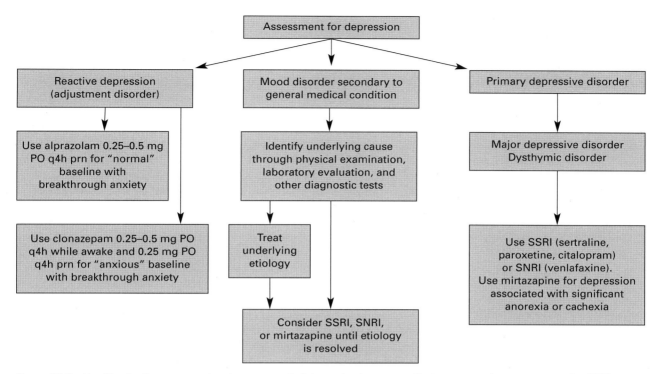

Figure 18–3. Algorithm for the assessment and management of depression in cancer patients. prn = as circumstances require; SNRI = serotonin/norepinephrine reuptake inhibitor; SSRI = selective serotonin reuptake inhibitor.

drug-drug interactions with other medications that are metabolized through that microenzyme (ie, opiates, many antibiotics, and antiarrhythmics).[117] The SSRIs as a class have relatively few adverse effects as compared to the TCAs. The primary side effects of sertraline are nausea, diarrhea, dyspepsia, tremor, dizziness, ejaculatory delay in men, and insomnia. Sertraline's shorter half-life allows for faster clearance and thus better control in patients with cancer.[118] Paroxetine has no active metabolites and is therefore excreted relatively quickly upon discontinuation; nausea, somnolence, and asthenia are common side effects.[119] Sertraline and paroxetine also may cause sexual dysfunction.[118,119] Because all of these drugs are strongly protein bound, consideration must be given to their ability to increase blood levels of coumadin, digoxin, and cisplatin.

Although SSRIs are the antidepressants that are most frequently used in the treatment of major depression in cancer patients, several newer antidepressants deserve mention and also have a place in the treatment of major depression in this population. Venlafaxine (150 to 225 mg of the long-acting form in the morning) is a selective norepinephrine and serotonin reuptake inhibitor (SNRI). As such, it possesses many of the attributes of the TCA class without the significant adverse effects. Because of its effect on norepinephrine reuptake, it has a particular niche in the treatment of the

anxiously depressed cancer patient.[120] Buproprion (150 to 300 mg of the long-acting form in the morning), a dopamine reuptake inhibitor, is useful for the patient who cannot tolerate SSRIs, such as the patient with carcinoid. The long-acting form of buproprion does not have the increased incidence of seizures that is associated with the short-acting form.[121] Nefazadone (100 to 200 mg twice daily), a heterocyclic, possesses many of the characteristics of its older cousin, trazodone.[122] It is potentially useful for the patient with depression and sleep disturbance. Along with the extended-release forms of buproprion and venlafaxine, nefazadone has a lower incidence of sexual side effects.[123,124] Last, mirtazapine (30 to 45 mg nightly) is a novel antidepressant that acts as an SSRI at lower doses and as an SNRI at higher doses,[125] making it useful in the treatment of the anxiously depressed patient as well as depressed patients with significant anorexia.

Although the starting doses of antidepressants for patients with cancer are typically lower than patients without cancer, these patients usually require the same doses as do healthy patients. Most antidepressants take 3 to 6 weeks to show efficacy. Therefore, it is usually not imperative to begin a medication immediately after recognizing depressive symptoms, so a medical work-up of possible causes can be done. A patient's prior response to a particular medication (or a family member's experience with an antidepressant) is a helpful predictor of response.[126] Patients who are unable to swallow pills may be able to take an antidepressant elixir (sertraline, paroxetine, citalopram), or immediate-release venlafaxine, mirtazapine, or nefazadone can be crushed and given in a liquid of choice.

Low doses of the psychostimulants methylphenidate, pemoline, and dextroamphetamine are useful for patients who are suffering from depressed mood, apathy, decreased energy, poor concentration, and weakness.[127,128] They promote a sense of well-being, decreased fatigue, and increased appetite. They produce a rapid effect in comparison with the other antidepressants. Side effects are infrequent but can include insomnia, euphoria, and mood lability. High doses and long-term use rarely produce anorexia, nightmares, insomnia, euphoria, or paranoid thinking. Pemoline is available as a chewable tablet; patients who have difficulty swallowing can therefore absorb the drug through the buccal mucosa. Pemoline appears to be as effective as the other psychostimulants, but it is not a controlled substance. Pemoline should be used with caution in patients with renal and/or hepatic impairment; patients under longer-term treatment should be monitored with liver function tests periodically.[129]

A useful strategy is to start patients who have significant depressive symptomatology as well as fatigue on a psychostimulant and antidepressant together. In this way, the psychostimulant provides immediate relief for the fatigue and increases the feeling of well-being; this also allows time for the antidepressant to have its effect. It would not be unusual to start methylphenidate at 5 mg orally twice daily (eg, at 8:00 am and 12:00 noon) and to add an SSRI or SNRI as well. The methylphenidate can be increased daily in increments of 5 mg per dose, to a final dose of 20 to 30 mg twice daily. The antidepressant can also be increased, as rapidly as tolerated, to the desired dose. For example, sertraline can be started at 12.5 to 25 mg once daily and increased by 12.5 to 25 mg per day to the desired dose of 150 to 200 mg per day.[118] If the patient develops troublesome diarrhea or nausea, the titration can be slowed. There is no reason to not try a rapid antidepressant titration (as tolerated by the patient) to relieve the suffering of major depression, even in a terminally ill patient.

SUICIDAL IDEATION AND SUICIDE

Assessment and Risk Factors

When suicidal ideation occurs, it is frightening for both the patient and the physician. Suicidal statements may range from an offhand comment resulting from frustration or disgust with the course of treatment ("I can't take the chemotherapy. If I have one more cycle, I'll jump out the window") to a reflection of significant despair and an emergent situation ("I can no longer bear what this disease is doing to my family, and I want all of this to end. Help me!"). Although exploring the seriousness of the thoughts is imperative, suicidal ideation is relatively infrequent in cancer patients. Nevertheless it has been established that cancer patients are at increased risk for suicidal ideation when compared with the general population,[110,130] and suicidal ideation occurs in up to 17% of cancer patients who have pain.[131]

Tables 18–15 and 18–16 describe an approach to the assessment of suicidal ideation in cancer patients. It is important to ask if the patient has made a definite plan. Is the patient stockpiling medication? Does he or she own or have access to a weapon? The factors leading patients to seek a hastened death that seem to have received the broadest empiric support are pain, depression, lack of social support, and cognitive dysfunction. The relationship between pain and the desire for death is often described as a relatively straightforward one: intractable or severe pain is thought to lead to a desire for hastened death and particularly to thoughts of suicide.[132] A recent study of terminally ill cancer patients showed that 76% of patients with moderate to severe pain had a "significant" desire for hastened death, compared to only 46% of patients with mild pain or no pain.[133] Thus, the presence of severe pain is likely to add significantly to a patient's desire for a hastened death.

Psychiatric disorders are frequently present in hospitalized cancer patients who are suicidal. In one review, up to one-third of suicidal cancer patients had a major depression, about 20% suffered from delirium, and 50% were diagnosed with an adjustment disorder with both anxious and depressed features at the time of evaluation.[131,134] The psychiatric consultation data on suicidal cancer patients showed that half of these patients had a diagnosable personality disorder.[134] Depression in the general population is a factor in 50% of all suicides, and those who suffer from depression have a risk of suicide that is 25 times greater than that of the general population.[135,136] The role depression plays in the suicide of cancer patients is equally significant. Among those with advanced illness and progressively impaired physical function, symptoms of severe depression rise to an incidence of 77%.[102] Hopelessness is the key variable that links depression and suicide in the general population. Furthermore, hopelessness is a significantly better predictor of completed suicide than is depression alone.[137,138] Being left to face illness alone creates a sense of isolation and abandonment that is critical to the development of hopelessness. In a recent study, up to 45% of patients had a slight to severe desire for death. Of those patients, 59% met the criteria for major depression and 38% of patients had had a prior episode of major depression. Importantly, 77% of patients had moderate to

TABLE 18–15. Questions to Ask to Assess Suicidal Risk in Cancer Patients

Open with following statement:
"Most patients with cancer have passing thoughts about suicide, such as 'I might do something if it gets bad enough.'"

Question*	Aspect Assessed
Have you ever had thoughts like that? Any thoughts of not wanting to live or that it would be easier if you were to die?	Acknowledgement
Do you have thoughts of suicide? Plan? Have you thought about how you might do it?	Seriousness of risk
Have you ever been depressed or made a suicide attempt?	Prior history
Have you ever been treated for other psychiatric problems, or were you been psychiatrically hospitalized before being diagnosed with cancer?	
Have you had a problem with alcohol or drugs?	Substance use
Have you lost anyone close to you recently (family, friends, co-patients)?	Bereavement

Adapted from Roth AJ, Holland JH.[126]
*Asking does not enhance risk.

severe pain, and overall, patients had lowered social support.[133] Another study documented that hopelessness predicted suicidal ideation above and beyond what might be predicted by the presence of major depression.[139]

It is important that 58% of terminally ill cancer patients classified as having a "significant" desire for death were simultaneously diagnosed with a major depressive episode. It appears that many terminally ill patients who express interest in a hastened death may be suffering from a depressive disorder.[133] It has also been shown that patients with lower levels of social support had more desire for a hastened death than patients with higher levels of social support.[133] In addition, delirium has been increasingly recognized as a factor that may substantially increase the likelihood of suicidal ideation or suicide attempts among medically ill individuals. Because delirium involves a general clouding of both consciousness and the ability to think rationally (as a result of an underlying medical condition), the potential for impulsive or irrational acts (such as a suicide attempt) is considerable.[134]

Other factors that may increase a cancer patient's vulnerability for suicide include fatigue, loss of control, and a sense of helplessness in the face of cancer. "Control" refers to the helplessness induced by symptoms or deficits due to cancer or its treatments, as well as to the excessive need on the part of some patients to be in control of all aspects of living or dying. Impairments or deficits induced by cancer or cancer treatments include loss of mobility, paraplegia, loss of bowel and bladder function, amputation, aphonia, sensory loss, and the inability to eat or swallow. Most distressing to patients is the sense that they are losing control of their minds, especially when they are confused or sedated by medications. The risk of suicide is increased in cancer patients with such physical impairments, especially when accompanied by psychological distress and disturbed interpersonal relationships due to these deficit factors.[140] On the other hand, patients who are accepting and adaptable are much less likely to commit suicide than are cancer patients who exhibit a need to be in control of even the

most minute details of their care. This controlling trait may be prominent in some patients and may cause distress with little provocation.[141]

Fatigue, in the form of the exhaustion of physical, emotional, spiritual, financial, familial, communal, and other resources, increases the risk of suicide for the cancer patient.[134] Cancer is now often a chronic illness. The increased survival is accompanied by increased hospitalizations, complications, and expense. Symptom control thus becomes a prolonged process with frequent advances and setbacks. The dying process also can become extremely long and arduous for all concerned. It is not uncommon for both family members and health care providers to withdraw prematurely from the cancer patient under these circumstances. A suicidal patient can thus feel even more isolated and abandoned. The presence of a strong support system for the patient that may act as an external control of suicidal behavior reduces the risk of cancer-related suicide significantly.

Management

Management of the cancer patient who is suicidal is based on developing and maintaining a supportive relationship and giving the patient a sense of control by helping him or her to focus on that which can still be controlled. It is important to convey the attitude that much can be done

TABLE 18–16. Evaluation of Suicidal Cancer Patients

Establish rapport with an empathic approach.
Ascertain patient's understanding of illness and present symptoms.
Assess mental status (internal control).
Assess vulnerability variables and pain control.
Assess support system (external control).
Obtain history of prior emotional/psychiatric problems.
Obtain family history.
Record prior suicide threats and/or attempts.
Assess suicidal thinking, intent, and plans.
Evaluate need for one-on-one nurse/companion in hospital/home.
Formulate immediate and long-term treatment plans.

Adapted from Breitbart.[131]

to improve the quality (if not the quantity) of life, even if the prognosis is poor. It is important to actively treat the symptoms of pain, nausea, insomnia, anxiety, and depression. If the patient is actively suicidal, a 24-hour companion should be used to monitor the suicidal risk, prevent a possible suicide attempt, and reassure the patient.

Suicide vulnerability factors should be used as a guide to evaluation and management. Once the setting has been made secure, assessment of relevant mental status and adequacy of pain control can begin. Analgesics, neuroleptics, or antidepressant drugs should be used when appropriate to treat agitation, psychosis, major depression, or pain. Underlying causes of delirium or pain should be addressed specifically when possible. Initiation of a crisis intervention–oriented psychotherapeutic approach, mobilizing as much of the patient's support system as possible, is important. A close family member or friend should be involved to support the patient, provide information, and assist in treatment planning. Psychiatric hospitalization can sometimes be helpful but is usually not desirable with the terminally ill patient. Thus, the hospital or home is the setting in which management most often takes place. Although it is appropriate to intervene when medical or psychiatric factors are clearly the driving force in a cancer-related suicide, there are circumstances when usurping control from the patient and family with overly aggressive intervention may be less helpful. This is most evident in the case of those with advanced illness, in which comfort and the control of symptoms are the primary concerns. The goal of the intervention should be to prevent suicide that is driven by desperation. Prolonged suffering due to poorly controlled symptoms leads to such desperation, and it is the consultant's role to provide effective management of such problems as an alternative to the cancer patient's suicide.

SUMMARY

Delirium, severe anxiety, depression, and suicidal ideation are among the most common psychiatric complications encountered in cancer patients. When severe, these disorders require attention as urgently and aggressively as other distressing physical symptoms, such as escalating pain. Early diagnosis and treatment can result in the effective management of these psychiatric emergencies.

REFERENCES

1. Breitbart W, Chochinov HM, Passik SD. Psychiatric aspects of palliative care. In: Doyle D, Hanks GW, MacDonald N, editors. Oxford textbook of palliative medicine. 2nd ed. Oxford: Oxford University Press; 1997. p. 933–54.
2. Portenoy RK, Thaler HT, Kornblith AB, et al. The Memorial symptom assessment scale: an instrument for evaluation of symptom prevalence, characteristics and distress. Eur J Cancer 1994;30A:1326–36.
3. Breitbart W. Psychiatric disorders in patients with progressive medical disease: the importance of diagnosis. Topics in palliative care. Vol. 3. New York (NY): Oxford University Press; 1998. p. 165–73.
4. Strain JJ. Adjustment disorders. In: Holland JC, Rowland JH, editors. Handbook of psychooncology. New York: Oxford University Press; 1989. p. 509–17.
5. Baxter S, Chodorkoff B, Underhill R. Psychiatric emergencies: Dispositional determinants and the validity of the decision to admit. Am J Psychiatry 1968;124:1542–8.
6. Lichter I, Hunt E. The last 24 hours of life. J Palliat Care 1990;6:7–15.
7. Stiefel F, Holland J. Delirium in cancer patients. Int Psychogeriatr 1991;3:333–6.
8. Trzepacz PT, Teague GB, Lipowski ZJ. Delirium and other organic mental disorders in a general hospital. Gen Hosp Psychiatry 1985;7:101–6.
9. Fainsinger RL, MacEachem T, Bruera E, et al. Symptom control during the last week of life in a palliative care unit. J Palliat Care 1991;7:5–11.
10. Bruera E, Fainsinger R, Miller MJ, Kuehn N. The assessment of pain intensity in patients with cognitive failure: a preliminary report. J Pain Symptom Manage 1992;7:267–70.
11. Coyle N, Breitbart W, Weaver S, Portenoy R. Delirium as a contributing factor to "crescendo" pain: three case reports. J Pain Symptom Manage 1994;9:44–7.
12. Breitbart W. Diagnosis and management of delirium in the terminally ill. In: Bruera E, Portenoy RK, editors. Topics in palliative care. Vol 5. New York: Oxford University Press; 2001. p. 303–21.
13. Stiefel F, Fainsinger R, Bruera E. Acute confusional states in patients with advanced cancer. J Pain Symptom Manage 1992;7:94–8.
14. Stiefel FC, Breitbart WS, Holland JC. Corticosteroids in cancer: neuropsychiatric complications. Cancer Invest 1989;7:479–91.
15. Inouye SK. Delirium and other mental status problems in the older patient. In: Goldman L, Bennett JC, editors. Cecil's textbook of medicine. 21st ed. St. Louis (MO): W.B. Saunders; 1999. p. 18–22.
16. Massie MJ, Holland JC, Glass E. Delirium in terminally ill cancer patients. Am J Psychiatry 1983;140:1048–50.
17. Pereira J, Hanson J, Bruera E. The frequency and clinical course of cognitive impairment in patients with terminal cancer. Cancer 1997; 79:835–42.
18. Tune LE. Post-operative delirium. Int Psychogeriatrics 1991;3:325–32.
19. Lipowski ZJ. Transient cognitive disorders (delirium, acute confusional states) in the elderly. Am J Psychiatry 1983;140:1426–36.
20. Knight EB, Folstein MF. Unsuspected emotional and cognitive disturbance in medical patients. Ann Intern Med 1977;87:723–4.
21. Hodkinson HM. Mental impairment in the elderly. J R Coll Physicians 1973;7:305–17.
22. Lipowski ZJ. Delirium: acute brain failure in man. Springfield (IL): Charles C. Thomas; 1980.
23. Lipowski ZJ. Delirium: acute confusional states. New York: Oxford University Press; 1990.
24. American Psychiatric Association. Diagnostic and statistical

manual of mental disorders (DSM-IV). 4th ed. Washington (DC): American Psychiatric Association; 1994.

25. Trzepacz PT, Wise MG. Neuropsychiatric aspects of delirium. In: Yudofsky SC, Hales RE, editors. Textbook of neuropsychiatry. 3rd ed. Washington (DC): American Psychiatric Press; 1997. p. 447–70.

26. Ross CA. CNS arousal systems: possible role in delirium. Int Psychogeriatr 1991;3:353–71.

27. Albert MA, Levkoff SE, Reilly C, et al. The delirium symptom interview: an interview for the detection of delirium symptoms in hospitalized patients. J Geriat Psychiatry Neurol 1991;5:14–21.

28. Inouye SK, Vandyck CH, Alessi CA, et al. Clarifying confusion: the confusion assessment method, a new method for detection of delirium. Ann Intern Med 1990;113:941–8.

29. Trzepacz PT, Baker RW, Greenhouse J. A symptom rating scale for delirium. Psychiatry Res 1988;23:89–97.

30. Trzepacz PT, Mittal D, Torres R, et al. Validity of the delirium rating scale—Revised—98 (DRS-R-98) A41. Proceedings of the 46th Annual Meeting of the Academy of Psychosomatic Medicine; 1999, November 18–21, New Orleans (LA).

31. Williams MA. Delirium/acute confusional states: evaluation devices in nursing. Int Psychogeriatr 1991;3:330–8.

32. Miller PS, Richardson JS, Jyu CA. Association of low serum anticholinergic levels and cognitive impairment by elderly presurgical patients. Am J Psychiatry 1988;145:342–5.

33. Breitbart W, Rosenfeld B, Roth A, et al. The Memorial Delirium Assessment Scale. J Pain Symptom Manage 1997;13:128–37.

34. Hart RP, Best AM, Sessler N, Levenson JL. Abbreviated cognitive test for delirium. J Psychosom Res 1997;43:417–23.

35. Folstein MF, Folstein SE, McHugh PR. "Mini mental state": a practical method of grading the cognitive state of patients for the clinician. J Psychiatr Res 1975;12:189–98.

36. Wolber G, Romaniuk M, Eastman E, Robinson C. Validity of the Short Portable Mental Status Questionnaire with elderly psychiatric patients. J Consult Clin Psychol 1984;52:712–3.

37. Jacobs JC, Bernhard MR, Delgado A, Strain JJ. Screening for organic mental syndromes in the medically ill. Ann Intern Med 1977;86:40–6.

38. Katzman R, Brown T, Fuld P, et al. Validation of a short orientation-memory-concentration test of cognitive impairment. Am J Psychiatry 1983;140:734–9.

39. Tombaugh TN, McIntyre NJ. The mini-mental state examination: a comprehensive review, J Am Geriatic Soc 1992;40:922–35.

40. Bruera E, MacMillan K, Kuehn N, et al. The cognitive effects of the administration of narcotics. Pain 1989;39:13–6.

41. Breitbart W, Cohen K. Delirium in the terminally ill. In: Chochinov HM, Breitbart W, editors. Handbook of psychiatry in palliative medicine. New York (NY): Oxford University Press; 2000. p. 75–90.

42. Tuma R, DeAngelis L. Altered mental status in patients with cancer. Arch Neurol 2000;57:1727–31.

43. Liepzig RM, Goodman H, Gray P, et al. Reversible narcotic-associated mental status impairment in patients with metastatic cancer. Pharmacology 1987;53:47–57.

44. Jellema JG. Hallucinations during sustained-release opioid and methadone administration. Lancet 1987; 2(8555):392.

45. Portenoy RK. Continuous intravenous infusions of opioid drugs. Med Clin North Am 1987;71:233–41.

46. Pereira J, Bruera E. Emerging neuropsychiatric toxicities of opioids. J Pharmaceut Care Pain Symptom Control 1997;5:3.

47. Abrahm JL. Advances in pain management for older adult patients. Clin Geriatr Med 2000;16:269–311.

48. Akechi T, Uchitomi Y, Okamura H, et al. Usage of haloperidol for delirium in cancer patients. Support Care Cancer 1996;4:390–2.

49. Olofsson SM, Weitzner MA, Valentine AD, et al. A retrospective study of the psychiatric management and outcome of delirium in the cancer patient. Support Care Cancer 1996;4:351–7.

50. Breitbart W, Marotta R, Platt MM, et al. A double-blind trial of haloperidol, chlorpramazine, and lorazepam in the treatment of delirium in hospitalized AIDS patients. Am J Psychiatry 1996;153:231–7.

51. Haloperidol prescribing information. Springhouse: McNeil Lab; 1998.

52. Breitbart W, Passik SD. Psychiatric aspects of palliative care. In: Doyle D, Hanks GW, MacDonald N, editors. Oxford textbook of palliative medicine. Oxford: Oxford University Press; 1993. p. 609–26.

53. Bieniek SA, Ownby RL, Penalver A, Dominguez RA. A double-blind study of lorazepam versus the combination of haloperidol and lorazepam in managing agitation. Pharmacotherapy 1998;18:57–62.

54. Battaglia J, Muss S, Rush J, et al. Haloperidol, lorazepam, or both for psychotic agitation: a multicenter, prospective double-blind emergency department study. Am J Emerg Med 1997;15:335–40.

55. Kloke M, Rapp M, Bosse B, Kloke O. Toxicity and/or insufficient analgesia by opioid therapy: risk factors and impact of changing the opioid. A retrospective analysis of 273 patients observed at a single center. Support Care Cancer 2000;8:479–86.

56. Bruera E, Franco JJ, Maltoni M, et al. Changing pattern of agitated impaired mental status in patients with advanced cancer: association with cognitive monitoring, hydration, and opioid rotation. J Pain Symptom Manage 1995;10:287–91.

57. Wilwerding MB, Loprinzi CL, Mailliard JA, et al. A randomized, crossover evaluation of methylphenidate in cancer patients receiving strong narcotics. Support Care Cancer 1995;3:135–8.

58. Modafinil prescribing information. Westchester: Cephalon; 1999.

59. D'Onofrio G, Rathlev NK, Ulrich AS, et al. Lorazepam for the prevention of recurrent seizures related to alcohol. N Engl J Med 1999:340:915–9.

60. Mayo-Smith MF. Pharmacological management of alcohol withdrawal. A meta-analysis and evidence-based practice guideline. American Society of Addiction Medicine Working Group on Pharmacological Management of Alcohol Withdrawal. JAMA 1997;278:144–51.

61. Palestine ML. Drug treatment of alcohol withdrawal syndrome with delirium tremens. A comparison of

haloperidol with mesoridazine and hydroxyzine. Q J Stud Alcohol 1973;34:185–93.

62. Derogatis L, Wise T. Anxiety and depressive disorder in the medical patient. Washington (DC): American Psychiatric Press; 1989.

63. Kessler R, McGonagle K, Zhao S, et al. Lifetime and 12 month prevalence of DSM-III-R psychiatric disorders in the United States. Arch Gen Psychiatry 1994;51:8–19.

64. Massie MJ, Holland JC. The cancer patient with pain: psychiatric complications and their management. Med Clin North Am 1987;71:243–58.

65. Derogatis LR, Morrow GR, Fetting J, et al. The prevalence of psychiatric disorders among cancer patients. JAMA 1983;249:751–7.

66. Maguire P, Lee E, Bevington D, et al. Psychiatric problems in the first year after mastectomy. BMJ 1978;1:963–5.

67. Brandenberg Y, Bolund C, Sigurdardottir V. Anxiety and depressive symptoms at different stages of malignant melanoma. Psychooncology 1992;1:71–8.

68. Shalev A, Screiber S, Galai T, McLoud R. Post-traumatic stress disorder following medical events. Br J Clin Psychol 1993;32:247–53.

69. Payne DK, Massie MJ. Anxiety in palliative care. In: Chochinov HM, Breitbart W, editors. Handbook of psychiatry in palliative medicine. New York (NY): Oxford University Press; 2000. p. 63–74.

70. Braun P, Greenberg D, Dasberg H, Lerer B. Core symptoms of PTSD improved by alprazolam treatment. J Clin Psychiatry 1990;51:236–8.

71. Roth AJ, Massie MJ, Redd WH. Consultation to the cancer patient. In: Jacobson JL, Jacobson AM, editors. Psychiatric secrets. Philadelphia: Hanley & Belfus; 1995.

72. Roth AJ, Breitbart W. Psychiatric emergencies in terminally ill cancer patients. Hematol Oncol Clin North Am 1996;10:235–59.

73. Koenig TW, Clark MR. Advances in comprehensive pain management. Psychiatr Clin North Am 1996;19:589–611.

74. Massie MJ, Gagnon P, Holland JC. Depression and suicide in patients with cancer. J Pain Symptom Manage 1994;9:325–40.

75. Goldberg RJ, Posner DA. Anxiety in the medically ill. In: Stoudemire A, Fogel BS, editors. Psychiatric care of the medical patient. Oxford: Oxford University Press; 1993. p. 87–104.

76. Noyes R, Holt CS, Massie MJ. Anxiety disorders. In: Holland JC, Breitbart WS, Jacobsen PJ, et al, editors. Textbook of psycho-oncology. New York (NY): Oxford University Press; 1998. p. 548–63.

77. Alter CL, Pelcovitz D, Axelrod A, et al. The identification of PTSD in cancer survivors. Psychosomatics 1996;37:137–43.

78. Jacobsen PB, Sadler IJ, Booth-Jones M, et al. Predictors of posttraumatic stress disorder symptomatology following bone marrow transplantation for cancer. J Consult Clin Psychol 2002;70:235–40.

79. Gorfinkle K, Redd WH. Behavioral control of anxiety, distress, and learned aversions in pediatric oncology. In: Breitbart W, Holland JC, editors. Psychiatric aspects of symptom management in cancer patients. Washington (DC): American Psychiatric Press; 1994. p. 129–46.

80. Teboul E, Chouinard G. A guide to benzodiazepine selection. Part I. Pharmacologic aspects. Can J Psychiatry 1990;35:700–10.

81. Hobbs WR, Rall TW, Verdoorn TA. Hypnotics and sedatives: ethanol. In: Hardman JG, Limbird LE, Molinoff PB, Ruddon RW, editors. Goodman and Gilman's the pharmacological basis of therapeutics. 9th ed. New York: McGraw-Hill; 1996. p. 361–96.

82. Verborgh C, De Coster R, D'Haese J, et al. Effects of chlordiazepoxide on opioid-induced antinociception and respiratory depression in restrained rats. Pharmacol Biochem Behav 1998;59:663–70.

83. Massie MJ, Holland JC. Depression and the cancer patient. J Clin Psychiatry 1990;51:12–7.

84. Juergens SM. Benzodiazepines and addiction. Psychiatr Clin North Am 1993;16:75–86.

85. Tanaka K, Shima Y, Kakinuma R, et al. Effect of nebulized morphine in cancer patients with dyspnea: pilot study. Jpn J Clin Oncol 1999;29:600–3.

86. Papiris S, Galavottii V, Sturani C. Effects of beta-agonists on breathlessness and exercise tolerance in patients with chronic obstructive pulmonary disease. Respiration 1986;49:101–8.

87. Colice GL. Nebulized bronchodilators for outpatient management of stable chronic obstructive pulmonary disease. Am J Med 1996;100:11S–8S.

88. Bruera E, MacEachern T, Ripamonti C, et al. Subcutaneous morphine for dyspnea in cancer patients. Ann Intern Med 1993;119:906–7.

89. Chandler S. Nebulized opioids to treat dyspnea. Am J Hosp Palliat Care 1999;16:418–22.

90. Cherry NI, Portenoy RK. Sedation in the treatment of refractory symptoms: guidelines for evaluation and treatment. J Palliat Care 1994;10:31–8.

91. Dumon JP, Catteau J, Lanvin F, Dupuis BA. Randomized, double-blind, crossover, placebo-controlled comparison of propranolol and betaxolol in the treatment of neuroleptic induced akathisia. Am J Psychiatry 1992;149:647–50.

92. Wells BG, Cold JA, Marken PA, et al. A placebo-controlled trial of nadolol in the treatment of neuroleptic-induced akathisia. J Clin Psychiatry 1991:52:255–60.

93. Fleishhacker WW, Roth SD, Kane JM. The pharmacologic treatment of neuroleptic induced akathisia. J Clin Psychopharmacol 1990;10:12–21.

94. Burke AL, Diamond PL, Hulbert J, et al. Terminal restlessness—its management and the role of midazolam. Med J Aust 1991;155:485–7.

95. McNamara P, Minton P, Twycross RG. The use of midazolam in palliative care. Palliat Med 1991;5:244–9.

96. Passik SD, Breitbart WS. Depression in patients with pancreatic carcinoma: diagnostic and treatment issues. Cancer 1996;78 Suppl 3:615–26.

97. Dunkel-Schetter C, Feinstein LG, Taylor SE, et al. Patterns of coping with cancer. Health Psychol 1992;11:79–87.

98. Harrison J, Maguire P. Predictors of psychiatric morbidity in cancer patients. Br J Psychiatry 1994;165:593–8.

99. Watson M, Green S, Rowden L, et al. Relationships between emotional control, adjustment to cancer and depression and anxiety in breast cancer patients. Psychol Med 1991;21:51–7.

100. Lynch ME. The assessment and prevalence of affective disorders in advanced cancer. J Palliat Care 1995;11:10–8.

101. Wilson KG, Chochinov HM, de Faye BJ, Breitbart W. Diagnosis and management of depression in palliative care. In: Chochinov HM, Breitbart W, editors. Handbook of psychiatry in palliative medicine. New York (NY): Oxford University Press; 2000. p. 25–49.

102. Bukberg J, Penman D, Holland JC. Depression in hospitalized cancer patients. Psychosom Med 1984;46:199–212.

103. Plumb MM, Holland JC. Comparative studies of psychological functioning patients with advanced cancer. Psychosom Med 1977;3 9:264–76.

104. Endicott J. Measurement of depression in patients with cancer. Cancer 1983;53:2243–8.

105. Passik SD, Dugan W, McDonald MV, et al. Oncologists' recognition of depression in their patients with cancer. J Clin Oncol 1998;16:1594–600.

106. Massie MJ, Holland JC, Straker N. Psychotherapeutic interventions. In: Holland JC, Rowland JH, editors. Handbook of psychooncology. New York: Oxford University Press; 1989. p. 455–69.

107. Spiegel D, Bloom JR. Group therapy and hypnosis reduce metastatic breast carcinoma pain. Psychosom Med 1983;4:333–9.

108. Spiegel D, Bloom JR, Yalom ID. Group support for patients with metastatic cancer: a randomized prospective outcome study. Arch Gen Psychiatry 1981;38:527–33.

109. Holland JC, Morrow GR, Schmale A, et al. A randomized clinical trial of alprazolam versus progressive muscle relaxation in cancer patients with anxiety and depressive symptoms. J Clin Oncol 1991;9:1004–11.

110. Massie MJ, Shakin EJ. Management of depression and anxiety. In: Breitbart W, Holland JC, editors. Psychiatric aspects of symptom management in cancer patients. Washington (DC): American Psychiatric Press; 1994.

111. Costa D, Mogos I, Toma T. Efficacy and safety of mianserin in the treatment of depression of women with cancer. Acta Psychiatr Scand 1985;72:85–92.

112. Popkin MK, Callie SAL, Mackenzie TB. The outcome of antidepressant use in the medically ill. Arch Gen Psychiatry 1985;42:1160–3.

113. Purohit DR, Navlakha PL, Modi R, et al. The role of antidepressants in hospitalized cancer patients. J Assoc Physicians India 1978;26:245–8.

114. Rifkin A, Reardon G, Siris SE, et al. Trimipramine in physical illness with depression. J Clin Psychiatry 1985;46:4–8.

115. Peretti S, Judge R, Hindmarch I. Safety and tolerability considerations: tricyclic antidepressants vs. selective serotonin reuptake inhibitors. Acta Psychiatr Scand Suppl 2000;403:17–25.

116. Kando JC, Wells BG, Hayes PE. Depressive disorders. In: Dipiro JT, Talbert R, Yee G, et al, editors. Pharmacotherapy: a pathophysiologic approach. 4th ed. Stamford: Appleton & Lange; 1999. p. 1141–60.

117. Fluoxetine prescribing information. Indianapolis: Dista Products; 1995.

118. Sertraline prescribing information. New York: Roerig Division of Pfizer; 1997.

119. Paroxetine prescribing information. Philadelphia: SmithKline Beecham Pharmaceuticals; 1995.

120. Venlafaxine prescribing information. Philadelphia: Wyeth-Ayerst Laboratories; 1995.

121. Buproprion prescribing information. Greenville: Glaxo Wellcome; 2000.

122. Nefazadone prescribing information. Wallingford (CT): Bristol-Myers Squibb; 1995.

123. Clayton AH, McGarvey EL, Abouesh AI, Pinkerton RC. Substitution of an SSRI with buproprion sustained release following SSRI-induced sexual dysfunction. J Clin Psychiatry 2001;62:185–90.

124. Montejo AL, Llorea G, Izquierdo JA, Rico-Villademoros F. Incidence of sexual dysfunction associated with antidepressant agents: a prospective multicenter study of 1022 outpatients. Spanish Working Group for the Study of Psychotropic-related Sexual Dysfunction. J Clin Psychiatry 2001;62(S3):10–21.

125. Mirtazipine prescribing information. West Orange (NJ): Organon; 2000.

126. Roth AJ, Holland JH. Treatment of depression in cancer patients. Prim Care Cancer 1994;14:23–9.

127. Pereira J, Bruera E. Depression with psychomotor retardation: diagnostic challenges and the use of psychostimulants. J Palliat Med 2001;4:15–21.

128. Macleod AD. Methylphenidate in terminal depression. J Pain Symptom Manage 1998;16: 193–8.

129. Breitbart W, Mermelstein H. Pemoline: an alternative psychostimulant for the management of depressive disorders in cancer patients. Psychosomatics 1992;33:352–6.

130. Hietanen P, Lonnqvist J. Cancer and suicide. Ann Oncol 1991;2:19–23.

131. Breitbart W. Cancer pain and suicide. In: Foley KM, Bonica JJ, Ventafridda V, editors. Second International Congress on Cancer Pain. Advances in pain research and therapy. Vol 16. New York: Raven Press; 1990. p. 399–412.

132. Foley K. Pain, physician-assisted suicide, and euthanasia. Pain Forum 1995;4:163–78.

133. Chochinov HM, Wilson KG, Enns M, et al. Desire for death in the terminally ill. Am J Psychiatry 1995;152:1185–91.

134. Breitbart W. Suicide in cancer patients. Oncology 1987;1:49–54.

135. Guze S, Robins E. Suicide and primary affective disorders. Br J Psychiatry 1970;117:437–8.

136. Robins E, Murphy G, Wilkinson RH, et al. Some clinical considerations in the prevention of suicide based on 134 successful suicides. Am J Public Health 1950;49:888–9.

137. Kovacs M, Beck AT, Weissman A. Hopelessness: an indication of suicidal risk. Suicide 1975;5:98–103.

138. Levine PM, Silberfarb PM, Lipowski ZJ. Mental disorders in cancer patients: a study of 100 psychiatric referrals. Cancer 1978;42:1385–90.

139. Chochinov HM, Wilson KG, Enns M, Lander S. Depression, hopelessness, and suicidal ideation in the terminally ill. Psychosomatics 1998;39:366–70.

140. Farberow NL, Ganzler S, Cuter F, et al. An eight year survey of hospital suicides. Suicide Life Threat Behav 1971;1:184–201.

141. Farberow NL, Schneiderman ES, Leonard CV. Suicide among general medical and surgical hospital patients with malignant neoplasms. Medical Bulletin, vol 9. Washington (DC): US Veterans Administration; 1963. p. 1–11.

CHAPTER 19

ORTHOPEDIC EMERGENCIES

SAI-CHING JIM YEUNG, MD, PHD, RPH

Skeletal complications of cancer and the treatment of cancer primarily consist of metastases to bones and metabolic bone diseases (osteoporosis and osteomalacia) and their manifestations as pain, fracture, loss of mechanical function, neurologic deficits, and vascular deficits. Cancer patients are also more susceptible to trauma from falls because of their debilitated weakened state or other complications of malignancy. In the presence of metastatic disease or decreased bone strength due to metabolic bone diseases, fractures can occur with minimal forces that are not traumatic to a normal person.

Musculoskeletal infections, especially in immunocompromised cancer patients, can present as emergent problems. This topic is also briefly discussed in this chapter.

SKELETAL COMPLICATIONS OF CANCER AND CANCER TREATMENT

Pathophysiology

Turnover of the bone matrix is the joint function of osteoblasts and osteoclasts. Osteoblasts develop from pluripotent mesenchymal stem cells.[1] Osteoblasts that are forming bone are polarized cuboidal mononuclear cells whereas those that are not actively forming bone become flat and elongated. The major products of osteoblasts are type I collagen and alkaline phosphatase. Matrix secretion determines the volume of bone, but bone density is determined by mineralization of the matrix by osteoblasts. Osteoclasts are large multinucleated cells.[2,3] The surface of normal bone is covered by a layer (1 to 2 microns thick) of unmineralized collagen matrix covered by bone lining cells. Osteoclasts cannot attach to this collagenous layer by themselves. Others cells must secrete collagenase to remove this layer before osteoclasts can attach and can dissolve the bone minerals in the acidic environment of the resorption site.

Bone is one of the most common sites of metastasis. Bone metastases are particularly common in certain types of cancer, such as myeloma and breast, prostate, and lung cancers. Growth factors in the bone marrow cavity during the normal bone remodeling process provide an environment that promotes colonization by metastatic tumor cells. The bone matrix acts as a rich store of immobilized growth factors that are released during bone resorption. Bone destruction is mediated by the osteoclast rather than by the tumor cells directly. A positive feedback cycle for the growth of osteolytic metastases has been described: cancer cells secrete osteoclast-stimulating factors through bone marrow stromal cells; bone resorption releases growth factors from the bone matrix; and locally released growth factors stimulate the growth of cancer cells.[4]

As a specific example, transforming growth factor beta (TGF-β) is released by osteoclastic bone resorption. Bone-derived TGF-β promotes osteolytic bone metastases by inducing cancer production of parathyroid hormone–related protein (PTHrP), an activator of osteoclasts.[5] In breast cancer cells, TGF-β stimulates PTHrP secretion through both Smad and p38 mitogen-activated protein (MAP) kinase signaling pathways. Other factors released from bone matrix may also act on tumor cells in bone in similar manners.[4]

For the cancer cells to metastasize to bone, the following processes must be involved: invasion of cancer into blood vessels, migration through the circulation to the bone, migration into the bone marrow cavity, and formation of cancer cell colonies. E-cadherin mediates cell-cell adhesion between identical cells and may play an important role in the detachment of cells from the primary tumor. Decreased E-cadherin expression in cancers (eg, breast cancer and prostate cancer) allows cancer cells to detach and metastasize. The cancer cells also release a variety of proteolytic enzymes, including metalloproteinases (MMPs),[6] serine proteases, and cysteine proteases, to break down the extracellular matrix.

Clinical Manifestations

Pain. Bone pain may result from the mechanical or chemical stimulation of pain receptors in the periosteum and endosteum. Pressure or stretching from expanding tumor mass, mechanical instability, pathologic fracture, invasion or compression of neurologic tissue, cytokine release, and microfractures are all contributory. Pain that is worsened by movement, weight bearing, or changes in body position or posture often results from metastasis involving the spine, pelvis, and femurs. This incidental pain is difficult to manage and often requires orthopedic or surgical stabilization.

Loss of Mechanical Function. Fractures result in the inability of muscles attaching to that piece of bone to perform normal mechanical functions. Losses of strength, support, and movements are observed. These symptoms are most obvious in fractures in the limbs.

Neurovascular Compromise. Displaced long-bone fractures may compress or injure the adjacent nerves or arteries and threaten the function and viability of the part of the limb distal to the fracture. Displacement of vertebral bodies into the spinal canal may lead to spinal-cord compression. Compression fractures of vertebral bodies may narrow the neural foramina and lead to spinal nerve root compression or radiculopathy.

Etiology

Metastasis. Among malignant diseases of the bone, bone metastasis is far more frequent than primary bone tumors.[7] Approximately one half to two thirds of metastatic breast, prostate, and lung cancer patients will develop bone metastases in the course of the disease.[8] Because of the high prevalence of breast, prostate, and lung cancers, these three cancers account for about 80% of cases of metastatic bone disease.[9,10] Radiologically, breast cancer metastases to the bone usually exhibit a mixed osteolytic and osteosclerotic appearance. In contrast, prostate cancer causes predominantly osteosclerotic lesions.

Fractures in long bones usually require surgical treatment. The survival rate after surgical treatment is about 30% at 1 year, but some patients may survive for more than 3 years.[11] For patients with breast cancer, the survival rate may be up to 20% at 5 years.[12] Because post-surgical survival is significant, surgical treatment is indicated in most cases.

Trauma. Cancer patients may become deconditioned cachectic, and have decreased muscle strength. They become at high risk for falls. Brain metastases can lead to seizures, muscle weakness, and impaired balance. Decreased oral intake and dehydration can lead to postural hypotension and syncope. All of these factors, which contribute to falls, may be associated with advanced malignancy, poor nutrition, senility, and the use of narcotic, antihypertensive, or sedative medications.[13]

Other than falls, motor vehicle accidents are perhaps the most common cause of trauma. Patients on narcotic treatments for pain related to cancer should be advised not to drive under the influence of narcotic or sedating medications.

Osteoporosis. Antineoplastic therapy may upset the balance of bone formation and bone resorption in a variety of ways.[14] The easiest of these ways to conceptualize is enhanced osteoclast resorption. Examples include cytokine (eg, interleukin-2)-stimulated osteoclast resorption or a premature menopause causing enhanced bone resorption. Although less easy to characterize, it seems likely that chemotherapy has direct toxic effects on osteoblast function, with consequent decreased bone formation. It is also important to recognize that these effects occur against a background of cancer and that the production of substances by the tumor (eg, PTHrP, lymphotoxin, or interleukin-1 and interleukin-6) may contribute to the clinical picture of bone loss.

In most cases, it is not clear whether bone loss is due to the therapy, the underlying disease process (including the impact of cachexia, malnutrition, and poor calcium and vitamin D intake), or a combination of the two.[15] Bone loss is prominent in patients with disorders affecting hematopoietic cells.[16] For instance, radiographic changes and bone pain are frequent presenting abnormalities of acute lymphocytic leukemia (ALL); this suggests a direct impact of ALL on bones.[17] In the absence of an adequate control group and control for nutritional variables, it is difficult to determine the relative importance of anticancer agents and the primary disease process in causing osteoporosis.

Effects of Methotrexate. Osteoporosis (generalized or localized) has been observed in children who are receiving methotrexate therapy for ALL.[18] The patients developed severe osteoporosis, distal-extremity pain, and associated fractures. The bone pain resolved promptly upon the discontinuation of methotrexate, but radiographic changes in bone persisted for longer periods. In general, the osteoporosis improves significantly after the cessation of methotrexate therapy.[19,20] Because ALL can cause osteopenia and bone pain independently[16] (perhaps by bone infiltration and cytokine secretion), it is difficult to assess the independent roles of disease and drug in these small study series.

Effects of Platinum Compounds. Of 16 ALL patients whose treatment included cisplatin or carboplatin, 11 evidenced bone pain, limping, and fracture and had bone mineral densities that averaged 2.3 standard deviations below normal.[21] The known effects of platinum compounds on calcium homeostasis include hypomagnesemia, hypocalcemia, and renal calcium wasting. These effects may enhance the bone loss that is associated with ALL.[22]

Effects of Combination Chemotherapy. Most combination regimens for hematopoietic malignancies include high-dose glucocorticoids or methotrexate; both agents affect bone formation and resorption. In one study, 29 men in complete remission following treatment for Hodgkin's disease had reduced cortical and trabecular bone mineral density. There was no correlation in this group with the time since chemotherapy, with the chemotherapeutic regimens, or with the number of cycles of chemotherapy.[23] Hypogonadism resulting from chemotherapy, high-dose glucocorticoid therapy, and Hodgkin's disease per se were cited as possible causes of bone loss in these men. In another study of Hodgkin's disease patients, no significant bone loss was found in men, but chemotherapy-induced menopause was associated with significant bone loss in women.[24] In young women who were treated for lymphoma, chemotherapy-induced menopause was a more important cause of osteoporosis than were cytotoxic agents and glucocorticoids.[25]

Adjuvant chemotherapy for breast carcinoma (usually involving 5-fluorouracil, cyclophosphamide, and doxorubicin or methotrexate) is associated with low bone mass. Chemotherapy-induced premature menopause appears to be a major factor. Women with adjuvant chemotherapy–induced ovarian failure have decreased cortical and trabecular bone mass when compared with age-matched controls without breast carcinoma.[26] The avoidance of estrogen replacement therapy in young women with breast carcinoma and premature ovarian failure compounds the problem and portends a major future health problem.

Effects of Bone Marrow Transplantation. Bone marrow transplantation has profound effects on the marrow-bone interface. Patients receive large doses of cytotoxic drugs[27] and irradiation[28] designed to eradicate all cells in the marrow. It is therefore not surprising that bone-forming cells are also affected. In study patients undergoing bone marrow transplantation, profound effects on bone biomarkers were observed. The serum osteocalcin and alkaline phosphatase levels, thought to be indicators of bone formation, were low. N-telopeptides, bone collagen degradation products thought to be indicative of bone resorption, were increased.[29]

Effects of Androgen and Estrogen Deficiency. Lack of sex hormone is a risk factor of osteoporosis in both males and females. Androgent deprivation therapy is given to male patients with androgen-dependent prostate cancer. Very often, cancer treatments lead to gonadal failure (eg, cytotoxic chemotherapy, orchiectomy for testicular cancer, oophorectomy for ovarian cancer, etc.). Contraindications to sex hormone replacement in hypogonadal patients with prostate cancer and breast cancer contribute to the development of osteoporosis.

Osteomalacia or Rickets. Osteomalacia results from the failure of the organic bone matrix to mineralize normally. Rickets is a unique variant in which there is abnormal mineralization and maturation of the growth plate at the epiphysis in children. The most common cause for these two conditions is a decrease in the concentration of serum calcium and/or in phosphorus concentration. Nutritional deficiency and renal wasting of phosphorus are common causes. Other contributing factors include systemic acidosis and drugs such as anticonvulsants and aluminum.

Effects of Ifosfamide. Ifosfamide causes tubular damage that leads to renal phosphate wasting, hypophosphatemia, and rickets.[30] The toxic effects of ifosfamide on renal tubular function include Fanconi's syndrome in adults and children.[31,32] Tubular damage is seen most commonly with doses of ≥ 50 g/m^2 or when ifosfamide is used in combination with cisplatin. Rickets is reported most commonly in the pediatric population.[33,34]

Effects of Estramustine. In a prospective trial which studied patients with prostrate cancer metastatic to bone and which compared treatment with estramustine and clodronate to treatment with estramustine and placebo, both treatment groups developed hypocalcemia, secondary hyperparathyroidism, hypophosphatemia, and osteomalacia, with normal vitamin D levels.[35] Bone resorption, quantitated by bone biopsy at 3 months, was decreased in both groups. The proposed mechanism for this striking clinical picture is the suppression of bone resorption by estramustine, alone or in combination with clodronate, leading to hypocalcemia, secondary hyperparathyroidism, with renal phosphate wasting.

Osteonecrosis. Avascular necrosis of bone has been reported as a complication of chemotherapy for ALL.[36] About 0.5 to 1% of study patients developed this complication within 3 years of the therapy,[36] but the incidence may be much higher in chemotherapy protocols with very high doses of glucocorticoids.[37] Osteonecrosis may also be induced by radiation. The differential diagnosis of bone pain in areas of prior external-beam irradiation includes metastatic disease to bone and radiation osteonecrosis. The failure to diagnose osteonecrosis with insufficiency fractures may lead to further irradiation, worsening the problem and causing prolonged morbidity.[38]

Diagnosis: Imaging and Tests

Bone Mineral Density Measurement. Bone mineral density measurement by dual-energy x-ray absorptiometry can give a risk assessment for the likelihood of fracture. This information can help determine the need and timing of therapy and determine the effectiveness of therapy.

Plain-Film Radiography. Radiographic diagnosis of fracture usually requires radiography of the affected bone in at least two views or planes. Full-length radiography of the affected bone may help identify concurrent lesions, and this information may have a significant impact on the planning of surgical repair.

Radiographic Computed Tomography. Computed tomography (CT) can evaluate the three-dimensional integrity of the bone and the soft-tissue component of the tumor. Fragments of bone in the spinal canal and pathologic acetabular fractures are ideally studied with CT.

Magnetic Resonance Imaging. Magnetic resonance imaging (MRI) is also a three-dimensional imaging study with good resolution, especially of soft tissue, and can help differentiate among malignancy, insufficiency fracture, infection, osteoporotic compression fracture, degenerative joint disease, and other benign bone diseases.[39] It is ideal for the evaluation of spinal-cord compression and solitary lesions that need to be treated with a wide excision.

Radionuclide Bone Scanning. Radionuclide bone scintigraphy is the first choice in the routine follow-up of asymptomatic cancer patients because of its sensitivity and the ease with which it can survey the whole skeleton.[39] Radionuclide bone scanning uses technetium 99m (^{99m}Tc). Preoperative bone scanning can identify occult bone metastasis. Areas of impending fracture can be identified by radiography and by "hot spots" on bone scans. Thus, fixation of the impending fracture and the pathologic fractures can be performed during one anesthetic administration.

Fine-Needle Biopsy. Because of overlap in diagnostic imaging characteristics, biopsy of affected areas is sometimes necessary to differentiate between malignant and nonmalignant lesions. Bone aspiration cytology performed by radiologists and cytopathologists together is highly accurate in diagnosing bone lesions.[39]

Angiography. Angiography is indicated for the evaluation of vascular tumors, and preoperative embolization may reduce blood loss and complications during surgical interventions.

Bone Metabolism Markers. Urinary excretions of calcium and hydroxyproline are the conventional markers of bone resorption. They can detect only large changes in bone resorption, and both lack sensitivity and specificity. Pyridinoline cross-links are more specific for bone turnover and are not influenced by collagen present in diet. For instance, breast cancer patients with bone metastasis have increased levels of pyridinium cross-links. Pyridinium cross-links excretion can also be increased because of the artificial menopause caused by chemotherapy. In breast cancer, serum osteocalcin can be used to detect the presence of bone metastasis, but the diagnostic value of osteocalcin is questionable. In multiple myeloma, osteocalcin correlates with bone formation. All patients with decreased osteocalcin levels have severe lytic bone lesions, and a low osteocalcin level is associated with poor survival. An increase in the osteocalcin during treatment is a good indicator of treatment efficacy, and a decreased level correlates with disease progression. In patients with prostate cancer and hormone-refractory disease, urinary deoxypyridinoline values with a cutoff at 38 picomolar/millimolar (pM/mM) creatinine can predict 51% of skeletal events with an 8% false-positive rate.[40]

Management

The management of orthopedic oncologic emergencies should take several factors into consideration. The stage of cancer, the life expectancy, the patient's functional status, the severity of symptoms, and the natural history of the underlying malignancy all affect the risks and benefits of surgical orthopedic interventions. The surgical treatment of terminal patients should be performed only when the intervention will improve the patient's quality of life. In the absence of acute fractures or other complications, metabolic bone diseases related to cancer or cancer treatments are seldom pessing issues in emergency centers, but they warrant referrals to endocrinologists for further evaluation and treatment.

Acute Management. Acute management of fracture usually occurs in an emergency center. Prompt relief of pain should be accomplished, and a rapid assessment of neurovascular integrity should be performed. Opiates are usually effective in controlling acute pain. The doses of opiates may need to be adjusted, based on whether or not the patient is already on high doses of opiates for chronic pain due to the underlying malignant disease. Nonsteroidal anti-inflammatory agents may also be used, provided that there is no need for emergent surgical intervention and that there is no active bleeding, thrombocytopenia, platelet dysfunction, or renal insufficiency. Immobilization and traction will help to decrease pain and further damage at the fracture site. If there is neurovascular compromise or active bleeding, emergent orthopedic consultation should be obtained.

Limb and Pelvic Fractures. About 90% of pathologic fractures that require surgery involve the femur (Figure 19–1), the humerus, or the hip joint (Figure 19–2). The survival time of patients with pathologic fractures may

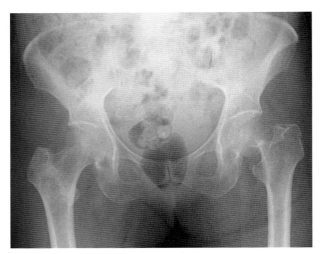

Figure 19–1. A left femoral neck fracture after a fall.

range from several months to over 2 years,[11] and a prompt restoration of full function should be attempted to improve the patient's quality of life. The restoration of function and pain relief can be achieved by the surgical stabilization of the fracture, which allows the patient to return to an ambulatory status, often without the need of external support. When the general condition of the patient is fairly good, complete resection of the metastases should be performed to avoid postoperative radiotherapy. In patients with advanced cancer and poor general condition, intramedullary nailing may be performed, without resection of the metastasis, to achieve pain relief and partial restoration of limb function.[41] Pathologic fracture is unusual when two-thirds (or less) of the diameter of a long bone is affected by a lytic lesion. Above two-thirds of the diameter, the fracture rate increases to about 80%. Prophylactic surgical fixation of a bone at risk (before the occurrence of a fracture) or prophylactic surgical intervention of an impending fracture is advisable if the patient does not have poor surgical risks. Two proposed criteria for prophylactic fixation of the femur include a lytic lesion > 2.5 cm or destroying > 50% of the femoral cortex and a lesion causing disabling local pain with weight bearing, despite radiotherapy.[42] The surgical fixation of pathologic fractures in long bones does not require excessive operative time or extended hospitalization (as compared with the surgical fixation of impending fractures) and has an acceptable risk-benefit ratio.[43]

The surgical techniques for internal fixation or prosthetic replacement take into consideration the fact that destructive bony lysis often extends well beyond the fracture site and that bony union may not occur after irradiation. Intramedullary fixation using an interlocking device, either proximally or distally, is preferable to the extramedullary fixation of fractures.[44] In the lower extremities, such fixation must be able to bear the weight of the body. The upper extremity must be able to withstand the distractive forces that are inherent in lifting and pulling and the heavy compressive forces in patients who require crutches or other assisting devices for walking. The fixation of upper- or lower-extremity long-bone fractures can usually be performed with minimal blood loss or morbidity. Pain relief can be achieved in 96% of patients after the internal fixation of pathologic long-bone fractures.[45]

In contrast, fractures and impending fractures that involve the acetabulum or periacetabular pelvis require extensive surgical intervention. The joint reconstruction is associated with increased risk for morbidity and complications. Therefore, the anticipated prognosis for survival based on the underlying malignancy should be greater for patients with acetabular or periacetabular fractures than for patients with long-bone fractures, so that the benefits can outweigh the risks. About 80% of patients with acetabular or periacetabular fractures attain good or excellent relief of pain after surgery.[45]

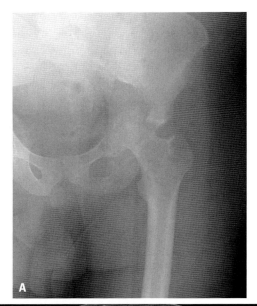

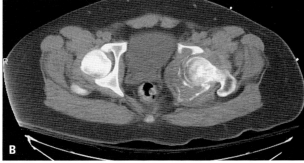

Figure 19–2. A: Radiograph showing a pathologic fracture of the left acetabulum. B: Computed tomography (CT) scan showing tumor involvement of the left acetabular region in the left pelvis.

Vertebral Fracture. Vertebral body fractures are common in patients with bone metastasis and osteoporosis. There is a loss of height of the vertebrae (Figure 19–3). Acute vertebral collapse is associated with severe pain, which is usually a combination of localized bone pain and the compression of nerve roots. A vertebral fracture with extension of tumor, displacement of the vertebral bodies (Figure 19–4), or retropulsion of bone into the spinal-canal can lead to spinal cord compression (see Chapter 11, Neurologic Emergencies). Vertebral fracture from metastatic disease is often difficult to distinguish from osteoporotic collapse. Most vertebral metastases can be managed conservatively. Those with progressive neurologic compromise require surgical decompression, and those with spinal instability require surgical stabilization. Surgical techniques must consider the adverse effect of local postoperative irradiation. About 80% of patients with neurologic compromise secondary to vertebral malignancy will have significant neurologic improvement after decompression and stabilization, and even more patients can experience good or excellent relief of spinal pain and can regain the ability to walk.[45] Vertebroplasty or kyphoplasty with methylmethacrylate injection (see Figure 19–3) may be helpful in relieving pain and improving posture when surgical intervention is not required.

Rib Fracture. Rib fractures are a common cause of chest pain (Figure 19–5). Such fractures rarely cause serious

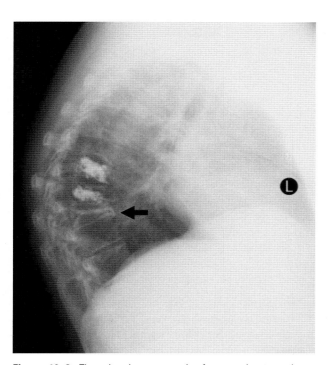

Figure 19–3. Thoracic spine compression fractures due to myeloma. Note that two of the vertebral bodies have been injected with methylmethacrylate for vertebroplasty.

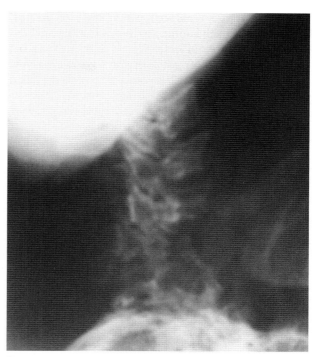

Figure 19–4. Pathologic fracture of the lower cervical vertebrae in a breast cancer patient who presented with acute neck pain and intermittent symptoms of spinal-cord compression.

sequelae and can be effectively treated by analgesics and a single course of radiotherapy. In extreme cases, multiple rib fractures can impair the integrity of the chest wall and result in impaired respiratory function. Radiation-induced necrosis of the bone following radiation therapy to the chest wall for breast cancer is another cause of rib fracture in addition to bone metastasis.

Tumor-Specific Treatment Considerations. In one report, breast cancer patients with pathologic fractures from metastatic carcinoma of the breast had a mean survival of about 2 years after the surgical management of their fractures.[45] Radiation therapy is indicated for those lesions that do not respond to endocrine therapy or chemotherapy, for sites of pathologic fracture after fixation, and for areas (such as the femoral neck and vertebral bodies) that are prone to complications in the event of tumor progression. Prophylactic surgery is recommended to avoid fracture in patients with large lesions of the hip or femur, especially those that remain symptomatic despite radiotherapy. Pathologic fractures of long bones are treated by a combination of methylmethacrylate and either intramedullary rods or plate fixation.

Renal Cell Carcinoma. Some patients with renal cell carcinoma and a solitary metastasis may have a 5-year survival rate of 20 to 30% after resection of the metastasis. However, the treatment modalities for patients with widely metastatic renal cell carcinoma are limited. Response rates to chemotherapy, hormonal therapy, and biologic response modifiers are low. Surgery or radiation therapy is indicated for patients with a reasonably long expected survival time. These tumors are very vascular; thus, preoperative embolization and proximal vascular control are important to avoid intraoperative hemorrhage.[46–48] Cryosurgery may also be used, to decrease bleeding and to achieve local tumor control.[49]

Colo-rectal Cancer. Gastrointestinal cancer metastases are rare, and pathologic fractures are rare. Radiation therapy is the most effective mode of palliation.

Lung Cancer. The average survival time of patients with lung cancer and bone metastasis is only a few months. Palliative radiotherapy usually provides pain relief. Surgical treatments of fractures are aimed at the quick restoration of function to improve the quality of life of the patient.

Thyroid Cancer. Bone metastasis occurs in about 10% of patients with thyroid cancer. Bone metastasis seems to be more common with cases of follicular thyroid carcinoma. Bone metastasis without fractures is treated primarily with radioactive iodide. Sites of severe bone pain can be managed with local external-beam radiation therapy to provide pain relief. Pathologic fractures are rare. Preoperative angiography and embolization may be warranted to reduce intraoperative bleeding.

Melanoma. Skeletal metastasis in melanoma patients carries a grave prognosis and a mean survival of less than 4 months. Palliative radiotherapy provides pain relief.

Prostate Cancer. Prostate cancer is the most common cause of bone metastasis in men. Prostate cancer patients have the longest survival rate among cancer patients with bone metastasis. Metastatic prostate cancer most often involves the spine and pelvis. Pathologic fractures are uncommon. Surgical management is guided by the extent and location of tumor involvement. Localized external-beam radiation will palliate skeletal disease at most sites. Pain from osteoblastic metastases can be significantly improved by both external radiotherapy and strontium 89 (^{89}Sr) whereas lytic metastases are responsive only to external irradiation.[50] In some cases, it may be difficult to distinguish Paget's disease from metastatic lesions or a solitary metastasis from a primary sarcoma.

Leukemia, Lymphoma, and Myeloma. Systemic therapy often relieves bone pain. However, localized radiotherapy is indicated for sites that are refractory to drug therapy and for metastases involving the spine. Radiation can provide excellent palliation for patients with symptomatic bony disease from multiple myeloma. Pathologic fractures are uncommon except with multiple myeloma.

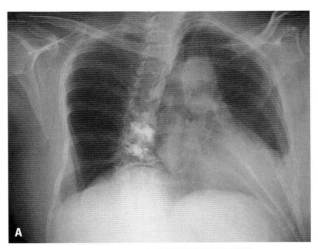

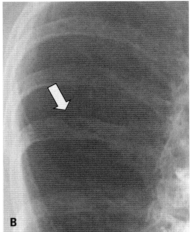

Figure 19–5. Pathologic fracture of the right ribs in a myeloma patient with right-sided chest pain after coughing.

Multiple myeloma tends to be highly vascular; therefore, angiography and embolization are often required before surgical intervention.

Sarcoma. Primary bone sarcomas occur in the same population that is at risk for metastatic disease. Therefore, a solitary bone lesion requires a biopsy before a decision on management is made. In general, a fracture through a spindle cell sarcoma requires amputation. A primary prosthetic replacement is preferable to internal fixation to avoid local disease progression. Radiotherapy generally offers good palliation for metastatic sarcoma.

Rehabilitation. Satisfactory outcomes of attempts to rehabilitate patients who have had recent surgical repair of pathologic or impending fractures have been demonstrated. The risk of producing pathologic fractures in cancer patients by increasing their mobility and function is low. Cancer patients with bone metastases can be safely rehabilitated with standard approaches.[51]

Other Palliative Measures. In many cases, bone metastases are too widespread or extensive to be eliminated through chemotherapy or radiotherapy. Several treatments are used in palliative care, including systemic radiopharmaceuticals, bisphosphonates, external-beam radiation, and chemotherapy.[8]

An alternative to this approach is the administration of radioisotopes that may localize to the sites of bone metastases either because they are tumor specific (eg, radioiodine for thyroid cancer) or bone seeking (eg, radioactive phosphorus [^{32}P] and strontium [^{89}Sr]).[52] Samarium-153 Lexidronam is a 1:1 complex of radioactive samarium (^{153}Sm) and a tetraphosphonate (ethylenediaminetetramethylene phosphonic acid). It has a high affinity for bone and concentrates by association with hydroxyapatite crystals. For the treatment of pain from bone metastasis, the current standards of care for cancer pain (analgesics and local radiation therapy) should not be displaced by bisphosphonates. Pamidronate (60 to 90 mg intravenously [IV] every 3 to 4 weeks) used concurrently with systemic chemotherapy and/or hormonal therapy can provide modest pain control in women who have pain caused by osteolytic metastasis. Zoledronic acid (4 mgIV over 5 minutes every month) has recently been approved for the treatment of osteolytic bone metastases. Bisphosphonates provide a meaningful supportive but non-life-prolonging benefit to many patients with bone metastases from cancer.[53]

Radiotherapy remains the palliative treatment of choice, and radiation treatment given in a single fraction has proven to be an efficient and cost-effective alternative to traditional multifraction radiotherapy courses. Analgesics are important in palliative therapy because they relieve pain while treatment is administered and while the patient awaits the relief of pain from treatment.[8]

MUSCULOSKELETAL AND JOINT INFECTIONS

Infections involving the limbs in cancer patients may require emergent consultations with orthopedic surgeons. Severe infections in ulcerated tumors on limbs may require amputation. Septic arthritis may require emergent drainage and irrigation. Necrotizing fasciitis and compartment syndromes also require emergent surgical interventions.

Clinical Manifestations

Localized redness, pain and swelling on a limb are signs of infection. Cellulitis, abscess, and osteomyelitis are in the differential diagnosis. Needle aspiration of purulent material will confirm the diagnosis of an abscess and decompress the abscess. Other systemic manifestations of infection, such as fever and chills, may also be present.

The symptoms of septic arthritis are pain, swelling, and decreased range of motion in the affected joints.

Pathophysiologic Mechanisms

There are several factors that may contribute to the development of musculoskeletal infections in cancer patients. Cancer patients may be immunocompromised because of the malignancy or the treatment of the malignancy. The immunocompromised state makes a cancer patient more susceptible to infections in general and to infection by opportunistic organisms. Many cancer patients have central venous catheters during the course of cancer therapy. Infection of central venous catheters can lead to bacteremia and to the hematogenous spread and seeding of microorganisms in the musculoskeletal system. Cancer patients are also prone to trauma and falls for various reasons, including debilitation, deconditioning, dehydration, seizures, and neurologic deficits. Abrasions, lacerations, and open fractures all may lead to the direct inoculation of microorganisms into the musculoskeletal system. The development of decubitus ulcers in an immobile cancer patient provides another way for microorganisms to gain access to the musculoskeletal system.

Etiology

Osteomyelitis of hematogenous origin usually involves one microorganism. In an immunocompetent patient, *Staphylococcus aureus* is the most common causative organism. Aerobic Gram-negative organisms are responsible for about 30% of cases. Intravenous drug abuse may be associated with organisms like *Pseudomonas aeruginosa* and *Serratia marcescens*. Osteomyelitis of direct inoculation usually involves multiple organisms. *Staphylococcus aureus* and coagulase-negative staphylococcal species are the most common. Gram-negative rods and anaerobic species are also frequently involved.

Staphylococcus and *Streptococcus* are the most common organisms causing septic arthritis. Gram-negative organisms, mycobacteria, and fungi are unusual. Other causes such as *Neisseria gonorrhoeae*, which is quite prevalent in the general adult population, should not be overlooked in the cancer patient population. *Streptococcus pneumoniae*[54,55] and *Neisseria meningitidis*[56] have been reported to cause septic arthritis in myeloma patients. *Streptococcus pneumoniae* septic arthritis has also been reported in bone marrow transplantation patients with skin graft-versus-host disease.[57,58]

Abscesses on extremities are most commonly caused by Gram-positive organisms. Gram-negative bacilli and anaerobes can also cause abscesses in immunocompromised cancer patients.

Group A *Streptococcus* is the most common organism causing necrotizing fasciitis. Other organisms causing this condition include *Staphylococcus aureus, Escherichia coli,*

Clostridium species, *Bacteroides*, and *Peptostreptococcus*. Many such infections are polymicrobial. Free air in the tissue is pathognomonic for a polymicrobial infection.

Diagnosis

Examination will show an inability to walk when a lower-extremity joint is involved. Guarding of the joint is seen when an upper-extremity joint is involved. Increased warmth with surrounding erythema and a joint effusion are common findings. The joint is held in a mildly flexed position to reduce intra-articular pressure and pain. Active and passive ranges of motion will produce severe pain. However, pain may be diminished in immunocompromised patients.

Arthrocentesis is indicated for the diagnostic evaluation of septic arthritis. Crystal arthritis (gout or pseudogout) may present with symptoms similar to those of septic arthritis and such symptoms must be properly diagnosed to be treated effectively. To prevent the introduction of organisms into the otherwise sterile joint, care should be taken to avoid unhealthy or suspected areas of skin or cutaneous tissue during the arthrocentesis procedure. Aspirated joint fluid should be sent for Gram's stain, culture, sensitivity, cell count and differential, chemical analysis, and microscopic examination for crystals. A white blood cell count of > 50,000 leukocytes/mL with > 80% neutrophils, low glucose, and high protein content are consistent with septic arthritis.

The infection of bone can be diagnosed by radiologic evidence of bone destruction. Radionuclide scanning can also be helpful in distinguishing cellulitis from osteomyelitis. Four-phase bone scanning with white blood cells (WBCs) tagged with technetium 99m (^{99m}Tc) is sensitive for detecting osteomyelitis. If this is not available, scanning with human immunoglobulin tagged with ^{99m}Tc can be used.[59]

Necrotizing fasciitis is an invasive infection of the fascia and causes progressive destruction of the skin, subcutaneous fat, and fascia. The characteristic feature is tissue necrosis along a single fascial plane, with widespread undermining of the skin. Swelling within the confines of the fascia can lead to the compression of neurovascular tissue, leading to compartment syndrome with peripheral-nerve dysfunction and ischemia in the limb distal to the compression site.

Management

For patients with osteomyelitis, the duration of antibiotic treatment is prolonged (ie, usually longer than 4 weeks). Local surgical débridement may be helpful. In patients with vascular insufficiency, hyperbaric oxygen may be helpful. Chronic suppressive antibiotic therapy may be indicated for cases in which amputation carries too much morbidity.

For abscesses, prompt drainage with aseptic precautions is indicated. Broad-spectrum antibiotics should be administered until the final cultures and sensitivities allow narrowing of the antibiotic spectrum.

If septic arthritis shows no signs of improvement after 24 to 48 hours of treatment with broad-spectrum antibiotics, surgical drainage should be performed. Patients with a long life expectancy should be treated with surgical drainage and synovectomy. A septic hip joint should be drained surgically because of a high incidence of femoral-head necrosis. Acutely inflamed joints should be initially immobilized, but once the acute symptoms resolve, the extremity should be mobilized.

When necrotizing fasciitis is likely, prompt exploration and thorough débridement of avascular skin and fascia is imperative. Aggressive surgical intervention allows the salvage of limbs in most patients; however, amputation may be necessary in some cases.

REFERENCES

1. Masi L, Brandi ML. Physiopathological basis of bone turnover. Q J Nucl Med 2001;45:2–6.
2. Greenfield EM. Bi Y, Miyauchi A. Regulation of osteoclast activity. Life Sci 1999;65:1087–102.
3. Filvaroff E, Derynck R. Bone remodelling: a signalling system for osteoclast regulation. Curr Biol 1998;8:R679–82.
4. Chirgwin JM, Guise TA. Molecular mechanisms of tumor-bone interactions in osteolytic metastases. Crit Rev Eukaryot Gene Expr 2000;10:159–78.
5. Guise TA. Molecular mechanisms of osteolytic bone metastases. Cancer 2000;88:2892–8.
6. Nemeth JA, Yousif R, Herzog M, et al. Matrix metalloproteinase activity, bone matrix turnover, and tumor cell proliferation in prostate cancer bone metastasis. J Natl Cancer Inst 2002;94:17–25.
7. Habermann ET, Lopez RA. Metastatic disease of bone and treatment of pathological fractures. Orthop Clin North Am 1989;20:469–86.
8. Janjan N. Bone metastases: approaches to management. Semin Oncol 2001;28:28–34.
9. Toma S, Venturino A, Sogno G, et al. Metastatic bone tumors. Nonsurgical treatment. Outcome and survival. Clin Orthop 1993;295:246–51.
10. Higinbotham NL, Marcove RC. The management of pathological fracture. J Trauma 1965;5:792–8.
11. Wedin R. Surgical treatment for pathologic fracture. Acta Orthopaed Scand 2001;72:1–29.
12. Scheid V, Buzdar AU, Smith TL, Hortobagyi GN. Clinical course of breast cancer patients with osseous metastasis treated with combination chemotherapy. Cancer 1986;58:2589–93.
13. Daniell HW. Osteoporosis due to androgen deprivation therapy in men with prostate cancer. Urology 2001;58:101–7.
14. Pfeilschifter J, Diel IJ. Osteoporosis due to cancer treatment: pathogenesis and management. J Clin Oncol 2000;18:1570–93.

15. Warner JT, Evans WD, Webb DK, et al. Relative osteopenia after treatment for acute lymphoblastic leukemia. Pediatr Res 1999;45:544–51.

16. Vassilopoulou-Sellin R, Ramirez I. Severe osteopenia and vertebral compression fractures after complete remission in an adolescent with acute leukemia. Am J Hematol 1992;39:142–3.

17. Halton JM, Atkinson SA, Fraher L, et al. Mineral homeostasis and bone mass at diagnosis in children with acute lymphoblastic leukemia. J Pediatr 1995;126:557–64.

18. Schwartz AM, Leonidas JC. Methotrexate osteopathy. Skeletal Radiol 1984;11:13–6.

19. Nesbit M, Krivit W, Heyn R, Sharp H. Acute and chronic effects of methotrexate on hepatic, pulmonary, and skeletal systems. Cancer 1976;37:1048–57.

20. D'Angelo P, Conter V, Di Chiara G, et al. Severe osteoporosis and multiple vertebral collapses in a child during treatment for B-ALL. Acta Haematol 1993;89:38–42.

21. Atkinson SA, Fraher L, Gundberg CM, et al. Mineral homeostasis and bone mass in children treated for acute lymphoblastic leukemia. J Pediatr 1989;114:793–800.

22. Atkinson SA, Halton JM, Bradley C, et al. Bone and mineral abnormalities in childhood acute lymphoblastic leukemia: influence of disease, drugs and nutrition. Int J Cancer Suppl 1998;11:35–9.

23. Holmes SJ, Whitehouse RW, Clark ST, et al. Reduced bone mineral density in men following chemotherapy for Hodgkin's disease. Br J Cancer 1994;70:371–5.

24. Kreuser ED, Felsenberg D, Behles C, et al. Long-term gonadal dysfunction and its impact on bone mineralization in patients following COPP/ABVD chemotherapy for Hodgkin's disease. Ann Oncol 1992;3:105–10.

25. Ratcliffe MA, Lanham SA, Reid DM, Dawson AA. Bone mineral density (BMD) in patients with lymphoma: the effects of chemotherapy, intermittent corticosteroids and premature menopause. Hematol Oncol 1992;10:181–7.

26. Bruning PF, Pit MJ, de Jong-Bakker M, et al. Bone mineral density after adjuvant chemotherapy for premenopausal breast cancer. Br J Cancer 1990;61:308–10.

27. Banfi A, Podesta M, Fazzuoli L, et al. High-dose chemotherapy shows a dose-dependent toxicity to bone marrow osteoprogenitors: a mechanism for post-bone marrow transplantation osteopenia. Cancer 2001;92:2419–28.

28. Kashyap A, Kandeel F, Yamauchi D, et al. Effects of allogeneic bone marrow transplantation on recipient bone mineral density: a prospective study. Biol Blood Marrow Transplant 2000;6:344–51.

29. Carlson K, Simonsson B, Ljunghall S. Acute effects of high-dose chemotherapy followed by bone marrow transplantation on serum markers of bone metabolism. Calcif Tissue Int 1994;55:408–11.

30. Kintzel PE. Anticancer drug-induced kidney disorders. Drug Saf 2001;24:19–38.

31. Ho PT, Zimmerman K, Wexler LH, et al. A prospective evaluation of ifosfamide-related nephrotoxicity in children and young adults. Cancer 1995;76:2557–64.

32. Rossi R, Pleyer J, Schafers P, et al. Development of ifosfamide-induced nephrotoxicity: prospective follow-up in 75 patients, Med Pediatr Oncol 1999;32:177–82.

33. Sweeney LE. Hypophosphataemic rickets after ifosfamide treatment in children. Clin Radiol 1993;47:345–7.

34. Pratt CB, Meyer WH, Jenkins JJ, et al. Ifosfamide, Fanconi's syndrome, and rickets. J Clin Oncol 1991;9:1495–9.

35. Taube T, Kylmala T, Lamberg-Allardt C, et al. The effect of clodronate on bone in metastatic prostate cancer. Histomorphometric report of a double-blind randomised placebo-controlled study. Eur J Cancer 1994;30A:751–8.

36. Vaidya S, Saika S, Sirohi B, et al. Avascular necrosis of bone—a complication of aggressive therapy for acute lymphoblastic leukemia. Acta Oncol 1998;37:175–7.

37. Chan-Lam D, Prentice AG, Copplestone JA, et al. Avascular necrosis of bone following intensified steroid therapy for acute lymphoblastic leukaemia and high-grade malignant lymphoma. Br J Haematol 1994;86:227–30.

38. Henry AP, Lachmann E, Tunkel RS, Nagler W. Pelvic insufficiency fractures after irradiation: diagnosis, management, and rehabilitation. Arch Phys Med Rehabil 1996;77:414–6.

39. Soderlund V. Radiological diagnosis of skeletal metastases. Eur Radiol 1996;6:587–95.

40. Berruti A, Dogliotti L, Bitossi R, et al. Incidence of skeletal complications in patients with bone metastatic prostate cancer and hormone refractory disease: predictive role of bone resorption and formation markers evaluated at baseline. J Urol 2000;164:1248–53.

41. Friedl W. Indication, management and results of surgical therapy for pathological fractures in patients with bone metastases. Eur J Surg Oncol 1990;16:380–96.

42. Harrington KD. New trends in the management of lower extremity metastases. Clin Orthop 1982;169:53–61.

43. Ampil FL, Sadasivan KK. Prophylactic and therapeutic fixation of weight-bearing long bones with metastatic cancer. South Med J 2001;94:394–6.

44. Harrington KD. Orthopaedic management of extremity and pelvic lesions. Clin Orthop 1995;312:136–47.

45. Harrington KD. Orthopedic surgical management of skeletal complications of malignancy. Cancer 1997;80:1614–27.

46. Rossi C, Ricci S, Boriani S, et al. Percutaneous transcatheter arterial embolization of bone and soft tissue tumors. Skeletal Radiol 1990;19:555–60.

47. Barton PP, Waneck RE, Karnel FJ, et al. Embolization of bone metastases. J Vasc Interv Radiol 1996;7:81–8.

48. Roscoe MW, McBroom RJ, St Louis E, et al. Preoperative embolization in the treatment of osseous metastases from renal cell carcinoma. Clin Orthop 1989;238:302–7.

49. Marcove RC, Miller TR. Treatment of primary and metastatic bone tumors by cryosurgery. JAMA 1969;207:1890–4.

50. De Ruysscher D, Spaas P, Specenier P. The treatment of osseous metastases of hormone-refractory prostate cancer with external beam radiotherapy and strontium-89. Acta Urol Belg 1996;64:13–9.

51. Bunting RW, Shea B. Bone metastasis and rehabilitation. Cancer 2001;92:1020–8.

52. Hoskin PJ. Radiotherapy in the management of bone pain. Clin Orthop 1995;312:105–19.

53. Hillner BE, Ingle JN, Berenson JR, et al. American Society of Clinical Oncology guideline on the role of bisphos-

phonates in breast cancer. American Society of Clinical Oncology Bisphosphonates Expert Panel. J Clin Oncol 2000;18:1378–91.

54. Cuesta M, Bernad M, Espinosa A, et al. Pneumococcal septic arthritis as the first manifestation of multiple myeloma. Clin Exp Rheumatol 1992;10:483–4.

55. Graham MP, Barzaga RA, Cunha BA. Pneumococcal septic arthritis of the knee in a patient with multiple myeloma. Heart Lung 1991;20:416–8.

56. Miller MI, Hoppmann RA, Pisko EJ. Multiple myeloma presenting with primary meningococcal arthritis. Am J Med 1987;82:1257–8.

57. Schwella N, Schwerdtfeger R, Schmidt-Wolf I, et al. Pneumococcal arthritis after allogeneic bone marrow transplantation, Bone Marrow Transplant 1993;12:165–6.

58. Sakata N, Yasui M, Kawa K. Pneumococcal arthritis affects performance status in patients with chronic GVHD of the skin following allogeneic bone marrow transplantation. Int J Hematol 2001;74:90–4.

59. Unal SN, Birinci H, Baktiroglu S, Cantez S. Comparison of Tc-99m methylene diphosphonate, Tc-99m human immune globulin, and Tc-99m-labeled white blood cell scintigraphy in the diabetic foot. Clin Nucl Med 2001;26:1016–21.

CHAPTER 20

DERMATOLOGIC EMERGENCIES

NARIN APISARNTHANARAX, MD
MADELEINE DUVIC, MD

Oncologic patients make up a unique patient population that presents with potentially complex combinations of medical problems. In addition to their inherent history of underlying malignancy, oncologic patients are susceptible to the problems of polypharmacy and the added risks of infection that are associated with immunosuppressive therapy and constant exposure to the nosocomial environment. In addition to the emergent dermatologic problems that are seen in the general patient population, the oncologic patient may suffer a higher incidence of dermatologic emergencies related to malignancy, infection, and drugs. Thus, in the face of a cutaneous eruption in a patient with cancer, consideration must be given to primary dermatologic diseases, cutaneous manifestations of malignancy, infectious processes, and reactions to drugs and treatments. Severe reactions that require emergent treatment often present with extensive erythroderma, desquamation, epidermal necrosis, or blistering. The presentation of fever and rash is also an emergency situation and requires evaluation for vasculitis, infections, severe drug reactions, acute graft-versus-host disease, fungemia, and cutaneous malignancies such as cutaneous T-cell lymphoma. Severe cutaneous reactions may present with systemic sequelae and may necessitate inpatient admission and management. These cases require expeditious diagnosis, which is complicated by their similarities in clinical manifestation. The most severe and life-threatening processes are discussed in this chapter (Table 20–1).

SEVERE CUTANEOUS DRUG REACTIONS

Cutaneous reactions to drug therapy occur frequently in hospitalized patients, with a 2 to 3% incidence.[1] While most cutaneous drug reactions involve a benign morbilliform or exanthematous eruption, approximately 2% of cutaneous drug reactions are serious, causing approximately 3% of nosocomial disabling injuries.[2,3] Drug eruptions can be expected in the oncologic patient population since these patients often present with coexisting medical diseases and disorders, along with a history of polypharmacy. If a drug reaction is suspected in the presence of urticaria, blisters, mucosal involvement, facial edema, ulcers, purpura, fever, or lymphadenopathy, the reaction is likely serious and requires prompt identification and discontinuation of the offending drug, and emergent care (Table 20–2).[4] Hypersensitivity responses are responsible for most cutaneous drug reactions, including hypersensitivity syndrome, small-vessel vasculitis, serum sickness, and angioedema. Furthermore, many oncologic patients, in their hypercoagulable and often bedridden state, require warfarin (Coumadin) for deep venous thrombosis prophylaxis and other medical problems and are at risk for anticoagulant-induced skin necrosis. These cutaneous disorders are discussed here at length; Stevens-Johnson syndrome and toxic epidermal necrolysis are discussed in another section.

TABLE 20–1. Life-threatening Dermatologic Conditions in the Onologic Patient

Severe Drug Reactions
    Hypersensitivity syndrome
    Vasculitis
    Angioedema
    Serum sickness
    Anticoagulant-induced skin necrosis
    Stevens-Johnson syndrome
    Toxic epidermal necrolysis
Paraneoplastic Pemphiqus
Graft-Versus-Host Disease
    Acute GVHD
    Chronic GVHD
Mysosis Fungoides and Sézary Syndrome
    Infectious complications
    Disease flare
Infectious Disease
    Meningococcemia
    Staphylococcal toxic shock syndrome
    Streptococcal toxic shock syndrome
    Disseminated varicella and herpes zoster
    Systemic candidiasis
    Disseminated aspergillosis and mucormycosis

TABLE 20–2. Servere Cutaneous Drug Reactions and Commonly Implicated Agents

Disease	Implicated Agents
Hypersensitivity syndrome	Anticonvulsants (phenytoin, cardamazepine, phenobarbital, lamotrigine), allopurinol, gold salts, dapsone, minocycline, amitriptyline, and sorbinil
Angioedema	ACE inhibitors, antibiotics (penicillin), anesthetics, radiocontrast dyes, NSAIDs, opiates, and curare
Serum sickness	Serum preparations, vaccines
Hypersensitivity vasculitis	Allopurinol, penicillin, aminopenicillins, sulfonamides, thiazides, pyrazolones, hydantoins, propylthiouracil, retinoids, quinolones, and immunotherapeautic agents
Stevens-Johnson syndrome/ Toxic epidermal necrolysis	Sulfonamides, anticonvulsants (phenytoin, barbiturates, carbamazepine), NSAIDs, allopurinol, other antibiotics, analgesics, antipyretics

Clinical Manifestation

Hypersensitivity Syndrome. Hypersensitivity syndrome is a reaction that occurs most often with aromatic antiepileptic agents and sulfonamides and usually presents with a pruritic rash, fever, lymphadenopathy, and sometimes hepatitis, arthralgias, or hematologic abnormalities.[5–8] In studies of antiepileptic drugs, fever and rash were the most common clinical signs, occurring in 87% of cases, and followed by lymphadenopathy in 75%, hepatitis in 51%, hematologic abnormalities (eosinophilia, atypical lymphocytosis) in 30%, and interstitial nephritis in 11% of cases.[5] The rash of hypersensitivity syndrome has a variety of manifestations, including morbilliform eruption, indurated and infiltrated confluent papules and plaques, erythroderma, exfoliative dermatitis, periorbital and facial edema, bullae, and purpura.[4,8] The rash usually begins on the trunk, face, and upper extremities, then spreads to the lower extremities. Cutaneous manifestations of erythema multiforme, Stevens-Johnson syndrome, or toxic epidermal necrolysis (the most severe manifestation) are also occasionally seen. Hypersensitivity syndrome occurs later than most other drug reactions, with an onset within 3 months of treatment; most reactions occur at between 2 and 6 weeks.[4,7] Whereas most patients experience a full recovery within weeks, mortality may occur and is related to severe hepatitis and liver failure (with aminotransaminase levels in the thousands).[9] Hepatitis portends a worse prognosis and has mortality rates of between 18 and 40%.[8,10] Complete resolution of hepatic dysfunction may take months to a year.

Drug-Induced Vasculitis. Drug-induced vasculitis typically involves small vessels and produces palpable purpura, usually on the lower extremities (Figure 20–1).[11,12] Hemorrhagic blisters, urticaria, ulcers, nodules, Raynaud's disease, and digital necrosis may also develop. Drug-induced vasculitis usually occurs between 1 and 3 weeks after the initiation of the offending agent. There is risk of mortality when multiorgan involvement develops, potential sites being the kidneys, liver, gastrointestinal (GI) tract, and nervous system.

Angioedema and Serum Sickness. Angioedema is an immediate hypersensitivity reaction that is characterized by erythema and edema, usually of the face. A burning or tingling sensation often accompanies the eruption. Angioedema is a severe variant of urticaria, in which the edematous process extends deeply into the dermis and subcutaneous tissue.[13] The erythematous raised wheals of urticaria also often appear in angioedema, as both angioedema and urticaria manifest in combination more often than they do alone.[14,15] The reaction becomes life threatening when the condition progresses to involve the pharyngeal and laryngeal passageways, causing respiratory distress and possible respiratory failure. The GI tract and cardiovascular systems may also be involved. The onset of angioedema depends on the specific drug; antibiotics, contrast medium, and anesthesia drugs usually induce the reaction within minutes to hours, whereas nonsteroidal anti-inflammatory drugs (NSAIDs) take up to a week and angiotensin-converting enzyme (ACE) inhibitors take up to 4 weeks.[4] Serum sickness is a similar systemic reaction that develops 7 to 20 days after the administration of foreign proteins and often begins as serpiginous erythema on the fingers, toes, and hands, followed by a morbilliform eruption, urticaria, or angioedema. Other symptoms that are usually present include fever, arthralgias, myalgias, and lymphadenopathy.[15,16]

Anticoagulant-Induced Skin Necrosis. Anticoagulant-induced skin necrosis results from thrombosis in dermal

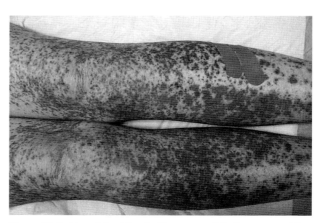

Figure 20–1. Vasculitis with palpable purpura of the lower extremities.

and subcutaneous vessels and initially appears as red and painful plaques that become necrotic.[17] The reaction is distributed over areas of the body with high amounts of adipose tissue, such as the breasts, hips, and buttocks. Priapism is an infrequent complication.[18] Onset of the reaction is usually 3 to 5 days after the initiation of therapy. Fortunately, anticoagulant-induced skin necrosis is uncommon. The incidence of the reaction is 1 in 10,000 patients undergoing warfarin therapy, or approximately 2% of patients with protein C deficiency.[19] Heparin may also induce necrosis at local injection sites although the reaction is occasionally widespread and affects other organs.[20,21] Heparin may induce thrombocytopenia on laboratory examination. Both reactions may be fatal if not properly recognized and treated.

Pathophysiologic Mechanisms

Hypersensitivity Syndrome. The mechanism of hypersensitivity syndrome is currently unknown although various hypotheses have been proposed. Hypersensitivity syndrome may be caused by abnormal metabolism of drugs. It has been shown that some individuals who develop the reaction may have a genetic limitation in the ability to detoxify the anticonvulsants' metabolic product arene oxide, which displays cellular toxicity and which may induce immunologic reactions.[5, 22, 23] The inability to metabolize these products may be due to abnormality or lack of the enzyme epoxide hydrolase.[24] Other hypotheses are geared towards ideas of allergic hypersensitivity, the development of autoantibodies, or a graft-versus-host effect.[8, 25]

Angioedema and Serum Sickness. Angioedema-immediate hypersensitivity occurs through a variety of pathways, including immunoglobulin E (IgE) (type I hypersensitivity), direct mast cell degranulation, complement (type III hypersensitivity), or arachidonic acid–mediated pathways.[13] Antibiotics and anesthetics are usually IgE mediated whereas opiates and radiocontrast dyes exert direct effects on mast cells, and NSAIDs work through cyclooxygenase inhibition and arachidonic acid production.[26,27] Angiotensin-converting enzyme inhibitor reactions are thought to be due to inhibition of kinin metabolism.[28] Invariably, mast cells are the major effector cell involved in angioedema and cause increased vascular permeability, vasodilation, and smooth-muscle contraction through the production of such mediators as histamine, heparin, neutral proteases, eosinophil chemotactic factor, neutrophil chemotactic factor, prostaglandin D_2, leukotrienes, platelet-activating factor, and thromboxane.[15,29] Serum sickness is induced by type III hypersensitivity, in which immune complexes are developed and deposited in small vessels, leading to the activation of complement and the recruitment of granulocytes.

Drug-Induced Vasculitis. There are different hypotheses on the pathophysiology of vasculitis although it is likely that antibodies are formed against drug-related haptens.[30] Damage to the vessels may also be incurred by direct drug toxicity, autoantibodies against vessel endothelial cells, and cell-mediated cytotoxic reactions.

Anticoagulant-Induced Skin Necrosis. The mechanisms of warfarin- and heparin-induced anticoagulation skin necroses are different. Warfarin induces a transient hypercoagulable state by decreasing protein C levels before affecting other vitamin K–dependent coagulation factors. In contrast, heparin-induced thrombosis is likely related to immune-complex deposition.[20,21] Heparin may also induce platelet aggregation, which is responsible for cases of widespread necrosis.

Etiology

Hypersensitivity Syndrome. Hypersensitivity syndrome is usually caused by aromatic anticonvulsants (such as phenytoin, carbamazepine, and phenobarbital) and has an estimated incidence of 1 per 5,000 patients.[6] Cross-reactivity between these drugs may run as high as 75%. Thus, a reaction to one agent signals a potential reaction to other aromatic anticonvulsants.[5,31] The relatively new anticonvulsant lamotrigine has been increasingly associated with hypersensitivity syndrome in a number of cases with severe cutaneous reactions.[32] Hypersensitivity syndrome has also been reported as occurring with the use of allopurinol alone or with thiazide diuretics, gold salts, dapsone, minocycline, amitriptyline, and sorbinil.[4,33,34] In a recent observation, re-activation of human herpesvirus 6 was associated with drug-induced hypersensitivity syndrome, which suggests this viral infection as a possible risk factor although a true association is still unclear.[35]

Angioedema and Serum Sickness. Angioedema is most often induced by antibiotics (especially penicillins), anesthetics, radiocontrast dyes, ACE inhibitors, NSAIDs, opiates, and curare.[26,27] The incidence varies between drugs, but penicillin-induced angioedema occurs in 1 per 10,000 courses, with a fatality occurring in 1 to 5 per 100,000 courses.[26,27] Angioedema induced by ACE inhibitors occurs even more frequently; its incidence is 2 to 10 per 10,000 patients, and it induces the most cases of angioedema that require hospital admission.[36,37] In addition, the use of ACE inhibitors during hemodialysis with high-flux dialysis membranes increases the risk of angioedema significantly, possibly due to the increased production of bradykinins during the procedure.[38] Radiocontrast agents are used with particularly high frequency during imaging studies in the oncologic population, and they elicit hypersensitivity reactions in 5 to 8% of patients.[13] Risk also varies during the course of treatment with different drugs. Patients receiving penicillin prophylaxis maintain a risk of angioedema during the course of treatment whereas reactions to ACE inhibitors are highest during the 1st 3 weeks of therapy and have incidence rates as high as 1 per 3,000 patients during the 1st week of therapy.[37] True serum sickness is usually seen with the use of serum preparations and vaccines. Antithymocyte globulin has continued to play an increasing role in cancer medicine and is a potential cause of serum sickness.[16]

Drug-Induced Vasculitis. Drugs that have been associated with producing acute cutaneous vasculitis include allopurinol, penicillin, aminopenicillins, sulfonamides, thiazides, pyrazolones, hydantoins, propylthiouracil, retinoids, quinolones, and immunotherapeutic agents.[4] Vasculitis may also occur as a result of cryoglobulins or cryofibrinogens related to hepatitis C or underlying malignancy.

Anticoagulant-Induced Skin Necrosis. There are several conditions that predispose an individual to anticoagulant-induced skin necrosis. Obesity, female gender, and the use of higher doses of warfarin predispose patients to the reaction.[39] The highest risk factor is heterozygous or homozygous hereditary protein C deficiency, even in the absence of a history of thrombosis.[17,39,40] Approximately one-third of patients with warfarin-induced skin necrosis have protein C deficiency.[41] Patients with protein S and antithrombin III deficiencies incur additional risk.[42]

Diagnosis

Hypersensitivity Syndrome. The diagnosis of the various drug-induced hypersensitivity reactions is made on the basis of medication history, clinical manifestations, and the results of skin biopsy and laboratory tests. A complete blood count with differentials, renal, and liver function tests can be used to assist in the diagnosis of hypersensitivity syndrome. Histopathology shows a dense superficial perivascular lymphocytic infiltrate with spongiotic or lichenoid features.[8] Lymph node biopsy specimens from lymphadenopathy usually show benign lymphoid hyperplasia although pseudolymphoma and (occasionally) frank lymphoma may appear.[43] Infectious causes (especially infectious mononucleosis) and other drug reactions (such as toxic epidermal necrolysis) should be excluded in considering a diagnosis of hypersensitivity syndrome.

Drug-Induced Vasculitis. Drug-induced hypersensitivity vasculitis is diagnosed by clinical history, histopathology, and laboratory data. On skin biopsy, vasculitis shows evidence of leukocytoclastic vasculitis, with fibrinoid necrosis of small dermal vessels and infiltration by polymorphonuclear leukocytes and nuclear dust.[12] Direct immunofluorescence may show capillary-wall deposition of immunoglobulin M (IgM) and C3 complement. Other

diseases and disorders that need to be considered in the differential diagnosis of palpable purpura include Henoch-Schönlein purpura (HSP), cryoglobulinemia or cryofibrinogenemia, polyarteritis nodosa (PAN), Wegener's granulomatosis, infections, and collagen vascular disorders.[44] Evidence of necrotizing systemic vasculitis on skin biopsy favors the diagnosis of PAN, Wegener's granulomatosis, or Churg-Strauss syndrome.[44] In addition to routine laboratory tests, immunologic tests may also aid in the diagnosis. Serum C3 and C4 levels are usually normal in hypersensitivity vasculitis, and antinuclear antibodies (ANAs) and rheumatoid factor, if positive, are usually present in low titers. Laboratory tests that are negative for cryoprecipitation and cryocrit exclude cryoglobulinemia. A chest roentgenography and hepatitis screening should be performed to exclude infectious causes, and urinalysis should be performed to screen for renal vasculitis. Hypersensitivity vasculitis and HSP may be difficult to differentiate although HSP patients are usually younger (age < 20 years) and will usually present with a greater number of signs and symptoms of multiorgan involvement, such as abdominal angina, GI bleeding, and hematuria.[45] Henoch-Schönlein purpura may also be associated with streptococcal infection. Secondary cutaneous vasculitis as a manifestation of malignancy must also be considered in the oncologic patient.

Angioedema and Serum Sickness. Angioedema is usually diagnosed through clinical suspicion. In addition to specific antigen causes such as drugs and foods, hereditary and acquired angioedema related to C1 esterase inhibitor deficiency must also be considered. Although a skin biopsy is rarely needed for the diagnosis of angioedema, histopathology shows edema of the deep dermis and subcutaneous tissues, with dilation of venules, mast cell degranulation, and a sparse or dense inflammatory infiltrate consisting of T cells, neutrophils, and eosinophils.[13] The diagnosis of serum sickness is likewise clinically based and is supported by laboratory tests showing decreased C3 and C4 complement.

Anticoagulant-Induced Skin Necrosis. The diagnosis of anticoagulant-induced skin necrosis is clinically based. Quick recognition of the characteristic lesions after warfarin and heparin administration is key. Tests for protein C deficiency may be required for the patient without a previous history of the disorder. Blood counts should also be drawn to assess for heparin-induced thrombocytopenia.

Treatment

The treatment of drug-induced hypersensitivity reactions invariably begins with the discontinuation of the offending agent. In most cases, rapid resolution of the reaction will be achieved by this action alone. Administration of

H_1 antihistamines is the therapy of choice for angioedema, and various classes and combinations of antihistamines, including H_1 and H_2 combinations, should be tried if one drug proves ineffective.[13] Systemic corticosteroids are sometimes used to treat hypersensitivity syndrome, inducing resolutions within 1 week although relapses may occur during steroid tapering.[46] The detoxifying properties of N-acetylcysteine have been used successfully in a few cases as well.[47,48] The use of corticosteroids does not appear to alter the course of severe hepatic involvement, however.[46,49] Corticosteroids may also be used for serum sickness, vasculitis, angioedema, and other hypersensitivity reactions, especially in severe cases. Warfarin-induced necrosis should be treated with vitamin K, heparin, and monoclonal antibody–purified protein C concentrate whereas heparin-induced necrosis may be treated with warfarin or antiplatelet therapy.[20,50] Surgical débridement and grafting may be required for the management of necrotic tissue.

STEVENS-JOHNSON SYNDROME AND TOXIC EPIDERMAL NECROLYSIS

Toxic epidermal necrolysis (TEN), Stevens-Johnson syndrome (SJS), and erythema multiforme (EM) are a spectrum of reaction patterns characterized by differing degrees of epidermal necrosis with the involvement of mucous membranes or glabrous skin. These reactions may occur with relatively high frequency in the oncologic patient, given their associations with infection and drugs. Through the years, there has been some confusion surrounding the relationship of these disorders to each other. Most authors now differentiate the diseases on the basis of clinical, pathologic, and etiologic differences.

Toxic epidermal necrolysis results in extensive detachment and death of full-thickness epidermis and is most commonly associated with an adverse drug reaction.[51] Stevens-Johnson syndrome and TEN are variants that occur on a continuous spectrum in which SJS represents the least severe and TEN the most severe form of disease.[52] By definition, the mucosal membranes are mostly affected in SJS. A consensus agreement has proposed a three-grade classification, which includes SJS, transitional SJS/TEN, and TEN.[53] Differentiation between the three grades is based upon the degree of epidermal detachment; the greatest degree of involvement occurs in TEN (Table 20–3). While EM-like target lesions may often appear in TEN, there are clinical, pathologic, and etiologic differences that separate SJS/TEN from the EM spectrum of EM majus and EM minor.[54–56] Erythema multiforme majus appears as a characteristic eruption of symmetrical acrally distributed target lesions, which may or may not have blisters but which may be accompanied by mucosal lesions. While SJS/TEN may also present with mucosal lesions, its target lesions manifest as widespread purpuric macules that are often confluent with epidermal detachment and display a positive Nikolsky sign. Erythema multiforme is usually associated with infection and causes low morbidity and no mortality whereas SJS/TEN is usually drug induced, has high morbidity, and may be fatal. Thus, this discussion is centered on the SJS/TEN spectrum because of its required emergent care.

Clinical Manifestation

Toxic epidermal necrolysis occurs worldwide in all ages and populations although it appears to occur with a higher incidence in women, elderly persons, and patients with human immunodeficiency virus (HIV) infection. This higher incidence may be related to higher medication use in these populations. The most recent epidemiologic study shows that TEN and SJS occur with an estimated incidence of 1.89 cases per million per year.[57] Thus, SJS and TEN remain relatively rare. In the oncologic population, one study has shown a high TEN incidence (6%) in bone marrow transplant recipients, and nearly the same number of cases were due to acute graft-versus-host disease as were due to adverse drug reactions.[58]

Toxic epidermal necrolysis begins with painful ill-defined macules with dark centers, usually beginning on the face, neck, and shoulders and spreading to the whole body, with predominance on the trunk and proximal extremities. The eruption then proceeds with the development of flaccid blisters and bullae, with loss of epidermis in sheets (Figure 20–2). Nikolsky's sign, which is the detachment of epidermis and the extension of bullae by lateral pressure, is positive. Trauma to the affected fragile skin causes denudation and exposes the deep red dermis. Epidermal detachment and sloughing may involve 100% of the cutaneous surface. Disruption of the skin barrier induces acute skin failure that is similar to that of the extensively burned patient. The resulting massive fluid losses lead to dehydration, prerenal azotemia, and elec-

TABLE 20–3. Comparison of SJS/Ten Spectrum Disease and Erythema Multiforme

Disease	Major Etiology	Mucosal Lesions	Epidermal Detachment	Clinical Appearance
Stevens-Johnson syndrome (SJS)	Drug	+	Less than 10%	Widespread purpuric macules
Transitional SJS/TEN	Drug	+	10–30%	Widespread purpuric macules
Toxic epidermal necrolysis	Drug	+	Greater than 30%	Widespread purpuric macules
Erythema multiforme	Infection	+	None	Acral, symmetrical target lesions

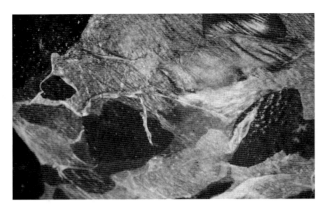

Figure 20–2. Toxic epidermal necrolysis with flaccid bullae and exposed red dermis.

trolyte imbalances.[56,59] Disruption of the skin barrier also places patients at high risk for infection and sepsis. *Staphylococcus aureus* colonization is common in early disease (Gram-negative rods in later disease) and can lead to sepsis and death.

Additional complications of TEN arise with the involvement of other organs. Epithelial necrosis may progress to involve the GI, genitourinary, and tracheobronchial tracts, inducing profuse diarrhea and respiratory distress, respectively.[60,61] Mucosal involvement is common in TEN and defines SJS. The oropharynx, eyes, genitalia, and anus are typically involved, leading to photophobia, dysuria, and the impairment of oral intake.[59] Conjunctival erosions may form synechiae between the eyelids and conjunctivae. These complications are responsible for severe morbidity. Laboratory alterations are nearly always present; anemia and lymphopenia are the most common and appear in almost all patients. Neutropenia occurs in 30% of patients and is a poor prognostic factor because it places patients at a higher risk for infection.[62] Thrombocytopenia also occurs in 15% of patients.

Toxic epidermal necrolysis is fatal in 30% of cases; most fatalities are related to infection with either *Staphylococcus aureus* or *Pseudomonas aeruginosa*.[63,64] At the less severe end of the spectrum, SJS is fatal in 5% of cases. Visceral involvement and increased age, percentage of denuded skin, and serum urea nitrogen level are associated with a poor prognosis.[59]

Pathophysiologic Mechanisms

The underlying mechanisms of SJS/TEN are unknown although it has been hypothesized that abnormal metabolism of TEN-inducing drugs and a cytotoxic immune-mediated response may be involved.[56] It has been shown that TEN patients are slow acetylators of sulfonamides by genotype, which may lead to a buildup of reactive metabolites.[65,66] These metabolites might then bind to carrier proteins on epidermal cell membranes and induce

an antigenic immune response, leading to a cell-mediated cytotoxic reaction against keratinocytes.[56,67] Immunohistologically, it appears that CD8-positive (CD8+) cytotoxic T-cell lymphocytes and macrophages may be involved in the epidermis of TEN patients whereas CD4+ T cells have predominance in the upper dermis.[68–70] Gelatinases and tumor necrosis factor alpha (TNF-α) may be involved in the inflammatory reaction of TEN lesions and may play roles in epidermal detachment.[71,72] Evidence of human leukocyte antigen (HLA) linkage may also support a genetic predisposition for TEN.[73,74] Ultimately, keratinocyte death likely occurs through apoptotic pathways.[75] A recent in vitro study suggested that nitric oxide may induce epidermal apoptosis and necrosis and play a role in apoptosis.[76] While evidence for the immunologic mechanisms of TEN are abundant, they have not been directly linked to the activity of reactive metabolites.

Etiology

The drugs most commonly implicated in causing TEN are the antibacterial sulfonamides, anticonvulsants, allopurinol, pyrazolone derivatives, and NSAIDs.[56,73] The most frequently implicated drugs, the sulfonamides, are responsible in 30% of cases of TEN. Long-acting sulfonamides such as sulfadoxine carry a greater risk although TEN induced by the short-acting drug trimethoprim/sulfamethoxazole is seen more often due to its frequent use.[77] The incidence of sulfonamide-induced TEN has become more common since the advent of sulfonamide therapy for opportunistic infections in acquired immunodeficiency syndrome (AIDS) patients.[78]

Anticonvulsants have been reported to induce TEN in patients, especially when patients are receiving concurrent radiotherapy or chemotherapy for malignant cerebral tumors.[79] Implicated agents include phenytoin, barbiturates, carbamazepine, and lamotrigine. Antiepileptic drugs are the most common inducers of TEN in children and account for 16% of SJS/TEN cases.[79] Furthermore, cross-reactions are possible between phenobarbital, phenytoin, and carbamazepine, due to common metabolic pathways, and all three drugs are contraindicated once TEN has occured from one drug.[80]

Other drugs that have been reported in association with TEN include NSAIDs (particularly long-acting), allopurinol, other antibiotics, other analgesics, and antipyretics. In addition to drug-induced TEN, idiopathic cases of TEN have occurred in patients without a medication history.[81] It is also thought that infection-induced TEN is a plausible though rare phenomenon.[82]

Diagnosis

The diagnosis of TEN or SJS can usually be made through clinical presentation and a careful drug history. In assessing a TEN patient's clinical history for culprit drugs, it is important to consider that the reported mean interval from the initiation of the implicated drug to the onset of TEN is 14 days. Thus, new drugs begun within 1 to 3 weeks before the onset of TEN should be considered the most likely suspects.[56] A skin biopsy specimen typically showing full-thickness necrosis of detached epidermis with sparing of the dermis can aid in the diagnosis, especially in excluding other bullous diseases that are unrelated to drug therapy, such as exfoliative dermatitis, staphylococcal scalded-skin syndrome, and acute exanthematous pustulosis.[56] A negative direct immunofluorescence study also serves to rule out paraneoplastic pemphigus, pemphigus vulgaris, and other bullous dermatoses, which may mimic TEN clinically. Other cutaneous disorders that are often confused with SJS/TEN are exfoliative dermatitis, acute graft-versus-host disease, staphylococcal scalded-skin syndrome, and acute exanthematous pustulosis. Evidence of oral involvement and full-thickness necrosis in SJS/TEN is a useful discriminating factor.[52]

Treatment

The key to the treatment of SJS/TEN is early diagnosis and discontinuation of the offending medication. Since it is often difficult to pinpoint a particular causative drug, it is prudent to discontinue all new drugs that have been started within 1 month of disease onset. Early discontinuation of the offending medication reduces the risk of death by approximately 30% per day.[83] Any drug that is not life sustaining should be withdrawn once the likelihood of a diagnosis of SJS/TEN is highly suspected. Acute treatment involves supportive care with intravenous fluids with macromolecules and saline. Admission into an intensive care or burn unit is optimal and may reduce mortality.[84,85]

Since infections are a major cause of morbidity and mortality in the SJS/TEN patient, appropriate prophylactic aseptic measures are required. Contact isolation is important to decrease transmission of infectious pathogens between health care workers and patients, especially since the transmission of infection occurs through bullous fluid as easily as through blood.[86] Likewise, environmental controls should be placed and room temperatures raised to 30°C. Intravenous access should be obtained through peripheral access, avoiding placement at affected areas of involvement. Central venous access should be avoided to minimize the risk of bacteremia and sepsis. Wound care should consist of topical antiseptic washes and wound dressings with 0.5% silver nitrate or 0.05% chlorhexidine on denuded skin.[87] Some authorities recommend the operative débridement of nonviable epidermis and the covering of the exposed dermis with biologic dressings such as cutaneous allografts or collagen-based skin substitutes. Appropriate systemic antibiotics should be administered if blood or skin cultures are positive for a large population of a bacterial strain, if there is a sudden drop in the patient's temperature, or if there is a deterioration in condition. Prophylactic antibiotics are not recommended due to the potential for cross-reactivity of SJS/TEN-inducing drugs and the risk of promoting the growth of antibiotic-resistant bacteria.[88]

Systemic corticosteroids have been controversial in the treatment of TEN because retrospective analysis suggests that they may be detrimental to TEN patients. Many authorities in the field recommend the avoidance of corticosteroids, especially in severe TEN, since they may be associated with higher rates of morbidity and mortality.[89,90] Systemic corticosteroids have also failed to prevent TEN in patients who are concomitantly receiving corticosteroid therapy for the treatment of their underlying disease.[91] Thalidomide has likewise been shown to be detrimental in a double-blinded randomized, placebo-controlled trial.[92] Plasmapheresis, cyclophosphamide, and N-acetylcysteine are reported as being beneficial by uncontrolled studies and anecdotal experiences.[47,93,94] Intravenous immunoglobulin (IVIG) is a promising treatment alternative, which targets CD95 and neutralizes Fas-Fas ligand-induced keratinocyte apoptosis and which has had efficacy in treating TEN in an open-labeled uncontrolled study.[95] Further investigation of these agents is required to elucidate their efficacy. Dialysis to remove the offending drug may also be indicated when appropriate.

PARANEOPLASTIC PEMPHIGUS

Among the numerous autoimmune blistering diseases, paraneoplastic pemphigus (PNP) is the most life threatening. In the group of autoimmune intraepidermal blistering diseases commonly referred to as pemphigus, PNP is a mucocutaneous blistering disorder that occurs in the setting of a benign or malignant neoplasm. While pemphigus vulgaris is the most common form of pemphigus in the general population, PNP may be of higher significance and relevance in oncology. Pemphigus has been a central topic for extensive immunofluorescence research over the recent decade, and many details of the pathophysiologic mechanisms of the disease have recently been elucidated. Despite this increased understanding, PNP remains a disease of severe debilitation, morbidity, and mortality and requires rapid recognition and treatment.

Clinical Manifestation

Manifestations of PNP are important to recognize in oncologic medicine as the disease may be more devastating and recalcitrant to therapy than the more common pemphigus vulgaris. Paraneoplastic pemphigus occurs over a wide geographic and ethnic distribution without gender predominance and may be seen in patients of all age groups. The mean age of onset is 51 years.[96] The first presenting (and most common) sign of PNP is intractable stomatitis, consisting of painful erosions and ulcerations of the oropharynx and vermilion border of the lips.[97] Pseudomembranous conjunctivitis is also often present. Mucosal lesions may involve any portion of the oral cavity, respiratory tract, and genital mucosa.[98,99] Progression to the respiratory tract may lead to bronchiolitis obliterans and respiratory failure.[100] Cutaneously, PNP is similar to pemphigus vulgaris and appears as fragile pruritic blisters affecting the head, neck, upper trunk, proximal extremities, and the palms and soles. Evidence of lesions on the palms and soles can be used to differentiate the disease from pemphigus vulgaris, which rarely affects these sites. Paraneoplastic pemphigus may also mimic lichen planus, bullous pemphigoid, or erythema multiforme with lichenoid papules, tense blisters, or target lesions. Atypical cases in which lichenoid eruptions occurred alone or at the sites of previous blistering have been reported.[101,102] In one-third of cases, the clinical manifestations of PNP precede those of the cancer and its diagnosis.[97] Thus, a diagnosis of PNP in the absence of obvious cancer calls for a full cancer work-up, including full-body computed tomography scans.

The prognosis for PNP associated with benign neoplasms is good, as the mucocutaneous lesions resolve once the tumors are excised. In contrast, there appears to be no correlation between tumor burden and the activity of PNP associated with malignant neoplasms, as it has been shown that lesions may persist despite neoplastic remission.[98] Thus, nearly all patients with this form of PNP experience a rapidly progressive and fatal course within 1 month to 2 years after diagnosis.[97] The longest reported survival cases were for 8 years in one patient, and more than 3 years in another patient.[101,103] Death is usually due to sepsis, GI bleeding, multiple organ failure, or respiratory failure.[97]

Pathophysiologic Mechanisms

Autoimmunity in PNP patients is developed when an immune response is directed against tumor protein antigens, which cross-react with normal epithelial proteins.[97,104] It is known that thymomas and Castleman's tumors express desmoplakins, which may explain their association with PNP. Cancers such as non-Hodgkin's lymphoma and chronic lymphocytic leukemia (CLL) may also produce desmosomes and desmoplakins anomalously.[96,104] Another hypothesis is based on the induction of autoimmunity through tumor-associated cytokine overexpression and dysregulation. Interleukin-6 (IL-6), which promotes B-cell differentiation and has been linked to autoimmune diseases, has been shown to be produced by certain cancers, including non-Hodgkin's lymphoma, CLL, and Castleman's tumors.[96,97,105]

Pathophysiologically, it is known that the autoantibodies in PNP are pathogenic and are responsible for initiating the changes of epidermal acantholysis and blister formation. Murine models have shown that transferring antidesmoglein-3 antibodies from PNP patients into mice induces the same histologic changes.[106] It is believed that the ensuing cell membrane damage that results from acantholysis allows the induction of autoantibodies against the plakin cytoplasmic proteins.

Etiology

Neoplasms are key to initiating the autoimmune response and the subsequent development of PNP. The most commonly reported type of cancer in association with PNP is non-Hodgkin's lymphoma.[96] Other commonly associated benign and malignant cancers are listed in Table 20–4.

Diagnosis

The diagnosis of PNP is based on characteristic clinical manifestations in the setting of an underlying neoplasm, histology, direct immunofluorescence (DIF), and detection of serum autoantibodies by indirect immunofluorescence and immunoblotting.[107] The major histologic features of PNP include epidermal changes such as suprabasal acantholysis, dyskeratotic keratinocytes, vacuolar changes of the basilar epidermis, suprabasilar cleft formation, and epidermal exocytosis of inflammatory cells.[108] Paraneoplastic pemphigus can be differentiated from other diseases by histology and immunofluorescence studies. Usually, pemphigus vulgaris features neutrophils and eosinophils in the papillary dermis along with eosinophilic epidermal spongiosis, which is absent in PNP. On DIF testing, PNP reveals immunoglobulin G (IgG) and C3 deposition in the epidermal intercellular spaces, as well as granular-linear complement deposition along the epidermal basement membrane zone.[107] The relatively high frequency of false-negative DIF studies may require repeated skin biopsies.

An indirect immunofluorescence examination can be used to detect the presence of serum autoantibodies with titers usually ranging between 1:320 to 1:5120.[96] Tests

TABLE 20–4. Most Common Neoplasms Associated with Paraneoplasic Pemphigus*

Non-Hodgkin's lymphoma
Chronic lymphocytic leukemia
Castleman's tumor
Thymoma
Poorly differentiated sarcoma
Waldenstrom's macroglobulinemia
Inflammatory fibrosarcoma
Bronchogenic squamous cell carcinoma
Round-cell liposarcoma
Hodgkins disease
T-cell lymphoma

*Decreasing order of frequency.

that are reactive to both monkey esophagus and rat urinary bladder are diagnostic of PNP whereas pemphigus vulgaris reacts only to monkey esophagus. Immunoblotting must be performed for the detection of PNP autoantigenic complexes, however, because indirect immunofluorescence on rat bladder epithelium has a false-negative rate as high as 25%.[109] The currently known autoantigens of PNP are cell structure components such as desmosomal antigens, cytoplasmic proteins of the plakin gene family, and a 170-kD transmembranous antigen.[96] Overall, the presence of a lymphoproliferative disorder, positive indirect immunofluorescence labeling of rat bladder, and the recognition of envoplakin and/or periplakin bands on immunoblotting have been shown to be the most sensitive and specific diagnostic criteria for PNP with sensitivities of 82 to 86% and specificities of 83 to 100%.[110]

Treatment

Improvement or resolution of PNP that is associated with benign tumors such as thymomas and Castleman's tumors usually occurs following the surgical excision of the cancer. Lesions usually resolve 6 to 18 months after excision.[107] Unfortunately, therapy for PNP induced by more malignant neoplasms is not as effective. Systemic corticosteroids may induce responses in cutaneous lesions, especially in less severe cases. On the other hand, stomatitis is usually refractory to therapy. There have been isolated reports of success with combination immunosuppressive therapy. Prednisone (0.75-1.0 mg/kg/d) and azathioprine (100 mg/d), or prednisone (35 mg/d) and cyclosporine (5 mg/kg/d) have produced improvements in both cutaneous and mucous lesions in isolated cases.[103, 111] Success was also found in the use of high-dose immunoablative cyclophosphamide (50 mg/kg) in a cyclosporine-refractory patient with oral involvement.[112] One modality that is particularly promising is plasmapheresis, which has been shown to decrease autoantibody titers and improve skin and mucosal lesions.[113] An immunoapheresis regimen using sheep anti-human immunoglobulin G (IgG) bead-formed agarose gel followed by high-dose immunoglobulin was used successfully for a PNP patient whose disease was refractory to tumor excision and corticosteroids.[114] The treatment led to the complete disappearance of circulating autoantibodies and to the patient's recovery.

GRAFT-VERSUS-HOST DISEASE

As bone marrow transplantation (BMT) has become more common in the area of cancer treatment, so has the incidence of graft-versus-host disease (GVHD), a frequent complication of BMT. Approximately 50% of BMTs result in GVHD.[115,116] In the setting of the post-BMT patient, vigilance is required in monitoring for symptoms of acute or chronic GVHD as the condition is associated with high morbidity and mortality. Based on the initial definition of Billingham, GVHD is a reaction that arises only when a donor organ containing immunologically competent cells is transplanted into an immunocompromised recipient with tissue antigens differing from the donor's antigens.[117,118] Allogeneic BMT exemplifies this description and is the most common cause of GVHD although it may also occur in solid-organ transplantation and blood transfusion.[116]

Graft-versus-host disease is classified as acute or chronic. Acute GVHD is characterized by dermatitis, hepatitis, and gastroenteritis and develops within 100 days after allogeneic BMT. There are four stages of cutaneous, liver, and GI involvement (Table 20–5). These four stages of organ involvement also determine the overall clinical grade (I to IV) of acute GVHD (Table 20–6). Patients with chronic GVHD present with multiorgan involvement that develops more than 100 days following BMT. Chronic GVHD occurs with a mean onset of 4 months after BMT; 32% of cases occur as a continuous disease process from acute GVHD, 36% of patients experience chronic GVHD as a relapse from acute GVHD in remission, and 30% of cases arise de novo.[118] Chronic GVHD is graded as either limited (with localized skin involvement, with or without liver dysfunction) or extensive (with generalized skin involvement). Extensive disease may also refer to localized skin involvement or liver dysfunction, with chronic aggressive liver disease, eye involvement, mucosalivary gland involvement, mucosal involvement, or involvement of other target organs.

Acute Graft-versus-Host Disease

Clinical Manifestation. The most frequent clinical manifestation of acute GVHD is a rash, followed by hepatic and GI involvement occurring at similar rates. In one large retrospective study of 740 acute GVHD patients, approxi-

TABLE 20–5. Skin, Liver, GI Performance Grading in Acute GVHD

Grade	Skin Involvement	Liver:Bilirubin (mg%)	GI	Performance Impairment
1+	Erythematous macules and papules, BSA < 25% involment	2–3	Diarrhea > 500 cc/day	1
2+	Erythematous macules and papules, 25% > BSA < 50%	3.1–6	Diarrhea > 1000 cc/day	2
3+	Generalized erythroderma, BSA > 50%	6.1 –15	Diarrhea > 1500 cc/day	3
4+	Bullae and epidermal necrolysis	> 15	Pain/Ileus	–

TABLE 20–6. Overall Clinical Grading of Acute Graft-versus-Host Disease

| Grade | Organ/System Involvement | | | |
	Skin	Liver	GI System	Performance
I	1+ to 2+	—	—	—
II	1+ to 3+	1+	1+	1+
III	2+ to 3+	2+ to 3+	2+ to 3+	2+
IV	2+ to 4+	2+ to 4+	2+ to 4+	3+

mately 80% had rash while 50% had hepatic and/or GI involvement.[119] The time of onset of acute GVHD ranges from 5 to 47 days (median 19 days) after BMT.[120] Acute GVHD usually appears as a maculopapular exanthem of sudden onset (Figure 20–3). The eruption may initially present with erythema limited to the palms and soles, which may mimic chemotherapy-induced acral erythema (Figure 20–4). Oral mucositis is also seen, with erythematous or erosive lesions. In its most severe form, acute GVHD (grade IV) may resemble (or be indistinguishable from) drug-induced TEN, with generalized erythroderma, epidermal necrosis, and blister formation.[116,120]

The liver is the next most frequent organ system to be affected by acute GVHD, with cholestatic jaundice being common.[121] However, in the BMT setting, hyperbilirubinemia from cyclosporine or tacrolimus hepatotoxicity must also be considered. Lower-GI involvement may also occur, affecting the distal small bowel and the colon. Signs and symptoms include abdominal pain, secretory diarrhea, intestinal bleeding, malabsorption, paralytic ileus, and ascites.[122] Enteric infection must be ruled out in the presence of these symptoms. In addition, upper-GI symptoms such as anorexia, nausea, vomiting, and dyspepsia may present in 13% of patients, especially in older patients. Hepatic and GI involvement may occur without cutaneous manifestations of GVHD.

A rare hyperacute form of GVHD also occurs, manifesting as severe generalized inflammation, high fever, hepatitis, fluid retention, vascular leakage, and shock.[116] In general, GVHD mortality is usually related to infectious complications. Prognosis is based on disease grade. While grade I disease has little effect on survival, grade IV GVHD mortality rates with TEN are very high, at 80 to 100%.[58]

Pathophysiologic Mechanisms. The signs and symptoms of acute GVHD are thought to be due to the activity of CD4 and/or CD8 T cells that are reactive against recipient cells.[118] Alloreactive T-cell activation occurs through stimulation by antigen-presenting cell (APC) secretion of inflammatory cytokines such as TNF-α and interleukin-1 (IL-1).[123–125] Under pro-inflammatory conditions, CD4+ and CD8+ cells clonally expand and differentiate into effector cells that are responsible for the GVHD reaction through the production of various cytokines, including

IL-2, IL-3, IL-4, interferon-γ (IFN-γ), and TNF-α.[115,126] These mediators activate additional lymphocytes, macrophages, and natural killer (NK) cells, which attack both host and donor tissue. After activation of effector cells, the expression of intercellular adhesion molecule 1 (ICAM-1) on keratinocytes may promote the retention of lymphocytes in the epidermis.[127] Keratinocyte death has been shown to occur ultimately by apoptosis.[128]

Etiology. Acute and chronic GVHD are essentially T cell–mediated diseases that are instigated through the mismatch of donor and recipient antigens. Mismatch of HLA is the dominant risk factor, and the degree of mismatch directly correlates with the severity of GVHD.[116] GVHD can occur even in HLA-matched related transplants and is also related to the mismatch of minor histocompatability antigens.[129] Acute GVHD occurs with high frequency (in up to 90% of allogeneic bone marrow transplants), depending on patient age, HLA type, sex of the donor and recipient, and prevention protocols.[118,130–132] Even when the donor is an HLA-identical sibling, acute GVHD occurs in 10 to 60% of BMT recipients.[115,120] Older age increases the incidence of GVHD by as much as three times that of younger patients.[116] Male recipients receiving HLA-identical related marrow from a female donor incur a higher risk of GVHD than do alternate cases (53% vs 42%). Current BMT procedures typically use combinations of tacrolimus (FK506), cyclosporine, methotrexate, and corticosteroids as prophylaxis against GVHD.[133,134] However, this prophylaxis lowers the incidence of acute GVHD by only 15 to 40%, and does not alter the incidence of chronic GVHD.

Diagnosis. Quick recognition and diagnosis of acute GVHD is important as the reaction requires immediate immunosuppressive therapy. However, the diagnosis of acute GVHD is often difficult to make. Both clinically and histologically, acute GVHD may mimic cutaneous reactions to chemotherapy, radiation therapy, other adverse drug reactions, and viral infections. Furthermore, when acute GVHD begins with palmoplantar erythema, the eruption may be difficult to distinguish from acral erythema or hand-foot-and-mouth syndrome, which has a 35% incidence in BMT patients.[135] While the two conditions can be distinguished by the progressive nature of acute GVHD, earlier diagnosis may be attained with serial biopsies at 3- to 5-day intervals. Another condition that complicates the diagnosis of grade IV acute GVHD is TEN, especially given the evidence that systemic corticosteroids, if inadvertently given for an incorrect diagnosis of acute GVHD, may be detrimental to the treatment of true TEN.

Even a histopathologic diagnosis is difficult to make, as findings may be similar to drug-induced or infectious processes and to the eruption of lymphocyte recovery.[116]

In a study of pathologic readings from three pathologists, there was consensus in only 31% of cases.[136] Generally, biopsy specimens show vacuolar degeneration of the basal layer, dyskeratotic keratinocytes, and superficial dermal lymphocytic infiltration. A grading system (grades 0 to 4) for the histopathologic findings of GVHD also exists and is of prognostic value. With this diagnostic difficulty, risks and benefits must be carefully considered when deciding on administering immunosuppressive therapies to the BMT patient with early symptoms of acute GVHD. The presence of extracutaneous symptoms may be of diagnostic aid. The diagnosis of GI involvement is made by the discovery of edema, mucosal sloughing, and crypt cell necrosis on endoscopic biopsy specimens.[122]

Treatment. The treatment of acute GVHD is required only for grade 2 to grade 4 disease and consists of the continuation of prophylactic therapies with the addition of high-dose systemic corticosteroids such as methylprednisolone (2 mg/kg/d for 10 to 14 days or until the disease is controlled).[137] A prolonged steroid taper of approximately 5 months has been associated with a shorter time (30-day median) to resolution of acute GVHD.[138] Less than half of treated patients will have a complete or partial response to initial therapy, and treatment failure portends an unfavorable outcome (a 70 to 80% mortality rate).[119] While some second-line therapies may induce responses, they rarely improve survival.[139] Second-line therapies include higher-dose corticosteroids and cyclosporine and other experimental therapies, including mycophenolate mofetil (Cellcept), extracorporeal photopheresis (ECP), anti-IL-2 receptor, and anti-TNF-α and IL-1 receptor antagonists.[140–144] A well-tolerated treatment, ECP was originally developed for the treatment of cutaneous T-cell lymphoma and has recently been shown to induce responses and remission of steroid-refractory acute GVHD.[145,146] A similar treatment, psoralen plus ultraviolet A (PUVA) therapy, may play a role in treating acute GVHD, possibly by improving cutaneous disease and by allowing the reduction of the corticosteroid dose.[147] In addition to these therapies, cases of grade 4 acute GVHD with epidermal necrosis require additional skin care treatment that is similar to the measures used for drug-induced TEN.

Chronic Graft-versus-Host Disease

Clinical Manifestation. Since T cells mediate a number of skin diseases, chronic GVHD may have features that are clinically similar to those of progressive systemic sclerosis, systemic lupus erythematosus (SLE), lichen planus, Sjögren's syndrome, eosinophilic fasciitis, rheumatoid arthritis, and primary biliary cirrhosis.[148–150] Chronic GVHD involves the skin in nearly all cases, and 90% of patients have oral involvement.[151] Disease may begin as erythema

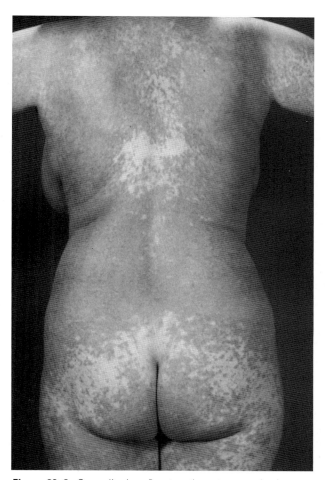

Figure 20–3. Generalized confluent erythematous papules in acute graft-versus-host disease.

in the malar area, mimicking cutaneous manifestations of SLE, or may appear as hypo- or hyperpigmentation.[148] Early on, chronic GVHD may resemble the acute condition, with a morbilliform eruption that evolves into ery-

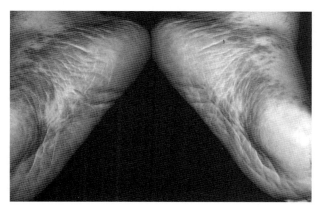

Figure 20–4. Plantar erythema of acute graft-versus-host disease mimicking acral erythema.

thematous or violaceous lichen planus–like papules or plaques, usually affecting the periorbital face, ears, palms, or soles (Figure 20–5). The eruption may become vesicular and may mimic dyshidrosis on the hands.

Later manifestations of chronic GVHD may mimic scleroderma by a sclerodermoid patchy hyperpigmentation (Figure 20–6). Retraction of digits and extremities may result from fibrosis around joints and ligaments. The nails and genitalia are also affected, creating phimosis and vaginal strictures. Fasciitis presenting as cellulitis with palpable subcutaneous infiltration and edema has been reported, preferentially affecting the sides of the body and proximal limbs.[152] Progression causes hardening and retraction of the cellulitis. Scleropathy may penetrate into deep tissues to cause peripheral entrapment neuropathy.[151]

Multisystem involvement is frequent and more extensive than in acute GVHD; commonly affected sites are the liver, mouth, eyes, lungs, and GI tract. Oral involvement occurs with atrophy of the mucosa and tongue and with painful ulcerations in severe cases.[153] Oral and ocular sicca syndrome occurs and may lead to candidal superinfection. Oral involvement may progress to esophagitis in one-third of patients.[116] Hepatic involvement manifests as cholestatic liver disease similar to primary biliary cirrhosis, with elevated alkaline phosphatase and obstructive jaundice. Pulmonary involvement causes bronchitis, bronchiolitis, and interstitial pneumonitis. Pulmonary involvement particularly increases mortality in chronic GVHD. Additionally, bone marrow hypocellularity, fibrosis, and plasmacytosis leads to peripheral anemia, thrombocytopenia, and eosinophilia.[116] Lymphocyte depletion also causes atrophy of lymphoid organs, including the lymph nodes, spleen, and thymus.[150]

Untreated, chronic GVHD carries a mortality of approximately 40%. Morbidity and mortality is highest in patients with progressive onset from acute GVHD and is lowest in patients with de novo onset. Death is most commonly due to infection followed by cachexia and liver dysfunction.[149,150] Chronic GVHD patients suffer immunodeficiency from functional asplenism, CD4 lymphopenia,

generation of nonspecific suppressor cells, hypogammaglobulinemia, and immunosuppression from GVHD therapy. Additionally, with the disruption of normal mucous and cutaneous protective barriers by atrophic and erosive lesions, infections tend to occur with an incidence of 34% in the ear, nose, and throat, 20% in the skin, and 7% in the blood. The distribution of pathogens is 42% viral, 30% bacterial, and 23% fungal; varicella zoster virus, *Pneumococcus*, *Staphylococcus*, and *Candida* are the most frequently isolated organisms. Late initiation of therapy, thrombocytopenia with a platelet count of < 100,000/μL, and onset as a progression from acute GVHD are factors that place a case of chronic GVHD in the high-risk category, which carries a worse prognosis.[154]

Pathophysiologic Mechanisms. In chronic GVHD patients, donor T cells from transplanted tissues display immunologic activity against host cells in the blood and skin.[155,156] Both alloreactive and autoreactive T-cell clones are persistent in chronic GVHD patients because of ineffective thymic selection and elimination due to advanced age, preceding acute GVHD, pretransplantation cytoreduction, and immunosuppressive therapies.[116] Epithelial cells suffer injury from CD8+ cytotoxic lymphocytes, NK cells, macrophages, and mast cells.[157] Cytokine mediators such as TNF-α induce major histocompatibility complex (MHC) molecules on target tissues and stimulate fibroblast proliferation and collagen production. Mast cells are chronically activated and contribute to the fibrosis of sclerodermoid GVHD. In addition, an autoimmune phenomenon is established in chronic GVHD, as polyclonal B-cell activation results in antibodies against donor cell lines, inducing hemolytic anemia, thrombocytopenia, and antilymphocyte activity.[158,159] Autoantibodies are also produced, targeting the nuclei, nucleoli, smooth muscle, thyroid, and skin of the host.

Etiology. Chronic GVHD occurs in 33% of HLA-matched sibling BMTs and in 80% of HLA-unmatched unrelated BMTs.[160] A history of prior acute GVHD increases the risk of developing the chronic form by 11

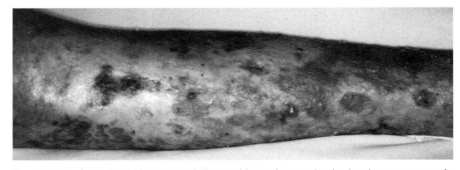

Figure 20–5. Sclerodermoid changes, vitiligo, and hyperpigmentation in chronic cutaneous graft-versus-host disease of the arm.

times and is the greatest risk factor.[161] Other risk factors are similar to those for acute GVHD and include recipient age greater than 20 years; sex mismatch, with a female donor (especially one who has undergone transfusion or pregnancy) and a male recipient; and the transplantation of non-T-cell depleted bone marrow.[162] In the presence of all three factors, there is a 55% chance of developing chronic GVHD within 3 years post-transplantation.

Diagnosis. The diagnosis of chronic GVHD can be made clinically by the identification of characteristic lichenoid or sclerodermatous lesions, but definitive diagnosis requires a skin biopsy. Other supportive evidence includes multiorgan involvement, histology, and a complete blood cell count showing evidence of eosinophilia or thrombocytopenia. Early chronic GVHD appears histologically similar to acute GVHD whereas the lichenoid form appears similar to classic lichen planus. In contrast, the late sclerodermatous phase is characterized by epidermal atrophy, destruction of adnexal structures, dense fibrosis, and a sparse inflammatory infiltrate.[158] Advanced sclerodermoid GVHD may be indistinguishable from systemic scleroderma. Granular IgM deposits are present at the dermoepidermal junction in 86% of chronic GVHD biopsy specimens.[163] The involvement of other organ systems can be diagnosed through biopsies showing histopathologic characteristics of primary biliary cirrhosis on liver biopsy or of bronchiolitis obliterans on bronchoscopic biopsy. In patients who do not display signs and symptoms of GVHD, screening studies with random skin biopsies may be performed between days 75 and 100 after BMT.[164]

Treatment. Similarly to acute GVHD, the chronic GVHD entails a high degree of morbidity and mortality and requires long-term systemic immunosuppressive therapy. The required first-line therapy is an alternating regimen of cyclosporine (12 mg/kg/d) and prednisone (1 mg/kg/d).[165–167] Approximately one-third of patients have a complete response to first-line therapy.[116] For oral involvement of chronic GVHD with lichen planus–like lesions, topical or oral cyclosporine may be used.[168] Topical steroids are also beneficial for oral, vaginal, or penile lesions.[148] Second-line therapy includes cyclophosphamide, methotrexate, or azathioprine.[118] Some studies have shown that thalidomide may be beneficial in cases that are refractory to initial therapy.[169,170] Phototherapy with PUVA provides a response in approximately 50% of patients and allows immunosuppressive dose reduction although this efficacy is limited to thereapy for oral and cutaneous disease.[171] As in the case of acute GVHD, studies demonstrate the efficacy of ECP in treating chronic GVHD, even cases with severe refractory sclerodermatous disease.[146,172,173] One study demonstrated complete cutaneous resolution in 80% of patients.[174]

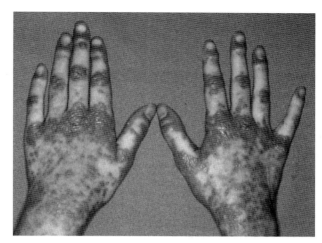

Figure 20–6. Lichenoid chronic cutaneous graft-versus-host disease of the dorsal hands.

Esophageal and pulmonary involvement also show significant improvement with ECP;[174] thus, improvement is not limited to the skin. Prophylactic antibiotics may decrease late infectious complications.

MYCOSIS FUNGOIDES AND SÉZARY SYNDROME

Mycosis fungoides (MF) and Sézary syndrome (SS) are subsets of cutaneous T-cell lymphoma (CTCL), which is a disease of malignant T-cell clones and which is primarily manifested in the skin. Mycosis fungoides is characterized by an epidermotropic skin infiltrate of atypical CD4+ helper T-cell clones, and SS is an erythrodermic variant that is characterized by leukemic involvement with peripherally circulating atypical T cells. While CTCL usually follows a relatively indolent course, life-threatening complications may occur and are usually related to secondary infection and septicemia from cutaneous lesions, indwelling intravenous catheters and lines, and immunosuppressive therapies. Cutaneous lesions, especially tumors and ulcers, may lead to a compromised cutaneous barrier (which places patients at risk of developing cellulitis) and to disseminated viral and bacterial infections. Cases of fulminant or acute exacerbations of cutaneous disease may also require emergent care.

Clinical Manifestation

The cutaneous manifestations of mycosis fungoides and Sézary syndrome (MF/SS) are polymorphic. The lesions, usually asymmetrically and variably distributed, appear as solitary, multiple, or confluent erythematous scaly patches in the earliest stages and may progress to plaques, tumors, or ulcerations. The nature of this progression is variable and unpredictable. The eruption may also be poikilodermatous, follicular, bullous, or hypopigmented.

Diffuse exfoliative erythroderma with keratoderma of the palms and soles may be seen, especially in cases of Sézary syndrome, the leukemic variant of MF (Figure 20–7). Flares of intense erythroderma are generally a sign of infection, especially infection with *Staphylococcus aureus*. Necrotic tumors are most commonly due to *Enterococcus* and *Pseudomonas*. Infections are the major cause of morbidity and mortality in MF/SS; sepsis and bacterial pneumonia account for 88% of infectious complications.[175] Advanced disease stages carry a higher risk of death from infection, and 50% of stage III deaths and 40% of stage IV deaths are due to infection.[175] Nodal involvement and visceral disease may also occur and are associated with a poor prognosis. The peripheral lymph nodes are the most common sites of extracutaneous spread, and the spleen, lung, and liver are the most common sites of visceral involvement.[176] Other indications of a poor prognosis include peripheral blood involvement with Sézary cells; elevated lactate dehydrogenase; elevated soluble IL-2 receptor (sIL-2R); and age greater than 60 years.[177–179]

Etiology

The etiology of mycosis fungoides is unknown although theories implicate infectious agents, oncogenes, cytokines, or environmental exposures.[180] One theory is that superantigens and chronic antigen stimulation may play a role in instigating clonal malignant transformation of reactive T cells.[181] Infectious agents such as *Staphylococcus aureus* may act as superantigens in MF/SS and may be capable of inducing acute exacerbations in disease.[182,183] Disease flares and rapid progression may also be related to large-cell transformation, which is associated with advanced disease and shortened median survival of only 2 to 19 months after transformation.[184,185]

Infectious complications in MF/SS are common; 23% of patients developed sepsis in one study, with *S. aureus,* other Gram-positive cocci, and *Pseudomonas aeruginosa* being the predominant pathogens.[180,186] Primary sites of infection include lymphomatous skin ulcers, intravenous-access sites, surgical-wound infections, sputum, and sites of invasive procedures. While *Staphylococcus aureus* accounts for approximately 20% of cases of septicemia, Gram-negative bacilli infections are associated with a higher rate of mortality (88%) than are Gram-positive cocci infections (22%), and most cases are due to nosocomial infections.[175] Herpesvirus infections, with or without cutaneous dissemination, are also common in MF/SS patients, but systemic dissemination is rare. Risk factors for infection include stage IV disease, generalized erythroderma, palpable lymphadenopathy, and involvement of the lymph nodes and peripheral blood.[186] Extracutaneous lymphomatous involvement is the most important factor for developing recurrent bacterial infections, disseminated herpesvirus infections, and blood stream infections.[175]

Diagnosis

The diagnosis of MF/SS is initially made through histologic findings of a dermal and epidermotropic atypical CD4+ T-cell infiltrate with hyperconvoluted cerebriform nuclei and Pautrier's microabscesses. Patients should be monitored for clinical signs and symptoms of infection and sepsis, such as impetiginization, erythrodermic flares, fever, hypothermia, tachycardia, tachypnea, hypotension, altered mental status, leukocytosis with left shift, thrombocytopenia, and coagulopathy. With the presentation of scaly and intensely erythematous lesions or erythroderma, skin cultures should be performed to evaluate for bacterial colonization and to guide antimicrobial therapy. A chest radiograph and laboratory data, including a complete blood count (CBC), liver function tests, urinalysis, blood cultures, levels of sIL-2R, and T-cell panel by flow cytometry, should be evaluated for evidence of infection and disease flare.[179]

Treatment

Management of the septic MF/SS patient should include supportive care and initial empiric broad-coverage systemic antibiotics, with combinations of cephalosporins, nafcillin, vancomycin, and aminoglycosides. The regimen should then be adjusted for specific organisms and

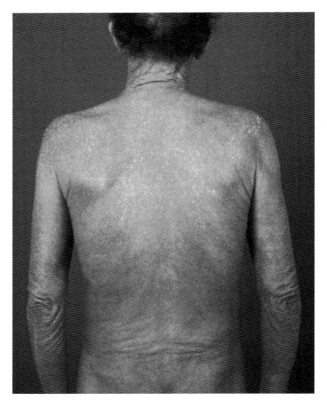

Figure 20–7. Erythroderma in Sézary syndrome.

sensitivities identified through culture. While cultures will grow Gram-positive cocci in most cases, consideration should be given to continuing Gram-negative coverage in patients with a severely compromised cutaneous barrier, since secondary nosocomial Gram-negative bacilli infections are common and rapidly fatal.[186] Skin care should include whirlpool therapy, baths of 20% acetic acid, moisturizers, and Silvadene Cream or Bactroban Cream on impetiginized or open wounds. For disease flare-ups with diffuse skin lesions or erythroderma, topical corticosteroids under wet wraps may offer temporary relief and palliation. Rapidly progressive tumors often require emergent local radiotherapy. Erythrodermic MF and SS patients may also benefit from ECP, which is well tolerated and has been shown to prolong survival when used as adjuvant therapy.[187]

INFECTIOUS DERMATOLOGIC EMERGENCIES

Infectious bacterial complications can become a major source of morbidity and mortality for many oncologic patients because these patients' cutaneous barriers are often disrupted by their disease and by the diagnostic tests and therapies that they undergo. Oncologic patients often have cutaneous lesions and tumors, and some undergo operative surgical explorations and resections of their cancers, as well as invasive diagnostic tests and biopsies that predispose them to the development of infection. It is important to monitor these patients for signs and symptoms of infection as they may become rapidly progressive and fatal if left undetected and untreated, especially in cases of staphylococcal and streptococcal toxic shock syndromes. Immunosuppression from both their cancer and chemotherapy also places them at risk for disseminated infections such as meningococcemia, systemic candidiasis, varicella zoster, and other viral and fungal infections.

Meningococcemia

Clinical Manifestation. Meningococcemia typically occurs during the winter and spring, usually in children or young adults. The infection manifests as fever, headache, nausea, vomiting, myalgia, mental status alterations, and meningeal signs, and it commonly presents with early cutaneous manifestations.[188] The eruption of meningococcemia typically appears on the distal extremities as geometric purpura or petechiae; this may be present in approximately 50 to 60% of patients and may be the first presenting sign of infection (Figure 20–8).[189] Petechiae may localize at areas of pressure. Maculopapular eruptions may also occur. Purpura fulminans, characterized by purpura with grey necrotic centers, large ecchymoses, hemorrhagic bullae, and (sometimes) ischemia progressing to

gangrene of the distal extremities, may develop in the setting of disseminated intravascular coagulation (DIC) in fulminant meningococcemia. Purpura fulminans in the presence of massive adrenal hemorrhage is referred to as Waterhouse-Friderichsen syndrome. Other complications of meningococcemia include myocardial failure, septic shock, meningococcal arthritis, nonpurulent pericarditis, and neurologic dysfunction. The mortality of meningococcal disease is 10 to 20% and usually occurs when diagnosis and treatment are delayed.[190] Poor prognostic factors include coma, shock, seizures, hyperventilation, thrombocytopenia ($< 100,000/\mu L$), metabolic acidosis (pH < 7.3), or extreme age.[189]

Pathophysiologic Mechanisms. Meningococcal lipopolysaccharide (LPS) endotoxin, which causes the release of cytokines such as TNF-α, IL-1, IL-6, and IFN-γ from monocytes, macrophages, and endothelial cells, is responsible for the systemic signs of meningococcemia.[189,191] The production of inflammatory mediators such as prostaglandins, leukotrienes, and platelet-activating factor increases capillary leakage and tissue damage and causes intravascular clotting and thrombosis.[192] These effects are thought to be responsible for the petechial and purpuric skin lesions, multiorgan failure, and shock.

Etiology. Meningococcemia is caused by *Neisseria meningitidis*, an encapsulated Gram-negative diplococcus, with serogroups A, B, and C being responsible in over 90% of worldwide cases of meningococcal disease.[189] Approximately 10 to 20% of the healthy population are nasopharyngeal carriers of this organism. Development of meningococcal disease is often linked to pneumonia, sinusitis, and tracheobronchitis.[193] Whereas most cases in healthy individuals occur because of a lack of bactericidal antibodies, individuals who are deficient in late complement components have a 50 to 60% risk of developing meningococcal disease.[189] Oncologic patients often fall into this category, as such acquired immunodeficiency

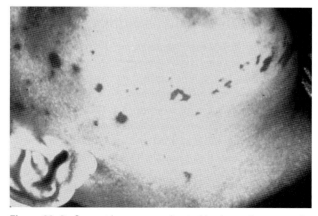

Figure 20–8. Geometric purpura and petechiae in meningococcemia.

occurs in patients with SLE, multiple myeloma, asplenia, immunoglobulin deficiency, severe hepatic disease, protein-losing enteropathies, and nephrotic syndromes.[189] In one population-based study, approximately two-thirds of the patients had one or more immunocompromising conditions.[193] Transmission occurs by contact through respiratory droplets, usually in crowded settings.

Diagnosis. The initial suspicion of meningococcemia is based on clinical findings of a petechial rash in the setting of fever and other characteristic constitutional symptoms. This clinical presentation should also spark suspicion of bacterial sepsis, Rocky Mountain spotted fever, endocarditis, disseminated gonococcal disease, typhus, and infections from viruses such as human parvovirus B19, Epstein-Barr virus, *Cytomegalovirus*, and hemorrhagic fever viruses.[189] Diagnosis is made through positive identification of the organism on Gram's stain and culture of the blood, in cerebrospinal fluid, and on skin biopsy specimens. Cultures and Gram's stain are positive in 60 to 70% of tissue cultures and scrapings of skin lesions, even after the start of antibiotics.[189,194] Histopathology shows organisms within endothelial cells and neutrophils, as well as vascular endothelial necrosis and thrombosis.[195]

Treatment. Meningococcemia requires early diagnosis and expeditious treatment to maintain a favorable prognosis. Under the suspicion of meningococcemia, penicillin G at a dose of 12 to 24 million units per day should be initiated immediately in divided doses every 4 hours.[196] Ceftriaxone (2 g every 12 hours) may be used for resistant organisms. All individuals who have been in close contact with or have been possibly exposed to the patient should receive chemoprophylaxis with rifampin, ciprofloxacin, or ceftriaxone. Patients should be managed in an intensive care setting and given appropriate intravenous fluids, oxygen and ventilatory support, and inotropic support. There have been anecdotal reports of benefit from using intravenous protein C concentrates and recombinant-tissue plasminogen activator in patients with purpura fulminans.[197,198]

Toxic Shock Syndromes

Clinical Manifestation. Staphylococcal toxic shock syndrome (TSS) manifests as fever, malaise, myalgia, nausea, vomiting, diarrhea, hypotension, and mental status alterations in the presence of diffuse erythroderma.[188] Desquamation subsequently follows within 5 to 14 days of erythroderma. Mucosal involvement also occurs, manifested as a strawberry tongue and as hyperemia of the conjunctivae, oral mucosa, and genital mucosa. Other cutaneous manifestations include edema of the hands and feet and a petechial rash. Multiorgan involvement occurs and affects the GI, hepatic, musculoskeletal, renal, cardiopulmonary, and central nervous systems. Mortality is less than 5% in cases related to menstruation and tampon use but is two- to threefold higher in cases related to other causes.[199]

While the influenza-like constitutional symptoms of streptococcal TSS are similar to those seen in *Staphylococcus*-induced infections, the initial cutaneous manifestations may be more subtle and localized. The infection usually appears at the site of cutaneous trauma as localized swelling, tenderness, and erythema. The portal of entry is identifiable in 60% of cases, and severe localized pain may precede cutaneous manifestations.[200] Desquamative erythroderma occurs less often than in *Staphylococcus*-induced infections. Violaceous bullae are common when the infection progresses deep into the subcutaneous tissue and develops into necrotizing fasciitis. Necrotizing fasciitis is a common complication that results in the progressive destruction of fat and fascia in approximately 50% of cases.[200] Initially, necrotizing fasciitis appears as inflamed indurated skin at the affected site; it may then develop blisters and bullae. If not treated early, the bullous stage of the condition evolves into cutaneous gangrene, with myonecrosis and extension along fascial planes. Shock and early-onset multiorgan involvement, with renal impairment, coagulopathy, hepatitis, and adult respiratory distress syndrome, are characteristic of streptococcal TSS. Hypotension develops in nearly all patients, usually following renal impairment, and is evident at presentation in 50% of cases.[200] Streptococcal TSS carries a 30 to 70% mortality rate.[199]

Pathophysiologic Mechanisms. Toxic shock syndromes are induced by bacterial toxins, which act as major virulence factors. Staphylococcal TSS is induced by the staphylococcal production of TSS toxin 1 (TSST-1) and staphylococcal enterotoxins, which exhibit pyrogenicity and superantigenicity. Staphylococcal toxins activate antigen-presenting cells and T-cell lymphocytes, which leads to a pro-inflammatory cytokine response, causing fever, hypotension, and shock.[201,202] The streptococcal pyrogenic exotoxins (particularly exotoxins A, B, and C) are thought to be involved in the mechanism of shock and multiorgan failure that is seen in TSS.[188,200] These toxins have superantigen activity in vitro, stimulating the synthesis and release of TNF, IL-1, IL-6, IL-2, and interferon-γ, which may be involved in the pathogenesis of shock.[203,204] Activation of the kallikrein/kinin system could also release bradykinin, contributing to the signs and symptoms of streptococcal TSS.[205]

Etiology. Staphylococcal TSS was originally associated with *Staphylococcus aureus* infections during tampon use by menstruating females.[206] Currently, however, nonmenstrual cases are more common and occur in association with influenza, childbirth, tracheitis, surgical-wound infections, nasal packing, barrier contraceptives, and localized staphylococcal infection. There is recurrence in up to 40% of cases, which may be related to an inability to produce appropriate antibodies.[206]

Streptococcal TSS is usually caused by group A streptococci or *Streptococcus pyogenes*. As with staphylococcal TSS, streptococcal TSS often begins with infection at sites of cutaneous trauma. However, streptococcal TSS has also been associated with streptococcal pneumonia, sinusitis, and pharyngitis without signs of overt cutaneous trauma, probably as a result of bacterial seeding into the soft tissues from transient bacteremia. While most cases of the "flesh-eating" bacterial syndrome are related to streptococcal necrotizing fasciitis, other causes are *Vibrio vulnificus*, *Escherichia coli*, *Staphylococcus aureus*, Enterobacteriaceae, and *Clostridium*, *Proteus*, and *Bacteroides* species. Advanced age, peripheral vascular disease, diabetes, renal disease, and alcohol or drug abuse are risk factors that are associated with the development of complications with necrotizing fasciitis.[195] In recent years, an association has been suggested between the use of ibuprofen and the development of necrotizing fasciitis in patients with varicella infections, possibly due to masking of initial symptoms and suppression of the immune response.[207] Furthermore, deficiency of specific bactericidal and antistreptococcal superantigen-neutralizing antibodies may predispose some patients to the development of invasive streptococcal infections.[208]

Diagnosis. Diagnosis of staphylococcal TSS relies heavily on the recognition of characteristic clinical signs and symptoms, especially since *Staphylococcus aureus* is only rarely identified from blood cultures. It is also important to exclude other etiologies of erythroderma, including Sézary syndrome, erythrodermic psoriasis, drug hypersensitivity, and pityriasis rubra pilaris.[209] Other diseases with similar systemic and cutaneous findings include TEN, staphylococcal scalded-skin syndrome (SSSS), Rocky Mountain spotted fever (RMSF), meningococcemia, Kawasaki syndrome, and systemic lupus erythematosus.[195]

In the diagnosis of streptococcal TSS, early necrotizing fasciitis must be differentiated from cellulitis so that appropriate treatment can be initiated. Radiographic imaging of the extremities is useful in excluding gas production from clostridial and anaerobic organisms, and magnetic resonance imaging can be used to locate and assess deep-seated infections.[210] Biopsies for culture, Gram's stains, and histopathology are also useful for definitive diagnosis and identification of the pathogen.[188,211] The organism may be isolated in more than 60% of cases.[199] The histopathology of TSS is similar to that of TEN, with splitting between the epidermis and dermis (although inflammatory patterns may distinguish TSS from TEN).[212] Muscle compartment pressure monitoring must be used when pain and swelling become progressive, as elevated compartment pressures may lead to myonecrosis. Common laboratory findings in

streptococcal TSS show a significant left shift in the white blood cell count differential, azotemia, hypocalcemia, hypoalbuminemia, thrombocytopenia, hematuria, and elevated creatine kinase.[199,200]

Treatment. Initial management of staphylococcal TSS involves removal of the infection source, such as tampons or nasal packing. Infected tissues may require surgical débridement. Supportive care and systemic antibiotics covering *Staphylococcus*, such as nafcillin or oxacillin, must be initiated as well.[195] Intravenous immunoglobulin (IVIG) may be used to neutralize circulating toxins.[213] Streptococcal TSS requires more aggressive surgical exploration and débridement of infected soft tissue. Depending on the extent and progression of involvement, surgical intervention may simply require drainage (under the least severe conditions) or may require limb amputation (under the most severe conditions). Empiric broad-spectrum antibiotics should be given until *Streptococcus* is identified, after which both penicillin G and clindamycin should be initiated.[200] The importance of clindamycin has become more apparent as studies have demonstrated its ability to suppress bacterial toxin and protein synthesis and to facilitate antibacterial phagocytic action.[199,214,215] Treatment with hyperbaric oxygen is an adjunctive option that has been shown to reduce mortality and the need for débridement.[216] There are an increasing number of reports documenting the efficacy of IVIG in neutralizing bacterial exotoxins when used as adjunctive treatment for streptococcal TSS.[213,217,218]

Disseminated Varicella and Herpes Zoster

Clinical Manifestation. Varicella infections may be classified by two separate clinical manifestations: primary varicella and herpes zoster. Primary varicella, or "chickenpox," usually appears in young children whereas herpes zoster tends to appear after the age of 50 years. In both, severe and disseminated cases occur in immunocompromised hosts. Primary varicella manifests as fever and a generalized rash with lesions in varying stages of evolution, starting from macules and papules and progressing to vesicles and crusts. The eruption appears predominantly on the trunk and proximal arms. Secondary bacterial infection is common and sometimes leads to severe conditions such as TSS. Severe disease and dissemination develop, with the most common extracutaneous complications being varicella pneumonia, occurring in 1 of 400 adults, and central nervous system (CNS) disease such as cerebellar ataxia, which occurs in 1 of 4,000 cases.[219] Varicella pneumonia results in death as a result of respiratory failure in 30% of immunocompromised patients.[220] Other commonly seen complications of disseminated varicella include hepatitis, necrotizing splenitis and lymphadenitis, esophagitis, enteritis, colitis, and pancreatitis.[221]

Disseminated herpes zoster (DHZ) presents as an extensive variation of herpes zoster, which classically appears as a painful eruption of grouped vesicles distributed in a dermatomal fashion (Figure 20–9). Disseminated herpes zoster is defined as the presence of 20 or more vesicles outside the primary and adjacent involved dermatomes.[195] Herpes zoster pain is often severe and precedes cutaneous manifestations by 1 to 3 days in 90% of cases. An eruption follows the neuralgia, beginning with erythematous macules and papules and progressing to vesicles, pustules, and finally to crusts. The evolution of cutaneous lesions is complete within 7 to 10 days.[222] Dissemination may take place 4 to 10 days after the onset of localized infection. A higher frequency of complications such as secondary bacterial infections, gangrene, prolonged healing time, and scarring characterizes DHZ. Life-threatening complications include multiorgan involvement of the lungs, liver, eyes, and brain and occur in 10% of DHZ patients. Varicella pneumonitis is the most common complication and the most frequent cause of mortality. Occasionally, severe varicella-zoster virus (VZV) infections with visceral or neurologic disease occur in immunocompromised patients without visible skin lesions.[223]

Pathophysiologic Mechanisms. Varicella usually infects individuals through the respiratory-tract mucosa and subsequently disseminates through the blood stream and into the skin, causing the cutaneous manifestations of primary varicella. After the resolution of primary varicella, VZV remains latent in the neurons and satellite cells of the dorsal root and cranial-nerve ganglia until re-activation. While not completely clear, the pathogenesis of herpes zoster is related to VZV re-activation by immunosuppression, specifically, impaired cell-mediated immunity. In this setting, VZV is allowed to replicate within sensory nerves, causing ganglionitis with inflammation and neuronal necrosis, resulting in neuralgia.[222] The infection spreads through direct neural extension or hematogenously to induce the cutaneous manifestations of herpes zoster.

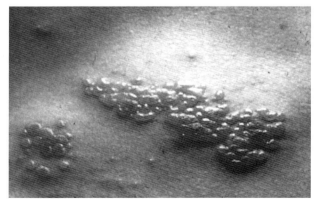

Figure 20–9. Grouped vesicles in herpes zoster.

Etiology. In general, oncologic patients have a high incidence of herpes zoster. The risk of dissemination of herpes zoster is significantly associated with the presence of active tumor and is highest among immunocompromised patients (as high as 40%).[222,224] Leukemia and lymphoma patients seem especially predisposed to developing the infection, and 20 to 50% of Hodgkin's disease patients are affected.[225] Herpes zoster eruptions in cancer patients typically appear within months after the initiation of chemotherapy (1 month) or radiotherapy (7 months).[224] Bone marrow transplantation also places patients at risk with a 30% probability of developing herpes zoster within 1 year after transplantation.[226] Acute or chronic GVHD adds additional risk of both infection and dissemination in affected patients.[226] Among other immunocompromised states, other associations with herpes zoster include other cancers, transplantation, HIV infection, immunosuppressive therapy, and advanced age.[195]

Diagnosis. The diagnosis of varicella infections can usually be made from the clinical presentation. A Tzanck test smear showing multinucleated giant cells and epithelial cells containing acidophilic intranuclear inclusions is diagnostic of either herpes simplex virus (HSV) or VZV infection. Viral cultures and direct immunofluorescence may also aid in the diagnosis although VZV is a labile virus that is more difficult to grow and isolate than HSV and is positive in only 30 to 60% of cases.[220,227] Direct fluoroscopy of VZV antigens, which is more sensitive, can also be performed on skin scrapings and can differentiate VZV from HSV. There are few mimics of dermatomal zoster, except for HSV infections. Disseminated herpes zoster may resemble other vesicular dermatoses such as dermatitis herpetiformis.

Treatment. Patients with disseminated varicella and herpes zoster require hospital admission for respiratory isolation, supportive care, and parenteral antiviral treatment. The recommended treatment for disseminated disease in the immunocompromised patient is acyclovir, 10 mg/kg intravenously every 8 hours for 10 days.[220] Resistant cases may be treated with foscarnet, 40 mg/kg every 8 hours for 14 days or until the infection is resolved. Less severe varicella and herpes zoster without dissemination may be treated with an oral antiviral regimen. Topical skin care consists of cool compresses followed by calamine lotion, topical antibiotics (such as Silvadene for nonallergic patients), and emollients. The neuralgic pain of herpes zoster is usually relieved by antiviral treatment although narcotic analgesics may be required for severe pain. Postherpetic neuralgia may be prevented by prednisone with H_2 blocker antihistamines. Postherpetic neuralgia is difficult to treat as there are no proven effective therapies. Capsaicin, tricyclic antidepressants, gabapentin, carbamazepine, topical anesthetics, and nerve blocks are options that may have some efficacy.[220]

Systemic Candidiasis, Aspergillosis, and Mucormycosis

Clinical Manifestation. Systemic candidiasis, aspergillosis, mucormycosis, and fusarium are prevalent in cancer patients because of the immunosuppression and neutropenia caused by cancer treatments. (Systemic candidiasis is the most common disseminated fungal infection and receives the most attention in this discussion.) In all three infectious diseases, systemic involvement is generally more common than cutaneous manifestations. Cutaneous lesions are seen in 10 to 15% of patients with systemic candidiasis, with *Candida tropicalis* infection exhibiting the highest frequency (23%) of cutaneous manifestations.[228] In addition to the typical mucocutaneous lesions of superficial candidiasis, the eruption of disseminated candidiasis manifests as palpable purpura (most common on the extremities), solitary or multiple erythematous papules with pale centers, subcutaneous abscesses, cellulitis, or ecthyma gangrenosum–like lesions.[229] Complications include meningitis, endocarditis, arthritis, pneumonitis, peritonitis, and endophthalmitis.[230] A clinical triad of fever, myalgias, and tender nodules is commonly seen in *Candida albicans* infections. If not appropriately diagnosed and treated, systemic candidiasis leads to significant morbidity and mortality.

Aspergillosis most commonly presents with sinusitis and with pulmonary and CNS involvement. Cutaneous emboli, which appear as erythematous indurated plaques evolving into hemorrhagic bullae and necrotic ulcers with eschars, are evident in 11% of patients with disseminated disease.[231,232] Lesions may also appear as molluscum-like papules, abscesses, cellulitis, subcutaneous granulomas, or vegetating plaques. (Figure 20–10) The mortality of disseminated aspergillosis is extremely high (80 to 100%) despite therapy.[232]

Mucormycosis may present with primary or secondary cutaneous lesions. Primary lesions appear as erythematous papules or pustules that evolve into necrotic ulcerations. Rhinocerebral mucormycosis, which is the most common primary manifestation, may involve the overlying skin of the nose and face, causing erythema, induration, and central purple-black discoloration. Cutaneous manifestations of hematogenous spread include violaceous subcutaneous nodules resembling ecthyma gangrenosum.[233] Pulmonary and GI involvement also occurs. Similarly to aspergillosis, the prognosis of mucormycosis is very poor, and mortality is frequent.

With the prevalence of myelosuppressive chemotherapy in the treatment of cancer, many previously nonpathogenic fungal organisms such as *Fusarium* have become an increasing source of disseminated fungal infections in oncologic patients. *Fusarium* has been isolated in 12% of bone marrow transplant patients (second to *Aspergillus*) who developed non-*Candida* disseminated fungal infections.[234] Patients with *Fusarium* infection usually have chemotherapy-induced neutropenia with intractable fever. Cutaneous manifestations occur early and affect 85% of patients with painful erythematous indurated papules and nodules that develop necrotic centers.[235] Unfortunately, disseminated *Fusarium* infections usually result in death (the mortality rate is > 70%), despite combination therapy.

Pathophysiologic Mechanisms. *Candida* species are known to produce virulence factors such as proteases, which are thought to play a pathogenic role. It is known that immunosuppression and alteration of the bacterial flora results in the proliferation of yeast. While deficiencies in T cell–mediated immunity results in a predisposition to superficial mucocutaneous candidiasis, patients with deficient or defective neutrophil and macrophage function are susceptible to both superficial and systemic candidiasis.[229] Thus, AIDS patients rarely develop systemic candidiasis whereas neutropenic cancer patients are at high risk of dissemination. Dissemination occurs through the GI tract, intravenous infusion lines, or skin lesions and areas of trauma.

Etiology. Systemic candidiasis is often seen in immunocompromised patients with cancer (particularly leukemia) although the incidence of yeast infections has decreased overall since the advent of fluconazole prophylaxis. Risk factors include neutropenia, systemic corticosteroid use, hyperglycemia, and broad-spectrum antibiotic use.[228] *Candida albicans* is the most frequently isolated organism in systemic candidiasis. Non–*Candida albicans* systemic infections have a high frequency (46%)

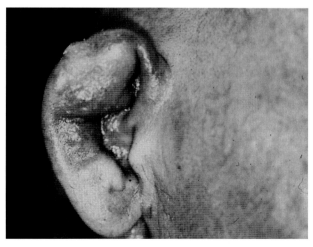

Figure 20–10. Aspergillus cellulitis of the ear.

in the oncologic population, particularly in patients with hematologic malignancies, with *Candida tropicalis* being responsible in 25% of cases, *Candida glabrata* in 8%, *Candida parapsilosis* in 7%, and *Candida krusei* in 4%.[236] Leukemia patients are particularly susceptible to *Candida albicans* or *Candida tropicalis* whereas *Candida glabrata* is more often pathogenic in other cancers.[235] Since its introduction in 1990, fluconazole prophylaxis has become a mainstay of management in BMT patients and has been associated with an increase in resistant *Candida* strains such as *Candida krusei, Candida lusitaniae,* and *Candida parapsilosis*.[236–238] Resistant strains of *Candida albicans* in cancer patients are uncommon, however.[237]

Aspergillosis is most often caused by the species *Aspergillus fumigatus* although *Aspergillus flavus* is most commonly isolated in primary cutaneous disease. Risk factors for aspergillosis include neutropenia, corticosteroid use, hematologic malignancy, broad-spectrum antibiotic use, AIDS, and immunosuppressive medication use. Mucormycosis is caused by molds of the Zygomycetes class, with *Rhizopus, Mucor,* and *Absidia* species being most frequently involved.[239] Risk factors of mucormycosis include hyperglycemia, neutropenia, systemic corticosteroid use, acidosis, malnutrition, extensive trauma and burns, receiving an organ transplant, and hematologic malignancies.[233] Disseminated *Fusarium* infection is most commonly caused by *Fusarium solani*.[235] Areas of local trauma (such as sites of indwelling venous catheters) are common ports of entry for *Fusarium* although the organism may also enter the respiratory tract, sinuses, or GI tract.

Diagnosis. The diagnosis of systemic candidiasis may be difficult as symptoms may be nonspecific and because cutaneous manifestations are often not present. The yeast organism is difficult to isolate from blood cultures, so cultures may be repeatedly negative.[229] Diagnosis can be made through skin biopsy specimens, with histology showing *Candida* cells in the dermis when lesions are present.[240] In some cases, the discovery of systemic candidiasis is not made until an autopsy is performed. Aspergillosis may be diagnosed by identification of the organism through tissue biopsy specimens and cultures and by staining with Gomori's methenamine silver stain or periodic acid–Schiff stain.[232] Blood cultures are rarely positive for aspergillosis although positive cultures with two or more colonies are associated with aggressive disease and poor outcome.[241] In contrast, *Fusarium* may be identified readily in cultures.

Treatment. The therapy of choice for systemic candidiasis, aspergillosis, mucormycosis, and *Fusarium* infecton is intravenous amphotericin B. Liposomal amphotericin B is an option that has been shown to be equal in efficacy and less nephrotoxic.[229] A combination of high-dose

amphotericin B and flucytosine may be effective in resistant cases. Surgical débridement may be required for adjunctive therapy of mucormycosis. High-dose amphotericin B is required for treatment of *Fusarium* infections, as the organism is usually resistant to conventional doses.[242] Generally, neutropenic recovery offers the best chance for the resolution of *Fusarium* infections.

REFERENCES

1. Bigby M, Jick S, Jick H, et al. Drug-induced cutaneous reactions: a report from the Boston Collaborative Drug Surveillance Program on 15,438 consecutive inpatients, 1975-1982. JAMA 1986;256:3358–63.

2. Leape LL, Brennan TA, Laird N, et al. The nature of adverse events in hospitalized patients: results of the Harvard Medical Practice Study II. N Engl J Med 1991;324:377–84.

3. Alanko K, Stubb S, Kauppinen K. Cutaneous drug reactions: clinical types and causative agents: a five-year survey of in-patients (1981–1985). Acta Derm Venereol 1989;69:223–6.

4. Roujeau JC, Stern RS. Medical progress: severe adverse cutaneous reactions to drugs. N Engl J Med 1994;331: 1272–85.

5. Shear NH, Spielberg SP. Anticonvulsant hypersensitivity syndrome: in vitro assessment of risk. J Clin Invest 1988;82:1826–32.

6. Pelekanos J, Camfield P, Camfield C, et al. Allergic rash due to antiepileptic drugs: clinical features and management. Epilepsia 1991;32:554–9.

7. Rapp NP, Norton JA, Young B, et al. Cutaneous reactions in head-injured patients receiving phenytoin for seizure prophylaxis. Neurosurgery 1983;13:272–5.

8. Vittorio CC, Muglia JJ. Anticonvulsant hypersensitivity syndrome. Arch Intern Med 1995;155:2285–90.

9. Parker WA, Shearer CA. Phenytoin hepatotoxicity: a case report and review. Neurology 1979;29:175–8.

10. Smythe MA, Umstead GS. Phenytoin hepatotoxicity: a review of the literature. Ann Pharmacother 1989;23: 13–7.

11. Ekenstam EAF, Callen JP. Cutaneous leukocytoclastic vasculitis: clinical and laboratory features of 82 patients seen in private practice. Arch Dermatol 1984;120:484–9.

12. Sanchez NP, Van Hale HM, Su WP. Clinical and histopathologic spectrum of necrotizing vasculitis: report of findings in 101 cases. Arch Dermatol 1985;15:665–70.

13. Leung DYM, Diaz LA, DeLeo V, et al. Allergic and immunologic skin disorders. JAMA 1997;278:1914–23.

14. Soter N. Acute and chronic urticaria and angioedema. J Am Acad Dermatol 1991;25:146–54.

15. Kulp-Shorten CL, Callen JP. Urticaria, angioedema, and rheumatologic disease. Rheum Dis Clin North Am 1996;22:95–115.

16. Bielory L, Yancey KB, Young NS, et al. Cutaneous manifestations of serum sickness in patients receiving antithymocyte globulin. J Am Acad Dermatol 1985;13:411–7.

17. Bauer KA. Coumarin-induced skin necrosis. Arch Dermatol 1993;129:766–8.

18. Zimbelman J, Lefkowitz J, Schaeffer C, et al. Unusual

complications of warfarin therapy: skin necrosis and priapism. J Pediatr 2000;137:266–8.

19. Miletich J, Sherman L, Broze G Jr. Absence of thrombosis in subjects with heterozygous protein C deficiency. N Engl J Med 1987;317:991–6.

20. MacLean JA, Moscicki R, Bloch KJ. Adverse reactions to heparin. Ann Allergy 1990;65:254–9.

21. Tuneau A, Moreno A, de Moragas JM. Cutaneous reactions secondary to heparin injections. J Am Acad Dermatol 1985;12:1072–7.

22. Spielberg SP, Gordon GB, Blake DA, et al. Anticonvulsant toxicity in vitro: possible role of arene oxides. J Pharmacol Exp Ther 1981;217:386–9.

23. Gennis MA, Vemuri R, Burns EA, et al. Familial occurrence of hypersensitivity to phenytoin. Am J Med 1991; 91:631–4.

24. Yoo JH, Kang DS, Chun WH, et al. Anticonvulsant hypersensitivity syndrome with an epoxide hydrolase defect. Br J Dermatol 1999;140:181–3.

25. Bedard K, Smith S, Cribb A. Sequential assessment of an antidrug antibody response in a patient with a systemic delayed-onset sulphonamide hypersensitivity syndrome reaction. Br J Dermatol 2000;142:253–8.

26. Bochner BS, Lichtenstein LM. Anaphylaxis. N Engl J Med 1991;324:1785–90.

27. Horan RF, Schneider LC, Sheffer AL. Allergic skin disorders and mastocytosis. JAMA 1992;268:2858–68.

28. Anderson MW, deShazo RD. Studies of the mechanism of angiotensin-converting enzyme (ACE) inhibitor-associated angioedema: the effect of an ACE inhibitor on cutaneous responses to bradykinin, codeine, and histamine. J Allergy Clin Immunol 1990;85:856–8.

29. Huston D, Bressler R. Urticaria and angioedema. Med Clin North Am 1992;76:805–40.

30. Wintroub BU, Stern R. Cutaneous drug reactions: pathogenesis and clinical classification. J Am Acad Dermatol 1985;13:167–79.

31. Beran RG. Cross-reactive skin eruption with both carbamazepine and oxcarbazepine. Epilepsia 1993;34:163–5.

32. Schlienger RG, Knowles SR, Shear NH. Lamotrigine-associated anticonvulsant hypersensitivity syndrome. Neurology 1998;51:1172–5.

33. MacNeil M, Haase DA, Tremaine R, et al. Fever, lymphadenopathy, eosinophilia, lymphocytosis, hepatitis, and dermatitis: a severe adverse reaction to minocycline. J Am Acad Dermatol 1997;36:347–50.

34. Milionis HJ, Skopelitou A, Elisaf MS. Hypersensitivity syndrome caused by amitriptyline administration. Postgrad Med J 2000;76:361–3.

35. Suzuki Y, Inagi R, Aono Y, et al. Human herpesvirus 6 infection as a risk factor for the development of severe drug-induced hypersensitivity syndrome. Arch Dermatol 1998;134:1108–12.

36. Hedner T, Samuelsson O, Lunde H, et al. Angio-oedema in relation to treatment with angiotensin converting enzyme inhibitors. BMJ 1992;304:941–6.

37. Slater EE, Merrill DD, Guess HA, et al. Clinical profile of angioedema associated with angiotensin converting-enzyme inhibition. JAMA 1988;260:967–70.

38. Brunet P, Jaber K, Berland Y, et al. Anaphylactoid reactions during hemodialysis and hemofiltration: role of associating AN69 membrane and angiotensin I-converting enzyme inhibitors. Am J Kidney Dis 1992;19:444–7.

39. Comp PC. Coumarin-induced skin necrosis: incidence, mechanisms, management, and avoidance. Drug Saf 1993;8:128–35.

40. Vigano D'Angelo S, Comp PC, Esmon CT, et al. Relationship between protein C antigen and anticoagulant activity during oral anticoagulation and in selected disease states. J Clin Invest 1986;77:416–25.

41. Sallah S, Thomas D, Roberts H. Warfarin and heparin-induced skin necrosis and the purple toe syndrome: infrequent complications of anticoagulant treatment. Thromb Haemost 1997;78:785–90.

42. Grimaudo V, Gueissaz F, Hauert J, et al. Necrosis of skin induced by coumarin in a patient deficient in protein S. BMJ 1989;298:233–4.

43. Charlesworth EN. Phenytoin-induced pseudolymphoma syndrome. Arch Dermatol 1977;113:477–80.

44. Blanco R, Martinez-Toboada VM, Rodriguez-Valverde V, et al. Cutaneous vasculitis in children and adults. Medicine 1998;77:403–18.

45. Michel BA, Hunder GG, Bloch DA, et al. Hypersensitivity vasculitis and Henoch-Schonlein purpura: a comparison between the 2 disorders. J Rheumatol 1992;19:721–8.

46. Chopra S, Levell NJ, Chowley G, et al. Systemic corticosteroids in the phenytoin hypersensitivity syndrome. Br J Dermatol 1996;134:1109–12.

47. Redondo P, deFelipe I, de la Pena A, et al. Drug-induced hypersensitivity syndrome and toxic epidermal necrolysis. Treatment with N-acetylcysteine. Br J Dermatol 1997;136:645–6.

48. Simonart T, Tugendhaft P, Vereecken P, et al. Hazards of therapy with high doses of N-acetylcysteine for anticonvulsant-induced hypersensitivity syndrome. Br J Dermatol 1998;138:553.

49. Gropper AL. Diphenylhydantoin sensitivity. Report of fatal case with hepatitis and exfoliative dermatitis. N Engl J Med 1956;254:522–3.

50. Schramm W, Spannagl M, Bauer KA, et al. Treatment of coumarin-induced skin necrosis with a monoclonal antibody purified protein C concentrate. Arch Dermatol 1993;129:753–6.

51. Lyell A. Toxic epidermal necrolysis: an eruption resembling scalding of the skin. Br J Dermatol 1956;68:35–61.

52. Roujeau JC. The spectrum of Stevens-Johnson syndrome and toxic epidermal necrolysis: a clinical classification. J Invest Dermatol 1994;102:S28–30.

53. Bastuji-Garin S, Rzany B, Stern RS, et al. Clinical classification of cases of toxic epidermal necrolysis, and erythema multiforme. Arch Dermatol 1993;129:92–6.

54. Assier H, Bastuji-Garin S, Revuz J, et al. Erythema multiforme major and Stevens-Johnson syndrome are clinically different disorders with distinct etiologies. Arch Dermatol 1995;131:539–43.

55. Rzany B, Hering O, Mockenhaupt M, et al. Histopathological and epidemiological characteristics of patients with erythema exudativum multiforme major, Stevens-Johnson syndrome and toxic epidermal necrolysis. Br J Dermatol 1996;135:6–11.

56. Wolkenstein P, Revuz J. Toxic epidermal necrosis. Dermatol Clin 2000;18:485–95.

57. Rzany B, Mockenhaupt M, Baur S, et al. Epidemiology of erythema exsudativum multiforme majus, Stevens-Johnson syndrome, and toxic epidermal necrolysis in Germany (1990–1992): structure and results of a population-based registry. J Clin Epidemiol 1996;49:769–73.

58. Villada G, Roujeau JC, Cordonnier C, et al. Toxic epidermal necrolysis after bone marrow transplantation: study of nine cases. J Am Acad Dermatol 1990;23:870–5.

59. Revuz J, Penso D, Roujeau JC, et al. Toxic epidermal necrolysis: clinical findings and prognosis factors in 87 patients. Arch Dermatol 1987;123:1160–5.

60. Lebargy F, Wolkenstein P, Lange F, et al. Pulmonary complications in toxic epidermal necrolysis: a clinical prospective study. Intensive Care Med 1997;23:1237–44.

61. Chosidow O, Delchier JC, Chaumette MT, et al. Intestinal involvement in drug-induced toxic epidermal necrolysis. Lancet 1991;337:928.

62. Westley ED, Wechsler HL. Toxic epidermal necrolysis: granulocytic leukopenia as a prognostic indicator. Arch Dermatol 1984;120:721–6.

63. Halebian PH, Corder VJ, Herndon D, et al. A burn center experience with toxic epidermal necrolysis. J Burn Care Rehabil 1983;4:176–83.

64. Ruiz-Maldonado R. Acute disseminated epidermal necrosis types 1, 2, and 3: study of sixty cases. J Am Acad Dermatol 1985;13:623–35.

65. Wolkenstein P, Carriere V, Charue D, et al. A slow acetylator genotype is a risk factor for sulphonamide-induced toxic epidermal necrolysis and Stevens-Johnson syndrome. Pharmacogenetics 1995;5:255–8.

66. Wolkenstein P, Charue D, Laurent Ph, et al. Metabolic predisposition to cutaneous adverse drug reactions: role in toxic epidermal necrolysis caused by sulfonamides and anticonvulsants. Arch Dermatol 1995;131:544–51.

67. Wolkenstein P, Tan C, Lecoeur S, et al. Covalent binding of carbamazepine reactive metabolites to P450 isoforms present in the skin. Chem Biol Interact 1998;113:39–50.

68. Villada G, Roujeau JC, Clerici T, et al. Immunopathology of toxic epidermal necrolysis. Arch Dermatol 1992;128:50–3.

69. Miyauchi H, Hosokawa H, Akaeda T, et al. T-cell subsets in drug-induced toxic epidermal necrolysis: possible pathogenic mechanism induced by CD8-positive T cells. Arch Dermatol 1991;127:851–5.

70. Correia O, Delgado L, Ramos JP, et al. Cutaneous T-cell recruitment in toxic epidermal necrolysis: further evidence of CD8+ lymphocyte involvement. Arch Dermatol 1993;129:466–8.

71. Paquet P, Nikkels A, Arrese JE, et al. Macrophage and tumor necrosis factor alpha in toxic epidermal necrolysis. Arch Dermatol 1994;130:605–8.

72. Paquet P, Nusgens BV, Pierard G, et al. Gelatinases in drug-induced toxic epidermal necrolysis. Eur J Clin Invest 1998;28:528–32.

73. Roujeau JC, Kelly JP, Naldi L, et al. Medication use and the risk of Stevens-Johnson syndrome or toxic epidermal necrolysis. N Engl J Med 1995;333:1600–7.

74. Roujeau JC, Huyn NT, Bracq C, et al. Genetic susceptibility to toxic epidermal necrolysis. Arch Dermatol 1987;123:1171–3.

75. Paul C, Wolkenstein P, Adle H, et al. Apoptosis as a mechanism of keratinocyte death in toxic epidermal necrolysis and Stevens-Johnson syndrome. Br J Dermatol 1996;134:710–4.

76. Lerner LH, Quereshi AA, Bhaskar V, et al. Nitric oxide synthase in toxic epidermal necrolysis and Stevens-Johnson syndrome. J Invest Dermatol 2000;114:196–9.

77. Hernborg H. Stevens-Johnson syndrome after mass prophylaxis with sulfadoxine for cholera in Mozambique. Lancet 1985;2:1072–3.

78. Porteous DM, Berger TG. Severe cutaneous reactions (Stevens-Johnson syndrome and toxic epidermal necrolysis) in human immunodeficiency infection. Arch Dermatol 1991;127:740–1.

79. Rzany B, Correia O, Kelly JP, et al. Risk of Stevens-Johnson syndrome and toxic epidermal necrolysis during first weeks of antiepileptic therapy: a case-control study. Lancet 1999;353:2190–4.

80. Shear NH, Spielberg SP. Anticonvulsant hypersensitivity syndrome. J Clin Invest 1988;82:1826–32.

81. Rasmussen JE. Update on the Stevens-Johnson syndrome. Cleve Clin Med J 1988;55:412–4.

82. Fournier S, Bastuji-Garin S, Mentec H, et al. Toxic epidermal necrolysis associated with mycoplasma pneumoniae infection [letter]. Eur J Clin Microbiol Infect Dis 1995;14:558–9.

83. Garcia-Doval I, LeCleach L, Bocquet H, et al. Toxic epidermal necrolysis and Stevens-Johnson syndrome: does early withdrawal of causative drugs decrease the risk of death? Arch Dermatol 2000;136:323–7.

84. McGee T, Munster A. Toxic epidermal necrolysis syndrome: mortality rate reduced with early referral to regional burn center. Plast Reconstr Surg 1998;102:1018–22.

85. Pruitt BA. Burn treatment for the unburned. JAMA 1987;257:2207–8.

86. Descamps V, Tattevin P, Descamps D, et al. HIV-1 infected patients with toxic epidermal necrolysis: an occupational risk for healthcare workers. Lancet 1999;353:1855–6.

87. Lehrer-Bell KA, Kirsner RS, Tallman PG, et al. Treatment of the cutaneous involvement in Stevens-Johnson syndrome and toxic epidermal necrolysis with silver nitrate-impregnated dressings. Arch Dermatol 1998;134:877–9.

88. Fine JD. Drug therapy: management of acquired bullous skin diseases. N Engl J Med 1995;333:1475–84.

89. Halebian PH, Corder VJ, Madden MR, et al. Improved burn center survival of patients with toxic epidermal necrolysis managed without corticosteroids. Ann Surg 1986;204:503–12.

90. Kelemen JJ, Cioffi WG, McManus WF, et al. Burn center care for patients with toxic epidermal necrolysis. J Am Coll Surg 1995;180:273–8.

91. Rzany B, Schmitt H, Schopf E. Toxic epidermal necrolysis in patients receiving glucocorticosteroids. Acta Derm Venereol 1991;71:171–2.

92. Wolkenstein P, Latarjet J, Roujeau JC, et al. Randomised comparison of thalidomide versus placebo in toxic epidermal necrolysis. Lancet 1998;352:1586–9.

93. Egan C, Grant W, Morris S, et al. Plasmapheresis as an

adjunct treatment in toxic epidermal necrolysis. J Am Acad Dermatol 1999;40:458–61.

94. Heng MC, Allen SG. Efficacy of cyclophosphamide in toxic epidermal necrolysis. J Am Acad Dermatol 1991; 25:778–86.

95. Viard I, Wehrli P, Bullani R, et al. Inhibition of toxic epidermal necrolysis by blockade of CD95 with human intravenous immunoglobulin. Science 1998;282:490–3.

96. Robinson ND, Hashimoto T, Amagai M. The new pemphigus variants. J Am Acad Dermatol 1999;40:649–71.

97. Anhalt GJ. Paraneoplastic pemphigus. Adv Dermatol 1997;12:77–96.

98. Fullerton SH, Wooley DT, Smoller BR, et al. Paraneoplastic pemphigus with autoantibody deposition in bronchial epithelium after autologous bone marrow transplantation. JAMA 1992;267:547–53.

99. Mutasim DF, Pelc NJ, Anhalt GJ. Paraneoplastic pemphigus. Dermatol Clin 1993;11:473–81.

100. Takahashi M, Shimatsu Y, Kazama T, et al. Paraneoplastic pemphigus associated with bronchiolitis obliterans. Chest 2000;117:603–7.

101. Camisa C, Helm TN, Liu YC, et al. Paraneoplastic pemphigus: a report of three cases including one long-term survivor. J Am Acad Dermatol 1992;27:547–53.

102. Stevens SR, Griffiths CEM, Anhalt GJ, et al. Paraneoplastic pemphigus presenting as a lichen planus pemphigoides-like eruption. Arch Dermatol 1993;129:866–9.

103. Perniciaro C, Kuechle MK, Colon-Otero G, et al. Paraneoplastic pemphigus: a case of prolonged survival. Mayo Clin Proc 1994;69:851–5.

104. Oursler JR, Labib RS, Ariss-Abdo L, et al. Human autoantibodies against desmoplakins in paraneoplastic pemphigus. J Clin Invest 1992;89:1775–82.

105. Biondi A, Rossi V, Bassan R, et al. Constitutive expression of the interleukin–6 gene in chronic lymphocytic leukemia. Blood 1989;73:1279–84.

106. Amagai M, Nishikawa T, Nousari HC, et al. Antibodies against desmoglein 3 (pemphigus vulgaris antigen) are present in sera from patients with paraneoplastic pemphigus and cause acantholysis in vivo in neonatal mice. J Clin Invest 1998;102:775–82.

107. Anhalt GJ, Kim S-C, Stanley JR, et al. Paraneoplastic pemphigus: an autoimmune mucocutaneous disease associated with neoplasia. N Engl J Med 1990;323:1729–35.

108. Horn TD, Anhalt GJ. Histologic features of paraneoplastic pemphigus. Arch Dermatol 1992;128:1091–5.

109. Helou J, Allbritton J, Anhalt GJ. Accuracy of indirect immunofluorescence testing in the diagnosis of paraneoplastic pemphigus. J Am Acad Dermatol 1995;32:441–7.

110. Joly P, Richard C, Gilbert D. Sensitivity and specificity of clinical, histologic, and immunologic features in the diagnosis of paraneoplastic pemphigus. J Am Acad Dermatol 2000;43:619–26.

111. Camisa C, Helm TN. Paraneoplastic pemphigus is a distinct neoplasia-induced autoimmune disease. Arch Dermatol 1993;129:883–6.

112. Nousari HC, Brodsky RA, Jones RJ, et al. Immunoablative high-dose cyclophosphamide without stem cell rescue in paraneoplastic pemphigus: report of a case and review of this new therapy for severe autoimmune disease. J Am Acad Dermatol 1999;40:750–4.

113. Izaki S, Yoshizawa Y, Kitamura K, et al. Paraneoplastic pemphigus: potential therapeutic effect of plasmapheresis. Br J Dermatol 1996;134:987–9.

114. Schoen H, Foedinger D, Derfler K, et al. Immunoapheresis in paraneoplastic pemphigus. Arch Dermatol 1998;134:706–10.

115. Ferrara JLM, Deeg HJ. Graft-versus-host disease. N Engl J Med 1991;324:667–74.

116. Johnson ML, Farmer ER. Graft-versus-host reactions in dermatology. J Am Acad Dermatol 1998;38:369–92.

117. Billingham R. The biology of graft versus host reactions. Harvey Lect 1966;62:21–73.

118. Aractingi S, Chosidow O. Cutaneous graft-versus-host disease. Arch Dermatol 1998;134:602–12.

119. Martin PJ, Schoch G, Fisher L, et al. A retrospective analysis of therapy for acute graft-versus-host disease: initial treatment. Blood 1990;76:1464–72.

120. Glucksberg H, Storb R, Buckner CD, et al. Clinical manifestation of graft-versus-host disease in human recipients of marrow from HLA-matched, sibling donor. Transplantation 1974;18:459–62.

121. McDonald GB, Shulman HM, Sullivan KM, et al. Intestinal and hepatic complications of human bone marrow transplantation. Part I. Gastroenterology 1986;90:460–77.

122. Weisdorf DJ, Snover DC, Haake R, et al. Acute upper gastrointestinal graft-versus-host disease: clinical significance and response to immunosuppressive therapy. Blood 1990;76:624–9.

123. McCarthy P, Abhyankar S, Neben S, et al. Inhibition of interleukin-1 by an interleukin-1 receptor antagonist prevents graft-versus-host disease. Blood 1991;78:1915–8.

124. Piguet P, Grau G, Allet B, et al. Tumor necrosis factor/cachectin is an effector of skin and gut lesions of the acute phase of graft-versus-host disease. J Exp Med 1987;166:1280–9.

125. Abhyankar S, Gilliland D, Ferrara J. Interleukin 1 is a critical effector molecule during cytokine dysregulation in graft versus host disease to minor histocompatibility antigen. Transplantation 1993;53:1518–23.

126. Jadus MR, Wepsic HT. The role of cytokines in graft-versus-host reactions and disease. Bone Marrow Transplant 1992;10:1–14.

127. Norton J, Sloane J. ICAM1 expression on epidermal keratinocytes in cutaneous graft-versus-host disease. Transplantation 1991;51:1203–6.

128. Langley R, Walsch N, Nevill T, et al. Apoptosis is the mode of keratinocyte death in cutaneous graft versus host disease. J Am Acad Dermatol 1996;35:187–90.

129. Goulmy E, Schipper R, Pool J, et al. Mismatches of minor histocompatibility antigens between HLA identical donors and recipients and the development of graft versus host disease after bone marrow transplantation. N Engl J Med 1996;334:281–5.

130. Bross DS, Tutschka PJ, Farmer ER, et al. Predictive factors for acute graft-versus-host disease in patients transplanted with HLA-identical bone marrow. Blood 1984;63:1265–70.

131. Nash RA, Pepe MS, Storb R, et al. Acute graft-versus-host disease: analysis of risk factors after allogeneic marrow

transplantation and prophylaxis with cyclosporine and methotrexate. Blood 1992;80:1838–45.

132. Weisdorf D, Hakke R, Blazar B, et al. Risk factors for acute graft-versus-host disease in histocompatible donor bone marrow transplantation. Transplantation 1991; 51:1197–203.

133. Przepiorka D. Practical considerations in the use of tacrolimus for allogeneic marrow transplantation. Bone Marrow Transplant 1999;24:1053–6.

134. Herve P, Tiberghien P, Racadot E, et al. Prevention and treatment of acute graft-versus-host disease: new modalities. Bone Marrow Transplant 1993;11 Suppl 1:103–6.

135. Crider MK, Jansen J, Norins AL, et al. Chemotherapy-induced acral erythema in patients receiving bone marrow transplantation. Arch Dermatol 1986;122:1023–7.

136. Sale G, Lerner K, Barker E, et al. The skin biopsy in the diagnosis of acute graft-versus-host disease in man. Am J Pathol 1977;89:621–36.

137. Deeg HJ, Henslee-Downee PJ. Management of acute graft-versus-host disease. Bone Marrow Transplant 1990;6:1–8.

138. Hings IM, Filipovich AH, Miller WJ, et al. Prednisone therapy for acute graft-versus-host disease: short versus long-term treatment. A prospective randomized trial. Transplantation 1993;56:577–80.

139. Martin PJ, Schoch G, Fisher L, et al. A retrospective analysis of therapy for acute graft-versus-host disease: secondary treatment. Blood 1991;77:1821–8.

140. Basara N, Blau W, Romer E, et al. Mycophenolate mofetil for the treatment of acute and chronic GVHD in bone marrow transplant patients. Bone Marrow Transplant 1998;22:61–5.

141. Ferrara JL, Holler E, Blazar B. Monoclonal antibody and receptor antagonist therapy for GVHD. Cancer Treat Res 1999;101:331–68.

142. Anasetti C, Hansen J, Waldmann T, et al. Treatment of acute graft versus host disease with humanized anti-Tac: an antibody that binds to IL2 receptor. Blood 1994;84:1320–7.

143. Przepiorka D. Daclizumab, a humanized anti-interleukin-2 receptor alpha chain antibody, for treatment of acute graft-versus-host disease. Blood 2000;95:83–9.

144. McCarthy PL, Williams L, Harris-Bacile M, et al. A clinical phase I/II study of recombinant human interleukin-1 receptor in glucocorticoid-resistant graft-versus-host disease. Transplantation 1996;62:626–31.

145. Richter HI, Stege H, Ruzicka T, et al. Extracorporeal photopheresis in the treatment of acute graft-versus-host disease. J Am Acad Dermatol 1997;36:787–9.

146. Greinix HT, Volc-Platzer B, Rabitsch W, et al. Successful use of extracorporeal photochemotherapy in the treatment of severe acute and chronic graft-versus-host disease. Blood 1998;92:3098–104.

147. Wiesmann A. Treatment of acute graft-versus-host disease with PUVA (psoralen and ultraviolet irradiation): results of a pilot study. Bone Marrow Transplant 1999;23:151–5.

148. Flowers ME, Kansu E, Sullivan KM. Pathophysiology and treatment of graft-versus-host disease. Hematol Oncol Clin North Am 1999;13:1091–112.

149. Sullivan KM, Shulman H, Storb R, et al. Chronic graft-

versus-host disease in 52 patients: adverse natural course and successful treatment with combination immunosuppression. Blood 1981;57:267–76.

150. Shulman H, Sullivan K, Weiden P, et al. Chronic graft-versus-host syndrome in man: a long-term clinicopathologic study of 20 Seattle patients. Am J Med 1980; 69:204–17.

151. Aractingi S, Socie G, Devergie A, et al. Localized sclerodermatous-like lesions on the legs in bone marrow transplant recipients: association polyneuropathy in the same distribution. Br J Dermatol 1993;129:201–3.

152. Janin-Mercier A, Socie G, Devergie A, et al. Fasciitis in chronic graft versus host disease. Ann Intern Med 1994;120:993–8.

153. Schubert M, Sullivan K, Morton T, et al. Oral manifestations of chronic graft-versus-host disease. Arch Intern Med 1984;144:1591–5.

154. Wingard JR, Piantadosi S, Vogelsang GB. Predictors of death from chronic graft versus host disease after bone marrow transplantation. Blood 1989;74:1428–35.

155. Tsoi M, Storb R, Dobbs S, et al. Cell-mediated immunity to non-HLA antigens of the host by donor lymphocytes in patients with chronic graft-versus-host disease. J Immunol 1980;125:2258–62.

156. Bunjes D, Theobald M, Nierle T, et al. Presence of host-specific interleukin 2-secreting T helper cell precursors correlates closely with active primary and secondary chronic graft-versus-host disease. Bone Marrow Transplant 1995;15:727–32.

157. Aractingi S, Gluckman E, LeGoue C, et al. Lymphocytes, cytokines, and adhesion molecules in chronic graft versus host disease. J Clin Pathol Mol Pathol 1996;49:M225–31.

158. Graze P, Gale R. Chronic graft-versus-host disease: a syndrome of disordered immunity. Am J Med 1979; 66:611–20.

159. Anasetti C, Rybka W, Sullivan K, et al. Graft-versus-host disease is associated with autoimmune-like thrombocytopenia. Blood 1989;73:1054–8.

160. Sullivan KM, Agura E, Anasetti C, et al. Chronic graft-versus-host disease and other late complications of bone marrow transplantation. Semin Hematol 1991;28:250–9.

161. Storb R, Prentice R, Buckner C, et al. Graft versus host disease and survival in patients with aplastic anemia treated by marrow grafts from HLA identical siblings. N Engl J Med 1983;98:461–6.

162. Atkinson K, Horowitz M, Gale R, et al. Risk factors for chronic graft-versus-host disease after HLA-identical sibling bone marrow transplantation. Blood 1990; 75:2459–64.

163. Tsoi M, Storb R, Jones E, et al. Deposition of IgM and complement at the dermoepidermal junction in acute and chronic cutaneous graft-versus-host disease in man. J Immunol 1978;120:1485–92.

164. Wagner JE, Flowers MED, Longton G, et al. The development of chronic graft-versus-host disease: an analysis of screening studies and the impact of corticosteroid use at 100 days after transplantation. Bone Marrow Transplant 1998;22:139–46.

165. Chosidow O, Bagot M, Vernant J, et al. Sclerodermatous chronic graft versus host disease. J Am Acad Dermatol 1992;26:49–55.

166. Sullivan KM, Witherspoon RP, Storb R, et al. Alternating-day cyclosporine and prednisone for treatment of high-risk chronic graft-v-host disease. Blood 1988;72:555–61.

167. Sullivan KM, Gooley T, Nims J, et al. Comparison of cyclosporine (CSP), prednisone (PRED) or alternating-day CSP/PRED in patients with standard and high-risk chronic graft-versus-host disease (GvHD) [abstract]. Blood 1993;82:215a.

168. Eisen D, Ellis C, Duell E, et al. Effect of topical cyclosporine rinse on oral lichen planus: a double-blind analysis. N Engl J Med 1990;323:290–4.

169. Vogelsang G, Farmer E, Hess A, et al. Thalidomide for the treatment of chronic graft versus host disease. N Engl J Med 1992;326:1055–8.

170. Parker P, Chao N, Nademanee A, et al. Thalidomide as salvage therapy for chronic graft versus host disease. Blood 1995;86:3604–9.

171. Volc-Platzer B, Honigsmann H, Hingerberger W, et al. Photochemotherapy improves chronic cutaneous graft versus host disease. J Am Acad Dermatol 1990;23:220–8.

172. Owsianowski M, Gollnick H, Siegert W, et al. Successful treatment of chronic graft-versus-host disease with extracorporeal photopheresis. Bone Marrow Transplant 1994;14:845–8.

173. Child FJ, Ratnavel R, Watkini P, et al. Extracorporeal photopheresis (ECP) in the treatment of chronic graft-versus-host disease (GVHD). Bone Marrow Transplant 1999;23:881–7.

174. Rossetti F, Zulian F, Dall'Amico R, et al. Extracorporeal photochemotherapy as single therapy for extensive, cutaneous chronic graft-versus-host disease. Transplantation 1995;59:49–51.

175. Axelrod PI, Lorber B, Vonderheid EC. Infections complicating mycosis fungoides and Sezary syndrome. JAMA 1992;267:1354–8.

176. Epstein EH Jr, Levin DL, Croft JD Jr, et al. Mycosis fungoides: survival, prognostic features, response to therapy, and autopsy findings. Medicine (Baltimore) 1972;51:61–72.

177. Diamandidou E, Colome M, Fayad L, et al. Prognostic factor analysis in mycosis fungoides/Sezary syndrome. J Am Acad Dermatol 1999;40:914–24.

178. Kim YH, Bishop K, Barghese A, et al. Prognostic factors in erythrodermic mycosis fungoides and the Sezary syndrome. Arch Dermatol 1995;131:1003–8.

179. Vonderheid EC, Zhang Q, Lessin SR, et al. Use of serum soluble interleukin-2 receptor levels to monitor the progression of cutaneous T-cell lymphoma. J Am Acad Dermatol 1998;38:207–20.

180. Diamandidou E, Cohen PR, Kurzrock R. Mycosis fungoides and Sezary syndrome. Blood 1996;88:2385–409.

181. Tan R, Butterworth C, McLaughlin H, et al. Mycosis fungoides: a disease of antigen persistence. Br J Dermatol 1974;91:607–16.

182. Tokura Y, Yagi H, Ohshima A, et al. Cutaneous colonization with staphylococci influences the disease activity of Sezary syndrome: a potential role for bacterial superantigens. Br J Dermatol 1995;133:6–12.

183. Jackow CM, Cather JC, Hearne V, et al. Association of erythrodermic cutaneous T-cell lymphoma, superantigen-positive *Staphylococcus aureus*, and oligoclonal T-cell receptor V-beta gene expansion. Blood 1997;89:32–40.

184. Dmitrovsky E, Matthews MF, Bunn PA, et al. Cytologic transformation in cutaneous T-cell lymphoma. A clinicopathologic entity associated with poor prognosis. J Clin Oncol 1987;5:208–15.

185. Diamandidou E, Colome-Grimmer M, Fayad L, et al. Transformation of mycosis fungoides/Sezary syndrome: clinical characteristics and prognosis. Blood 1998;92:1150–9.

186. Posner LE, Fossieck BE, Eddy JL, et al. Septicemic complications of the cutaneous T-cell lymphoma. Am J Med 1981;71:210–6.

187. Wilson LD, Jones GW, Kim D, et al. Experience with total skin electron beam therapy in combination with extracorporeal photopheresis in the management of patients with erythrodermic (T4) mycosis fungoides. J Am Acad Dermatol 2000;43:54–60.

188. Drage LA. Life-threatening rashes: dermatologic signs of four infectious diseases. Mayo Clin Proc 1999;74:68–72.

189. Salzman MB, Rubin LG. Meningococcemia. Infect Dis Clin North Am 1996;10:709–25.

190. Kirsch EA, Barton RP, Kitchen L, et al. Pathophysiology, treatment, and outcome of meningococcemia: a review and recent experience. Pediatr Infect Dis J 1996;15:967–78.

191. Brandtzaeg P, Kierulf P, Gaustad P, et al. Plasma endotoxin as a predictor of multiple organ failure and death in systemic meningococcal disease. J Infect Dis 1989;159:195–204.

192. Jafari HS, McCracken GH. Sepsis and septic shock: a review for clinicians. Pediatr Infect Dis J 1992;11:739–48.

193. Stephens DS, Hajjeh RA, Baughman WS, et al. Sporadic meningococcal disease in adults: results of a 5-year population-based study. Ann Intern Med 1995;123:937–40.

194. Van Deuran M, Van Dijke BJ, Koopman RJ, et al. Rapid diagnosis of acute meningococcal infection by needle aspiration or biopsy of skin lesions. BMJ 1993;306:1229–32.

195. Callahan EF, Adal KA, Tomecki KJ. Cutaneous (non-HIV) infections. Dermatol Clin 2000;18:497–508.

196. Quagliarello VJ, Scheld WM. Treatment of bacterial meningitis. N Engl J Med 1997;336:708–16.

197. Aiuto LT, Barone SR, Cohen PS, et al. Recombinant tissue plasminogen activator restores perfusion in meningococcal purpura fulminans. Crit Care Med 1997;25:1079–82.

198. Rivard GE, David M, Farrell C, et al. Treatment of purpura fulminans in meningococcemia with protein C concentrate J Pediatr 1995;126:646–52.

199. Stevens DL. The toxic shock syndromes. Infect Dis Clin North Am 1996;10:727–46.

200. Bisno AL, Stevens DL. Streptococcal infections of skin and soft tissues. N Engl J Med 1996;334:240–5.

201. Dinges MM, Orwin PM, Schlievert PM. Exotoxins of *Staphylococcus aureus*. Clin Microbiol Rev 2000;13:16–34.

202. Krakauer T. Immune response to staphylococcal superantigens Immunol Res 1999;20:163–73.

203. Stevens DL. Streptococcal toxic shock syndrome associated with necrotizing fasciitis. Ann Rev Med 2000;51:271–88.

204. Norrby-Teglund A, Newton D, Kotb M, et al. Superantigenic properties of the group A streptococcal exotoxin SpeF (MF). Infect Immun 1994;62:5227–33.

205. Sriskandan S, Cohen J. Kallikrein-kinin system activation in streptococcal toxic shock syndrome. Clin Infect Dis 2000;30:961–2.

206. Manders SM. Toxin-mediated streptococcal and staphylococcal disease. J Am Acad Dermatol 1998;39:383–98.

207. Zerr DM, Alexander ER, Duchin JS, et al. A case-control study of necrotizing fasciitis during primary varicella. Pediatrics 1999;103:783–90.

208. Basma H, Norrby-Teglund A, Guedez Y, et al. Risk factors in the pathogenesis of invasive group A streptococcal infections: role of protective humoral immunity. Infect Immun 1999;67:1871–7.

209. Rothe MJ, Bialy TL, Grant-Kels JM. Erythroderma. Dermatol Clin 2000;18:405–15.

210. Zittergruen M, Grose C. Magnetic resonance imaging for early diagnosis of necrotizing fasciitis. Pediatr Emerg Care 1993;9:26–8.

211. Stamenkovic I, Lew PD. Early recognition of potentially fatal necrotizing fasciitis: the use of frozen-section biopsy. N Engl J Med 1984;310:1689–93.

212. Hurwitz RM, Ackerman AB. Cutaneous pathology of the toxic shock syndrome. J Dermatopathol 1985;7:563–78.

213. Barry W, Hudgins L, Donta ST, et al. Intravenous immunoglobulin therapy for toxic shock syndrome. JAMA 1992;267:3315–6.

214. Stevens DL, Maier KA, Mitten JE. Effect of antibiotics on toxin production and viability of Clostridium perfringens. Antimicrob Agents Chemother 1987;31:213–8.

215. Gemmell CG, Peterson PK, Schmeling D, et al. Potentiation of opsonization and phagocytosis of Streptococcus pyogenes following growth in the presence of clindamycin. J Clin Invest 1981;67:1249–56.

216. Riseman JA, Zamboni WA, Curtis A, et al. Hyperbaric oxygen therapy for necrotizing fasciitis reduces mortality and the need for debridements. Surgery 1990;108:847–50.

217. Cawley MJ, Briggs M, Haith LR Jr, et al. Intravenous immunoglobulin as adjunctive treatment for streptococcal toxic shock syndrome associated with necrotizing fasciitis: case report and review. Pharmacotherapy 1999;19:1094–8.

218. Kaul R, McGeer A, Norrby-Teglund A, et al. Intravenous immunoglobulin therapy for streptococcal toxic shock syndrome—a comparative observational study. The Canadian Streptococcal Study Group. Clin Infect Dis 1999;28:800–7.

219. Guess HA, Broughton DD, Melton LJ III, et al. Population-based studies of varicella complications. Pediatrics 1986;78:723–7.

220. Cohen JI, Brunell PA, Straus SE, et al. Recent advances in varicella-zoster virus infection. Ann Intern Med 1999;130:922–32.

221. Miliauskas JR. Disseminated varicella at autopsy in children with cancer. Cancer 1984;53:1581–25.

222. McCrary ML, Severson J, Tyring SK. Varicella zoster virus. J Am Acad Dermatol 1999;41:1–14.

223. Stemmer SM, Kinsman K, Tellschow S, et al. Fatal noncutaneous visceral infection with varicella-zoster virus in a patient with lymphoma after autologous bone marrow transplantation. Clin Infect Dis 1993;16:497–9.

224. Rusthoven JJ, Ahlgren P, Elhakim T, et al. Varicella-zoster infection in adult cancer patients: a population study. Arch Intern Med 1988;148:1561–6.

225. Reboul F, Donaldson SS, Kaplan HS. Herpes zoster and varicella infections in children with Hodgkin's disease: an analysis of contributing factors. Cancer 1978;41:95–9.

226. Locksley RM, Flournoy N, Thomas ED. Infection with varicella-zoster virus after bone marrow transplantation. J Infect Dis 1985;152:1172–81.

227. Schmidt NJ, Gallo D, Delvin V, et al. Direct immunofluorescence staining for detection of herpes simplex and varicella zoster virus antigen in vesicular lesions and certain tissue specimens. J Clin Microbiol 1980;12:651–5.

228. Horn R, Wong B, Kiehn TE, et al. Fungemia in a cancer hospital: changing frequency, earlier onset, and results of therapy. Rev Infect Dis 1985;7:646–55.

229. Hay RJ. Yeast infections. Dermatol Clin 1996;14:113–24.

230. Radentz WH. Opportunistic fungal infections in immunocompromised hosts. J Am Acad Dermatol 1989;20:989–1003.

231. Watsky KL, Eisen RN, Bolognia JL. Unilateral cutaneous emboli of aspergillosis. Arch Dermatol 1990;126:1214–7.

232. Isaac M. Cutaneous aspergillosis. Dermatol Clin 1996;14:137–40.

233. Chapman SW, Daniel CR III. Cutaneous manifestations of fungal infection. Infect Dis North Am 1994;8:879–910.

234. Morrison VA, Haake RJ, Weisdorf DJ. The spectrum of non-Candida fungal infections following bone marrow transplantation. Medicine 1993;72:78–89.

235. Bushelman SJ, Callen JP, Roth DN, Cohen LM. Disseminated Fusarium solani infection. J Am Acad Dermatol 1995;32:346–51.

236. Wingard JR. Importance of Candida species other than C. albicans as pathogens in oncology patients. Clin Infect Dis 1995;20:115–25.

237. Wingard JR. Infections due to resistant Candida species in patients with cancer who are receiving chemotherapy. Clin Infect Dis 1994;19 Suppl 1:49–53.

238. Wingard JR, Merz WG, Rinaldi MG, et al. Increase in Candida krusei infection among patients with bone marrow transplantation and neutropenia treated prophylactically with fluconazole. N Engl J Med 1991;325:1274–7.

239. Myskowski PL, White MH, Ahkami R. Fungal disease in the immunocompromised host. Dermatol Clin 1997;15:295–305.

240. Slater DN, Wylde P, Harrington CI, et al. Systemic candidiasis: diagnosis from cutaneous manifestations J R Soc Med 1982;75:875–8.

241. Brown RS Jr, Lake JR, Katzman BA, et al. Incidence and significance of Aspergillus cultures following liver and kidney transplantation. Transplantation 1996;61:666–9.

242. Walsh TJ, Hiemenz JW, Anaissie E. Recent progress and current problems in treatment of invasive fungal infections in neutropenic patients. Infect Dis North Am 1996;10:365–400.

CHAPTER 21

OPHTHALMOLOGIC EMERGENCIES IN CANCER PATIENTS

BITA ESMAELI, MD
SINA SAFAR, BS
JULIE BETH YELIN, MD
M. AMIR AHMADI, MD

While there are few ophthalmologic emergencies that are life threatening, there are a number of ocular conditions in cancer patients that require immediate diagnosis and management. This chapter reviews the differential diagnosis and management of common ocular or visual symptoms encountered in a cancer hospital–based emergency center, including acute visual loss, diplopia, red eye, proptosis, epiphora, and ptosis. A discussion of trauma-related ocular emergencies is outside the scope of this textbook, and the reader is referred to other texts for a detailed discussion of non-cancer-related ocular emergencies.[1,2]

ACUTE VISUAL LOSS

Probably the most distressing ophthalmologic symptom is a sudden loss of vision. The many different causes of acute visual loss may be classified as those involving the optic nerve, those involving the retina, and those that involve the retinal vasculature.

Acute visual loss secondary to optic-nerve disease in cancer patients is usually due to a mass effect, either from metastatic disease or from the direct extension of tumor from paranasal sinuses or the nasal cavity. Paranasal sinus tumors can commonly extend into the orbit or the skull base to involve the optic nerve (Figure 21–1). Primary malignancies of the optic nerve include optic-nerve glioma, meningioma, craniopharyngioma, and medulloblastoma.[3] The optic nerve can also be infiltrated by leukemic or lymphomatous cells (Figure 21–2).[4] In immunocompromised hosts, the possibility of orbital cellulitis or fungal infections such as mucormycosis of the orbit should also be considered. Optic-nerve toxicity secondary to chemotherapeutic agents is another possible cause of optic neuropathy in cancer patients.

The primary symptoms associated with optic-nerve disease may include decreased visual acuity associated with a central visual field defect, decreased color vision and contrast sensitivity, and ocular pain on eye movement. A sensitive clinical sign for the presence of asymmetric optic-nerve disease is a relative afferent pupillary defect (Marcus-Gunn pupil) on the affected side.[5] On ophthalmoscopy, the optic-nerve head may appear swollen or pale. Magnetic resonance imaging (MRI) can usually demonstrate the extent of optic-nerve disease although in the case of leptomeningeal disease, the MRI scan may be normal in the early stages.[6]

Optic neuritis (optic-nerve swelling) in the general population is most often due to multiple sclerosis; however, it may also result from inflammatory conditions, such as Wegener's granulomatosis, systemic lupus erythematosus, and sarcoidosis, or it may be idiopathic. Infectious etiologies (including syphilis and Lyme disease) may also produce similar findings. In the elderly population or in patients with atherosclerosis, hypertension, or diabetes, the most common cause of acute visual loss of optic-nerve origin is an ischemic optic neuropathy. Giant cell arteritis is an important form of ischemic optic neuropathy that is sometimes associated with polymyalgia rheumatica.[7] Giant cell arteritis requires prompt diagnosis and treatment with high-dose systemic steroids to prevent progressive and sometimes bilateral visual loss.

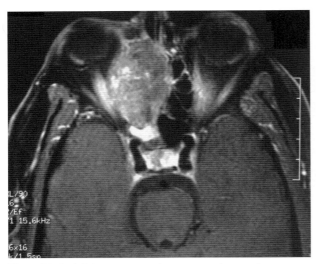

Figure 21–1. Axial post-contrast, fat-suppressed magnetic resonance image of paranasal sinus squamous cell carcinoma with extension into the right orbit and compression of the optic nerve.

The management of optic-nerve disease depends on the etiology. In cancer patients, the initial management may include systemic antibiotics or antifungals, chemotherapy, external-beam radiation therapy, high-dose steroids, or surgery.[8–10]

Retinal disease (particularly if it involves the macula, where visual acuity is most sensitive) may cause acute visual loss. Serous retinal detachment may result from leukemic or lymphomatous infiltration of the choroid or subretinal space. Opportunistic infections such as those with *Cytomegalovirus* (CMV), herpes simplex virus (HSV), herpes zoster virus (HZV), and candida may cause retinitis in immunocompromised patients (Figure 21–3). Retinitis due to HSV or HZV may cause rapid visual loss to "no light perception" within 24 hours.[11] It is

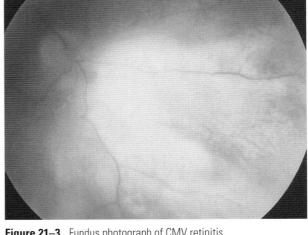

Figure 21–3. Fundus photograph of CMV retinitis.

important to diagnose the infectious forms of retinitis in a timely fashion so that the appropriate systemic therapy can be initiated as soon as possible. Another very common cause of visual loss among cancer patients is retinal hemorrhage secondary to thrombocytopenia (Figure 21–4).[12] A dilated fundus examination is necessary to correctly diagnose the retinal causes of acute visual loss.

Obstruction of the retinal vasculature can cause acute visual loss. Retinal vascular obstruction usually results from thrombi or emboli and is more likely to occur in patients with hypertension, atherosclerosis, or diabetes. However, cancer patients have the added risk of neoplasm-associated hypercoagulability.[13] Central retinal artery occlusion (CRAO) or central retinal vein occlusion (CRVO) may lead to devastating visual loss. Involvement of the smaller vessels may lead to partial visual acuity or visual field loss. Most occlusive vascular events are not reversible although they require proper diagnosis and fol-

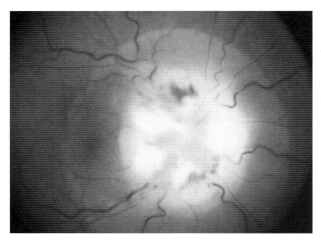

Figure 21–2. Fundus photograph demonstrating leukemic infiltration of the optic nerve head.

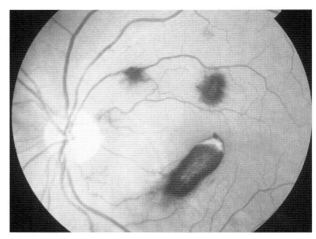

Figure 21–4. Fundus photograph of multiple retinal hemorrhages secondary to thrombocytopenia.

low-up to address the underlying medical problems and to prevent future ocular complications from ischemic retinopathy. The visual prognosis depends on the extent of retinal ischemia. Particularly, the ischemic variety of CRVO (Figure 21–5) can be complicated by secondary neovascular glaucoma and may require panretinal photocoagulation.[14] Prompt referral to an ophthalmologist is recommended when a retinal vascular event is suspected.

DIPLOPIA

Diplopia (double vision) is a common symptom in cancer patients. The first thing to establish is whether diplopia is monocular or binocular and whether it is horizontal or vertical. In addition, true diplopia must be distinguished from blurred vision, in which the image is blurred but is not in fact double. If diplopia persists after one eye is covered, the patient has monocular diplopia, which is almost certainly not a neurologic problem. The usual causes of monocular diplopia are either a refractive error, or media opacity (eg, a cataract). In contrast, if diplopia is present only when both eyes are open, it is binocular in nature, and there is usually an underlying neurologic or extraocular motility problem. Binocular diplopia can be horizontal, vertical, or torsional.[15] Specific neurologic causes of binocular diplopia include cranial nerve III, IV, or VI palsies, or a mechanical process that may limit the function of the extraocular muscles. While cranial-nerve palsies can be secondary to an ischemic event (particularly in patients with hypertension, diabetes, or atherosclerosis), in cancer patients, the most common etiology is tumor extension in the orbital apex or cavernous sinus. Another important but less common cause of palsy of the third cranial nerve, particularly if pupillary fibers are involved, is a cerebral aneurysm. Extraocular muscles may also be compressed or entrapped by a mass, or they may be infiltrated by inflammatory or neoplastic processes. If only one cranial nerve or extraocular muscle is affected, then a simple noncomitant diplopia may develop. In contrast, any space occupying lesion in the orbital apex, superior orbital fissure, or the cavernous sinus may affect multiple cranial nerves at the same time, resulting in a more complex pattern of diplopia (Figure 21–6, A). Opportunistic infections, particularly fungal infections secondary to mucormycosis or aspergillosis, may extend into the orbit from the paranasal sinuses. A high index of suspicion for fungal cellulitis or pansinusitis is necessary to make the correct diagnosis and initiate therapy for these potentially fatal infections in immunocompromised hosts.[16]

In the emergency evaluation of a patient with an acute onset of diplopia, an imaging study (ideally, an MRI) is often necessary to rule out or establish the extent of orbital or cavernous sinus disease (see Figure 21–6, A and B). The treatment of diplopia depends on the underlying cause and (usually in cancer patients) entails treatment of the underlying tumor or infectious etiology. The

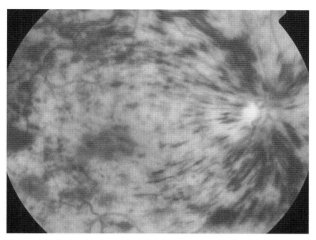

Figure 21–5. Fundus photograph of a central retinal vein occlusion.

patching of one eye or temporary Fresnel prisms may help the patient symptomatically until the exact cause and treatment for diplopia is determined.

RED EYE

There are many possible causes of a red eye in cancer patients. It is helpful to classify the causes of a red eye on the basis of intraocular structures that may be the cause of inflammation on the surface of the globe. Any disease process that can cause inflammation in the conjunctiva, cornea, iris, anterior chamber, ciliary body, or sclera can present as a red eye. Therefore, it is important to perform a comprehensive ophthalmologic examination to identify the correct cause.

Conjunctivitis is probably the most common cause of a red eye. Conjunctivitis can be due to infectious etiology such as bacteria (*Staphylococcus aureus*, *Streptococcus pneumonia*, *Pseudomonas aeruginosa*, *Chlamydia*, *Neisseria gonococcus*) or viruses (adenovirus, herpes simplex virus [HSV]).[17] However, occasionally, the cause is not infectious. The inflammatory causes of conjunctivitis include toxic conjunctivitis secondary to the excessive or inappropriate use of topical antibiotics (medicamentosa), allergic conjunctivitis, and acute or chronic ocular graft-versus-host disease.

Superficial keratopathy secondary to ocular graft-versus-host disease or as a side effect of cancer chemotherapeutic agents such as arabinosylcytosine (ara-C) can cause a red eye.[18,19] Superficial keratopathy secondary to ara-C use is treated with topical steroid, lubricating eye drops, and a lowering of the dose of ara-C. The management of conjunctival or corneal problems secondary to graft-versus-host disease entails the use of topical lubricants, cyclosporine drops, and the systemic administration of immunomodulatory agents such as steroids.[20] Infectious keratitis is another important cause of red eye

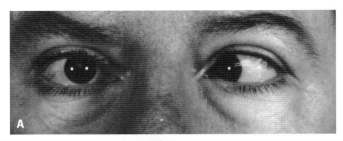

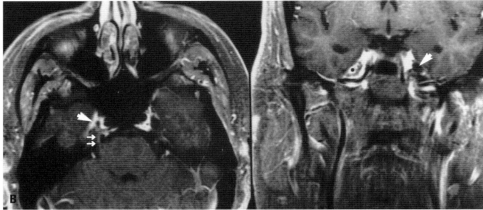

Figure 21–6. A: A 51-year-old man with a right sixth nerve palsy (abduction deficit in the right eye) secondary to squamous cell carcinoma with perineural invasion of Meckle's cave. B: Axial (left) and coronal (right) post-contrast, fat-suppressed magnetic resonance image through the level of Meckle's cave. Left, there is subtle abnormal thickening and enhancement along the lateral wall of Meckle's cave on the right side (*arrowhead*). Right, note the abnormal enhancement centrally within Meckle's cave on the right side (black dot). This is never normal and is not present on the left side (*arrowhead*).

and can be caused by bacterial (*Staphylococcus aureus, Streptococcus pneumonia, Neisseria gonococcus, Moraxella, Pseudomonas aeruginosa*), viral (adenovirus, HSV, HZV) (Figure 21–7, A and B), or fungal (*Candida, Aspergillus*) organisms.[21] The diagnosis and management of infectious keratitis requires the direct involvement of an ophthalmologist. Management often involves obtaining corneal cultures and instituting topical fortified antibiotics or antifungal agents. Another common cause of superficial keratopathy in cancer patients is exposure keratopathy secondary to facial palsy. Facial paralysis secondary to the compressive effects of a parotid mass or due to ablative surgery for malignancies in the parotid area can result in inadequate eyelid closure and chronic corneal exposure.[22] The immediate treatment of exposure keratopathy includes the use of lubricating ointments and artificial tears inside the eye. If facial paralysis is expected to last longer than a few weeks, periocular surgery, such as placement of a gold weight in the upper eyelid and a lateral tarsorrhaphy, should be considered.[23]

Acute angle-closure glaucoma can cause a red eye. It occurs in patients who have narrow angles that become blocked by the iris (Figure 21–8). Anticholinergic or sympathomimetic medications dilate the iris and lead to crowding of the anterior chamber angle peripherally.[24] A mass in the ciliary body or choroid can also push the iris forward and cause angle closure.[25] Primary intraocular tumors such as uveal melanomas or medulloepitheliomas may be present in the angle and may obstruct the aqueous outflow. Signs and symptoms of acute angle-closure glaucoma are pain, a red eye, blurred or "steamy" vision from corneal edema, halos around lights, and a mid-dilated pupil. The intraocular pressure can rise to 50 to 60 mm Hg, and urgent medical treatment to lower the pressure is necessary to avoid permanent vision loss. The medical management of angle-closure glaucoma in the emergency department includes the use of topical antiglaucoma medications, particularly pilocarpine, that can constrict the pupil and decrease the crowding of the angle. Additional topical antiglaucoma medications and systemic carbonic anhydrase inhibitors are often necessary to bring the intraocular pressure down to a safe level. For primary acute angle-closure glaucoma, the patient should be referred to an ophthalmologist for consideration of a laser peripheral iridotomy, after the intraocular pressure has been brought down to a safer level with medications.[26]

Inflammation of the iris, ciliary body, or choroid is referred to as uveitis. In addition to red eye, uveitis can present with pain, photophobia, blurred vision, and miosis of the pupil. Anterior chamber cells and flare noted during slit-lamp biomicroscopy are the hallmarks of iritis or uveitis. Uveitis is thought to be idiopathic in about 50% of cases or can be associated with various autoimmune processes such as rheumatoid arthritis, lupus, ankylosing spondylitis, and Wegener's granulomatosis.[27] In an immunocompromised host, the infectious causes of uveitis must be considered. The most severe form of intraocular infection, endogenous endophthalmitis, can initially present as mild but progressive uveitis (see Figure 21–7B).[28] Once the diagnosis of endogenous endophthalmitis is suspected, a vitreous biopsy is often necessary to identify the causative infectious organism. Broad-spectrum antimicrobial therapy is administered until sensitivity results are available from the vitreous cultures. For uveitis due to noninfectious causes, the judicious use of topical steroids may be helpful in decreasing the inflammation in the anterior chamber.

EPIPHORA

True epiphora (excessive tearing) results from an obstruction of the tear drainage apparatus. Epiphora must be differentiated from pseudoepiphora, which may be caused by ocular-surface irritation due to conditions such as dry-eye syndrome, ocular graft-versus-host disease, and exposure keratopathy. The most common cause of epiphora in the general population is obstruction of the nasolacrimal duct at its junction with the lacrimal sac.[29] Primary nasolacrimal-duct blockage is the most common form of obstruction of the nasolacrimal duct and occurs more frequently in women and as a result of senescence. In cancer patients, however, the most common etiology for epiphora is likely to be (a) mechanical blockage of the tear drainage pathway secondary to the extension of tumors from the paranasal sinus or nasal cavity or (b) canalicular and nasolacrimal-duct stenosis secondary to chemotherapeutic agents. Common chemotherapeutic agents that are known to cause canalicular stenosis include 5-fluorouracil and docetaxel (Taxotere).[30,31] Because timely diagnosis of early canalicular stenosis in patients receiving these agents can lead to early insertion of silicone tubing in the nasolacrimal duct and therefore prevention of further narrowing of the canaliculi, appropriate referral to an ophthalmologist early in the course of therapy with these agents is crucial.

Acute dacryocystitis is another important cause of epiphora. The infectious causes for acute or chronic dacryocystitis include *Staphylococcus aureus, Streptococcus pneumonia,* and *Haemophilus influenzae*.[32] Clinical signs associated with dacryocystitis are epiphora, mucopurulent discharge upon pressure over the lacrimal sac, and erythema and edema over the lacrimal sac. Treatment for infectious dacryocystitis involves systemic antibiotics and

warm compresses. A dacryocystorhinostomy may be necessary to prevent future episodes of dacryocystitis, particularly in an immunocompromised host.[33]

PROPTOSIS

Proptosis (outward protrusion of the eye) may be caused by an orbital mass or a diffuse inflammatory or infiltrative process involving the retrobulbar space. Other possible associated signs may include diplopia, decreased vision, and multiple cranial neuropathies secondary to involvement of the orbital apex. The most common malignancy affecting the orbit in adults is lymphoma (Figure 21–9).[34] Orbital lymphoma can be the extranodal manifestation of systemic lymphoma or may be the only site of lymphomatous involvement.[35] Another important cause of proptosis, particularly if associated with pain and inflammatory signs, is orbital pseudotumor. The diagnosis of orbital inflammatory syndrome (orbital pseudotumor) should be made only after an orbital biopsy specimen proves to be negative for malignancy.[36] Other benign or malignant tumors that can cause proptosis include optic-nerve glioma, meningioma, and metastatic lesions.[37] Management of propto-

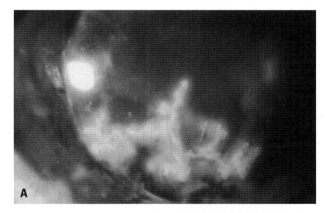
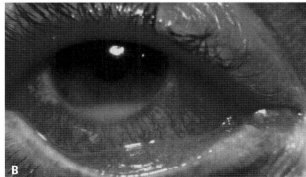

Figure 21–7. A: A dendritic lesion on the cornea, brightly-staining with fluorescein in a patient with herpes simplex keratitis. B: Infectious endophthalmitis with conjunctival injection, anterior chamber cells, and a layered hypopyon inferiorly.

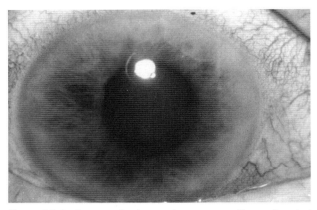

Figure 21–8. Acute angle-closure glaucoma revealing conjunctival injection, mid-dilated pupil, and edematous cornea.

sis consists of treatment of the underlying cause. It is important to avoid the administration of systemic steroids until the diagnosis is clearly established, ideally on the basis of an orbital biopsy to rule out lymphoma, orbital metastasis, or rhabdomyosarcoma as the underlying cause of proptosis. The use of anti-inflammatory agents can mask the clinical signs and symptoms, delay diagnosis, and lead to a lower yield for an orbital biopsy.

The most important cause of sudden and progressive proptosis in children is orbital rhabdomyosarcoma.[38] Timely diagnosis of this malignancy on the basis of an orbital biopsy is important for institution of appropriate therapy.

Orbital cellulitis can present as proptosis, decreased extraocular movement, and visual loss. Orbital cellulitis usually results from the direct extension of infection from the paranasal sinuses, especially the ethmoidal sinus.[39] However, direct inoculation from trauma, extension of an eyelid infection, and septicemia may also cause orbital cellulitis.[40] The causative infectious organisms are typically *Staphylococcus aureus, Haemophilus influenzae, Streptococcus pneumonia,* or fungi such as *Candida* or *Aspergillus.*[41] Orbital cellulitis may be complicated by the formation of an orbital abscess or by direct extension of infection into the cavernous sinus and the brain, a complication with a high risk of mortality.[42] Immediate treatment with systemic antibiotics and antifungals is prudent when orbital cellulitis or an orbital abscess are suspected. An orbital abscess can be diagnosed by computed tomography (CT) or MRI and usually requires immediate surgical drainage, particularly if it is associated with progressive visual loss or proptosis.[43]

Proptosis can be caused by orbital hemorrhage. Possible causes include postoperative hemorrhage, trauma, and hematologic disorders.[44] The patient's vision and intraocular pressure (IOP) should be immediately assessed because retrobulbar hemorrhage may cause a compressive optic neuropathy. If the vision is decreased or the IOP is elevated above 30 to 35 mm Hg, a lateral canthotomy and cantholysis should be performed in the emergency department to evacuate the hemorrhage and decompress the optic nerve.[45] Orbital emphysema can yield findings similar to those of orbital hemorrhage. The usual cause of orbital emphysema is trauma or a history of tracheal or thoracic surgery.[46]

PTOSIS

Ptosis (droopiness of the upper eyelid) can be gradual or sudden in onset. As with other symptoms discussed in this chapter, determining the underlying cause is the most important aspect of the management of this condition in the emergency department. The most common cause of ptosis in adults in the general population is involutional ptosis. In children, a congenital abnormality of the levator muscle is the most common cause of ptosis. In cancer patients, the most common cause of ptosis is neurologic. A palsy of the third cranial nerve due to primary or metastatic tumors of the base of the skull can cause blepharoptosis, decreased extraocular movement, and a dilated pupil. If pupillary fibers are involved, consideration should be given to a cerebral aneurysm as the possible cause of a third-nerve palsy.[47] Perineural invasion secondary to squamous cell carcinoma of the facial skin can also cause multiple cranial neuropathies, including a third-nerve palsy.[48]

Another neurologic cause of ptosis is Horner's syndrome. Horner's syndrome refers to the triad of mild ptosis ($\leq$ 2 mm), miosis of the pupil, and anhydrosis on one side of the face.[49] A mass effect anywhere along the path of sympathetic fibers can cause Horner's syndrome. This three-neuron chain originates in the hypothalamus. The second-order neurons originate in Budge's center (C8–T2) and wind over the lung apex. The third-order neurons originate in the superior cervical ganglion, where they follow the carotid artery and then the fifth and sixth cranial nerves before they accompany the third cranial nerve to the eye. When ipsilateral miosis is associated with ptosis, Horner's syndrome must be ruled out. Associated signs and symptoms may be helpful in determining the location of the lesion causing Horner's syndrome. For example, ataxia, nystagmus, and weakness may indicate a first-order Horner syndrome from a brain tumor whereas coughing, hemoptysis, or shoulder pain may indicate a pancoast tumor and thus a second-order Horner syndrome. Heterochromia usually indicates congenital Horner's syndrome and does not require any work-up or treatment. Pharmacologic testing with cocaine and hydroxyamphetamine drops may also help localize the lesion.[50]

Another cause of ptosis may be mechanical. For example, inflammatory changes in the upper eyelid due to orbital or paranasal sinus infection, surgical trauma,

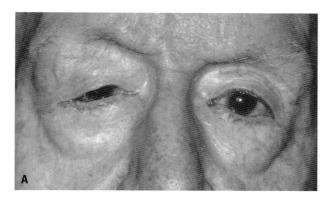

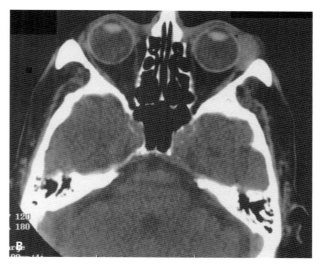

Figure 21–9. A: A 91-year-old man with left orbital lymphoma, causing proptosis and mechanical ptosis of the right upper eyelid. B: Axial computed tomography scan with lymphomatous mass involving the lacrimal gland in the lateral orbit.

or external-beam radiation therapy may cause temporary ptosis. An isolated tumor in the upper eyelid, such as a lacrimal-gland lymphoma or plexiform neurofibroma, may also lead to mechanical ptosis of the upper eyelid.

FLASHES AND FLOATERS

Flashes of light and "showers of floaters" can be ominous symptoms of vitreoretinal traction, a possible retinal tear, or retinal detachment. Various forms of retinitis, endogenous endophthalmitis, and posterior uveitis may also present with the same initial symptoms. "Masquerade syndrome" refers to vitritis (inflammation of the vitreous gel) caused by intraocular neoplasms, most commonly leukemia, lymphoma, retinoblastoma, and melanoma; it can present with the onset of floaters and gradual loss of vision.[51] A common benign condition that can also cause the acute onset of flashes and floaters is acute vitreous detachment, which is mostly secondary to senescence or trauma.[52,53] A thorough dilated funduscopic examination is necessary to determine the exact nature of vitreoretinal pathology in patients who complain of an acute onset of flashes and floaters, particularly if these symptoms are associated with a loss of vision.

TABLE 21–1. Essential Components of Ocular Examination before Consultation with an Ophthalmologist

Visual acuity, with prescription if necessary
Pupils: note size, reactivity to light; rule out an afferent pupillary defect
Extraocular muscles
Ocular adnexa
Confrontation visual fields
Anterior-segment examination with penlight
Intraocular pressure
Direct ophthalmoscopy

CONCLUSION

Ophthalmologic emergencies in cancer patients are multifaceted. In most instances, consultation with an ophthalmologist is necessary to insure the timely diagnosis and management of these conditions. A general understanding of the different components of an eye examination (Table 21–1) and the differential diagnosis for common ocular presentations may help the oncologist with work-up and treatment until the patient can be examined by an ophthalmologist.

REFERENCES

1. MacCumber MW. Management of ocular injuries and emergencies. Lippincott, Williams & Wilkins; 1998.
2. Rhee DJ. The Wills eye manual: office and emergency room diagnosis and treatment of eye disease. Lippincott, Williams & Wilkins; 1999.
3. Liu GT, Volpe NJ, Galetta SJ. Neuro-ophthalmology: diagnosis and management. W.B. Saunders; 2001.
4. Esmaeli B, Medeiros LJ, Myers J, et al. Orbital mass secondary to precursor T-cell acute lymphoblastic leukemia: a rare presentation. Arch Ophthalmol [In press].
5. Thompson HS, Corbett JJ, Cox TA. How to measure the relative afferent pupillary defect. Surv Ophthalmol 1981;26:39–42.
6. Bianchi-Marzoli S, Brancato R. Tumors of the optic nerve and chiasm. Curr Opin Ophthalmol 1994;5:11–7.
7. Fauci AS, Braunwald E, Isselbacher K, et al. Harrison's principles of internal medicine. McGraw-Hill (Health Professions Division); 1998. p. 120.
8. Christmas NJ, Mead MD, Richardson EP, Albert DM. Secondary optic nerve tumors. Surv Ophthalmol 1991; 36:196–206.
9. Mack HG, Jakobiec FA. Isolated metastases to the retina or optic nerve. Int Ophthalmol Clin 1997;37:251–60.
10. Albert DM, Jakobiec FA. Principles and practice of ophthalmology. W.B. Saunders; 2000.
11. Duker JS, Nielsen JC, Eagle RC Jr, et al. Rapidly progressive

acute retinal necrosis secondary to herpes simplex virus, type 1. Ophthalmology 1990;97:1638–43.

12. Black RL, Terry JE. Ocular manifestations of thrombotic thrombocytopenic purpura. J Am Optom Assoc 1991; 62:457–61.

13. Sallah S, Ahmad O, Kaiser HE. Pathogenesis of thrombotic disorders in patients with cancer. In Vivo 2000; 14:251–3.

14. Kohner EM, Laatikainen L, Oughton J.The management of central retinal vein occlusion. Ophthalmology 1983;90:484–7.

15. Leigh RJ, Zee DS. The neurology of eye movement. Philadelphia: F.A. Davis; p. 227–31.

16. Rizk SS, Kraus DH, Gerresheim G, Mudan S.Aggressive combination treatment for invasive fungal sinusitis in immunocompromised patients. Ear Nose Throat J 2000;79:278–80, 282, 284–5.

17. Dawson CR, Hanna L, Wood TR, et al. Adenovirus type 8 keratoconjunctivitis in the United States. Am J Ophthalmol 1970;69:473–80.

18. Kiang E, Tesavibul N, Yee R, et al. The use of topical cyclosporin A in ocular graft-versus-host-disease. Bone Marrow Transplant 1998;22:147–51.

19. Higa GM, Gockerman JP, Hunt AL, et al. The use of prophylactic eye drops during high-dose cytosine arabinoside therapy. Cancer 1991;68:1691–3.

20. Lass JH, Lazarus HM, Reed MD, Herzig RH.Topical corticosteroid therapy for corneal toxicity from systemically administered cytarabine. Am J Ophthalmol 1982; 94:617–21.

21. Wilhelmus KR.The red eye. Infectious conjunctivitis, keratitis, endophthalmitis, and periocular cellulitis. Infect Dis Clin North Am 1988;2(1):99–116.

22. Kartush JM, Linstrom CJ, McCann PM, Graham MD. Early gold weight eyelid implantation for facial paralysis. Otolaryngol Head Neck Surg 1990;103:1016–23.

23. Patipa M. Ophthalmic surgical management of facial paralysis. J Fla Med Assoc 1990;77:839–42.

24. Mapstone R. Closed-angle glaucoma: theoretical considerations. Br J Ophthalmol 1974;58:36–40.

25. Reddy SC, Madhavan M, Mutum SS. Anterior uveal and episcleral metastases from carcinoma of the breast. Ophthalmologica 2000;214:368–72.

26. Lam DS, Lai JS, Tham CC. The management of acute angle-closure glaucoma. Eye 2000;14(Pt 3a):412.

27. Dick AD. Immune mechanisms of uveitis: insights into disease pathogenesis and treatment. Int Ophthalmol Clin 2000;40(2):1–18.

28. Romero CF, Rai MK, Lowder CY, Adal KA. Endogenous endophthalmitis: case report and brief review. Am Fam Physician 1999;60:510–4.

29. Wobig JL, Wirta DL. Clinical and radiologic lacrimal testing in patients with epiphora. Ophthalmology 1998; 105:1574.

30. Esmaeli B, Valero V, Ahmadi MA, Booser D. Canalicular fibrosis secondary to docetaxel (taxotere): a newly recognized side effect. Ophthalmology. [In press].

31. Caravella LP Jr, Burns JA, Zangmeister M. Punctal-canalicular stenosis related to systemic fluorouracil therapy. Arch Ophthalmol 1981;99:284–6.

32. Easty DL, Sparrow JM. Oxford textbook of ophthalmology. Oxford and New York: Oxford University Press; 1999.

33. Cahill KV, Burns JA. Management of acute dacryocystitis in adults. Ophthal Plast Reconstr Surg 1993;9(1):38–42.

34. Margo CE, Mulla ZD. Malignant tumors of the orbit. Analysis of the Florida Cancer Registry. Ophthalmology 1998;105(1):185–90.

35. Mills P, Parsons CA. Primary orbital lymphoma: staging by computed tomographic scanning. Br J Radiol 1989; 62:287–9.

36. Weber AL, Romo LV, Sabates NR. Pseudotumor of the orbit. Clinical, pathologic, and radiologic evaluation. Radiol Clin North Am 1999;37(1):151–68.

37. Calcaterra TC, Trapp TK. Unilateral proptosis. Otolaryngol Clin North Am 1988;21(1):53–63.

38. Sindhu K, Downie J, Ghabrial R, Martin F. Aetiology of childhood proptosis. J Paediatr Child Health 1998; 34:374–6.

39. Lessner A, Stern GA. Preseptal and orbital cellulitis. Infect Dis Clin North Am 1992;6:933–52.

40. Rumelt S, Rubin PA. Potential sources for orbital cellulitis. Int Ophthalmol Clin 1996;36:207–21.

41. Klapper SR, Lee AG, Patrinely JR, et al. Orbital involvement in allergic fungal sinusitis. Ophthalmology 1997; 104:2094–100.

42. Tole DM, Anderton LC, Hayward JM. Orbital cellulitis demands early recognition, urgent admission and aggressive management. J Accid Emerg Med 1995;12: 151–3.

43. Hornblass A, Herschorn BJ, Stern K, Grimes C. Orbital abscess. Surv Ophthalmol 1984;29:169–78.

44. Dallow RL . Evaluation of unilateral exophthalmos with ultrasonography: analysis of 258 consecutive cases. Laryngoscope 1975;85(11 pt 1):1905–19.

45. Goodall KL, Brahma A, Bates A, Leatherbarrow B. Lateral canthotomy and inferior cantholysis: an effective method of urgent orbital decompression for sight threatening acute retrobulbar haemorrhage. Injury 1999;30:485–90.

46. Muhammad JK, Simpson MT. Orbital emphysema and the medial orbital wall: a review of the literature with particular reference to that associated with indirect trauma and possible blindness. J Craniomaxillofac Surg 1996 ;24:245–50.

47. Jacobson DM, Trobe JD.The emerging role of magnetic resonance angiography in the management of patients with third cranial nerve palsy. Am J Ophthalmol 1999; 128(1):94–6.

48. Esmaeli B, Ginsberg L, Goepfert H, Deavers M. Squamous cell carcinoma with perineural invasion presenting as a Tolosa-Hunt-like syndrome: a potential pitfall in diagnosis. Ophthal Plast Reconstr Surg 2000;16:450–2.

49. Parkinson D. Bernard, Mitchell, Horner syndrome and others? Surg Neurol 1979;11:221–3.

50. Wilhelm H, Ochsner H, Kopycziok E, et al. Horner's syndrome: a retrospective analysis of 90 cases and recommendations for clinical handling. Ger J Ophthalmol 1992;1:96–102.

51. Shields JA. Diagnosis and management of intraocular tumors. St Louis: C.V. Mosby; 1983.

52. Rothova A, Coijam F, Kerknoff F. Uveitis masquerode syndromes. Ophthalmology 2001;108:386–99.

53. Classe JG. Clinicolegal aspects of vitreous and retinal detachment. Optom Clin 1992;2:113–25.

CHAPTER 22

OBSTETRIC AND GYNECOLOGIC EMERGENCIES IN CANCER PATIENTS

DIANE C. BODURKE, MD
THOMAS W. BURKE, MD

PREGNANT CANCER PATIENT

The diagnosis of cancer is often overwhelming, especially for the pregnant patient. Medical decision making can become extremely complex, as both the health of the mother and safety of the fetus must be considered. Appropriate treatment planning is influenced by the indication for treatment, as well as by the patient's feelings regarding the continuation of the pregnancy once she has been properly counseled regarding the risks and benefits of therapy.

Recent estimates indicate that maternal cancer complicates approximately 1 in 1,000 to 1 in 5,000 live births in the United States annually[1] and that there are approximately 4,000 cases of concurrent pregnancy and maternal malignancy in the United States each year.[2] In 1985, in an effort to gather more data about this topic, the National Cancer Institute established a national registry for in utero exposure to chemotherapeutic agents.[3] Twenty-nine abnormal outcomes and a total of 52 birth defects were reported in the first 210 cases studied. While these numbers are small, it seems somewhat reassuring that only two abnormal outcomes were identified in women with exposure after the first trimester. However, significant potential for reporting bias exists since participation in the registry is voluntary.

The most frequently diagnosed cancer in pregnancy is cervical cancer, followed by breast cancer, melanoma, ovarian cancer, thyroid cancer, leukemia, lymphoma, and colorectal cancer. Pregnancy does not increase the risk of malignancy, and the incidence of specific malignancies in pregnant women is similar to that in nonpregnant women of the same age range. The incidence of cancer complicating pregnancy may increase as more women delay pregnancy and childbearing until later in life.

Chemotherapy and Pregnancy

All chemotherapeutic regimens are potentially teratogenic and mutagenic. Although controlled studies have been performed on pregnant laboratory animals, one must be cautious when extrapolating animal data to human pregnancies. Since there are no large prospective studies which evaluate chemotherapy during pregnancy, treatment regimens are frequently based on case reports or small retrospective reviews.

Both the mother and the fetus may be affected by chemotherapy. When evaluating the potential effect of a specific antineoplastic agent upon the developing fetus, it is important to consider both the maternal physiologic processes during pregnancy as well as the developmental stage at which the fetus is exposed to the cancer treatment.

Pregnancy may affect the absorption, distribution, and excretion of chemotherapeutic agents.[4] The increase in maternal blood volume affects the distribution of antineoplastic agents, while the absorption of oral agents may be influenced by changes in gastrointestinal motility. An increase in glomerular filtration rate changes the rate of renal excretion of chemotherapeutic agents. Virtually all chemotherapeutic agents cross the placenta.

The developmental stages of the embryo and fetus have been well-defined. These stages are divided into the preimplantation period (fertilization to implantation), the embryonic period (gestational weeks 2 through 8), and the fetal period (week 9 to term). Several principles based upon these stages apply to the effects of chemotherapy on the fetus.

The first trimester is the most crucial time period and, in terms of impact on the fetus, is best characterized by the "all-or-none" principle. Since its circulation has not yet been established, the blastocyst is resistant to teratogens in the preimplantation period. After this time, an exposed blastocyst may be severely damaged and may result in a spontaneous abortion. Conversely, the blastocyst may survive without abnormalities from this exposure.

During the period of organogenesis (gestational weeks 5 through 10), the fetal stem cell population is limited. This is the period of maximal susceptibility to teratogenic insults. Several small studies have reported that 10 to 20% of fetuses exposed to cytotoxic agents during this time period have major malformations, as opposed to a rate of 3% in the general population.[5] Although the underlying rates of spontaneous abortion and birth defects in the general population are large enough to potentially confound data from small series, it is generally recommended that chemotherapy administration be delayed until after the first trimester.

Organogenesis is completed by the end of the twelfth gestational week, with the exception of that of the brain and the gonadal tissue. During the fetal period, fetal growth restriction due to chemotherapy surpasses the risk of structural birth defects. Since the central nervous system continues to develop throughout the fetal period, the cortical brain function of the child may be affected by chemotherapeutic agents.[4]

Both maternal and fetal physiology during the final weeks of gestation must be taken into consideration when planning and administering chemotherapy. Chemotherapy administration should also be coordinated with the anticipated time of delivery. In an effort to decrease potential maternal chemotherapy-related complications from delivery, myelosuppressive regimens that may cause neutropenia or thrombocytopenia should be avoided for approximately 3 weeks prior to the anticipated delivery.

Since the placenta functions as a route of drug delivery and excretion, the timing of chemotherapy administration may also affect the neonate. Elevated drug levels due to a lack of elimination may be seen in the newborn if neoplastic agents are administered close to delivery. Additionally, a limited ability of the neonatal liver and kidneys to metabolize and excrete specific agents may also elevate blood levels of these drugs, especially in the preterm infant. Several authors have reported that children born to mothers who were receiving chemotherapy during pregnancy experienced no physical, neurologic, psychological, hematologic, or cytogenetic defects.[6,7] However, premature birth and low birth weight for gestational age are likely to be the most common complications associated with maternal chemotherapy administration, and these rates are most likely under-reported.[8]

Many chemotherapeutic agents, including cisplatin, cyclophosphamide, doxorubicin, hydroxyurea, and methotrexate, can be found in breast milk. Because of this, breast-feeding is contraindicated for women who are receiving chemotherapy.[9,10]

Effects of Specific Chemotherapeutic Agents

Antimetabolites. The folic acid antagonists methotrexate and aminopterin are the most commonly reported agents associated with birth defects when administered in the first trimester. Methotrexate is a teratogen and abortifacient. Infants of women treated with methotrexate in the first trimester have been reported to have multiple birth defects, including malformed extremities and cranial defects.[11] Children of mothers treated with aminopterin in the first trimester may develop the aminopterin syndrome, characterized by cranial dysostosis, anomalies of the external ears, hypertelorism, micrognathia, and cleft palate.[12] Multiple congenital anomalies have been reported in a neonate exposed to 5-fluorouracil (5-FU), a pyrimidine antagonist, in the first trimester.[13]

Antibiotics. Doxorubicin and daunorubicin (anthracycline antibiotics) have been administered to pregnant women, several of whom were in the first trimester. No fetal malformations have been reported with these drugs, nor with the administration of actinomycin D in the second and third trimesters.[14]

Although no adverse effects have been reported with the administration of bleomycin to pregnant women, bleomycin is known to cause maternal pulmonary toxicity. The common practice of increasing oxygen concentration during delivery (to optimize fetal oxygenation) may cause significant pulmonary toxicity in women exposed to bleomycin. Additionally, oxygen should be given at room air concentrations to women exposed to bleomycin who require general anesthesia.

Taxanes. Paclitaxel has been reported to cause increased fetal deaths in rat models.[15] To date, there have been no adequate controlled studies of paclitaxel in pregnant women. This drug is highly teratogenic in pregnant laboratory animals.

Cisplatin. There are no outcome data on exposure of pregnant women to cisplatin during the first trimester. Cisplatin has been associated with fetal growth retardation, persistent hearing loss, and transient neonatal leukopenia and alopecia when given during the second and third trimesters.[16]

Vinca Alkaloids. Several small reviews have reported no anomalies in neonates exposed to vinca alkaloids during the first trimester.[17,18] Vincristine and vinblastine are known to cause malformations in animals.

Etoposide. No data have been published regarding first-trimester exposure to etoposide. An association with neonatal pancytopenia has been reported for second-trimester chemotherapy regimens that include this drug.[19]

Radiation Therapy and the Pregnant Patient

As with chemotherapy, the administration of radiation during pregnancy requires careful consideration of therapeutic, moral, and ethical issues. Due to a lack of clinical trials in this area, it is difficult to establish accurate estimates of risks. Most available data regarding radiation and pregnancy outcomes are extrapolated from animal models or reported in small retrospective series. And as with chemotherapy, the period of fetal development influences the impact of in utero radiation exposure.

The blastocyst is most sensitive to the in utero lethal effects of ionizing radiation during preimplantation and early implantation (the first 10 days after conception). Doses as low as 10 cGy have been shown to increase prenatal death and embryonic resorption in laboratory mice. Virtually all animal experiments, however, reveal that survivors of radiation exposure during this time period develop no congenital anomalies.[2,20]

The greatest incidence of malformations in animals irradiated in utero occurs during organogenesis. Note that this time period is also the time of maximal susceptibility to chemotherapy-induced teratogenicity. Human exposure to radiation during this time period results in intrauterine growth retardation and central nervous system–related anomalies such as eye abnormalities, severe mental retardation, and microcephaly. Structural abnormalities are not usually seen from radiation therapy. A dose threshold of 5 to 10 cGy has been suggested for the above anomalies, based on data from Japanese survivors of the atomic bomb.[2] However, this analysis is somewhat compromised by a lack of accurate dosimetry on which to base risk estimates.

The central nervous system (CNS) continues to develop until term, and it remains very sensitive to radiation through approximately 25 weeks after conception. Milder forms of microcephaly and other CNS anomalies can be seen, as opposed to the more severe anomalies associated with radiation exposure earlier in gestation.[21] Growth retardation may be seen with doses > 50 cGy.[2]

The level of a threshold dose below which radiation would not be likely to adversely affect a pregnancy has not yet been determined. While several authors suggest that doses < 10 cGy do not cause adverse effects, any dose of radiation is capable of inducing genetic mutations that may not be expressed until future generations.[22] It has been estimated that in utero radiation of 1 cGy may double the risk of childhood malignancies, especially leukemias, during the first 10 years of life.[20] Despite this increase in risk, the absolute risk of future cancers remains low. Table 22–1[20,22,23] presents the estimated fetal dose of radiation from several common diagnostic procedures.

It has been suggested that in utero exposure to 10 cGy be used as a cutoff point for consideration of therapeutic abortion.[20] However, case reports of 50 cGy administered during the first trimester have not demonstrated a substantial risk of malformation.[2] Radiation therapy directed to the abdomen or pelvis during pregnancy will result in high doses of radiation to the fetus and should be avoided unless fetal loss due to spontaneous abortion or evacuation is expected. Issues regarding radiation exposure of the pregnant patient, including the topic of therapeutic abortion, require the consideration of all factors affecting the mother and the fetus.

VAGINAL HEMORRHAGE

The appropriate initial management of the patient who presents with vaginal bleeding requires a stepwise approach to determining the etiology of the bleeding. Vaginal bleeding in postmenopausal women is strongly suggestive of malignancy. In premenopausal women, bleeding may be due to pregnancy-related disease and should be further evaluated with a pregnancy test.

If the pregnancy test is positive, the differential diagnosis includes spontaneous abortion, missed abortion, molar pregnancy, gestational trophoblastic disease, and ectopic pregnancy (discussed later in this chapter). If the patient is bleeding vigorously, large-bore intravenous access should be obtained, fluids should be administered, and blood should be sent for evaluation of hematologic as well as clotting parameters. Blood should be typed and screened in preparation for possible transfusion. Careful physical and pelvic examinations should be performed. No biopsy should be performed on any visible vaginal

TABLE 22–1. Estimated Fetal Dose from Common Diagnostic Radiologic Exposures

Radiologic Procedure	Fetal Dose (cGy [rad])
Chest radiography	0.00006
Abdomen flat plate examination	0.15–0.26
Lumbar spine examination	0.65
Pelvic examination	0.2–0.35
Hip examination	0.13–0.2
Intravenous pyelography	0.47–0.82
Upper GI series	0.17–0.48
Barium enema	0.82–1.14
Mammography	Essentially undetectable
CT of head	0.007
CT of upper abdomen	0.04 *
CT of pelvis	2.5
99mTc bone imaging	0.15 †

Adapted from Hall EJ;[20] Gaulden ME;[23] Hall EJ.[24]

CT = computed tomography; GI = gastrointestinal; 99mTc = technetium 99m.

* For early pregnancy with uterus confined to the pelvis.

†Based on an ovarian dose of 0.015 cGy per mCi of 99mTc, with a typical injected dose of 10 mCi. Bladder drainage should be used due to the high local dose retained from urinary excretion of the radiopharmaceutical.

lesion that may appear bluish, as this may precipitate hemorrhage from choriocarcinoma. An obstetrician/gynecologist should be consulted for further evaluation and management.

Women with gestational trophoblastic disease present with vaginal bleeding and a positive pregnancy test. Although a high index of suspicion is required to diagnose this disease, women may present with a history of multiple emergency-room visits for threatened abortion, a uterus larger than usual at the reported gestational age, and no fetal movement. They may also experience significant nausea, vomiting, and hypertension. On pelvic examination, the cervical os is usually closed, and the uterus larger than expected for the gestational age. An ultrasound examination of the pelvis should be performed; pathognomonic findings include a heterogeneous echogenic pattern and the absence of fetal parts. Chest radiography should be performed, and the quantitative serum β–human chorionic gonadotropin level should be assessed. The patient should be admitted to the hospital. An obstetrician/gynecologist should be consulted for appropriate evaluation, evacuation of the pregnancy, and follow-up.

If the pregnancy test is negative and the patient is bleeding heavily, resuscitative measures with intravenous fluid and blood products should be implemented. Thorough physical and pelvic examinations should again be performed, with careful attention given to the visualization and inspection of the vagina and cervix. If the bleeding is due to an exophytic cervical lesion, a vaginal pack with Monsel's solution should be placed. The patient should be admitted to the hospital for more definitive diagnosis and potential emergent therapy. Treatment options for hemorrhage that is not controlled by packing include hypogastric artery embolization, transvaginal radiation, and hypogastric artery ligation.

If the cervix is normal in gross appearance, consideration should be given to an endometrial biopsy if the biopsy can be performed. Also, a biopsy should be performed on any vaginal lesion. If the patient is not bleeding heavily, she may be discharged, with immediate referral to a gynecologist or to a gynecologic oncologist if malignancy is suspected. The vulva and vagina should also be inspected, especially in older women. Packing and hospital admission may be required to establish a definitive diagnosis and begin appropriate treatment.

Premenopausal cancer patients often experience significant vaginal bleeding. If this bleeding is related to treatment, the underlying cause (such as thrombocytopenia) should be corrected. Intravenous conjugated estrogen (Premarin IV) may be given at a dose of 25 mg every 4 hours for 24 hours or until bleeding stops. Alternatively, oral contraceptives (eg, Ovral) may be given three times daily (tid) for 3 days, then twice daily (bid) for 3 days, then daily.

ECTOPIC PREGNANCY

Ectopic pregnancy is the leading cause of pregnancy-related death during the first trimester. The diagnosis and treatment of tubal pregnancy prior to tubal rupture significantly decreases the risk of maternal death. Early detection of tubal pregnancy increases treatment options, and some patients may be able to receive medical intervention rather than surgical intervention.

The incidence of ectopic pregnancy has tripled since the early 1970s. In 1992, there were an estimated 109,000 ectopic pregnancies, representing approximately 20 per 1,000 pregnancies and almost 10% of all pregnancy-related deaths.[24] Current Centers for Disease Control and Prevention data do not include ectopic pregnancies that are diagnosed or treated in physicians' offices; the true incidence of ectopic pregnancy is thereby underestimated.

Several factors have been identified as contributing to the increased incidence of ectopic pregnancy. These include the rising incidence of acute and chronic salpingitis, tubal ligation, tubal reconstructive surgery, and conservative management of tubal pregnancy, all of which cause structural damage to the tube; an increase in the use of contraceptive intrauterine devices (IUDs), which increase the risk of ectopic pregnancy by a factor of 4; and improved technology, which allows for more definitive diagnosis of some patients whose condition may have been undetected in the past.

Many retrospective studies have shown that patients with an ectopic pregnancy may be evaluated by a physician on several occasions before the correct diagnosis is made. This delay in diagnosis is usually related to a low index of suspicion on the part of the clinician. An awareness of the risk factors associated with ectopic pregnancy is critical to a prompt diagnosis. Significant risk factors are as follows: (1) a history of tubal infection (this increases the rate of ectopic pregnancy from 1 in 200 to 1 in 24), (2) prior ectopic pregnancy (there is a 15 to 50% increase in the incidence of ectopic pregnancy in subsequent pregnancies), (3) a history of tubal reconstructive surgery, (4) a history of tubal sterilization within the previous 2 years, and (5) pregnancy occurring with an IUD in place or with a history of IUD use. While there are no pathognomonic symptoms of ectopic pregnancy, the classic triad consists of amenorrhea, vaginal bleeding, and abdominal pain.

Amenorrhea or a history of an abnormal last menstrual period is associated with 75 to 90% of ectopic pregnancies. Vaginal bleeding, which may consist of light spotting or which may be as heavy as a menstrual period, results from a low production of human chorionic gonadotropin (hCG) by the ectopic trophoblast; this occurs in 50 to 80% of patients with an ectopic pregnancy. Abdominal pain is present in more than 90%

of cases. Arriving at the correct diagnosis in a patient with an acutely ruptured ectopic pregnancy is fairly straightforward. The patient usually presents with symptoms of abdominal pain and distention, as well as with hypovolemia (tachycardia, orthostatic blood pressure changes, diaphoresis, etc). Shoulder pain may be present due to irritation of the phrenic nerve from blood in the peritoneal cavity.

The diagnosis of an unruptured ectopic pregnancy is more difficult to make. Physical examination findings in these patients are extremely variable. While 90% of patients have abdominal tenderness, only 45% have rebound tenderness. Fifty percent of patients have a palpable adnexal mass. In half of these cases, the mass is actually contralateral to the ectopic pregnancy and is actually the corpus luteum.[25]

Several critical diagnostic tests should be performed in patients suspected of having an ectopic pregnancy. These include a rapid serum or urine hCG test, transvaginal ultrasonography, and a quantitative β-hCG test. The rapid hCG test result is obtained to diagnose pregnancy. The β-hCG should be drawn at the time of presentation, then repeated as necessary. The doubling time of β-hCG in the serum varies from 1.2 days immediately following implantation to 3.5 days at 2 months after the last menstrual period. It is important to understand that ectopic gestations may be associated with a normal rise in hCG levels as well as with plateauing or decreasing titers. If serial quantitative levels of β-hCG do not fall into the normal range, ultrasonography should be performed to attempt to locate the pregnancy. As early as 5 weeks of amenorrhea, transvaginal ultrasonography permits the identification of an intrauterine gestational sac (2 mm in diameter), which virtually rules out an ectopic pregnancy.

The management of ectopic pregnancy has changed significantly in recent years. Therapeutic options vary from medical therapy to emergent laparotomy. The appropriate treatment depends on the medical status of the patient as well as on the characteristics of the pregnancy. A laparotomy is indicated in a patient with an unstable cardiovascular status, in whom vaginal ultrasonography identifies a gestational sac > 3.5 cm, and whose β-hCG level is > 15,000 mIU/dL (or in whom fetal cardiac activity is identified). A patient with stable cardiac status, an ultrasonographically identified gestational sac < 3.5 cm, and a β-hCG level < 15,000 mIU/dL is an appropriate candidate for a laparoscopic procedure. Methotrexate therapy is also an option for this subgroup of patients, but other criteria, such a willingness to return for follow-up care, must be discussed by the patient and her physician.

The key to the successful management of ectopic pregnancy is early diagnosis. Although the number of cases of ectopic pregnancy have steadily increased, the mortality has declined significantly in the past 10 years.[26]

A high index of suspicion and vigorous efforts at an early diagnosis must be made by all physicians evaluating women of reproductive age who present to the emergency room with abdominal pain and a positive pregnancy test.

SEXUALLY TRANSMITTED DISEASES

Patients with vaginal or vulvar infections often present to emergency rooms complaining of nonbloody vaginal discharge. The characteristics of the discharge can often be useful in making the diagnosis. The pH should be determined with litmus paper; the normal adult pH is 4.0. To evaluate the discharge definitively, a wet-mount smear preparation should be made. (An adequate sample of vaginal discharge should be obtained with a cotton-tipped applicator and suspended in 2 mL of normal saline. A drop of this solution should then be placed on a glass slide, covered with a coverslip, and examined under the microscope.) If a mycotic infection is suspected (as in patients recently treated with antibiotics), some of the discharge should be suspended in 10% potassium hydroxide (KOH) and examined in the same manner under the microscope. Aerobic and anaerobic cultures, chlamydial cultures, and mycotic cultures may be indicated in complicated cases. Immunofluorescent studies for *Trichomonas* or *Chlamydia* may also be required.

Trichomonas Vaginitis

Trichomonas vaginitis is caused by the protozoan flagellate *Trichomonas vaginalis*. It is usually transmitted by sexual intercourse.

Although symptoms may vary from mild to severe, 25% of patients are asymptomatic. Symptoms include vaginal discharge, vaginal and vulvar pruritus, burning, dyspareunia, and frequent urination.

The vaginal discharge is bubbly, thin, and pale gray or green, with a pH of 5 to 6.5. *Trichomonas vaginalis* produces a foul odor and a frothy-appearing discharge due to the fermentation of carbohydrates. The vulva and vagina may be erythematous, and petechiae may be seen on the cervix and vaginal mucosa.

The diagnosis is made by identifying the organism on a wet-mount smear. *Trichomonas vaginalis* is pear-shaped and motile, with a flagellum. It is larger than a white blood cell. Culture techniques may confirm the diagnosis but are seldom indicated.

The treatment is oral metronidazole (Flagyl) in a single oral dose of 1,500 to 2,000 mg or a 250-mg dose three times a day for 7 days. The single-dose regimen may not be as effective but improves patient compliance. The side effects of this drug include nausea, occasional vomiting, and dark amber urine. The patient must abstain from alcohol intake while taking this drug, since the drug acts like disulfiram (Antabuse) and causes a significant reaction. The patient's consort must also be treated, since failures are usually due to re-infection. Metronidazole gel (MetroGel) is an alternative treatment; it is applied to the vagina twice a day for 5 days. The consort must also be treated with oral metronidazole.

Candidiasis

Candidiasis is primarily caused by *Candida albicans*. The incidence of yeast infections not caused by *Candida albicans* has increased over the last decade; *Candida tropicalis* and *Torulopsis glabrata* are the main organisms responsible. Populations at increased risk for developing yeast infections include pregnant women, diabetic women, women using oral contraceptives, and immunosuppressed women.

Symptoms include pruritus, burning, dyspareunia, and a cottage cheese–like or thick white discharge.

The duration of the infection influences the signs. If the infection is diagnosed early, a thick discharge may be the only sign. Conversely, the vulva and vagina may be excoriated, edematous, and exquisitely tender if the infection is of long-standing duration.

Candidiasis is diagnosed by identifying pseudohyphae and yeast forms on a KOH wet-mount preparation. To identify the strain of yeast present in patients who complain of recurrent infections, a culture should be obtained.

The most common cause for failure of treatment is noncompliance. While vaginal preparations such as miconazole may be prescribed for 3 to 7 nights, new oral regimens are now available. Fluconazole (Diflucan) may be given in a single dose of 150 mg, then repeated in 1 week.

Bacterial Vaginosis

Bacterial vaginosis has previously been called nonspecific vaginitis, *Gardnerella vaginalis* vaginitis, and *Haemophilus vaginalis* vaginitis. It is found in more than half of patients presenting to sexually transmitted disease clinics.

The most common symptom is a moderate-to-profuse malodorous vaginal discharge, ivory to gray in color, with a pH of 5 to 6.5. It has a distinct fishy odor that may be enhanced by adding 10% KOH to the specimen. This odor is caused by amines, the metabolic by-products of anaerobes.

The diagnosis can be made by the following findings: a pH of 5 to > 6.5, a positive odor test, clue cells (squamous cells covered by small coccobacilli, especially at the edges) in a saline wet-mount preparation, and the absence of irritation of the vaginal or vulvar epithelium.

The preferred treatment is metronidazole, 500-mg twice daily for 7 days. Since most physicians recommend that the consort be treated, a single dose of 2 g to each party may be less effective but may yield more compliance in the setting of prolonged therapy. Topical metronidazole and clindamycin are alternative therapies. Patients with

recurrent bacterial vaginosis should be screened for *Chlamydia* infection and gonorrhea. If either is present, the patient should also be tested for hepatitis B, syphilis, and human immunodeficiency virus (HIV).

Herpes Genitalis

Herpes genitalis is a sexually transmitted disease caused by herpes simplex virus type II in 90% of cases and herpes simplex virus type I in 10% of cases. Patients who have had oral herpes (type I virus) may have some protection against subsequent infections with genital herpes (type II virus).

The symptoms of a primary herpes infection usually appear within 3 to 7 days of exposure. The infection may be asymptomatic, or the patient may experience prodromal symptoms including mild paresthesia and burning in the perineal area before lesions become visible. The initial lesions may cause severe vulvar pain and tenderness. Patients may also have inguinal adenopathy, a low-grade fever, and generalized malaise.

Physical findings are dependent on the stage of the lesions at presentation. Clear vesicles that involve the labia majora, labia minora, and perineal skin may be present. These vesicles usually rupture in 1 to 7 days and form ulcers. These ulcers are shallow and painful and may be surrounded by an area of erythema. They usually heal within a week to 10 days.

The diagnosis of herpes genitalis is made by recognizing the typical appearance of the vesicles and ulcers, as well as the tender vulva. Immunofluorescent staining or viral cultures are helpful in the first 3 to 5 days of symptoms. Fluorescent antibody staining performed on short-term tissue culture provides a diagnosis within 48 hours.

Acyclovir is prescribed for the treatment of herpes genitalis. This drug is not curative, and lesions recur once treatment is discontinued.

Syphilis

Syphilis is caused by *Treponema pallidum*, a motile anaerobic spirochete that invades moist but intact mucosa.

In females, the vulva is the most frequent site of entry for the spirochete. A chancre appears on the vulva, cervix, or vagina 10 to 60 days after innoculation, thereby heralding the stage of primary syphilis. The chancre is a firm painless lesion with a punched-out base and rolled edges. Painless inguinal adenopathy is also usually present.

The diagnosis of syphilis is made by identifying the spirochete in material scraped from the base of the chancre by dark-field microscopy. The chancre will heal spontaneously within 3 to 9 weeks, even if left untreated. A serologic test for syphilis should be performed at this time; it will be negative, but it can be used as a baseline.

The patient usually develops systemic manifestations of secondary syphilis 8 weeks after infection or about 3 to

6 weeks after the chancre develops. These symptoms include headache, malaise, anorexia, and a generalized maculopapular rash. The patient may also develop condylomata lata, or broad exophytic excrescences that ulcerate and are highly contagious. These lesions appear on the vulva, perianal area, and upper thighs. Dark-field microscopic examination of material from these lesions reveals numerous spirochetes. Serologic tests for syphilis are positive at this stage.

The failure to treat primary or secondary syphilis places the patient at risk for the development of tertiary syphilis, which may affect any organ in the body. Patients may also develop a gumma of the vulva, a rare manifestation of tertiary syphilis. This nodule enlarges, ulcerates, and becomes necrotic.

Primary and secondary syphilis are treated with benzathine penicillin G, 2.4 million units given intramuscularly. Tetracycline may also be given to treat these stages of syphilis: a 500-mg dose is prescribed four times daily for 15 days. The treatment of tertiary syphilis is weekly penicillin for 3 weeks or tetracycline for 30 days.[27]

Pelvic Inflammatory Disease

Pelvic inflammatory disease (PID) is the most serious and costly sexually transmitted bacterial infection affecting women. While this term traditionally refers to ascending reproductive-tract infections in nonpregnant women, infections following pelvic instrumentation (dilatation and curettage, cesarean section, etc) have a similar presentation and treatment. The disease affects approximately 1% of young sexually active women yearly. The most frequently identified pathogens are *Neisseria gonorrhoeae* and *Chlamydia trachomatis*. Both types of infection are sexually transmitted and can be traced to recent sexual exposure to an infected partner, often within the previous 2 weeks (gonorrhea) to 2 months (*Chlamydia*).

Criteria for the diagnosis of PID include abdominal tenderness, cervical motion tenderness, and adnexal tenderness. One of the following confirmatory findings must also be present: fever $\geq 38°C$, leukocytosis, purulent cervical discharge, or an elevated erythrocyte sedimentation rate.[28]

The Centers for Disease Control and Prevention (CDC) guidelines for the treatment of PID are presented in Table 22–2. Outpatient regimens may be prescribed for women who will return if there is no improvement in their condition within 24 to 48 hours and who are likely to comply with these regimens. Hospitalization is required for women with severe infections or who are unable to tolerate an oral regimen.

Women should be tested for gonococcal and chlamydial infections prior to beginning treatment with antibiotics. Tests of cure should be initiated 3 to 4 weeks after therapy is begun. A pelvic examination should be performed at a follow-up visit, and repeat counseling on prevention strategies for sexually transmitted diseases and HIV infection should be offered. Contraception counseling should also be provided.

Consorts for the 2 months prior to a diagnosis of PID should be identified, screened, and treated either on the basis of test results or empirically. Suggested treatment regimens include azithromycin (1 g orally) for chlamydial infection, and ofloxacin (400 mg orally) for gonorrhea.[29]

TABLE 22–2. Centers for Disease Control and Prevention Guidelines for Treatment of Pelvic Inflammatory Disease

Recommended Treatment	Alternative Treatments
Hospitalized Patients	
Cefoxitin, 2 g IV q6h, or Cefotetan, 2g IV q12h, plus doxycycline, 100 mg IV q12h until improved, followed by doxycycline, 100 mg orally bid, to complete 14 days	Clindamycin, 600 mg IV q8h, plus gentamcin, 2 mg/kg IV once, followed by 1.5 mg IV q8H until improved, followed by doxycycline, 100 mg orally bid, to complete 14 days
Nonhospitalized Patients	
Ceftriaxone, 250 mg IM or Cefoxitin, 2 g IM, plus probenecid, 1 g orally; either one followed by doxycycline, 100 mg bid, to complete 14 days	Ofloxacin, 400 mg orally for 14 days, plus metronidazole, 500 mg bid orally for 14 days or clindamycin, 450 mg orally qid for 14 days

Adapted from Centers for Disease Control and Prevention.[26]
IM = intramuscularly; IV = intravenously.

REFERENCES

1. Waalen J. Pregnancy poses tough questions for cancer treatment. J Natl Cancer Inst 1991;83:900.
2. Stovall M, Blackwell RC, Cundiff J, et al. Fetal dose from radiotherapy with photon beams: report of AAPM Radiation Therapy Committee Task Group No. 36. Med Phys 1995;22:63.
3. Randall T. National registry seeks scarce data on pregnancy outcomes during chemotherapy. JAMA 1993;269:323.
4. Cunningham FG, MacDonald PC, Gant NF, et al. Neoplastic diseases. In: Cunningham FG, MacDonald PC, Gant NF, et al, editors. Williams obstetrics, 19th ed. Norwalk (CT): Appleton & Lange; 1993. p. 1267–9.
5. Caligiuri MA, Mayer RJ. Pregnancy and leukemia. Semin Oncol 1989;16:388.
6. Aviles A, Diaz-Magneo JC, Talavera A, et al. Growth and development of children of mothers treated with chemotherapy during pregnancy: current status of 43 children. Am J Hematol 1991;36:243.
7. Berry DL, Theriault RL, Holmes FA, et al. Management of breast cancer during pregnancy using a standardized protocol. J Clin Oncol 1999;17:3.

8. Garber JE. Long-term follow-up of children exposed in utero to antineoplastic agents. Semin Oncol 1989;16:437.

9. Ben-Baruch G, Menczer J, Goshen R, et al. Cisplatin excretion in human milk. J Natl Cancer Inst 1992;84:451.

10. Egan PC, Costanza M, Dadion P, et al. Doxorubicin and cisplatin excretion into human breast milk. Cancer Treat Rep 1985;69:1387.

11. Kozlowski RD, Steinbrunner JF, MacKenzie AH, et al. Outcome of first trimester exposure to low-dose methotrexate in eight patients with rheumatic disease. Am J Med 1990;88:59.

12. Doll RC, Ringenberg OS, Yarbo JW. Antineoplastic agents and pregnancy. Semin Oncol 1989;16:337.

13. Stephens JD, Golbus MS, Miller TR, et al. Multiple congenital anomalies in a fetus exposed to 5-fluorouracil during the first trimester. Am J Obstet 1980;137:746.

14. Turchi JJ, Villasis C. Anthracyclines in the treatment of malignancy in pregnancy. Cancer 1988;61:425.

15. Kai S, Kohmura H, Hiraiwa E, et al. Reproductive and developmental toxicity studies of paclitaxel (III). J Toxicol Sci 1994;19(Suppl 1):93–111.

16. Tomlinson MW, Tredwell MC, Deppe G. Platinum based chemotherapy to treat recurrent Sertoli-Leydig cell ovarian carcinoma during pregnancy. Eur J Gynecol Oncol 1997;18:44–6.

17. Schapira DV, Chudley AE. Successful pregnancy following continuous treatment with combination chemotherapy before conception and throughout pregnancy. Cancer 1983;54:800.

18. Gililland J, Weinstein L. The effects of cancer chemotherapeutic agents on developing fetus. Obstet Gynecol Surv 1983;3:6.

19. Hsu KF, Chang CH, Chou CY. Sinusoidal fetal heart pattern during chemotherapy in a pregnant woman with acute myelogenous leukemia. J Formos Med Assoc 1995;94:562–5.

20. Hall EJ. Effects of radiation on the embryo and fetus. In: Hall EJ, editor. Radiobiology for the radiologist. 4th ed. Philadelphia: J.B. Lippincott; 1994.

21. Dekabon AS. Abnormalities in children exposed to x-radiation during various stages of gestation: tentative timetable of radiation injury to the human fetus, part I. J Nucl Med 1968;9:471.

22. Gaulden ME. Possible effects of diagnostic x-rays on the human embryo and fetus. J Ark Med Soc 1974;70:424.

23. Hall EJ. Diagnostic radiology and nuclear medicine: risk versus benefit. In: Hall EJ, editor. Radiobiology for the radiologist. 4th ed. Philadelphia: J.B. Lippincott; 1994.

24. Centers for Disease Control and Prevention. Ectopic pregnancy–United States, 1990–1992. MMRW Morb Mortal Wkly Rep 1995;44:46–8.

25. Breen JL. A 21 year study of 645 ectopic pregnancies. Am J Obstet Gynecol 1970;106:104.

26. Centers for Disease Control. Ectopic pregnancy in the USA. MMWR Morb Mortal Wkly Rep 1989;38:481.

27. Centers for Disease Control and Prevention. Vestibular papillomatosis: report of ISSVD Committee on Sexually Transmitted Diseases, treatment guidelines. MMWR Morb Mortal Wkly Rep 1993;42:111.

28. Hager WD, Eschenbach DA, Spence MR, et al. Criteria for diagnosis and grading of salpingitis. Obstet Gynecol 1983;61:113.

29. McCormack W. Current concepts in pelvic inflammatory disease. N Engl J Med 1994;330:115.

CHAPTER 23

MISCELLANEOUS ONCOLOGIC EMERGENCIES

MARTIN LEVETT, MD

MARGARET ROW, MD

SAI-CHING JIM YEUNG, MD, PhD, RPH

CARDIOPULMONARY ARREST

Cardiopulmonary arrest is the usual terminal event at the end of life. However, cardiopulmonary arrest can also be caused by acute reversible conditions, and a significant number of patients who experience cardiopulmonary arrest and are resuscitated go on to experience many more years of high-quality life. This is just as true in patients with non-end-stage cancer as it is in the general population.

A patient with cancer who experiences cardiopulmonary arrest while he or she still has significant therapeutic options should be resuscitated just like any other patient without cancer. In patients with cancer, just as in other patients, cardiopulmonary arrest is often caused by potentially reversible processes or events, such as pulmonary emboli, cardiac arrhythmias, choking, and aspiration. With the major advances in cancer therapy in recent years, the survival rates for many types of cancer now exceed the survival rate for severe (class IV) congestive heart failure. Even gravely ill cancer patients can have remarkable improvement or meaningful survival after being stabilized and treated, either definitively or with palliative intent. However, when cardiac arrest comes as the expected final event of a gradual failure of bodily functions due to cancer, resuscitation will not succeed.

Resuscitation of Patients in Cardiac Arrest

Importance of Do-Not-Resuscitate Orders. Oncologists should be diligent in writing do-not-resuscitate (DNR) orders and in explaining these orders to patients and their families. Do-not-resuscitate orders do not imply that efforts to control or palliate the disease will be decreased or that the level of care will be decreased.

Rather, they ensure that treatment will be discontinued if continued efforts to treat the cancer would be fruitless and would only cause suffering. A nationwide study found that many well-informed patients would readily sign living wills[1] or appoint a health care proxy. Many patients, particularly elderly patients and those who have a realistic understanding of their disease, are willing to discuss DNR orders and make an informed decision not to be resuscitated. Oncologists should communicate in advance and frequently update their recommendations concerning the advisability of resuscitative efforts for each particular patient. Timely recommendations help to avoid unnecessary emotional trauma to the patient and unnecessary anguish for the surviving family members; they also allow time to settle any disagreements with the patient or family.

Deciding whether to Resuscitate a Patient in the Emergency Room. When a cancer patient presents with cardiopulmonary arrest or impending arrest to an emergency physician who has never seen the patient before, the assessment of prognosis is difficult and often virtually impossible. The decision whether to begin or continue resuscitative efforts requires the physician to rapidly assess the patient's physical condition, the events leading to or immediately preceding the cardiopulmonary arrest, and the considerations outlined in Table 23–1 if that information is available.

The fact that emergency medical services were called to transport the patient to the emergency room may indicate that death or impending death is unexpected or that the family has not come to terms with the patient's prognosis. Another possibility is that the patient or family is seeking relief of the patient's symptoms or suffering at the last moments of life. Resuscitation of patients with

TABLE 23–1. Factors Influencing the Decision to Resuscitate

Duration of cardiopulmonary arrest
Initial cardiac rhythm
Rigor mortis
Expressed directives of the patient or family
Type, stage, and prognosis of cancer
History and prospects of therapy for the cancer
Comorbid conditions
Age
Performance status and nutritional status
Potential quality of life if patient survives

Adapted from Morris JC and Holland JF.[11]

advanced refractory cancers may not be appropriate. Intubation and resuscitation of a patient with end-stage cancer will only prolong the patient's pain and suffering and waste health care resources without affecting outcome. However, if it is decided that resuscitation of the cancer patient is appropriate under the circumstances, the patient should be treated with the same vigorous level of support that is given to patients without cancer.

In cancer patients, as in patients with other types of disease, resuscitation is successful mainly when cardiac arrest is the consequence of an acute reversible insult.[2] The rate of successful resuscitation of cancer patients is about 65%,[3] and about 10% of these resuscitated patients are able to be discharged from the hospital.[3] These rates are not significantly different from those for patients with noncancer diagnoses who undergo cardiopulmonary resuscitation.[4,5] A meta-analysis of inpatient resuscitation showed that the overall likelihood of surviving resuscitation is 1:3 and that the likelihood of being discharged alive is 1:8.[6] The mortality rate of cancer patients in the intensive care unit is about 50% and is comparable to that of severely ill patients without cancer.[7] Reluctance to resuscitate a cancer patient or to admit a cancer patient to an intensive care unit cannot be justified if the patient has good performance status and if death is unexpected.

Special Considerations in the Resuscitation of Patients with Cancer. Most physicians follow the resuscitation procedures outlined in the advanced cardiac life support protocols (<http://www.acls.net>). However, the identification of the specific causes of the cardiopulmonary arrest may allow the physician to tailor resuscitative care to the individual patient. For example, an uncommon but preventable cause of acute cardiopulmonary arrest in cancer patients is the acute carcinoid syndrome. Acute carcinoid syndrome (also termed carcinoid crisis) is precipitated by the anesthesia, biopsy surgery, adrenergic drugs (eg, dopamine or epinephrine), or chemotherapy. Patients with secreting carcinoid tumors may develop refractory hypotension, bronchospasm, and arrhythmias

due to massive release of serotonin and other vasoactive peptides from the carcinoid tumor.[8,9] Acute carcinoid syndrome can be treated effectively with octreotide acetate (Sandostatin), a somatostatin analogue. Octreotide (150 to 500 μg), injected intravenously, rapidly terminates or aborts a carcinoid crisis.[10] Another example of a case in which knowledge of the precipitating event would help the physician to tailor cardiopulmonary resuscitation to the patient is that of pulseless electrical activity due to cardiac tamponade caused by malignant pericardial effusion. In this case, resuscitative attempts will not be effective until pericardiocentesis is performed to relieve the pressure on the cardiac chambers.

Causes of Cardiac Arrest in Cancer Patients

The pathophysiologic mechanisms precipitating cardiopulmonary arrest in cancer patients may be (1) a direct consequence of the neoplastic process, (2) a consequence of antineoplastic therapy, or (3) completely unrelated to the cancer. The various causes of cardiac arrest in cancer patients have been reviewed by Morris and Holland.[11] An undiagnosed neoplasm is rarely a cause of sudden death. Sudden cardiopulmonary arrest is often the result of underlying heart disease, ventricular dysrhythmia being the most common event. Inagaki and colleagues reported that 4% of cancer patients died of cardiac disease and that 90% of these deaths were due to coronary atherosclerosis.[12]

Tumor-Related Causes. Cardiac symptoms due to the tumor itself are usually the result of pericardial involvement; neoplastic pericarditis and cardiac tamponade are good examples. Tumors can also cause arrhythmias due to the mediators they secrete (eg, pheochromocytoma secreting catecholamines, or carcinoid tumors secreting serotonin) or to direct mechanical irritation of the heart or pericardium.[13] Causes of sudden cardiopulmonary arrest in cancer patients also include arrhythmias due to metastases in myocardium, heart block due to metastases to the conduction system, outflow-tract abstruction by intracardiac tumor, and massive tumor embolization.[14–19] Cardiac amyloidosis may cause congestive heart failure, arrhythmias, and sudden death.[20–24] Other tumor-related causes of cardiopulmonary arrest include tumor- or malignancy-induced hemorrhage, malignancy-induced loss of lung function (lymphangitic spread of tumor, airway obstruction, or tumor embolism in the pulmonary arterial system),[25] and loss of brain stem function.[26,27]

Treatment-Related Causes. *Chemotherapy.* Antineoplastic therapy can cause complications that can lead to cardiopulmonary arrest.[13] Hypotension, angina, myocardial infarction, tachycardia, congestive heart failure, and sudden death have been reported as complications of treatment with interleukin-2, interferons, monoclonal antibodies, and several cytotoxic chemotherapy drugs. Anthracyclines (doxorubicin, daunorubicin, idarubicin) and (to a lesser extent) mitoxantrone and mitomycin can injure cardiomyocytes and cause cardiomyopathy. The long-term cardiotoxicity of anthracyclines is dependent on the cumulative dose.[28] However, these drugs also cause acute side effects, and all kind of dysrhythmias have been reported in up to 41% of patients treated with doxorubicin.[29–33] Sudden cardiopulmonary arrest was reported in almost 1% of patients receiving doxorubicin in studies done in the 1970's and the early 1980's. With advances in prevention of anthracycline-induced cardiomyopathy, antracycline-related sudden cardiac arrest is probably much less common.[34–36] High-dose cyclophosphamide may cause acute ventricular arrhythmia, cardiomyopathy, pericardial effusion, and cardiac arrest.[37] Fluorouracil has been associated with acute coronary vasospasm leading to angina and myocardial infarction.[38,39] Vasospasm or worsening angina in a patient receiving fluorouracil can be treated with calcium channel blockers.[40] Chemotherapy-induced thrombocytopenia also puts the patients at risk for sudden catastrophic events, such as massive pulmonary hemorrhage, intracranial hemorrhage, or massive gastrointestinal hemorrhage, leading to cardiopulmonary arrest.

Radiotherapy. Radiotherapy to the chest also affects the pericardium and the heart.[13,41–43] Pericarditis may occur acutely or months to years after radiation exposure. Radiotherapy to the chest can also cause pericardial effusion, tamponade, or pericardial fibrosis. The direct effect of radiation on the heart can lead to electrocardiographic changes, including T-wave changes and atrial arrhythmias. Cardiac exposure to radiation is also associated with coronary endarteritis, intimal proliferation, atherosclerosis, myocardial infarction, and sudden death.[41–44] Restrictive cardiomyopathy[41] and valvular diseases[45,46] are also significant problems after radiotherapy of the chest.

Summary

In conclusion, cardiopulmonary resuscitation is appropriate in any cancer patient whose death is not expected. Cancer patients should be treated with the same high level of support that is given to patients without cancer. On the other hand, intubation and resuscitation of a patient with end-stage cancer will only prolong the patient's pain and suffering and waste health-care resources without changing the inevitable outcome. Family demands for resuscitation may be motivated by lack of acceptance of or denial of the patient's terminal condition. In the absence of clear documentation of previous directives from the patient, resuscitation may be needed to give the family the peace of mind and closure that comes from knowing that everything possible was done.

HYPERSENSITIVITY REACTIONS

Like all drugs, the chemotherapeutic agents used in the treatment of cancer have the potential to cause hypersensitivity reactions. Certain agents, because of the frequency or severity of the reactions they cause, are widely known to cause hypersensitivity reactions. However, any drug or biologic-response modifier used in the treatment of cancer should be viewed as having the potential to cause reactions ranging from mild hypersensitivity reactions to severe anaphylactic responses.

This section reviews the various types of hypersensitivity reactions, describes the specific reactions that can be caused by individual chemotherapeutic agents, and offers recommendations for preventing and treating these reactions. Table 23–2 lists the most common chemotherapeutic agents according to their relative potential for causing hypersensitivity reactions.

Types of Hypersensitivity Reactions

Hypersensitivity reactions are pathologic processes that occur when an antigenic stimulant or antigen (allergen) interacts with humoral antibodies or sensitized lympho-

TABLE 23–2. Common Chemotherapeutic Agents That Cause Hypersensitivity Reactions

High Potential for Hypersensitivity Reactions
    L-Asparaginase
    Docetaxel
    Procarbazine
    Paclitaxel
    Teniposide
Low to Moderate Potential for Hypersensitivity Reactions
    Anthracyclines
    Bleomycin
    Carboplatin
    Chlorambucil
    Cisplatin
    Cyclophosphamide
    Cytarabine
    Dacarbazine
    Etoposide
    Fluorouracil
    Gemcitabine
    Hydroxyurea
    Infosfamide
    Interleukin-2
    Interferons
    Mechlorethamine
    Melphalan
    6-Mercaptopurine
    Methotrexate
    Mitomycin
    Mitoxantrone
    Pentostatin
    PEG-Asparaginase
    Vinca alkaloids

PEG = polyethylene glycol.

cytes, causing an excessive and inappropriate response from the immune system. The Gell and Coombs[47] classification consists of four types and is the most widely used classification for hypersensitivity reactions.

Type I Reactions. The type of hypersensitivity reaction most commonly observed with oncologic agents is the humoral type I reaction, in which antigens combine with specific immunoglobulin E (IgE) antibodies bound to membrane receptors on tissue mast cells and blood basophils, causing the rapid release of potent vasoactive and inflammatory mediators, which may be preformed (eg, histamine) or newly generated from membrane lipids (eg, leukotrienes and prostaglandins). Over hours, mast cells and basophils also release pro-inflammatory cytokines (eg, interleukin-4 [IL-4] and IL-13). These mediators produce vasodilation, increased capillary permeability, glandular hypersecretion, smooth-muscle spasm, and tissue infiltration by eosinophils and other inflammatory cells. Reaction to L-asparaginase is a good example of type I hypersensitivity reaction.

Type IV Reactions. The next most commonly observed hypersensitivity reaction produced by cancer treatment agents is the cellular type IV cell-mediated delayed reaction, which is caused by sensitized T lymphocytes after contact with a specific antigen. Contact dermatitis from the intravesicular administration of mitomycin may be an example of this type of hypersensitivity reaction.

Type II and III Reactions. Type II hypersensitivity reactions, which are cytotoxic, occur when an antibody reacts with antigenic components of a cell or tissue or with an antigen or hapten that is coupled to a cell or to tissue. The rare hemolytic reaction of teniposide may be an example of this type of hypersensitivity reaction. Type III reactions are immune-complex reactions resulting from the deposition of soluble circulating antigen-antibody immune complexes in vessels or tissue, causing acute inflammation as a result of complement-activated polymorphonuclear cell migration and the release of lysosomal proteolytic enzymes and permeability factors in tissues. Allergic alveolitis due to procarbazine and vasculitis due to methotrexate may be examples of type III hypersensitivity reactions.

Anaphylaxis. Anaphylaxis (meaning "without protection," from Portier and Richter in 1902) is an acute, rapid, and life-threatening systemic reaction mediated by IgE in a person previously sensitized to a specific foreign antigen. This reaction may occur immediately but most often occurs within the first 30 minutes of exposure to an antigen and lasts up to 24 hours in some cases. The more immediate the reaction, the greater the severity of the reaction. The risk of sensitization is increased with increasing intermittent exposures to the antigens and increasing doses of antigens.

Chemical mediators (previously mentioned in the description of type I hypersensitivity reactions) are released in very large quantities from mast cells and basophils, causing severe smooth-muscle contractions and severe vascular dilatation, characteristics of anaphylaxis.

The most common manifestations of anaphylaxis are urticaria and angioedema, which occur in 90% of anaphylactic reactions. The next most common manifestations are chest tightness, bronchospasm, upper-airway obstruction, abdominal pain, and hypotension. Laryngeal edema leading to upper-airway obstruction is the leading cause of death in anaphylaxis, followed by hypotension.[48,49] The most life-threatening and immediate anaphylactic reactions are caused by parenterally administered drugs. The other routes of administration of chemotherapeutic agents, in order of decreasing severity of associated reactions, are the intravenous, intra-arterial, intramuscular, subcutaneous, intradermal, oral, vaginal, rectal, and trans-dermal routes.[48] The three most critical elements of the treatment of anaphylaxis are early recognition, airway maintenance, and the administration of epinephrine. Recommendations for the treatment of anaphylaxis are given in Table 23–3.[50–53]

Specific Chemotherapeutic Agents and Hypersensitivity Reactions

The treatment of hypersensitivity reactions and anaphylaxis due to chemotherapeutic agents is based on the pathophysiology of these reactions. Due to the reversibility of these reactions, when patients with cancer or patients receiving chemotherapeutic agents experience a hypersensitivity reaction or anaphylaxis, they should be managed as aggressively as any other patient with a similar medical emergency unless there are known overriding circumstances.

Factors known to affect the incidence or severity of hypersensitivity reactions include the class of drug being used, the dose, the rate of infusion, the route of administration, the interval between doses, previous exposure to the drug, the cumulative dose, the total number of times a patient is exposed to the drug, and administration of prophylactic agents (ie, the dosing and timing of administration of the prophylactic agents and the thoroughness of the prevention plan). Additional factors include the excipient used to make an agent soluble for administration (eg, Cremophor EL) and the patient's age. Recommendations for pretreatment regimens depend on various factors, such as the severity of observed and potential reactions and the typical time delay from administration of the drug to the onset of reactions.

L-Asparaginase. L-Asparaginase is a polypeptide of bacterial origin that can stimulate the production of immunoglobulins, especially IgE, through multiple anti-

TABLE 23–3. Treatment of Anaphylaxis

1. Remove the antigen or delay the absorption of the antigen.
2. Maintain an adequate airway and oxygenation; intubate if there is evidence of laryngeal edema or impending severe airway obstruction.
3. Administer epinephrine.
   - In case of a mild episode:
     0.3 mg SQ (0.01 mg/kg in a child), 1 mg/mL
     Repeat at 10- to 20-minute intervals.
   - In case of a more severe episode:
     0.3–0.5 mg IM, 1 mg/mL
     Repeat at 5 to 10-minute intervals.
   - In case of shock or incipient airway obstruction:
     1 mg/100 mL IV, 0.01–0.02 mg/min, up to a total of 0.1 mg
   - In case of persistent shock:
     May repeat dose or start a drip. Add 1 mg to 500 mL normal saline and infuse at 2–10 μg/min.
   - If patient is over 50 years old or has a cardiac history and life-threatening symptoms exist:
     Test dose of 0.1–0.15 mg SQ or IM.
   - If shock is resistant to other measures or there is imminent airway closure:
     Consider a drip, as noted previously.
4. Expand intravascular volume with IV normal saline or lactated Ringer's solution.
   - In case of shock, use the following dosages:
     Adult: 1 L over 15 minutes, then reassess
     Child: 20 mL/kg bolus, then reassess
5. Administer methylprednisolone.
   - 125 mg IV push; may repeat every 4 hours if symptoms persist (alternative: hydrocortisone, 500 mg, or other potent corticosteroid).
   - If discharging the patient home, prescribe prednisone, 40 mg per day for 2 to 3 days.
6. Administer diphenhydramine.
   - 25–50 mg IV, IM, or orally. Repeat every 2–4 hours as needed.
   - If the patient is being discharged, prescribe 50 mg every 6 hours as needed for 3 days.
7. In case of resistant hypotension:
   - MAST and Trendelenburg's position (may be helpful).
   - Infuse dopamine, 5–15 μg/kg/min IV.
   - Administer naloxone 0.4 - 2.0 mg IV every 2 minutes (maximum, 10 mg).
   - Administer cimetidine, 300 mg IV.
8. In case of β-blocker-accentuated epinephrine-resistant anaphylaxis:
   - Administer glucagon, 1–5 mg IV over 2–5 minutes.
   - Administer terbutaline, 0.25 mg SQ.
   - Administer isoproterenol, 2–10 μg/min IV.

Adapted from Schwartz GR, et al.,[50] Murrant T, Bihari D.,[51] Gavalas M, et al.;[52] Brown AF.[53]

IM = intramuscularly; IV = intravenously; MAST = military antishock trousers; SQ = subcutaneously.

genic sites. Hypersensitivity reactions have been reported in 6 to 43% of patients treated with this drug.[54,55] The risk of hypersensitivity reactions increases by 5 to 8% with each subsequent dose and reaches 33% with the fourth dose.[56] Anaphylactic reactions can occur with both the *Escherichia coli* and *Erwinia chrysanthemi* forms of L-asparaginase.[56,57] However, fewer than 10% of treated patients suffer from anaphylaxis, and fatal reactions occur in less than 1% of patients.[58] A modified form of asparaginase with covalently attached polyethyl-ene glycol (PEG-asparaginase or pegaspargase), does not appear to cause anaphylactic reactions.[59]

Risk factors for adverse reactions to L-asparaginase include administration of a higher dose (> 6,000 IU/m^2/d),[60] previous exposure to L-asparaginase, intravenous administration,[61] a history of atopy or other drug allergy,[62] and single-agent treatment with L-asparaginase.[63,64] Intradermal skin testing[65] and test dosing[57] are of no value in predicting adverse reactions to L-asparaginase.

L-Asparaginase–induced hypersensitivity reactions generally occur during the 2nd week of treatment or later.[58] Clinical manifestations occur within 1 hour of administration and are typical of a type I hypersensitivity reaction. Pruritus, dyspnea, and agitation are initially observed. Urticaria (in up to 66% of reactions),[60] rash, nausea and vomiting, angioedema, pain in the abdomen and extremities, nasal congestion, hypotension, and laryngospasm or bronchospasm may also occur.[62,66]

Although reactions to L-asparaginase usually occur during the 2nd week of treatment or later,[58] preparations for the immediate treatment of hypersensitivity reactions must be in place before every dose, including the first dose. Intramuscular administration is recommended because it is associated with a lower incidence of anaphylactic reactions than is intravenous administration.[61] Reactions to one form of L-asparaginase should prompt a change to another less immunogenic preparation.

Taxanes. In early studies, the taxanes (paclitaxel and docetaxel) caused major hypersensitivity reactions in approximately 10 to 30% of treated patients and minor reactions in approximately 40%.[67,68] Since reactions can occur with the first treatment, a nonimmunologic mechanism is likely. Further studies are needed to fully understand this mechanism. These major hypersensitivity reactions to the taxanes form a syndrome that is very similar to anaphylaxis and thus have been called anaphylactoid reactions.

Risk factors for hypersensitivity reactions with taxane infusion include shorter infusion schedules and faster infusion rates. Since the taxanes are insoluble, excipients are used to maintain their solubility; Cremophor EL is used with paclitaxel, and Tween 80 is used with docetaxel. The question of hypersensitivity reactions being caused by these vehicles is still open for discussion since these vehicles can induce similar reactions in dogs.[69]

Minor reactions to the taxanes include erythematous rash, flushing, low back pain, and chest tightness. Minor reactions do not increase in severity with repeated administrations[70] nor do they predict future major reactions.[67,68] Most major reactions occur within the first two doses, but major reactions may appear in later cycles as well. Reactions begin within 2 to 10 minutes of the initiation of treatment and resolve within 15 minutes of the discontinuation of treatment. Manifestations of major hypersensitivity reactions consistent with type I reactions include dyspnea, bronchospasm, hypotension, urticaria, and angioedema.

Methods studied for their potential to prevent hypersensitivity reactions to the taxanes include prophylactic medication schedules[71] and reducing the rate of infusion. One study showed that infusion of paclitaxel over 96 hours without prior premedication resulted in no major hypersensitivity reactions.[72] However, with the shorter infusion times of 24 hours and 3 hours, prophylaxis with appropriate premedications reduced the incidence of major hypersensitivity reactions to 1 and 2%, respectively.[73–75] Pretreatment regimens of steroids and histamine (H_1 and H_2) receptor antagonists have reduced the incidence of major hypersensitivity reactions to 1 to 3%.[68]

Teniposide and Etoposide. In adults, hypersensitivity reactions occur in up to approximately 7% of patients treated with teniposide[76,77] and in about 3% of patients treated with etoposide.[78,79] In children, especially those with acute lymphocytic leukemia, reactions to etoposide may occur more frequently than in adults.[79,80]

The mechanism of reactions to the epipodophyllotoxins is still not fully understood. That reactions can occur during the first exposure to these agents[76] suggests a nonimmunologic mechanism, but increased rates of reaction are seen with increased cumulative doses,[81] which suggests the development of an antibody-mediated reaction.[80] Excipients such as benzyl alcohol, Tween 80, and Cremophor EL are used to solubilize etoposide and teniposide. As is the case for the taxanes, further studies are needed to determine what role (if any) these excipients have in hypersensitivity reactions to the epipodophyllotoxins. There are no known risk factors for teniposide- or etoposide-induced reactions.

Reactions most often occur during the first 10 minutes of infusion, sometimes after only a few milligrams have been infused,[77] but reactions can also occur hours after administration.[76,82] The hypersensitivity reactions seen are typically type I reactions, with the development of urticaria, bronchospasm, hypotension, angioedema, flushing, and rashes. One case of a type II hemolytic reaction due to teniposide has been reported.[83] No hypersensitivity reactions have been reported with oral etoposide.[80] Patients who develop severe reactions to the epipodophyllotoxins or whose symptoms are slow to resolve should not be rechallenged with these agents.

Procarbazine. Procarbazine causes a type I hypersensitivity reaction in approximately 6 to 18% of patients treated[84,85] and may cause a type III reaction consisting of pulmonary side effects in the form of allergic alveolitis.[86] The mechanism of these reactions is unknown. There are no known risk factors for procarbazine-induced reactions. Manifestations are the development of a maculopapular rash and urticaria typical of type I

reactions. Skin testing is not predictive of reactions. Patients who have a hypersensitivity reaction to procarbazine are unable to continue treatment. Rechallenging such patients will cause the recurrence of symptoms.

Cisplatin and Cisplatin Analogues. Cisplatin produces type I hypersensitivity reactions and type II hypersensitivity reactions resulting in hemolytic anemia.[87] The incidence of hypersensitivity reactions appears to be between 1 and 20%[88,89] when cisplatin is given intravenously and between 10 and 25% with intravesicular administration.[90,91] Carboplatin also produces type I hypersensitivity reactions.[92,93] The type I reactions of both cisplatin and carboplatin appear to be IgE mediated and may be caused by the platinum in these compounds.[94] One review suggested that six or more doses may be necessary to produce a hypersensitivity reaction.[66] Cross-reactivity among analogues is possible.[95–97] The manifestations of hypersensitivity reactions caused by cisplatin and its analogues include the development of rashes, urticaria, anxiety, bronchospasm, and hypotension. Anaphylaxis may occur in 5% of patients treated.

Cytarabine. Type I reactions to cytarabine are uncommon. However, cytarabine syndrome,[98] palmar-plantar erythema,[99,100] and neutrophilic eccrine hidradenitis[101–103] also can occur with administration of this drug. There are no known risk factors for cytarabine-induced reactions. The manifestations of cytarabine-induced reactions that are IgE-mediated include dyspnea, chest pain, fever, angioedema, urticaria, and hypotension.

Methotrexate. Methotrexate can produce type I hypersensitivity reactions and possibly type III reactions in the form of acute pneumonitis or cutaneous vasculitis. The type III reaction is of sudden onset and is not related to the dose or duration of treatment. There are no known risk factors for methotrexate-induced reactions. The type I reactions produce rashes, urticaria, angioedema, generalized pruritus, and hypotension. The type III reactions produce lung eosinophilia, pleural effusions, hilar adenopathy, and rashes.

Cyclophosphamide and Ifosfamide. Both oral and intravenous administration of cyclophosphamide can produce type I reactions, which appear to be IgE mediated. Ifosfamide may also produce type I reactions. Since mesna is given with ifosfamide and since mesna alone can cause these type I reactions, there is uncertainty regarding the cause of such reactions. Reactions to cyclophosphamide and ifosfamide may occur with the first dose or with subsequent doses. Reported manifestations of cyclophosphamide- and ifosfamide-induced reactions include rashes, angioneurotic edema, urticaria, and anaphylaxis.[104–107]

Anthracycline Antibiotics. Daunorubicin and doxorubicin are capable of producing type I reactions when given intravenously,[108,109] and doxorubicin can produce type I reactions when given intravesically.[110] Idarubicin has not been reported to produce type I reactions when given orally or intravenously. Cross-reactivity between anthracycline antibiotics appears to be uncommon. Reported manifestations of reactions induced by anthracycline antibiotics include erythema, pruritus, urticaria, hypotension, and anaphylaxis.

Melphalan and Chlorambucil. Melphalan given orally or intravenously can cause type I hypersensitivity reactions. Reactions are uncommon when the drug is given orally, but approximately 2 to 4% of patients treated intravenously have hypersensitivity reactions.[111] The reason for the difference in the rates of hypersensitivity reactions between the oral and intravenous routes is unclear. Chlorambucil has produced rare cases of type I hypersensitivity reactions.[112] However, toxic epidermal necrolysis,[113,114] hemolysis,[115] and pneumonitis[116] have been reported with chlorambucil treatment. There are no known risk factors for melphalan- and chlorambucil-induced hypersensitivity reactions. Reactions to intravenous melphalan occur after at least 2 doses have been administered. Manifestations include urticaria and angioedema but not hypotension or bronchospasm.[117,118]

Mitomycin C. Mitomycin C may cause a generalized rash when given intravenously. When given intravesically, mitomycin C causes hypersensitivity reactions in up to 10% of treated patients.[119] Most of these patients receive five or more doses before the reactions occur. This delayed hypersensitivity reaction develops through drug contact with the bladder epithelium and appears to be a type IV reaction that is not mediated by IgE.[120] Manifestations of reactions induced by mitomycin C include rashes, angioedema, and pruritus. These skin rashes are erythematous, vesicular, and pruritic, eventually resulting in desquamation. Skin testing with mitomycin C has a high positive predictive value for skin reactions.[119,120]

Miscellaneous Antineoplastics. The drugs listed in this paragraph are either relatively new (so little is known about their potential to cause hypersensitivity reactions) or relatively unlikely to cause hypersensitivity reactions. Fluorouracil causes rare cases of angioedema and hypotension consistent with type I hypersensitivity reactions.[121] Pentostatin, an antibiotic produced by *Streptomyces antibioticus,* causes erythematous and pruritic rashes,[122] angioedema, fever, and eosinophilia.[123] Diaziquone causes hypersensitivity reactions in 1 to 2% of patients; the reactions manifest as urticaria, bronchospasm, hypotension, and anaphylaxis.[124] (These are possibly IgE-mediated type I hypersensitivity reactions.

It is still unclear whether diaziquone itself or the diluent dimethylacetamide is the cause of the observed hypersensitivity reactions). Bleomycin causes urticaria, periorbital edema, and bronchospasm.[125] (In rare instances, hypersensitivity reactions to bleomycin have been fatal.[126] Test dosing with 1 mg of bleomycin is suggested prior to the initial treatment dose and prior to doses of 5 to 15 U/m^2 given on a weekly or biweekly schedule.) Mitoxantrone has been reported to cause diffuse erythematous rashes and angioedema;[127,128] rechallenge caused a recurrence of these symptoms.

Treatment Recommendations

General recommendations for the treatment of hypersensitivity reactions are given in Table 23–4. General recommendations for prophylaxis regimens are given in Table 23–5. Prophylaxis for rechallenge with paclitaxel is outlined in Table 23–6.

SYSTEMIC REACTIONS TO CYTOKINES AND MONOCLONAL ANTIBODIES

Cytokines are soluble proteins that are produced by mononuclear cells of the immune system. Cytokines exert a regulatory action on other cells or on target cells involved in an immune reaction. Several cytokines, including interferons, interleukins, and monoclonal antibodies, have been approved for the treatment of solid and hematologic malignancies. The toxic effects associated with individual cytokines and monoclonal antibodies are discussed in this section.

Interferon

Interferons (IFNs) are a family of proteins produced by cells in response to various stimuli. Interferon-α is produced by macrophages and lymphocytes, IFN-β is produced by fibroblasts and epithelial cells, and IFN-γ is produced by natural killer cells, CD4- or CD8-positive lymphocytes, and lymphokine-activated killer

TABLE 23–4. Treatment of Hypersensitivity Reactions

- Discontinue the drug immediately.
- Although corticosteroids have no effect on the initial reaction, they can block late allergic symptoms; therefore, administer methylprednisolone, 125 mg (or its equivalent) IV.
- Administer diphenhydramine, 50 mg IV.
- Administer epinephrine, 0.35 to 0.5 mg of 1 mg/mL solution IV every 15 to 20 minutes until the reaction subsides or a total of 6 doses have been administered.
- If hypotension is present and does not respond to epinephrine, administer crystalloid fluids IV.
- If wheezing is present and does not respond to epinephrine, administer 0.30 mL (2.5 mg) of nebulized albuterol solution or other inhaled β-agonists.

Adapted from Weiss RB.[66]
IV = intravenously.

TABLE 23–5. Prophylaxis of Hypersensitivity Reactions From Antitumor Drugs

Premedication
- 20 mg dexamethasone orally 12 hours and 6 hours before treatment and 20 mg IV just before chemotherapy treatment.
- 50 mg diphenhydramine orally or IV 30 minutes before treatment.
- H$_2$ receptor antagonist (famotidine 20 mg, ranitidine 150 mg, or cimetidine 300 mg) IV 30 minutes before treatment.
- Consider 25 mg ephedrine sulfate orally 1 hour before treatment unless contraindicated by unstable angina or hypertension.
- Slowly withdraw patient (if possible) from any β-blockers that could potentiate a reaction or make management of a reaction difficult.

Treatment setting
- IV access must be established.
- Blood pressure monitoring must be available.
- Have epinephrine and IV diphenhydramine readily available.

Observation
- Observe the patient for up to 2 h after antitumor drug administration is completed.

Adapted from Weiss RB.[66]
IV = intravenous(ly).

cells. Recombinant forms of IFNs are used worldwide as therapy for viral infections, malignancies, and autoimmune diseases. Interferons can regulate gene expression, modulate cell surface antigen expression, and induce new enzyme synthesis. On a cellular basis, these effects translate into alterations in the differentiation, proliferation rate, cell death, and functional activity of many types of cells.

Acute adverse effects of IFNs occur within the first 2 to 8 hours after treatment, but they rarely limit treatment. Flulike symptoms (including myalgia, headache, and low-grade fever),[129] nausea, vomiting, hypo- or hypertension, and tachycardia are the most common side effects. Subacute and chronic adverse effects develop after 2 to 4 weeks of therapy. With chronic administration of IFNs, fatigue and anorexia can be dose limiting, and weight loss may be significant (> 10% of body weight).[130] Neurologic side effects including behavioral and cognitive changes may limit treatment. In general,

TABLE 23–6. Paclitaxel Rechallenge Prophylactic Regimen*

- Dexamethasone, 20 mg IV every 6 hours for 4 doses, with the last dose administered 30 minutes before rechallenge
- Diphenhydramine, 50 mg IV, 30 minutes before rechallenge
- Cimetidine, 300 mg IV, 30 minutes before rechallenge
- Administer paclitaxel at 10% of the rate required to deliver the solution over 24 hours. If no major reactions occur within the first 2 hours, the infusion rate should be gradually increased over the next 2 hours to the original 24-hour infusion rate.

Adapted from Peereboom DM, et al.[71]
IV = intravenously.
*For patients with a prior hypersensitivity reaction to paclitaxel.

younger patients tolerate these side effects better than do older patients. Anxiety, agitation, seizures, and coma have been reported with high-dose schedules and are reversible. Mild granulocytopenia (reduction in counts by approximately 50%) develops gradually after the 1st week of treatment and rapidly resolves upon discontinuation of the drug. Autoimmune and immune hemolytic anemias, myelosuppression, and thrombocytopenias may also be seen, but these side effects are rare.

Management of flulike side effects with aspirin, acetaminophen, or nonsteroidal anti-inflammatory drugs is recommended. Other supportive care may be provided, based on the symptoms. In most patients, symptoms lessen with subsequent doses of IFN.

Interleukin-2

Through interaction with specific receptors located on T cells, B cells, macrophages, and natural killer cells, interleukin-2 (IL-2) plays a major role in the maturation and development of lymphocytes and monocytes. Interleukin-2 is approved by the Food and Drug Administration (FDA) for the treatment of patients with metastatic renal cell carcinoma and melanoma. High-dose IL-2 therapy is associated with a wide spectrum of cardiovascular and hemodynamic toxic effects that resemble septic shock. Hypotension, vascular leak syndrome, and respiratory insufficiency are seen with high-dose intravenous therapy. High-dose intravenous therapy must be given in a hospital setting, and intensive care monitoring is sometimes necessary. Hemodynamic support with pressors, endotracheal intubation, and fluid resuscitation may be necessary during therapy. Acute central nervous system side effects such as behavioral changes, psychosis, disorientation, and confusion may be seen with high-dose IL-2 therapy. Abnormalities usually require 48 to 72 hours after the discontinuation of IL-2 to resolve. Other central nervous system side effects, such as seizures and coma, have been reported in patients with brain metastases. At the first sign of neurologic toxicity, IL-2 should be discontinued.

Lower-dose intravenous and subcutaneous IL-2 regimens can be given in an outpatient setting, but patients may require several hours of observation after administration. The side effects of lower-dose therapy are dose dependent. Myelosuppression and anemia are uncommon. Common symptoms include nausea, vomiting, anorexia, fever, chills, malaise, fatigue, myalgias, arthralgias, and pruritus.

Prophylaxis against acute toxic effects includes acetaminophen (650 to 1,000 mg 1 hour before therapy and every 3 hours, for two doses), and histamine (H$_1$ and H$_2$) receptor antagonists (eg, diphenhydramine, 50 mg by mouth 1 hour before therapy and every 3 hours for 3 doses, plus cimetidine, 800 mg by mouth before therapy). Antiemetics may be given as needed, and intravenous meperidine (25 to 50 mg) may be given as needed for chills during therapy.

Monoclonal Antibodies

Monoclonal antibodies are becoming more widely used in the treatment of cancer. A potential serious side effect of these antibodies is the induction of a massive release of cytokines, which may lead to fever, rigor, dyspnea, hypoxia, hypotension, or even death. Strategies for decreasing the incidence of this severe cytokine release syndrome include fractionated schedules of infusion and pretreatment with corticosteroids. Monoclonal antibodies can also produce a range of hypersensitivity reactions, which are described below.

Rituximab. Rituximab is a humanized murine monoclonal antibody directed against the CD20 molecule. Rituximab is commonly used to treat B-cell lymphomas.[131] Rituximab is also being investigated for use in the treatment of other malignancies (including chronic lymphocytic leukemia, intermediate- and high-grade lymphomas, and Waldenström's macroglobulinemia) and for use in combination with other chemotherapeutic agents.[132–134] The CD20 molecule is a B-cell-specific surface molecule that is involved in cellular differentiation and growth. It is not expressed on hematopoietic stem cells, plasma cells, or cells of other lineage. Rituximab is very effective for in vivo B-cell depletion. Circulating B cells become undetectable after a single 375-mg/m^2 infusion of rituximab. Recovery of B-cells begins 6 to 9 months after treatment, and counts normalize by 9 to 12 months.[135]

In the phase III trial of the antibody, adverse reactions were seen in approximately 84% of patients. Most toxic effects were seen with the first infusion and consisted of minor reactions. An infusion syndrome consisting of transient fever, chills, nausea, headache, and fatigue is commonly seen with the first dose. Other side effects reported included rash, pain at the tumor site, hypotension, arrhythmias, bronchospasm, and angioedema, which may reflect immune responses to the murine immunoglobulin.[136,137] Rituximab also causes an expected depletion of normal B cells; recovery occurs within 9 to 12 months, but there was no depletion of mean serum immunoglobulin levels in the trial.[138] Pretreatment with acetaminophen and diphenhydramine may attenuate the symptoms of the infusion syndrome. In preapproval clinical studies, corticosteroids were not used for pretreatment. Reactions occur within 30 to 120 minutes after starting the infusion and resolve with the slowing or interruption of the infusion. The standard management of reactions to rituximab is to interrupt the infusion and to restart at 50% of the previous infusion rate when symptoms resolve. The treatment of reactions should be supportive after stopping the infusion.

Trastuzumab. Trastuzumab is a recombinant humanized monoclonal antibody whose antigen is the HER-2/neu (c-erb B2) protein, a glycoprotein receptor with intrinsic tyrosine kinase activity and partial homology with the epidermal growth factor receptor.[139] Up to 35% of breast cancers overexpress the HER-2 proto-oncogene.[140] Trastuzumab is approved by the FDA for the treatment of metastatic breast cancer refractory to chemotherapy and is also approved as part of a combination with paclitaxel for first-line treatment of metastatic breast cancer.

Treatment with trastuzumab is generally well tolerated. The side effects are usually mild to moderate and include fever, chills, pain at the tumor site, diarrhea, nausea, and vomiting. Fever and chills during the first infusion are the most prominent symptoms.

Campath-1H. Campath-1H is a human immunoglobulin G1 monoclonal antibody directed against CD52 that binds to nearly all B-cell and T-cell lymphomas. Campath-1H has received orphan drug status from the FDA for use in chronic leukemias and is under investigation as therapy for non-Hodgkin's lymphoma and for multiple sclerosis. Campath-1H has been associated with a variety of side effects, some of which are life threatening. The first three or four antibody infusions in each patient are associated with side effects such as rigor, fever, facial flushing, nausea, vomiting, hives, wheezes, hypotension, and diarrhea. However, these side effects were less severe or were absent with gradually escalated dosages. Pretreatment with acetaminophen and diphenhydramine can attenuate infusion reactions.

Gemtuzumab Ozogamicin. Gemtuzumab ozogamicin (Mylotarg) is a monoclonal antibody bound to a cytotoxic antibiotic that is approved by the FDA for the treatment of patients with CD33-positive acute myeloid leukemia in first relapse who are more than 60 years old and who may not be able to tolerate cytotoxic chemotherapy.[141] The CD33 antigen is expressed on normal and leukemic myeloid progenitor cells but not on hematopoietic stem cells. Gemtuzumab is a humanized anti-CD33 antibody-calcheamicin conjugate. Calcheamicin, a small molecule that is 1,000 times more potent than doxorubicin, forms free radical intermediates intercellularly and is a deoxyribonucleic acid (DNA) minor groove binder that causes double-strand breaks and apoptosis.[142]

Twenty percent of 40 patients with acute myeloid leukemia in first relapse treated with gemtuzumab had a complete remission or a complete remission without platelet recovery. The dosage recommended for gemtuzumab is 9 mg/m^2 given by intravenous infusion over 2 hours, with a second dose given 14 days later. The most common side effect is a postinfusion syndrome of fever and chills. Other infusion-related effects, which usually occur within 4 hours of administration, include nausea, hypotension, and shortness of breath. Prophylaxis with acetaminophen (650 mg) and diphenhydramine (25 to 50 mg) 15 to 30 minutes before infusion is recommended.[143]

Denileukin Diftitox. Denileukin diftitox (Ontak) is a fusion protein of IL-2 attached to diphtheria toxin. The IL-2 portion of the molecule binds to the IL-2 receptor on the surface of lymphoma cells, thus delivering the diphtheria toxin to the lymphoma cells. The diphtheria toxin inhibits cellular protein synthesis, leading to cell death within hours. Denileukin diftitox is approved by the FDA for the treatment of persistent or recurrent cutaneous T-cell lymphoma whose malignant cells express CD25.

In a trial, significant side effects included fever and flulike symptoms, nausea and vomiting, infections, cytokine release syndrome, and vascular leak syndrome.[144] Acute reactions usually occurred on the 1st day of dosing and included hypotension, back pain, difficulty in breathing, vasodilation, rashes, chest pain, tachycardia, difficulty in swallowing, and syncope. Only 2% of patients experienced severe reactions. Treatment of the reactions included slowing the infusion rate, terminating the infusion, and administering intravenous antihistamines, corticosteroids, and epinephrine. Resuscitative equipment and the aforementioned drugs should be readily available during the infusion of denileukin diftitox.

Vascular (or capillary) leak syndrome is characterized by hypotension, edema, pleural effusion, and hypoalbuminemia. The onset of symptoms occurs within the first 2 weeks of therapy, and symptoms can persist or worsen after the drug is discontinued. The condition is self-limiting. Medical management may be necessary and should include diuretics, albumin infusion, and intravenous fluids. Patients with low albumin levels are at risk for the syndrome, and in these patients, the administration of denileukin diftitox should be delayed until the patient's serum albumin level is at least 3.0 g/dL. Premedication with systemic corticosteroids is recommended to avoid vascular leak syndrome.[145,146]

DRUG EXTRAVASATION

Drug extravasation is a well-known adverse event associated with the administration of chemotherapy. Extravasation occurs when a drug escapes from a vessel into the surrounding tissues, either by leakage or by direct infiltration. Many factors increase the risk of extravasation, including fragile, small, or sclerosed veins; lymphedema; peripheral neuropathy; superior vena cava syndrome; and altered mental status. Extravasation has been reported to occur in 0.1 to 6.5% of chemotherapy infusions.[147]

Clinical Manifestations

The clinical manifestations of extravasation injury range from minor discomfort and erythema to painful skin ulceration and necrosis of underlying tissues. Increased erythema, pain, discoloration of the surrounding skin, induration, blistering, and desquamation may occur within 48 to 72 hours after extravasation. Necrosis, eschar formation, and ulceration may appear over the next several weeks, depending on the amount of agent released into the surrounding tissues. Cellulitis, abscess formation, and systemic manifestations are rarely seen.[148] Extravasation may also cause damage to underlying nerves and tendons, leading to loss of neurologic and joint function. The extent of damage from drug extravasation depends largely on the concentration of the drug, the volume that escapes, and the type of drug.[149] Continuous infusion of chemotherapeutic drugs increases the risk of extravasation.

Drug Classification and Types of Extravasation Injury

On the basis of the potential for local injury upon extravasation, chemotherapeutic agents can be classified as nonvesicants, irritants, and vesicants. Nonvesicants cause no damage when they escape from a vein. Irritants cause inflammatory reactions, pain, aching, tightness, or phlebitis at the injection site or along the involved vein.[150] Tissue damage is immediate with an irritant, but the drug is quickly metabolized and degraded, limiting the extent of damage. The injury produced by irritants is similar to a burn and is followed by normal healing processes. Gross necrosis and ulceration do not occur.[151] Vesicants cause immediate injury and also remain in the tissue, usually binding DNA, causing a prolonged course of injury. It has been postulated that the prolonged course of damage from vesicants is due to "recycling" of the drug in the tissue. According to this concept, when one cell dies, the vesicant within is released and taken up by another cell (endocytolysis). The early manifestations of vesicant reactions may be subtle and can appear immediately or after several days or weeks. The initial signs and symptoms may include a local burning sensation or tingling at the infusion site, mild erythema, swelling, and pruritus. Many chemotherapeutic drugs can act as both irritants and vesicants (Table 23–7).

The most devastating and well-known vesicant injuries are seen with the anthracyclines. Vinca alkaloids are also well-known vesicants. Only one-third of vesicant reactions produce ulceration when local conservative management is employed. With certain chemotherapeutic drugs, extravasation at the site of previous drug extravasation or previous radiotherapy can cause "recall soft-tissue injury," a form of dermatitis.[152] These so-called recall injuries are a rare complication of chemotherapeutic extravasation; they occur most often with anthracycline chemotherapy but also with paclitaxel. In these cases, the reaction includes a low-grade skin reaction with no noted ulcerations. The etiology and pathophysiology of recall dermatitis are unclear. Histologic examination of

TABLE 23–7. Classification of Chemotherapeutic Agents Commonly Seen in Extravasation Reactions

Irritant	Vesicant	Irritant/Vesicant	
Carboplatin	Vindesine	Amsacrine	Idarubicin
Cyclophosphamide	Idarubicin	Bleomycin	Mechlorethamine
Ifosfamide	Melphalan	Carmustine	Mitomycin
Thiotepa	Vincristine	Cisplatin	Mitoxantrone
	Teniposide	Dacarbazine	Paclitaxel
		Dactinomycin	Plicamycin
		Daunorubicin	Streptozocin
		Doxorubicin	Teniposide
		Epirubicin	Vinblastine
		Etoposide	Vinorelbine
		Fluorouracil	

Adapted from Susser et al.[151]

tissues after the occurrence of recall dermatitis has suggested several possible etiologies, ranging from skin necrosis to mixed inflammatory infiltration.[153]

Management

Most cases of drug extravasation can be prevented with the systematic implementation of carefully planned drug administration techniques. Central venous catheters (CVCs) are recommended when vesicants are administered by continuous infusion. However, drug extravasation can occur even with CVCs and ports because of (for example) poor needle placement in the port or because of breakage or fracture of a catheter.

All personnel who administer chemotherapeutic agents should be trained in handling extravasation and in the proper management of acute reactions. During administration of chemotherapeutic drugs, nursing personnel must monitor for signs of extravasation (eg, changes in the rate of infusion or the absence of blood return on aspiration).

Conservative management of an acute episode is recommended.[62] The infusion should be stopped immediately. If an antidote is to be given intravenously, residual drug must be aspirated from the needle and tubing prior to administering the antidote. Specific antidotes are discussed in detail later in this section. Trained nursing personnel should carefully document the episode, and the patient should be evaluated by a physician. The affected extremity should be placed in a sling or elevated by other means, to minimize edema. Application of ice for 20 minutes four times a day for the first 3 days is recommended. Cold has been shown to ameliorate the locally destructive effects of certain chemotherapeutic agents, such as the anthracyclines and mitomycin.[154] Except in cases treated with hyaluronidase (discussed below), the use of heat should be avoided because it could increase the metabolic rate and damage tissue. Evaluation for plastic surgery may be necessary when conservative management fails to pre-

vent tissue ulceration. The clinician must also be aware of the possibility of late local reactions and must educate the patient about the possible associated symptoms. Proper education of the patient is imperative in the first 48 hours to carefully monitor the site, and prompt physician follow-up after 3 to 4 days, to re-evaluate the extravasation site, is recommended. Pain and ulceration are the most common complaints that should prompt consultation with a plastic surgeon.

The use of antidotes in the case of extravasation injuries produced by chemotherapeutic agents is controversial. There are few clinical studies that have demonstrated benefit from specific antidotes. Empiric guidelines for the use of antidotes after the extravasation of chemotherapeutic drugs have been published by the Oncology Nursing Society.[155]

Antidotes that appear useful include hyaluronidase, sodium thiosulfate, and dimethyl sulfoxide (Table 23–8).[62] Hyaluronidase may be helpful in cases of vinblastine, vincristine, or etoposide extravasation. The recommended treatment is an injection of 150 to 900 units in 1 to 3 mL of saline through the original needle, followed by the application of a warm pack without pressure. Sodium thiosulfate may be helpful in cases of alkylating-agent extravasation. The recommended treatment is an injection of 2 mL of sodium thiosulfate solution (4 mL of a 10% solution mixed with 5 mL of sterile water) at the extravasation site. Dimethyl sulfoxide is recommended in the case of anthracycline or mitomycin extravasation. The patient may apply 1.5 mL topically on the extravasation site every 6 to 8 hours for 14 days.[62]

TABLE 23–8. Guidelines for the Use of Antidotes for Extravasation of Chemotherapeutic Drugs

Drug	Antidotes	Comments
Anthracyclines	DMSO; ice packs	Apply topically and allow to dry, repeating every 6 to 8 hours for at least a few days.
Mitomycin	DMSO	Apply topically and allow to dry, repeating every 6 to 8 hours for at least a few days.
Mechlorethamine	Sodium thiosulfate	Prepare a 0.17 mol/L solution by mixing 4 mL of sodium thiosulfate 10% wt/vol with 6 mL sterile water for injections. Inject 2 mL into the extravasation site.
Vinca alkaloids*	Hyaluronidase; warm packs	Reconstitute with normal saline and inject 150 to 900 U into the extravasation site.
Paclitaxel	Hyaluronidase; ice packs	As for vinca alkaloids.

Adapted from Albanell J, Baselga J.[62]
DMSO = dimethyl sulfoxide.
*And epipodophyllotoxins when concentrated drugs are extravasated.

REFERENCES

1. Hanson LC, Rodgman E. The use of living wills at the end of life. A national study. Arch Intern Med 1996;156:1018–22.

2. Sculier JP, Markiewicz E. Cardiopulmonary resuscitation in medical cancer patients: the experience of a medical intensive-care unit of a cancer centre. Support Care Cancer 1993;1:135–8.

3. Vitelli CE, Cooper K, Rogatko A, Brennan MF. Cardiopulmonary resuscitation and the patient with cancer. J Clin Oncol 1991;9:111–5.

4. Hendrick JM, Pijls NH, van der Werf T, Crul JF. Cardiopulmonary resuscitation on the general ward: no category of patients should be excluded in advance. Resuscitation 1990;20:163–71.

5. Rozenbaum EA, Shenkman L. Predicting outcome of inhospital cardiopulmonary resuscitation. Crit Care Med 1988;16:583–6.

6. Ebell MH, Becker LA, Barry HC, Hagen M. Survival after in-hospital cardiopulmonary resuscitation. A meta-analysis. J Gen Intern Med 1998;13:805–16.

7. Staudinger T, Stoiser B, Mullner M, et al. Outcome and prognostic factors in critically ill cancer patients admitted to the intensive care unit. Crit Care Med 2000;28:1322–8.

8. Bissonnette RT, Gibney RG, Berry BR, Buckley AR. Fatal carcinoid crisis after percutaneous fine-needle biopsy of hepatic metastasis: case report and literature review. Radiology 1990;174:751–2.

9. Mehta AC, Rafanan AL, Bulkley R, et al. Coronary spasm and cardiac arrest from carcinoid crisis during laser bronchoscopy. Chest 1999;115:598–600.

10. Kvols LK. Therapy of the malignant carcinoid syndrome. Endocrinol Metab Clin North Am 1989;18:557–68.

11. Morris JC, Holland JF. Oncologic Emergencies. In: Bast RC, Kufe DW, Pollock RE, et al., editors. Holland-Frei Cancer Medicine. 5th ed. Hamilton: BC Decker Inc; 2000. p. 2433–2453.

12. Inagaki J, Rodriguez V, Bodey GP. Proceedings: causes of death in cancer patients. Cancer 1974;33:568–73.

13. Keefe DL. Cardiovascular emergencies in the cancer patient. Sem Oncol 2000;27:244–55.

14. Buck M, Ingle JN, Giuliani ER, et al. Pericardial effusion in women with breast cancer. Cancer 1987;60:263–9.

15. Burke AP, Afzal MN, Barnett DS, Virmani R. Sudden death after a cold drink: case report. Am J Forensic Med Pathol 1999;20:37–9.

16. Chan GS, Ng WK, Ng IO, Dickens P. Sudden death from massive pulmonary tumor embolism due to hepatocellular carcinoma. Forensic Sci Int 2000;108:215–21.

17. Bussani R, Silvestri F. Images in cardiovascular medicine. Sudden death in a woman with fibroelastoma of the aortic valve chronically occluding the right coronary ostium. Circulation 1999;100:2204.

18. Idir M, Oysel N, Guibaud JP, et al. Fragmentation of a right atrial myxoma presenting as a pulmonary embolism. J Am Soc Echocardiogr 2000;13:61–3.

19. Ottaviani G, Rossi L, Ramos SG, Matturri L. Pathology of the heart and conduction system in a case of sudden death due to a cardiac fibroma in a 6-month-old child. Cardiovasc Pathol 1999;8:109–12.

20. King D, Sheard JD, Silas JH. Cardiac amyloidosis in the presence of Bence-Jones proteinuria and normal serum immunoglobulins. Br J Clin Pract 1993;47:336–7.

21. Skadberg BT, Bruserud O, Karwinski W, Ohm OJ. Sudden death caused by heart block in a patient with multiple myeloma and cardiac amyloidosis. Acta Med Scand 1988;223:379–83.

22. Kyle RA, Bayrd ED. Amyloidosis: review of 236 cases. Medicine 1975;54:271–99.

23. Wahlin A, Olofsson BO, Eriksson A, Backman C. Myeloma-associated cardiac amyloidosis. A case report. Acta Med Scand 1984;215:189–92.

24. Schoen FJ, Berger BM, Guerina NG. Cardiac effects of noncardiac neoplasms. Cardiol Clin 1984;2:657–70.

25. Rees H, Ang LC. Massive pulmonary tumor emboli in a sarcoma. An unusual cause of sudden death. Am J Forensic Med Pathol 1996;17:146–50.

26. Sanchez-Hermosillo E, Sikirica M, Carter D, Valigorsky JM. Sudden death due to undetected mediastinal germ cell tumor. Am J Forensic Med Pathol 1998;19:69–71.

27. Opeskin K, Ruszkiewicz A, Anderson RM. Sudden death due to undiagnosed medullary-pontine astrocytoma. Am J Forensic Med Pathol 1995;16:168–71.

28. Steinherz L, Steinherz P. Delayed cardiac toxicity from anthracycline therapy. Pediatrician 1991;18:49–52.

29. Bristow MR, Billingham ME, Mason JW, Daniels JR. Clinical spectrum of anthracycline antibiotic cardiotoxicity. Cancer Treat Rep 1978;62:873–9.

30. Dindogru A, Barcos M, Henderson ES, Wallace HJ Jr. Electrocardiographic changes following Adriamycin treatment. Med Pediatr Oncol 1978;5:65–71.

31. Sarubbi B, Orditura M, Ducceschi V, et al. Ventricular repolarization time indexes following anthracycline treatment. Heart Vessels 1997;12:262–6.

32. Nousiainen T, Vanninen E, Rantala A, et al. QT dispersion and late potentials during doxorubicin therapy for non-Hodgkin's lymphoma. J Intern Med 1999;245:359–64.

33. Friess GG, Boyd JF, Geer MR, Garcia JC. Effects of first-dose doxorubicin on cardiac rhythm as evaluated by continuous 24-hour monitoring. Cancer 1985;56:2762–4.

34. Wortman JE, Lucas VS Jr, Schuster E, et al. Sudden death during doxorubicin administration. Cancer 1979;44:1588–91.

35. Couch RD, Loh KK, Sugino J. Sudden cardiac death following Adriamycin therapy. Cancer 1981;48:38–9.

36. Keefe DL. Anthracycline-induced cardiomyopathy. Semin Oncol 2001;28:2–7.

37. Mills BA, Roberts RW. Cyclophosphamide-induced cardiomyopathy: a report of two cases and review of the English literature. Cancer 1979;43:2223–6.

38. Ensley JF, Patel B, Kloner R, et al. The clinical syndrome of 5-fluorouracil cardiotoxicity. Invest New Drugs 1989;7:101–9.

39. Gradishar W, Vokes E, Schilsky R, et al. Vascular events in patients receiving high-dose infusional 5-fluorouracil-

based chemotherapy: the University of Chicago experience. Med Pediatr Oncol 1991;19:8–15.

40. Oleksowicz L, Bruckner HW. Prophylaxis of 5-fluorouracil-induced coronary vasospasm with calcium channel blockers. Am J Med 1988;85:750–1.

41. Vallebona A. Cardiac damage following therapeutic chest irradiation. Importance, evaluation and treatment. Minerva Cardioangiol 2000;48:79–87.

42. Benoff LJ, Schweitzer P. Radiation therapy-induced cardiac injury. Am Heart J 1995;129:1193–6.

43. Stewart JR, Fajardo LF, Gillette SM, Constine LS. Radiation injury to the heart. Int J Radiat Oncol Biol Phys 1995;31:1205–11.

44. Gyenes G. Radiation-induced ischemic heart disease in breast cancer—a review. Acta Oncol 1998;37:241–6.

45. Knight CJ, Sutton GC. Complete heart block and severe tricuspid regurgitation after radiotherapy. Case report and review of the literature. Chest 1995;108:1748–51.

46. Raviprasad GS, Salem BI, Gowda S, Leidenfrost R. Radiation-induced mitral and tricuspid regurgitation with severe ostial coronary artery disease: a case report with successful surgical treatment. Cathet Cardiovasc Diagn 1995;35:146-8.

47. Gell PHG, Coombs RRA. Clinical aspects of immunology. Oxford: Blackwell Scientific Publications; 1975.

48. Smith PL, Kagey-Sobotka A, Bleecker ER, et al. Physiologic manifestations of human anaphylaxis. J Clin Invest 1980;66:1072–80.

49. Silverman HJ, Van Hook C, Haponik EF. Hemodynamic changes in human anaphylaxis. Am J Med 1984;77:341–4.

50. Schwartz GR, Cayton CG, Mayer T, Mangelsen MA. Principles and practice of emergency medicine, 3rd ed. Philadelphia: Lee and Sebiger Publications; 1992. p. 1925.

51. Murrant T, Bihari D. Anaphylaxis and anaphylactoid reactions. Int J Clin Pract 2000;54:322–8.

52. Gavalas M, Sadana A, Metcalf S. Guidelines for the management of anaphylaxis in the emergency department. J Accid Emerg Med 1998;15:96–8.

53. Brown AF. Anaphylactic shock: mechanisms and treatment. J Accid Emerg Med 1995;12:89–100.

54. Schneider SM, Distelhorst CW. Chemotherapy-induced emergencies. Semin Oncol 1989;16:572–8.

55. Haskell CM. L-Asparaginase: human toxicology and single agent activity in nonleukemic neoplasms. Cancer Treat Rep 1981;65:57–9.

56. Dellinger CT, Miale TD. Comparison of anaphylactic reactions to asparaginase derived from *Escherichia coli* and from *Erwinia* cultures. Cancer 1976;38:1843–6.

57. Evans WE, Tsiatis A, Rivera G, et al. Anaphylactoid reactions to *Escherichia coli* and *Erwinia asparaginase* in children with leukemia and lymphoma. Cancer 1982;49:1378–83.

58. Jones B, Holland JF, Glidewell O, et al. Optimal use of L-asparaginase (NSC-109229) in acute lymphocytic leukemia. Med Pediatr Oncol 1977;3:387–400.

59. Holle LM. Pegaspargase: an alternative? Ann Pharmacother 1997;31:616–24.

60. Oettgen HF, Stephenson PA, Schwartz MK, et al. Toxicity of E. coli L-asparaginase in man. Cancer 1970;25:253–78.

61. Nesbit M, Chard R, Evans A, et al. Evaluation of intramuscular versus intravenous administration of L-asparaginase in childhood leukemia. Am J Pediatr Hematol Oncol 1979;1:9–13.

62. Albanell J, Baselga J. Systemic therapy emergencies. Semin Oncol 2000;27:347–61.

63. Peterson RG, Handschumacher RE, Mitchell MS. Immunological responses to L-asparaginase. J Clin Invest 1971;50:1080–90.

64. Capizzi RL, Bertino JR, Skeel RT, et al. L-asparaginase: clinical, biochemical, pharmacological, and immunological studies. Ann Intern Med 1971;74:893–901.

65. Land VJ, Sutow WW, Fernbach DJ, et al. Toxicity of L-asparaginase in children with advanced leukemia. Cancer 1972;30:339–47.

66. Weiss RB. Hypersensitivity reactions. Semin Oncol 1992;19:458–77.

67. Weiss RB, Donehower RC, Wiernik PH, et al. Hypersensitivity reactions from Taxol. J Clin Oncol 1990;8:1263–8.

68. Rowinsky EK, Eisenhauer EA, Chaudhry V, et al. Clinical toxicities encountered with paclitaxel (Taxol). Semin Oncol 1993;20:1–15.

69. Lorenz W, Reimann HJ, Schmal A, et al. Histamine release in dogs by Cremophor E1 and its derivatives: oxethylated oleic acid is the most effective constituent. Agents Actions 1977;7:63–7.

70. Onetto N, Canetta R, Winograd B, et al. Overview of Taxol safety. J Natl Cancer Inst Monogr 1993;131–9.

71. Peereboom DM, Donehower RC, Eisenhauer EA, et al. Successful re-treatment with Taxol after major hypersensitivity reactions. J Clin Oncol 1993;11:885–90.

72. Seidman AD, Hochhauser D, Gollub M, et al. Ninety-six-hour paclitaxel infusion after progression during short taxane exposure: a phase II pharmacokinetic and pharmacodynamic study in metastatic breast cancer. J Clin Oncol 1996;14:1877–84.

73. DeVore RF 3rd, Jagasia M, Johnson DH. Paclitaxel by either 1-hour or 24-hour infusion in combination with carboplatin in advanced non-small cell lung cancer: preliminary results comparing sequential phase II trials. Semin Oncol 1997;24:S12–29.

74. Seidman AD, Hudis CA, Albanel J, et al. Dose-dense therapy with weekly 1-hour paclitaxel infusions in the treatment of metastatic breast cancer. J Clin Oncol 1998;16:3353–61.

75. Greco FA, Thomas M, Hainsworth JD. One-hour paclitaxel infusions: review of safety and efficacy. Cancer J Sci Am 1999;5:179–91.

76. O'Dwyer PJ, King SA, Fortner CL, Leyland-Jones B. Hypersensitivity reactions to teniposide (VM-26): an analysis. J Clin Oncol 1986;4:1262–9.

77. Hayes FA, Abromowitch M, Green AA. Allergic reactions to teniposide in patients with neuroblastoma and lymphoid malignancies. Cancer Treat Rep 1985;69:439–41.

78. Ogle KM, Kennedy BJ. Hypersensitivity reactions to etoposide. A case report and review of the literature. Am J Clin Oncol 1988;11:663–5.

79. de Souza P, Friedlander M, Wilde C, et al. Hypersensitivity reactions to etoposide. A report of three cases and review of the literature. Am J Clin Oncol 1994;17:387–9.

80. Kellie SJ, Crist WM, Pui CH, et al. Hypersensitivity reactions to epipodophyllotoxins in children with acute lymphoblastic leukemia. Cancer 1991;67:1070–5.

81. Cersosimo RJ, Calarese P, Karp DD. Acute hypotensive reaction to etoposide with successful rechallenge: case report and review of the literature. DICP 1989;23:876–7.

82. O'Dwyer PJ, Weiss RB. Hypersensitivity reactions induced by etoposide. Cancer Treat Rep 1984;68:959–61.

83. Habibi B, Lopez M, Serdaru M, et al. Immune hemolytic anemia and renal failure due to teniposide. N Engl J Med 1982;306:1091–3.

84. Weiss RB, Bruno S. Hypersensitivity reactions to cancer chemotherapeutic agents. Ann Intern Med 1981;94: 66–72.

85. Glovsky MM, Braunwald J, Opelz G, Alenty A. Hypersensitivity to procarbazine associated with angioedema, urticaria, and low serum complement activity. J Allergy Clin Immunol 1976;57:134–40.

86. Brooks BJ Jr, Hendler NB, Alvarez S, et al. Delayed life-threatening pneumonitis secondary to procarbazine. Am J Clin Oncol 1990;13:244–6.

87. Getaz EP, Beckley S, Fitzpatrick J, Dozier A. Cisplatin-induced hemolysis. N Engl J Med 1980;302:334–5.

88. Zweizig S, Roman LD, Muderspach LI. Death from anaphylaxis to cisplatin: a case report. Gynecol Oncol 1994;53:121–2.

89. Cheng E, Cvitkovic E, Wittes RE, Golbey RB. Germ cell tumors (II): VAB II in metastatic testicular cancer. Cancer 1978;42:2162–8.

90. Blumenreich MS, Needles B, Yagoda A, et al. Intravesical cisplatin for superficial bladder tumors. Cancer 1982;50:863–5.

91. Denis L. Anaphylactic reactions to repeated intravesical instillation with cisplatin. Lancet 1983;1:1378–9.

92. Markman M, Kennedy A, Webster K, et al. Clinical features of hypersensitivity reactions to carboplatin. J Clin Oncol 1999;17:1141.

93. Planner RS, Weerasiri T, Timmins D, Grant P. Hypersensitivity reactions to carboplatin. J Natl Cancer Inst 1991;83:1763–4.

94. Khan A, Hill JM, Grater W, et al. Atopic hypersensitivity to cis-dichlorodiammineplatinum(II) and other platinum complexes. Cancer Res 1975;35:2766–70.

95. Shlebak AA, Clark PI, Green JA. Hypersensitivity and cross-reactivity to cisplatin and analogues. Cancer Chemother Pharmacol 1995;35:349–51.

96. Allen JC, Walker R, Luks E, et al. Carboplatin and recurrent childhood brain tumors. J Clin Oncol 1987;5:459–63.

97. Bacha DM, Caparros-Sison B, Allen JA, et al. Phase I study of carboplatin (CBDCA) in children with cancer. Cancer Treat Rep 1986;70:865–9.

98. Castleberry RP, Crist WM, Holbrook T, et al. The cytosine arabinoside (Ara-C) syndrome. Med Pediatr Oncol 1981;9:257–64.

99. Baack BR, Burgdorf WH. Chemotherapy-induced acral erythema. J Am Acad Dermatol 1991;24:457–61.

100. Burgdorf WH, Gilmore WA, Ganick RG. Peculiar acral erythema secondary to high-dose chemotherapy for acute myelogenous leukemia. Ann Intern Med 1982;97:61–2.

101. Kanzaki H, Oono T, Makino E, et al. Neutrophilic eccrine hidradenitis: report of two cases. J Dermatol 1995;22: 137–42.

102. Flynn TC, Harrist TJ, Murphy GF, et al. Neutrophilic eccrine hidradenitis: a distinctive rash associated with cytarabine therapy and acute leukemia. J Am Acad Dermatol 1984;11:584–90.

103. Hurt MA, Halvorson RD, Petr FC, et al. Eccrine squamous syringometaplasia. A cutaneous sweat gland reaction in the histologic spectrum of "chemotherapy-associated eccrine hidradenitis" and "neutrophilic eccrine hidradenitis." Arch Dermatol 1990;126:73–7.

104. Jones JB, Purdy CY, Bailey RT. Cyclophosphamide anaphylaxis. DICP 1989;23:88–9.

105. Lakin JD, Cahill RA. Generalized urticaria to cyclophosphamide: type I hypersensitivity to an immunosuppressive agent. J Allergy Clin Immunol 1976;58:160–71.

106. Ross WE, Chabner BA. Allergic reaction to cyclophosphamide in a mechlorethamine-sensitive patient. Cancer Treat Rep 1977;61:495–6.

107. Legha SS, Hall S. Acute cyclophosphamide hypersensitivity reaction: possible lack of cross-sensitivity to mechlorethamine and isophosphamide. Cancer Treat Rep 1978;62:180–1.

108. Collins JA. Hypersensitivity reaction to doxorubicin. Drug Intell Clin Pharm 1984;18:402–3.

109. Solimando DA, Wilson JP. Doxorubicin-induced hypersensitivity reactions. Drug Intell Clin Pharm 1984;18: 808–11.

110. Crawford ED, McKenzie D, Mansson W, et al. Adverse reactions to the intravesical administration of doxorubicin hydrochloride: report of 6 cases. J Urol 1986;136:668–9.

111. Cornwell GG, Pajak TF, McIntyre OR. Hypersensitivity reactions to IV melphalan during treatment of multiple myeloma: Cancer and Leukemia Group B experience. Cancer Treat Rep 1979;63:399–403.

112. Hitchins RN, Hocker GA, Thomson DB. Chlorambucil allergy—a series of three cases. Aust N Z J Med 1987; 17:600–2.

113. Barone C, Cassano A, Astone A. Toxic epidermal necrolysis during chlorambucil therapy in chronic lymphocytic leukaemia. Eur J Cancer 1990;26:1262.

114. Pietrantonio F, Moriconi L, Torino F, et al. Unusual reaction to chlorambucil: a case report. Cancer Lett 1990;54:109–11.

115. Thompson-Moya L, Martin T, Heuft HG, et al. Allergic reaction with immune hemolytic anemia resulting from chlorambucil. Am J Hematol 1989;32:230–1.

116. Crestani B, Jaccard A, Israel-Biet D, et al. Chlorambucil-associated pneumonitis. Chest 1994;105:634–6.

117. Millard LG, Rajah SM. Cutaneous reaction to chlorambucil. Arch Dermatol 1977;113:1298.

118. Peterman A, Braunstein B. Cutaneous reaction to chlorambucil therapy. Arch Dermatol 1986;122:1358–60.

119. de Groot AC, Conemans JM. Systemic allergic contact dermatitis from intravesical instillation of the antitumor antibiotic mitomycin C. Contact Dermatitis 1991;24:201–9.

120. Colver GB, Inglis JA, McVittie E, e al. Dermatitis due to intravesical mitomycin C: a delayed-type hypersensitivity reaction? Br J Dermatol 1990;122:217–24.

121. Sridhar KS. Allergic reaction to 5-fluorouracil infusion. Cancer 1986;58:862–4.

122. Johnston JB, Eisenhauer E, Corbett WE, et al. Efficacy of 2'-deoxycoformycin in hairy-cell leukemia: a study of the National Cancer Institute of Canada Clinical Trials Group. J Natl Cancer Inst 1988;80:765–9.

123. O'Dwyer PJ, King SA, Eisenhauer E, et al. Hypersensitivity reactions to deoxycoformycin. Cancer Chemother Pharmacol 1989;23:173–5.

124. Posada JG, O'Dwyer PJ, Hoth DF. Anaphylactic reactions to diaziquone. Cancer Treat Rep 1984;68:1215–7.

125. Blum RH, Carter SK, Agre K. A clinical review of bleomycin—a new antineoplastic agent. Cancer 1973; 31:903–14.

126. Levy RL, Chiarillo S. Hyperpyrexia, allergic-type response and death occurring with low-dose bleomycin administration. Oncology 1980;37:316–7.

127. Taylor WB, Cantwell BM, Roberts JT, Harris AL. Allergic reactions to mitoxantrone. Lancet 1986;1:1439.

128. Anderson KC, Cohen GI, Garnick MB. Phase II trial of mitoxantrone. Cancer Treat Rep 1982;66:1929–31.

129. Vial T, Descotes J. Immune-mediated side-effects of cytokines in humans. Toxicology 1995;105:31–57.

130. Jones TH, Wadler S, Hupart KH. Endocrine-mediated mechanisms of fatigue during treatment with interferon-alpha. Semin Oncol 1998;25:54–63.

131. Leget GA, Czuczman MS. Use of rituximab, the new FDA-approved antibody. Curr Opin Oncol 1998;10: 548–51.

132. Green MC, Murray JL, Hortobagyi GN. Monoclonal antibody therapy for solid tumors. Cancer Treat Rev 2000;26:269–86.

133. White CA. Rituximab immunotherapy for non-Hodgkin's lymphoma. Cancer Biother Radiopharm 1999;14:241–50.

134. Czuczman MS, Grillo-Lopez AJ, White CA, et al. Treatment of patients with low-grade B-cell lymphoma with the combination of chimeric anti-CD20 monoclonal antibody and CHOP chemotherapy. J Clin Oncol 1999;17:268–76.

135. McLaughlin P, Grillo-Lopez AJ, Link BK, et al. Rituximab chimeric anti-CD20 monoclonal antibody therapy for relapsed indolent lymphoma: half of patients respond to a four-dose treatment program. J Clin Oncol 1998; 16:2825–33.

136. Oldham RK. Monoclonal antibodies in cancer therapy. J Clin Oncol 1983;1:582–90.

137. Levy R, Miller RA. Tumor therapy with monoclonal antibodies. Fed Proc 1983;42:2650–6.

138. McLaughlin P, Hagemeister FB, Grillo-Lopez AJ. Rituximab in indolent lymphoma: the single-agent pivotal trial. Semin Oncol 1999;26:79–87.

139. Stern DF. Tyrosine kinase signalling in breast cancer: ErbB family receptor tyrosine kinases. Breast Cancer Res 2000;2:176–83.

140. Stebbing J, Copson E, O'Reilly S. Herceptin (trastuzamab) in advanced breast cancer. Cancer Treat Rev 2000; 26:287–90.

141. Gemtuzumab for relapsed acute myeloid leukemia. Med Lett Drugs Ther 2000;42:67–8.

142. Bernstein ID. Monoclonal antibodies to the myeloid stem cells: therapeutic implications of CMA-676, a humanized anti-CD33 antibody calicheamicin conjugate. Leukemia 2000;14:474–5.

143. Sievers EL, Appelbaum FR, Spielberger RT, et al. Selective ablation of acute myeloid leukemia using antibody-targeted chemotherapy: a phase I study of an anti-CD33 calicheamicin immunoconjugate. Blood 1999; 93:3678–84.

144. Olsen E, Duvic M, Frankel A, et al. Pivotal phase III trial of two dose levels of denileukin diftitox for the treatment of cutaneous T-cell lymphoma. J Clin Oncol 2001;19:376–88.

145. Railan D, Fivenson DP, Wittenberg G. Capillary leak syndrome in a patient treated with interleukin 2 fusion toxin for cutaneous T-cell lymphoma. J Am Acad Dermatol 2000;43:323–4.

146. Piascik P. FDA approves fusion protein for treatment of lymphoma. J Am Pharm Assoc (Wash) 1999;39:571–2.

147. Clamon GH. Extravasation. In: Perry MC, editor. The chemotherapy source book. 2nd ed. Baltimore: Williams & Wilkins; 1996, p. 607–11.

148. Beason R. Antineoplastic vesicant extravasation. J Intraven Nurs 1990;13:111–4.

149. Rudolph R, Larson DL. Etiology and treatment of chemotherapeutic agent extravasation injuries: a review. J Clin Oncol 1987;5:1116–26.

150. Boyle DM, Engelking C. Vesicant extravasation: myths and realities. Oncol Nurs Forum 1995;22:57–67.

151. Susser WS, Whitaker-Worth DL, Grant-Kels JM. Mucocutaneous reactions to chemotherapy. J Am Acad Dermatol 1999;40:367–98.

152. du Bois A, Kommoss FG, Pfisterer J, et al. Paclitaxel-induced "recall" soft tissue ulcerations occurring at the site of previous subcutaneous administration of paclitaxel in low doses. Gynecol Oncol 1996;60:94–6.

153. Larson DL. Treatment of tissue extravasation by antitumor agents. Cancer 1982;49:1796–9.

154. Wood LS, Gullo SM. IV vesicants: how to avoid extravasation. Am J Nurs 1993;93:42–6.

155. Dorr RT. Antidotes to vesicant chemotherapy extravasations. Blood Rev 1990;4:41–60.

CHAPTER 24

PEDIATRIC CANCER PATIENTS IN THE EMERGENCY ROOM

KENAN ONEL, MD, PhD
PAUL A. MEYERS, MD

Once a child survives his or her 1st year, in the absence of an underlying congenital condition, he or she is generally healthy, and accidents and infections are the leading causes of morbidity and mortality. Nevertheless, malignancy remains the leading cause of death due to disease for children between the ages of 1 and 15 years.

As a group, the pediatric cancers are quite rare, accounting for only about 2% of all cancer diagnoses. The annual incidence of new cases of cancer in children less than 15 years of age in the United States is about 10,000. Of this group of children, roughly 33% are children newly diagnosed with leukemia while another 25% are children with central nervous system tumors.[1] In contrast, the annual incidence of new cases of lung cancer in the United States is about 150,000, and that of colon cancer in the United States is also 150,000.

Because of the rarity of pediatric cancers, it has long been recognized that coordinated large-scale clinical trials are required to achieve the statistical power necessary to define appropriate treatment regimens for these diseases. This led to the formation of the Childrens' Cancer Group (CCG) and the Pediatric Oncology Group (POG), which recently combined to form the Childrens' Oncology Group (COG). As a result, more than 90% of all children diagnosed with cancer are enrolled in prospective multicenter clinical trials. The treatment of children with cancer has evolved to more aggressive therapies with modalities including surgery, radiation therapy, both external-beam radiation and various forms of brachytherapy, and high-dose multiagent chemotherapeutic regimens. As a result of these more intensive therapies and their wide dissemination through the cooperative groups, there have been remarkable advances in the treatment of a number of the pediatric-onset cancers over the past 30 years. Over 75% of all children diagnosed with cancer in the United States can expect to survive at least 5 years.[2] Paralleling this success, however, has been an increase in both the acute and long-term potential toxicities to which children with cancer are exposed and a concomitant increase in visits to the emergency room by children with cancer.

Emergency department management of children with cancer overlaps considerably with that of adults with cancer. The most common presenting complaint in the emergency room of children with cancer is febrile neutropenia. Tumor lysis syndrome can complicate the treatment of tumors with the extremely high proliferative index and tumor burden seen in certain pediatric tumors such as acute lymphoblastic leukemia (ALL) or Burkitt's lymphoma. The management of these emergencies, however, is not specific to the pediatric population and is discussed at length elsewhere in this text.

However, there are several problems and considerations unique to the emergency-room evaluation and management of pediatric patients with cancer. Both developmentally and physiologically, children are different from adults. Likewise, there are significant pharmacologic differences between children and adults. Children cannot be assessed in the same way as adults, and there are significant limitations in the ability of the emergency-room physician to evaluate the pediatric patient. These and other issues distinct to the pediatric population are the focus of this chapter.

EVALUATION OF THE PEDIATRIC CANCER PATIENT

One of the great successes of the war against cancer has been the strides made in the treatment of the pediatric cancers. Because most children diagnosed with cancer are entered into large-scale clinical trials, a considerable amount of data have accrued in regard to multidrug combinations and the maximally tolerated dosages of different chemotherapeutic agents. The bone marrow of a child recovers more quickly following treatment than that of an adult, and a child is more likely to recover from a serious infection. It has been possible, therefore, to treat children with high-dose multiagent and multimodality regimens that might not be tolerated by adults. Although the result has been that many children are cured of their disease, one consequence has been that children are more likely than adults to suffer serious side effects from their therapy. These side effects include prolonged periods of neutropenia and the concomitant risk of infection; hemorrhagic cystitis from high-dose cyclophosphamide or ifosfamide; severe mucositis and pain; decreased renal function because of prior treatment with renal toxic chemotherapeutic agents and aminoglycoside antibiotics; and impaired cardiac function due to anthracycline exposure.

The ability to rapidly and effectively evaluate a patient in an emergency-room setting is both a skill and an art. The physician's assessment is based on both subjective and objective data. However, assessment of the pediatric patient is often complicated by both the physiologic and developmental immaturity of the patient. Infants, in particular, are unable to localize symptoms and may show sepsis or pain only as increased irritability. Often, babies and small children either are unable to speak or have limited vocabularies. They have difficulty both in describing their complaints and in ordering events temporally. Because they may be unable to comprehend and follow commands or directions, the physical examination may be limited. Given the facts that tumors of the central nervous system (CNS) are the second most common group of pediatric tumors and that ALL may involve the CNS, this inability is of particular importance with respect to the assessment of neurologic function. Further, if a patient is taking opiates for pain control, the assessment of both level of consciousness and mental status, as well as the neurologic examination, may be obscured.

Commonly, information and histories are obtained from the parents of a patient, and are therefore secondhand accounts. In addition, information conveyed by a parent is often colored or biased by the mechanisms by which the parent copes with having a sick child. Some parents may downplay the significance or severity of a child's symptoms whereas to other parents, every unexpected incident warrants a trip to the emergency room or oncology clinic.

Many of the severe toxicities seen in the treatment of pediatric cancers, as well as the other emergencies associated with pediatric cancers, demand immediate assessment and intervention, often before the results of tests can be obtained. This, combined with the difficulties inherent in evaluating a child, frequently mandates the initiation of empiric therapy in the emergency room and admission to a major tertiary care hospital or cancer center for observation, continued treatment, and completion of the work-up initiated in the emergency room.

Pediatric History

Despite the above obstacles, a rapid and thorough evaluation of the pediatric oncology patient's condition is possible in the emergency-room setting. While a complete history may not be obtainable, the physician should determine the following:

- Age of the patient
- Underlying diagnosis
- Approximate date of diagnosis and (if appropriate) relapse or transplantation, as well as type of transplant
- Chief complaint and (for ongoing problems) reason the patient was brought to the emergency room at that moment
- Number of previous cycles of chemotherapy and dates of surgery
- Dates of last chemotherapeutic treatment and medications given
- Presence of indwelling catheters and central lines, ventricular shunts, Omaya reservoirs, allografts, or internal prostheses
- Past infections and their causative organisms
- Current medications
- Known drug allergies
- Other ongoing medical problems

If the parent or caregiver is unable to provide this information, then it is incumbent upon the emergency-room physician to contact the patient's oncologist. These facts will serve to direct the physical examination, as well as specific diagnostic and therapeutic interventions.

With particular respect to babies and small infants. the physician should inquire about activity level. Decreased activity, lethargy, missed feedings, or increased sleepiness may be the only indicators of sepsis. Because of their small size and their high ratio of surface area to volume, children are also far more sensitive to hydration status than adults. Hence, it is important to ask whether a child is eating normally, how many cups or bottles the child has had in the past 24 hours, the degree of vigor and interest shown in feeding, and the time and amount of the last urination. Not only decreased input but also increased output can rapidly result in dehydration in a child. Especially immediately after chemotherapy treatments or surgery, there may be increased stooling and diarrhea, as well as bouts of emesis. Poor feeding may also be an indication of other underlying problems. Painful oral mucositis or esophagitis may manifest as irritability and the inability to feed. Respiratory infections and aspiration pneumonias in infants may also present as only poor feeding, either with or without associated emesis.

One medical emergency commonly encountered in oncology patients is febrile neutropenia. Fever in a neutropenic patient is defined as a core temperature $\geq 38°C$ and is best determined by either an oral or a rectal thermometer. Rectal temperatures are contraindicated in neutropenic patients because of the risk for infection, and it is often difficult or impossible to take oral temperatures in infants and small children. Most parents, therefore, will check the temperature of their child with either an axillary or a tympanic-membrane thermometer. Axillary temperatures are about 1°C below core temperature. Digital tympanic-membrane temperatures can be reliable, but an accurate measurement is dependent on a number of variables. The proper size of ear adaptor must be used, and the thermometer must be positioned properly and be in contact with the membrane long enough to actually read the temperature. Hence, when obtaining a history from a parent, especially in a child without fever, it is important to know how the temperature was taken and also whether and when anti-pyretics were given prior to assessment in the emergency room.

Pediatric Physical Examination

The clearest window into the physical status of a child is based on observation. Children (even children with cancer) are by nature active, curious, and interactive. Although a child may not be able to describe his or her complaints, he or she will provide clues as to underlying etiologies by his or her actions and interactions with parents and other trusted adults. A lethargic child or a child who wants only to be held and comforted is cause for concern. If a child who is positioned on a bed holds a leg in a flexed and externally rotated position, then that child is effectively localizing his or her symptoms. While all babies and small children cry, especially in the context of an unfamiliar and chaotic setting such as an emergency room, they can usually be consoled by a parent or trusted caregiver. The only sign of sepsis or uncontrolled pain in an infant may be that he or she cannot be comforted. The astute emergency-room physician can learn a great deal simply by closely watching the behavior of a child.

As with adult patients, vital signs provide an index of a pediatric patient's metabolic activity, hydration status, and ability to maintain homeostasis. Vital signs, however, vary as a function of age; adult norms are not attained until physiologic maturity. Resting heart rates and respiratory rates are higher in children than in adults whereas blood pressures in children are lower. Normal values (by age) are listed in Table 24–1.[3] When evaluating a child, it must be remembered that there can be considerable variability in these values, which partly reflect the level of activity of the child. If a child is crying, for example, his or her vital signs will be elevated. A tachycardic child who is sleeping, on the other hand, may be septic or dehydrated. It is important, therefore, to interpret these values within the context of the child.

Fever in a child with cancer, especially when the child is neutropenic, is assumed empirically to be secondary to infection and is treated as such. Infants, however, are notoriously poor at regulating their core temperature. With little body fat, limited metabolic reserves, and a large exposed surface area, they are also prone to hypothermia, especially when stressed. Therefore, sepsis must be considered in an infant with low body temperature, even if he or she is otherwise warm and well perfused.

Because of the difficulties of obtaining history and localizing details from children, as complete a physical examination as is possible must be performed upon presentation to the emergency room. Small children and infants must be completely undressed (including diapers) and completely inspected. In particular, attention should be paid to the following:

1. Warmth of the patient's extremities; strength of pulses (ie, whether strong, bounding, or thready); paleness of nailbeds; and capillary refill (whether < 2 seconds). These observations provide insight into the overall cardiac and circulatory status of the patient.
2. The mucous membranes, as an index of hydration.
3. The oropharynx, for signs of mucositis; breakdown of barriers to infection, in particular anaerobic or polymicrobial; evidence of stomatitis or oral herpes.
4. The skin, which should be thoroughly examined for evidence of cellulitis or breakdown suggestive of other infection; desquamation, particularly of the palms and soles (suggestive of a drug reaction); and turgor.
5. Sites of recent surgery, for dehiscence (especially following chemotherapy, when healing is impaired); abscesses; gas gangrene.
6. Perianal area, for abscesses or fistulae.
7. All central lines, ports, indwelling catheters, reservoirs, and shunts (for skin breakdown, exudates or discharge at the site, cellulitis, or tunnel infections).

In pediatrics, the examination of the respiratory system is of special importance. In the absence of congenital

TABLE 24–1. Mean Age-Specific Vital Signs

| Age | Weight (kg) | Vital Signs | | | |
		Heart Rate*	Respiratory Rate†	Systolic Blood Pressure	Diastolic Blood Pressure
2 mo–1 yr	3–10	110–140	25–40	70–90	40–60
1–2 yr	10–14	90–130	22–30	80–105	45–60
2–4 yr	12–18	80–120	20–30	85–105	50–65
4–7 yr	16–28	80–120	20–25	90–120	50–70
7–13 yr	26–50	70–110	16–22	100–130	55–75
Adult	> 50	60–100	12–18	100–130	60–80

Adapted from Barone MA.[3]
*Beats per minute
†Breaths per minute

malformations, it is extremely unusual for children to suffer from compromised cardiac function of primary cardiac etiology. Chest pain in a child, for example, is usually either musculoskeletal in origin or costochondral, both of which can be diagnosed by the fact that the pain can be reproduced by deep palpation at the site of the pain or by deep inspiration. In general, children who suffer a cardiopulmonary arrest do so not because of cardiac failure but because of respiratory failure. The respiratory system in children is particularly vulnerable because the cross-sectional area of the bronchial tree varies as a function of the square of the radius. Hence, for each unit increase in the radius, the area increases by a factor of four. Because children are smaller than adults, their medium and small bronchioles are especially susceptible to insults. Likewise, because they are often unable to generate strong coughs, they are less able to clear their airways.

The respiratory examination in a child begins with the observation of the child breathing at rest. This cannot be accomplished if a child is crying, so it is often advantageous to examine the child while he or she is in the arms of a parent. The resting respiratory rate of a child is normally higher than that of an adult (see Table 24–1), and it is not uncommon for infants to breathe in a disorganized manner, with pauses lasting several seconds interspersed with rapid breaths. To determine the respiratory rate, the child must be watched for a full minute. In the presence of an obstructive lesion or decreased lung compliance, the work of breathing is increased. The use of accessory respiratory muscles (such as the sternocleidomastoids and the intercostals) leading to the presence of intercostal, subcostal, or suprasternal retractions will be noted on examination, as will nasal flaring. Expiratory grunting is another sign of dyspnea in children. Because of painful mucositis, children often experience difficulty swallowing their mucus after chemotherapy treatments. As a result, they are at risk for aspiration pneumonia, most frequently in the upper and middle lobes. In particular, the right lung is at risk because the right main stem bronchus is a direct continuation of the trachea. Auscultation in children, because of their size, is often less precise than in adults. However, it is of particular importance to listen to the upper lung fields as well as the lingular area and the right middle lobe, because of the risk of aspiration. Although pathologic breath sounds may be difficult to hear in children (because they may not be able to take deep breaths), it is often possible to bring out abnormal sounds. Infants will occasionally take deep breaths, and gentle compression of the diaphragm at the xiphoid process will generate a forced expiration in children, which can unmask pathology.

Although heart disease is very rare in children, it is important to keep in mind that children exposed to anthracyclines or cyclophosphamide can have decreased cardiac output and may manifest signs of heart failure.

Hence, dependent edema, hepatomegaly, and even pulmonary edema, may be seen in such children. Although angina and myocardial infarctions in such children are unusual, chest pain in children who have received treatment with these agents warrants a thorough cardiac examination as well as a chest radiograph, and electrocardiogram, and an echocardiogram.

Most children being treated for cancer have ports, Broviac catheters, or other central venous access devices, both for the delivery of chemotherapeutic agents and to facilitate the frequent blood drawing required for monitoring the child during treatment. The tip of these catheters sits in the right atrium, near the sinoatrial (SA) node. In the context of palpitations, arrhythmias, or a pulmonary embolism, both catheter tip irritation of the SA node and a clot at the catheter's tip must be considered in the differential diagnosis. More ominously, in the case of an acute cardiovascular decompensation (especially if accompanied by a new heart murmur), bacterial endocarditis must be considered.

MANAGEMENT OF PEDIATRIC PATIENTS IN THE EMERGENCY DEPARTMENT

Pharmacologic Considerations

Because there are so many variables that may limit the ability of the physician to assess and monitor the pediatric patient, laboratory investigation (eg, CBC, electrolytes, urinalysis, etc.) and symptom-guided radiologic tests are often helpful. By and large, treatment algorithms for the various oncologic emergencies routinely encountered in pediatrics are no different than those used to treat adult patients. There are, however, certain important distinctions. The most obvious of these is that the dosage of medications given and the volume of intravenous fluids used are not uniform but are instead usually dosed per kilogram. This reflects a number of factors. Pediatric patients range in size, from infants to fully mature young adults, and drug dosing is scaled to reflect this. Likewise, the percentage of water in infants is considerably greater than in adults. Hence, the volume of distribution of a drug differs in children. Children, and particularly infants, have a much faster gastrointestinal (GI) transit time than do adults. This, combined with a smaller gut surface area, results in the fact that children are less able to absorb enterally administered drugs effectively than are adults.

Elimination of drugs is also not as efficient in the pediatric population as it is in adults. The metabolic inactivation of drugs by the liver, involving both phase I nonsynthetic processes (such as the cytochrome P-450 system) and phase II synthetic reactions, (such as uridine diphosphate [UDP] glucuronidation), attains adult levels of activity by about 6 months of age. In contrast, renal function lags considerably. Clearance of drugs by the kidneys increases throughout the first two decades of life. The glomerular filtration rate, corrected for body surface area, does not achieve the adult norm until the child is about 3 years of age.

Children will differ from adults in their ability to absorb drugs, in the effective volume of distribution of the drugs, and in their ability to clear drugs. Although dosing by weight can minimize the effects of most of these variables, certain drugs (such as the aminoglycosides, vancomycin, and cyclosporine) have narrow therapeutic windows. Because many of these drugs are renally cleared, one of their major toxicities is kidney damage. The aminoglycosides and vancomycin are also associated with significant ototoxicity. This is of concern because the learning of language is dependent on hearing. A child with cancer can expect to survive his diagnosis by many years; hence, it is of great importance to dose these drugs within their peak and trough levels, both to preserve organ function and to maximize the likelihood of normal development. Tables 24–2 list the initial pediatric dosing of common antibiotics (assuming normal renal function) and miscellaneous medications in use at Memorial

Sloan-Kettering Cancer Center. Table 24–3 lists dosing of other drugs commonly used in children as antipyretic agents, antiometics, and for analgesia. Note that ibuprofen and other nonsteriodal anti-inflammatory agents are centraindicated because of their antiplatelet effects. In the emergency room, this initial dosing should be adjusted to reflect antecedent kidney dysfunction, with further dose adjustments to be made on the basis of levels obtained when steady-state concentrations of the drugs have been achieved. Serum creatinine reflects glomerular filtration and therefore renal function. Creatinine is a breakdown product of muscle. Until late puberty, the muscle mass of children remains a smaller fraction of body mass than is seen in adults. Serum creatinine, then, is lower in children than in adults (Table 24–4). If no previous dosing of these drugs is available for a particular patient, then adjustments of the initial dose can be determined from the serum creatinine, using tables that are available in standard reference manuals.

Fluid Support and the Management of Blood Products in the Emergency Room

As has already been discussed, infants and children are extremely sensitive to the effects of dehydration. Any combination of decreased intake and increased output puts a child at risk, and the increased metabolic demands and insensible losses of either fever or anemia exacerbate this condition. Children, even when treated with anthracyclines, generally have good cardiac function. Hence, fluid resuscitation and intravascular volume expansion is a very important part of the emergency-room management of children. Although it may not be possible to assess whether or not a small child is orthostatic, hydra-

TABLE 24–2. Recommended Initial Pediatric Treatment Dosages for Common Antibiotics*

Antibiotic	Dosage
Acyclovir	750 mg/m^2/d IV divided q8h (Herpes simplex)
	1,500 mg/m^2/d IV divided q8h (Herpes zoster)
Amikacin	15–22.5 mg/kg/d IV divided q8h (levels to be checked following 5th dose)
Amphotericin	1 mg/kg/d IV
(Liposomal Formulation)	(5 mg/kg/d IV)
Ampicillin	100–200 mg/kg/d IV divided q4-6h; for meningitis, 200–400 mg/kg/d IV divided q4–6h (max: 12 gr/d)
Azithromycin	10 mg/kg/d PO/IV on day 1 (max: 500 mg)
	5 mg/kg/d PO/IV on days 2–5 (max: 250 mg)
Cefazolin	100 mg/kg/d IV divided q8h
Cefipime	150 mg/kg/d IV divided q8h (max: 2 g/dose)
Ceftriaxone	50–75 mg/kg/d IV divided q12-24h; for meningitis, 100 mg/kg/d IV divided q12h (max: 4 g/d)
Ciprofloxacin	15–20 mg/kg/d IV divided q12h (max: 800 mg/d)
	20–30 mg/kg/d PO divided q12h
	(max: 1,500 mg/d)
Clindamycin	40 mg/kg/d IV divided q6–8h (max: 2,700 mg/d)
	30 mg/kg/d PO divided q6–8h (max: 1,800 mg/d)
Ganciclovir	Induction: 7.5 mg/kg/d IV divided q8–12h (must ensure adequate hydration)
Gentamycin	5–7.5 mg/kg/d IV divided q6h (levels to be checked following 5th dose)
Metronidazole	30 mg/kg/d IV divided q6h. C. diff: 15–35 mg/kg/d PO divided q8h
Timentin	300 mg/kg/d IV divided q4h (max: 3.1 g/dose)
Tobramycin	5–7.5 mg/kg/d IV divided q6h (levels to be checked following 5th dose)
Vancomycin	40 mg/kg/d IV divided q6–12h (levels to be checked following 5th dose)

C. diff = *clostridiumdifficile*; IV = intravenously; max = maximum; PO = by mouth.
*Recommendations from Memorial Sloan-Kettering Cancer Center.

TABLE 24–3. Recommended Pediatric Dosages of Miscellaneous Medications*

Antipyretic
   Acetaminophen: 15 mg/kg/dose PO q4h

Pain (in opioid-naive patient)
   Codeine: 0.5 mg/kg/dose PO q4h
   Fentanyl: 1–2 µg/kg/dose IV q30–60 min
   Hydromorphone: 0.015 mg/kg/dose IV q4h
   Morphine: 0.1–0.2 mg/kg/dose IV q4h
   Oxycodone: 0.05–0.15 mg/kg/dose PO q4h

PCA: Divide hourly dose as 50% continuous infusion and 50% bolus infusion. Titrate to effect.

Antiemetic
   Hydroxyzine: 1 mg/kg/dose IV/PO q4h
   Granisetron: 20 µg/kg/dose IV qday or PO q12h to max. of 1 mg/dose (for chemoassociated anticipatory nausea)
   Lorazepam: 0.04–0.08 mg/kg/dose IV q6h
   Metoclopramide: 1–2 mg/kg/dose IV q2h
   Ondansetron: 0.15 mg/kg/dose IV

IV = intravenously; PCA = patient-controlled analgesia; PO = by mouth.
*Recommendations from Memorial Sloan-Kettering Cancer Center.

tion status can be ascertained from both the history and the physical examination of a patient. From the history, it should be determined whether a child is eating or drinking, when the last feed was, the quantity that was taken in, and whether this deviates from the child's norm. Likewise, urine output over 24 hours, the number of wet diapers, and the time of the last urination should all be assessed, as should the presence or absence of emesis or increased stooling. On physical examination, cool extremities, dry mucous membranes, the absence of tears when crying, and decreased skin turgor all suggest dehydration, as does persistent resting tachycardia and bounding pulses.

Initial volume expansion should involve the rapid intravenous infusion of an isotonic crystalloid bolus, followed by a reassessment of the patient and his or her vital signs. Continuous intravenous fluids at 1.5 to 2 times the maintenance rate should also be initiated. *Pediatric Advanced Life Support* teaches that the standard bolus infusion is 20 mL/kg of normal saline, given over 20 minutes (Table 24–5).[4] Patients who cannot tolerate the fluid infusion because of cardiac or renal dysfunction will manifest signs of fluid overload. They may develop

TABLE 24–4. Normal Serum Creatinine Levels, by Age Group

Age Group	Serum Creatinine Range (mg/dL)
Infants	0.2–0.4
Children	0.3–0.7
Adolescents	0.5–1.0
Adult males	0.5–1.3
Adult females	0.5–1.2

Adapted from Barone MA.[3]

TABLE 24–5. Recommended Dosages for Fluid and Blood Product Support in Pediatric Patients*

Rapid calculation of maintenance fluids[†]
  0–10 kg: 4 mL/kg/h
  10–20 kg: 2 mL/kg/h
  > 20 kg: 1 mL/kg/h

Initial composition of intravenous fluids[‡]
  < 10 kg: D51/4NS + 10 mEq/L KCl
  > 10 kg: D51/2NS + 20 mEq/L KCl

Volume expansion and blood product support
  NS bolus: 20 mL/kg, to be infused over 20 min
  Packed red blood cells: 15 mL/kg (expect increase in Hgb of 3–5 g/dL)
  Platelets: 1 unit/10 kg, rounding up (expect increase of 50,000/mm^3)
  Fresh frozen plasma: 10 mL/kg

Diuretic
  Furosemide, 0.5–1.0 mg/kg IV q6h

D = dextrose; Eq = equivalents; Hgb = hemoglobin; IV = intravenously; KCl = potassium chloride; NS = normal saline.
*Recommendations from Memorial Sloan-Kettering Cancer Center.
[†]For each kilogram of body weight.
[‡]Assuming normal electrolytes and renal function.

evidence of pulmonary edema, such as increased respiratory rate, decreasing blood oxygen saturation, or new crackles on physical examination; dependent edema in their extremities and encircling the orbits; or increasing hepatosplenomegaly. Fliud overload can effectively be treated by decreasing the rate of infusion and by diuresis with furosemide (0.5 to 1 mg/kg, to be repeated every 6 hours as needed). Furosemide must be used with extreme caution in this setting. Furosemide promotes diuresis by removing fluid from the intravascular compartment. If a child is truly volume depleted, the use of furosemide can further deplete the intravascular volume, leading to a further decrease in perfusion.

While fluid replacement will increase intravascular volume, it will also dilute the hematocrit. Following chemotherapy treatments, the hemoglobin falls. Adequate oxygenation of tissues, particularly in the brain and the heart, requires a hemoglobin level of at least 8 g/dL. Hence, an alternative form of volume replacement, which serves to increase not only perfusion but also oxygenation, is the transfusion of packed red blood cells (15 mL/kg, infused over 2 to 4 hours). At Memorial Sloan-Kettering Cancer Center, this is routinely done for hemoglobin < 8 g/dL. In the emergency room, even for an initial hemoglobin of > 8 g/dL, following bolus infusions totaling 40 to 60 mL/kg of crystalloid, pediatric patients will also receive packed red blood cell transfusions of 15 mL/kg. This is expected to increase the hemoglobin by about 3 g/dL (see Table 24–5).

Oncology patients require platelet support to facilitate clotting and to protect against intracerebral hemorrhage. The concern with platelet transfusions is that patients eventually develop antiplatelet antibodies and become refractory to the transfusions. It has been shown that spontaneous hemorrhage is rare with a platelet count of > 5,000/mm^3. In the absence of active bleeding, pediatric patients are transfused 1 unit of platelets per 10 kg of body weight, rounding up to the next highest unit for a platelet count of < 10,000/mm^2 (see Table 24-5). The exception to this rule is that children with CNS tumors (the vasculature of which can be quite friable) or who have CNS shunts or reservoirs are maintained between 30,000 to 50,000/mm^2. In contrast to packed red blood cells, platelets can be given rapidly. It is expected that this dosage will result in an increase in the platelet count of about 50,000/mm^3 in naive patients. Platelet transfusions contain considerable serum as well as platelets. Hence, these transfusions provide not only volume but also albumin. They generate oncotic pressure, which draws fluid intravascularly, and can further aid in volume expansion.

Management of the Febrile Pediatric Oncology Patient

A theme repeated throughout this chapter has been that when faced with an ill-appearing or febrile child with cancer, the prudent course of action is to treat empirically because it cannot be determined *a priori* whether that child is infected; when a child looks sick, he or she must be admitted for observation, daily surveillance cultures, and intravenous antibiotic therapy. Almost as significant is the idea that all infections should be treated initially through the central line. Because the central line is a direct connection between the outside world and the blood supply of a patient, the most conservative hypothesis is that every fever in a pediatric patient with a central access device results from a bacteremia introduced through the device. Virtually every child diagnosed with cancer in the United States has a central venous access device. Because the available sites for these devices are limited in children by their size, every effort is made to treat the patient through the device, thereby sterilizing it and preserving it.

A child being brought to the emergency room with fever and suspected neutropenia should be regarded as a true medical emergency (Figure 24–1). Arrangements should be made to admit the child, and work-up and empiric therapy must be initiated without delay. The child, even if happy and playful appearing, is potentially quite unstable and should be monitored closely, especially prior to the completion of his or her first dose of broad-spectrum intravenous antibiotics. Upon arrival at the emergency room, the child should be immediately assessed, and a thorough history and physical examination should be performed, as described above. Both aerobic and anaerobic blood cultures should be drawn from each lumen of the central line. In addition to blood cultures, laboratory studies should include a complete blood count (CBC) with differential, as well as studies of serum electrolytes, blood urea nitrogen (BUN), creatinine, glucose, calcium, magnesium, phosphorous, prothrombin time (PT) and partial thromboplastin time (PTT), transaminases, bilirubin, and lactate dehydrogenase (LDH). A chest radiography should be performed. In patients under 2 years of age, a urine culture should be obtained because the urine is a common source for infection in this age group. Any other cultures taken should be directed by the history and the physical examination. Any area of skin breakdown, for example, should be cultured. Likewise, if the patient has diarrhea or loose stools, a stool specimen should be obtained for microbiologic evaluation and should also be tested for *Rotavirus* and adenovirus if these tests are available. Ideally, all cultures (particularly the blood cultures) should be obtained before initiating antibiotic therapy. Broad-spectrum intravenous antibiotic therapy through all lumens of the central access device, however, should not be delayed until the completion of this initial work-up.

In addition to undergoing this initial evaluation and laboratory work-up, all children presenting to the emergency room with febrile neutropenia should have at least

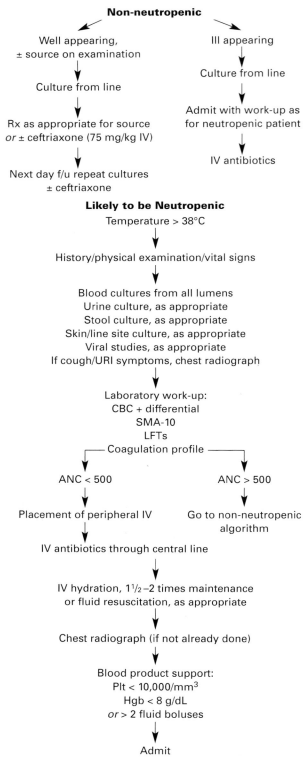

Figure 24–1. An algorithm for the assessment and maintenance of a febrile pediatric oncologic patient with a central line. (ANC = absolute neutrophil count; CBC = complete blood count; f/u = follow-up; Hgb = hemoglobin; IV = intravenous; LFT = liver function tests; Plt = platelets; Rx = drugs; SMA = Sequential Multiple Analyzer; URI = upper respiratory infection.)

one large-bore peripheral intravenous (IV) device immediately placed for emergency access. Because the central line is the most likely source of infection, use of the line or flushing of the line may result in the bolus injection of microorganisms into the patient's blood stream. Hence, a patient may appear to be warm and well perfused, but upon handling of the line, he or she may very quickly appear ill, become peripherally vasoconstricted, and even go into shock. Further, the introduction of antibiotics through the central line can result in the synchronized lysis of bacteria in the line, thereby releasing endotoxin or lipopolysaccharide (LPS) into the blood stream, again potentially resulting in hypotension or shock. In these settings, the central line should be temporarily capped, and both fluid resuscitation and antibiotic therapy should be given through the peripheral IV device. In an emergent setting in children under 6 years of age, interosseus access, either through the proximal tibia or through the anterior iliac crest, may also be considered.

To minimize the possibility of shock in a child with febrile neutropenia, blood pressure and tissue perfusion and oxygenation are aggressively supported with intravenous fluids and blood products. Rates of initial intravenous fluid should be 1.5 to 2 times the rates of maintenance fluids, both to maintain intravascular volume and to replace the increased insensible losses secondary to fever. Electrolyte abnormalities should also be corrected with the intravenous fluid. It is critical to recognize impending shock and to intervene before the patient develops hypotension. Signs of inadequate perfusion and impending shock include tachycardia, cool extremities, capillary refill prolonged beyond seconds, dry mucous membranes, and decreased urine output. The treatment for impending shock should include rapid volume expansion. Guidelines from *Pediatric Advanced Life Support* (PALS) call for boluses of isotonic crystalloid. These boluses should be 20 mL/kg, administered over no more than 20 minutes.[4] If the first bolus does not improve the status of the patient, the bolus should be repeated up to a total of three boluses, or 60 mL/kg. To maintain tissue oxygenation, patients with a hemoglobin (Hgb) level of < 8 g/dL should receive packed red blood cell transfusions, as should patients requiring fluid bolus infusions of > 40 mL/kg, so as to prevent hemodilution. If the patient is unable to maintain adequate perfusion despite this vigorous fluid and blood product support, then a dopamine infusion at an inotropic dose (10 µg/kg/min) should be considered, along with arrangements to monitor the patient in an intensive care unit (ICU) setting.

The initial choice for antibiotic therapy should include coverage for Gram-negative bacilli, Gram-positive cocci, and *Pseudomonas* species. The choice of specific antibiotics should reflect both the microorganisms and resistance patterns indigenous to a specific hospital, as well as the past infection history of a patient. In general, the combination of an aminoglycoside and an extended-spectrum penicillin with a β-lactamase inhibitor or a fourth-generation cephalosporin is recommended. There is considerable debate in the literature on the need for empiric double coverage against Gram-negative bacilli. At Memorial Sloan-Kettering Cancer Center, double coverage is routinely used; the current first-line combination is cefepime (50 mg/kg/dose every 8 hours) and amikacin (22.5 mg/kg per 24 hours, divided every 8 hours), both for synergy and to prevent the emergence of resistant organisms. It is also critical to modify the choice of empiric antibiotic therapy based on actual or potential toxicity related to chemotherapy. For example, when cisplatin is part of the chemotherapy regimen, patients are at risk for nephro- and ototoxicity. To reduce the risk of renal and hearing impairment, initial empiric therapy for these patients should avoid the use of aminoglycoside antibiotics.

Although this empiric antibiotic regimen adequately covers many of the bacterial organisms most likely to cause fever in a patient with central venous access, this initial regimen may be expanded as a result of data obtained by the history or the physical examination. From shortly after birth, coagulase-negative staphylococci colonize the skin and mucous membranes of virtually every individual. At best, community-acquired strains of coagulase-negative staphylococci are heterogeneous in their sensitivity to the semisynthetic penicillins and the cephalosporins. Many nosocomially acquired strains are completely methicillin resistant. Over time, children with cancer become colonized with resistant coagulase-negative staphylococci species that can invade the blood stream at sites of breaks in the skin (such as Broviac catheter sites) or at unhealed decubitus sores and mouth sores. If there is an indication that the portal of entry for a bloodborne infection is the skin or mucous membranes (eg, chills when a central line is accessed), then the patient should be started empirically on vancomycin.

While on chemotherapy, children are functionally immunocompromised. During periods of neutropenia, they also lack the inflammatory cells necessary to manifest both the physical and radiographic findings of pneumonia. They are exposed to a variety of nosocomial pathogens. If they manifest any respiratory symptoms at all, an antibiotic such as the macrolide azithromycin should be added to their antibiotic coverage, to treat atypical infections. When patients are neutropenic, they are unable to wall off anaerobic infections and form abscesses. Hence, they rarely manifest signs of anaerobic infections other than fever until their neutrophil count begins to recover. However, if a patient complains of pain when moving his or her bowels, then an antibiotic such as metronidazole should be empirically added to improve anaerobic coverage.

A number of chemotherapeutic regimens directed against solid tumors in pediatrics use the deoxyribonucleic acid (DNA) cross-linking agent cisplatin as one element of multidrug-containing treatments. These courses of therapy are marrow suppressive and result in prolonged periods of neutropenia. A major long-term toxicity of cisplatin is renal insufficiency due to both direct glomerular and tubular toxicity. Aminoglycosides are also nephrotoxic, and repeated exposure to both agents can increase the risk of toxicity. At Memorial Sloan-Kettering Cancer Center, the broad-spectrum fluoroquinolone ciprofloxacin is often substituted for an aminoglycoside as empiric antibiotic therapy for patients treated with cisplatin-containing regimens. The fluoroquinolones as a class have been associated with cartilage damage in numerous juvenile animal models at dosages equivalent to those needed to be therapeutic. However, there is extensive experience with the use of ciprofloxacin in the pediatric population. It is well tolerated, and has not been associated with arthropathy in humans. Therefore, the Committee on Infectious Diseases of the American Academy of Pediatrics (AAP) recommends that following a careful appraisal of the risks and benefits, the use of ciproflaxacin in the pediatric population be at the discretion of the responsible physician.[5]

When fever develops in the non-neutropenic pediatric cancer patient, a thorough history and physical examination must be performed, and surveillance cultures must be obtained from all lumens. The child need not be admitted unless he or she appears to be ill. In particular, the assessing physician should carefully look for evidence of illnesses typical of childhood, such as otitis media and pharyngitis, and which may not be specifically related to the child's cancer. If a source for the fever is identified, it should be treated, if possible, with oral antibiotics, and appropriate follow-up should be arranged. If the child appears to be well and is without an obvious source for the fever, then the patient should be discharged, with follow-up by telephone the next day. Empiric antibiotic coverage with ceftriaxone (75 mg/kg IV) is an option in the febrile non-neutropenic patient without an identifiable source of infection. If still febrile or unwell on follow-up, the patient should return to the emergency room or oncology clinic for re-evaluation and repeat blood cultures (see Figure 24–1).

DIAGNOSIS OF CANCER IN THE PEDIATRIC POPULATION

Overview

Given that there are only about 10,000 new cases diagnosed each year in the United States, the incidence of cancer in children is exceedingly low. Further, many of the signs and symptoms suggestive of cancer in children are either nonspecific or extremely subtle. Often, they are misdiagnosed, resulting in a delay in the diagnosis of cancer and the initiation of therapy. As much as 7% of all pediatric cancer is diagnosed in the emergency room,[6] and unless cancer is specifically part of the differential diagnosis formulated by the assessing physician, it is often overlooked. Only rarely (as in case of the metabolic derangements associated with tumor lysis syndrome) is it necessary to initiate therapy at the moment the diagnosis of cancer is suspected. More commonly, the role of the assessing physician in the emergency department is to recognize that a particular symptom may represent cancer and to then ensure that the child is referred for the appropriate work-up and biopsy-proven diagnosis.

In the pediatric population, the most common cancers are acute lymphoblastic leukemia, central nervous system tumors, and sarcomas (Table 24–6). There are, however, age-specific variations in the incidence of the pediatric cancers, which can help the emergency-room physician determine (a) the likelihood that a particular constellation of symptoms in a patient represents a malignant process and (b) which process is most likely. This will allow the physician to ensure that the most appropriate and informative studies are undertaken.

Many of the common presenting signs of adult-onset malignancies (such as changes in bowel habits, persistent cough or hoarseness, and non-healing skin ulcerations) are rare in the pediatric population. Likewise, paraneoplastic syndromes are infrequently associated with cancers in children. The exception is neuroblastoma, in which there may be seen wide blood pressure fluctuations, as well as stereotypical eye movements, opsoclonus, and myoclonus.

This section discusses some of the most common presenting signs and symptoms that might be seen in the emergency room and that should serve to alert the physician of the possibility of cancer in a child. The goal is not to catalogue a comprehensive list of complaints associated with cancer in children seen in the emergency room. Rather, it is to highlight several examples of symptoms suggestive of malignancy but that are commonly mistaken for benign processes. It is hoped that this will ensure that the assessing physician will consider malignancy when evaluating children with these particular complaints and can gather appropriate information from the history and physical examination to determine with confidence the likelihood of malignancy. If there is any question as to whether a child may have a malignancy, a pediatric oncology specialist must be consulted immediately.

Specific Symptoms Suggestive of Malignancy

Headache is a complaint frequently encountered in the emergency room. It is often nonspecific. In the setting of school anxiety or the stresses associated with adolescence

TABLE 24–6. Annual Incidence of Common Pediatric Cancers in the United States

Leukemia (30% of all pediatric malignancies)
  Acute leukemias
- > 95% of all leukemias
- Peak incidence: 2–5 years of age
- 1:25,000 incidence under 14 years
- ALL = 75–80% of acute leukemias
- AML = 20% of acute leukemias
  Chronic leukemia (3% of all leukemias)

Brain tumors (20–25% of all pediatric malignancies)
  Most common pediatric solid tumor
  60% infratentorial
  65:1,000,000 incidence under 14 years
  Medulloblastoma
- 20–30% of all brain tumors
- Peak incidence: under age 15 years
  Astrocytomas
- 10–20% of all brain tumors
- Peak incidence: under age 10 years

Lymphoma (11% of all pediatric malignancies)
  Non-Hodgkin's
- 60% of all lymphomas
- Peak incidence: 5–15 years
- Male:female = 2.5:1
  Hodgkin's
- Bimodal peaks of incidence; pediatric age peak 15–35 years
- Incidence of 1–10:100,000
- Male:female hr =hr 3:1

Neuroblastoma (7% of all pediatric malignancies)
  Most common tumor of infancy
  Incidence of 10:1,000,000
  Peak incidence of 2 years of age
  75% diagnosed under 4 years of age
  75% with metastatic disease at diagnosis

Wilms' tumor (6% of all pediatric malignancies)
  9:1,000,000 incidence
  Peak incidence: 3–4 years of age

Rhabdomyosarcoma (3–5% of all pediatric malignancies)
  Two-thirds diagnosed in under 6 years of age
  Second smaller peak at 15–19 years of age
  Incidence of 7–8: 1,000,000 in white children
  Incidence of 4:1,000,000 in black children

Primary bone tumors (5% of all pediatric malignancies)
  Osteosarcoma
- 2.6% of all pediatric malignancies
- Incidence of 3:1,000,000
- Peak incidence during growth spurt years
- Previous history of irradiation at site strongly correlated with OS
- History of retinoblastoma is strongly correlated with OS
  Ewing's sarcoma
- 2% of all pediatric malignancies
- Peak incidence in second decade of life
- 80% of cases diagnosed before age of 20
- Incidence of 2.1:1,000,000 in whites
- Incidence of 0.2:1,000,000 in blacks

Data from Gurney JG, et al.[1]
ALL = acute lymphoblastic leukemia; AML = acute myelogenous leukemia; OS = osteosarcoma.

in particular, it is often thought to be functional in nature. There are several clues, however, that might suggest an organic etiology. A persistent headache, one that does not resolve as perceived stresses are resolved, is of concern. If it awakens the child from sleep, then it is unlikely to be functional. Likewise, the temporal nature of the headache is important. Most brain tumors in childhood are infratentorial and block the outflow of cerebrospinal fluid. As such, they result in increased intracranial pressure (ICP), which manifests as a headache, most commonly when the child is lying flat. Hence, early morning headaches, especially when associated with morning vomiting, are suggestive of increased ICP and warrant further investigation. In an infant, headache may be noted only as increased irritability. If a brain tumor is suspected, the history should focus on eliciting other evidence for an ongoing CNS process, such as personality changes, a drop-off in school performance, worsening handwriting, seizures (including those thought to be febrile seizures), or increased lethargy and drowsiness. The neurologic examination is especially important if a brain tumor is suspected; 95% of children with brain tumors have focal findings on examination.[7] When examining infants, the physician must measure head circumference and determine the percentile for age. Head circumference reflects underlying brain size in infants. Hence, an unusually large head or a change in the rate of increase in head size is a potentially ominous sign. Computed tomography (CT) and magnetic resonance imaging (MRI) evaluations are the appropriate studies if a brain tumor is suspected. To ensure adequate resolution in small children, it is often necessary to perform these studies with the child under sedation.

Children, especially those just starting school or day care, frequently fall prey to a variety of infectious agents, most commonly viruses. Infections are often passed around a classroom, particularly during the winter months, when the children are mostly kept indoors and in enclosed spaces. In fact, it is not uncommon for a young child to have as many as six cases of otitis media in 1 year. Hence, a very common complaint encountered in the emergency room is fever. The sudden onset of high spiking fevers in the context of upper respiratory infection (URI) symptoms most likely does represent a viral syndrome or other acute infection. Although fever from a viral infection can last up to several weeks, the persistence of fever can be an ominous sign, suggestive of the cytokine disregulation associated with leukemia. The context in which the fever appears (ie, the constellation of signs, symptoms, and physical findings associated with the fever) becomes important in assessing the likelihood of cancer. Weakness, fatigue, and lethargy, as well as generalized achiness and myalgias, are often associated with febrile infections. Lethargy and fatigue may also be signs of anemia and should be well characterized. It should be determined whether these symptoms are new in onset, whether it is noted only at certain times of the day (such as before school) or are persistent. It should be asked whether there are times of the day in which the child is happy and playful, and whether the fatigue prevents the child from playing or participating in his or her daily activities.

It is also important that the physician investigate the true nature of any aches and pains described by the child. Children have difficulty localizing pain, but whereas muscle aches may be associated with viral syndromes or simply aggressive play, a pain may represent bone pain if the child describes the pain as tracking along the long bones (such as the tibia or femur) or the ribs. This may be the result of bone marrow replacement and marrow compartment expansion by leukemic cells. Children may also report leg pain at night (that is commonly referred to as "growing pains"); this pain is distinguished from the bone pain associated with leukemia by the fact that it only occurs at night, and it is usually described as occurring either at the knees or on the soles of the feet. Despite the fact that what usually brings children with growing pains to medical attention is that the pain is so severe that it wakes them from sleep, such pain never occurs during the day, and there are no associated physical findings.

Leukemia is a malignant process in which the normal precursor cells of the bone marrow are replaced by a malignant clone. Consequently, the child will often present with evidence of low counts in more than one lineage. Not only may there be signs of anemia, but there may also be evidence of thrombocytopenia. Children frequently have bruises. The distribution of the bruises is stereotypical; they occur where children fall. Hence, they are most commonly noted on bony prominences and along the long bones of the legs. On physical examination, deviation from this distribution is unusual and warrants investigation. In particular, bruising on the trunk is unusual. Likewise, the presence of petechiae is indicative of thrombocytopenia. The presence of hepatosplenomegaly should be noted on examination, as well as diffuse lymphadenopathy (defined as an enlargement of two or more noncontiguous lymph nodes).

If there is evidence, either by history or on physical examination, that two lines are decreased or that there are physical findings consistent with leukemia, then a CBC with differential and reticulocyte count should be performed. If two cell lines are actually low, the child should be evaluated by a pediatric oncologist immediately. Likewise, a complete chemistry panel should be performed, including (a) studies for phosphorus and uric acid, to determine whether the child is manifesting signs of electrolyte abnormalities and tumor lysis; (b) an LDH study, to evaluate tumor burden; and (c) liver function tests. In addition, PT/PTT and fibrinogen should be evaluated to determine whether the child is in disseminated intravascular coagulopathy (DIC), and a blood culture should be done because children newly diagnosed with leukemia (even if they are not neutropenic) are functionally immunocompromised and often present with concomitant infections.

Fractures are another pediatric problem often encountered in the emergency room. Given the active lifestyle of most children as well as their general inability or unwillingness to consider the consequences of risky behaviors, the tendency is to attribute virtually all fractures to trauma, a direct blow, or an indirect stress to the fractured bone. A fracture may also be indicative of structural weakness in a bone. Such structural weakness may be the result of a primary bone tumor, a soft-tissue sarcoma invading the bone, or bony metastases from lymphoma. The key to the diagnosis of these pathologic fractures is that the injury is disproportionate to the stress or that the injury occurs in a location that is unusual for the given mechanism. So, for example, a teenager who fractures her distal femur while stepping off a curb should undergo radiologic evaluation to rule out a tumor.

Radiographic evaluation of the fracture should initially include both anteroposterior (AP) and lateral plain-film views, on which evidence of a mass may be seen. Regions of active disregulated bone remodeling (especially in the metaphysis) with both lytic lesions and areas of new bone formation and calcification are suggestive of osteosarcoma. Ewing's sarcoma is classically a destructive lesion in the diaphysis of a long bone with radiation to the metaphysis. A periosteal reaction may also be noted. Frequently associated with both of these tumors are prominent soft-tissue extensions. Plain films should also be examined for evidence of cortical thinning or marrow-space widening, which may be indicative of a marrow infiltrative process. For patients in whom a malignancy is suspected, an MRI of the site is mandatory, as MRI allows optimal visualization of bony lesions. As well as undergoing imaging studies of the primary site, these patients should also undergo plain-film radiography and CT of the chest, to detect lung metastases. Ultimately, the diagnosis of malignancy is made not by radiographic means but by biopsy, which should be scheduled without delay. A biopsy is of particular significance also because a major component of the differential diagnosis is osteomyelitis, the antibiotic treatment of which will be delayed by a delayed biopsy diagnosis.

Finally, otitis media is one of the most common pediatric diagnoses. Children will often present to an emergency room with only the complaint of fever, irritability, or decreased peroral intake. According to the AAP Committee on Infectious Diseases, first-line therapy for otitis in a child who is not allergic to penicillin is a 10-day course of amoxicillin.[5] Not infrequently, a child will require a second or even a third course of antibiotics to clear the infection. In addition, the infection may become supperative. Despite the fact that these potential complications of otitis media are not rare, a persistently suppurative otitis or an otitis refractory to appropriate antibiotic therapy is cause for concern. The orbit is a common site of occurrence for embryonal rhabdomyosarcomas and osteosarcomas, and persistent infections may reflect an underlying destructive process. Hence, CT of the head and orbits is an appropriate intervention.

SUMMARY

In conclusion, pediatric patients with cancer present a unique set of challenges to the emergency-department physician. While the management of these patients overlaps considerably with the management of adult patients, there are certain issues specific to the child with cancer. Paramount among these is the concept that because it is frequently difficult to assess a pediatric patient rapidly and accurately, admission to the hospital for observation and the immediate initiation of empiric therapy is the most conservative and appropriate management strategy.

Although it can be difficult to evaluate a child's condition, observation of the child and close monitoring of vital signs open subtle windows into the physiologic and homeostatic status of the child. The assessing physician, however, must be cognizant of both the physiologic and developmental immaturity of the child, as well as the age-specific norms for vital signs. The preceding text has presented a framework for the evaluation of a child's condition in the emergency room.

Finally, pediatric cancers are rare diseases. In certain contexts, common pediatric complaints may be suggestive of underlying malignancies. However, for these malignancies to be diagnosed and for therapy to be initiated, it must be recognized that malignancy is among the possible etiologies for the complaint. Thus, common pediatric complaints that are encountered in the emergency room and that might be indicative of malignancies were also discussed in this chapter.

REFERENCES

1. Gurney JG, Severson RK, Davis S, Robison LL. Incidence of cancer in children in the United States. Sex-, race-, and 1-year age-specific rates by histologic type. Cancer 1995;75:2186.
2. Ries LA, Hankey BF, Miller BA, et al, editors. Cancer statistics review 1973–1988. NIH Publication no. 91-2789. Bethesda: National Cancer Institute; 1991.
3. Barone MA, editor. The Harriet Lane handbook. 14th ed. St. Louis: Mosby; 1996.
4. Chameides L, Hazinski MF, editors. Pediatric advanced life support. Dallas: American Heart Association; 1997. p. 6-1–6-19.
5. The Committee on Infectious Diseases, American Academy of Pediatrics. Red book 2000. 25th ed. Elk Grove Village (IL): American Academy of Pediatrics; 2000. p. 645–62.
6. Barkin RM, Rosen P, editors. Emergency pediatrics. 4th ed. St. Louis: Mosby; 1994.
7. Honig PJ, Charney EB. Children with brain tumor headaches. Am J Dis Child 1982;136:121.

CHAPTER 25

ONCOLOGIC EMERGENCIES IN THE ELDERLY PATIENT

LODOVICO BALDUCCI, MD

As cancer in the older-aged person is the most common form of cancer, the management of oncologic emergencies in older individuals is becoming increasingly common.[1–3] Already, 60% of all neoplasms occur in persons aged 65 years and older,[1,2] and this percentage is expected to increase with the simultaneous expansion of the older population and shrinkage of the younger population in the Western world.[1,2]

To explore the effects of aging on oncologic emergencies, we must first analyze the clinical meaning of aging and then consider two nonmutually exclusive possibilities: (1) age may effect a change in the clinical presentation and course of common oncologic emergencies, and (2) age may be associated with oncologic emergencies exclusive of older individuals.

OVERVIEW OF AGING

In general terms, aging involves physiologic, functional, medical, and social changes, leading to a progressively reduced ability to withstand stress.[3] From this universally accepted observation, one may expect that oncologic emergencies become more common and severe for elderly persons.

Aging is highly individualized and is poorly reflected in chronologic age; the reduction in stress tolerance occurs at different rates in different persons and varies for different forms of stress within the same person. Diversity is the hallmark of the older population, and the ability to account for this diversity is essential to individualized treatment.

Age-related changes in different domains are interwoven and may result synergistically in the genesis of an emergency. For example, a neutropenic infection may be more often life threatening in an older person both because the neutropenia is more severe and prolonged and because the patient has no independent transportation to seek timely emergency care. Likewise, blunted perception of pain and inadequate access to care may result in more frequent paraplegia from spinal-cord compression.

Physiology

Aging is associated with a progressive decline in the functional reserve of many organ systems (Figure 25–1). The rate of this decline varies from system to system; while there is no appreciable difference in fasting blood sugar between ages 30 and 80 years, the average maximal respiratory capacity drops more than 40% during the same time span.[4] Of special interest are physiologic changes that make clinical emergencies more likely and more serious (Table 25–1).

Of the changes in body composition, decline in lean body weight and in protein synthesis may be associated with delayed wound repair and inadequate immune response to infections, as well as with delayed recovery of normal tissues destroyed by chemotherapy and radiotherapy. Also, reduction in total body water makes older patients particularly susceptible to volume depletion from mucositis and diarrhea.[5,6] In addition, a decreased volume of distribution of water-soluble agents may lead to enhanced toxicity of these drugs.[7]

Cardiovascular changes may lead to an increased risk of thromboembolic phenomena associated with cancer, cancer chemotherapy,[8] and hormonal therapy;[9] enhanced risk of anoxia (particularly myocardial anoxia) in the presence of anemia; and cardiac failure from cardiotoxic drugs.[8]

The gastrointestinal mucosae undergo changes that make them more vulnerable to chemotherapy and radiotherapy.[10] These changes include increased proliferation of the cryptal cells, which portends increased destruction by cycle-active agents, and depletion of mucosal stem cells, which results in delayed repair of mucosal damage. Of the hepatic changes, a decline in the activity of phase-1 cytochrome P-450–dependent-reactions is probably the most relevant, as it implies an increased risk of drug-drug interactions that is further enhanced in elderly persons by polypharmacy.[11,12]

While a decline in glomerular filtration rate (GFR) is probably the most consistent of age-related physio-

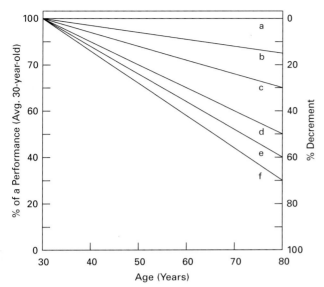

Figure 25–1. Age decrements in physiological performance. Average values for 30-year-old subjects taken as 100%. Decrements shown are schematic. A: Fasting blood glucose. B: Nerve conduction velocity and some cellular enzyme activities. C: Resting cardiac index. D: Vital capacity and renal blood flow. E: maximum breathing capacity. F: Maximum work rate and maximum oxygen uptake. Adapted from Yancik R.[1]

logic alterations, its contribution to oncologic emergencies is probably negligible and is limited to the complications of reduced renal excretion of drugs and their active metabolites.[8,13]

Hemopoiesis is of special concern because the hematopoietic system is an almost universal target of cytotoxic agents and because hematopoietic suppression may follow the irradiation of large flat bone surfaces, such as the pelvic bones. The risk and severity of the most common oncologic emergencies (ie, infection and bleeding) are enhanced in older individuals by deeper and more prolonged myelodepression than in younger patients.[14] The following findings constitute abundant experimental and clinical evidence that the hematopoietic reserve is compromised with advanced age:

- Reduced concentration of pluripotent hematopoietic progenitors in the bone marrow of aging animals[15]
- Reduced telomerase activity and telomere length in hematopoietic progenitors of aging animals[16–17]
- Reduced ability of aging animals and aging humans to increase the concentration of hematopoietic progenitors following hematopoietic stress[18–22]
- Decreased production of hematopoietic cytokines and increased production of hemopoiesis-inhibiting cytokines in the marrow of aging animals and humans[22–24]
- Progressive reduction in active hematopoietic tissue in aging humans[25]

TABLE 25–1. Physiologic Changes of Age That May Influence the Occurrence of Oncologic Emergencies

Change	Consequences

Body composition
    Decline in protein and water
    Decreased protein synthesis
    Possible increase in adipose tissue
	Decreased volume of distribution of water soluble drugs → increased serum concentration → increased toxicity
	Increased susceptibility to malnutrition from cancer and chemotherapy
	Increased susceptibility to volume depletion

Circulatory system
    Decreased number of myocardic sarcomeres
    Arteriosclerosis of peripheral vessels
    Venous pooling and decreased venous circulation
	Increased risk of myocardial toxicity from chemotherapy
	Increased risk of tissue anoxia that may lead to perforation of viscera, cerebral, myocardial, and renal ischemia
	Increased risk of thromboembolic phenomena connected with cancer, chemotherapy, and hormonal therapy
	Increased risk of fluid retention with hormonal therapy

Genitourinary system
    Decreased glomerular filtration rate
    Prostate hypertrophy
    Neurogenic bladder dysfunctions
	Decreased excretion of drugs and active drug metabolites
	Increased risk of urinary retention

Gastrointestinal system
    Gastrointestinal atrophy and dysmotility
    Increased proliferation of mucosal cells, with depetion of mucosal stem cells
	Decreased absorption of drug and food → increased risk of malnutrition
	Increased risk of chemotherapy-related diarrhea and mucositis, leading to dehydration

Hematologic system
    Depletion of hematopoietic stem cell reserve
    Decreased production of hematopoietic cytokines and increased concentration of cytokines that inhibit hematopoietic
    Decreased sensitivity of stem cells and hematopoietic progenitors to the stimulatory effects of hematopoietic cytokines
	Increased risk of neutropenia, infections, and infectious death
	Increased risk of thrombocytopenia and bleeding
	Increased risk, prevalence, and incidence of anemia, which may enhance the risk of chemotherapy-induced myelodepression, of fatigue and functional dependence, and of delirium

Central nervous system
    Decreased number of neurons
    Increased prevalence of degenerative changes
	Increased susceptibility to cognitive complications of chemotherapy
	Increased risk of delirium
	Altered perception of pain

Peripheral nervous system
    Decreased number of neurons
    Demyelinization and decreased conduction rate
	Altered perception of pain
	Increased susceptibility to neurologic complications of chemotherapy
	Increased risk of autonomic dysfunctions (postural hypotension, urinary retention and incontinence, impotence)

Systemic effects
(endocrine and immune system)
    Decline in cellular immunity
    Increased production of inflammatory cytokines
    Decreased production of growth hormone, insulin-like growth factor 1, and gonadotropins
	Increased risk of intracellular (fungal, viral, and mycobacterial) infection
	Decreased protein synthesis
	Decreased hemopoiesis
	Fatigue

- Increased risk of anemia of unknown cause in aging humans, which has been associated with decreased production of erythropoietin in some cases[26]
- Increased risk of neutropenia and neutropenic infections in older individuals treated with cytotoxic chemotherapy[14,27–36]

It is important to add that the hematopoietic response to pharmacologic doses of hematopoietic growth factors does not seem to be compromised in the aged,[28,33,36,37] and these factors may represent an effective bulwark against deadly infections.

The number of neurons in the central nervous system decline approximately by 20% between the ages of 20 and 80 years. This decline is accompanied by an increased prevalence of degenerative changes, such as neurofibrillary plaque formation and amyloidosis.[38,39] These changes underlie an increased prevalence of cognitive disorders (from benign forgetfulness to full-blown dementia[40] to a propensity to delirium),[41] and disturbances of perception that may increase the threshold for pain and other symptoms.[42] These changes seemingly predispose older individuals to the cognitive complications of chemotherapy and radiotherapy[43] and may delay the recognition of catastrophic complications such as spinal-cord compression or visceral perforation.

Changes in the peripheral nervous system may predispose older individuals to neuropathic complications of cytotoxic drugs such as vinca alkaloids, epipodophyllotoxins, cisplatin, and taxanes.[44,45] Although these complications are generally chronic in nature, they may precipitate a functional dependence that is devastating and costly. In addition, peripheral neuropathy may also alter the perception of pain.

Decline in vision and hearing are common in older individuals and are almost universal after the age of 85 years.[46] These changes are due to a complex of factors, including peripheral nerve degeneration and may lead to some degree of functional dependence, especially in regard to transportation and telephone use.

A number of systemic changes in the aged person may reduce the tolerance to cancer and its treatment and may precipitate an emergency. These changes include

- endocrine changes (such as a decline in the production of sexual hormones, growth hormone, and insulin-like growth factor 1) that may lead to fatigue and reduced anabolism;[47,48]
- increased production of inflammatory cytokines (including interleukin-6 and tumor necrosis factor) that may inhibit hemopoiesis, and protein synthesis, and generally lead to a prevalently catabolic status;[49–51] and
- immune senescence, which involves prevalently cell-mediated immunity and which may predispose to fungal, viral, parasitic, and more general infections by intracellular microorganisms.[52–54]

An emerging clinical concept, somatopause, attempts to encompass the systemic changes of aging. Somatopause signifies a catabolic status due to the simultaneous exhaustion of growth hormone and increased concentrations of inflammatory cytokines in the circulation.[49,50] Somatopause may become a clinical landmark of aging, beyond which anabolic processes and the ability to repair injuries are progressively and irreversibly impaired. Whereas somatopause is a real condition, the clinical criteria to recognize somatopause are still wanted.

Functional Aging

The incidence of functional dependence increases with age. Different degrees of functional dependence are recognized according to a person's ability to perform activities of daily living (ADL) and instrumental activities of daily living (IADL) (Table 25–2).[55,56] A fully independent person is able to perform both IADL and ADL; a person dependent in one or more IADL needs home help and supervision; and a person dependent in ADL needs total care by a live-in caregiver. Persons dependent in ADL are generally considered frail and do not receive aggressive antineoplastic treatment. Dependence in IADL is particularly significant in relation to emergencies because such individuals bear an increased risk of developing complications of cytotoxic chemotherapy[57] and have a lessened ability to seek timely medical treatment in an emergency.

Dependence in IADL is more common than generally thought. This author and colleagues found that approximately 70% of cancer patients aged 70 years and older and attending the senior adult oncology program at the H. Lee Moffitt Cancer Center and Research Institute in Tampa (FL) were dependent in at least one IADL.[58] As patients who attend a tertiary care cancer center seem to be selected in terms of better function and higher wealth, the prevalence of IADL dependence may be even higher in the general population.

TABLE 25–2. Activities of Daily Living and Instrumental Activities of Daily Living

ADL	IADL
Continence	Use of transportation
Grooming	Shopping
Dressing	Providing own meals
Using the bathroom	Taking medications
Eating	Using the telephone
Transferring	Money management
	Housekeeping and laundering

ADL = activities of daily living; IADL = instrumental activities of daily living.

Medical changes

Two medical aspects of aging may influence oncologic emergencies: (1) the increased prevalence of comorbidity with age,[59] and (2) the emergence of a number of disorders that are more typical of (if not specific to) older age and that are referred to as " geriatric syndromes." These include severe dementia, delirium in the presence of mild infection or drug ingestion, severe depression, falls, total incontinence, spontaneous bone fractures, neglect and abuse, and failure to thrive.[60]

Comorbidity and geriatric syndromes may modulate medical emergencies in different ways that render the emergencies more likely and more serious. First, there is an increased susceptibility to complications of cancer and cancer treatment, due to a reduction in function of a specific organ system. For example, anemia may enhance the risk of myelodepression from chemotherapy;[61–65] coronary artery disease may enhance the risk of cardiomyopathy from anthracyclines;[66] degenerative brain disease may enhance the risk of delirium;[43,67] and pre-existing heart disease, reduced lean body weight, and restricted hematopoietic reserve may contribute to enhanced risks from emergency surgery.[68]

Second, the increased vulnerability of certain organ systems may transform simple complications of cancer and cancer treatment into emergencies. For example, diarrhea from fluorinated pyrimidines may lead to hypovolemic shock in older individuals.[7]

Third, pre-existing diseases may delay the recognition of emergencies; this may occur through a number of mechanisms, including *masking* and *summation*.[69] Masking implies that symptoms of a pre-existing disease mask the symptoms of a new condition. For example, back pain from pre-existing spinal stenosis may mask the pain of impending spinal-cord compression, or pre-existing chronic disease or an inadequate immune response from medication may prevent the recognition of visceral perforation. Summation implies that the effects of two coexisting diseases are summed up in producing a syndrome that is unrelated to either. For example, delirium may result from a number of conditions unrelated to the central nervous system, such as the coexistence of congestive heart failure and upper respiratory infection.

Finally, pre-existing diseases and geriatric syndromes may prevent timely access to care. For example, a fall on the way to the phone by a patient who lives alone may delay that patient's admission to the hospital for neutropenic infection by hours or days.

Social Aspects

Several demographic and social aspects of aging may influence the management of emergencies. These aspects include the following:

- The prevalence of women in the population increases with age because of the longer life expectancy of women. The majority of these older women live alone, which does not mean that they are fully independent or (especially) that they can react to an emergency in a timely and appropriate way.
- Disease may precipitate functional dependence in persons who previously were fully dependent; this occurrence is most common after hospitalization, especially if prolonged.[70,71]
- The prevalence of functional dependence increases with age. At least 70% of persons over 70 years of age are dependent in one or more IADL; by age 85 years, at least 50% of the population is dependent in one or more ADL.[56] Progressive decline in vision and hearing may contribute to dependence even in persons who are cognitively intact.[55]
- The individuals who supervise the care of older individuals at home (ie, caregivers) are often inadequate. In many cases, the caregiver is an elderly spouse with health problems of his or her own; or the caregiver is an adult son or daughter who is already committed to a profession and/or to his or her own family.[72,73]
- The majority of older persons have limited resources. This may interfere with their ability to buy oral medications (eg, antibiotics to prevent Gram-negative sepsis during neutropenia) or to pay for repeated visits to clinics for the administration of growth factors or for control of blood counts. Likewise, financial restrictions may prevent the hiring of adequate home help or admission to an assisted-living facility.[74]
- Admission to an assisted-living facility or to a nursing home may be associated with adaptive reactions that may compromise the administration of antineoplastic treatment.[75]

Clinical Assessment

Two aspects of aging were emphasized in the previous discussion, namely, that aging is multidimensional and that aging is highly individualized. The questions faced by the practitioner who is managing older cancer patients are, Is this person going to die of cancer? and Is this person going to tolerate the treatment of cancer? Clearly, a purely medical evaluation of the older person is insufficient to provide the answers; it is of no use to prescribe lifesaving medications if the patient is unable to pay for medications, take the medications without supervision, or react in time to complications of treatment. Furthermore, the risks of treatment need to be balanced by a gain in longevity and quality of life; thus, an estimate of life expectancy is necessary. The diversity of the older population may be accounted for by a comprehensive geriatric assessment exploring the functional, medical, emotional, cognitive, and social status of the patient (Table 25–3).[55] A number

TABLE 25–3. Model of a Comprehensive Geriatric Assessment

Domain	Assessment Methods
Functional	
Performance status (PS)	Karnofsky or Zubrod scale
IADL	IADL scale
ADL	ADL scale
Medical	
Comorbidity	Number of comorbid conditions
	Comorbidity Scales (Charlson or CIRS-G)
Geriatric syndromes	Assessment for the presence of specific syndrome
Pharmacologic	Number of medications, duplication, risk of drug interaction
Cognitive	Mental status (Folstein Mini-Mental Status or equivalent tests)
Emotional	Geriatric Depression Scale or equivalent test
Socioeconomic	
Income	Resources
Caregiver	Adequacy
	Availability
	Caregiver function scales
Nutritional status	Absence of protein-calorie malnutrition
	Nutritional history
	Nutritional risk (by mininutritional assessment)

ADL = activities of daily living; CIRS-G = _____ ; IADL = instrumental activities of daily living.

of issues related to geriatric assessment are still unresolved. These include the importance of rating housekeeping and laundering in the IADL (since the inability to perform either of these activities does not seem to have prognostic significance); the most meaningful way to assess comorbidity; the point at which dementia and depression should be considered geriatric syndromes; and the clinical definitions of neglect, abuse, and failure to thrive. Even with these limitations, the Comprehensive Geriatric Assessment (CGA) has improved the function and survival of older individuals and has decreased their hospitalization and institutionalization rate.[76–79] In addition, the CGA has helped to prevent a number of adverse events, such as falls and in-hospital delirium.[80–82]

Most relevant to the issues of clinical oncology, the CGA has allowed the recognition of different stages of aging.[50] Of the various staging systems, the system proposed by Hemerman is one of the more accepted and is most applicable to the management of cancer. This system is based on the rehabilitation needs of older individuals (Table 25–4). The secondary stage implies that the functional reserve of a person is almost completely exhausted and the tolerance of stress very limited. Figure 25–2 presents an algorithm, based on this staging system, for the antineoplastic chemotherapeutic treatment of older persons. In applying this algorithm to older cancer patients, one should remember that frailty is a chronic condition; rapid changes in the functional status are common, due to reduced functional reserve, but do not represent frailty. For example, this author recently had the opportunity to manage an 84-year-old woman who had come to the hospital in a hypotensive and confused state but who had been living alone and fully independent up until 1 week prior to presenting. The patient had a large-cell lymphoma of the stomach and had become volume depleted due to having vomited for 3 days. After appropriate fluid resuscitation, the patient received combined cyclophosphamide, hydroxy-daunomycin, vincristine (Oncovin), and prednisone (CHOP) in full doses and experienced a complete recovery. It would have been unfortunate if her treatment had been compromised by a wrong determination of frailty.

A CGA prior to antineoplastic treatment goes a long way in preventing oncologic emergencies by accomplishing the following:

- Patients at increased risk of treatment complications are recognized, and special precautions are taken; these may include initial reduction of chemotherapy doses, closer observation, and provision of adequate caregiver services.

TABLE 25–4. Stages of Aging*

Stages	Rehabilitation Needs	Clinical Characteristics	2-yr Mortality
Primary	No rehabilitation needs besides preservation of function	Independent in ADL and IADL No serious comorbidity No geriatric syndromes	8%
Intermediate	Need of functional rehabilitation that may be fully successful	Dependent in one or more IADL (with exclusion of housekeeping and laundering) Presence of some incapacitating comorbidity No geriatric syndromes	16–30%
Secondary (frailty)	Functional rehabilitation probably ineffective Main goal is to delay further functional deterioration	Dependent in one or more ADL Presence of one or more geriatric syndromes Serious comorbid conditions	~40%
Tertiary (near death)	Further functional deterioration unavoidable	Immediately life-threatening condition	> 95%

ADL = activities of daily living; IADL = instrumental activities of daily living.
*Adapted from Hemerman's staging system.

- Unrecognized comorbidity or functional dependence is brought to light and managed.
- Malnutrition is possibly prevented.
- Cognitive and emotional problems are recognized and addressed.
- The social situation of the patient is optimized (this includes provision of an adequate caregiver and regular access to care and daily meals).

Although functional age is poorly reflected by chronologic age, two chronologic landmarks are helpful: ages 70 and 85 years. Age of 70 years may be considered the lower border of senescence as the prevalence of age-related changes increases steeply between the ages of 70 and 75 years. Age of 85 years represents a "red flag" for frailty, as the prevalence of this condition increases steeply after the age of 85 years.[55,60]

A number of means besides the CGA have been studied for the determination of aging; these include physical performance[83,84] and laboratory tests, such as those assessing serum levels of interleukin-6, the ratio between circulating cystein and thiolic groups (s/d ratio), and the D dimer.[85–87] Although helpful for specific purposes (eg, tests of physical performance identify persons at risk for disability), none of these tests have the wide scope of the CGA and can substitute for the CGA. Seemingly, the clin-

ical determination of somatopause may represent an important landmark in the future.

The importance of a CGA in the management of the older cancer patient has been recognized by the National Cancer Center Network (NCCN).[88] The panel on guidelines for the management of older persons has recommended that some form of geriatric assessment be performed in all cancer patients aged 70 years and older. Ideally, the assessment should be performed by a primary care provider and communicated to the oncologist as part of patient information. In the absence of a primary care provider, the oncologist should be able to perform and interpret the CGA.

With this outline of aging as background, specific oncologic emergencies in aged persons can now be examined.

ONCOLOGIC EMERGENCIES IN OLDER INDIVIDUALS

Neutropenic Infections

The risk of chemotherapy-induced neutropenia increases with age.[14,15,28–37] However, this statement needs to be qualified: six retrospective studies of patients treated in cooperative oncology groups and major cancer centers showed that the risk of neutropenia was not significantly increased among people aged 70 years and

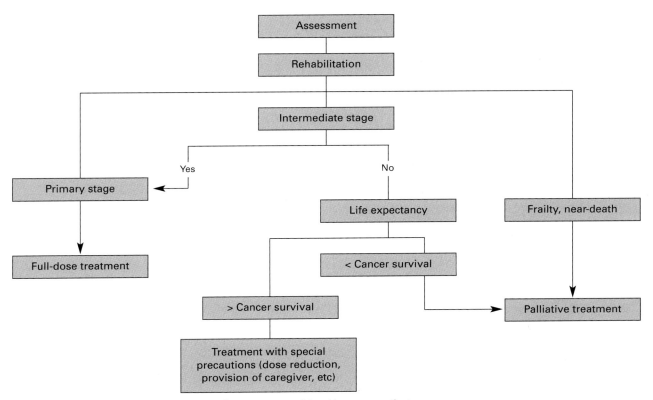

Figure 25–2. Algorithm for the chemotherapeutic management of the older cancer patient.

older.[89–94] These studies had several limitations, including the following:

- Patients were highly selected to meet the exacting eligibility conditions of clinical trials.
- Only a minority of patients were older than 65 years.
- The treatment regimens used in these studies had lesser dose intensities than current regimens.

A number of other studies suggested quite a different picture. First, Dees and colleagues showed that the risk and the severity of myelodepression following adjuvant treatment with cyclophosphamide and doxorubicin increase with the age of the patients.[14] Of special interest is that after four courses of treatment, myelotoxicity appeared to be cumulative in women aged 65 years and older but not in younger women, suggesting a restriction of hematopoietic reserve with age. Second, in the majority of studies of acute myeloid leukemia, age of over 55 years is a poor prognostic factor, and the risk of dying from neutropenic infections increases with the age of the patient.[95–100] Third, in nine studies of older patients with large-cell non-Hodgkin's lymphoma who were treated with CHOP or CHOP-like chemotherapy, the risk of grade III and grade IV neutropenia was consistently 50% or higher and the risk of death from neutropenic infection also varied between 5 and 30%[28–36] (Table 25–5). With the now obsolete regimen of methotrexate, doxorubicin (Adriamycin), cyclophosphamide, vincristine (Oncovin), prednisone, and bleomycin (MACOP-B), the risk of infectious death was 3% among patients younger than 60 years and 11% for the older patients.[101] The study of Gomez and colleagues, involving 260 patients aged 60 years and older, found that 63% of 35 deaths occurred during the first course of chemotherapy.[30] In a subsequent study, these authors showed that the risk of complications was higher after the age of 70 years, especially in persons with poor functional status.[102] Also, a number of pre-existing conditions may contribute to infection in neutropenic elderly patients, including urinary incontinence and retention, diverticulosis, constipation, chronic bronchitis, and poor oral care. On the basis of these data, it is reasonable to conclude that the risk of neutropenic infections increases in older individuals, especially after the age of 70 years.

Timely diagnosis in older individuals may be hampered by unusual presentation and late recognition of the infection, as well as by inadequate access to health care.

In addition to the common presentation of fever, chills, general malaise, and organ-specific symptoms, infections in older individuals may be heralded by delirium (encompassing a number of manifestations, from somnolence to agitation), absence of fever, or hypothermia.[103–106] To compensate for the absence of fever, some authors have proposed that any increment in body temperature (2°F or 1°C) be considered fever in older individuals.[103]

Another peculiarity of infections in older individuals is the high degree of colonization of the upper airways, the oropharynx, and the urine, which may be source of sepsis by unusual and antibiotic-resistant organisms. This occurrence is particularly common in elderly residents in adult living facilities.

Infection may lead to functional dependence. Older individuals who are completely independent may suddenly become unable or unwilling to provide their own meals, go shopping, manage their money, talk on the telephone, or take their medications regularly. Patients who

TABLE 25–5. Incidence of Life-Threatening Neutropenia and Neutropenic Infections in Older Individuals with Large-Cell Non-Hodgkin's Lymphomas

Study Author	No. of Patients	Drug Regimen	Age of Patients (yr)	Neutropenia (%)	Neutropenic Fever (%)	Treatment Related Deaths (%)	Growth Factor
Zinzani	161	VNCOP-B	60+	44	32	1.3	—
Sonneveld	148	CHOP	60+	NR	NR	14	—
		CNOP	60+	NR	NR	13	—
Gomez	26	CHOP	60+	24	8	0	GM-CSF
			70+	73	42	20	GM-CSF
Tirelli	119	VMP	70 +	50	21	7	—
		CHOP	70+	48	21	5	—
Bastion	444	CVP	70+	9	7	12	—
		CTVP	70+	29	13	15	—
O'Reilly	63	POCE	65+	50	20	8	—
Armitage	20	CHOP	70+	NR	NR	30	—

CHOP = cyclophosphamide, hydroxydaunomycin, vincristine (Oncovin), and prednisone; CNOP = Cyclophosphamide, mitoxantrone, vincristine, and prednisone; CTVP = cyclophosphamide, pirarubicin, vincristine, and prednisone; CVP = cyclophosphamide, vincristine, and prednisone; GM-CSF = granulocyte-macrophage colony-stimulating factor; NR = not recorded; POCE = etoposide, vincristine, cyclophosphamide, and epirubicin; VMP = VP16, mitoxantrone, and prednimustine; VNCOP-B = etoposide, mitoxantrone, cyclophosphamide, vincristine, prednisone, and bleomycin.

are independent in ADL may suddenly need help eating, getting dressed, or grooming, or they may develop incontinence. Thus, with older individuals receiving chemotherapy, it is important to consider any sudden change in cognitive or functional status as a possible sign of infection.

Clinical Course. With age, the risk of dying of infections increases, and so do the duration of antibiotic treatment and hospitalization and the risk of long-term consequences such as disability and functional dependence.[103–106] Although there are no specific data for neutropenic infections, it is reasonable to apply the data related to older patients in general to neutropenic patients. So, infections may impair the ability of the patient to receive timely cancer treatment and may compromise the patient's long-term independence and quality of life, even when recovery from infection occurs.[106–108]

Management. Once the infection is diagnosed, its management is the same as in younger patients and involves fluid resuscitation and broad-spectrum antibiotic treatment until the specific organism is isolated. Two special issues related to older individuals are the suitability of oral outpatient treatment and rehabilitative procedures.

Oral outpatient antibiotic treatment has been increasingly used for neutropenic fever in patients who are considered to be at low risk.[109–111] Criteria for low risk include the absence of sepsis and of radiologic evidence of pneumonia, and normal serum blood urea nitrogen (BUN), creatinine, and liver enzymes.

Outpatient treatment is very appealing for older individuals as it may obviate the risk of hospitalization, which entails delirium and functional deterioration in addition to nosocomial infections. Although specific studies related to older individuals are lacking, it is reasonable to follow the same approach that is used for younger patients, at least for those individuals who live close to a treatment facility (less than an hour's drive) and who have a caregiver available on short notice 24 hours a day. It may also be advisable to connect these patients to some form of home care.

In addition to the rehabilitative measures used with all hospitalized patients, it is important to provide older patients with conditions that maintain their independence; these include beds that can be lowered enough so that patients can get in and out on their own; help and encouragement with feeding, grooming, and use of the bathroom; daily walks; airway control; and aggressive management of depression.[107] When patients are confused, physical and chemical restraints should be used to a minimum and only to prevent the patient from hurting him- or herself. Phenotiazines should be used preferentially over benzodiazepines; if benzodiazepines are used, those with the shortest half-life should be chosen, such as lorazepam.[41] In general, proper review of the patient's medications (especially pain medications and anticholinergic drugs) and adequate antibiotic and fluid management should suffice.

Prevention. Perhaps the most important form of management of neutropenic infections in older individuals is prevention; this should include the following measures:

1. Proper patient selection for chemotherapy, based on the algorithm provided in Figure 25–2.
2. Prophylactic use of hematopoietic growth factors in all patients aged 70 years and older receiving chemotherapy with dose intensity comparable to CHOP. This recommendation, unanimously supported by the NCCN panel on guidelines for the management of older cancer patients,[88] is based on the following considerations:
   - There is a high risk of neutropenia, neutropenic infections, and mortality in these patients (see Table 25–5).
   - More than half of the infectious deaths occur during the first course of chemotherapy, in the absence of growth factors. If the American Society of Clinical Oncology (ASCO) guidelines for the use of hematopoietic growth factors were applied to older individuals, these deaths could not be prevented (these guidelines call for the institution of hematopoietic growth factor treatment only after one episode of neutropenic infection).[112]
   - Hematopoietic growth factors do reduce (by 50 to 75%), the risk of life-threatening neutropenia and neutropenic infections in older individuals, according to four randomized controlled studies (Table 25–6).
   - Dose reduction may compromise the antineoplastic effects of treatment (according to five randomized controlled studies and a retrospective analysis), at least in patients with lymphoma.[29,31,32,113,114]
   - The value of alternative forms of infection prevention, such as the use of oral antibiotics, has not been as well established; prophylactic antibiotics may be complementary to the use of growth factors.[115]
   - Given the fact that hospitalization is more prolonged in older individuals and may be associated with long-term functional complications, the use of growth factors does not appear to increase the cost of treatment and may even reduce costs.
3. Maintenance of hemoglobin levels ≥ 12 g/dL with erythropoietin. This recommendation is also unanimously supported by the NCCN panel for the management of cancer in the older person and is based on the following considerations:
   - Five studies demonstrated that low hemoglobin level is an independent risk factor for myelotoxicity.[61–65] A number of antineoplastic agents, espe-

cially the anthracyclines and the epipodophyllo-toxins, are heavily bound to red blood cells; consequently, a decline in hemoglobin levels may lead to an increased concentration of free drug in the circulation and an increased risk of toxicity. The risk is particularly high in older individuals, in whom lean body weight is also decreased and cannot buffer the effects of lower hemoglobin as it does in younger persons.

- Anemia is associated with fatigue[116–120] (which may also precipitate functional dependence) and with other complications, such as iatrogenic delirium.[121]
- Anemia represents an independent risk factor for death in the course of serious infections.[15]

4. Management of coexisting problems, identified during the geriatric assessment, that may contribute to the seriousness of the infections. This management includes the following:

- Provision of an adequate caregiver. This is essential for the persons who are at Hemerman's intermediate stage (ie, those who are already dependent in one or more IADL, have one or two comorbid conditions that make them more susceptible to infections, or present mild dementia, vision, or hearing impairments that prevent timely access to care). A caregiver is highly desirable also for those elderly patients who live alone and are fully independent, because moderately toxic chemotherapy may precipitate functional dependence. (This author observed the case of a 74-year-old man with mantle cell lymphoma, previously fully independent, who became hypotensive during an episode of neutropenic fever, fell close to the heating system, and developed third-degree burns before being found by a neighbor, 24 hours later. He recovered but spent almost a month in the intensive care unit.) If an adequate caregiver cannot live with the patient, the patient should at least wear an alarm system connecting him or her to the caregiver. The ideal caregiver should be fully independent, own personal transportation, and be able to help the patient on short notice.
- Optimal management of pre-existing conditions that may favor the development of infections. These include poorly controlled diabetes, poor oral or skin hygiene, serious constipation, inadequate mobility, and depression.
- Aggressive nutritional management in patients at high risk for malnutrition. For example, prophylactic gastrostomy of jejunostomy may be indicated in persons for whom a combination of chemotherapy and radiation therapy to the upper airways is planned. Close supervision of food intake is indicated for patients with swallowing

TABLE 25–6. Studies Demonstrating Benefits of Hematopoietic Growth Factors in Older Patients with Large-Cell Lymphoma Receiving Combination Chemotherapy

Study and Drug Regimen	No. of Patients	Neutropenia Incidence* (%)	Neutropenic Infection Incidence (%)
Zinzani			
VNCOP-B	350	—	—
G-CSF	—	23	5
No G-CSF	—	56	21
Zagonel			
CHOP	—	—	—
G-CSF	—	4.8	4.8
No G-CSF	—	27.7	15.6
Bertini			
VEPBC	90	—	—
G-CSF	—	22	2
No G-CSF	—	44	9

CHOP = cyclophosphamide, hydroxydaunomycin, vincristine (Oncovin), and prednisone; G-CSF = granulocyte colony-stimulating factor; VEPBC = VP16, epirubicin, prednisone, bleomycin, and cyclophosphamide; VNCOP-B = etoposide, mitoxantrone, cyclophosphamide, vincristine, prednisone, and bleomycin. *Grades III and IV.

disorders, depression, confusion, or mild dementia, who may neglect nutrition in the course of chemotherapy. Management of constipation may also reduce the risk of anorexia.

- Pharmacologic management, to avoid drug interactions and to minimize the use of medication that may cause confusion, nausea, or constipation.

Volume Depletion

Volume depletion may lead to hypovolemic shock in older individuals more rapidly than in younger individuals because of limited body water and decreased sympathetic control of small vessels, especially capacitance vessels. Among the several causes of volume depletion, chemotherapy-induced mucositis and diarrhea deserve special mention. The susceptibility of older individuals to mucositis is increased due to the underlying conditions of the gastrointestinal mucosae. Gelman and Taylor demonstrated that adjusting the doses of methotrexate and cyclophosphamide in older women with metastatic breast cancer reduced the risk of myelotoxicity but not the risk of mucositis, suggesting that mucositis was mainly due to the enhanced vulnerability.[93] Likewise, Stein and colleagues showed that age over 70 years was an independent risk factor for mucositis induced by fluorinated pyrimidines.[7] In the initial study by the Gastrointestinal Tumor Study Group (GITSG) of fluorouracil and leucovorin, 10 patients aged 65 years and older, but only one of those younger, died as a direct consequence of volume depletion from mucositis, thereby indicating that mucositis may quickly become an emergency in older individuals.[7]

The presentation of volume depletion may be delayed for a number of reasons, including poor appreciation of the initial symptoms of mucositis, inadequate fluid replacement (from swallowing disorders), and inadequate access to transportation.

The management of fluid depletion includes aggressive fluid resuscitation. As in the case of infectious neutropenia, early management may prevent both death and chronic complications, including functional dependence and the delay of further chemotherapy. Thus, it is very important to instruct both the patient and the caregiver to report diarrhea (even when it appears to be only moderate) and any condition that may prevent fluid intake. Aggressive fluid replacement, together with aggressive management of nausea and vomiting and of dysphagia, should start as soon as oral fluid intake appears to be inadequate.

Prevention is the best management of fluid depletion. Unfortunately, no effective prevention of chemotherapy-induced mucositis exists. While it is effective in relieving the discomfort of mucositis, sucralfate failed to ameliorate the risk of this complication.[122] Despite anecdotal reports that granulocyte-macrophage colony-stimulating factor (GM-CSF) may prevent mucositis, the efficacy of this compound was not conclusively demonstrated.[123] Ongoing studies are exploring the use of oral interleukin-11 (IL-II) (oprelvekin) and of keratinocyte proliferating factor.[124]

In addition to educating patients about oral hygiene and about reporting diarrhea and mucositis, reducing the initial dose of fluorinated pyrimidines by 25% may be prudent (especially in patients with some functional dependence and comorbidity), and the use of leucovorin should be avoided.

Visceral Perforation

The risk of spontaneous visceral perforation increases with age because of a number of factors, including ischemia, muscular atrophy, and a higher prevalence of colonic diverticuli and constipation.[125] Also, the presentation of visceral perforation may be less dramatic and acute in older patients than in the young because the inflammatory reaction may be less intense, the perception of pain may be blunted by cognitive disorders or peripheral nerve dysfunction, and some degree of abdominal distention is not uncommon, even in normal circumstances. In the older cancer patients, the administration of chemotherapy or radiation therapy may both increase the risk of perforation and further delay the recognition of the syndrome.

Although visceral perforation is most commonly fatal, early diagnosis may allow lifesaving treatment. The key to early diagnosis is a high degree of suspicion, involving frequent checks of patients at high risk, such as patients with intraluminal or intraperitoneal cancer, patients treated with corticosteroids for a prolonged

time, and patients who experience prolonged neutropenia. In these individuals, rapid changes in mental status, a drop in blood pressure, or a sudden drop in neutrophil counts may herald visceral perforation, even in the presence of a benign physical examination of the abdomen, and should prompt upright radiography of chest and abdomen to look for free air.

EMERGENCIES TYPICAL OF AGING: DELIRIUM

Features, Diagnosis, and Assessment

Delirium is probably the most vexing emergency for the patient, the family, and the care provider and is also one of the most common. The definition of delirium, according to the *Diagnostic and Statistical Manual of Mental Disorders,* 4th edition (DSM-IV), involves an acute alteration of consciousness, with waxing and waning orientation and disturbed cognition, developing over a short period of time (hours or days) and accompanied by neurovegetative signs including fever, tachypnea, and tachycardia.[41] Delirium is always associated with an underlying organic disorder. The causes of delirium can be briefly reviewed by using the acrostic shown in Figure 25–3.

Whereas the pathogenesis of delirium is complex, recent evidence suggests that the development of delirium is favored by high concentrations of cytokines.[126]

In older individuals with pre-existing dementia, it is important to distinguish delirium from acute exacerbations of dementia, the so-called catastrophic reactions that are particularly common during the last phases of dementia and during which delusions and hallucinations may occur. The differentiation of these conditions, which requires considerable experience, is based on the capacity of attention: the patient with delirium experiences a continuous variation in focus whereas the patient with a catastrophic reaction is generally well focused on his or her delusions or inappropriate endeavor.

The occurrence of delirium has two important clinical implications

1. The patient has a serious and acute underlying disease.
2. The patient is frail.

The differential diagnosis of delirium in the older cancer patient needs to be related to the specific conditions. A number of common pictures include the following:

* An older patient who is feverish has received cancer chemotherapy in the previous 2 weeks. In this case, the delirium should be considered the consequence of an infection unless proved otherwise. Management includes blood, urine, and sputum cultures, chest radiography, a complete blood count, and broad-spectrum antibiotic coverage.

- Delirium in a patient with intra-abdominal cancer. This should suggest the possibility of visceral perforation.

Delirium in a patient in whom new medications were originally administered, especially pain medications or corticosteroids, suggests drug-related delirium. The management of pain in older patients may be problematic for the following reasons:[127,128]

1. Pharmacodynamic alteration in the central nervous system can result in a decline in the u/delta receptor ratio and may lead to increased susceptibility to delirium.
2. Unpredictable pharmacokinetics. The glucoronide forms of opioids, especially the 6 glucoronide, is an active metabolite and is excreted through the kidneys; in older individuals, this compound may have a prolonged half-life, which may lead to accumulation due to a decline in creatinine clearance.

In the realm of drug-related delirium, one should always consider drug withdrawal. Older individuals may forget to take their pain medication or may deliberately fail to take them because of nausea or constipation.

Metabolic delirium should be considered in a patient with a recent history of prolonged nausea and vomiting, diarrhea, or a simply reduced food intake. Some medications, including corticosteroids and diuretics, may unmask diabetes.

In the presence of cancer, delirium may always be a manifestation of central nervous system involvement, especially with those neoplasms with a high likelihood of metastasizing to the central nervous system or of producing neoplastic meningitis. Such neoplasms include large-cell lymphoma, melanoma, and small-cell cancer of the lung .

Finally, in older individuals with multiple comorbidities, delirium may also be a manifestation of a coexisting condition, especially cardiovascular disease, and may be totally independent from cancer.

Upon presentation of delirium it is necessary to review the recent medical history, including the dates of chemotherapy, the most recent complete blood counts, any recent change of medications (especially involving opioid analgesics and glucocorticoids), changes in bowel habits, reduced food intake, and recent episodes of nausea and vomiting. The physical examination should assess the patient for fever, postural hypotension, signs of volume depletion (such as decreased skin turgor and lack of jugular vein distention when the patient lies supine), new cardiac abnormalities suggesting coronary artery disease (such as an S4 gallop and a pansystolic murmur of mitral regurgitation), signs of pulmonary infections (including rales, pleural effusion, and bronchial breathing), signs of

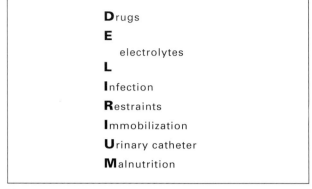

Figure 25–3. Acrostic summarizing the differential diagnosis of delirium.

acute abdomen (including rebound tenderness and the disappearance of bowel sounds), and the presence of focal neurologic signs (suggesting a recent cerebrovascular accident). Immediate laboratory tests should include complete blood counts; assessments of serum glucose, BUN, serum creatinine, electrolytes (including magnesium and calcium), hepatic and cardiac enzymes, and serum troponin levels; blood cultures and sensitivity; urine culture; radiography of the thorax; and electrocardiography.

Additional tests, including magnetic resonance imaging (MRI) of the brain, lumbar puncture, ventilation-perfusion scanning of the chest, and abdominal computed tomography (CT), should be performed if dictated by the clinical situation and if no diagnosis emerged from the initial evaluation.

Management and Prevention

Management includes rapid control of the causes of delirium, alleviation of agitation, and prevention.

Once the diagnosis of delirium is established, emergency admission to the hospital is mandatory because the patient needs to be prevented from harming him or herself or other individuals and needs to receive intravenous fluids and medications. Furthermore, emergency interventions that are available only in the hospital may be required. Whereas the diagnostic work-up may be initiated in the outpatient department, outpatient management of delirium should be discouraged.

While the cause of the delirium is sought, it is prudent to establish a venous access, with intravenous fluid running, and to start broad-spectrum antibiotics in patients who are at risk for neutropenic infections.

The management of agitation should be exclusively to prevent personal harm. As stated earlier, it is ethically unacceptable to use physical or pharmacologic methods of restraint simply because the patient disturbs other patients or because the hospital is understaffed. One-on-one supervision should be instituted as necessary.[106] If medications are used to resolve agitation, haloperidol or droperidol are preferred.[106]

Prevention of delirium includes prevention and early detection of the causes of delirium (such as infections, volume depletion, hyperglycemia, and anemia), as well as a multidisciplinary effort to manage conditions that may lead to delirium, such as depression, loneliness, family tensions, poor food intake, and polypharmacy. Multidisciplinary intervention has proved to be effective in preventing delirium in hospitalized older patients and appears to be the most promising strategy for the prevention of delirium in the older patient with cancer.

CONCLUSION

Oncologic emergencies in older individuals are common. Age is generally associated with increased risk and severity of neutropenic infections, volume depletion, and visceral perforation. In the older patient, delirium as presentation of an emergency is more common than in younger individuals.

Prevention is the most effective management of emergencies in older individuals and includes the prophylactic use of hematopoietic growth factors in patients treated with moderately toxic chemotherapy, maintenance of hemoglobin values at ≥ 12 g/dL, lower initial doses of fluorinated pyrimidines, aggressive fluid replacement in the presence of diarrhea and mucositis, prevention of malnutrition, and good mouth, skin, and bowel hygiene.

More generally, a multidisciplinary assessment of the older cancer patient seems the key to emergency prevention, because such an assessment allows

- recognition of patients at high risk for chemotherapy complications;
- evaluation of the adequacy of the caregiver;
- proper management of coexisting conditions that may enhance the risk of treatment complications;
- rehabilitation of functional disability; and
- prevention of malnutrition and polypharmacy.

Ideally, older individuals should have a primary care provider to coordinate their care and to direct them in the case of an emergency. In the absence of this provider, it behooves the oncologist to assume this role.

REFERENCES

1. Yancik R, Ries LAG. Aging and cancer in America: demographic and epidemiologic perspectives. Hematol Oncol Clin North Am 2000;14:17–24.
2. Yancik RM, Ries L. Cancer and age: magnitude of the problem. In: Balducci L, Lyman GH, Ershler WB, editors. Comprehensive geriatric oncology. London: Harwood Academic Publishers; 1998. p. 95–104.
3. Balducci L, Extermann M. Cancer and aging: an evolving panorama. Hematol Oncol Clin North Am 2000;14:1–16.
4. Duthie E. Physiology of aging: relevance to symptom perceptions and treatment tolerance. In: Balducci L, Lyman GH, Ershler WB, editors. Comprehensive geriatric oncology. London: Harwood Academic Publishers; 1998. p. 247–62.
5. Melton LJ, Khosla S, Crowson CS, et al. Epidemiology of sarcopenia. J Am Geriatr Soc 2000;48:625–30.
6. Baumgartner RN, Heymsfield SB, Roche SF. Human body composition and the epidemiology of chronic diseases. Obes Res 1995;3:73–95.
7. Stein BN, Petrelli NJ, Douglass HO, et al. Age and sex are independent predictors of 5-fluorouracil toxicity. Cancer 1995;75:11–7.
8. Cova D, Beretta G, Balducci L. Cancer chemotherapy in the older patients. In: Balducci L, Lyman GH, Ershler WB, editors. Comprehensive geriatric oncology. London, England: Harwood Academic Publishers; 1998. p. 429–42.
9. Fisher B, Costantino JP, Wickerham DL, et al. Tamoxifen for prevention of breast cancer: report from the National Adjuvant Breast and Bowel Project. J Natl Cancer Inst 1998;90:1371–88.
10. Atillasoy E, Holt PR. Gastrointestinal proliferation and aging. J Gerontol 1993;48:B43–9.
11. Vestal RE. Aging and pharmacology. Cancer 1997;80:1302–10.
12. Corcoran MB. Polypharmacy in the older patient. In: Balducci L, Lyman GH, Ershler WB, editors. Comprehensive geriatric oncology. London: Harwood Academic Publishers; 1998; p. 525–32.
13. Balducci L, Corcoran MB. Antineoplastic chemotherapy of the older cancer patient. Hematol Oncol Clin North Am 2000;14:193–212.
14. Dees EC, O'Reilly S, Goodman SN, et al. A prospective pharmacologic evaluation of age-related toxicity of adjuvant chemotherapy in women with breast cancer. Cancer Invest 2000;18:521–9.
15. Balducci L, Hardy CL, Lyman GH. Hematopoietic reserve in older cancer patients: clinical and economical considerations. Cancer Control 2000;7:539–47.
16. Van Zant G. Stem cells and genetics in the study of development, aging and longevity. Results and problems in cell differentiation. Vol. 29. Berlin and Heidelberg: Springer-Verlag; 2000. p. 203–35.
17. Marley SB, Lewis JL, Davidson RJ, et al. Evidence for a continuous decline in hematopoietic cell function from birth: application to evaluating bone marrow failure in children. Br J Haematol 1999;106:162–6.
18. Lipschitz DA. Age-related declines in hematopoietic reserve capacity. Semin Oncol 1995;22(1 Suppl):3–5.
19. Price TH, Chatta GS, Dale DC. Effect of recombinant granulocyte colony-stimulating factor on neutrophil kinetics in normal young and elderly humans. Blood 1996;88:335–40.
20. Chatta DS, Dale DC. Aging and haemopoiesis. Implications for treatment with haemopoietic growth factors. Drugs Aging 1996;9:37–47.
21. Chatta GS, Price TH, Allen RC, et al. Effects of "in vivo"

recombinant methionyl human granulocyte colony-stimulating factor on the neutrophil response and peripheral blood colony-forming cells in healthy young and elderly adult volunteers. Blood 1994;84:2923–9.

22. Baraldi-Junkins CA, Beck AC, Rothstein G. Hematopiesis and cytokines: relevance to cancer and aging. Hematol Oncol Clin North Am 2000;14:45–51.

23. Bagnara GP, Bonsi L, Strippoli P, et al. Hemopoiesis in healthy old people and centenarian; well maintained responsiveness of CD34+ cells to hematopoietic growth factors and remodeling of cytokine network. J Gerontol A Biol Sci Med Sci 2000;55:B61–70.

24. Kumagai T, Morimoto K, Saitoh H, et al. Age-related changes in myelopoietic response to lipopolysaccharide in senescence-accelerated mice. Mech Ageing Dev 2000;112:153–7.

25. Moscinsky LC. Hemopoiesis and aging. In: Balducci L, Lyman GH, Ershler WB, editors. Comprehensive geriatric oncology. London: Harwood Academic Publisher; 1998. p. 399–412.

26. Balducci L, Hardy CL. Anemia of aging: a model of cancer-related anemia. Cancer Control. 1998;5(2 Suppl):17–21.

27. Balducci L, Hardy CL, Lyman GH. Hematopoietic growth factors and age in the older cancer patient. Curr opin Hematol 2001;8:170–87.

28. Zinzani PG, Storti S, Zaccaria A, et al. Elderly aggressive histology non-Hodgkin's lymphoma: first line VNCOP-B regimen: experience on 350 patients. Blood 1999;94:33–8.

29. Sonneveld P, de Ridder M, van der Lelie H, et al. Comparison of doxorubicin and mitoxantrone in the treatment of elderly patients with advanced diffuse non-Hodgkin's lymphoma using CHOP vs CNOP chemotherapy. J Clin Oncol 1995;13:2530–9.

30. Gomez H, Mas L, Casanova L, et al. Elderly patients with aggressive non-Hodgkin's lymphoma treated with CHOP chemotherapy plus granulocyte-macrophage colony-stimulating factor: identification of two age subgroups with differing hematologic toxicity. J Clin Oncol 1998;16:2352–8.

31. Tirelli U, Errante D, Van Glabbeke M, et al. CHOP is the standard regimen in patients ≥ 70 years of age with intermediate and high grade Non-Hodgkin's lymphoma: results of a randomized study of the European Organization for the Research and Treatment of Cancer Lymphoma Cooperative Study. J Clin Oncol 1998;16:27–34.

32. Bastion Y, Blay J-Y, Divine M, et al. Elderly patients with aggressive non-Hodgkin's lymphoma: disease presentation, response to treatment and survival. A Groupe d'Etude des Lymphomes de l'Adulte Study on 453 patients older than 69 years. J Clin Oncol 1997;15:2945–53.

33. Bertini M, Freilone R, Vitolo U, et al. The treatment of elderly patients with aggressive non-Hodgkin's lymphomas: feasiblity and efficacy of an intensive multidrug regimen. Leuk Lymphoma 1996;22:483–93.

34. O'Reilly SE, Connors JM, Howdle S, et al. In search of an optimal regimen for elderly patients with advanced-stage diffuse large-cell lymphoma: results of a phase II study of P/DOCE chemotherapy. J Clin Oncol 1993;2250–7.

35. Armitage JO, Potter JF. Aggressive chemotherapy for diffuse histiocytic lymphoma in the elderly. J Am Geriatr Soc 1984;32:269–73.

36. Bjorkholm M, Osby E, Hagberg H, et al. Randomized trial of R-methu granulocyte colony stimulating factors as adjunct to CHOP or CNOP treatment of elderly patients with aggressive non-Hodgkin's lymphoma. Proc ASH. Blood 1999;94(Suppl):599a [abstract 2665].

37. Zagonel V, Babare R, Merola MC, et al. Cost-benefit of granulocyte colony-stimulating factor administration in older patients with non-Hodgkin's lymphoma treated with combination chemotherapy. Ann Oncol 1994;5(Suppl 2):127–32.

38. De-Toledo Morrell L, Goncharova I, Dickerson B, et al. From healthy aging to early Alzheimer's disease: in vivo detection of entorhinal cortex atrophy. Ann N Y Acad Sci 2000;911:240–53.

39. Weller RO, Massey A, Kuo YM, et al. Cerebral amyloid angiopathy: accumulation of A beta in intercerebral fluid drainage pathway in Alzheimer's disease. Ann N Y Acad Sci 2000;903:110–7.

40. Kinosian BP, Stallard E, Lee JH, et al. Predicting 10-year care requirements for older people with suspected Alzheimer disease. J Am Geriatr Soc 2000;48:631–8.

41. Inouye SK, Schlesinger MJ, Lydon TJ. Delirium: a symptom of how hospital care is failing older persons and a window to improve quality of care. Am J Med 1999;106:565–73.

42. Kugler CFA. Interrelations of age, sensory functions and human brain signaling process. J Gerontol 1999;54A:B231–8.

43. Schagen SB, Van Dam FSAM, Muller MJ, et al. Cognitive deficit after postoperative adjuvant chemotherapy for breast carcinoma. Cancer 1999;85:640–50.

44. Longo DL, Young RC, Wesley M, et al. Twenty years of MOPP therapy for Hodgkin's disease. J Clin Oncol 1986;8:1157–9.

45. Apfel SC. Managing the neurotoxicity of paclitaxel and docetaxel with neurotrophic factors. Cancer Invest 2000;18:564–673.

46. Hogan DB, Ebly EM, Fung TS. Disease, disability, and age in cognitively intact seniors: results from the Canadian Study of Health and Aging. J Gerontol 1999;54A:M77–82.

47. Rosen CJ. Growth hormone and aging. Endocrine 2000;12:197–201.

48. Martin F. Frailty and the somatopause. Growth Horm IGF Res 1999;9:3–10.

49. Hamermann D, Berman JW, Albers GW, et al. Emerging evidence for inflammation in conditions frequently affecting older adults: report of a symposium. J Am Geriatr Soc 1999;47:995–9.

50. Hamermann D. Toward an understanding of frailty. Ann Intern Med 1999;130:945–50.

51. Yeh SS, Schuster MW. Geriatric cachexia: the role of cytokines. Am J Clin Nutr 1999;70:183–97.

52. Burns EA, Goodwin JS. Immunological changes of aging. In: Balducci L, Lyman GH, Ershler WB, editors. Comprehensive geriatric oncology. London: Harwood Academic Publishers; 1998. p. 213–22.

53. Franceschi C, Bonafe M, Valnesiu S, et al. Inflamm-aging: an evolutionary perspective on immunosenescense. Ann N Y Acad Sci 2000;908:244–54.

54. Ershler WB. The influence of an aging immune system on cancer incidence and progression. J Gerontol 1993;48:B3–7.

55. Balducci L, Beghe' C. The application of geriatric principles to the management of the older cancer patient. Crit Rev Hematol Oncol 2000;35:147–55.

56. Cassel CK. Money, medicine and Metusalah. Mt Sinai J Med 1998;65:237–45.

57. Monfardini S, Ferrucci L, Fratino L, et al. Validation of a multidimensional evaluation scale for use in elderly cancer patients. Cancer 1996;77:395–401.

58. Extermann M, Overcash J, Lyman GH, et al. Comorbidity and functional status are independent in older cancer patients. J Clin Oncol 1998;16:1582–7.

59. Extermann M. Measurement and impact of comorbidity in older cancer patients. CRC Hematol Oncol 2000;35:181–200.

60. Balducci L, Stanta G. Cancer in the frail patient: a coming epidemic. Hematol Oncol Clin North Am 2000;14:235–50.

61. Pierelli L, Perillo A, Greggi S, et al. Erythropoietin addition to granulocyte-colony stimulating factor abrogates life-threatening neutropenia and increases peripheral blood progenitor-cell mobilization after epirubicin, paclitaxel and cisplatin in combination chemotherapy. J Clin Oncol 1999;17:1288–96.

62. Ratain MJ, Schilsky RL, Choi KE, et al. Adaptive control of etoposide administration: impact of interpatient pharmacodynamic variability. Clin Pharmacol Ther 1989;45:226–33.

63. Silber JH, Fridman M, Di Paola RS, et al. First-cycle blood counts and subsequent neutropenia, dose reduction or delay in early stage breast cancer therapy. J Clin Oncol 1998;16:2392–400.

64. Extermann M, Chen A, Cantor AB, et al. Predictors of toxicity from chemotherapy in older patients. Proc Am Soc Clin Oncol 2000;19:617a.

65. Schijvers D, Highley M, DeBruyn E, et al. Role of red blood cell in pharmakinetics of chemotherapeutic agents. Anticancer Drugs 1999;10:147–53.

66. Von Hoff DD, Layard MW, Basa P, et al. Risk factors for doxorubicin induced congestive heart failure. Ann Intern Med 1979;91:710–7.

67. Brezden CB, Phillips KA, Abdollel M, et al. Cognitive function in breast cancer patients receiving adjuvant chemotherapy. J Clin Oncol 2000;18:2695–70.

68. Kemeny MM, Busch-Devereaux E, Merriam LT, et al. Cancer surgery in the elderly. Hematol Oncol Clin North Am 2000;14:169–92.

69. Balducci L. Quality of life in the older cancer patient. Drugs Aging 1994;4:313–24

70. Leape LL, Brennan TA, Laird NM, et al. The nature of adverse events in hospitalized patients: results of the Harvard medical practice study II. N Engl J Med 1991;324:377–84.

71. Wu AW, Yasui Y, Alzola C, et al. Predicting functional status outcomes in hospitalized patients 80 years and older. J Am Geriatr Soc 2000;48(Suppl 5):S6–15.

72. Weitzner MA, Haley WE, Chen H. The family caregiver of the older cancer patient. Hematol Oncol Clin 2000;14:269–82.

73. Haley WE, Ehrbar L, Schonwetter RS. Family caregiving issues. In: Balducci L, Lyman GH, Ershler WB, editors. Comprehensive geriatric oncology. London: Harwood Academic Publishers; 1998. p. 805–12.

74. Lewis ME. An economic profile of American older women. J Am Med Womens Assoc 1997;52:107–12.

75. Haight BK, Michel Y, Hendrix S. The extended effects of life review in nursing home residents. Int J Aging Hum Dev 2000;50:151–68.

76. Bernabei R, Landi F, Gambassi G, et al. Randomised trial of impact of model of integrated care and case management for older people living in the community. BMJ 1998;316:1348–51.

77. Alessi CA, Stuck AE, Aronow HU, et al. The process of care in preventive "in home" comprehensive geriatric assessment. J Am Geriatr Soc 1997;45:1044–50.

78. Reuben DB, Effros RB, Hirsch SH, et al. An in-home nurse-administered geriatric assessment for hypoalbuminemic older persons: development and preliminary experience. J Am Geriatr Soc 1999;47:1244–8.

79. Reuben DB, Rubenstein LV, Hirsch SH, et al. Value of functional status as predictor of mortality. Am J Med 1992;93:663–9.

80. Inouye SK, Peduzzi PN, Robison JT, et al. Importance of functional measures in predicting mortality among older hospitalized patients. JAMA 1998;279:1187–93.

81. Inouye SK, Bogardus ST, Charpentier PA, et al. A multicomponent intervention to prevent delirium in hospitalized older patients. N Engl J Med 1999;340:669–74.

82. Tinetti ME, McAvay G, Claus G, et al. A multifactorial intervention to reduce the risk of falling among elderly people living in the community. N Engl J Med 1994;331:821–7.

83. Ostchega Y, Harris TB, Hirsch R, et al. Reliability and prevalence of physical performance examination assessing mobility and balance in older persons in the US: Data from the third National Health and Nutrition Examination Survey. J Am Geriatr Soc 2000;48:1136–41.

84. Ferrucci L, Penninx BWJH, Leveille SG, et al. Characteristics of nondisabled older persons who perform poorly in objective tests of lower extremities function. J Am Geriatr Soc 2000;48:1102–10.

85. Hack V, Breitkreutz R, Kinscherf R, et al. The redox status as a correlate of senescence and wasting and as a target for therapeutic intervention. Blood 1998;54:59–67.

86. Hager K, Platt D. Fibrin degeneration product concentration (D-dimer) in the course of aging. Gerontology 1995;41:159–65.

87. Reuben DB, Ferrucci L, Wallace R, et al. The prognostic value of serum albumin in healthy older persons with low and high serum interleukin 6 (Il-6) levels. J Am Geriatr Soc 2000;48:1404–7.

88. Balducci L. A proposal for guidelines for the management of older persons with cancer. Oncology. [In press].

89. Christman K, Muss HB, Case D, et al. Chemotherapy of metastatic breast cancer in the elderly. JAMA 1992; 268:57–62.

90. Ibrahim N, Frye DK, Buzdar AU, et al. Doxorubicin based combination chemotherapy in elderly patients with metastatic breast cancer. Tolerance and outcome. Arch Intern Med 1996;156:882–8.

91. Begg CB, Carbone P. Clinical trials and drug toxicity in the elderly. The experience of the Eastern Cooperative Oncology Group. Cancer 1983;52:1986–92.

92. Giovannozzi-Bannon S, Rademaker A, Lai G, et al. Treatment tolerance of elderly cancer patients entered onto phase II clinical trials. An Illinois Cancer Center study. J Clin Oncol 1994;12:2447–52.

93. Gelman RS, Taylor SG. Cyclophosphamide, methotrexate and 5-fluorouracil chemotherapy in women more than 65 years old with advanced breast cancer. The elimination of age trends in toxicity by using doses based on creatinine clearance. J Clin Oncol 1984;2:1406–14.

94. Ibrahim NK, Buzdar AU, Asmar L, et al. Doxorubicin based adjuvant chemotherapy in elderly breast cancer patients: the M.D. Anderson experience with long term follow-up. Ann Oncol 2000;11:1–5.

95. Rowe JM, Andersen JW, Mazza JJ, et al. Randomized placebo-controlled phase III study of granulocyte-macrophage colony stimulating factor in adult patients (> 55–70 years) with acute myelogenous leukemia: a study of the Eastern Cooperative Oncology Group (E1490). Blood 1995;86:457–62.

96. Heil D, Hoelzer D, Sanz MA, et al. A randomized double blind placebo controlled phase III study of filgrastim in remission induction and consolidation therapy for patients with "de novo" acute myeloid leukemia. The International Acute Leukemia Study Group. Blood 1997;90:4710–8.

97. Tilly H, Castaigne S, Bordessoule D, et al. Low-dose cytarabine versus intensive chemotherapy in the treatment of acute non-lymphocytic leukemia in the elderly. J Clin Oncol 1990;8:272–9.

98. Cheson BD, Jasper DM, Simon R, et al. A critical appraisal of low-dose cytosine arabinoside in patients with acute non-lymphocytic leukemia and myelodysplastic syndromes. J Clin Oncol 1986;40:1857–64.

99. Meyer RJ, Davis RB, Schiffer CH, et al. Intensive postremission chemotherapy in adult with acute myeloid leukemia. N Engl J Med 1994;31:896–903.

100. Bloomfield CD, Lawrence D, Byrd JC, et al. Frequency of prolonged remission duration after high-dose cytarabine intensification in acute myeloid leukemia varies with cytogenetics subtype. Cancer Res 1998;58:4173–9.

101. Fisher RI, Gaynor ER, Dahlberg S, et al. A phase III comparison of CHOP vs m_BACOD vs ProMACE-CytaBOM vs MACOP-B in patients with intermediate or high grade non-Hodgkin's lymphoma: results of SWOG-8516. Ann Oncol 1994;5(Suppl 2):91–5.

102. Gomez H, Hidalgo M, Casanova L, et al. Risk factors for treatment-related death in elderly patients with aggressive non-Hodgkin's lymphoma: result of a multivariate analysis. J Clin Oncol 1998;16:2065–9.

103. Yoshikawa TT. Perpectives: aging and infectious diseases: past, present and future. J Infect Dis 1997;176:1053–7.

104. Norman DC. Fever and aging. Infect Dis Clin Pract 1998; 7:387–90.

105. Yoshikawa TT. Epidemiology and unique aspects of aging and infectious diseases. Clin Infect Dis 2000;30:931–3.

106. Chan DC, Brennan NJ. Delirium: making the diagnosis, improving the prognosis. Geriatrics 1999;54:28–42.

107. Deulofeu F, Cervello B, Capell S, et al. Mortality of patients with bacteremia: the importance of functional status. J Am Geriatr Soc 1998;46:14–8.

108. von Sternberg T, Hepburn K, Cibuzar P, et al. Post-hospitalization subacute care: an example of managed care model. J Am Geriatr Soc 1997;45:87–91.

109. Rolston KVI, Talcott JA. Ambulatory antimicrobial therapy for hematologic malignancies. Oncology 2000;14 (6 Suppl):17–22.

110. Freifeld AG, Pizzo PA. The outpatient management of febrile neutropenia in cancer patients. Oncology 1996;10:599–612.

111. Rolston KV. New trends in patient management: risk-based therapy for febrile patients with neutropenia. Clin Infect Dis 1999;29:2561–8.

112. Ozer H, Armitage JO, Bennett CL, et al. 2000 updated recommendations for the use of hematopoietic colony-stimulating factors. Evidence-based clinical practice guidelines. J Clin Oncol 2000;18:3558–85.

113. Dixon DO, Neilan B, Jones SE, et al. Effect of age on therapuetic outcome in advanced diffuse histiocytic lymphoma: the Southwest Oncology Group experience. Clin Oncol 1986;4:295–305.

114. Meyer RM, Browman GP, Samosh ML, et al. Randomized phase II comparison of standard CHOP with weekly CHOP in elderly patients with non-Hodgkin's lymphoma. J Clin Oncol 1995;13:2386–93.

115. Bow EJ, Rayner E, Louie TJ. Comparison of norfloxacin and cotrimoxazole for infection prophylaxis in acute leukemia. Am J Med 1988;84:847–54.

116. Curt GA, Breitbart W, Cella D, et al. Impact of cancer-related fatigue on the lives of patients: new findings from the fatigue coalition. Oncologist 2000;5:353–60.

117. Cleeland CS, Demetri GD, Glaspy J, et al. Identifying hemoglobin levels for optimal quality of life. Results of an incremental analysis. Proc Am Soc Clin Oncol 1999; 16:Abstr 2215.

118. Gabrilove JL, Einhorn LH, Livingston RB, et al. Once weekly dosing of epoietin alfa is similar to three-times weekly dosing in increasing hemoglobin and quality of life. Proc Am Soc Clin Oncol 1999;18:574A.

119. Glaspy J, Bukowski R, Steinberg C, et al. Impact of therapy with epoietin alfa on clinical outcomes in patients with non-myeloid malignancies during cancer chemotherapy in community oncology practices. J Clin Oncol 1997;5:1218–34.

120. Demetri GD, Kris M, Wade J, et al. Quality of life benefits in chemotherapy patients treated with epoietin alfa is independent from disease response and tumor type. Result of a prospective community oncology study. The procrit study group. J Clin Oncol 1998;16:3412–20.

121. Marcantonio ER, Flacker JM, Michaels M, et al. Delirium is independently associated with poor functional recovery after hip fracture. J Am Geriatr Soc 2000;48:618–24.

122. Carl W, Havens J. The cancer patient with severe mucositis. Curr Rev Pain 2000;4:192–202.

123. Gordon B, Spadinger A, Hodges E, et al. Effect of granulocyte-macrophage colony-stimulating factor on oral mucositis after hematopoietic stem cell transplantation. J Clin Oncol 1994;12:1917–22.

124. Symonds RP. Treatment induced mucositis: an old problem with new remedies. Br J Cancer 1998;77:1689–95.

125. Maurer CA, Renzulli P, Mazzucchelli L, et al. Use of accurate diagnostic criteria may increase the incidence of stercoral perforation of the colon. Dis Colon Rectum 2000;43:991–8.

126. Flacker JM, Lipsitz LA. Neural mechanisms of delirium: current hypotheses and evolving concepts. J Gerontol 1999;54:B239–46.

127. Mulder GJ. Glucuronidation and its role in regulation of biological activities of drugs. Ann Rev Pharmacol Toxicol 1990;32:25–43.

128. Abbott FV, Palmour RM. Morphine 6-glucuronide. Analgesic effects and receptor binding profile in rats. Life Sci 1988;43:1685–91.

CHAPTER 26

DIAGNOSTIC IMAGING IN ONCOLOGIC EMERGENCIES

RICHARD J. HATCHETT, MD
CHRISTOPHER J. KRIPAS, MD

Cancer patients frequently have complicated medical histories, are at risk for complications relating both to their underlying malignancies and to the treatments they receive, and often present with nonspecific symptoms such as dyspnea or back pain. The evaluation of such patients in emergency or urgent care settings, therefore, is facilitated by and often requires the use of diagnostic imaging. Additionally, certain diagnoses for which cancer patients are at greater-than-usual risk, such as venous thromboembolism or bowel obstruction, cannot be reliably established on clinical grounds alone; and certain (especially the neurologic) manifestations of malignancy require prompt diagnosis and intervention to avoid negative outcomes. In practical terms, then, the threshold for the use of diagnostic imaging studies in most cancer patients is quite low, and the importance of using such studies in a reasoned and judicious way cannot be overemphasized.

We have organized this chapter by body region; under each region, we discuss the use of imaging procedures in the evaluation and management of patients with specific clinical syndromes or symptom complexes. We have chosen this approach to make the chapter as relevant as possible to the concerns of physicians encountering cancer patients in emergency or urgent care settings. We assume that the reader is familiar with the techniques of plain radiography and begin with some general remarks about more advanced modalities, specifically ultrasonography, computed tomography (CT), and magnetic resonance imaging (MRI).

IMAGING METHODS

Ultrasonography

Ultrasonographic imaging is rapid and noninvasive, and it is the only advanced technique that may be performed at the patient's bedside. The tissue of interest reflects sound, and the returning echoes are reconstructed into an image. Echogenic structures produce echoes and appear white while anechoic structures do not produce echoes, allow the unreflected transmission of sound waves, and appear black. The usefulness of ultrasonography is consequently limited by the ability of anatomic structures to conduct and reflect sound waves. Soft tissues conduct sound more efficiently than liquid or air; thus, in practical terms, ultrasonography is not useful for assessing lungs or gas-filled bowel loops. This fact also explains why a full bladder is necessary to image deeper pelvic structures when an external transducer is used. To overcome this inherent limitation, intracavitary transducers are being used increasingly for endovaginal, transrectal, and transesophageal imaging. The development of Doppler technology has substantially increased the usefulness of diagnostic ultrasonography. Doppler shift occurs when returning echoes undergo changes in frequency as they are reflected off moving structures (eg, circulating red blood cells). Such shifts, represented graphically, can be used to evaluate for the presence or absence of flow.[1]

Computed Tomography

Computed tomography uses ionizing radiation, but unlike conventional plain-film radiography, the x-ray tube and opposing photon detectors rotate around the patient while collecting data. The digital information collected is subsequently reconstructed to form cross-sectional images at the level of interest.[2] As with plain radiographs, the density of the recorded image relates to the ability of any given tissue to absorb the ionizing radiation. Air absorbs little radiation and appears black (hypodense) on the CT image whereas bone, which is highly absorptive, appears white (hyperdense). Between these extremes, the CT reconstruction can distinguish density differences as small as 4%, yielding images that demonstrate subtle changes in tissue composition. Plain-film radiography, by contrast, can resolve changes in tissue density of no less than 10%.[3] The index of attenuation is stated in Hounsfield units (HU) and generally ranges from 1,000 (bone) to 0 (water) to −1,000 (air).[4] The range of the scale used in a given reconstruction can be adjusted to maximize the resolution of specific types of tissue, as with the so-called bone and lung windows, according to the needs of the interpreter. The spectrum of an image is defined by the "window width" and "level." The window width is the number of Hounsfield units spanned by the gray scale while the level is the Hounsfield unit assigned to the center of the gray scale. For example, a window width of 500 is often used for imaging the mediastinum, with a window level of 39. In this case, all pixels within the range of −211 to 289 HU will be displayed. Most lungs (largely air) will have an index of attenuation of < −211 HU and therefore appear black on the final image.

The spacing between cross sections (ie, collimation) will vary according to the information being sought. Helical or spiral CT technology permits scanning while the table top moves continuously during a single breath-hold. Faster data aquisition results in superior vascular opacification and allows the study of the larger pulmonary and systemic vessels as an alternative to conventional angiography. Helical CT technology minimizes respiratory artifacts, decreases contrast volume requirements and scan time, and allows more sophisticated image reconstruction with three-dimensional reformations.[5]

Intravenous (IV) contrast opacifies blood vessels and identifies areas of relatively decreased vascularity by its absence. In cranial imaging, contrast demonstrates areas of blood-brain-barrier breakdown by leaking across the defect. Contrast media are available in ionic (high osmolality [several thousand mOsm/kg]) and nonionic (low osmolality [600 to 1,500 mOsm/kg]) formulations. Minor adverse reactions to IV contrast include flushing, nausea and vomiting, and pain at the injection site. The most common severe adverse effects of IV contrast are hypersensitivity reactions, ranging from urticaria to life-threatening anaphylaxis, and nephrotoxicity. In general, acute renal failure following the administration of radiocontrast is more common in patients who are elderly, volume depleted, or already afflicted with renal insufficiency. Radiocontrast should be used cautiously in patients suffering from diabetic nephropathy or advanced heart failure. Cancer patients receiving nephrotoxic chemotherapy are at increased risk of developing acute renal failure with radiocontrast, as are those who have had other recent radiocontrast studies, and acute renal failure is a potential although infrequent (< 1.5%) complication of radiocontrast administration in patients with multiple myeloma.[6] Patients at risk who require studies with IV contrast should be well hydrated prior to the administration of contrast. Of note, the risk of death from adverse reactions from either ionic or nonionic contrast is identical (0.9 per 100,000) but the risk of severe reactions has been reported as 157 and 126 per 100,000 uses, respectively.[7] Informed consent is required for IV contrast, and a prior severe reaction is a contraindication for administration. If CT with contrast is required, patients who have had prior non-life-threatening hypersensitivity reactions may be premedicated with corticosteroids and antihistamines. Protocols for premedication vary from institution to institution and may be implemented after discussion with the consulting radiologist.

Oral contrast opacifies the bowel. While gas and stool provide natural contrast within the large bowel, the small bowel normally does not contain much air or liquid. Water-soluble oral contrast is preferable to barium in most cases because aspiration or extravasation of barium into the peritoneum can lead to significant complications. The most commonly used water-soluble oral contrast agent is meglumine diatrizoate (Gastrografin [Bristol-Meyers Squibb, Wallingford, CT]). In certain circumstances, rectal and bladder contrast may also be helpful.

Magnetic Resonance Imaging

Magnetic resonance imaging uses no ionizing radiation, relying instead on the behavior of atomic nuclei (usually hydrogen) after excitation in a magnetic field in the tissue of interest. Magnetic resonance (MR) techniques allow for multiplanar imaging, do not produce bone artifacts, and are extremely useful for the evaluation of the central nervous and musculoskeletal systems. Magnetic resonance imaging is clearly better than CT in detecting and defining the extent of recurrent or residual lesions in the central nervous system, and magnetic resonance images of the posterior fossa are superior to those of CT in that they are not degraded by bone artifacts.

Magnetic resonance imaging is contraindicated in patients with cardiac pacemakers, implanted neurostimulators, metallic foreign bodies in or near the orbits, cochlear implants, non-MR-compatible metallic surgical clips (eg, aneurysm clips) and tissue expanders. Conventional "closed" MRI causes significant claustrophobia in some patients. Where it is available, such patients may tolerate "open" MRI better; alternatively, they can be premedicated with anxiolytics. Claustrophobia is seldom a complete contraindication for MRI.

Standard MRI provides T1- and T2-weighted precontrast and T1-weighted postcontrast images. Chelated gadolinium, the contrast agent used in MRI, increases T1 relaxation. When used to image the central nervous system, it leaks through defects in the blood-brain barrier; lesions collecting gadolinium then appear as hyperintense or white on postcontrast T1-weighted images. Gadolinium is also used to evaluate liver lesions that are not adequately depicted with other imaging techiques.[8] Gadolinium has few side effects, and hypersensitivity reactions are rare. Gadolinium compounds are well tolerated in patients with hepatic and renal insufficiency. The use of gadolinium contrast is contraindicated only in patients who have had earlier hypersensitivity reactions to gadolinium or gadolinium compounds.

Recent technologic advances in MRI are well outlined elsewhere.[9,10] Fluid-attenuated inversion recovery (FLAIR), magnetization transfer (MT), diffusion-weighted imaging (DWI), perfusion imaging (PI), magnetic resonance angiography (MRA), and magnetic resonance spectroscopy (MRS) are among the techniques that will play an increasing role in the evaluation and management of patients with cancer. As studies of cost-effectiveness and outcome accumulate, MRI may replace CT as the mode of choice for imaging patients with acute stroke[10] and may also come to play a more prominent role in the evaluation of acute complaints in patients with cancer.

IMAGING OF THE BRAIN AND SPINAL CORD

Nontraumatic central nervous system (CNS) dysfunction is one of the most common reasons patients come to the emergency department. The causes of CNS dysfunction are numerous, and a wide differential diagnosis must be considered for any given patient.[11] Altered mental status is cited as a reason for admission in approximately 10% of all hospitalized patients, and CNS dysfunction is especially common in patients with cancer.[12] Central and peripheral neurologic disorders have been reported to affect roughly 15% of patients with cancer at some point in their disease.[13] At Memorial Sloan-Kettering Cancer Center, the most common neurologic diagnoses in patients seen for neurologic symptoms are brain metastases (16% of all consultations), metabolic encephalopathy (10%), pain associated with bone metastases (10%), and epidural tumor (8%).[14] These complications usually occur in patients with advanced disease, but 10% of patients with lung cancer first present with symptomatic brain metastases, and approximately 20% of patients developing epidural spinal-cord compression present with that condition as the initial manifestation of their malignancy.[15,16] Neurologic abnormalities in patients with cancer may be caused by metastatic deposits, paraneoplastic syndromes, infection, or metabolic derangements; they can also be an adverse consequence of therapy or be coincidental.[17]

Epidural spinal-cord compression, raised intracranial pressure, status epilepticus, and intracerebral hemorrhage are the most common true neurologic emergencies in the cancer patient.[18] Although any primary tumor can metastasize to any part of the nervous system, some tumors have a predilection for causing specific complications. Leukemia and lymphoma, for example, commonly involve the leptomeninges whereas prostate cancer often metastasizes to the vertebral column (leading to cauda equina compression and epidural spinal-cord compression) but seldom metastasizes to the leptomeninges or brain.[19,20] Likewise, vertebral metastases from lung and breast carcinoma are frequent causes of epidural spinal-cord compression.[21] The full evaluation of patients presenting with seizures, mental status change, focal neurologic abnormalities, or signs or symptoms of spinal-cord compression is described in Chapter 12.

In the emergency setting, CT and MRI are by far the most important tools for evaluating dysfunction of the central nervous system. Both techniques can be performed with or without the administration of intravenous contrast material, depending on the nature of the patient's symptoms. It is usually wise to confer with the neurology and/or radiology consultants before ordering any particular study.

Intracranial Masses

Each year in the United States, an estimated 17,500 people are diagnosed with a primary brain malignancy while 66,000 others develop brain metastases.[22,23] Lung, breast, melanoma, genitourinary, and gastrointestinal malignancies are among those that commonly metastasize to the brain. Pelvic and gastrointestinal tumors, for unknown reasons, have a predilection for the cerebellum rather than the cerebral hemispheres.[24] Roughly one of every five patients with systemic cancer eventually develops evidence of brain metastases, and expanding masses in the cranial vault may precipitate fatal cerebral herniation when untreated.

Headache is often the presenting complaint. Seventy percent of patients with an intracranial neoplasm report headaches.[25] Other causes of headache that must be considered include migraine, cluster or tension headache, sinusitis, temporal arteritis, meningitis, abscess, hypertensive crisis, and intracranial hemorrhage or hematoma. Patients with cancer may be at increased risk of venous sinus thrombosis because of hypercoagulability or direct compression from the tumor.[26]

Worrisome signs and symptoms include new-onset or first severe headache; persistent or unilateral headache; a change in the frequency, intensity, or location of headache; and concomitant meningismus, vomiting, fever, or focal neurologic deficits. In the absence of headache, other presenting complaints in patients with the subsequent diagnosis of brain metastases include focal weakness, mental disturbances, seizures, and gait ataxia.[15] The evaluation of patients with cancer and any of these signs or symptoms should include neurologic imaging. Likewise, patients with known brain metastases who present with a sudden change of mental status require immediate neuroimaging. Lumbar puncture, when indicated, should be considered only after the risk of cerebral herniation has been assessed.

Neuroimaging usually begins with unenhanced CT of the brain. Unenhanced CT is fast, is widely available, and has no absolute contraindications. Also, the configuration of the scanner permits continuous monitoring and (if necessary) mechanical ventilation of critically ill patients. Computed tomography is more sensitive than MRI for cranial fractures and adequately demonstrates intracranial bleeding, hydrocephalus, cerebral edema and mass effect. Unenhanced CT may miss smaller or bilateral metastatic lesions and frequently underestimates the number of lesions present. The use of IV contrast improves the sensitivity of CT by increasing the density of most metastatic tumors. The administration of IV contrast, however, also lowers the seizure threshold. If brain metastases are strongly suspected, premedication with a benzodiazepine should be considered.

Magnetic resonance imaging with gadolinium enhancement is the best diagnostic test for brain metastases but is not usually available in the emergency setting. Compared with CT, MRI is more sensitive in revealing small lesions, particularly in the brain stem and cerebellum. On T2-weighted images, free water (cerebrospinal fluid [CSF]) has the highest signal intensity and appears brightest, followed by edematous parenchyma and then normal parenchyma.[27] Thus, on T2-weighted images, the edema that commonly circumscribes tumor deposits appears hyperintense when compared with normal parenchyma.[15] Contrast enhancement with gadolinium further increases the sensitivity of MRI in diagnosing brain lesions, by highlighting areas of blood-brain-barrier breakdown. Almost all tumors appear hyperintense on T1-weighted postgadolinium images (Figure 26–1).[28]

Intracranial Hemorrhage

Falls are common in patients with cancer. The side effects of medication, general debilitation, and neurologic deficits (when present) all increase the risk of falls in this population. Coagulopathies related to anticoagulation, hepatic insufficiency, vitamin K deficiency, and/or thrombocytopenia may increase the risk of bleeding with minor trauma. While most subdural hematomas are due to head trauma, they also occur in association with dural metastases and carry a significant risk of mortality in any circumstance. Patients with a subdural hematoma may present with symptoms that have evolved hours to months after the initial insult.[29] The imaging technique of choice is noncontrast CT. Depending on the chronicity of the hematoma, the image may vary in density. Computed tomographic images depict acute subdural hematomas as high-density masses adjacent to the cal-

varium. In subacute subdural hematomas (which develop 2 to 6 weeks after the precipitating trauma), the hematoma adjacent to the brain may be isodense with normal parenchyma, so that the only sign of the hematoma is parenchymal shift. If bilateral isodense hematomas are present, the offsetting compression may cause the CT image to appear normal. A normal CT image with small ventricles in an elderly patient suggests the diagnosis of bilateral isodense hematomas. Chronic subdural hematomas may appear hypodense with an enhancing membrane and may appear loculated. Magnetic resonance imaging is reliable for further evaluation of a suspected subacute or chronic subdural hematoma. Using MR FLAIR sequencing increases sensitivity for subdural hematoma from 21% (using standard T2-weighted images) to 79%.[30]

Because of their abnormal vasculature, intracranial tumors introduce a risk of bleeding. This catastrophic complication occurs most frequently with melanoma, renal, and germ cell (especially choriocarcinoma) metastases.[31] Patients with acute myeloid leukemia who develop hyperleukocytosis (white blood cell count [WBC] > 100,000/mm^3) also have an increased risk of intracerebral hemorrhage;[32] such patients present with the sudden onset of headache, vomiting, and/or neurologic deficits that worsen over a period of 30 to 90 minutes. Acute intraparenchymal hemorrhage is most easily documented with noncontrast CT. Acute intracerebral hemorrhage manifests radiographically as a homogenous high-attenuation lesion.[33] The center of the hematoma may appear hypodense. Mass effect and surrounding hypodense parenchymal edema may be noted, particularly with large hematomas.

Patients with brain metastases, meningiomas, or primary brain tumors occasionally present with subarachnoid hemorrhage (SAH). Tumor, coagulopathy, and vasculitis account for 15 to 20% of all cases of SAH.[11] Again, non-enhanced CT is the first imaging study. Computed tomography of patients with SAH demonstrates hyperdense blood within the cisterns or ventricles. Fluid-attenuated inversion-recovery MR imaging is also highly sensitive for the detection of SAH.[34] The sensitivity of CT for SAH has been reported to be 92% within 24 hours of the ictus, so a negative result does not definitively exclude this condition.[35] When patients present with histories suggestive of SAH but their imaging studies are normal, lumbar puncture is recommended.[33]

Ischemic Stroke

Ischemic stroke is a common nontraumatic neurologic emergency and has been well reviewed elsewhere.[36,37] In the patient with cancer, direct effects of tumor and indirect effects of treatment may increase the risk of embolic stroke or thrombotic complications. Radiation therapy that

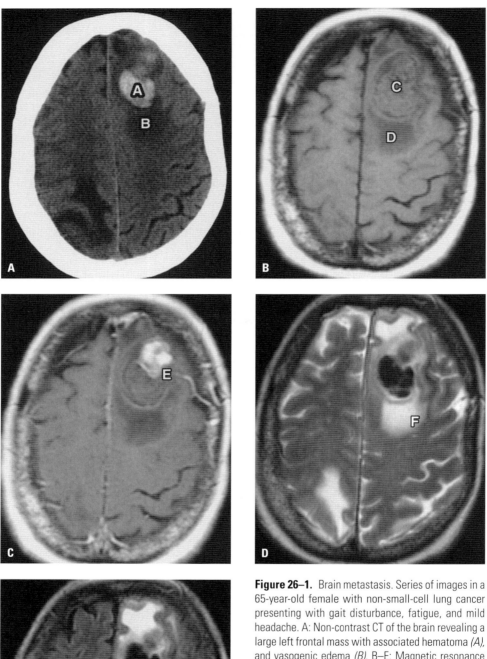

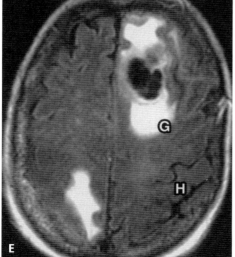

Figure 26–1. Brain metastasis. Series of images in a 65-year-old female with non-small-cell lung cancer presenting with gait disturbance, fatigue, and mild headache. A: Non-contrast CT of the brain revealing a large left frontal mass with associated hematoma *(A)*, and vasogenic edema *(B)*. B–E: Magnetic resonance imaging of the brain with and without gadolinium enhancement. B: Pre-contrast T1-weighted image reveals left frontal mass *(C)*, and associated cerebral edema *(D)*. C: Post-gadolinium enhanced T1-weighted image shows contrast-enhancement of frontal metastasis *(E)*. D: T2-weighted image outlines areas of vasogenic edema *(F)*. E: Fluid attenuated inversion recovery (FLAIR), image showing the effective CSF nulling effect of this technique. Compared with plate D, area of edema *(G)*, is made more conspicuous by eliminating signal from CSF *(H)*.

includes cervical or cerebral vessels, for example, can lead to accelerated atherosclerosis and stenosis months or years after radiation therapy.[17] Patients with certain malignancies (eg, acute promyelocytic leukemia and some adenocarcinomas) are at increased risk of developing disseminated intravascular coagulation, which may result in cerebrovascular thrombosis.[38] Emboli from opportunistic infections (usually fungal) as well as from nonbacterial thrombotic endocarditis can also cause cerebral infarction.[31] Cerebral venous thrombosis occasionally occurs as a consequence of tumor-associated coagulopathy or direct compression by tumor.[17,26] Thrombotic stroke and superior sagittal sinus thrombosis are frequently reported in patients treated with L-asparaginase.[39] Ipsilateral hemispheric infarction has been reported following trigeminal or segmental herpes zoster infection.[40]

Stable patients with symptoms suggesting nonhemorrhagic stroke may be evaluated by using MRI of the brain, without gadolinium. With the use of DWI, areas of infarction will be evident within minutes (Figure 26–2).[37] Emergency MRI that includes DWI, perfusion-weighted imaging, MRA, T2-weighted imaging, and susceptibility-weighted MR for hemorrhage detection can rule out intracranial hemorrhage and confirm ischemic pathology in one scanning session. Emergency MRI may thus soon become the imaging modality of choice for patients with acute stroke.[41] For patients who are unstable, or when emergent MRI is not available, noncontrast CT is recommended. Computed tomographic scans obtained within the first 6 hours are normal approximately 60% of the time and may need to be repeated sequentially to identify the infarct.[37]

Seizure

Seizure is the presenting complaint in 15 to 20% of patients with brain metastases and occurs at some point in 25 to 56% of patients with known metastatic disease.[15] In the patient with cancer, the possible precipitants of seizure are numerous.[18] The decision to pursue emergent scanning depends on a variety of factors. It is recommended that scans be performed in all patients with seizure and new focal deficits, persistent altered mental status, fever, recent trauma, persistent headache, coagulopathy, or suspicion of acquired immunodeficiency syndrome (AIDS).[42] In patients with status epilepticus, seizure activity must be controlled before radiologic images are obtained. Because most of the life-threatening causes of seizure involve mass effect, hemorrhage, or cerebral edema, noncontrast CT is recommended as the first study after the patient is stabilized. If recommended by the neurologic consultant, follow-up MRI can be performed subsequently.

Diffuse Cerebral Edema Not Specifically Related to Brain Metastases

Diffuse cerebral edema sometimes develops during radiation therapy, but this complication is rare with the doses used in conventional external-beam radiation.[43] Cerebral edema as a consequence of hypertensive encephalopathy is sometimes observed after treatment with immunosuppressive agents (eg, cyclosporin A).[44] Non-enhanced CT of such patients demonstrates global diffuse low attenuation, effacement of sulci, and compression of the ventricular system.[11] Thrombosis of the cortical veins or venous sinus is an uncommon cause of diffuse cerebral edema. Magnetic resonance imaging is substantially superior to CT at identifying dural sinus thrombosis and shows abnormal signal intensity in the dural sinus or major veins.[26]

Infection of the Central Nervous System

Patients with cancer are at increased risk of CNS infection.[45] Patients with primary brain tumors or brain metastases may be at increased risk of meningitis because of immune compromise, defects in the blood-brain barrier, the presence of Ommaya reservoirs, or the placement of ventriculoperitoneal shunts to alleviate hydrocephalus. The causative organisms, diagnosis, and treatment of meningitis have been well outlined elsewhere.[46] Noncon-

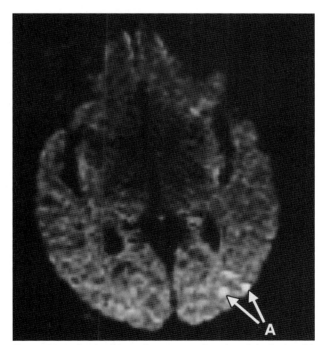

Figure 26–2. Stroke. Magnetic resonance imaging of the brain with diffusion-weighted imaging (DWI), in a 67-year-old female with multiple myeloma presenting with intermittent visual changes. Diffusion weighted image reveals punctate areas of restricted diffusion in left occipital area *(A)*, representing probable recent cortical infarction.

trast CT in patients with suspected meningitis is typically obtained prior to lumbar puncture, to identify those at risk of cerebral herniation due to increased intracranial pressure as a consequence of abscess or empyema. The presence of a concomitant intracranial malignancy may increase the risk of this catastophic complication and mandates imaging prior to lumbar puncture.

Brain abscesses may evolve in the setting of bacterial, fungal, protozoan, and even helminthic infection. Patients may present with symptoms of acute cerebritis, or they may report symptoms evolving over weeks to months.[47] Central nervous system dysfunction relates to the mass effect of the lesion as well as to direct neuronal damage from the inflammatory response. In patients with cancer of the head and neck, abscesses may develop because of contiguous extension of infection in the mastoid process, middle ear, or paranasal sinuses. Brain abscess may also evolve hematogenously from a distant focus, beginning as a cerebritis that later becomes encapsulated. Neovascularization occurs at the border of the cerebritis. The blood-brain barrier is not fully developed in these vessels, however, so a contrast-enhancing rim is easily visualized. Thus, contrast-enhanced CT is the study of choice in patients with suspected cerebritis or abscess (Figure 26–3).

Evaluation of Spinal-Cord Compression and Leptomeningeal Carcinomatosis

Epidural spinal cord compression (ESCC) is the compression of the thecal sac by tumor in the epidural space anywhere along the spinal cord or the cauda equina. Tumor is usually confined to the epidural space, with intradural involvement noted in only 2 to 4% of cases.[48] Epidural disease commonly reflects extension from metastases in the vertebral bodies, and vertebral-body metastases occur in 25 to 70% of patients with stage IV disease.[49] The distribution of metastases is in rough proportion to the vertebral-body volumes: approximately 50% occur in the thoracic spine, 35% occur in the lumbar and sacral spine, and 15% occur in the cervical spine.[21] One-third of patients with ESCC have multiple sites of epidural metastases.[50] Pain is present in 95% of patients with ESCC and typically precedes any other symptom by 1 to 2 months. A sudden worsening of pain in a patient with known vertebral metastases suggests the development of a pathologic compression fracture. The differential diagnosis for patients with symptoms suggestive of ESCC also includes intramedullary metastasis, disc herniation, suppurative bacterial infections, tuberculosis, hemorrhage, chordoma, and (in those patients who have been previously irradiated) chronic progressive radiation myelopathy.[51] Chronic progressive radiation myelopathy typically develops 9 to 15 months after radiotherapy and is dependent on the total radiation dose and length of cord irradiated.

The presentation is one of progressive myelopathy with pain.[52] Intramedullary spinal metastases occur about one-fifteenth as often as ESCC and are usually associated with lung cancer (particularly small-cell lung cancer).[53] Approximately one-third to one-half of patients with intramedullary disease present with Brown-Séquard's or pseudo–Brown-Séquard's syndrome (hemiparaplegia and hyperesthesia, with ipsilateral loss of joint and muscle sense and contralateral hemianesthesia).[53] Rarely, paraplegia (the pathogenesis of which is unknown) can also be caused by intrathecal chemotherapy with methotrexate or cytosine arabinoside (ara-C).[54,55]

The importance of early diagnosis and prompt initiation of therapy for ESCC cannot be overemphasized. Poor clinical outcomes are the rule once neurologic function has deteriorated, but 80 to 98% of patients who are ambulatory at the start of therapy will remain ambulatory. Patients with tumors known to be radiosensitive have a higher chance of regaining some neurologic function and are less likely to relapse at the site of treatment.[56,57]

In cancer patients with back pain and suspected spinal column involvement but without neurologic compromise, plain-film radiography of the spine is the initial diagnostic test. Plain films carry a high false-negative rate and are helpful only when abnormal. Findings that can

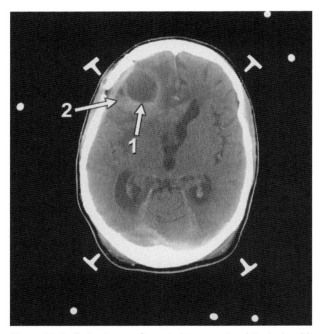

Figure 26–3. Brain abscess. Computed tomography of the brain with intravenous contrast in a 39-year-old female with oligodendroglioma. The patient presented 15 months after craniotomy with signs and symptoms of meningitis. The patient's head is in a stereotactic frame. Underlying the previous craniotomy site the CT scan shows (1) abscess with peripheral enhancement as well as (2) surrounding cerebritis. Also notable is the dilated ventricular system consistent with hydrocephalus.

be documented by plain-film radiography include the destruction or collapse of vertebral bodies, erosion of the pedicles, and (occasionally) the presence of paravertebral soft-tissue masses. In the neurologically intact patient, a normal plain-film series can be followed by outpatient bone scanning. In one retrospective study, 12% of patients with symptomatic epidural disease (pain or neurologic dysfunction) had no plain-film findings but had abnormal results on bone scintigraphy.[58]

Any patient with neurologic complaints, radiculopathy, myelopathy, severe or progressive pain, or suspected pathology found by plain-film radiography is a candidate for more definitive studies. Because of its ability to image the entire spine and to demonstrate intramedullary lesions, MRI is now the study of choice in most patients. Magnetic resonance imaging without contrast enhancement should be done when ESCC is suspected (Figure 26–4). Studies with gadolinium enhancement should be performed if other causes of myelopathy are being considered (eg, leptomeningeal disease, radiation myelopathy, transverse myelopathy, intramedullary tumor, or intradural tumor). Computed tomographic myelography may occasionally be necessary when MRI is contraindicated; CT myelography additionally allows for the simultaneous collection of CSF. In general, however, lumbar puncture should be avoided as the release of spinal fluid caudal to a partial blockage can

lead to herniation of the spinal cord and result in paraplegia.[59] A useful algorithm for the management of back pain in patients with cancer has been published previously.[49]

Leptomeningeal metastases occur when tumor cells seed the meninges either diffusely or multifocally. Leptomeningeal carcinomatosis, or carcinomatous meningitis, generally carries a poor prognosis and will relentlessly progress if left untreated, leading to neurologic dysfunction and death within weeks. The incidence of this complication varies with different types of malignancy but approximates 8% overall.[60] Any malignancy can involve the meninges, but certain malignancies (such as non-Hodgkin's lymphoma, acute lymphoblastic, acute myelogenous, and chronic lymphocytic leukemias [ALL, AML, and CLL], breast cancer, small-cell lung cancer, and melanoma) are more likely to do so.[17] Typically, patients with leptomeningeal disease present with multiple neurologic complaints and findings that suggest disease at multiple sites of the neuroaxis. Certain findings (such as headache without evidence of metastasis on CT or MRI, multiple cranial nerve palsies, radicular symptoms in any of the extremities without spinal pain, and asymmetric leg weakness with decreased reflexes but without a sensory component) should lead the clinician to consider the diagnosis.[17]

The diagnosis typically requires documentation of malignant cells in the CSF. False-positives are rare except

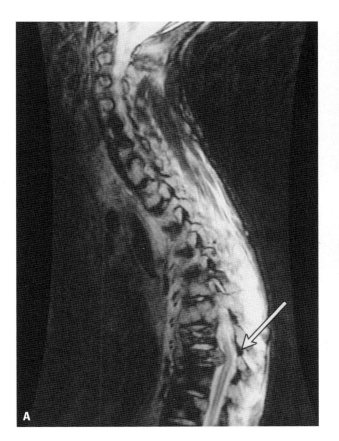

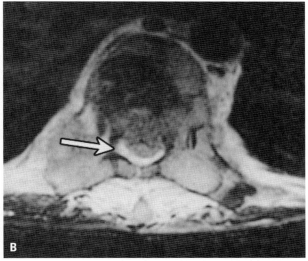

Figure 26–4. Spinal cord compression. Magnetic resonance imaging of spine without gadolinium enhancement in a 22-year-old patient with metastatic nasopharyngeal carcinoma presenting with back pain. A: Sagittal view, shows pathologic compression fracture at T8 level with moderately severe spinal cord compression *(arrow)*. B: T2-weighted axial view at this level shows retropulsion of the collapsed vertebral body and compression of spinal cord *(arrow)* with loss of ventral thecal space.

in leukemia and lymphoma. Imaging may serve as an adjunct to diagnosis and entails a gadolinium-enhanced MRI evaluation of the entire neuroaxis. Contrast-enhanced MRI of the brain may demonstrate communicating hydrocephalus, enhancement of the leptomeninges, or cortical or ependymal nodularity; however, the result can be normal. Spinal MRI with gadolinium, which can also yield normal results in patients with documented disease, may show enhancement of the leptomeninges, and nodular or diffuse thickening of nerve roots (Figure 26–5). Gadolinium-enhanced MRI showing enhancement of the basal cisterns, cauda equina, or ependyma provides sufficient confirmation for treatment of symptomatic patients, even in the absence of malignant cells in the CSF.[61] Further, in cases in which leptomeningeal disease is likely, diagnostic MRI can obviate the need for lumbar puncture.

IMAGING OF THE CHEST AND EVALUATION OF SUSPECTED VENOUS THROMBOEMBOLISM

Common thoracic complications of malignancy include pleural, pulmonary, myocardial, and pericardial metastases; malignant pleural and pericardial effusions; obstruction of the superior vena cava; pneumonitis related to radiation or the use of certain chemotherapeutic agents; congestive heart failure, with or without pulmonary edema; noncardiogenic pulmonary edema; bacterial, viral, or fungal pneumonia; and pulmonary embolism. These conditions, as well as their evaluation and management, are described at length in Chapter 10, Chapter 11, and Chapter 14. This section describes strategies for the use of diagnostic imaging in cancer patients who present with chest pain (with or without pleurisy, dyspnea, cough, or hemoptysis) and/or with physical examination findings suggestive of pneumonia, pulmonary edema, or pleural effusion. Because the diagnosis is based on radiologic confirmation of a clot in the pulmonary or peripheral vasculature, this section also describes an approach to the evaluation of patients with suspected venous thromboembolic disease. The use of echocardiography in patients suspected of having myocardial ischemia, cardiomyopathy, or pericardial tamponade is described in Chapter 14.

Plain-Film Radiography and Pulmonary Infiltrates in Patients with Cancer

Chest radiography is a useful imaging method in any patient presenting with symptoms of cardiopulmonary

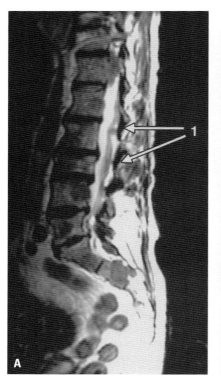
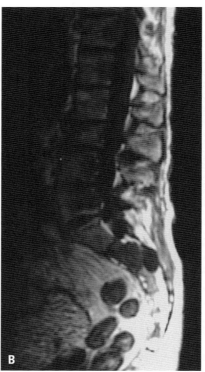
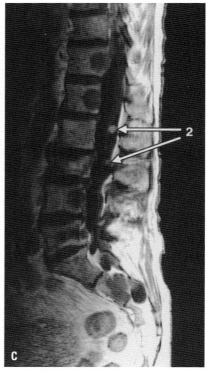

Figure 26–5. Leptomeningeal disease. A–C: Magnetic resonance imaging of total spine with and without gadolinium enhancement in a 76-year-old man with metastatic adenocarcinoma of unknown primary. A: Sagittal T2-weighted image showing multiple sites of leptomeningeal disease at L2 and L3 levels *(1)*. B: Pre-contrast T1-weighted sagittal image of similar section. C: T1-weighted post gadolinium enhancement of revealing leptomeningeal deposits at L2 and L3 levels *(2)*.

disease. It provides information about the size and configuration of the heart and great vessels and is the cornerstone of the work-up of patients with suspected pulmonary disease. Pathophysiologic alterations of pulmonary vascular pressures may be reflected in the dilatation of the pulmonary artery and its central branches, the pruning of the distal pulmonary arteries, or the development of perivascular, interstitial, and (ultimately) alveolar pulmonary edema. Plain-film radiography may also visualize abnormalities of thoracic structure; pulmonary, mediastinal, and pleural masses; consolidated and interstitial infiltrates; cysts and other bronchiectatic changes; pleural effusions; and abscesses (Figure 26–6). Many of the cardiopulmonary complications of cancer or its therapy produce changes visible in the chest radiograph (Table 26–1), and the most important of these findings are discussed below. Patients with cancer frequently suffer from coexisting but unrelated chronic cardiopulmonary conditions, and of course, they may develop any form of acute cardiopulmonary disease found in patients without cancer, but it is beyond the scope of this section to discuss the associated radiographic findings in these circumstances.

Pulmonary infiltrates in cancer patients are usually infectious, iatrogenic, or neoplastic in origin. Miscellaneous causes of pulmonary infiltrates include diffuse alveolar hemorrhage, sarcoidosis or sarcoidlike reactions, bronchiolitis obliterans with organizing pneumonia (BOOP), and (occasionally) pulmonary embolus.[62–66] In patients with leukemia, infiltrates will sometimes reflect leukostasis, the syndrome of leukemic cell lysis pneumonopathy, or hyperleukocytic reactions.[67] The findings from chest radiography, in conjunction with a careful history and physical examination, will narrow the differential in any particular case although additional imaging studies, fiberoptic bronchoscopy with bronchoalveolar lavage, and (occasionally) open lung biopsy may be required for definitive diagnosis.

Infiltrates Related to Infection. The infiltrates of infection may be focal or diffuse. Focal infiltrates represent bacterial infection in the majority of cases.[68] Diffuse infiltrates occur more commonly in immunocompromised hosts and have an infectious and usually opportunistic etiology in the plurality in this setting (up to 75% in some series).[69,70] Focal infiltrates may reflect pneumonia caused by any of the usual community-acquired or nosocomial pathogens. In patients who are neutropenic or suffering from hematologic malignancies, focal infiltrates often denote infection with gram-negative organisms such as *Pseudomonas aeruginosa*, *Escherichia coli*, and *Klebsiella pneumoniae*.[67] Mycobacteria, viruses (mainly *Cytomegalovirus*), *Pneumocystis carinii*, and fungal pathogens such as *Aspergillus, Can-*

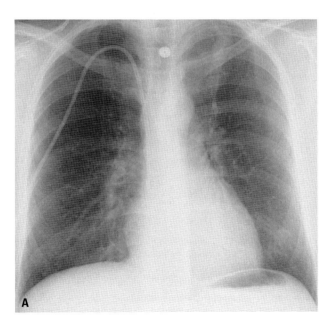 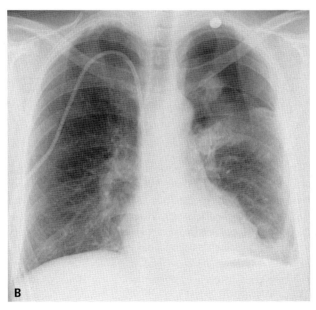

Figure 26–6. Pre- and postoperative posteroanterior radiographs of the chest in a 41-year-old man with refractory acute lymphoblastic leukemia. Panel A demonstrates a vague opacity at the left apex initially thought to represent recurrent fungal pneumonia. A left upper lobe wedge resection the day after this radiograph was taken revealed lobar pneumonia with focal areas of organization and abscess formation. Culture of biopsy specimens revealed infection with *Pseudomonas aeruginosa*. Ten days postoperatively, and 7 days after the patient's chest tubes were removed, the patient complained of intense pain in the left chest. Panel B demonstrates the development of a new large left hydropneumothorax with extensive atelectasis of the upper lung. An air-fluid level is visible at the left base.

TABLE 26–1. Radiographic Appearance Associated with Common Pulmonary Disorders in Cancer Patients

Radiographic Appearance	Pulmonary Disorders

Localized infiltrates	• Pneumonia
	  • Bacterial
	  • Mycobacterial
	  • Fungal
	• Cancer – lung
	• Radiation pneumonitis
	• Pulmonary infarct

Diffuse infiltrates	• Pneumocystis carinii pneumonia • Viral pneumonia • Cardiogenic and noncardiogenic pulmonary edema • Metastatic disease • Drug toxicity • Nonspecific pneumonitis
Hilar and/or mediastinal adenopathy	• Tuberculosis and atypical mycobacterial pneumonia • Fungal pneumonia (histoplasmosis, coccidiosis) • Lymphomas • Solid tumors (lung, breast, head and neck, germ cell) • Drugs (methotrexate)
Cavitation	• Bacterial pneumonia (gram-negatives, anaerobes, Legionella, Actinomyces, Nocardia) • Tuberculosis and atypical mycobacterial pneumonia • Septic emboli (bacterial or fungal) • Tumors (squamous lung carcinoma)
Pleural effusions	• Bacterial pneumonia (parapneumonic or empyema) • Tuberculosis • Tumors (lung, breast, ovarian) • Congestive heart failure • Pericardial disease (left-sided pleural effusion) • Pulmonary embolism
Nodules	• Bacterial pneumonia (Nocardia, Actinomyces, Haemophilus influenzae) • Atypical mycobacterial pneumonia • Metastatic cancer • Bronchiolitis obliterans with organizing pneumonia

Reproduced with permission from Stover DE, Kaner RJ. Pulmonary complications in cancer patients. CA Cancer J Clin 1996;46:303–20.

dida, and the agents of mucormycosis may also cause focal infiltrates in this population.[71,72] Cancer patients with impaired cell-mediated immunity due to leukemia, lymphoma, AIDS, or the ingestion of corticosteroids are highly predisposed to severe infections with *Pneumocystis,* which occasionally presents as a focal pulmonary infiltrate.[73–75] Such patients are also at risk of contracting *Legionella pneumophila,* typical or atypical mycobacteria, *Cryptococcus* or other opportunistic fungi, and *Nocardia.* These organisms have variable radiographic presentations but sometimes present as focal infiltrates. Noninfectious causes of localized infiltrates include radiation pneumonitis, pulmonary infarcts, and malignancy. These are discussed at greater length below.

Diffuse infiltrates are associated with high mortality rates, especially when they occur in immunocompro-

mised patients.[68,69,72,76] The causes of diffuse infiltrates are numerous and often multiple; among infectious agents, opportunistic pathogens such as *Pneumocystis, Cytomegalovirus, Candida* species, and *Aspergillus* predominate while hemorrhage, cardiogenic and noncardiogenic pulmonary edema, diffuse involvement of the lungs with tumor, and drug toxicity may contribute to or be wholly causative of the same picture. Mixed infections occur but are not usual (Figure 26–7).[69,72] All of the opportunistic pathogens mentioned in the preceding paragraph can present as diffuse pulmonary infiltrates. Massive invasion of the lungs by larval forms of *Strongyloides stercoralis* has been described in patients with lymphoma, leukemia, and human immunodeficiency virus (HIV) infection as well as in those who are taking large doses of corticosteroids, and such invasion should be suspected in susceptible patients who have lived or traveled in the tropics.[77] Pulmonary toxoplasmosis is uncommon but may present as an interstitial or necrotizing pneumonitis, with or without consolidation, in patients with AIDS, Hodgkin's disease, and other lymphomas.[78] Because of the diversity of infectious agents that cause diffuse infiltrates and due to the rapid decline many patients experience

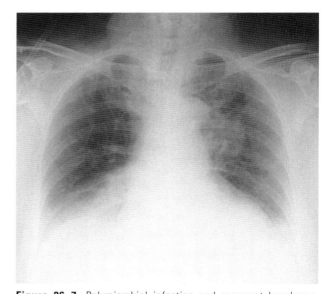

Figure 26–7. Polymicrobial infection and recurrent lymphoma. Anteroposterior radiograph of the chest demonstrating marked worsening of previously noted bibasilar opacities, a new left pleural effusion, and a new masslike opacity in the left suprahilar region in a 75-year-old woman with a history of diffuse large cell lymphoma of the small bowel resected two years previously. Expectorated sputum grew *Candida albicans.* Culture of bronchial brushings and washings were positive for *Pseudomonas aeruginosa* and *Cytomegalovirus.* Transbronchial biopsy of the mass in the left upper lobe revealed diffuse large B-cell lymphoma. The patient's condition improved after she received 21 days of antibiotics (ciprofloxacin, ceftazidime, clindamycin, and ganciclovir) and appropriate chemotherapy.

once diffuse infiltrates appear, early invasive procedures for determining a diagnosis are probably indicated.[68]

Infiltrates Related to Therapy. Iatrogenic pulmonary infiltrates occur in patients exposed to radiation and numerous chemotherapeutic agents and (occasionally) after pleurodesis. Clinical presentations vary and are often insidious, but the vast majority of patients report dyspnea and fever. Acute presentations can be fulminant, with severe respiratory insufficiency and cyanosis progressing quickly to acute cor pulmonale. There are no radiographic findings pathognomonic of drug-related injury, but the finding of patchy infiltrates that coalesce to form a relatively sharp edge that demarcates the radiation port rather than the lung's normal anatomic borders is typical of acute radiation pneumonitis. A diffuse haze in the treatment zone is often the earliest radiographic finding. Subsequently, air bronchograms in areas of increased density, elevation of the ipsilateral diaphragm, pleural effusions (representing a syndrome of radiation pleuritis), and a shift of the mediastinum toward the damage may also be noted. It must be emphasized, however, that acute radiation pneumonitis is a clinical rather than a radiographic diagnosis. Symptoms often precede changes seen in the chest radiograph, and radiologic changes usually do not correlate with symptoms. Of note, the damaging effects of radiation may be potentiated by a number of cytotoxic drugs, including bleomycin, dactinomycin, cyclophosphamide, vincristine, and doxorubicin, especially when these agents and radiation are administered concurrently.[79] Radiation pneumonitis typically develops 2 to 6 months after the completion of radiation therapy. Patchy migratory alveolar infiltrates suggestive of BOOP and findings outside the radiation field and even in the contralateral lung are also occasionally reported.[80,81] Radiation fibrosis, a more indolent process developing 6 months to 2 years after irradiation, produces linear interstitial infiltrates, volume loss, and (occasionally) pleural thickening and tenting of the diaphragm on the affected side.[81] Studies suggest that CT is probably more sensitive for the acute and chronic sequelae of radiation and may detect it earlier than chest radiography.[82,83] Nevertheless, it may be difficult or impossible to differentiate lung injury due to radiation from the recurrence of malignancy or infectious pneumonia even when clinicians have accurate knowledge of the radiation field and access to prior films.

The radiographic manifestations of toxic drug injury are extremely diverse, reflecting the variety of pathophysiologic mechanisms at play. Bleomycin toxicity, for example, classically causes bibasilar reticular or fine nodular infiltrates (Figure 26–8), often limited to the costophrenic-angle area, but also may present with peripheral subpleural infiltrates, patchy alveolar infiltrates, lobar consolidation,

pleural thickening, and/or large nodules. Findings are usually bilateral but may be asymmetric or focal. Volume loss, reflecting the restrictive nature of the underlying interstitial fibrosis, and diaphragmatic elevation are noted in up to 88% of cases.[84] Diverse abnormalities are seen with other agents as well. Reticular or reticulonodular infiltrates have been reported in association with the use of ara-C, busulfan, cyclophosphamide, gemcitabine, mitomycin, methotrexate, procarbazine, and vinblastine. Mitomycin, ara-C, and vinblastine can also cause focal, lobar, or diffuse alveolar infiltrates, and ara-C, cyclophosphamide, gemcitabine, mitomycin, and methotrexate have been known to precipitate acute noncardiogenic pulmonary edema.[85–89] Bleomycin, busulfan, carmustine (BCNU), cyclophosphamide, and many other agents cause pulmonary fibrosis.[85] The combination of these drugs with radiation, colony-stimulating factors, or each other in multiagent chemotherapy regimens may enhance their toxicity. Thoracic irradiation prior to or simultaneous with the administration of bleomycin, for example, increases the likelihood of pulmonary complications.[84] A syndrome of acute respiratory distress, associated in most cases with diffuse

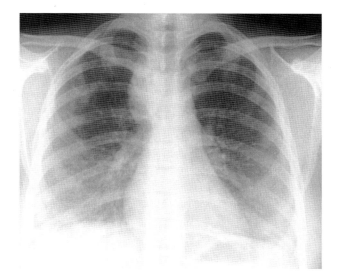

Figure 26–8. Bleomycin toxicity. Posteroanterior radiograph of the chest demonstrating bibasilar infiltrates and small bilateral pleural effusions in a 19-year-old woman with stage 2A nodular sclerosing Hodgkin's disease. The patient had completed her fifth cycle of a bleomycin-containing regimen 10 days prior to this radiograph and presented with complaints of low-grade fevers, cough, and shortness of breath. Bilateral dry rales were noted on physical examination. Throat culture was positive for *Haemophilus influenzae*, combined bronchial washings demonstrated *Candida*, and culture of bronchial washings grew *Staphylococcus aureus*. Pulmonary function tests showed a reduced diffusing capacity and moderate restrictive ventilatory defect, consistent with bleomycin pneumonitis. The patient's condition improved with intravenous azithromycin, intravenous trimethoprim-sulfamethoxazole, and oral prednisone.

or focal interstitial infiltrates, has likewise been described in patients receiving combined chemotherapy with mitomycin and vindesine or vinblastine.[90] The role of colony-stimulating factors in the potentiation of pulmonary toxicity has not been precisely delineated, but they have been cited in numerous case reports as a contributing and possibly causative factor.[91,92]

With bleomycin-induced interstitial pneumonitis or fibrosis, radiographic abnormalities typically follow but can also precede the onset of symptoms. As with radiation pneumonitis, CT is probably more sensitive for the acute and chronic sequelae of bleomycin-induced pulmonary toxicity and may detect them earlier than may chest radiography.[93] Clearing of chest radiography and CT images over several months after the discontinuation of bleomycin or in response to corticosteroid therapy is not uncommon, but infiltrates may recur as steroids are tapered. Of note, oxygen potentiates bleomycin-induced pulmonary toxicity, and infiltrates may develop or recur when patients receive supplemental oxygen even for very brief periods.[84] The timing of the development and resolution of the abnormalities induced by the other agents mentioned are described in the appropriate references. Table 26–2 lists the characteristics, radiographic findings, and incidence of pulmonary injury associated with commonly used cytotoxic medications.

A few other causes of iatrogenic pulmonary infiltrates should be mentioned in passing. Intravesical bacille Calmette-Guérin immunotherapy, used in the management of superficial transitional cell carcinoma of the bladder, is sometimes associated with the development of interstitial pneumonitis and even frank miliary tuberculosis.[94,95] Roentgenographic abnormalities (including pleural effusions, diffuse infiltrates representing a noncardiogenic pulmonary edema, and focal infiltrates of uncertain significance) have been reported in up to 72% of patients receiving high-dose interleukin-2 (Figure 26–9).[96] Approximately 50% of patients with acute promyelocytic leukemia (APL) receiving all-*trans* retinoic acid and at least 30% of such patients retreated

TABLE 26–2. Radiographic Abnormalities Associated with Selected Cytotoxic Agents

Drug	Plain Radiographic Findings	Incidence (%)	Time Course
Bleomycin	Bibasilar reticular or fine nodular infiltrates, with a predilection for the costophrenic angles	3-11	4-10 weeks after completion of therapy
Busulfan	Bibasilar reticular infiltrates	4	6 weeks to 120 months
Chlorambucil	Interstitial infiltrates; pulmonary fibrosis	Rare	1-2 weeks after administration
Cyclophosphamide	Bilateral reticulonodular infiltrates (early); bilateral reticulonodular infiltrates, frequently with pleural thickening, sparing costophrenic angles (late)	Rare	Within 6 months (early); 1.5-13 years (late)
Carmustine	Bibasilar reticular infiltrates; also apical peripheral or patchy infiltrates, fibrosis and contraction of upper lung fields	20-30, dose-related (patients receiving > 1400 mg/m^2 at greatest risk)	30-371 days after initiation of drug; occasionally late (up to 17 years)
Cytosine arabinoside (ara-C)	Bilateral pulmonary infiltrates, with or without pleural effusions, consistent with noncardiogenic pulmonary edema	7-22	2-21 days after administration
Docetaxel	Interstitial infiltrates; CHF, effusions	Rare; fluid retention syndrome in 6%	After median dose of 705 mg/m^2
Gemcitabine	Diffuse interstitial infiltrates; noncardiogenic pulmonary edema (with docetaxel and cytosine arabinoside)	Unknown	Within weeks of starting therapy
Melphalan	Upper lobe infiltrates; pulmonary fibrosis	Rare	Within weeks
Mitomycin	Bilateral reticular infiltrates, occasionally with acinar infiltrates or fine nodules; noncardiogenic pulmonary edema with hemolytic-uremic syndrome	< 10, but higher when given with other toxic agents; edema/HUS: rare	2-4 months into therapy
Mitomycin/vinca alkaloids	Diffuse interstitial infiltrates in most patients; occasionally focal infiltrates	4	Within 4 hours of vinca alkaloid dose
Methotrexate	Diffuse bilateral reticular, acinar, or nodular infiltrates; occasionally pleural effusions, bibasilar atelectasis	7	Usually within weeks of starting therapy; occ. late
Paclitaxel	Transient interstitial infiltrates	Rare	2-14 days after dose
Procarbazine	Interstitial infiltrates	Rare	Hours to 1 week

CHF = congestive heart failure; HUS = hemolytic uremic syndrome.

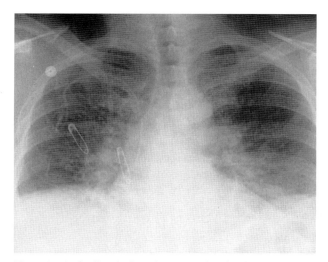

Figure 26–9. Capillary leak syndrome associated with aldesleukin, an interleukin-2 analog. Posteroanterior radiograph of the chest demonstrating extensive perihilar infiltrates and blunting of the right costophrenic angle in a 62-year-old man with metastatic melanoma. The patient developed acute shortness of breath on the fourth day of his first cycle of biochemotherapy with vinblastine, dacarbazine, cis-platinum, recombinant interferon-alpha, and aldesleukin, a recombinant analog of interleukin-2 that has been associated with a capillary leak syndrome. The patient's symptoms improved after the administration of intravenous furosemide and albuterol nebulizers.

with arsenic trioxide develop a "retinoic acid syndrome" characterized by the development of fever, interstitial infiltrates, and pleural effusions.[97,98] Finally, talc pleurodesis, a procedure that is generally well tolerated, is associated with the development of diffuse bilateral pulmonary infiltrates and the adult respiratory distress syndrome in up to 9% of patients.[99,100]

Infiltrates Related to Malignancy. Bronchogenic carcinomas and thoracic metastases of solid tumors usually manifest as slowly enlarging nodules or masses. Occasionally, however, they show rapid progression and can mimic other causes of acute air space disease. Bronchoalveolar carcinoma, for example, can present as a focal consolidation or a diffuse alveolar process with air bronchogram formation.[101] Mucoid impaction due to the accumulation of inspissated secretions occurs in patients with bronchial obstructions and presents radiographically as a fusiform or branching density radiating distally from the obstruction.[101] Invasion of the pulmonary arteries can lead to infarction and the development of dumbbell-shaped opacities on chest radiographs, with the central mass of each "dumbbell" representing the tumor and with the peripheral mass representing the infarction.[101] Many tumors (notably carcinomas of the lung and breast) have a predilection for lymphangitic spread, the radiographic presentation of which is diffuse interstitial infiltrates.

Hematologic malignancies involving the lung also present variably. Enlarged mediastinal lymph nodes are a common finding on chest radiographs from patients with lymphoma, but lymphomas also frequently invade the lung parenchyma, where they present radiographically as nodules or focal consolidation, as lymphangitic spread, or as a diffuse alveolar, interstitial, or mixed process. Lymphomatous infiltrates may progress rapidly and may thereby be confused with infectious processes (Figure 26–10).[102,103] A good rule of thumb is that a new pulmonary process in patients with lymphoma represents the lymphoma in approximately half of the cases.[70] The most common cause of noninfectious pulmonary infiltrates in leukemic patients, on the other hand, is hemorrhage (followed closely by parenchymal infiltration with leukemic cells).[71]

Several unique (albeit rare) causes of infiltrates in patients with leukemia should also be mentioned. The first, pulmonary leukostasis, occurs when the peripheral blood contains more than 40% blast cells and in almost all patients with leukocyte counts of $> 200,000/mm^3$; the clinical and radiographic presentation is that of an acute or subacute diffuse pneumonitis.[70] The second, "leukemic cell lysis pneumonopathy," is sometimes precipitated by chemotherapy in patients with acute myelogenous leukemia; the radiographic manifestations include vascular engorgement, progressive patchy nodular or alveolar infiltrates, and pleural effusions.[104,105] Finally, a "hyperleukocytic reaction" associated with pulmonary hemorrhage and the development of alveolar edema has been observed in patients with rapidly rising leukocyte counts and hyperblastemia.[67]

Infiltrates of Miscellaneous Etiology. Miscellaneous causes of pulmonary infiltrates in patients with cancer include diffuse pulmonary hemorrhage, sarcoidlike reactions, and BOOP. Diffuse alveolar hemorrhage, a life-threatening complication of autologous bone marrow transplantation, presents at an average of 11 days after transplantation with diffuse interstitial (73% of cases) or alveolar (27% of cases) infiltrates involving the central portion of the lung. Hemoptysis is uncommon. The radiographic findings evolve rapidly, and the majority of patients (nearly 80%) develop diffuse bilateral radiographic abnormalities involving all lung zones. The syndrome occasionally presents late, up to a month after transplantation, but it seems unlikely that it would ever be encountered in an outpatient population.[62] Sarcoidlike reactions (noncaseating granulomas developing in the lung parenchyma or thoracic lymph nodes in the absence of systemic signs of sarcoidosis) have been reported in patients with various solid tumors and lymphoma and may occur while patients are in remission. Common radiographic findings include hilar or mediastinal lymphadenopathy and bilateral lung nodules in perivascular

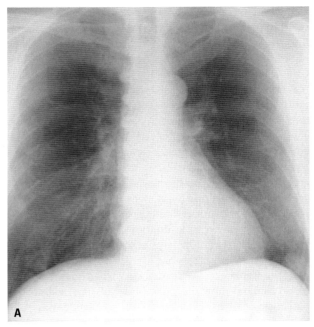

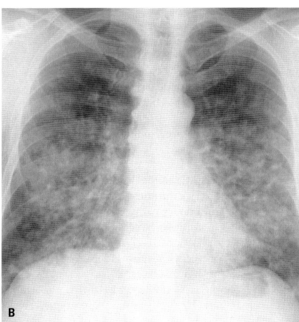

and peribronchial distributions. Parenchymal nodules may also be subpleural or random in distribution and range from 1 mm to several centimeters in diameter.[64] A variety of insults, including viral or bacterial infections, radiation, and chemotherapy, may precipitate BOOP. The radiographic pattern typically consists of diffuse, patchy, "ground glass," or alveolar densities, but nodules, interstitial infiltrates, and emphysematous changes have also been reported (Figure 26–11). As with many of the processes described above, the radiographic findings are suggestive rather than specific, and the diagnosis must be confirmed by biopsy.[65,106]

Suspected Venous Thromboembolism

Patients with certain types of malignancy (eg, lung, brain, ovarian, pancreatic, and gastric cancers) are at increased risk of developing deep venous thrombosis (DVT) and pulmonary embolism (PE) (these are collectively referred to hereafter as venous thromboembolism [VTE]) independent of the presence or absence of other risk factors. Cancer patients may also be at risk for VTE because of deconditioning, immobility, recent surgery, pathologic

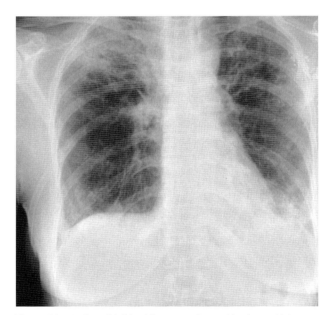

Figure 26–10. Rapidly progressive lymphoma. Posteroanterior radiograph of the chest (Panel B) demonstrating extensive bilateral nodular parenchymal infiltrates in a 58-year-old man with diffuse large B-cell lymphoma presenting to the emergency room with fever, shortness of breath, a cough productive of blood-tinged sputum, new renal insufficiency, and diffuse abdominal pain. The infiltrates showed dramatic interval change when compared to a study obtained nine days previously (Panel A). Sputum and blood cultures and bronchial washings obtained at bronchoalveolar lavage were negative for all viral, bacterial, and fungal pathogens. A CT-guided biopsy of similarly progressive lesions in the liver revealed diffuse large B-cell lymphoma. Despite aggressive supportive care and the administration of appropriate chemotherapy, the patient expired 30 days after the second study was obtained.

Figure 26–11. Bronchiolitis obliterans and organizing interstitial pneumonitis (BOOP). Anteroposterior radiograph of the chest demonstrating mixed interstitial and reticulonodular infiltrates in the right upper lobe, left upper lobe, and left base of a 67-year-old woman with malignant melanoma. The patient presented with fever, cough productive of yellow-tinged sputum, and progressive dyspnea. Cultures of bronchial washings were negative for bacterial, fungal, or viral pathogens. Wedge resection of the left upper and lower lobes revealed extensive BOOP, a few non-necrotizing granulomata, and bronchiectatic changes. The patient had been receiving high dose interferon-alpha therapy for several months as part of an experimental protocol. Her symptoms improved with oral prednisone.

fracture of a lower extremity, or the use of implanted venous access and constant infusion delivery systems. While explicit clinical criteria can reliably separate patients with suspected DVT or PE into high, moderate, and low pretest probability categories, objective testing is required to establish either diagnosis with certainty.[107–109] Contrast venography and pulmonary angiography remain the "gold standards" for the evaluation of DVT and PE, respectively, but these tests are moderately invasive, require the use of contrast material, and are not universally available. As a result (and also because pulmonary angiography in particular is associated with a low but not negligible risk of serious complications, including death), most clinicians reserve these tests for patients with whom other and less invasive tests are inconclusive.[110] Fortunately, diagnostic algorithms that rely primarily on noninvasive procedures have now been validated, so invasive vascular imaging is seldom necessary.[109,111,112] The evolution of highly sensitive and specific but noninvasive techniques of imaging the pulmonary vasculature represents an important advance,[113–115] but whether such studies can be used to rule out the diagnosis of clinically significant pulmonary embolism remains controversial.[116–119]

Evaluation of Patients with Normal Chest Radiographs. Because of their pre-existing risk for VTE, cancer patients presenting with unexplained dyspnea, chest discomfort, or syncope should be regarded as having a moderate or high clinical likelihood of having PE. In patients without underlying lung disease, primary lung cancer, known parenchymal metastasis, or pleural effusion, the best initial screening test for the work-up of suspected PE is perfusion lung scanning. In the multicenter Prospective Investigation of Pulmonary Embolism Diagnosis (PIOPED) trial, a high-probability perfusion lung scan had no less positive predictive value for acute PE than a high-probability combined ventilation-perfusion (V/Q) lung scan whereas near-normal and normal perfusion scans excluded PE with no less validity than equivalently interpreted V/Q scans.[120] In the absence of a high index of suspicion for PE, near-normal or normal studies effectively exclude the diagnosis and are almost never associated with recurrent embolism. Unfortunately, nuclear imaging studies provide a definitive diagnosis in only a minority of patients (in the PIOPED trial, for example, only 41% of patients with positive angiograms had high-probability V/Q scans).[121] In the PIOPED trial, the sensitivity of V/Q scintigraphy for the detection of clinically significant PE exceeded 90% only when scans of high, intermediate, and low probability were lumped together (at the cost of a drastic reduction in the test's specificity).

Historically, experts have recommended that pulmonary angiography be performed in patients with a moderate or high clinical likelihood of PE but with non-diagnostic V/Q scans. In recent years, numerous authors have advocated the use of serial noninvasive tests for lower-extremity DVT in such patients, since DVT and PE are treated identically. The safety of this approach has been demonstrated for both impedance plethysmography (IPG) and compression ultrasonography (US); in 1999, the American Thoracic Society endorsed the use of either modality as an alternative to pulmonary angiography in selected stable patients.[109,112,122] Serial testing is inconvenient, however, and it may not be cost-effective.[123] Moreover, some authors have expressed concern about this approach because less than one-half of patients with angiographic evidence of PE have demonstrable DVT.[124]

Unfortunately, serial testing for DVT is the only proven alternative to pulmonary angiography for patients whose diagnosis is unresolved after scintigraphy. Despite their advantages, neither MRA nor helical (spiral) CT should be substituted for pulmonary angiography in such patients.[112,125] Although these tests are sensitive and specific for the detection of PE in the proximal pulmonary vasculature (ie, in the main, lobar, or segmental vessels), they do not reliably detect subsegmental emboli.[118,126–128] This limitation is significant because the overall prevalence of isolated subsegmental emboli in the PIOPED trial was 6%, and such emboli rarely correlated with high-probability V/Q scans.[129] Other researchers have reported a higher prevalence of subsegmental PE. Oser and associates, reviewing 76 of 88 consecutive positive pulmonary angiograms, found that the largest occluded artery was subsegmental or smaller in 23 (30%).[130] Goodman and associates, in a study of 20 patients with nondiagnostic V/Q scans, reported that 4 of the 11 patients with positive angiograms had PE in subsegmental vessels only.[126] To substitute either MRA or helical CT for pulmonary angiography in the evaluation of patients with suspected PE is to assume that small emboli are clinically insignificant. Some authors have asserted that in otherwise healthy individuals, this may actually be the case.[131,132] The latest statement of the American College of Chest Physicians Consensus Committee on Pulmonary Embolism rejects this assumption, however, stating explicitly that "any patient who has a proven diagnosis of PE needs to be treated unless there are extenuating circumstances such as terminal carcinoma."[125]

In the setting of nondiagnostic V/Q scanning, clinicians often pursue noninvasive imaging of the pulmonary vasculature before proceeding to pulmonary angiography, but the cost-effectiveness of this strategy has not been determined.[133] Where helical CT is the option, one must also consider the consequences of the load of radiographic contrast material. If there are concerns about the amount of contrast that can be given to a particular patient, one should proceed directly to conventional pulmonary angiography.

Evaluation of Patients with Abnormal Chest Radiographs or with Underlying Lung Disease. The diagnosis of PE in patients with underlying lung disease is particularly challenging. The symptoms of PE are nonspecific and mimic those of other cardiopulmonary illnesses. In patients with lung cancer, for example, it is often difficult to discriminate between acute PE and progression of dyspnea related to the patient's malignancy. Chest radiography may be performed to screen for postobstructive pneumonia, pathologic rib fracture, or pneumothorax. Subsequently, it is best to proceed directly to helical CT in patients with neoplasms of the lung, pulmonary metastases, chronic lung disease, pleural effusion, or other conditions that limit the usefulness of V/Q scintigraphy. Pooled data suggest that the sensitivity, specificity, and positive and negative predictive values of helical CT exceed 90% for the detection of central PE and are superior to those of V/Q scintigraphy (Figures 26–12 and 26–13).[125,134,135] The chief advantage of helical CT for such patients, however, is that it provides high-quality cross-sectional images of the mediastinum, lung parenchyma, and chest wall. The images obtained may suggest or confirm alternate diagnoses such as pneumonia, pulmonary hypertension, pulmonary fibrosis, radiation pneumonitis, iatrogenic lung injury, or pericardial effusion.[136] The versatility and power of the technique are formidable; rare causes of acute thoracic pain and dyspnea, such as cardiac or lobar torsion (complications of pneumonectomy and lobectomy, respectively), have been documented with helical CT, and experienced radiographers can often distinguish acute and chronic thromboembolic disease.[137]

Helical CT or Conventional Angiography? The optimization of radiocontrast injection protocols and technologic advances in CT scanners that permit subsecond scanning times and 2- to 3-mm collimation have resulted in improved visualization of the peripheral pulmonary arteries, and the percentage of analyzable subsegmental arteries in the most recent studies approaches that reported for pulmonary angiography.[138–140] In fact, numerous studies suggest that pulmonary angiography may be no more precise than helical CT for the evaluation of subsegmental PE. Interobserver agreement for patients with PE limited to subsegmental arteries, for example, varies tremendously, and reported co-positivity rates range between 13 and 79%.[141–143] Baile and associ-

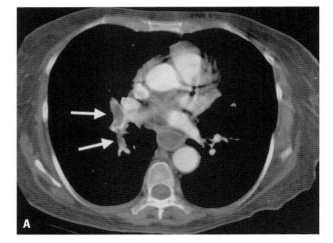

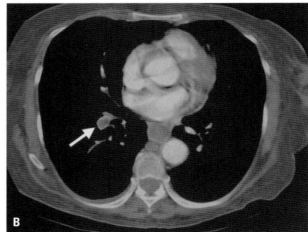

Figure 26–13. Pulmonary embolus. Helical CT of the chest with nonionic intravenous contrast demonstrating extensive bilateral pulmonary emboli in a 69-year-old woman with metastatic endometrial carcinoma. The patient presented with increasing lower extremity edema (right greater than left), calf tenderness, dyspnea on exertion, and a room-air oxygen saturation of 92%. Panel A reveals emboli in the main lobar branches of the right pulmonary artery; Panel B shows an embolus in a segmental artery of the right lower lobe.

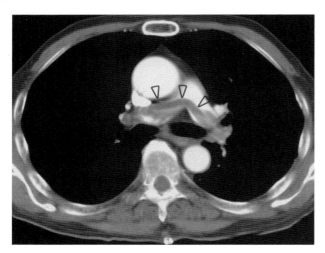

Figure 26–12. Pulmonary embolus. Helical CT of the chest with nonionic intravenous contrast demonstrating a large saddle embolus (*open arrowheads*) extending into the right and left main pulmonary arteries and segmental arterial branches in a 66-year-old man with non-small-cell lung cancer. The patient presented with dyspnea 3 weeks after surgical stabilization of a vertebral compression fracture.

ates, comparing helical CT and conventional angiography to an independent gold standard (postmortem methacrylate casts of porcine pulmonary vessels), found that helical CT may actually be equivalent to angiography in detecting subsegmental-sized PE.[144]

The value of a helical CT scan is dependent on its quality. If the subsegmental vasculature is clearly identified and the scan is interpeted as negative, the usefulness of subsequent conventional angiography is debatable. On the other hand, image quality may be compromised in patients who are hemodynamically unstable or severely dyspneic. Scanning times and collimation must be adjusted (with adverse effects on image quality and percision) to accommodate patients who are significantly short of breath, and motion artifacts due to shallow breathing or abrupt expiration can degrade otherwise adequate

studies. Suboptimal enhancement of specific vessels (usually in the middle or upper lobes) and partial-volume effects have also been cited as causes of indeterminate studies.[134,135,140] Clinical circumstances will dictate which patients are or are not appropriate for evaluation by helical CT. Contrast-enhanced electron beam CT, which allows shorter acquisition times, does not require breath holding, and is at least equivalent to helical CT in depicting peripheral pulmonary arteries, may be advantageous in certain cases.[114,139,145] At present, however, electron beam CT scanners are not widely available. Thus, unstable patients who are strongly suspected of having PE may occasionally be best served by being routed directly to conventional angiography.

A reasonable algorithm for the evaluation of suspected PE in cancer patients is outlined below (Figure 26–14).

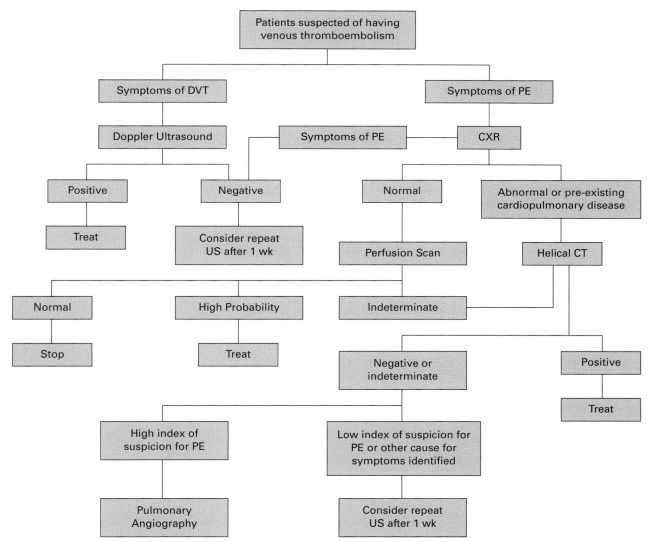

Figure 26–14. Algorithm for the evaluation of suspected thromboembolic disease in patients with cancer. CT = computed tomography; CXR = chest radiograph; DVT = deep venous thrombosis; PE = pulmonary embolism; US ultrasonography.

IMAGING OF THE ABDOMEN

Patients with cancer, regardless of the primary malignancy, are at increased risk of abdominal pain, nausea and vomiting, diarrhea, constipation, jaundice, and gastrointestinal hemorrhage. These conditions may be malignant, benign, or iatrogenic in etiology and are among the most common reasons patients with cancer seek medical attention in emergency or urgent care settings. Radiographic evaluation is frequently essential for the proper management of these patients. The discussion that follows focuses on the radiographic work-up of adult patients with cancer and assumes the taking of a detailed history, a physical examination, and the performance of appropriate laboratory studies.

Abdominal pain is a common chief complaint on the part of patients presenting to general emergency departments, and one should remember that patients with cancer may develop pain for the same reasons as patients without cancer. More frequently, however (at least in our experience), their complaints will relate in some way to their underlying malignancy or its therapy. Patients with malignancy may have direct intra-abdominal effects from mass or tissue invasion. Peritoneal tumor implants, for example, increase the likelihood of adhesion formation and bowel obstruction whereas visceral malignancies occasionally cause perforation of the involved viscera. Malignant ascites may complicate any intra-abdominal malignancy and can also cause abdominal distension and pain. Coagulopathies develop in patients with cancer for a multitude of reasons, increasing the risk of spontaneous hemorrhage and complicating surgical interventions where they are indicated. Opiate and anticholinergic use, dehydration, inactivity, and electrolyte abnormalities commonly result in constipation or obstipation manifesting as abdominal pain. On the other hand, the use of corticosteroids, antiemetics, and opiates may blunt symptoms of pain, fever, and nausea and significantly delay the recognition of more severe processes. Steroid use may also increase the risk of bowel perforation and gastrointestinal bleeding.

Chemotherapy and radiation often have significant direct abdominal effects.[146] Vincristine administration, for example, has been associated with the development of paralytic ileus, and radiation therapy can cause strictures and sometimes results in fistula formation, perforation, and enteropathy. Irinotecan and 5-fluorouracil cause significant diarrhea, and numerous chemotherapeutic agents are associated with emesis (some agents, notably cisplatin, can provoke vomiting for days after administration). Therapy with myelosuppressive agents, steroids, or growth factors may alter the white blood cell count and limit its usefulness in clinical evaluation, and myelosuppressive therapy, immunomodulation, and primary hematologic malignancy can compromise the body's ability to fight intra-abdominal infection.

Imaging Techniques

Imaging of the abdomen usually begins with plain-film radiography. The diagnostic power of plain-film radiography is actually rather limited, but the technique may provide useful information in patients with obstruction, perforation, and stool impaction.[147,148] Patients with limited disease and no known intra-abdominal involvement or prior surgery can be approached conservatively. In these patients, plain-film abdominal radiography is not indicated for abdominal pain associated with isolated nausea, vomiting, or diarrhea and should be reserved for patients with moderate or severe tenderness, suspected perforation or obstruction, and prior abdominal surgery.[149] Obtaining supine and erect views facilitates the evaluation of bowel gas patterns and usually permits the identification of extraluminal air. In critically ill or debilitated patients who are unable to stand, a left decubitus view may be substituted for the upright view. The use of portable abdominal imaging spares ill patients from being transported but usually results in technically inferior images and potentially exposes other patients and hospital staff to ionizing radiation. Supplementary views should be ordered only after the initial films are reviewed. Cross-table lateral views are rarely necessary but may be helpful in delineating ventral abdominal hernias. In some patients, right decubitus and prone views may allow the differentiation of colonic obstruction and adynamic ileus (see below).

Because the diagnostic yield of plain-film radiography is low, the evaluation of abdominal pain with CT has become commonplace. The many complicating features of malignancy and its treatment generally lower the threshold for ordering CT in patients with cancer and unexplained abdominal pain. Computed tomography performed in the emergency department has been reported to increase physicians' level of diagnostic certainty, reduce hospital admission rates, and lead to more timely surgical intervention.[150] Computed tomography is the method of choice for imaging patients with abdominal pain associated with fever, acidosis, leukocytosis, and/or signs and symptoms of peritoneal irritation (rebound tenderness, involuntary guarding, rigidity, or absent bowel sounds) for which preliminary plain-film radiography may not be helpful and may often be misleading.[151] Computed tomography is also invaluable when plain films are nondiagnostic but the patient's presentation suggests any of several diagnoses requiring immediate intervention, such as obstruction or perforation of the bowel, appendicitis, diverticulitis, abscess, mesenteric ischemia, intra-abdominal bleeding, or a dissecting abdominal aortic aneurysm.

Magnetic resonance imaging currently plays a negligible role in evaluating patients with acute abdominal pain although magnetic resonance cholangiopancreatography (MRCP) is becoming an important tool for the evaluation of pancreaticobiliary disease (see below).

Intestinal Obstruction

The diagnosis of intestinal obstruction is based largely on radiographic confirmation. (The presentation and clinical evaluation of patients with bowel obstruction is described in Chapter 9). Bowel obstruction may be partial or complete and can develop at any point along the small or large intestine. In closed-loop obstructions (usually associated with strangulation), a section of bowel is occluded at both ends whereas obturation obstruction is caused by an intraluminal mass such as a bezoar or gallstone.

Cases of intestinal obstruction can represent up to 20% of surgical admissions and account for as many as one-third of emergent surgical procedures in the cancer patient.[152,153] Ovarian, pancreatic, colonic, and gastric cancers are the primary tumors most frequently associated with the development of intestinal obstruction. In patients with advanced metastatic disease, the obstruction may reflect extrinsic luminal occlusion resulting from an enlarging primary or recurrent tumor, mesenteric masses, surgical adhesions, or postradiation fibrosis; intraluminal occlusion by a polypoid lesion; or infiltration of intestinal muscle.[154] Nonmalignant causes of intestinal obstruction include the strangulation of bowel in ventral and inguinal hernias, inflammatory processes, volvulus, intussusception, diverticulitis, and stool impaction.[155–158] Obstruction of the large bowel usually reflects primary or recurrent malignancy. Pseudo-obstruction (eg, paralytic ileus and Ogilvie's syndrome) is most frequently encountered in the postoperative setting but has been associated with a large variety of causes.[159]

In general, flat and erect abdominal radiography should be performed in clinically stable patients whenever the diagnosis of bowel obstruction is entertained. Plain-film radiography is estimated to be diagnostic in 50 to 60% of cases, equivocal in 20 to 30% of cases, and normal, nondiagnostic, or even misleading 10 to 20% of the time.[158] Plain-film radiography has a marginal negative predictive value but is a mainstay in the evaluation of suspected bowel obstruction because of its sensitivity for high-grade obstruction, its availability, and its relatively low cost.[160] Air-fluid levels and extraluminal air are best visualized by radiography done when the patient is standing erect. If the patient is too ill to stand, left decubitus views may be substituted; in the case of pneumoperitoneum, however, the false-negative rate for this view exceeds 50% when compared with CT.[161]

Plain-film radiographic findings of mechanical small-bowel obstruction include dilated air-filled loops of small bowel with multiple air-fluid levels and decreased distal bowel gas and fecal material (Figure 26–15). Gastric-outlet obstruction should be suspected when a large left-upper-quadrant air-fluid level (stomach bubble) is observed on plain films of patients who report vomiting undigested food. The incidence of malignancy in adult patients presenting with gastric-outlet obstruction is > 50%.[162] For more distal blockages, dilatation of small bowel to a diameter of > 2.5 cm suggests obstruction.[163] Differential air-fluid levels (distinct air-fluid interfaces at different heights within a single loop of bowel) may be observed in both mechanical and ady-

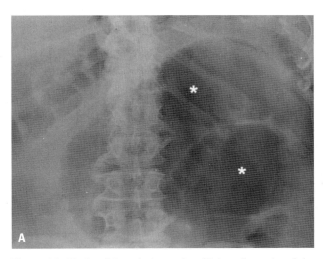
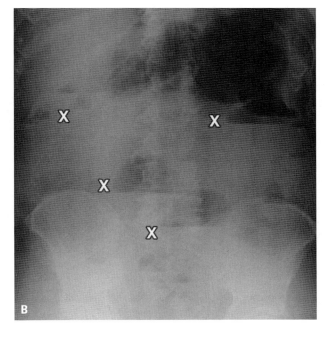

Figure 26–15. Small bowel obstruction. Plain radiographs of the abdomen in a 57-year-old man with metastatic colorectal cancer presenting with abdominal distension, nausea and vomiting. A: Supine view reveals markedly dilated loop of small bowel (*). B: Upright view shows multiple differential air-fluid levels (x).

namic obstructions, but a difference in height of ≥ 20 mm is moderately suggestive (with a positive predictive value of 0.86) of mechanical obstruction.[164] Up to five air-fluid levels of < 2.5 cm in length may be seen in normal individuals.[165] An absence of distal bowel gas suggests complete obstruction, but residual colonic air may be seen in early complete obstruction or partial obstruction.[147] A complete lack of intestinal gas is abnormal, suggests proximal obstruction, and results from either static fluid-filled bowel or significant vomiting.[147,166] Linear collections of small gas bubbles between the valvulae conniventes in a fluid-filled small bowel (the string-of-beads sign) is pathognomonic for small-bowel obstruction.[165]

The degree of colonic dilatation in large-bowel obstruction depends on the competency of the ileocecal valve. Cecal diameters of > 10 cm correlate with an increased risk of perforation.[166] Colonic air-fluid levels are seldom diagnostic and are frequently seen in diarrhea. There are no absolute radiographic criteria by which to distinguish mechanical bowel obstruction and adynamic ileus. The demonstration of nondifferential air-fluid levels is suggestive of adynamic ileus but must be interpreted in light of other clinical data. The absence of mechanical obstruction can sometimes be demonstrated by having the patient lie with his or her right side down for 10 to 15 minutes before obtaining a right decubitus view. In patients with adynamic ileus, this maneuver may promote the passage of gas into the left colon and rectum.[167] Similarly, a prone view may allow air from a dilated but unobstructed sigmoid colon to percolate to the rectum. One should remember that adynamic ileus can be generalized or localized. Localized ileus sometimes develops in patients with acute pancreatitis, acute cholecystitis, and/or retroperitoneal hemorrhage, but the finding is nonspecific in and of itself. Volvulus, whether sigmoid or cecal, manifests radiographically as a large dilated loop of bowel extending from the pelvis to the upper abdomen.[168]

Plain-film abdominal radiographs, as mentioned above, are frequently not completely normal but are nondiagnostic. The term "nonspecific abdominal gas pattern" is often used by radiologists to describe such films and can be confusing. Sixty-five percent of radiologists surveyed perceived this phrase to mean that the image to which it was applied was normal or probably normal; 22% interpreted it to mean that there was uncertainty about whether the image was normal or abnormal; and 13% interpreted it to mean that the image was abnormal but nondiagnostic of obstruction or ileus.[169] Where there is any uncertainty, the radiologist using this term should be queried as to the denotation he or she intends.

Abdominal and pelvic CT play an important role in the evaluation of suspected bowel obstruction and are the techniques of choice for patients presenting with signs and symptoms of obstruction and systemic toxicity. Computed tomography reveals the cause of obstruction in 73 to 95% of cases although its specificity, sensitivity, and accuracy vary according to the degree or grade of obstruction.[170–172] Mechanical and functional obstruction can usually be differentiated, and CT facilitates the diagnosis of strangulation with intestinal ischemia, which is an indication for emergent surgical intervention.[173] Abrupt changes in lumen caliber demarcate the

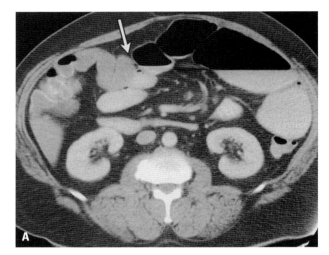

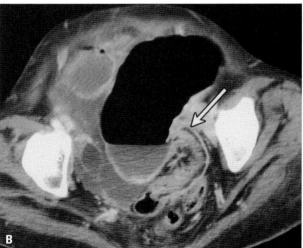

Figure 26–16. Computed tomographic images depicting transition zone in small and large bowel obstruction. A: A 57-year-old man with metastatic colorectal cancer presented complaining of abdominal distension. Computed tomography of the abdomen shows partial small bowel obstruction and transition zone *(arrow)*. Loops of bowel proximal to the point of obstruction are conspicuously dilated, while loops distal to the obstruction are of normal caliber. B: A 54-year-old woman with metastatic ovarian carcinoma presented with increasing abdominal distension. Computed tomography of the pelvis reveals large bowel obstruction with a transition zone *(arrow)* at the level of the sigmoid colon.

so-called transition zone, with dilated bowel proximal to the point of obstruction and normal or collapsed bowel distal to it (Figure 26–16).

Oral contrast enhances the visualization of the bowel wall and facilitates the detection of edema, hematoma, mass lesions, and the point of obstruction, but it should be administered carefully to patients with small-bowel obstruction as the volume of intraluminal fluid is already high and because these patients are likely to regurgitate. It may be helpful to administer the contrast agent through a nasogastric tube, in which case time must be alotted for the contrast to reach the point of obstruction. Water-soluble contrast is preferred because barium may cause chemical peritonitis or permanently stain the retroperitoneum if there is perforation. Intravenous contrast should be used whenever possible to maximize the amount of information obtained from a given scan. Opacification of blood vessels and parenchymal enhancement facilitates the assessment of bowel wall thickness and may provide evidence of infarction. Scans without IV contrast should be performed first if nephrolithiasis is included in the differential diagnosis.

When plain-film radiography and CT examinations are nondiagnostic, or if additional information is desired, enteroclysis or a fluoroscopically-guided barium small-bowel study can be performed. In the acutely ill patient, conventional upper gastrointestinal barium studies with a small-bowel follow-through are of little value. Enteroclysis, however, objectively gauges the severity of obstruction and may be used to evaluate low-grade obstructions, intraluminal tumors, small ulcerations, and mucosal inflammatory changes. In ambiguous cases, enteroclysis may provide data that determine whether patients require immediate surgical intervention.[160]

Contrast enemas may be diagnostic of colonic obstruction and are often employed therapeutically in the treatment of volvulus (Figure 26–17).[174]

Gastrointestinal Perforation

Gastrointestinal perforation in patients with cancer may be due to primary or metastatic deposits and has been reported in association with a wide variety of tumors. Non-Hodgkin's lymphoma accounts for nearly half of the cases, but melanoma and carcinoma of the colo-rectum, stomach, ovary, lung, and breast have also been associated with perforation.[175] In patients with lymphoma, perforation typically occurs when chemotherapy or radiation causes necrosis of the tumor penetrating the bowel. With other types of tumors, rupture may occur proximal to malignant obstructions or in the setting of severe radiation enteritis. Typhlitis and other intra-abdominal infections for which patients with cancer are at greater-than-usual risk may be complicated by perforation. The association of glucocorticosteroid adminis-

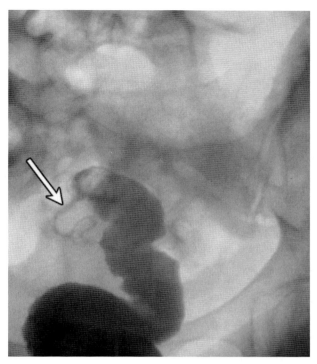

Figure 26–17. Contrast enema in large bowel obstruction. A 47-year-old woman with metastatic cervical cancer presented with abdominal pain and distension. A Gastrograffin enema was diagnostic of complete large bowel obstruction showing obstruction of flow at the level of the lesion *(arrow)*.

tration and gastroduodenal perforation is well documented, and high-dose glucocorticosteroid therapy (defined as ≥ 20 mg of prednisone daily) alters the presentation of peritonitis to the extent that its recognition is often delayed.[176] Perforation may occur in patients with peptic ulcers or mesenteric ischemia and as a complication of surgery or endoscopy. The identification of extraluminal air on plain abdominal films indicates a perforated abdominal viscus requiring prompt surgical intervention in all but a few circumstances (eg, when air is retained postoperatively, after peritoneal dialysis, and occasionally in the setting of recent endoscopy, mechanical ventilation, or pneumothorax).[177,178]

Visceral perforation does not always result in visualized free air on a plain-film radiograph; in fact, the sensitivity of plain-film radiography for pneumoperitoneum may be as low as 50%.[161,178] Free air is usually noted as a crescentic lucency under the diaphragm on upright chest or abdominal radiographs. It may be visualized under either hemidiaphragm, but is typically easier to identify on the right. Upright chest radiography has been found to be more sensitive than erect abdominal films for the detection of free intraperitoneal air. As little as 1 to 2 mL of air can be detected by upright chest films whereas it is seldom possible to discern less than 5 mL on the upright abdominal radiograph.[147] For patients for whom obtaining erect views is infeasible or when upright views are suspicious but nondiagnostic, left decubitus views of the abdomen may be obtained. On these views, free air may be visualized as a linear lucency in the least dependent portions of the abdomen or pelvis (Figure 26–18). Remember that for free air to be perceived in any view, it must first percolate to the least dependent portion of the abdomen. Having a patient maintain a given position (upright or decubitus) for at least 10 minutes prior to performing the study will maximize the chances of detecting small amounts of free air. In patients too ill to tolerate decubitus views, supine abdominal radiography may demonstrate signs of free intraperitoneal air when large amounts (≥ 1L) of extraluminal gas are present. The most common of these signs are the right-upper-quadrant (air surrounding the liver) and double-wall (or Rigler's) signs (air on both sides of the intestinal wall). Air outlining the falciform ligament, the peritoneal cavity ("football" sign), and medial umbilical folds (inverted-V sign) occur less frequently. One or more of these signs are present in 59% of pneumoperitoneum cases, but all are prone to misinterpretation (Figure 26–19).[179]

Oral or rectal contrast may be useful for identifying and delineating the site of perforation.[180] Because of the risks associated with extraluminal barium, only water-soluble contrast should be used in such studies, and rectal contrast should not be given to patients suspected of having ischemic bowel, neutropenic colitis, or toxic megacolon. Examination with contrast has been reported to have a sensitivity of 100% for the diagnosis of perforation of the stomach, duodenum, and colon.[178]

Any question of extraluminal air or perforation on plain-film radiography can be settled definitively with CT. Abdominal and pelvic CT is extremely sensitive and detects extraintestinal gas in quantities as low as 0.3 mL.[161]

Pneumoretroperitoneum may develop in patients with abscess, perforation of a retroperitoneal portion of the gastrointestinal tract, or pneumomediastinum. Retroperitoneal air tends to remain unilateral, can often be seen under the diaphragm, and may outline the psoas muscle, kidney, or other retroperitoneal structures (see Figure 26–19).[147]

Biliary Obstruction, Cholecystitis, and Cholangitis

The normal gallbladder is generally 7 to 8 cm by 2 to 3 cm in dimension and is best imaged after the patient has fasted for 8 hours. In the emergency department, 5 to 10% of emergent examinations of the gallbladder will be limited by the patient's having eaten prior to the study.[181] Ultrasonography is the study of choice for diagnosing cholecystitis and should be performed in most patients with right-upper-quadrant pain, nausea, fever, and leukocytosis. Ultrasonographic findings suggestive of cholecystitis include pericholecystic fluid, wall thickening > 4 mm, the presence of an ultrasonographic Murphy sign, and a tense distended gallbladder.[182] Gallstones and biliary sludge, which typically play a role in the pathogenesis of cholecystitis, are commonly visualized. Approximately 10% of patients with acute cholecystitis, however,

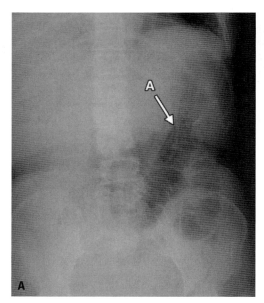
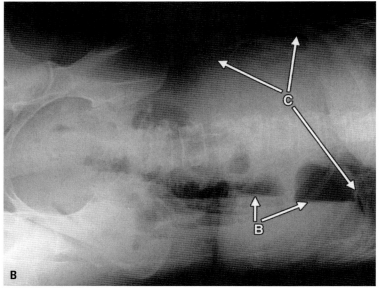

Figure 26–18. Bowel perforation evident on plain lateral decubitus view of the abdomen. A 60-year-old female with metastatic lung cancer presented with constipation and abdominal pain. A: Supine view reveals mildly dilated loops of small bowel *(A)*. B: Left lateral decubitus view shows multiple air-fluid levels *(B)* and free intraperitoneal air *(C)*.

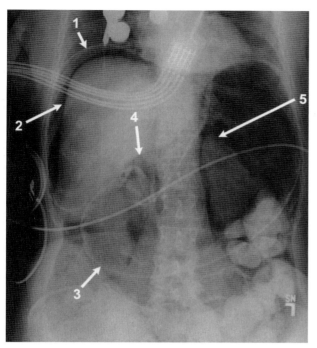

Figure 26–19. Plain film findings of free intra- and retroperitoneal air. A 47-year-old woman with metastatic esophageal cancer presented with abdominal pain following endoscopy for feeding tube placement. The patient was noted to have an esophageal perforation during the procedure. On this supine view the diaphragm *(1)* is evident, with underlying free air displacing the liver medially *(2)*. The greater curvature of the stomach demonstrates the "double-wall sign" *(3)* and the inferior margin of the liver is also outlined *(4)*. The left kidney is evident, outlined by free retroperitoneal air *(5)*.

develop disease (acalculous cholecystitis) without having gallstones. Ultrasonography of patients with acalculous cholecystitis demonstrates thickening of the gallbladder wall and an enlarged tender gallbladder. Acalculous cholecystitis often results in rupture of the gallbladder and carries a higher risk of mortality than calculous cholecystitis.[183] Radionuclide hepatobiliary hydroxy-iminodiacetic acid (HIDA) scans, with or without cholecystokinin administration, are recommended for the evaluation of patients with thickening of the gallbladder wall and with stones but no ultrasonographic Murphy sign and for patients with a positive Murphy sign but no other ultrasonographic findings.

Jaundice often reflects obstruction of the intra- or extrahepatic biliary tree. The most common causes of malignant obstruction are carcinoma of the head of the pancreas, carcinoma of the bile duct, and metastatic lymphadenopathy in the hepatoduodenal ligament. Obstructive and hepatocellular causes of jaundice can be differentiated by using US or CT to assess the hepatobiliary system for evidence of dilatation. Endoscopic US is unparalleled at depicting stones in the common bile duct.[184] In general, however, endoscopic retrograde cholangiopancreatography (ERCP) remains the gold standard for the complete evaluation of the biliopancreatic ducts and the definitive method for excluding stenoses or stones. By definition, endoscopic US and ERCP are invasive and expose patients to the inherent risks of endoscopy. Moreover, ERCP also carries the risk of precipitating cholangitis and pancreatitis. Magnetic resonance cholangiopancreatography has been reported to provide a diagnostic accuracy equivalent to that of ERCP.[185,186] For most patients with malignant biliary stenosis, MRCP combined with MRA provides effective staging and spares patients endoscopy, vascular cannulation, and unnecessary surgery.[187,188] Magnetic resonance cholangiopancreatography also aids in the identification of patients who require percutaneous stenting or who have anatomically complex lesions.[189] Patients with internal biliary stents who present with fever and suspected cholangitis require emergent imaging with US or CT to assess stent patency.

In general, acute pancreatitis is most often a consequence of alcohol ingestion or biliary tract disease. In patients with cancer, pancreatitis may also develop because of direct invasion of the pancreas by tumor (eg, from the stomach) or as a complication of surgical or endoscopic manipulation of the bile ducts. Pancreatitis may also be precipitated by malignancy-related hypercalcemia and by various agents, including L-asparaginase, 6-mercaptopurine, azathioprine, pentamidine, and (possibly) corticosteroids. Plain-film radiographic findings that are sometimes associated with pancreatitis include localized ileus, with the "sentinel loop" or the colon cutoff sign, and pancreatic calcifications (seen in chronic pancreatitis). An isolated left pleural effusion may be noted on the chest radiograph. Further abdominal imaging with US in thin patients and with CT in obese or critically ill patients is recommended to evaluate for calcifications, dilatated pancreatic ducts, and pancreatic necrosis. In the future, MRCP may replace contrast-enhanced CT as the technique of choice for evaluating pancreatic disease.[189,190]

Intra-abdominal Hemorrhage

The evaluation of gastrointestinal bleeding in patients with cancer is well outlined elsewhere.[175] Briefly, although slow bleeding from gastrointestinal tumors is common, frank hemorrhage is rare. Hemorrhage may occur, however, as a complication of treatment (because of thrombocytopenia, anticoagulation, or gastritis related to the use of nonsteroidal anti-inflammatory drugs [NSAIDs]), and esophageal varices may develop in patients with extensive liver metastases. Patients who vomit or retch violently may develop lacerations of the esophagogastric junction (Mallory-Weiss lesions) and hematemesis. Lower-gastrointestinal hemorrhage, as in patients without cancer, is most often related to diverticular disease, vascular malformations, or colitis. Nuclear scanning or angiography may be helpful in patients with active bleeding, but specific diagnoses are usually established with endoscopy.

Right-upper-quadrant pain suggestive of acute cholecystitis in patients with malignancies may represent hemorrhage into a hepatic tumor or metastasis. Similarly, in patients with hematologic malignancies or splenic metastases, left-upper-quadrant pain may indicate spontaneous rupture of the spleen. Retroperitoneal bleeding associated with coagulopathy or retroperitoneal tumor deposits may be occult. Patients may present with an unexplained drop in hematocrit and may be otherwise asymptomatic, or they may report lower-back pain and new ecchymoses of the flank or back. Rectus sheath hematomas sometimes occur in patients with coagulopathy or thrombocytopenia and are usually associated with muscular strain such as from coughing or twisting. Patients who develop rectus sheath hematomas present with acute abdominal pain with or without an associated mass of the anterior abdominal wall.[191] Contrast-enhanced CT of the abdomen and pelvis should be performed in most patients with suspected extraluminal intra-abdominal bleeding.[192] Unenhanced CT is adequate for the evaluation of patients with retroperitoneal hemorrhage. Bleeding into pre-existing metastases can usually be managed conservatively, but surgical intervention or arterial embolization is indicated for patients with uncontrolled hemorrhage.[193]

Intra-abdominal Infections

Neutropenic enterocolitis (an inflammatory enteritis of the terminal ileum and right colon) occurs almost exclusively in patients with cancer and carries a significant mortality (30 to 50% in some series), even in aggressively treated patients.[194,195] Typhlitis (neutropenic enterocolitis limited to the cecum) occurs in association with prolonged neutropenia, principally in patients with leukemia, myelodysplastic syndrome, and aplastic anemia but also occasionally in patients with solid tumors after aggressive therapy. Plain-film radiography is nonspecific but sometimes shows an ileus with a distended cecum. Computed tomography and US are more sensitive and typically show thickened bowel wall and pericolic fluid.[196] Endoscopy and enema contrast studies should be deferred because patients with neutropenic enterocolitis are already at increased risk for perforation.

Abscess formation occurs relatively frequently in the postoperative setting and may complicate any intra-abdominal infection. Depending on the location of the abscess, patients may complain of pain or symptoms referable to the compression of adjacent structures. Fever may be intermittent and low-grade, or it may be associated with rigors and night sweats. Related constitutional symptoms (fatigue, weight loss, etc) may be mistakenly attributed to the patient's underlying malignancy. Perirectal infection is a relatively common complication of prolonged neutropenia, especially in the setting of proctitis or localized radiotherapy. Plain-film radiography in patients with an abscess may reveal atypical collections, displacement of organs, or abnormal tissue densities. Imaging with CT is the best way to identify and characterize intra-abdominal abscesses. Fortunately, most abscesses are amenable to percutaneous draining (Figure 26-20).[197]

Ascites

Ascites is a frequent complication of intra-abdominal malignancy. With massive ascites, pressure on the stomach and diaphragm may cause pain, early satiety, vomiting, and dyspnea. Therapeutic paracentesis provides significant palliation for most patients. Ultrasonographic guidance of paracentesis is recommended for patients with peritoneal carcinomatosis, bulky disease, or a history of prior surgery as adhesions and/or organomegaly are common in such patients. Ultrasonographic guidance minimizes the risks of the procedure in these patients and identifies areas of loculated ascites that are unsuitable for drainage.

Vascular Emergencies

Mesenteric ischemia occasionally develops in patients with intra-abdominal desmoid and ileal carcinoid tumors. Rarely, it develops in patients with other primary

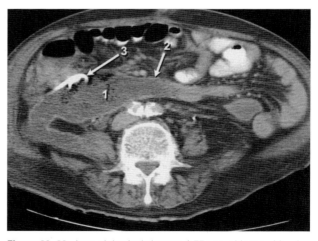

Figure 26–20. Intra-abdominal abscess. A 75-year-old man with colon cancer presented with fever and abdominal pain approximately 3 weeks after hemicolectomy, was found to have intra-abdominal abscess, and a percutaneous drainage catheter was placed. This follow-up contrast-enhanced abdominal CT image depicts the abscess containing air *(1)*, the wall of the abscess *(2)*, and the tip of the percutaneous drainage catheter *(3)*.

malignancies, because of arterial embolization of tumor fragments.[198–200] Risk factors for mesenteric ischemia in other patients include a history of arterial emboli, cardiac valvular disease, cardiac arrhythmias, and aortic atherosclerosis.[201] Emboli affect vessels in the watershed of the superior mesenteric artery 80% of the time. Patients with mesenteric ischemia classically present with abdominal pain that is "out of proportion" to the findings on physical examination. Leukocytosis, acidosis, and elevated serum amylase are nonspecific findings. Plain-film radiographic findings are also usually nonspecific but may include bowel gas patterns that are suggestive of ileus or that do not change on serial examination. Signs of bowel wall thickening, pseudotumor "thumbprinting" (caused by submucosal edema or hemorrhage), intestinal emphysema (pneumatosis intestinalis), air in mesenteric veins, air in the portal system, and free intraperitoneal air are late manifestations of bowel infarction. Ultrasonography, CT, and MRI are not diagnostic in patients with mesenteric ischemia but may rule out other causes of abdominal pain. Mesenteric angiography is diagnostic of thromboembolism, and patients in whom the diagnosis is established may be moved on to embolectomy. Complete recovery is possible if normal circulation is promptly restored, but in practice, transmural infarction and necrosis have usually already occurred by the time patients are brought to surgery.

Abdominal venous thrombosis is uncommon and has been reviewed elsewhere.[202] Plain-film radiographs are usually normal, they may be consistent with bowel ischemia. Contrast-enhanced CT is diagnostic of this uncommon entity.

IMAGING OF THE GENITOURINARY TRACT

Emergent radiographic assessment of the genitourinary tract is indicated for patients with acute renal failure of unclear etiology or with suspected urinary-tract infection (UTI), in patients with signs or symptoms of acute ureteral obstruction or urolithiasis, and in certain patients with hemorrhage. Patients with indwelling ureteral stents or stents with exteriorized catheters are subject to a variety of complications that may necessitate uroradiographic assessment, including stent migration or fragmentation, encrustation with urinary sediment, infection, pain, and erosion of the underlying tissue bed. The most important imaging techniques for the physician treating patients in an emergency setting are intravenous urography (IVU), US, and helical CT, which has emerged in recent years as an alternative to IVU for the evaluation of renal colic and other urologic disorders. Palliative interventional procedures are frequently used. Obstruction of the urinary tract, for example, may obligate external decompression, and emergent urinary diversion via percutaneous nephrostomy is indicated for patients with pyonephrosis or obstruction otherwise complicated by infection when endourologic decompression is unfeasible. Percutaneous nephrostomy has also been used to treat complicated malignant obstructions that are not amenable to retrograde stenting.

Urinary-Tract Obstruction

The causes of acute renal failure in patients with cancer are reviewed in Chapter 13. If a careful history and physical examination do not suggest prerenal azotemia or intrinsic renal disease as the basic disorder, the most likely explanation for declining glomerular filtration is an obstructive uropathy, especially if back or flank pain or signs or symptoms of infection are prominent. The causes of obstructive uropathy in cancer patients (also reviewed in Chapter 13) include malignant obstruction of the ureters, bladder neck, or urethra due to primary or metastatic cancer; calculi; blood clots; failure of indwelling stents; retroperitoneal fibrosis; accidental surgical ligation of the ureter; ureteral or urethral stricture; and papillary necrosis with sloughing due to analgesic nephropathy.[203] Bladder neck or urethral obstruction due to mechanical or neurophysiologic factors should be suspected in patients with suprapubic pain, a palpable bladder, and/or symptoms of hesitancy, dribbling, overflow incontinence, and incomplete bladder emptying. Such obstructions can usually be relieved by the passage of a small Foley catheter.[204] Radiologic tests are generally reserved for the evaluation of obstruction at or above the level of the ureters. For decades, IVU was the most commonly used method of investigating suspected renal obstruction, but clinical practice has evolved in recent years, and US and CT are now favored.

Findings on excretory urography that are suggestive of acute obstruction include (1) a persistently dense nephrogram, (2) renal enlargement, (3) moderate dilatation of the collecting system, (4) a delayed pyelogram, (5) ureteric dilatation, and (6) pyelosinus extravasation.[205] Concerns about contrast-induced nephrotoxicity (and the fact that IVU sometimes takes several hours to delineate the point of obstruction) have resulted in a reduction in the use of IVU.[206] Retrograde pyelography is an alternative when excretory urography is likely to be suboptimal because of poor renal function, but it requires anesthesia in most patients and exposes the patient to the risk of infection.

Renal US has several advantages over IVU and retrograde pyelography: It is noninvasive, quick, safe, and relatively inexpensive. Moreover, it excels at identifying hydronephrosis, with a sensitivity approaching 100%. Unfortunately, hydronephrosis does not always indicate obstruction, nor does obstruction always result in demonstrable hydronephrosis. It should be remembered that hydronephrosis is a *sign* of obstruction, with a specificity ranging from 75 to 90%.[207] Renal cystic disease, papillary necrosis, acute and chronic pyelonephritis, overhydration, diabetes insipidus, vesicoureteral reflux, a full bladder, and the use of diuretics have all been reported to cause nonobstructive hydronephrosis.[207] False-negative scan results, on the other hand, while rare, sometimes occur early in the course of obstruction or when acute obstruction causes pyelosinus backflow, leading to spontaneous decompression; they may also occur in patients with retroperitoneal tumors or fibrosis encasing the collecting system, in volume-depleted patients with partial or intermittent obstruction, and in patients in whom obesity or adjacent bowel gas limit the quality of the study.[207] An important refinement of renal US in this regard has been the application of Doppler technology. Doppler analysis reliably distinguishes vascular structures that cause separation of sinus echoes from true mild hydronephrosis, and it sometimes detects asymmetric jets of urine into the bladder, a finding consistent with unilateral obstruction.[208,209] The resistive index (a measure of renal arterial resistance) calculated with or without diuretic challenge, has been advocated as a "separate and distinct parameter from collecting-system dilatation" in the evaluation of urinary obstruction, but other authors have noted serious limitations in its usefulness, and its place in clinical practice is as a supportive or adjunctive tool rather than as a primary tool.[206,210,211] With relief of obstruction, the resistive index typically returns quickly to baseline levels, even if pyelocaliectasis persists, which is often the case after surgical intervention or stent placement. Doppler analysis thus appears to be valuable as a noninvasive method of assessing stent patency.[212]

The increasing availability and high sensitivity and specificity of unenhanced helical CT make it an attractive alternative to renal US for the evaluation of acute flank pain or azotemia of unclear etiology in patients with malignancy. The great advantage of this technique is its ability to determine not only the presence or absence of obstruction but also the obstruction's level and cause. (Renal US, by comparison, is poor at identifying the causes of hydronephrosis because bowel gas and bone often obscure the regions of interest.) Most intrinsic and extrinsic causes of ureteral obstruction, as well as extraurinary causes of acute flank pain, can be identified.[213,214] The sensitivity and specificity of the technique in identifying stone disease (the most extensively studied application) is greater than 95%, and helical CT appears to be accurate and effective for other purposes as well, such as the assessment of suspected acute appendicitis.[213–215] The use of IV contrast is avoided, eliminating the risk of adverse reactions and nephrotoxicity, and image acquisition takes less than a minute. Finally, at centers where the procedure is performed regularly, it may cost less than excretory urography.[216] Collectively, these advantages make helical CT the study of choice for the evaluation of suspected ureteral obstruction.

Urinary-Tract Infections and Pyelonephritis

Obstructive uropathies causing urinary stasis or vesicoureteral reflux, the frequent use of urinary catheters, the presence of indwelling stents and percutaneous nephrostomies, prolonged and repeated hospitalizations, immunocompromise, dehydration, and the liberal use of steroids and prophylactic antibiotics have put cancer patients at increased risk of developing UTIs with atypical or resistant organisms. Even infections caused by the usual pathogens can be difficult to eradicate in such patients. The standard teaching is that patients with UTIs that do not respond to appropriate antibiotic therapy require radiologic assessment to exclude complications such as septic ureteral obstruction, renal or perinephric abscess, emphysematous pyelitis or pyelonephritis, and pyonephrosis.[217–219] Once identified, these complications mandate aggressive intervention in all but the most terminally ill patients. Percutaneous drainage, as opposed to surgical intervention, is recommended for the initial management of renal and perinephric abscesses. It substantially reduces the duration of hospitalization and convalescence in such patients and may be curative in two-thirds of these cases.[220,221] Percutaneous aspirates also permit the tailoring of antibiotic or antifungal therapy to the specific pathogens involved. In a recent retrospective review of 315 patients receiving percutaneous nephrostomy for pyonephrosis, Watson and colleagues found that for 116 (37%) of the patients, the culture of aspirated material identified organisms disparate or additional to those that were isolated in blood and urine cultures, leading to a significant change of antibiotics and/or antifungal agents for 84 patients (27%).[222] Similar findings have been reported for renal and perinephric abscesses.[221] Contrast-enhanced CT appears to be the test of highest yield in patients with complicated renal infections.[218,219,223] Although less sensitive and less accurate, US can depict abscess and pyonephrosis and may be substituted for CT in patients who are unable to receive intravenous contrast. It sometimes misses and often underestimates the extent of emphysematous complications, but these rarely evolve in nondiabetic patients.[219,224] Finally, plain-film radiography of the abdomen and IVU are occasionally used to screen for calculi, changes in renal contour, and abnormal gas collections, but these findings are usually nonspecific and require confirmation by other imaging techniques.[217]

Percutaneous Nephrostomy

Interventional uroradiologic procedures now play an important role in the management of patients with cancer. Their use in patients with complicated renal infections has been mentioned, but the most common reason for performing percutaneous nephrostomy in cancer patients is to relieve malignant ureteral obstructions. The risks and benefits of urinary diversion should be carefully weighed before proceeding with percutaneous nephrostomy in patients with obstructed collecting systems, however. Creating a nephrostomy tract causes significant immediate complications (including renal hemorrhage, sepsis, injury of adjacent bowel or vascular structures, pneumo- and/or hemothorax, and death) in about 4% of patients. Minor complications (such as transient hematuria) occur in another 15 to 25% of patients.[225] Urinary diversion demonstrably benefits patients with nonmalignant obstruction as a complication of surgery or radiotherapy and appears to be beneficial in patients with malignant obstruction when there is a viable treatment option or when an improvement in renal function would facilitate the use of effective chemotherapy.[204,226] Percutaneous nephrostomy is probably unwarranted, however, in patients who have no conventional treatment option; Watkinson and colleagues reported that such patients have a median survival of just 38 days.[226]

Recent studies have clarified the role of ureteral decompression in patients with advanced malignancy. Donat and Russo reported significant morbidity (50%) and a median survival of fewer than 7 months for patients with advanced nonurologic malignancies undergoing endoscopic or percutaneous decompression of malignant ureteral obstructions. In only 2 of 40 patients did subsequent therapy permit removal of the devices before death, and 36 patients were known to have died with a stent or percutaneous nephrostomy tube in place. Of note, patients with gastric or pancreatic cancer survived a median of just 1.4 months after decompression, so decisions regarding decompression in such patients should be highly individualized.[227] In a study of 103 patients with advanced malignancies and undergoing endourologic diversion (stent or nephrostomy), Shekarriz and colleagues reported a median survival of 112 days, a complication rate of 68%, and prolonged hospitalization (> 50% of survival) between the procedure and death for most patients. A trend toward better survival and quality of life was noted in patients with obstructions caused by prostate carcinoma, but the differences noted lacked statistical significance. Patients with unilateral obstruction had prolonged survival (mean, 293 days), spent less time in the hospital (11% of survival), and reported resolution of flank pain after urinary diversion.[228] The benefits (if any) of urinary diversion in asymptomatic patients with unilateral ureteral obstruction and stable contralateral renal function, however, have not been defined. In general, patients with poor performance status or with disease that is progress-

ing despite maximal therapy should undergo decompression only when the procedure will substantially and immediately improve their welfare.

It is reasonable to attempt endoscopic stenting in most patients with cancer for whom decompression is appropriate, as the procedure will be successful in 40 to 70% of cases.[227–229] The most common complications of stent placement are infection and recurrent obstruction or encrustation. Pain, stent migration or fragmentation, and hematuria can also occur.[227] Unfortunately, approximately 50% of silicone and polyurethane stents deployed in patients with extrinsic compression of the ureters fail within 30 days of placement.[230] Improvements in stent design and the evolution of better biomaterials promise that future stents will be more durable and have a higher resistance to infection and encrustation than currently available models.[231] Extra-anatomic stents connecting the kidney and bladder via a subcutaneous tunnel have functioned well in selected patients; in the future, such stents may become an alternative to percutaneous nephrostomy for patients in whom conventional stents fail.[232,233]

IMAGING OF BONE AND SOFT TISSUES

The general principles of imaging primary or metastatic tumors in bone and soft tissue have been reviewed elsewhere in the literature.[234–240] Cancer patients who present to emergency or urgent care settings require orthopedic imaging when pathologic fracture is suspected or when severe pain suggests the presence of undocumented metastases. Compression of the spinal cord must be ruled out when progressive back pain is associated with signs or symptoms of neurologic dysfunction (see above). Vertebral fractures may result in spinal instability, neurologic deficits, and severe mechanical back pain and must be ruled out in the appropriate clinical setting.[241] Imaging is also appropriate for patients who report pain that is worse with weight bearing and is relieved by inactivity (to screen for impending pathologic fracture) and when the diagnosis of necrotizing fasciitis is entertained. The point of obtaining radiographic images is to confirm suspected diagnoses and to aid orthopedic consultants in their decision making. Treating physicians should remember that while the management of pathologic fractures in patients with cancer may differ from that of pathologic or usual traumatic fractures in other types of patient, the principles of imaging are the same.

Bone Metastases

Bone metastases have traditionally been classified as lytic, blastic, or mixed, based on their radiographic appearance (Figure 26–21). Lytic metastases are associated with breast, lung, thyroid, renal, and gastrointestinal malig-

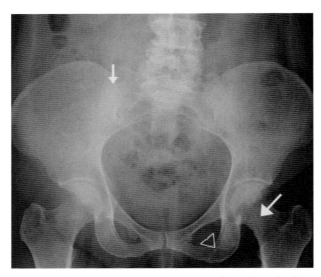

Figure 26–21. Bone metastases. Anteroposterior radiograph of the pelvis in a 62-year-old woman with metastatic breast cancer demonstrating blastic *(small arrow)*, mixed *(large arrow)*, and lytic *(open arrowhead)* lesions of right iliac wing, left femoral neck, and left inferior pubic ramus respectively.

nancies as well as multiple myeloma and melanoma whereas blastic metastases occur primarily in patients with bronchial carcinoid or prostate or bladder carcinoma. Mixed lesions are observed in patients with breast, ovarian, cervical, testicular, and some lung carcinomas.[236,237] Osteolytic lesions develop when bone resorption predominates over osteoblastic activity in the area of metastasis whereas osteoblastic (or sclerotic) lesions evolve when the situation is reversed. According to this schema, mixed lesions reflect the simultaneous acceleration of both processes within a single area of metastasis. This method of classification oversimplifies the pathophysiology of metastatic bone disease but has proved to be clinically useful in that patients with lytic or mixed lesions are thought to have a generally higher risk of fracture than patients with purely blastic lesions.[242,243] Although practical, this rule of thumb should be applied cautiously, for contradictory data have been reported. In a study of 203 women with 516 metastatic lesions in the proximal femur, for example, Keene and colleagues found no difference in the rate of fracture among lytic, blastic, and mixed lesions.[244] Whether or not they are stronger than bones with lytic metastases, bones with blastic metastases undoubtedly lack the strength and plasticity of normal bone. In a recent study of 112 men with hormone-refractory prostate cancer metastatic to bone who were followed for a median of 13.3 months, 30 (27%) suffered pathologic fracture or vertebral deformity or collapse requiring spinal orthosis. In 99 of these men, the bone mestastases were described as blastic (n = 73) or mixed (n = 26) in appearance.[245]

Pathologic Fractures

Patients with suspected fractures require radiography of the region in question, to define the fracture pattern and architecture of the surrounding bone, and full-length radiography of the affected bone in two planes, to screen for synchronous lesions. In patients with symptoms suggesting compression of the spinal cord or cauda equina, plain-film radiography may help to identify the level of vertebral collapse and deformity, but MRI better delineates the degree of cord compression and is vastly more sensitive in detecting significant vertebral and paravertebral metastases.[246] Computed tomography with or without myelography is the best alternative for patients with suspected cord compression when MRI is unavailable or contraindicated (see discussion above). Certain other types of fracture, including fractures of the pelvis, acetabulum, and sacrum, can also be difficult to visualize by plain-film radiography. Specialized views of particular areas may allow adequate visualization (eg, three-quarter internal and external oblique [Judet] views may be obtained to evaluate for acetabular fractures in patients with known acetabular metastases), but CT is generally more sensitive, especially in detecting subtle fractures (Figure 26–22). Computed tomography is demonstrably better than routine radiography at detecting fractures of the sacrum, the quadrilateral surface of the ilium, the acetabular roof, and the posterior acetabular lip; evaluating comminution of the acetabular dome; and discerning intra-articular bone fragments.[247] Magnetic resonance imaging is reported to have a sensitivity and specificity of 100% in diagnosing minimally impacted nondisplaced hip fractures and is clearly useful in the emergency setting.[248,249] When the field of view is expanded to include the pelvis, MRI reliably detects other lesions as well; radiographically occult pelvic fractures and soft-tissue injuries, for example, have been respectively demonstrated in 23% and 74% of patients referred for the assessment of hip pain (Figure 26–23).[250] Historically, because of its exquisite sensitivity, scintigraphy was the test of choice for patients with suspected hip or pelvic fracture and negative or equivocal radiographs. However, MRI permits the immediate diagnosis and precise characterization of such fractures and is currently favored.

Impending Pathologic Fractures

Because of the pain and morbidity associated with pathologic fracture, numerous attempts have been made to identify factors common to the lesions that are at greatest risk. It is argued that treating such lesions prophylactically is the best way to minimize pain and disability, decrease rehabilitation time, and prevent emergent hospitalization and surgery.[251] The findings most commonly cited as indicators of high risk are defects > 2.5 cm in dimension

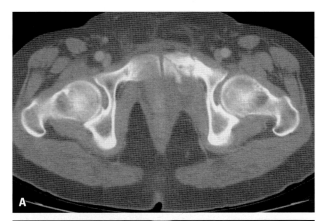

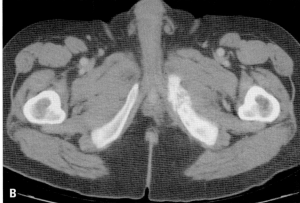

Figure 26–22. CT scan of the pelvis in a 62-year-old man with metastatic prostate cancer demonstrating extensive metastatic involvement and pathologic fractures of the left superior (Panel A) and inferior (Panel B) pubic rami with an associated extraosseous soft tissue component.

and lesions causing > 50% destruction of the cortex at any given level.[252] Unfortunately, these parameters permit only an approximate assessment of the risk any given lesion confers. The 2.5-cm criterion has been associated with a false-negative rate approaching or exceeding 40%, was derived from a retrospective analysis of femoral defects only, and has not been validated for metastases at other anatomic locations. Even when such lesions occur in the femur, their significance will vary considerably, depending on the size of the patient, the presence or absence of osteoporosis, and the lesion's degree of eccentricity (lesions at the point of maximal bending stress producing relatively greater loss of integrity than more central lesions) (Figure 26–24).[252] Moreover, accurately assessing the percentage of cortical involvement is difficult under the best of circumstances, and errors of greater than 100% can occur when measuring diaphyseal defect size from radiographs that are not optimally aligned with respect to the defect.[253] In one study using cadaveric femurs with simulated lytic defects in the intertrochanteric region, three highly trained orthopedic oncology surgeons were incapable of estimating either

the load-bearing capacity of the femurs or the strength reductions caused by the defects when compared with the intact contralateral femur, and they achieved only modest agreement regarding the maximum size of the simulated defects. The radiographs and CT scans the surgeons reviewed in making their estimates were obtained under optimal conditions after the femurs had been stripped of soft tissue, so their quality was better than that which can be achieved clinically. The authors concluded that predicting the risk of pathologic fracture on the basis of radiographic features alone was fraught with hazard.[252] Most of the current systems for predicting the risk of pathologic fracture use radiographic and clinical findings in some combination. Mirels' scoring system for long-bone metastases that have not been previously irradiated assigns one, two, or three points for each of four variables according to the degree of associated risk: site (upper limb, lower limb, or peritrochanter), pain (mild, moderate, or functional), type of lesion (blastic, mixed, or lytic), and size ($< 1/3$, $1/3$ to $2/3$, or $> 2/3$ of the diameter of the involved bone). Mirels found that lesions with a score of ≤ 7 had a 4% probability of fracture within 6 months of irradiation, lesions with a score of 9 had a probability of 57%, and lesions with a score of ≥ 10 had a probability of 100%. The most significant indicator of impending fracture was functional pain.[243] Harrington's indications for prophylactic fixation of impending long-

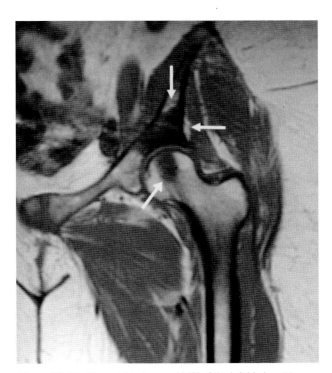

Figure 26–23. T1–weighted coronal MRI of the left hip in a 54-year-old woman with metastatic breast cancer demonstrating low signal intensity lesions in the ilium, acetabulum, and femoral head *(arrows)*.

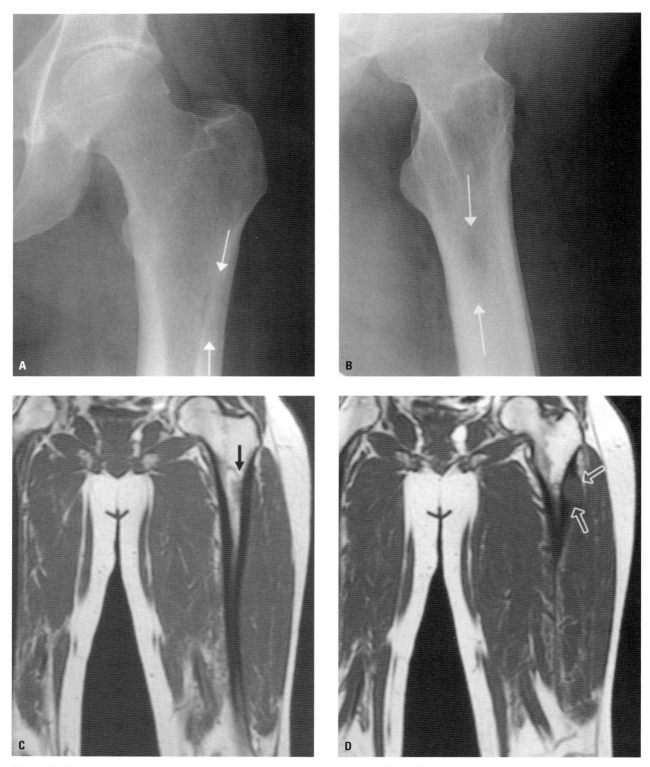

Figure 26–24. Impending fracture with associated soft tissue mass. Anteroposterior (Panel A) and lateral (Panel B) radiographs of the left hip in a 30-year-old man with metastatic renal cell carcinoma demonstrating a lytic lesion *(arrows)* involving the lateral aspect of the proximal femur with associated cortical destruction. This lesion (Panel C; *arrow*) and an associated 3.4 × 2.3 × 2.0 cm soft tissue mass in the proximal portion of the left vastus intermedius muscle (Panel D; *open arrows*) are better visualized on spin echo T1-weighted coronal MRI of the left lower extremity. The patient underwent excision of the soft tissue tumor and prophylactic resection of the head and neck of the femur with insertion of a long stem bipolar prosthesis 11 days after the MRI was obtained.

bone fractures include (1) cortical bone destruction of > 50%; (2) lesions of the proximal femur measuring ≥ 2.5 cm in any view; (3) pathologic avulsion fracture of the lesser trochanter; and (4) persistent pain with stress or weight bearing, despite irradiation.[254] At Memorial Sloan-Kettering Cancer Center, prophylactic fixation is performed when (1) painful medullary lytic lesions occupy more than 50% of the cross-sectional bone diameter, (2) painful lytic lesions involve cortex greater than the cross-sectional diameter of the bone, (3) painful cortical lesions exceed 2.5 cm in length, or (4) lesions produce mechanical pain after radiation therapy.[251]

Assessing the Response of Bone Metastases to Medical Therapy and Radiation

Assessing the response of bone metastases to chemotherapy or irradiation can be difficult, especially in the acute setting. Where prior radiographs are available for comparison, the development of new lytic lesions or the enlargement of existing ones obviously indicates progression of disease, but new sclerotic lesions may represent either progression of disease or the healing of previously inapparent lytic metastases (in which case referring to prior scintigrams can be helpful). In general, the development of a sclerotic rim or sclerosis in a treated lytic lesion signifies a response to therapy. Healing lesions fill centripetally until they become uniformly sclerotic, after which (over several months to years) they may regress completely. On the other hand, if a lesion with a sclerotic rim enlarges or if the sclerotic response diminishes prematurely, then progression has occurred. Blastic metastases demonstrate response by gradually fading away whereas enlarging areas of sclerosis imply progression. Serial scintigraphy may be useful in assessing the response to therapy for any type of metastasis, but the scintigrams should not be read in isolation. During the first 4 to 12 weeks, successful therapy can actually cause an increase in radionuclide uptake, but this "false flare" will be followed by a prolonged period of decreased uptake with a loss of anatomic detail. Diminished uptake, however, is also sometimes observed in patients with rapidly progessive disease, presumably because the disease is so aggressive that there is little chance of new bone formation. In ambiguous cases, MRI or CT can be helpful.[234]

Necrotizing Fasciitis and Other Soft-Tissue Infections

Necrotizing fasciitis, crepitant cellulitis, and streptococcal gangrene are uncommon but potentially devastating infections of the skin and subcutaneous tissues. Group A *Streptococcus* is the most common organism isolated from culture, and patients with cancer are at increased risk of infection with this pathogen for a variety of reasons (eg, general debilitation, malnutrition, immunosuppression, regional lymph node dissections, the presence of edema, and injuries, ranging from needle sticks to surgery, disrupting the integrity of the skin).[255] Necrotizing fasciitis, by definition, represents the extension of infection from whatever source to the superficial (and often the deep) fascia. Prompt diagnosis is crucial because of the rapidity with which these infections can progress but may be difficult because the initial signs, which include pain, edema, and erythema, are not distinctive. Subcutaneous gas is pathognomonic of the polymicrobial form of necrotizing fasciitis and was the basis of early attempts to use radiographic techniques as an aid to diagnosis. Fisher and colleagues found roentgenographic studies to be more sensitive than physical examination for crepitus for the detection of gas in soft tissues, and scrotal US has been used to identify skin thickening and subcutaneous air in cases of Fournier's gangrene.[256,257] Deeper fascial gas, however, is rarely identified on plain-film radiographs, and gas does not develop in the soft tissues of every patient with necrotizing fasciitis. For these reasons and because of the increasing prevalence of invasive soft-tissue infections, CT and MRI have been investigated as adjuncts to diagnosis. Computed tomography depicts abnormal gas in soft tissues with high resolution, may provide information about coexisting deep fluid collections, and can distinguish necrotizing fasciitis from myonecrosis. Asymmetric fascial thickening and fat stranding are noted in up to 80% of patients, and correspond to the extent of disease as confirmed by surgery.[258] With MRI, the absence of gadolinium contrast enhancement on T1-weighted images reliably detects fascial necrosis and thereby identifies patients who require operative débridement.[259] Using different criteria in a retrospective review of 17 patients with clinically suspected necrotizing fasciitis, Schmid and colleagues reported a sensitivity of 100%, a specificity of 86%, and an accuracy of 94% for MRI in differentiating necrotizing fasciitis from cellulitis. This high sensitivity was mainly due to the ability of MRI to detect fluid collections along deep fascial sheaths. Such fluid collections were characterized by high signal intensity and thickening of the fascial planes on T2-weighted images and enhancement (presumably because of early extravasation of gadolinium into areas of necrosis) on T1-weighted images. When compared to the findings at surgery, however, this method tended to overestimate the extent of infection and resulted in the overstaging of 1 of 6 cases of cellulitis. Nevertheless, the authors concluded that MRI should be the technique of choice for differentiating necrotizing fasciitis from cellulitis.[260] Magnetic resonance imaging has also been shown to be more helpful than CT in planning operative intervention in patients with infections of the chest or abdominal wall.[261]

We would like to thank Dr. Anita Wu, for sharing materials, and Dr. Susan Hilton, Dr. Nina Luxenberg, and Dr. Jeffrey Raizer, for reviewing sections of the manuscript.

REFERENCES

1. Kremkau FW. Diagnostic ultrasound: principles, instruments and exercises. Philadelphia: W.B. Saunders; 1989.

2. Colby JM. Contrast imaging. In: Harwood-Nuss AL, Linden CH, Luten RC, et al, editors. The clinical practice of emergency medicine. 2nd ed. Philadelphia: Lippincott-Raven; 1996. p. 1598.

3. Knorr JR, Davidoff A. Computed tomography. In: Harwood-Nuss AL, Linden CH, Luten RC, et al, editors. The clinical practice of emergency medicine. 2nd ed. Philadelphia: Lippincott-Raven; 1996. p. 1589.

4. Grossman RI, Yousem DM. Neuroradiology: the requisites. St. Louis: Mosby-Year Book; 1994.

5. Ibukuro K, Charnsangavej C, Chasen MH, et al. Helical CT angiography with multiplanar reformation: techniques and clinical applications. Radiographics 1995;15:671–82.

6. McCarthy CS, Becker JA. Multiple myeloma and contrast media. Radiology 1992;183:519–21.

7. Caro JJ, Trindade E, McGregor M. The risks of death and of severe nonfatal reactions with high- vs. low-osmolality contrast media: a meta-analysis. AJR Am J Roentgenol 1991;156:825–32.

8. Rubin RA, Mitchell DG. Evaluation of the solid hepatic mass. Med Clin North Am 1996;80:907–28.

9. Vezina LG. Diagnostic imaging in neuro-oncology. Pediatr Clin North Am 1997;44:701–19.

10. Prichard JW, Grossman RI. New reasons for early use of MRI in stroke. Neurology 1999;52:1733–6.

11. Araiza, J, Araiza B. Neuroimaging. Emerg Med Clin North Am 1997;15:507–26.

12. Barish RA, Young J, Whye D. Altered consciousness and syncope. In: Rosen P, Doris PE, Barkin RM, Markovchick VJ, editors. Diagnostic radiology in emergency medicine. St. Louis: Mosby-Year Book; 1992. p. 391.

13. Posner JB. Overview. In: Neurologic complications of cancer. Philadelphia: F.A. Davis; 1995. p. 5–14.

14. Clouston PD, DeAngelis LM, Posner JB. The spectrum of neurologic disease in patients with systemic cancer. Ann Neurol 1992;31:268–73.

15. Posner JB. Intracranial metastases. In: Neurologic complications of cancer. Philadelphia: F.A. Davis; 1995. p. 77–110.

16. Schiff D, O'Neill BP, Suman VJ. Spinal epidural metastasis as the initial manifestation of malignancy: clinical features and diagnostic approach. Neurology 1997;49:452–6.

17. DeAngelis LM, Posner JB. Neurologic complications. In: Bast RC, Holland JF, Pollock RE, et al, editors. Cancer medicine. 5th ed. Vol. 5. Hamilton: B.C. Decker,; 2000. p. 2251–78.

18. Quinn JA, DeAngelis LM. Neurologic emergencies in the cancer patient. Semin Oncol 2000;27:311–21.

19. Suzuki T, Shimizu T, Kurokawa K, et al. Pattern of prostate cancer metastasis to the vertebral column. Prostate 1994;25:141–6.

20. Zachariah B, Casey L, Zachariah SB, et al. Case report: brain metastasis from primary small cell carcinoma of the prostate. Am J Med Sci 1994;308:177–9.

21. Byrne TN. Spinal cord compression from epidural metastases. N Engl J Med 1992;327:614–9.

22. Lesser GJ, Grossman S. The chemotherapy of high-grade astrocytomas. Semin Oncol 1994;21:220–35.

23. Posner JB. Brain metastases: 1995. A brief review. J Neurooncol 1996;27:287–93.

24. Delattre JY, Krol G, Thaler HT, Posner JB. Distribution of brain metastases. Arch Neurol 1988;45:741–4.

25. Wen PY. Diagnosis and management of brain tumors. In: Black PM, Loeffler JS, editors. Cancer of the nervous system. Cambridge: Blackwell Science; 1997. p. 106–27.

26. Provenzale JM. Centennial dissertation. Honoring Arthur W. Goodspeed, MD and James B. Bullitt, MD. CT and MR imaging and nontraumatic neurologic emergencies. AJR Am J Roentgenol 2000;174:289–99.

27. Seung SK, Shu HK, McDermott MW, et al. Stereotactic radiosurgery for malignant melanoma to the brain. Surg Clin North Am 1996;76:1399–411.

28. Kirchin MA, Pirovano GP, Spinazzi A. Gadobenate dimeglumine (Gd-BOPTA): an overview. Invest Radiol 1998;33:798–809.

29. Ropper AH. Trauma of the head and spinal cord. In: Braunwald E, Isselbacher KJ, Petersdorf RG, et al, editors. Harrison's principles of internal medicine. 11th ed. New York: McGraw Hill; 1987. p. 1960–8.

30. Ashikaga R, Araki Y, Ishida O. MRI of head injury using FLAIR. Neuroradiology 1997;39:239–42.

31. Graus F, Rogers LR, Posner JB. Cerebrovascular complication in patients with cancer. Medicine 1985;64:16–35.

32. Bunin NJ, Pui CH. Differing complications of hyperleukocytosis in children with acute lymphoblastic or acute nonlymphoblastic leukemia. J Clin Oncol 1985;3:1590–5.

33. Stieg PE, Kase CS. Intracranial hemorrhage: diagnosis and emergency management. Neurol Clin 1998;16:373–90.

34. Noguchi K, Ogawa T, Seto H, et al. Subacute and chronic subarachnoid hemorrhage: diagnosis with fluid attenuated inversion-recovery MR imaging. Radiology 1997;203:257–62.

35. Kopitnik TA, Samson DS. Management of subarachnoid hemorrhage. J Neurol Neurosurg Pysch 1993;56:947–59.

36. Beauchamp NJ, Bryan RN. Acute cerebral ischemic infarction: a pathophysiologic review and radiologic perspective. AJR Am J Roentgenol 1998:171:73–84.

37. Wityk RJ, Beauchamp NJ. Diagnostic evaluation of stroke. Neurol Clin 2000;18:357–78.

38. Shimamura K, Oka K, Nakazawa M, Kojima M. Distribution patterns of microthrombi in disseminated intravascular coagulation. Arch Pathol Lab Med 1983;107:543–7.

39. Feinberg WM, Swenson MR. Cerebrovascular complication of L-asparaginase therapy. Neurology 1988; 38:127–33.

40. Eidelberg D, Sotrel A, Horoupian DS, et al. Thrombotic cerebral vasculopathy associated with herpes zoster. Ann Neurol 1986;19:7–14.

41. Hacke W, Warach S. Diffusion-weighted MRI as an evolving standard of care in acute stroke. Neurology 2000; 54:1548–9.

42. American Academy of Neurology. Practice parameter: neuroimaging in the emergency patient presenting with seizure – summary statement. Quality Standards Subcommittee of the American Academy of Neurology in cooperation with American College of Emergency Physicians, American Association of Neurological Surgeons, and American Society of Neuroradiology. Neurology 1996;47:288–91.

43. Delattre JY, Posner JB. Neurological complications of chemotherapy and radiation therapy. In: Aminoff MJ, editor. Neurology and general medicine. New York: Churchill Livingstone; 1995. p. 421–45.

44. Schwartz RB, Bravo SM, Klufas RA, et al. Cyclosporine neurotoxicity and its relationship to hypertensive encephalopathy: CT and MR findings in 16 cases. AJR Am J Roentgenol 1995;165:627–31.

45. Posner JB. Central nervous system infections. In: Neurologic complications of cancer. Philadelphia: F.A. Davis; 1995. p. 230–63.

46. Harter DH, Petersdorf RG. Pyogenic infections of the central nervous system. In: Braunwald E, Isselbacher KJ, Petersdorf RG, et al, editors. Harrison's principles of internal medicine. 11th ed. New York: McGraw Hill; 1987. p. 1980–7.

47. Enzmann DR, Britt RH, Placone R. Staging of human brain abscess by computed tomography. Radiology 1983;146:703–8.

48. Wagner R, Jagoda A. Spinal cord syndromes. Emerg Med Clin North Am 1997;15:699–711.

49. Posner JB. Spinal metastases. In: Neurologic complications of cancer. Philadelphia: F.A. Davis; 1995. p. 111–42.

50. Helweg-Larsen S, Hansen SW, Sorensen PS. Second occurrence of symptomatic metastatic spinal cord compression and findings of multiple spinal epidural metastases. Int J Radiat Oncol Biol Phys 1995;33:595–8.

51. Schultheiss TE, Stephens LC. Invited review: permanent radiation myelopathy. Br J Radiol 1992;65:737–53.

52. Glantz MJ, Burger PC, Friedman AH, et al. Treatment of radiation-induced nervous system injury with heparin and warfarin. Neurology 1994;44:2020–7.

53. Schiff D, O'Neill BP. Intramedullary spinal cord metastases: clinical features and treatment outcome. Neurology 1996;47:906–12.

54. Graus F. Acute meningospinal syndromes: acute myelopathy and radiculopathy. In: Hildebrand J, editor. European School of Oncology monographs. Neurological adverse reactions to anticancer drugs. Berlin: Springer-Verlag; 1990. p. 87–92.

55. McLean DR, Clink HM, Enst P, et al. Myelopathy after intrathecal chemotherapy. A case report with unique magnetic resonance imaging changes. Cancer 1994;73: 3037–40.

56. Maranzano E, Latini P. Effectiveness of radiation therapy without surgery in metastatic spinal cord compression: final results from a prospective trial. Int J Radiat Oncol Biol Phys 1995;32:959–67.

57. Gilbert RW, Kim JH, Posner JB. Epidural spinal cord compression from metastatic tumor: diagnosis and treatment. Ann Neurol 1978;3:40–51.

58. Portenoy RK, Galer BS, Salamon O, et al. Identification of epidural neoplasm. Radiography and bone scintigraphy in the symptomatic and asymptomatic spine. Cancer 1989;64:2707–13.

59. Johnston RA. The management of acute spinal cord compression. J Neurol Neurosurg Psychiatry 1993;56: 1046–54.

60. Van Oostenbrugge RJ, Twijnstra A. Presenting features and value of diagnostic procedures in leptomeningeal metastases. Neurology 1999;53:382–5.

61. Posner JB. Leptomeningeal metastases. In: Neurologic complications of cancer. Philadelphia: F.A. Davis; 1995. p. 143–71.

62. Witte RJ, Gurney JW, Robbins RA, et al. Diffuse pulmonary alveolar hemorrhage after bone marrow transplantation: radiographic findings in 39 patients. AJR Am J Roentgenol 1991;157:461–4.

63. Reich JM, Mullooly JP, Johnson RE. Linkage analysis of malignancy-associated sarcoidosis. Chest 1995;107: 605–13.

64. Hunsaker AR, Munden RF, Pugatch RD, Mentzer SJ. Sarcoidlike reaction in patients with malignancy. Radiology 1996;200:255–61.

65. Tietjen PA, Lukeso D, Vander Els NJ, et al. Bronchiolitis obliterans with organizing pneumonia (BOOP) in cancer patients [abstract]. Chest 1994;106 (Suppl 2):156S.

66. Elliott CG, Goldhaber SZ, Visani L, DeRosa M. Chest radiographs in acute pulmonary embolism. Chest 2000;118:33–8.

67. Hildebrand FL, Rosenow EC, Tazelaar HD. Pulmonary complications of leukemia. Chest 1990;98:1233–9.

68. Wardman AG, Milligan DW, Child JA, et al. Pulmonary infiltrates and adult acute leukaemia: empirical treatment and survival related to the extent of pulmonary radiological disease. Thorax 1984;39:568–71.

69. Singer C, Armstrong D, Rosen PP, et al. Diffuse pulmonary infiltrates in immunosuppressed patients. Prospective study of 80 cases. Am J Med 1979;66:110–20.

70. Rosenow EC. Diffuse pulmonary infiltrates in the immunocompromised host. Clin Chest Med 1990;11:55–64.

71. Tenholder MF, Hooper RG. Pulmonary infiltrates in leukemia. Chest 1980;78:468–73.

72. Pennington JE, Feldman NT. Pulmonary infiltrates and fever in patients with hematologic malignancy. Assessment of transbronchial biopsy. Am J Med 1977;62:581–7.

73. Santamauro JT, Stover DE. *Pneumocystis carinii* pneumonia. Med Clin North Am 1997;81:299–318.

74. Sepkowitz KA, Brown AE, Telzak EE, et al. *Pneumocystis carinii* pneumonia among patients without AIDS at a cancer hospital. JAMA 1992;267:832–7.

75. Kennedy CA, Goetz MB. Atypical roentgenographic manifestations of *Pneumocystis carinii* pneumonia. Arch Intern Med 1992;152:1390–8.

76. Ewig S, Torres A, Riquelme R, et al. Pulmonary complications in patients with haematological malignancies treated at a respiratory ICU. Eur Respir J 1998;12:116–22.

77. Mahmoud AAF. Intestinal nematodes (roundworms). In:

Mandell GL, Bennett JE, Dolin R, editors. Principles and practice of infectious diseases. 4th ed. New York: Churchill Livingstone; 1995. p. 2526–31.

78. Pomeroy C, Filice GA. Pulmonary toxoplasmosis: a review. Clin Infect Dis 1992;14:863–70.

79. Movsas B, Raffin TA, Epstein AH, Link CJ Jr. Pulmonary radiation injury. Chest 1997;111:1061–76.

80. Crestani B, Kambouchner M, Soler P, et al. Migratory bronchiolitis obliterans organizing pneumonia after unilateral radiation therapy for breast carcinoma. Eur Respir J 1995;8:318–21.

81. Rosiello RA, Merrill WW. Radiation-induced lung injury. Clin Chest Med 1990;11:65–71.

82. Pagani JJ, Libshitz HI. CT manifestations of radiation-induced change in chest tissue. J Comput Assist Tomogr 1982;6:243–8.

83. Ikezoe J, Takashima S, Morimoto S, et al. CT appearance of acute radiation-induced injury in the lung. AJR Am J Roentgenol 1988;150:765–70.

84. Jules-Elysee K, White DA. Bleomycin-induced pulmonary toxicity. Clin Chest Med 1990;11:1–20.

85. Twohig KJ, Matthay RA. Pulmonary effects of cytotoxic agents other than bleomycin. Clin Chest Med 1990;11:31–54.

86. Taylor CR. Diagnostic imaging techniques in the evaluation of drug-induced pulmonary disease. Clin Chest Med 1990;11:87–94.

87. Buzdar AU, Legha SS, Luna MA, et al. Pulmonary toxicity of mitomycin. Cancer 1980;45:236–44.

88. Malik SW, Myers JL, DeRemee RA, Specks U. Lung toxicity associated with cyclophosphamide use. Two distinct patterns. Am J Respir Crit Care Med 1996;154:1851–6.

89. Vander Els NJ, Miller V. Successful treatment of gemcitabine toxicity with a brief course of oral corticosteroid therapy. Chest 1998;114:1779–81.

90. Rivera MP, Kris MG, Gralla RJ, White DA. Syndrome of acute dyspnea related to combined mitomycin plus vinca alkaloid chemotherapy. Am J Clin Oncol 1995;18:245–50.

91. Yokose N, Ogata K, Tamura H, et al. Pulmonary toxicity after granulocyte colony-stimulating factor-combined chemotherapy for non-Hodgkin's lymphoma. Br J Cancer 1998;77:2286–90.

92. Lei KI, Leung WT, Johnson PJ. Serious pulmonary complications in patients receiving recombinant granulocyte colony-stimulating factor during BACOP chemotherapy for aggressive non-Hodgkin's lymphoma. Br J Cancer 1994;70:1009–13.

93. Bellamy EA, Husband JE, Blaquiere RM, Law MR. Bleomycin-related lung damage: CT evidence. Radiology 1985;156:155–8.

94. Jasmer RM, McCowin MJ, Webb WR. Miliary lung disease after intravesical bacillus Calmette-Guérin immunotherapy. Radiology 1996;201:43–4.

95. Israel-Biet D, Venet A, Sandron D, et al. Pulmonary complications of intravesical bacille Calmette-Guérin immunotherapy. Am Rev Respir Dis 1987;135:763–5,

96. Vogelzang PJ, Bloom SM, Mier JW, Atkins MB. Chest roentgenographic abnormalities in IL-2 recipients. Incidence and correlation with clinical parameters. Chest 1992;101:746–52.

97. Frankel SR, Eardley A, Lauwers G, et al. The "retinoic acid syndrome" in acute promyelocytic leukemia. Ann Intern Med 1992;117:292–6.

98. Camacho LH, Soignet SL, Chanel S, et al. Leukocytosis and the retinoic acid syndrome in patients with acute promyelocytic leukemia treated with arsenic trioxide. J Clin Oncol 2000;18:2620–5.

99. Rinaldo JE, Owens GR, Rogers RM. Adult respiratory distress syndrome following intrapleural instillation of talc. J Thorac Cardiovasc Surg 1983;85:523–6.

100. Rehse DH, Aye RW, Florence MG. Respiratory failure following talc pleurodesis. Am J Surg 1999;177:437–40.

101. Woodring JH. Unusual radiographic manifestations of lung cancer. Radiol Clin North Am 1990;28:599–618.

102. Kennedy P, Buck M, Joshua DE, Kronenberg H. Rapidly progressive fatal pulmonary infiltration by lymphoma. Aust N Z J Med 1985;15:62–5.

103. Cathcart-Rake W, Bone RC, Sobonya RE, Stephens RL. Rapid development of diffuse pulmonary infiltrates in histiocytic lymphoma. Am Rev Respir Dis 1978;117:587–93.

104. Myers TJ, Cole SR, Klatsky AU, Hild DH. Respiratory failure due to pulmonary leukostasis following chemotherapy of acute nonlymphocytic leukemia. Cancer 1983;51:1808–13.

105. Tryka AF, Godleski JJ, Fanta CH. Leukemic cell lysis pneumonopathy. A complication of treated myeloblastic leukemia. Cancer 1982;50:2763–70.

106. Epler GR, Colby TV, McLoud TC, et al. Bronchiolitis obliterans organizing pneumonia. N Engl J Med 1985;312:152–8.

107. Wells PS, Hirsh J, Anderson DR, et al. Accuracy of clinical assessment of deep-vein thrombosis. Lancet 1995;345:1326–30.

108. Landefeld CS, McGuire E, Cohen A. Clinical findings associated with acute proximal deep vein thrombosis: a basis for quantifying clinical judgment. Am J Med 1990;88:382–8.

109. Wells PS, Ginsberg JS, Anderson DR, et al. Use of a clinical model for safe management of patients with suspected pulmonary embolism. Ann Intern Med 1998;129:997–1005.

110. Zuckerman DA, Sterling KM, Oser RF. Safety of pulmonary angiography in the 1990s. J Vasc Interv Radiol 1996;7:199–205.

111. Anderson DR, Wells PS. Improvements in the diagnostic approach for patients with suspected deep vein thrombosis or pulmonary embolism. Thromb Haemost 1999;82:878–86.

112. American Thoracic Society Clinical Practice Committee. The diagnostic approach to acute venous thromboembolism. Am J Respir Crit Care Med 1999;160:1043–66.

113. Rémy-Jardin M, Rémy J, Wattinne L, Giraud F. Central pulmonary thromboembolism: diagnosis with spiral volumetric CT with the single-breath-hold technique—comparison with pulmonary angiography. Radiology 1992;185:381–7.

114. Teigen CL, Maus TP, Sheedy PF II, et al. Pulmonary embolism: diagnosis with electron-beam CT. Radiology 1993;188:839–45.

115. Meaney JFM, Weg JG, Chenevert TL, et al. Diagnosis of pulmonary embolism with magnetic resonance angiography. N Engl J Med 1997;336:1422–7.

116. Garg K, Sieler H, Welsh C, et al. Clinical validity of helical CT being interpreted as negative for pulmonary embolism: implications for patient treatment. AJR Am J Roentgenol 1999;172:1627–31.

117. Goodman LR, Lipchik RJ, Kuzo RS, et al. Subsequent pulmonary embolism after a negative helical CT pulmonary angiogram—prospective comparison with scintigraphy. Radiology 2000;215:535–42.

118. Rathbun SW, Raskob GE, Whitsett TL. Sensitivity and specificity of helical computed tomography in the diagnosis of pulmonary embolism: a systematic review. Ann Intern Med 2000;132:227–32.

119. Yucel EK. Pulmonary MR angiography: is it ready now? Radiology 1999;210:301–3.

120. Stein PD, Terrin ML, Gottschalk A, et al. Value of ventilation/perfusion scans compared to perfusion scans alone in acute pulmonary embolism. Am J Cardiol 1992;69:1239–41.

121. The PIOPED Investigators. Value of the ventilation/perfusion scan in acute pulmonary embolism: results of the Prospective Investigation of Pulmonary Embolism Diagnosis (PIOPED). JAMA 1990;263:2753–9.

122. Hull RD, Raskob GE, Ginsberg JS, et al. A noninvasive strategy for the treatment of patients with suspected pulmonary embolism. Arch Intern Med 1994;154:289–97.

123. Hillner BE, Philbrick JT, Becker DM. Optimal management of suspected lower-extremity deep vein thrombosis. An evaluation with cost assessment of 24 management strategies. Arch Intern Med 1992;152:165–75.

124. Goodman LR, Lipchik RJ. Diagnosis of acute pulmonary embolism: time for a new approach. Radiology 1996;199:25–7.

125. ACCP Consensus Committee on Pulmonary Embolism. Opinions regarding the diagnosis and management of venous thromboembolic disease. Chest 1998;113:499–504.

126. Goodman LR, Curtin JJ, Mewissen MW, et al. Detection of pulmonary embolism in patients with unresolved clinical and scintigraphic diagnosis: helical CT versus angiography. AJR Am J Roentgenol 1995;164:1369–74.

127. Meaney JFM, Weg JG, Chenevert TL, et al. Diagnosis of pulmonary embolism with magnetic resonance angiography. N Engl J Med 1997;336:1422–7.

128. Gupta A, Frazer CK, Ferguson JM, et al. Acute pulmonary embolism: diagnosis with MR angiography. Radiology 1999;210:353–9.

129. Stein PD, Henry JW. Prevalence of acute pulmonary embolism in central and subsegmental pulmonary arteries and relation to probability interpretation of ventilation/perfusion lung scans. Chest 1997;111:1246–8.

130. Oser RF, Zuckerman DA, Gutierrez FR, Brink JA. Anatomic distribution of pulmonary emboli at pulmonary angiography: implications for cross-sectional imaging. Radiology 1996;199:31–5.

131. Gurney JW. No fooling around: direct visualization of pulmonary embolism. Radiology 1993;188:618–9.

132. Dalen JE. When can treatment be withheld in patients with suspected pulmonary embolism? Arch Intern Med 1993;153:1415–8.

133. Van Erkel AR, Van Rossum AB, Bloem JL, et al. Spiral CT angiography for suspected pulmonary embolism: a cost-effectiveness analysis. Radiology 1996;201:29–36.

134. Mayo JR, Rémy-Jardin M, Muller NL, et al. Pulmonary embolism: prospective comparison of spiral CT with ventilation-perfusion scintigraphy. Radiology 1997;205:447–52.

135. Rémy-Jardin M, Rémy J, Deschildre F, et al. Diagnosis of pulmonary embolism with spiral CT: comparison with pulmonary angiography and scintigraphy. Radiology 1996;200:699–706.

136. Kim K, Muller NL, Mayo JR. Clinically suspected pulmonary embolism: utility of spiral CT. Radiology 1999;210:693–7.

137. Rémy-Jardin M, Rémy J. Spiral CT angiography of the pulmonary circulation. Radiology 1999;212:615–36.

138. Rémy-Jardin M, Rémy J, Artaud D, et al. Peripheral pulmonary arteries: optimization of the acquisition protocol. Radiology 1997;204:157–63.

139. Schoepf UJ, Helmberger T, Holzknecht N, et al. Segmental and subsegmental pulmonary arteries: evaluation with electron-beam versus spiral CT. Radiology 2000;214:433–9.

140. Rémy-Jardin M, Baghaie F, Bonnel F, et al. Thoracic helical CT: influence of subsecond scan time and thin collimation on evaluation of peripheral pulmonary arteries. Eur Radiol 2000;10:1297–303.

141. Quinn MF, Lundell CJ, Finck EJ, et al. Reliability of selective pulmonary arteriography in the diagnosis of pulmonary embolism. AJR Am J Roentgenol 1987;149:469–71.

142. Diffin DC, Leyendecker JR, Johnson SP, et al. Effect of anatomic distribution of pulmonary emboli on interobserver agreement in the interpretation of pulmonary angiography. AJR Am J Roentgenol 1998;171:1085–9.

143. Stein PD, Henry JW, Gottschalk A. Reassessment of pulmonary angiography for the diagnosis of pulmonary embolism: relation of interpreter agreement to the order of the involved pulmonary arterial branch. Radiology 1999;210:689–91.

144. Baile EM, King GG, Muller NL, et al. Spiral computed tomography is comparable to angiography for the diagnosis of pulmonary embolism. Am J Respir Crit Care Med 2000;161:1010–5.

145. Goldin JG, Yoon HC, Greaser LE, Nishimura EK. Detection of pulmonary emboli at the segmental and subsegmental level with electron-beam CT: validation in a porcine model. Acad Radiol 1998;5:503–8.

146. Lowenthal RM, Eaton K. Toxicity of chemotherapy. Hematol Oncol Clin North Am 1996;10:967–90.

147. Shaffer HA. Perforation and obstruction of the gastrointestinal tract. Assesment by conventional radiology. Radiol Clin North Am 1992:30:405–26.

148. Fainsinger RL. Integrating medical and surgical treat-

ments in gastrointestinal, genitourinary, and biliary obstruction in patients with cancer. Hematol Oncol Clin North Am 1996;10:173–88.

149. Rothrock SG, Green SM, Harding M, et al. Plain abdominal radiography in the detection of acute medical and surgical disease in children: a retrospective analysis. Pediatr Emerg Care 1991;7:281–5.

150. Rosen MP, Sands DZ, Longmaid HE, et al. Impact of abdominal CT on the management of patients presenting to the emergency department with acute abdominal pain. AJR Am J Roentgenol 2000;174:1391–6.

151. Nagurney JT, Brown DF, Novelline RA, et al. Plain abdominal radiographs and abdominal CT for nontraumatic abdominal pain—added value? Am J Emerg Med 1999;17:668–71.

152. Welch JP. General considerations and mortality. In: Welch JP, editor. Bowel obstruction: differential diagnosis and clinical management. Philadelphia: W.B. Saunders; 1990. p. 59–95.

153. Turnbull AD. Abdominal and upper gastrointestinal emergencies. In: Turnbull AD, editor. Surgical emergencies in the cancer patient. Chicago: Mosby-Year Book; 1987. p. 152.

154. Ripamonti C. Management of bowel obstruction in advanced cancer patients. J Pain Symptom Manage 1994;9:193–200.

155. Mucha P. Small intestinal obstruction. Surg Clin North Am 1987;67:597–620.

156. Brolin RE, Krasna MJ, Mast BA. Use of tubes and radiographs in the management of small-bowel obstruction. Ann Surg 1987;206:126–33.

157. Bizer LS, Leibling RW, Delany HM, Gliedman ML. Small-bowel obstruction: the role of nonoperative treatment in simple intestinal obstruction and predictive criteria for strangulation obstruction. Surgery 1981;89:407–13.

158. Maglinte DD, Balthazar EJ, Kelvin FM, et al. The role of radiography in the diagnosis of small-bowel obstruction. AJR Am J Roentgenol 1997;168:1171–80.

159. Anuras S, Shirazi SS. Colonic pseudoobstruction. Am J Gastroenterol 1984;79:525–32.

160. Maglinte DD, Reyes BL, Harmon BH, et al. Reliability and role of plain film radiography and CT in the diagnosis of small-bowel obstruction. AJR Am J Roentgenol 1996;167:1451–5.

161. Earls JP, Dachman AH, Colon E, et al. Prevalence and duration of postoperative pneumoperitoneum: sensitivity of CT vs left lateral decubitus radiography. AJR Am J Roentgenol 1993;161:781–5.

162. Shone DN, Nikoomanesh P, Smith-Meek MM, et al. Malignancy is the most common cause of gastric outlet obstruction in the era of H2 blockers. Am J Gastroenterol 1995;90:1769–70.

163. Plewa MC. Emergency abdominal radiography. Emerg Med Clin North Am 1991;9:827–52.

164. Harlow CL, Stears RL, Zeligman BE, et al. Diagnosis of bowel obstruction on plain abdominal radiographs: significance of air-fluid levels at different heights in the same loop of bowel. AJR Am J Roentgenol 1993; 161:291–5.

165. Gammill SL, Nice CM. Air fluid levels: their occurrence in normal patients and their role in the analysis of ileus. Surgery 1972;71:771–80.

166. Loberant N, Rose C. Imaging considerations in the geriatric emergency department patient. Emerg Med Clin North Am 1990;8:361–97.

167. Sloyer AF, Panella VS, Demas BE, et al. Ogilvie's syndrome: successful management without colonoscopy. Dig Dis Sci 1988;33:1391–6.

168. Sternbach GL, Barkin SZ. Acute abdominal pain. In: Rosen P, Doris PE, Barkin RM, Markovchick VJ, editors. Diagnostic radiology in emergency medicine. St. Louis: Mosby-Year Book; 1992. p. 359–78.

169. Patel NH, Lauber PR. The meaning of a nonspecific abdominal gas pattern. Acad Radiol 1995;2:667–9.

170. Maglinte DD, Gage SN, Harmon BH, et al. Obstruction of the small intestine: accuracy and role of CT in diagnosis. Radiology 1993;188:61–4.

171. Megibow AJ, Balthazar EJ, Cho DC, et al. Bowel obstruction: evaluation with CT. Radiology 1991;180:313–8.

172. Fukuya T, Hawes DR, Lu CC, et al. CT diagnosis of small-bowel obstruction: efficacy in 60 patients. AJR Am J Roentgenol 1992;158:765–72.

173. Taourel PG, Fabre JM, Pradel JA, et al. Value of CT in the diagnosis and management of patients with suspected acute small-bowel obstruction. AJR Am J Roentgenol 1995;165:1187–92.

174. Mellor MR, Drake DG. Colonic volvulus in children: value of barium enema for diagnosis and treatment in 14 children. AJR Am J Roentgenol 1994;162:1157–9.

175. Schwartzentruber DJ. Surgical emergencies. In: DeVita VT Jr, Hellman S, Rosenberg SA, editors. Cancer principles and practice of oncology. 5th ed. Philadelphia and New York: Lippincott-Raven; 1997. p. 2500–11.

176. ReMine SG, McIlrath DC. Bowel perforation in steroid-treated patients. Ann Surg 1980;192:581–6.

177. Mularski RA, Sippel JM, Osborne ML. Pneumoperitoneum: a review of nonsurgical causes. Crit Care Med 2000;28:2638–44.

178. Roh JJ, Thompson JS, Harned RK, Hodgson PE. Value of pneumoperitoneum in the diagnosis of visceral perforation. Am J Surg 1983;146:830–3.

179. Levine MS, Scheiner JD, Rubesin SE, et al. Diagnosis of pneumoperitoneum on supine abdominal radiographs. AJR Am J Roentgenol 1991;156:731–5.

180. Ericksen AS, Krasna MJ, Mast BA, et al. Use of gastrointestinal contrast studies in obstruction of the small and large bowel. Dis Colon Rectum 1990;33:56–64.

181. Heller M, Jehle D. Ultrasound in emergency medicine. Philadelphia: W.B. Saunders; 1995. p. 1–165.

182. Madrazo BL. Emergency applications of abdominal sonography. In: Tintinalli JE, Kriome RL, Ruiz E, editors. Emergency medicine: a comprehensive study guide. 3rd ed. New York: McGraw-Hill; 1992. p. 1120–2.

183. Billittier AJ, Abrams BJ, Brunetto A. Radiographic imaging modalities for the patient in the emergency department with abdominal complaints. Emerg Med Clin North Am 1996;14:789–850.

184. Prat F, Amouyal G, Amouyal P, et al. Prospective randomized study of endoscopic ultrasonography and endo-

scopic retrograde cholangiopancreatography in patients with suspected common-bileduct lithiasis. Lancet 1996;347:75–9.

185. Soto JA, Barish MA, Yucel EK, et al. Magnetic resonance cholangiography: comparison with endoscopic retrograde cholangiopancreatography. Gastroenterology 1996;110:589–97.

186. Vaghese JC, Farrell MA, Courtney G, et al. A prospective comparison of magnetic resonance cholangiopancreatography with endoscopic retrograde cholangiopancreatography in the evaluation of patients with suspected biliary tract disease. Clin Radiol 1999;54:513–20.

187. Trede M, Rumstadt B, Wendl K, et al. Ultrafast magnetic resonance imaging improves the staging of pancreatic tumors. Ann Surg 1997;226:393–407.

188. Matos C, Deviere J, Nicaise N, et al. Magnetic resonance cholangiopancreatography (MRCP): a perspective on potential clinical applications. Acta Gastroenterol Belg 1997;60:268–73.

189. Deviere J, Matos C, Cremer M. The impact of magnetic resonance cholangiopancreatography on ERCP. Gastrointest Endosc 1999;50:136–43.

190. Werner J, Schmidt J, Warshaw AL, et al. The relative safty of MRI contrast agent in acute necrotizing pancreatitis. Ann Surg 1998;227(1):105–11.

191. Edlow JA, Juang P, Margulies S, Burstein J. Rectus sheath hematoma. Ann Emerg Med 1999;34:671–5.

192. Jeffrey RB, Cardoza JD, Olcott EW. Detection of active intraabdominal arterial hemorrhage: value of dynamic contrast-enhanced CT. AJR Am J Roentgenol 1991;156:725–9.

193. Okazaki M, Higashihara H, Koganemaru F, et al. Intraperitoneal hemorrhage from hepatocellular carcinoma: emergency chemoembolization or embolization. Radiology 1991;180:647–51.

194. Sloas MM, Flynn PM, Kaste SC, Patrick CC. Typhlitis in children with cancer: a 30-year experience. Clin Infect Dis 1993;17;484–90.

195. Mower WJ, Hawkins JA, Nelson EW. Neutropenic enterocolitis in adults with acute leukemia. Arch Surg 1986;121:571–4.

196. Ettinghausen SE. Collagenous colitis, eosinophilic colitis, and neutropenic colitis. Surg Clin North Am 1993;73:993–1016.

197. Fry DE. Noninvasive imaging tests in the diagnosis and treatment of intra-abdominal abscesses in the postoperative patient. Surg Clin North Am 1994;74:693–709.

198. Church JM. Mucosal ischemia caused by desmoid tumors in patients with familial adenomatous polyposis: report of four cases. Dis Colon Rectum 1998;41:601–3.

199. Strobbe L, D'Hondt E, Ramboer C, et al. Ileal carcinoid tumors and intestinal ischemia. Hepatogastroenterology 1994;41:499–502.

200. Low DE, Frenkel VJ, Manley PN, et al. Embolic mesenteric infarction: a unique initial manifestation of renal cell carcinoma. Surgery 1989;106:925–8.

201. Schneider TA, Longo WE, Ure T, Vernava AM. Mesenteric ischemia. Acute arterial syndromes. Dis Colon Rectum 1994;37:1163–74.

202. Cappell MS. Intestinal (mesenteric) vasculopathy. I. Acute superior mesenteric arteriopathy and venopathy. Gastroenterol Clin North Am 1998;27:783–825.

203. Black RM. Rose & Black's clinical problems in nephrology. 1st ed. Boston: Little, Brown and Company; 1996.

204. Russo P. Urologic emergencies in the cancer patient. Semin Oncol 2000;27:284–98.

205. Cronan JJ. Contemporary concepts in imaging urinary tract obstruction. Radiol Clin North Am 1991;29:527–42.

206. Koelliker SL, Cronan JJ. Acute urinary tract obstruction. Imaging update. Urol Clin North Am 1997;24:571–82.

207. Amis ES, Cronan JJ, Pfister RC, Yoder IC. Ultrasonic inaccuracies in diagnosing renal obstruction. Urology 1982;19:101–5.

208. Scola FH, Cronan JJ, Schepps B. Grade I hydronephrosis: pulsed Doppler US evaluation. Radiology 1989;171:519–20.

209. Burge HJ, Middleton WD, McClennan BL, Hildebolt CF. Ureteral jets in healthy subjects and in patients with unilateral ureteral calculi: comparison with color Doppler US. Radiology 1991;180:437–42.

210. Platt JF. Urinary obstruction. Radiol Clin North Am 1996;34:1113–29.

211. Lee HJ, Kim SH, Jeong YK, Yeun KM. Doppler sonographic resistive index in obstructed kidneys. J Ultrasound Med 1996;15:613–8.

212. Platt JF, Ellis JH, Rubin JM. Assessment of internal ureteral stent patency in patients with pyelocaliectasis: value of renal duplex sonography. AJR Am J Roentgenol 1993;161:87–90.

213. Smith RC, Verga M, McCarthy S, Rosenfield AT. Diagnosis of acute flank pain: value of unenhanced helical CT. AJR Am J Roentgenol 1996;166:97–101.

214. Dalrymple NC, Verga M, Anderson KR, et al. The value of unenhanced helical computerized tomography in the management of acute flank pain. J Urol 1998;159:735–40.

215. Lane MJ, Katz DS, Ross BA, et al. Unenhanced helical CT for suspected acute appendicitis. AJR Am J Roentgenol 1997;168:405–9.

216. Dretler SP. Editorial comment. The value of unenhanced helical computerized tomography in the management of acute flank pain. J Urol 1998;159:740.

217. Merenich WM, Popky GL. Radiology of renal infection. Med Clin North Am 1991;75:425–69.

218. Papanicolaou N, Pfister RC. Acute renal infections. Radiol Clin North Am 1996;34:965–95.

219. Baumgarten DA, Baumgartner BR. Imaging and radiologic management of upper urinary tract infections. Urol Clin North Am 1997;24:545–69.

220. Deyoe LA, Cronan JJ, Lambiase RE, Dorfman GS. Percutaneous drainage of renal and perirenal abscesses: results in 30 patients. AJR Am J Roentgenol 1990;155:81–3.

221. Lang EK. Renal, perirenal, and pararenal abscesses: percutaneous drainage. Radiology 1990;174:109–13.

222. Watson RA, Esposito M, Richter F, et al. Percutaneous nephrostomy as adjunct management in advanced upper urinary tract infection. Urology 1999;54:234–9.

223. Soulen MC, Fishman EK, Goldman SM, Gatewood OM.

Bacterial renal infection: role of CT. Radiology 1989; 171:703–7.

224. Huang JJ, Tseng CC. Emphysematous pyelonephritis: clinicoradiological classification, management, prognosis, and pathogenesis. Arch Intern Med 2000;160:797–805.

225. Dyer RB, Assimos DG, Regan JD. Update on interventional uroradiology. Urol Clin North Am 1997;24:623–52.

226. Watkinson AF, A'Hern RP, Jones A, et al. The role of percutaneous nephrostomy in malignant urinary tract obstruction. Clin Radiol 1993;47:32–5.

227. Donat SM, Russo P. Ureteral decompression in advanced nonurologic malignancies. Ann Surg Oncol 1996;3:393–9.

228. Shekarriz B, Shekarriz H, Upadhyay J, et al. Outcome of palliative urinary diversion in the treatment of advanced malignancies. Cancer 1999;85:998–1003.

229. Zadra JA, Jewett MA, Keresteci AG, et al. Nonoperative urinary diversion for malignant ureteral obstruction. Cancer 1987;60:1353–7.

230. Docimo SG, Dewolf WC. High failure rate of indwelling ureteral stents in patients with extrinsic obstruction: experience at 2 institutions. J Urol 1989;142:277–9.

231. Denstedt JD, Reid G, Sofer M. Advances in ureteral stent technology. World J Urol 2000;18:237–42.

232. Minhas S, Irving HC, Lloyd SN, et al. Extra-anatomic stents in ureteric obstruction: experience and complications. BJU Int 1999;84:762–4.

233. Nissenkorn I, Gdor Y. Nephrovesical subcutaneous stent: an alternative to percutaneous nephrostomy. J Urol 2000;163:528–30.

234. Galasko CS. Diagnosis of skeletal metastases and assessment of response to treatment. Clin Orthop 1995;312:64–75.

235. Traill Z, Richards MA, Moore NR. Magnetic resonance imaging of metastatic bone disease. Clin Orthop 1995;312:76–88.

236. Coleman RE. Skeletal complications of malignancy. Cancer 1997;80:1588–94.

237. Rosenthal DI. Radiologic diagnosis of bone metastases. Cancer 1997;80:1595–607.

238. Marcantonio DR, Weatherall PT, Berrey BH. Practical considerations in the imaging of soft tissue tumors. Orthop Clin North Am 1998;29:1–17.

239. Jaovisidha S, Subhadrabandhu T, Siriwongpairat P, Pochanugool L. An integrated approach to the evaluation of osseous tumors. Orthop Clin North Am 1998; 29:19–39.

240. Hage WD, Aboulafia AJ, Aboulafia DM. Incidence, location, and diagnostic evaluation of metastatic bone disease. Orthop Clin North Am 2000;31:515–28.

241. Galasko CSB, Norris HE, Crank S. Spinal instability secondary to metastatic cancer. J Bone Joint Surg 2000; 82:570–6.

242. Zickel RE, Mouradian WH. Intramedullary fixation of pathologic fractures and lesions of the subtrochanteric region of the femur. J Bone Joint Surg Am 1976;58: 1061–6.

243. Mirels H. Metastatic disease in long bones. A proposed scoring system for diagnosing impending pathologic fractures. Clin Orthop 1989;249:256–64.

244. Keene JS, Sellinger DS, McBeath AA, Engber WD. Metastatic breast cancer in the femur. A search for the lesion at risk of fracture. Clin Orthop 1986;203:282–8.

245. Berruti A, Dogliotti L, Bitossi R, et al. Incidence of skeletal complications in patients with bone metastatic prostate cancer and hormone refractory disease: predictive role of bone resorption and formation markers evaluated at baseline. J Urol 2000;164:1248–53.

246. Godersky JC, Smoker WR, Knutzon R. Use of magnetic resonance imaging in the evaluation of metastatic spinal disease. Neurosurgery 1987;21:676–80.

247. Kricun ME. Fractures of the pelvis. Orthop Clin North Am 1990;21:573–90.

248. Mlinek EJ, Clark KC, Walker CW. Limited magnetic resonance imaging in the diagnosis of occult hip fractures. Am J Emerg Med 1998;16:390–2.

249. Eustace S, Adams J, Assaf A. Emergency MR imaging of orthopedic trauma. Current and future directions. Radiol Clin North Am 1999;37:975–94.

250. Bogost GA, Lizerbram EK, Crues JV. MR imaging in evaluation of suspected hip fracture: frequency of unsuspected bone and soft-tissue injury. Radiology 1995;197:263–7.

251. Manglani HH, Marco RAW, Picciolo A, Healey JH. Orthopedic emergencies in cancer patients. Semin Oncol 2000;27:299–310.

252. Hipp JA, Springfield DS, Hayes WC. Predicting pathologic fracture risk in the management of metastatic bone defects. Clin Orthop 1995;312:120–35.

253. Hipp JA, Katz G, Hayes WC. Local demineralization as a model for bone strength reductions in lytic transcortical metastatic lesions. Invest Radiol 1991;26:934–8.

254. Harrington KD. Impending pathologic fractures from metastatic malignancy: evaluation and management. Instr Course Lect 1986;35:357–81.

255. Davies HD, McGeer A, Schwartz B, et al. Invasive group A streptococcal infections in Ontario, Canada. Ontario Group A Streptococcal Study Group. N Engl J Med 1996;335:547–54.

256. Fisher JR, Conway MJ, Takeshita RT, Sandoval MR. Necrotizing fasciitis. Importance of roentgenographic studies for soft-tissue gas. JAMA 1979;241:803–6.

257. Begley MG, Shawker TH, Robertson CN, et al. Fournier gangrene: diagnosis with scrotal US. Radiology 1988;169:387–9.

258. Wysoki MG, Santora TA, Shah RM, Friedman AC. Necrotizing fasciitis: CT characteristics. Radiology 1997; 203:859–63.

259. Brothers TE, Tagge DU, Stutley JE, et al. Magnetic resonance imaging differentiates between necrotizing and non-necrotizing fasciitis of the lower extremity. J Am Coll Surg 1998;187:416–21.

260. Schmid MR, Kossmann T, Duewell S. Differentiation of necrotizing fasciitis and cellulitis using MR imaging. AJR Am J Roentgenol 1998;170:615–20.

261. Sharif HS, Clark DC, Aabed MY, et al. MR imaging of thoracic and abdominal wall infections: comparison with other imaging procedures. AJR Am J Roentgenol 1990;154:989–95.

INDEX